ENCYCLOPEDIA
OF
HUMAN NUTRITION

ENCYCLOPEDIA
OF
HUMAN NUTRITION

Editor-in-Chief

MICHELE J. SADLER

Editors

J.J. STRAIN

BENJAMIN CABALLERO

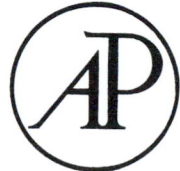

ACADEMIC PRESS

Harcourt Brace & Company Publishers

San Diego   London   Boston   New York
Sydney   Tokyo   Toronto

90054

ACADEMIC PRESS
525 B Street, Suite 1900,
San Diego, CA 92101–4495, USA
http://www.apnet.com

ACADEMIC PRESS
24-28 Oval Road
London NW1 7DX, UK
http.hbuk.co.uk/ap/

ISBN 0-12-226694-3

A catalogue record for this Encyclopedia is available from the British Library

Access for a limited period to an on-line version of the Encyclopedia of Human Nutrition is included in
the purchase price of the print edition.
This on-line version has been uniquely and persistently identified by the Digital Object Identifier (DOI)

10.1006/0127995110

By following the link

http://dx.doi.org/10.1006/0127995110

from any Web Browser, buyers of the Encyclopedia of Human Nutrition will find instructions on how to
register for access.

Typeset by Photo·graphics, Honiton, Devon, UK.
Printed and bound in Great Britain by The Bath Press, Bath, Avon, UK.

EDITORIAL ADVISORY BOARD

FOREWORD

Why an encyclopedia? The original Greek word means 'the circle of arts and sciences essential for a liberal education', and such a book was intended to embrace all knowledge. That was the aim of the famous Encyclopédie produced by Diderot and d'Alembert in the middle of the 18th century, which contributed so much to what has been called the Enlightenment. It is recorded that after all the authors had corrected the proofs of their contributions, the printer secretly cut out whatever he thought might give offence to the king, mutilated most of the best articles and burnt the manuscripts! Later, and less controversially, the word 'encyclopedia' came to be used for an exhaustive repertory of information on some particular department of knowledge. It is in this class that the present work falls.

In recent years the scope of Human Nutrition as a scientific discipline has expanded enormously. I used to think of it as an applied subject, relying on the basic sciences of physiology and biochemistry in much the same way that engineering relies on physics. That traditional relationship remains and is fundamental, but the field is now much wider. At one end of the spectrum epidemiological studies and the techniques on which they depend have played a major part in establishing the relationships between diet, nutritional status and health, and there is greater recognition of the importance of social factors. At the other end of the spectrum we are becoming increasingly aware of the genetic determinants of ways in which the body handles food and is able to resist adverse influences of the environment. Nutritionists are thus beginning to explore the genome.

In parallel with this widening of the subject there has been an increase in opportunities for training and research in nutrition, with new departments and new courses being developed in universities, medical schools and schools of public health, along with a greater involvement of schoolchildren and their teachers. Public interest in nutrition is intense and needs to be guided by sound science. Governments are realizing more and more the role that nutrition plays in the prevention of disease and the maintenance of good health, and the need to develop a nutrition policy that is integrated with policies for food production.

The appearance of this encyclopedia at the present time is therefore welcome and timely. It is as comprehensive as the present state of knowledge allows, but is not overly technical and is well supplied with suggestions for further reading. All the articles have been carefully reviewed and although some of the subjects are controversial and sensitive, the publishers have not exerted the kind of political censorship that so infuriated Diderot.

John Waterlow.

J.C. Waterlow
Emeritus Professor of Human Nutrition
London School of Hygiene and Tropical Medicine
July 1998

PREFACE

The science of nutrition is a diverse and complex subject. To attempt to draw together the many different elements of this rapidly developing science into a comprehensive encyclopedia has been a particularly daunting task.

The inspiration for taking on this task and the central elements of the work were borne out of the highly acclaimed Encyclopaedia of Food Science, Food Technology and Nutrition which was published in 1993. That the content of this new work is considerably different mainly reflects the rapid developments that have occurred in nutrition since the early 1990s.

The Editors have aimed to include a balance of material of interest to many readers, including those of different nationalities where the applications of nutritional science may be very different. Those with a clinical and medical background, those with a role in producing and processing food, and those involved in applying the science to public health policy, including educating the public about the importance of sound nutrition, should find much of interest in this work.

At a time when there is a continuing increase in the general public's interest in diet and health, there is not always agreement between different groups about the advice that should be given. Moreover, topics are increasingly debated in the media at a very early stage in the scientific exploration. The public look to nutritionists for advice concerning a number of current public health problems, and this Encyclopedia should prove helpful in providing summaries of the scientific background for those who are less familiar with particular subject areas.

The extent of coverage is wide and broad-based. It includes: physiological aspects of nutrient and energy requirements by different population groups; measurement of dietary intake and nutritional status; nutrient composition of the main food groups; associations between diet, lifestyle and disease; clinical applications of nutrition to improve health; topical issues relating to the food processing industry; influences on food choice and eating behaviour; nutritional guidelines and public health policies in both developed and developing countries; international aspects of food labelling, and a range of related topics in between these key subject areas.

It has not been possible to cover every aspect of the subject in minute detail; there has been the restraint of size, and for a large work of this nature, with considerable commitment required from all of the contributors, it has been understandably difficult to ensure that every article that had been ambitiously commissioned at the outset was received. Naturally there are some gaps, but we have endeavoured to keep these to a minimum. Full guidance for further reading is given and we are satisfied that we have delivered coverage that should easily meet the requirements of most readers.

Our thanks are due to all who contributed to this project.

M.J. Sadler, J.J. Strain, B. Caballero
Editors

INTRODUCTION

"Nutrition is not a discipline to be studied but a problem to be solved". This phrase, attributed to Jean Mayer, underscores the importance of nutritional science in addressing major public health problems. The statement also epitomizes the role that nutrition plays in linking basic biomedical disciplines with operational, problem-solving activities.

Our ability to develop effective responses to major health issues can only be as good as our understanding of those issues. In the case of nutrition, that knowledge involves a staggering number of disciplines, from molecular biology to agriculture and food science, from social sciences and human behaviour to clinical medicine. Few, if any, individuals can claim to master all these disciplines but, in order for a multi-disciplinary team to communicate and be effective, each member needs to be familiar with all the relevant disciplines. Hence the need for this encyclopedia. By combining up-to-date information on fundamental nutrition science with practical, operational issues, we hope these volumes will facilitate the necessary dialogue between the many branches of modern nutrition practice.

The effects of the globalization of modern life are particularly apparent for nutrition. Food production and food availability in individual countries are highly dependent on the world market, and rapid changes in agricultural policies in a few key nations can have a major global impact on food prices and availability.

Urbanization and industrialization of developing countries are creating new, rapidly increasing nutritional problems, particularly among the urban poor, while in some cases causing significant reductions in usable land. While the declining trends in infant mortality and childhood malnutrition in many areas of the world are encouraging, the threat posed by non-communicable diseases such as obesity, diabetes, and cardiovascular diseases is increasing. Worldwide data from 1990 show that 47 per cent of deaths in the developing world were due to chronic diseases, most of them associated with unhealthy diet and lifestyle. By the year 2020, it is predicted that 67 per cent of years lost to disability (a major index of population health) in developing countries will be related to chronic non-communicable diseases. How to bring the benefits of industrialization and modern technology to large population groups while preserving their health and nutrition status will be one of the major challenges for the next decades.

In the realm of basic science, continuing discoveries of the genetic mechanisms of physiological and pathological processes are just beginning to shape the nutritional practice of the future. The contrast between deceptively simple preventive measures (such as dietary change) and sophisticated, high-tech therapies could not be sharper. And yet, there is no question that advances in molecular genetics will continue to play a major role in our understanding of nutritional disorders and in the development of novel preventive strategies, from increasing crop yields to modulating host response to illness.

This encyclopedia builds on a distinguished tradition of comprehensive, systematic information delivery, of which all Academic Press encyclopedias are excellent examples. The editors acknowledge the commitment of the authors and of the outstanding staff of the Major Reference Works division of Academic Press in enabling this encyclopedia to come to fruition. We are confident that the many authors who contributed their work are among the best that today's global nutritional science has to offer.

We trust this encyclopedia – and its electronic version – will be a valuable resource to inform and provide practical support to readers in their daily tasks, be it caring for the nutritional needs of a patient, teaching a nutrition course, advising policy makers, or communicating the science of nutrition to the general public.

GUIDE TO USE OF THE ENCYCLOPEDIA

Structure of the Encyclopedia

The material in the Encyclopedia is arranged as a series of entries in alphabetical order. Some entries comprise a single article, whilst entries on more diverse subjects consist of several articles that deal with various aspects of the topic. In the latter case the articles are arranged in a logical sequence within an entry.

To help you realize the full potential of the material in the Encyclopedia we have provided three features to help you find the topic of your choice.

1. Contents Lists

Your first point of reference will probably be the contents list. The complete contents list appearing in each volume will provide you with both the volume number and the page number of the entry. On the opening page of an entry a contents list is provided so that the full details of the articles within the entry are immediately available.

Alternatively you may choose to browse through a volume using the alphabetical order of the entries as your guide. To assist you in identifying your location within the Encyclopedia a running headline indicates the current entry and the current article within that entry.

You will find 'dummy entries' where obvious synonyms exist for entries or where we have grouped together related topics. Dummy entries appear in both the contents list and the body of the text. For example, a dummy entry appears for AIDS which directs you to HIV Disease: Nutritional Management, where the material is located.

Example

If you were attempting to locate material on Sugar via the contents list.

SUGAR *see* CARBOHYDRATES: Chemistry and Classification (including Dietary Fibre (Fiber));
  Regulation of Carbohydrate Metabolism; Requirements and Dietary Importance; GALACTOSE:
  Absorption and Metabolism; GLUCOSE: Chemistry, Dietary Sources and Glycaemic Index; Metabolism
  and Maintenance of Blood Glucose Level; Glucose Tolerance; SUCROSE: Nutritional Role, Absorption
  and Metabolism; Dietary Sucrose and Disease

At the appropriate location in the contents list, the page numbers for articles under Carbohydrates are given.

If you were trying to locate the material by browsing through the text and you looked up Sugar then the following information would be provided.

Sugar *see* **Carbohydrates**: Chemistry and Classification (including Dietary Fibre); Regulation of Carbohydrate Metabolism; Requirements and Dietary Importance. **Galactose**: Absorption and Metabolism. **Glucose**: Chemistry, Dietary Sources and Glycaemic Index; Metabolism and Maintenance of Blood Glucose Level; Glucose Tolerance. **Sucrose**: Nutritional role, Absorption and Metabolism; Dietary Sucrose and Disease.

Alternatively, if you were looking up Carbohydrates the following information would be provided.

CARBOHYDRATES

Contents
Chemistry and Classification (including Dietary Fibre)
Regulation of Carbohydrate Metabolism
Requirements and Dietary Importance
Resistant Starch and Oligosaccharides

2. Cross References

All of the articles in the Encyclopedia have been extensively cross referenced.
 The cross references, which appear at the end of an article, have been provided at three levels:

i. To indicate if a topic is discussed in greater detail elsewhere.

ANTIOXIDANTS/Diet and Antioxidant Defence.
See also: **Arthritis**: Dietary Aspects of Aetiology and Nutritional Management. **Ascorbic Acid**: Physiology, Dietary Sources and Requirements. **Cancer**: Epidemiology and Associations Between Diet and Cancer. **Carotenoids**: Chemistry, Sources and Physiology; Epidemiology. **Copper**: Physiology, Dietary Sources and Requirements. **Coronary Heart Disease**: Prevention. **Diabetes Mellitus**: Dietary Management. **Dietary Guidelines**: International Perspectives. **Folic Acid**: Physiology, Dietary Sources and Requirements. **Magnesium**: Physiology, Dietary Sources and Requirements. **Manganese**: Physiology, Dietary Sources and Requirements. **Phytochemicals**: Classification and Occurrence. **Riboflavin**: Physiology. **Selenium**: Physiology, Dietary Sources and Requirements. **Tocopherols**: Physiology. **Vitamin Supplementation**: Role. **Zinc**: Physiology.

ii. To draw the reader's attention to parallel discussions in other articles.

> **ANTIOXIDANTS/Diet and Antioxidant Defence.**
> *See also:* **Arthritis**: Dietary Aspects of Aetiology and Nutritional Management. **Ascorbic Acid**: Physiology, Dietary Sources and Requirements. **Cancer**: Epidemiology and Associations Between Diet and Cancer. **Carotenoids**: Chemistry, Sources and Physiology; Epidemiology. **Copper**: Physiology, Dietary Sources and Requirements. **Coronary Heart Disease**: Prevention. **Diabetes Mellitus**: Dietary Management. **Dietary Guidelines**: International Perspectives. **Folic Acid**: Physiology, Dietary Sources and Requirements. **Magnesium**: Physiology, Dietary Sources and Requirements. **Manganese**: Physiology, Dietary Sources and Requirements. **Phytochemicals**: Classification and Occurrence. **Riboflavin**: Physiology. **Selenium**: Physiology, Dietary Sources and Requirements. **Tocopherols**: Physiology. **Vitamin Supplementation**: Role. **Zinc**: Physiology.

iii. To indicate material that broadens the discussion.

> **ANTIOXIDANTS/Diet and Antioxidant Defence.**
> *See also:* **Arthritis**: Dietary Aspects of Aetiology and Nutritional Management. **Ascorbic Acid**: Physiology, Dietary Sources and Requirements. **Cancer**: Epidemiology and Associations Between Diet and Cancer. **Carotenoids**: Chemistry, Sources and Physiology; Epidemiology. **Copper**: Physiology, Dietary Sources and Requirements. **Coronary Heart Disease**: Prevention. **Diabetes Mellitus**: Dietary Management. **Dietary Guidelines**: International Perspectives. **Folic Acid**: Physiology, Dietary Sources and Requirements. **Magnesium**: Physiology, Dietary Sources and Requirements. **Manganese**: Physiology, Dietary Sources and Requirements. **Phytochemicals**: Classification and Occurrence. **Riboflavin**: Physiology. **Selenium**: Physiology, Dietary Sources and Requirements. **Tocopherols**: Physiology. **Vitamin Supplementation**: Role. **Zinc**: Physiology.

3. Index

The index will provide you with the volume number and page number of where the material is to be located, and the index entries differentiate between material that is a whole article, is part of an article or is data presented in a table. On the opening page of the index detailed notes are provided.

4. Colour Plates

The colour figures for each volume have been grouped together in a plate section. The location of this section is cited both in the contents list and before the *See also* list of the pertinent articles.

5. Contributors

A full list of contributors appears at the beginning of each volume.

CONTRIBUTORS

Adel Abi-Hanna
Division of Gastroenterology/Nutrition
Johns Hopkins School of Medicine
Brady 320 - 600 N. Wolfe Street
Baltimore MD 21287
USA

P B Acosta
Ross Products Division
Abbott Laboratories
625 Cleveland Avenue
Columbus OH 43215-1724
USA

J Akré
Programme of Nutrition
World Health Organization
CH-1211 Geneva 27
Switzerland

A J Alberg
Epidemiology
Johns Hopkins University
School of Hygiene and Public Health
615, North Wolfe Street, Baltimore MD 21205
USA

L Albon
Medical Unit, St Bartholemew's and the Royal London
School
of Medicine and Dentistry
Queen Mary and Westfield College
Whitechapel London E1 2AD
UK

L Allen
Department of Nutrition
University of California - Davis
3113 Meyer Hall
Davis CA 95616-8669
USA

D Alnwick
Health Section, Programme Division
UNICEF, 633 Third Avenue
TA 24A New York
NY 10017
USA

Ross Andersen
Johns Hopkins School of Medicine
Division of Geriatric Medicine and Gerontology
5501 Hopkins Bayview Circle/JHAAC 5B:81
Baltimore MD 21224
USA

D Anderson
BIBRA International
Woodmansterne Road
Carshalton
Surrey SM5 4DS
UK

J J B Anderson
University of North Carolina at Chapel Hill
Schools of Public Health & Medicine
Chapel Hill
NC 27599-7400
USA

R A Anderson
Research in Chemistry
USDA Beltsville Human Nutrition Research Center
Bldg 307, room 224
Beltsville MD 20705
USA

U Arens
British Nutrition Foundation
52-54 High Holborn
London
WC1V 6RQ
UK

M J Arnaud
Water Institute Perrier Vittel
BP 101 - 88804 Vittel Cedex
France

E W Askew
Division of Foods & Nutrition
University of Utah
Salt Lake City
UT 84112
USA

Richard L Atkinson
Medicine and Nutrition Sciences
University of Wisconsin at Madison
1415 Linden Drive, Madison
WI 53706-1571
USA

C Baldwin
Dunn Clinical Nutrition Centre
Hills Road
Cambridge
CB2 2DH
UK

D J P Barker
MRC Environmental Epidemiology Unit
Southampton General Hospital
Southampton
SO16 6YD
UK

Y A Barnett
Cancer & Ageing Research Group
Senior Lecturer in School of Biomedical Sciences
University of Ulster
Coleraine BT52 1SA
Northern Ireland UK

S Bartlett
The Johns Hopkins Bayview Medical Center
Division of Digestive Diseases
A Building, 4940 Eastern Avenue
Baltimore MD 21224
USA

C J Bates
MRC Dunn Nutrition Unit
Milton Road
Cambridge
CB4 1XJ
UK

A E Bender
2 Willow Vale
Fetcham
Leatherhead
Surrey KT22 9TE
UK

D A Bender
Department of Biochemistry & Molecular Biology
University College London
Gower Street
London WC1E 6BT
UK

I F F Benzie
Department of Nursing and Health Sciences
The Hong Kong Polytechnic University
Hung Hom
Kowloon
Hong Kong

Zulfiqar A Bhutta
Department of Paediatrics
The Aga Khan University
Stadium Road, PO Box 3500
Karachi-74800
Pakistan

J Bines
Head of Clinical Nutrition
Department of Gastroenterology and Clinical Nutrition
Royal Children's Hospital
Parkville, Victoria 3052
Australia

S A Bingham
Dunn Clinical Nutrition Centre
Hills Road
Cambridge
CB2 2DH
UK

A Bird
Institute of Food Research
Earley Gate
Whiteknights Road
Reading Berkshire RG6 6BZ
UK

George L Blackburn
Harvard Medical School
Beth Israel Deaconess Medical Center
194 Pilgrim Road
Boston MA 02115
USA

R E Blum
Channing Laboratory
181 Longwood Avenue
Boston
MA 02115
USA

J E Blundell
Biopsychology Group, Psychology Department
The University of Leeds
Leeds
LS2 9JY
UK

C Boreham
Sport and Exercise Sciences
The University of Ulster
Jordanstown
Co. Antrim BT37 0QB
Northern Ireland UK

J Brand-Miller
Department of Biochemistry
University of Sydney
NSW 2006
Australia

Ronette R Briefel
Centers for Disease Control and Prevention
National Center for Health Statistics
6525 Belcrest Road
Hyattsville, Maryland 20782
USA

H R Brunner
Division d'Hypertension et de Médecine Vasculaire
Centre Hospitalier Universitaire Vaudois
1011 Lausanne
Switzerland

A Burke
Gastroenterology Division
Dulles 3, University of Pensylvania
3400 Spruce Street
Philadelphia PA 19143
USA

V Burley
Nuffield Institute for Health
University of Leeds
Leeds LS2 9PL
UK

M L Burr
Centre for Applied Public Health Medicine
University of Wales College of Medicine
Temple of Peace and Health
Cathays Park, Cardiff CF1 3NW
Wales UK

D H Buss
5 Howard Close
Fleet, Hampshire
GU13 9ER
UK

J Buttriss
British Nutrition Foundation
High Holborn House
52-54 High Holborn
London WC1V 6RQ
UK

B Caballero
Center for Human Nutrition
Johns Hopkins University
615 North Wolfe Street
Baltimore, MA 21205-2179
USA

J E Casterline
University of California at Davis
CA, USA

A E Cathcart
Northern Ireland Centre for Diet and Health
University of Ulster, Coleraine
Co L'Derry BT52 1SA
Northern Ireland UK

Samuel Chan
BIDMC/Harvard Medical School
194 Pilgrim Road
Boston MA 02215
USA

Lawrence Cheskin
Johns Hopkins Weight Management Center
Johns Hopkins University School of Medicine
4940 Eastern Avenue
Baltimore MD 21224
USA

F S Chu
Food Research Institute
Department of Food Microbiology & Toxicology
University of Wisconsin
Madison WI 53706-1187
USA

G A Clugston
Nutrition
World Health Organisation
1211 Geneva 27
Switzerland

L Cobiac
CSIRO Human Nutrition
PO Box 10041
Gouger Street
Adelaide 5000
Australia

Miriam Coelho de Souza
Departamento de Nutrição, Universidade de Mogi das Cruzes
Av Dr Candido Xavier de Almeida Souza, 200
Mogi das Cruzes - São Paulo
CEP 08780-911
Brazil

G A Colditz
Channing Laboratory
Harvard Medical School
181 Longwood Avenue
Boston MA 02115
USA

M Collins
Muckamore Abbey Hospital
1 Abbey Road
Muckamore
Antrim BT41 4SH
Northern Ireland UK

Kim G Conner
Johns Hopkins Hospital
Children Center
600 North Wolfe Street, Brady 306
Baltimore, Maryland 21205-2179
USA

B Corridan
Department of Nutrition
University College Cork
Ireland

R Cottrell
The Sugar Bureau
Duncan House
Dolphin Square
London SW1V 3PW
UK

J Coutts
Formerly of Willink Laboratory
Royal Manchester Children's Hospital
Pendlebury
Near Manchester M27 1HA
UK

B D'Avanzo
Istituto di Ricerche Farmacologiche
Mario Negri
Via Eritrea 62
20157 Milano
Italy

G Davey
Department of Epidemiology and Population Health
London School of Hygiene and Tropical Medicine
Keppel Street
London WC1E 7HT
UK

T J David
Department of Child Health
Booth Hall Children's Hospital
Charlestown Road
Blackley Manchester M9 7AA
UK

C P Day
Department of Medicine
Floor 4 William Leech Building
The Medical School, Framlington Place
Newcastle upon Tyne NE2 4HH
UK

C P G M de Groot
Division of Human Nutrition and Epidemiology
Wageningen Agricultural University
Bomenweg 2
6703 HD Wageningen
The Netherlands

M de Onis
Programme of Nutrition
World Health Organization
1211 Geneva 27
Switzerland

S C Dennis
Bioenergetics of Exercise Research Unit
Sports Science Institute of South Africa
University of Cape Town, Boundary Road
115 Newlands 7725
South Africa

Nikhil V Dhurandhar
University of Wisconsin at Madison
1415 Linden Drive
Madison
WI 53706-1571
USA

B D Dimitrov
Department of Social Medicine
Faculty of Medicine, Higher Medical Institute
15A V Aprilov Blvd
Plovdiv 4000
Bulgaria

E Dowler
Public Health Nutrition Unit
Dept of Epidemiology and Population Health
London School of Hygiene and Tropical Medicine
Keppel Street, London WC1E 7HT
UK

J Dowsett
St Vincent's Hospital
Elm Park
Dublin 4
Ireland

A Draper
Public Health Nutrition Unit
Dept of Epidemiology & Population Health
London School of Hygiene and Tropical Medicine
Keppel Street, London WC1E 7HT
UK

H D Duncan
Department of Gastroenterology
Queen Alexandra Hospital
Southwick Hill Road
Cosham, Portsmouth PO6 3LY
UK

Jacqueline L Dupont
Department of Nutrition, Food and Movement Sciences
Florida State University
Tallahassee
FL 32306-1490
USA

Johanna T Dwyer
Tufts University School of Medicine and Nutrition
Frances Stern Nutrition Center
New England Medical Center, #783
750 Washington Street, Boston MA 02111
USA

M A Eastwood
Gastrointestinal Unit, Department of Medicine
University of Edinburgh
Western General Hospital
Edinburgh EH4 2XU
Scotland UK

J Eaton-Evans
Northern Ireland Centre for Diet and Health
University of Ulster
Coleraine
BT52 1SA
Northern Ireland UK

C Edwards
Department of Human Nutrition
University of Glasgow
Yorkhills Hospital
Glasgow G3 8SJ
UK

B Eley
Dept of Paediatrics and Child Health
University of Cape Town
Red Cross War Memorial Children's Hospital
Rondesbosch, Cape 7700
South Africa

Gloria Elfert
Johns Hopkins Diabetes Center
601 North Caroline St
Room 2008
Baltimore MD 21287-0760
USA

M Elia
Dunn Clinical Nutrition Centre
Hills Road
Cambridge
CB2 2DH
UK

L J Elsas
Division of Medical Genetics
Department of Pediatrics, Emory Uni School of Medicine
2040 Ridgewood Drive NE
Atlanta GA 30322
USA

P Emery
Department of Nutrition and Dietetics
King's College London
Campden Hill Road
Kensington London
UK

J L Ensunsa
Department of Nutrition
University of California at Davis
Meyer Hall 3rd Floor
Davis CA 95616
USA

C I Ewing
Booth Hall Children's Hospital
Manchester
M9 7AA
UK

S Fairweather-Tait
Institute of Food Research
Norwich Research Park
Colney
Norwich NR4 7UA
UK

A Fehily
Company Nutritionist
HJ Heinz Ltd
Kitt Green, Wigan
Lancashire WN5 0JL
UK

Lawrence Feinman
Mount Sinai School of Medicine
Section of Gastronenterology
Veterans Affairs Medicine Center (111D)
130 West Kingsbridge Road, Bronx NY 10468-3992
USA

A Ferro-Luzzi
Human Nutrition Unit
Via Ardeatina 546
Rome
I-00179
Italy

F Fidanza
Istituto di Scienza dell'Alimentazione
Universita degli Studi di Perugia
via S. Costanzo, CP 333
I 06100 Perugia
Italy

P Fieldhouse
Faculty of Nursing
The University of Manitoba
Winnipeg
Manitoba
Canada R3T 2N2

N Finer
Centre for Obesity Research
Luton and Dunstable Hospital NHS Trust
Luton LU4 0DZ
UK

Marta L Fiorotto
Children's Nutrition Research Center at
Baylor College of Medicine
1100 Bates
Houston, Texas 77030 - 2600
USA

Josef E Fischer
Department of Surgery
University of Cincinnati Medical Center
231 Bethesda Avenue, Cincinnati
OH 45267-0558
USA

D J Flint
Hannah Research Institute
Ayr
KA6 5HL
Scotland UK

C Ford
Human Nutrition Research Centre
University of Newcastle
Department of Biological and Nutritional Sciences
University of Newcastle upon Tyne
Newcastle upon Tyne, NE1 7RU
UK

R Fraser
Department of Obstetrics and Gynaecology
University Clinical Sciences Centre
Northern General Hospital, Herries Road
Sheffield S5 7AU
UK

R E Frisch
Harvard Center for Population and Development
Studies
9 Bow Street
Cambridge
MA 02138
USA

R Fuller
59 Ryeish Green
Reading
RG7 1ES
UK

H C Furr
Department of Nutritional Sciences
U-17, University of Connecticut
Storrs
CT 06269-4017
USA

S C Garner
Division of General Surgery
Duke University, 103A Bell Building
Box 3826 Medical Centre
Durham, NC 27710
USA

J Garrow
European Journal of Clinical Nutrition
Dial House, 93 Uxbridge Road
Rickmansworth
Hertfordshire WD3 2DQ
UK

S Gatenby
SmithKline Beecham
Consumer Healthcare
11 Stoke Poges Lane
Slough SL1 3NW
UK

J M Gaziano
Brigham and Women's Hospital
Division of Preventative Medicine
900 Commonwealth Avenue East
Boston, MA 02215-1204
USA

C Geissler
Department of Nutrition and Dietetics
Kings College London
Campden Hill Road
London W8 7AH
UK

G Gibson
Microbiology Department
Institute of Food Research
Earley Gate
Reading Berkshire RG6 6BZ
UK

T Gill
Rowett Research Institute
Greenburn Road
Bucksburn
Aberdeen AB2 9SB
Scotland UK

W S Gilmore
School of Biomedical Sciences
University of Ulster
Coleraine
BT52 1SA
Northern Ireland UK

G R Goldberg
Dunn Clinical Nutrition Centre
Hills Road
Cambridge
CB2 2DH
UK

J Gray
6 Kingswood Close
Guildford
Surrey
GU1 2SD
UK

J P Greaves
2 The Plantation
Blackheath
London
SE3 0AB
UK

S Greely
North Dakota State University
Department of Foods and Nutrition
Fargo
ND 58102
USA

C J Green
Nutricia Corporate Research
PO Box 1
2700 MA Zoetermeer
The Netherlands

J Green
Formerly of Department of Nutrition and Dietetics
Royal Marsden NHS Trust
London SW3
UK

C Greenwood
Department of Nutritional Sciences
Faculty of Medicine
University of Toronto
Toronto, Ontario, M5S 2E3
Canada

R Grimble
Institute of Human Nutrition
University of Southampton
Southampton
SO16 7PX
UK

R Gross
Deutsche Gesellschaft für
Tecnische Zusammenarbeit (GTZ) GmbH
PO Box 5180
D - 65726 Eschborn
Germany

S M Grundy
Center for Human Nutrition
University of Texas, 5323 Harry Hines Blvd
Southwestern Medical Center at Dallas
Dallas TX 75235-9052
USA

J C G Halford
Department of Psychology
University of Central Lancashire
Preston
Lancashire PR1 2HE
UK

B M Hannigan
School of Biomedical Sciences
University of Ulster
Coleraine
BT52 1SA
Northern Ireland UK

R Harding
Formerly of Nutrition, Biotechnology and Scientific
Services Unit, Food Science Division II
Ministry of Agriculture, Fisheries and Food
Ergon House, 17 Smith Square, London SW1P 3JR
UK

Edward D Harris
Department of Biochemistry and Biophysics
Texas A&M University
College Station
TX 77843-2128
USA

M Harris
UNC School of Public Health
2103 D McGarvan-Greenberg Hall
CB 7400
Chapel Hill NC 27599-7400
USA

N P Hays
USDA-Human Nutrition Research Center on Aging
Energy Metabolism Laboratory
Tufts University, 711 Washington Street
Boston MA 02111-1524
USA

C J K Henry
School of Biological and Molecular Sciences
Oxford Brookes University
Gipsy Lane
Headington, Oxford OX3 0BP
UK

J Higgs
Nutrition and Dietetic Manager
Meat and Livestock Commission
PO Box 44, Winterhill House
Snowdon Drive, Milton Keynes MK6 1AX
UK

A J Hill
Division of Psychiatry and Behavioural Sciences
School of Medicine, University of Leeds
15 Hyde Terrace
Leeds, LS2 9JT
UK

S A Hill
Southampton General Hospital
Tremona Road
Southampton
SO16 6YD
UK

G A Hitman
Medical Unit, St Bartholemew's and the Royal London
School of Medicine and Dentistry
The Royal London Hospital, Whitechapel
London E1 1BB
UK

J Hodgson
University Department of Medicine
Box X2213 GPO
Perth
WA 6000
Australia

Daniel J Hoffman
Department of Endocrine Physiology
Federal University of São Paulo, Escola Paulista de
Medicina
Rua Botucatu 862, 2 Andar
V Clementiona 04023-900, São Paulo
Brazil

M F Holick
Boston University School of Medicine
715 Albany Street
Boston
MA 02118-2394
USA

L Houghton
Ross Products Division
Abbott Laboratories
625 Cleveland Avenue
Columbus OH 43215-3453
USA

R Houston
Program Against Micronutrient Malnutrition (PAMM)
Emory University Rollins School of Public Health
and Department of International Health
1518 Clifton Road NE, Atlanta GA 30322
USA

Barbara V Howard
Medlantic Research Institute
108 Irving Street NW
Washington
DC 20010
USA

L Howard
Department of Medicine
Albany Medical College
47 New Scotland Avenue
Albany NY 12208-3479
USA

Y-S Huang
Medical Nutritional R&D
Ross Products Division, Abbott Laboratories
3300 Stelzer Road
Columbus, Ohio 43219
USA

D Hughes
The Rowett Research Institute
Greenburn Road
Bucksburn
Aberdeen AB2 9SB
Scotland UK

K F A M Hulsof
TNO Nutrition and Food Research Institute
PO Box 360
3700 AJ Zeist
The Netherlands

C Hunt
Department of Food and Nutrition
University of Huddersfield
Queensgate
Huddersfield HD1 3DH
UK

M A Hunt
Food and Drink Federation
6 Catherine Street
London WC2B 5JJ
UK

G D Hussey
Child Health Unit, Dept of Pediatrics and Child Health
University of Cape Town
46 Sawkins Road
Rondesbosch 7700
South Africa

D Hutton
Bioprocessing Limited
Medomsley Road
Consett, County Durham DH8 6SZ
UK

A A Jackson
Institute of Human Nutrition
Bassett Cres East
University of Southampton
Highfield Southampton SO16 7PX
UK

W P T James
Rowett Research Institute
Greenburn Road
Bucksburn
Aberdeen AB21 9SB
Scotland UK

Alan G Jardine
Department of Medicine and Therapeutics
University of Glasgow
Gardiner Institute
Western Infirmary
Glasgow G11 6NT
Scotland UK

David J A Jenkins
Clinical Nutrition and Risk Factor Modification Center
St Michael's Hospital
61 Queen Street East
Toronto, Ontario M5C 3E2
Canada

I Johnson
Institute of Food Research
Norwich Laboratory
Colney Lane
Norwich NR4 7UA
UK

J M Johnson
Department of Human Nutrition, Foods and Exercise
Virginia Polytechnic Institute and State University
Blacksburg
VA 24061-0426
USA

M A Johnson
Department of Foods and Nutrition
College of Family and Consumer Sciences
Dawson Hall, University of Georgia
Athens, GA 30602
USA

A M Johnstone
The Rowett Research Institute
Greenburn Road
Bucksburn
Aberdeen AB2 9SB
Scotland UK

P A Judd
Department of Nutrition and Dietetics
King's College London
Campden Hill Road
London W8 7AH
UK

S Katayama
The Fourth Department of Medicine
Saitama Medical School
38 Morohongo, Moroyama-cho
Iruma-gun, Saitama 350-0495
Japan

Festo P Kavishe
Tanzania Food and Nutrition Center
PO Box 977
Dar es Salaam
Tanzania

C L Keen
Department of Nutrition
University of California at Davis
3135 Meyer Hall, One Shields Avenue
Davis CA 95616
USA

G T Keusch
New England Medical Center
Division of Geographical Medicine/Infectious Diseases
Box 041, 750 Washington Street
Boston MA 02111
USA

A A Kielmann
Deutsche Gesellschaft für Technische
Zusammenarbeit (GTZ) GmbH
BP 26, F-83570 Cotignac, Var
France

Eric S Kilpatrick
Royal Infirmary
Oxford Road
Manchester
M13 9WL UK

J C King
Western Human Nutrition Research Center
PO Box 29997, San Francisco
CA 94129
USA

P Kirk
NICHE
School of Biomedical Sciences
University of Ulster at Coleraine
BT52 1SA
Northern Ireland

S F Kirk
Division of Public Health
Nuffield Institute of Health
71-75 Clarendon Road
Leeds LS2 9LT
UK

P Kirke
Child Health Department
The Health Research Board
73 Lower Baggot Street
Dublin 2
Ireland

C Kjolhede
Research Institute
The Mary Imogene Bassett Hospital
One Atwell Road
Cooperstown NY 13326-1394
USA

D M Klurfeld
Department of Nutrition and Food Science
Wayne State University
Detroit MI 48202
USA ·

G S Knight
University Department of Surgery
Auckland Hospital
Private Bag 92019
Auckland
New Zealand

Lenore Kohlmeier
Departments of Nutrition and Epidemiology
School of Public Health, CB #7400
University of North Carolina
Chapel Hill, NC 27599-7400
USA

M Kohlmeier
Department of Nutrition
University of North Carolina at Chapel Hill
McGavran-Greenberg Hall
2205A Chapel Hill
NC 27514
USA

P Kopelman
Medical Unit, St Bartholemew's and the Royal London
School of Medicine and Dentistry
Queen Mary and Westfield College
Whitechapel London E1 2AD
UK

A Kouris-Blazos
Department of Medicine
Level 5 Block E, Monash Medical Center
246 Clayton Road
Clayton Victoria
Australia 3168

Jackie Krick
Division of Nutrition
Kennedy-Krieger Institute
707 North Broadway
Baltimore MD 21205
USA

Norman I Krinsky
Department of Biochemistry
Tufts University School of Medicine
136 Harrison Avenue
Boston MA 02111-1837
USA

D Kritchevsky
Wistar Institute
3601 Spruce Street
Philadelphia PA 19104-4268
USA

C La Vecchia
Istituto di Ricerche Farmacologiche
Mario Negri
20157 Milan
Via Eritrea 62
Italy

V Lakin
The Rowett Research Institute
Greenburn Road
Bucksburn,
Aberdeen AB2 9SB
UK

A Laviano
Department of Surgery
University Hospital
SUNY Health Science Center
Syracuse, NY
USA

James B Lee
State University of New York
Buffalo
New York
USA

A R Leeds
Department of Nutrition
Kings College London
Campden Hill Road
London W8 7AH
UK

J Leiper
Department of Biomedical Sciences
University Medical School
Forester Hill
Aberdeen AB9 2ZD
Scotland UK

Claus Leitzmann
Institute of Nutrition
Justus-Liebig University
D-35392 Giessen
Wilhelmstrasse 20
Germany

A H Lichtenstein
Lipid Metabolism Laboratory
USDA Human Nutrition Research Center on Aging
Tufts University
711 Washington Street, Boston MA 02111-1524
USA

C S Lieber
Alcohol Research and Treatment Center
Veterans Affairs Medical Center (151-2)
Mount Sinai School of Medicine
130 West Kingsbridge Road, Bronx NY 10468-3904
USA

J-W Liu
Medical Nutritional R&D
Ross Products Division, Abbott Laboratories
3300 Stelzer Road
Columbus, Ohio 43219
USA

M B E Livingstone
Northern Ireland Centre for Diet and Health
University of Ulster
Coleraine
BT52 1SA
Northern Ireland UK

Michiel R H Löwik
TNO Nutrition and Food Research Institute
PO Box 360
3700 AJ Zeist
The Netherlands

M J Luetkemeier
Department of Exercise and Sport Science
300S 1850E Room 259, University of Utah
Salt Lake City
UT 84112
USA

P G Lunn
Dunn Nutrition Laboratory
Downhams Lane
Milton Road
Cambridge
UK

S R Lynch
Eastern Virginia Medical School
Hampton Veterans Affairs Medical Center
Hampton
VA 23667
USA

A MacDonald
Birmingham Children's Hospital
Steelhouse Lane
Birmingham
B4 6NH
UK

I Macdonald
University of London
Hillside
Fountain Drive
London SE19 1UP
UK

GA MacGregor
Blood Pressure Unit
Department of Medicine
St George's Hospital Medical School
Cranmer Terrace, London SW17 0RE
UK

M Malone
Albany College of Pharmacy
Albany
New York 12208
USA

J I Mann
Human Nutrition
University of Otago
PO Box 56
Dunedin
New Zealand

B Margetts
Institute of Human Nutrition
University of Southampton
Southampton General Hospital
Southampton SO16 6YD
UK

V Marks
European Institute of Health and Medical Sciences
University of Surrey, Stirling House Campus, Stirling Road
Guildford, Surrey GU2 5RF
UK

R J Maughan
Department of Biomedical Sciences
University Medical School
Foresterhill
Aberdeen AB25 2ZD
Scotland UK

Susan McAreavey
Nutrition Services
Beth Israel Deaconess Medical Center
330 Brookline Avenue
Boston, MA 02215
USA

K C McCowen
Joslin Diabetes Center
Harvard Medical School
Boston MA 02215-5397
USA

Margaret A McDowell
Centers for Disease Control and Prevention
National Center for Health Statistics
6525 Belcrest Road
Hyattsville, Maryland 20782
USA

P McKeigue
Department of Epidemiology and Population Health
London School of Hygiene and Tropical Medicine
Keppel Street
London WC1E 7HT
UK

D McLaren
Nutritional Blindness Prevention Programme
International Centre for Eye Health
Institute of Ophthalmology, 11–43 Bath Street
London EC1V 9EL
UK

S McLaren
Faculty of Healthcare Sciences
Kingston Hill Campus
Kingston Hill, Kingston-Upon-Thames
Surrey KT2 7LB
UK

Donald J McNamara
Egg Nutrition Center
1819 H Street, NW, Suite 520
Washington DC 20006
USA

Joseph McPartlin
Department of Clinical Medicine
Trinity College, Faculty of Health Sciences
St James' Hospital
Dublin 8
Ireland

M Meguid
Department of Surgery
SUNY Health Science Center at Syracuse
750 E Adams Street
Syracuse NY 13210
USA

D Mela
Consumer Sciences Department
Institute of Food Research
Earley Gate
Reading RG6 6BZ
UK

R P Mensink
Department of Human Biology
Maastricht University
PO Box 616
6200 MD Maastricht
The Netherlands

A R Michell
Animal Health Trust
Centre for Small Animal Studies
Lanwades Park, Kentford
Suffolk CB8 7UU
UK

D J Millward
Center for Nutrition and Food Safety
School of Biological Sciences
University of Surrey, Guildford
Surrey GU2 5XH
UK

N Minaur
Royal National Hospital for Rheumatic Diseases
Upper Borough Walls
Bath BA1 1RL
UK

D M Mock
Division of Gastroenterology, Hepatology and Nutrition
Department of Pediatrics, University of Arkansas for
Medical Sciences
Arkansas Children's Hospital
800 Marshall St 512-7, Little Rock AR 72205
USA

A Ayesh Molla
Faculty of Allied Health Sciences
Kuwait University
PO Box 31470 Sulaibikaat 90805
Kuwait

A Majid Molla
Department of Pediatrics
Faculty of Medicine
Kuwait University
PO Box 24923 Safat 13110
Kuwait

J B Morgan
School of Biological Sciences
University of Surrey
Guildford
Surrey GU2 5XH
UK

T Morgan
Department of Physiology
University of Melbourne
Parkville 3052
Australia

John E Morley
Saint Louis University Health Sciences Center
Division of Geriatric Medicine
1402 S Grand Boulevard, Room M238
St Louis MO 63104-1079
USA

P A Morrisey
Department of Nutrition
University College Cork
Cork
Ireland

M Murphy
Sport and Exercise Sciences
The University of Ulster
Jordanstown
Co. Antrim BT37 0QB
Northern Ireland UK

M Stephen Murphy
Institute of Child Health
Whittal Street
Birmingham
B4 6NH
UK

Patricia Murphy-Miller
Division of Nutrition
Kennedy-Krieger Institute
707 North Broadway
Baltimore MD 21205
USA

M P Navarro
Estación Experimental del Zaidin CSIC
Departamento de Nutricion
Prof. Albereda 1
18008 Granada
Spain

M Nelson
Department of Nutrition and Dietetics
Kings College London
Campden Hill Road
London W8 7AH
UK

M C Neville
Departments of Physiology and Cell and Structural
Biology
University of Colorado
Health Science Center
4200 E 9th Avenue, Denver CO 80262-0001
USA

R Nicolosi
Center for Cardiovascular Disease Control
University of Massachusetts Lowell
Weed Hall, Rolfe St, Lowell, MA 01854
USA

F Nielsen
USDA, ARS
Grand Forks Human Nutrition Research Center
Grand Forks
ND 58202-9034
USA

C O'Brien
The Sugar Bureau
Duncan House
Dolphin Square
London SW1V 3PW
UK

K O'Brien
Johns Hopkins University
School of Hygiene and Public Health
Center for Human Nutrition
615 North Wolfe Street
Baltimore MD 21205
USA

D L O'Connor
Ross Products Division
Abbott Laboratories
625 Cleveland Avenue
Columbus OH 43215-3453
USA

M O'Neill
Northern Ireland Center for Diet and Health (NICHE)
School of Biomedical Sciences
University of Ulster, Coleraine
Co. L'Derry BT52 1SA
Northern Ireland UK

J M Ordovas
The Lipid Metabolism Laboratory
JM USDA Human Nutrition Research Center on Aging
Tufts University
Boston MA 02111
USA

L Patel
Booth Hall Children's Hospital
Manchester
M9 7AA
UK

J P Pearson
Department of Physiological Sciences
University of Newcastle
Newcastle-upon-Tyne
NE1 7RU
UK

F Pender
Queen Margaret College
Corstorphine Campus
Clewood Terrace
Edinburgh EH12 8TS
Scotland UK

J C Phillips
BIBRA International
Woodmansterne Road
Carshalton
Surrey SM5 4DS
UK

Barry M Popkin
Dept of Nutrition and Carolina Population Center
University of North Carolina, University Square
CB #8120
123 W Franklin Street
Chapel Hill, NC 27516-3997
USA

S D Poppitt
Department of Medicine
University of Auckland
Private Bag 92019
Auckland
New Zealand

E M Poskitt
Medical Research Council
Dunn Nutrition Group
Keneba
PO Box 273, Banjul
The Gambia

A D Postle
Child Health
School of Medicine
Southampton General Hospital
Southampton SO16 6YD
UK

J Pratt
Meat and Livestock Commission
PO Box 44, Winterhill House
Snowdon Drive, Milton Keynes MK6 1AX
UK

K R Price
Institute of Food Research
Norwich Laboratory, Norwich Research Park
Colney
Norwich NR4 7UA
UK

N D Priest
School of Environmental Science
Middlesex University
Bounds Green Rd
London N11 2NQ
UK

J Pryer
Public Health Nutrition Unit
Dept of Epidemiology and Population Health
London School of Hygiene and Tropical Medicine
49/51 Bedford Square, London WC1B 3DP
UK

Laura C Rall
School of Human Development and Nutritional
Sciences
University of Wisconsin
Stevens Point WI 54481-3897
USA

S Reddy
Department of Health
Skipton House
80 London Road
SE1 6LW
UK

C Reilly
10 Litchfield Close
Enstone
Chipping Norton
Oxon OX7 4LB
UK

M Rhodes
Institute of Food Research
Norwich Laboratory, Norwich Research Park
Colney
Norwich NR4 7UA
UK

R Rice
The Fish Foundation
PO Box 24
Tiverton
Devon EX16 4QQ
UK

D P Richardson
Nestle UK Ltd
St George's House
Croydon, Surrey CR9 1NR
UK

S B Roberts
USDA Human Nutrition Research Center on Aging
Energy Metabolism Laboratory
Tufts University, 711 Washington Street
Boston MA 02111-1524
USA

C L Rock
Dept of Family and Preventive Medicine
Cancer Prevention and Control Program
9500 Gilman Drive, University of California
San Diego, La Jolla, CA 92093-0901
USA

P J Rogers
Institute of Food Research
Earley Gate
Whiteknights Road
Reading RG6 6BZ
UK

Arturo R Rolla
Beth Israel Deaconess Medical Center
Harvard Medical School
110 Francis Street, Suite 2-F
Boston MA 02215
USA

J L Rombeau
Department of Surgery
Silverstein 4, University of Pennsylvania
3400 Spruce Street
Philadelphia PA 19143
USA

Pedro Rosso
Department of Pediatrics, Obstetrics and Gynecology
Facultad de Medicina
Pontificia Universidad Catolica de Chile
Casilla 114-D, Santiago
Chile

R Roubenoff
USDA Human Nutrition Research Center
Tufts University
711 Washington Street
Boston MA 02111
USA

Sharon Rubinstein
Center for Human Nutrition
Johns Hopkins University
615 North Wolfe Street
Baltimore, MA 21205-2179
USA

RDE Rumsey
Department of Biomedical Sciences
University of Sheffield
Firth Court, Western Bank
Sheffield S10 2TN
UK

C H S Ruxton
The Sugar Bureau
Duncan House
Dolphin Square
London SW1V 3PW
UK

Jose M Saavedra
Department of Pediatrics
Johns Hopkins University
School of Medicine, 300 N. Wolfe Street - Brady 320
Baltimore MD 21237
USA

Michèle J Sadler
Institute of Grocery Distribution
Grange Lane
Letchmore Heath
Watford, Hertfordshire WD2 8DQ
UK

Sofia P Salas
Department of Pediatrics, Obstetrics and Gynecology
Facultad de Medicina
Pontificia Universidad Catolica de Chile
Casilla 114-D, Santiago
Chile

M Saltmarsh
53 Blackberry Lane
Four Marks
Alton
Hants GU34 5DF
UK

J Samet
Department of Epidemiology
Johns Hopkins University
School of Hygiene and Public Health
615 North Wolfe Street
Baltimore MD 21205
USA

Patricia Queen Samour
Nutrition Services
Beth Israel Deaconess Medical Center
One Deaconess Road, Farr B
Boston, MA 02215
USA

C P Sánchez-Castillo
Department of Physiology of Nutrition
General Subdirection of Nutrition
National Institute of Nutrition "Salvador Zubirán"
Vasco de Quiroga # 15, Tlalpan 14000, Mexico DF
Mexico

Christopher D Saudek
Clinical Research Center
Osler 576, Johns Hopkins Hospital
500 North Wolfe Street
Baltimore MD 21205
USA

Sally Savidge
Division of Nutrition
Kennedy-Krieger Institute
707 North Broadway
Baltimore MD 21205
USA

G S Savige
Department of Medicine
Level 5 Block E, Monash Medical Center
246 Clayton Road
Clayton, Victoria
Australia 3168

Ana Lydia Sawaya
Department of Endocrine Physiology
Federal University of São Paulo, Escola Paulista de
Medicina
Rua Botucatu 862, 2 Andar
V Clementiona 04023-900, São Paulo
Brazil

W Schultink
Deutsche Gesellschaft fuer
Tecnische Zusammenarbeit (GTZ) GmbH
PO Box 5180
D - 65726 Eschborn
Germany

J M Scott
Department of Biochemistry
Trinity College
Dublin 2
Ireland

C J Seal
Human Nutrition Research Centre
University of Newcastle
Wellcome Research Laboratories
Royal Victoria Infirmary, Queen Victoria Road
Newcastle upon Tyne NE1 4LP
UK

C E Shaw
Royal Marsden NHS Trust
Fulham Road
London SW3
UK

D J Shaw
112 Kenwood Road
Beckenham
Kent
BR3 6RB
UK

T Sheehy
Department of Nutrition
University College Cork
Cork
Ireland

R Shepherd
Consumer Sciences Department
Institute of Food Research
Earley Gate, Whiteknights Road
Reading RG6 6BZ
UK

P S Shetty
Department of Epidemiology and Public Health
London School of Hygiene and Tropical Medicine
49/51 Bedford Square
London WC1B 3DP
UK

S M Shirreffs
Department of Biomedical Sciences
University Medical School
Foresterhill
Aberdeen AB25 2ZD
Scotland UK

D Shrimpton
Cambridge, UK

D B A Silk
Department of Gastroenterology & Nutrition
Central Middlesex Hospital NHS Trust
Acton Lane, Park Royal
London NW10 7NS
UK

H A Simmonds
Purine Research Laboratory
Guy's and St Thomas's United Medical and
Dental School
Floor 5 Thomas Guy House, Guy's Hospital
London Bridge, London SE1 9RT
UK

R J Smith
Metabolism Section
Joslin Diabetes Center
Harvard Medical School
One Joslin Place, Boston MA 02215-5397
USA

N W Solomons
Center for Studies of Sensory Impairment,
Aging and Metabolism (CeSSIAM)
Zone 11
Guatemala City
01011 Guatemala

D A T Southgate
8 Penryn Close
Norwich
Norfolk
NR4 7LY
UK

June Stevens
Departments of Nutrition and Epidemiology
UNC School of Public Health
CB 7400
Chapel Hill NC 27599-7400
USA

L Stockley
Timberland
Mill Hill
Brockweir
Near Chepstow NP6 7NN
UK

J J Strain
Northern Ireland Center for Diet and Health (NICHE)
University of Ulster, Coleraine
BT52 1SA
Northern Ireland UK

J Stubbs
The Rowett Research Institute
Greenburn Road
Bucksburn
Aberdeen AB2 9SB
Scotland UK

C Summerbell
Department of Primary Care and Population Sciences
Royal Free Hospital School of Medicine
University of London
Rowland Hill Street
London NW3 2PF UK

J F Sutcliffe
Department of Radiotherapy/Oncology
Palmerston North Hospital
Private Bag 11036
Palmerston North
New Zealand

E H M Temme
University of Leuven
Capucnenvoer 35
B-3000 Leuven
Belgium

R Tester
Department of Biological Sciences (Food Science)
Glasgow Caledonian University
Southbrae Campus, Southbrae Drive
Glasgow G13 1PP
UK

Briony Thomas
Elmers Farmhouse
Ockley
Dorking
Surrey RH5 5TQ
UK

R L Thompson
Institute of Human Nutrition
University of Southampton
Southampton General Hospital
Southampton, SO16 6YD
UK

B M Thomson
Rowett Research Institute
Grenburn Road
Bucksburn
Aberdeen AB2 9SB
Scotland UK

M Thorogood
Health Promotion Research Unit
London School of Hygiene and Tropical Medicine
Keppel Street
London WC1E 7HT
UK

D I Thurnham
Northern Ireland Centre for Diet and Health
School of Biomedical Sciences
University of Ulster, Coleraine
Co L'Derry BT52 1SA
Northern Ireland UK

D Topping
CSIRO Human Nutrition
Gate 13
Kintore Avenue
Adelaide SA 5000
Australia

Benjamin Torun
Clinical Nutrition and Metabolism
Division of Nutrition and Health
Institute of Nutrition of Central America and Panama
Apartado Postal 1188
Guatemala City
Guatemala

S U Toverud
University of North Carolina at Chapel Hill
School of Medicine
Chapel Hill
NC 27599-7455
USA

T R Trinick
Ulster Hospital
The Laboratories
Dundonald
Belfast
BT16 0RH
Northern Ireland UK

E Turley
The Northern Ireland Centre for Diet and Health
(NICHE)
Human Nutrition Research Group
University of Ulster, Coleraine BT52 1SA
Northern Ireland
UK

W H Turnbull
Centre for Nutrition and Food Research
Department of Dietetics and Nutrition
Queen Margaret College, Corstophine Campus
Clerwood Terrace, Edinburgh EH12 8TS
Scotland UK

B Underwood
International Union of Nutritional Sciences (IUNS)
Food and Nutrition Board
Institute of Medicine, NAS
2101 Constitution Avenue NW (FO 3049)
Washington DC 20418
USA

W A van Staveren
Wageningen Agricultural University
Division of Human Nutrition and Epidemiology
Bomenweg 2
6703 HD Wageningen
The Netherlands

M P Vaquero
Instituto de Nutricion y Bromatologia
CSIC-UCM, Facultad de Farmacia
Ciudad Universitaria
28040 Madrid
Spain

RG Vernon
Hannah Research Institute
Ayr
KA6 5HL
Scotland UK

M Wahlqvist
Department of Medicine
Level 5 Block E, Monash Medical Center
246 Clayton Road
Clayton Victoria
Australia 3168

Ann F Walker
Hugh Sinclair Unit of Human Nutrition
Food Science and Technology Dept, Reading University
Whiteknights Reading, PO Box 226
RG6 6AP
UK

A R P Walker
Human Biochemistry Research Unit
South African Institute for Medical Research
PO Box 1038
Johannesburg
South Africa

Donald G Weir
Department of Clinical Medicine
Trinity College Centre for Health Sciences
St James's Hospital
Dublin 8
Ireland

R W Welch
Northern Ireland Centre for Diet and Health
School of Biomedical Sciences
University of Ulster
Coleraine BT52 1SA
Northern Ireland UK

A West
Department of Food and Nutrition
University of Huddersfield
Queensgate
Huddersfield HD1 3DH
UK

K West
Johns Hopkins University
School of Hygiene and Public Health
615 North Wolfe Street
Baltimore, Maryland 21205-2179
USA

A B Williams
Department of Surgery
University of Cincinnati Medical Center
Cincinnati
OH 45267-0558
USA

D H Williamson
Metabolic Research Laboratory
Radcliffe Infirmary
Oxford
OX2 6HE
UK

D Wilmore
Brigham and Women's Hospital
Harvard Medical School
75 Francis Street
Boston MA 02115
USA

A Wilson
Department of Nutrition
University College Cork
Ireland

M-M G Wilson
Division of Geriatric Medicine
Saint Louis University Health Sciences Center
1402 South Grand Boulevard, Room M238
St Louis MO 63104-1028
USA

H Wiseman
Department of Nutrition and Dietetics
King's College London
Campden Hill Road
London W8 7AH
UK

T Wolever
Department of Nutritional Sciences
150 College Street
University of Toronto
Toronto
Canada M5S 3E2

M Wolraich
Director of the Division of Child Development
Vanderbilt University
2100 Pierce Avenue, Nashville
Tennessee 37232-3573
USA

J E Wraith
Willink Laboratory
Royal Manchester Children's Hospital
Pendlebury
Near Manchester M27 1HA
UK

Jacqueline D Wright
Centers for Disease Control and Prevention
National Center for Health Statistics
6525 Belcrest Road
Hyattsville, Maryland 20782
USA

A Wynne
Microbiology Department
Institute of Food Research
Earley Gate
Reading, Berkshire RG6 6BZ
UK

Steven H Zeisel
Department of Nutrition
University of North Carolina at Chapel Hill
2212 McGavran-Greenberg Hall
Chapel Hill, NC 27599-7400
USA

Aglaia Zellos
Division of Gastroenterology and Nutrition
Johns Hopkins School of Medicine
Brady 314 - 600 N Wolfe Street
Baltimore MD 21287
USA

S Zidenberg-Cherr
Department of Nutrition
University of California at Davis
Meyer Hall 3rd Floor
Davis CA 95616
USA

CONTENTS

VOLUME 1

A

VOLUME 2

E

F

I

K

L

VOLUME 3

Biochemical Aspects   *J Bines*   1779

STEATORRHOEA

Nutritional Management   *A Burke, J L Rombeau*   1786

STOMACH *see* GASTROINTESTINAL TRACT: Structure and Function of the Stomach

STROKE

Nutritional Management   *S McLaren*   1795

SUCROSE

Nutritional Role, Absorption and Metabolism   *J Brand-Miller*   1802

Dietary Sucrose and Disease   *I Macdonald*   1810

SUGAR *see* CARBOHYDRATES: Chemistry and Classification (Including Dietary Fibre (Fiber));
Regulation of Carbohydrate Metabolism; Requirements and Dietary Importance; GALACTOSE:
Absorption and Metabolism; GLUCOSE: Chemistry, Dietary Sources and Glycaemic Index; Metabolism
and Maintenance of Blood Glucose Level; Glucose Tolerance; SUCROSE: Nutritional Role, Absorption
and Metabolism; Dietary Sucrose and Disease

SURGERY

Perioperative Feeding   *S A Hill*   1815

Long-term Nutritional Management of Patients   *D W Wilmore*   1822

T

TEA *see* CAFFEINE: Chemistry and Physiological Effects

TEETH *see* DENTAL DISEASE: Aetiology and Epidemiology

THERAPEUTIC DIETETICS

Lung Diseases   *A MacDonald*   1831

Intensive Care Management   *Susan McAreavey, Patricia Queen Samour*   1839

Short Bowel Syndrome   *L Howard, M Malone*   1846

THIAMIN

Physiology   *A E Cathcart, D I Thurnham*   1858

Beriberi   *A E Cathcart, David I Thurnham*   1863

THIRST

Physiology   *J Leiper*   1870

TOCOPHEROLS

Physiology   *T Sheehy, P A Morrissey*   1878

TRACE ELEMENTS *see* CHROMIUM: Physiology, Dietary Sources and Requirements; COPPER:
Physiology, Dietary Sources and Requirements; IMMUNITY: Role of Iron and Zinc; IODINE: Physiology,
Dietary Sources and Requirements; IRON: Physiology, Dietary Sources and Requirements;
MANGANESE: Physiology, Dietary Sources and Requirements; SELENIUM: Physiology, Dietary
Sources and Requirements; ZINC: Physiology

TRANS-FATTY ACIDS *see* FATTY ACIDS: Health Effects of *trans* Fatty Acids

TUMOUR *see* CANCER: Epidemiology and Associations Between Diet and Cancer; Epidemiology of
Breast Cancer; Epidemiology of Colorectal Cancer; Epidemiology of Lung Cancer; Epidemiology of
Gastrointestinal Cancers other than Colorectal Cancers

U

ULTRATRACE ELEMENTS

Physiology   *F Nielsen*   1884

UNITED NATIONS CHILDREN'S FUND

History and Role   *D Alnwick, J P Greaves*   1897

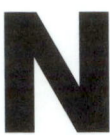

NIACIN

Contents
Physiology, Dietary Sources and Requirements
Pellagra

Physiology, Dietary Sources and Requirements

C J Bates, MRC Dunn Nutrition Unit, Cambridge, UK

Absorption, Transport and Storage

Niacin is a B vitamin that is essential for health in humans and also in most other mammals that have been investigated. Niacin is associated with a characteristic deficiency disease in humans known as pellagra. Pellagra has been described and identified in various communities, notably in Spain and North America in the last century and the early years of this century. It has persisted in Yugoslavia, Egypt, Mexico and some African countries to the middle of the present century and beyond. Pellagra is characteristically associated with maize-based diets. The skin lesions found in pellagra are most severe during the summer months because of the effects of the exacerbating sun exposure. However, some countries with a maize diet (e.g. Guatemala) avoid pellagra by means of the niacin present in roasted coffee (**Table 1**). Others avoid it by lime treatment, e.g. in the preparation of tortillas.

Preformed niacin occurs in foods either as nicotinamide (niacinamide) or as the pyridine nucleotide coenzymes derived from it, or as nicotinic acid, without the amide nitrogen, which is the form known as 'niacin' in North America. Both nicotinamide and nicotinic acid are equally effective as the vitamin, but in large doses they exert markedly different pharmacological effects, so it is important, at least in that context, to make and maintain the distinction. In addition to the preformed vitamin, an important *in vivo* precursor is the amino acid L-tryptophan, obtained from dietary protein. Because the human total niacin supply, and hence niacin status,

depends on the dietary tryptophan supply as well as on the amount of preformed dietary niacin and its bioavailability, it has become the accepted practice to express niacin intakes as 'niacin equivalents', which is a combination of mg preformed dietary niacin and mg niacin which can become available by conversion from tryptophan within the body. As discussed later, this calculation involves several assumptions, and is therefore only an approximation to the actual supply to the body for any particular individual; however, it is considered adequate for most practical purposes.

It appears likely that the most important ultimate sources of preformed niacin in most foods, particularly those of animal foods, are the pyridine nucleotides: $NAD(H_2)$ and $NADP(H_2)$. Hydrolases and pyrophosphatases present in biological tissues convert these coenzymes to partly degraded products, which are then available as sources of the vitamin. NAD glycohydrolase and pyrophosphatase enzymes are present in the gut mucosa to assist hydrolysis and absorption of the hydrolysed products, and these are likely to include both nicotinamide and nicotinamide ribonucleotide, the latter being further degraded to the riboside. Absorption of nicotinamide or nicotinic acid by the mammalian intestine has been shown to consist of a saturable transport component, dominant at low intakes, which is dependent on sodium, energy and pH, and a nonsaturable component, which becomes dominant at high doses or intake levels. Absorption is efficient even at such high discrete doses as 3 g or more: as much as 85% of such a dose is subsequently excreted into the urine. Absorption of test niacin doses introduced directly into the human upper ileum is rapid, with peak levels appearing in blood plasma within 5–10 min.

Transport of niacin between the liver and the

Table 1 Niacin equivalents in selected foods[a]

	Niacin equivalents from preformed niacin[b] (mg per 100 g, wet)	Niacin equivalents from tryptophan[c] (mg per 100 g, wet)	Total niacin equivalents (mg per 100 g, wet)
Milk	0.1	0.8	0.9
Raw beef	5.0	4.7	9.7
Raw white fish	2.4	3.4	5.8
Raw eggs	0.1	3.7	3.8
Raw potatoes	0.6	0.5	1.1
Raw peas	2.5	1.1	3.6
Raw peanuts	13.8	5.5	19.3
White bread	0.8	1.7	2.5
Polished rice	0.2	1.5	1.7
Maize	0.1	0.9	1.0
Cornflakes (fortified)	16.0	0.9	16.9
Coffee[d]	24.1	2.9	27.0

[a,d]Data adapted from: Paul AA (1969) The calculation of nicotinic acid equivalents and retinol equivalents in the British diet. *Nutrition (London)* **23**: 131–136,[a] and supplements to *McCance and Widdowson's The Composition of Foods* (Holland B, Welch AA, Unwin ID, Buss DH, Paul AA and Southgate DAT (1991), The Royal Society of Chemistry and MAFF),[a] and from Bressani R *et al.* (1961) Effect of processing method and variety on niacin and ether extract content of green and roasted coffee. *Food Technology* **15**: 306–308.[a,d]
  Niacin is released from trigonelline in coffee beans by the roasting process.
[b]Amount available for absorption. In the case of bread, rice and maize, the total amounts present are 1.7, 1.5 and 1.2 mg per 100 g, but apart from the niacin added in the fortification of white flour, 90% of this is unavailable for utilization by humans.
[c]Assuming that 60 mg tryptophan yields 1 mg niacin equivalent.

intestine can occur *in vivo*, as indicated by radioactive probes in animals, and the liver appears to be a major site of conversion of niacin to its ultimate functional products: the nicotinamide nucleotide coenzymes. Nicotinamide can pass readily between the cerebrospinal fluid and the plasma, thus ensuring a supply also to the brain and spinal cord. Liver contains greater niacin coenzyme concentrations than most other tissues, but all metabolically active tissues contain these essential metabolic components. Both facilitated diffusion (which is sodium- and energy-dependent and saturable), and passive diffusion (which is nonsaturable) contribute to tissue uptake from the bloodstream. With the exception of muscle, brain and testis, within the body nicotinic acid is a better precursor of the coenzyme form than is nicotinamide. The liver appears to be the most important site of conversion of tryptophan to the nicotinamide coenzymes.

Of the two pyridine nucleotide coenzymes, NAD is present mainly as the oxidized form in the tissues, whereas NADP is principally present in the reduced form, $NADPH_2$. There are important homeostatic regulation mechanisms which ensure and maintain an appropriate ratio of these coenzymes in their respective oxidized or reduced forms in healthy tissues. Once converted to coenzymes within the cells, the niacin therein is effectively trapped, and can only diffuse out again after degradation to smaller molecules. This implies, of course, that the synthesis of the essential coenzyme nucleotides must occur within each tissue and cell type, each of which must possess the enzymatic apparatus for their synthesis from the precursor niacin. Loss of nicotinamide and nicotinic acid into the urine is minimized (except when the intake exceeds requirements) by means of an efficient reabsorption from the glomerular filtrate.

Metabolism and Excretion

The conversion of tryptophan to nicotinic acid *in vivo* is depicted in **Fig. 1**. The rate of conversion of tryptophan to niacin and the pyridine nucleotides is controlled by the activities of tryptophan dioxygenase (known alternatively as tryptophan pyrrolase), kynurenine hydroxylase and kynureninase. These enzymes are, in turn, dependent on factors such as other B vitamins, glucagon, glucocorticoid hormones and oestrogen metabolites, and there are various competing pathways which also affect the rate of conversion. For these reasons, a variety of nutrient deficiencies, toxins, genetic and metabolic abnormalities, etc. can influence niacin status and requirements.

For practical purposes, on the basis of studies performed in the 1950s, 60 mg tryptophan is deemed to give rise to 1 mg nicotinic acid; hence 60 mg

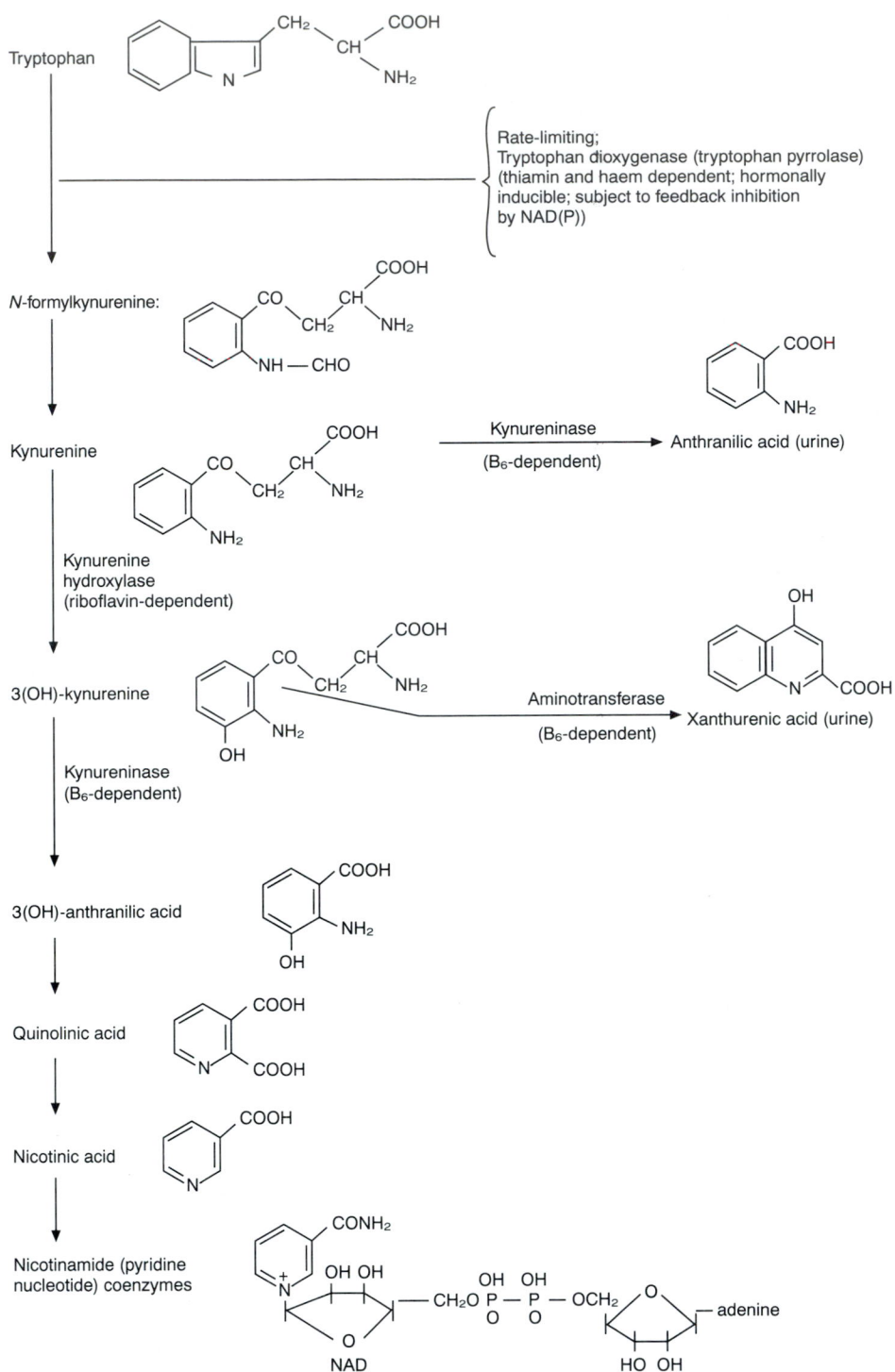

Figure 1 *In vivo* conversion of tryptophan to nicotinic acid.

tryptophan contributes 1 mg niacin equivalent, for dietary intake calculations and food tables (see Table 1).

The two pyridine nucleotide coenzymes, formerly known as 'coenzymes I and II', then for a period as 'DPN and TPN', and known nowadays as 'NAD' and 'NADP' (nicotinamide adenine dinucleotide and nicotinamide adenine dinucleotide phosphate), are involved in hundreds of enzyme-catalysed redox reactions *in vivo*. Although a minority of these diverse reactions can use either of the two niacin-derived cofactors, most are highly specific for one or the other.

Catabolism of the pyridine nucleotide coenzymes

in vivo is achieved by four classes of enzymes: NAD glycohydrolase, ADP ribosyl transferases and poly (ADP ribose) synthetases, (all of which liberate nicotinamide), and NAD pyrophosphatase (which liberates nicotinamide mononucleotide which is then further hydrolysed to nicotinamide). Turnover of nicotinamide then results in the formation of 1-methylnicotinamide (usually described as N^1-methyl nicotinamide or NMN), an excretory product which is excreted in the kidney and appears in the urine, together with some further oxidation products, typically the 1-methyl-2-pyridone-5-carboxamide and 1-methyl-4-pyridone-3-carboxamide (usually referred to as '2-pyridone' and '4-pyridone', respectively). These excretory turnover products can be used as indicators of whole body niacin status (see below). At high intakes of niacin, as much as 85% of the intake may be excreted unchanged; however the excretion of nicotinamide always predominates over that of nicotinic acid.

Hydrolysis of hepatic NAD to yield nicotinamide allows the release of niacin for utilization by other tissues. Four key enzyme classes – NAD glycohydrolase, NAD pyrophosphatase, ADP ribosyltransferase and poly (ADP ribose) synthetase – control this turnover process. Relative protection of the pyridine nucleotide within certain key enzymes such as glyceraldehyde 3-phosphate dehydrogenase confers a protection on certain key metabolic pathways, thus ensuring good homeostatic control. By contrast, there is evidence that the enzymes which catalyse pyridine nucleotide turnover may be hyperactivated within cells that have been damaged by carcinogens, including mycotoxins, thus starving these damaged cells of essential cofactors and causing their death, presumably to protect the rest of the organism. This effect may help to explain the otherwise puzzling observation that mouldy grain in the diet can increase the risk of pellagra when niacin and tryptophan intakes are marginal. In normal, healthy cells, the compartmentalization of hydrolytic enzymes prevents unwanted coenzyme turnover, and this compartmentalization seems to become breached in damaged or dying cells.

Other urinary excretion products of niacin include nicotinuric acid (nicotinoyl glycine); nicotinamide N-oxide, and trigonelline (N^1-methyl nicotinic acid); the latter may arise from bacterial action in the gut or from the absorption of this substance from foods. The pattern of the different turnover metabolites varies between species, between diets (depending partly on the ratio of nicotinamide to nicotinic acid in the diet), and partly with niacin status; thus there are complex regulatory mechanisms to be considered.

Metabolic Function and Essentiality

The best-known functions of niacin are derived from the functions of its coenzymes: NAD and NADP in the hydrogen/electron transfer redox reactions in living cells. Like most B vitamins, niacin is not extensively stored in forms or in depots that are usually metabolically inactive, but rather those that can become available during dietary deficiency. However, some 'storage' of the coenzymes NAD and NADP in the liver is thought to occur. An inadequate dietary intake leads rapidly to significant tissue depletion within 1–2 months, and then successively to biochemical abnormalities, followed by clinical signs of deficiency, and eventually to death. As with the other B vitamins, rates of turnover and hence the rates of excretion of coenzyme breakdown products decline progressively as dietary deficiency becomes more severe and prolonged, so that the tissue levels are relatively protected and spared. In adult humans a severe deficiency may take many months to develop before it results in the clinical signs of pellagra.

Some of the most important and characteristic functions of NAD manifest in the principal cellular catabolic pathways, responsible for liberation of energy during the oxidation of energy-producing fuels. NADP, however, functions mainly in the reductive reactions of lipid biosynthesis, and the reduced form of this coenzyme is generated via the pentose phosphate cycle. NAD is essential for the synthesis and repair of DNA. NAD has, in addition, a role in supplying ADP ribose moieties to lysine, arginine and asparagine residues in proteins such as histones, DNA lyase II and DNA-dependent RNA polymerase, and to polypeptides such as the bacterial diphtheria and cholera toxins. In the nucleus, poly (ADP ribose) synthetase is activated by binding to DNA breakage points and is involved in DNA repair. It is also concerned with condensation and expansion of chromatin during the cell cycle and in DNA replication. Niacin status affects the level of ADP ribolysation of proteins. A high level of poly (ADP ribose) synthetase activity, which is found in some tumours, can result in low levels of NAD. A chromium dinicotinate complex found in yeast extracts may function as a glucose tolerance factor or in detoxification, but this has not yet been proven.

Because the electron transport functions of NAD frequently involve flavin coenzymes, and because both flavin coenzymes and vitamin B_6 coenzymes are involved in the conversion of tryptophan to niacin *in vivo*, there are important metabolic interactions between these B vitamins. A similarity of clinical deficiency signs, making it difficult to distinguish between them, may be encountered in population studies of deficiency.

Because the body's need for niacin can be met completely by dietary tryptophan, it is not, strictly speaking, an essential vitamin. In this respect it resembles carnitine, which can be synthesized entirely from lysine, but for which in some circumstances a dietary requirement exists. Traditionally, however, niacin is classified as an essential vitamin, because some human diets have tended to be lacking in niacin and its precursor, tryptophan. Some animals such as sheep and cattle appear to be able to synthesize sufficient niacin for their needs from tryptophan, and do not therefore need preformed niacin in their diets.

Assessment of Niacin Status

Whereas the measurement of B vitamin status has, in recent years, tended to focus on blood analysis, perhaps mainly because of the convenience of sample collection, the development of blood-based status analysis for niacin has lagged behind that of the other components of the B complex. Recent studies have indeed suggested that the erythrocyte concentration of the niacin-derived coenzyme NAD may provide useful information about the niacin status of human subjects; that a reduction in the ratio of NAD to NADP to below 1.0 in red cells may provide evidence of niacin deficiency; and that a decline in plasma tryptophan levels may indicate a more severe deficiency than a decline in red cell NAD levels. These claims now need to be tested in naturally deficient human populations. The niacin coenzymes can be quantitated either by enzyme-linked reactions or by making use of their natural fluorescence in alkaline solution.

At present, niacin status is most commonly assessed by the assay of some of the breakdown products of niacin coenzymes in the urine. Of these, N^1-methyl nicotinamide (NMN) is the easiest to measure, because of a convenient conversion *in vitro* to a fluorescent product, which can then be quantitated without the need for separation. However, more definitive and reliable information can be obtained by the measurement of urinary NMN in conjunction with one or more of the urinary pyridone turnover products (N^1-methyl-2-pyridone-5-carboxamide and N^1-methyl-4-pyridone-3-carboxamide), which can be detected and quantitated by UV absorption following high-pressure liquid chromatography. The Interdepartmental Committee on Nutrition for National Defense (USA) selected the criterion of niacin deficiency in humans as an NMN excretion rate of <5.8 μmol (0.8 mg) NMN per day in 24 h urine samples. More recently, the ratio of NMN to 2-pyridone excretion was proposed as a convenient alternative, applicable to casual urine samples, but this approach has been criticized, and a more recent study has suggested that <8.8 μmol per day (1.2 mg per day) of either NMN or 2-pyridone, or both, can be used as evidence of niacin intakes less than 6 mg nicotinic acid equivalents per day, which is likely to lead to deficiency in adult subjects. It is of interest that the catabolic pathways for niacin differ markedly between mammalian species: thus 2-pyridone is not an important catabolite for the rat, cat or dog.

Requirements and Signs of Deficiency

As for most other micronutrients, the requirement of niacin to prevent or reverse the clinical deficiency signs is not known very precisely, and probably depends on ancillary dietary deficiences or other insults occurring in natural human populations. For the purpose of estimating niacin requirements for RDAs or Dietary Reference Values, the criterion of restoration of urinary excretion of NMN during controlled human depletion–repletion studies has been selected, and on this basis, the average adult requirement has been estimated as 5.5 mg (45 μmol) of niacin equivalents per 1000 kcal (4200 kJ). Adding a 20% allowance for individual variation, so as to cover the mean ± 2 SD of requirements, this needs to be increased to 6.6 mg (54 μmol) per 1000 kcal, (4200 kJ), which is the current RDA (USA) or Reference Nutrient Intake (UK). Niacin requirements are, by convention, expressed as a ratio to energy expenditure. For subjects with very low energy intakes, the daily intake of niacin should not fall below 13 mg, however. Provided that dietary protein levels are reasonable, as is the case for most Western diets, the tryptophan content alone is likely to be sufficient to provide at least 6.6 mg niacin per 1000 kcal (4200 kJ) without the need for any performed dietary niacin. For this reason, niacin is generally considered to be adequately, indeed generously, supplied in Western diets, and there is now relatively little concern about possible endemic deficiency of niacin in developed countries.

The appearance of severe niacin deficiency as endemic pellagra, especially in North America in the nineteenth and early twentieth centuries, has been ascribed to the very poor availability of bound forms of niacin (in niacytin, a polysaccharide/ glycopeptide/polypeptide-bound form, which is 90% indigestible), together with the relatively low content of tryptophan occurring in grains (see Table 1). However, the lack of available niacin and tryptophan may not have been the whole story, since coexisting deficiencies or imbalances of other nutrients, including riboflavin, may also have contributed to this endemic disease. It appears also that the choice of cooking methods may have been critical, since the Mexican custom of cooking maize with lime in the preparation of tortillas helps to release the bound niacin from its carbohydrate complex and to increase the bioavailability of tryptophan-containing proteins, and thus to reduce the prevalence of clinical deficiency disease. In parts of India, pellagra has been encountered in communities whose main staple is a form of millet known as 'jowar', which is rich in leucine. It was proposed, and evidence was obtained from animal and *in vitro* studies, that high intakes of leucine can increase the requirements for niacin. However other evidence is conflicting (this interaction is not fully understood). In parts of South Africa, iron overload has been reported to complicate the metabolic effects of low niacin intakes.

The average content of niacin in human breast milk is 8 mg (65.6 μmol) per 1000 kcal (4200 kJ), and this is the basis for the recommendations (and dietary reference values) for infants up to 6 months. In the UK, the Reference Nutrient Intake niacin increment during pregnancy is nil, and during lactation it is 2 mg per day.

The most characteristic clinical signs of severe niacin deficiency in humans are dermatosis (hyperpigmentation, hyperkeratosis, desquamation – especially where exposed to the sun), anorexia, achlorhydria, diarrhoea, angular stomatitis, cheilosis, magenta tongue, anaemia, neuropathy (headache, dizziness, tremor, neurosis, apathy). In addition to the pellagra caused by dietary deficiency or imbalance, there are also reports of disturbed niacin metabolism associated with phenylketonuria, acute intermittent porphyria, diabetes mellitus, some types of cancer (carcinoid syndrome), thyrotoxicosis, fever, stress, tissue repair, renal disease, iron overload, etc. The picture in other species is not radically different; however, deficient dogs and cats typically exhibit 'black tongue' (pustules in the mouth, excessive salivation), and bloody diarrhoea: pigs exhibit neurological lesions affecting the ganglion cells; rats exhibit damage to the peripheral nerves (cells and axons); fowl exhibit inflammation of the upper gastrointestinal tract, dermatitis, diarrhoea and damage to the feathers. All species exhibit reduction of appetite and loss of weight; however it is of interest that the skin lesions seen in humans are rare in most other species.

Dietary Sources, High Intakes and Antimetabolites

As can be seen from Table 1, different types of foods differ considerably, not only in their total contribution to nicotinic acid equivalents, but also in the ratio of the contribution from preformed niacin and from tryptophan. In a typical Western diet, it has been calculated that if the 60 mg tryptophan = 1 mg niacin formula is applied, then preformed niacin provides about 50% of the niacin supply in the diet. In practice it seems possible for all of the niacin requirement to be provided by dietary tryptophan in Western diets. As is the case for the other B vitamins, meat, poultry and fish are excellent sources of niacin equivalents, followed by dairy and grain products, but as noted above, certain grains such as maize, and whole highly polished rice, can be very poor sources and may be associated with clinical deficiency if the diets are otherwise poor and monotonous.

In recent years, both nicotinamide and nicotinic acid have been proposed and tested for possibly useful pharmacological properties at high intake levels. This new phase of interest in the vitamin has, in turn, raised concerns about the possible side effects of high intakes, and the definition of maximum safe intakes.

The greatest interest, in pharmacological terms, has been centred around nicotinic acid, which has been shown to have marked antihyperlipidaemic properties at daily doses of 2–6 g. Nicotinamide does not share this particular pharmacological activity. Large doses of nicotinic acid reduce the mobilization of fatty acids from adipose tissue by inhibiting the breakdown of triacylglycerols through lipolysis. They also inhibit hepatic triacylglycerol synthesis, thus limiting the assembly and secretion of very low-density lipoproteins from the liver and reducing serum cholesterol levels. Large doses of nicotinic acid also lower the serum level of lipoprotein (a), which is a risk factor for cardiovascular disease, and increase plasma high-density lipoprotein. The ratio of HDL_2 to HDL_3 is increased by nicotinic acid; there is a reduced rate of synthesis of apolipoprotein A-II and a transfer of some apolipoprotein A-I from HDL_3 to HDL_2. These changes are all considered potentially beneficial in reducing the risk of cardiovascular disease. If given intravenously, large doses of nicotinic acid can, however, produce side effects such as temporary vasodilatation and hypotension. Other side effects can include nausea, vomiting, diarrhoea and general gastrointestinal disturbance, headache, fatigue, difficulty in focusing, skin discoloration, dry hair, sore throat, etc. A large trial for secondary prevention of myocardial infarction, with a 15 year period of follow-up, produced convincing evidence for moderate but significant protection against mortality, which was attributed either to the cholesterol-lowering effect or an early effect on nonfatal reinfarction, or both. Nicotinic acid is still the treatment of choice for some classes of high-risk hyperlipidaemic patients, although newer drugs may have fewer side effects and therefore be preferred.

The potential benefits of the lipid-lowering effects of nicotinic acid have to be considered in the light of possibly toxic effects, particularly for the liver. These may manifest as jaundice, changes in liver function tests, changes in carbohydrate tolerance, and changes in uric acid metabolism including hyperuricaemia. There may also be accompanying ultrastructural changes. Hyperuricaemia may result from effects on intestinal bacteria and enzymes, and from effects on renal tubular function. Such toxic effects are especially severe if sustained release preparations of nicotinic acid are used.

Nicotinamide does not share with nicotinic acid these effects on lipid metabolism or the associated toxicity. However, it has been shown to be an inhibitor of poly (ADP ribose) synthetase in pancreatic β cells in animal studies, A high-risk group of children aged 5–8 years in New Zealand, given large doses of nicotinamide daily for up to 4.2 years had only half the predicted incidence of insulin-dependent diabetes. This promising result clearly requires confirmation, and an international trial is now being carried out.

Other claims for megadoses of nicotinic acid or nicotinamide, such as the claim that abnormalities associated with schizophrenia, Down syndrome, hyperactivity in children, etc. can be reduced, have so far failed to win general acceptance. Clearly niacin deficiency or dependency can exacerbate some types of mental illness such as depression or dementia. There have been a number of attempts to treat depression with tryptophan or niacin, or both, on the basis that the correction of depressed brain levels of serotonin would be advantageous. However, these have met with only limited success. Schizophrenics have been treated with nicotinic acid on the basis that their synthesis of NAD is impaired in some parts of the brain, and that the formation of hallucinogenic substances such as methylated indoles may be controlled. Another type of intervention has been to give vitamin B_6 supplements, to attempt to stimulate the conversion of tryptophan to NAD.

There are various medical conditions and drug interactions that can increase the requirement for niacin. Examples are Hartnup disease, in which tryptophan transport in the intestine and kidney is impaired; carcinoid syndrome, in which tryptophan turnover is increased; and isoniazid treatment, which causes B_6 depletion and hence interference with niacin formation from tryptophan. Hartnup disease (the name of the first patient being Hartnup) is a rare genetic disease in which the conversion of tryptophan to niacin is reduced, partly as a result of impaired tryptophan absorption. Affected subjects exhibit the classical skin and neurological lesions of pellagra, which can be alleviated by prolonged treatment with niacin. Another genetic disease which may respond to niacin supplements is Fredrikson type I familial hypercholesterolaemia; nicotinic acid is effective in reducing the raised blood cholesterol levels associated with this abnormality. Although self-medication with large doses of niacin cannot be recommended for genetically normal people, it clearly retains a place as a useful therapeutic drug for some medical conditions.

There are several analogues and antimetabolites of niacin that are of potential use or metabolic interest. The closely related isoniazid is commonly used for treatment of tuberculosis; indeed, nicotinamide itself has been used for that purpose. Nicotinic acid diethylamide ('nikethamide') is used as a stimulant in cases of central nervous system depression after poisoning, trauma or collapse. Possible antineoplastic analogues include 6-dimethylaminonicotinamide and 6-aminonicotinamide; however, the latter is also highly teratogenic. These latter compounds inhibit several key enzymes whose substrates are NAD or NADP, by being converted *in vivo* to analogues of these coenzymes. The compound 3-acetyl pyridine, which also forms an analogue of NAD, can have either antagonistic or niacin-replacing properties, depending on the dose used. Commonly used drugs such as metronidazole are also niacin antagonists.

See also: **Bioavailability**: Definition and General Aspects. **Energy Metabolism**: Tricarboxylic Acid Cycle and Oxidative Phosphorylation. **Hyperlipidaemia (Hyperlipidemia)**: Overview; Nutritional Management. **Riboflavin**: Physiology. **Vitamin B_6**: Physiology.

Further Reading

Bender DA (1992) Niacin. In: *Nutritional Biochemistry of the Vitamins*, chap. 8, pp 184–222. Cambridge: Cambridge University Press.

Carpenter KJ (1981) *Pellagra: Benchmark Papers in the History of Biochemistry/II*. Stroudsburg, Pennsylvania: Dowden, Hutchinson & Ross Publ. Co.

Di Palma JR and Thayer WS (1991) Use of niacin as a drug. *Annual Review of Nutrition* 11:169–187.

Fu CS, Swendseid ME, Jacob RA and McKee RW (1989) Biochemical markers for assessment of niacin status in young men: levels of erythrocyte niacin coenzymes and plasma tryptophan. *Journal of Nutrition* 119:1949–1955.

Hankes LV (1984) Nicotinic acid and nicotinamide. In: Machlin LJ (ed.) *Handbook of Vitamins*, chap. 8, pp 329–377. New York: Marcel Dekker Inc.

Henderson LM (1983). Niacin. *Annual Review of Biochemistry* 3:289–307.

Horwitt MK, Harvey CC, Rothwell WS, Cutler JL and Haffron D (1956) Tryptophan–niacin relationship in man. *Journal of Nutrition* 60 (supplement 1):1–43.

Jacob RA, Swendseid ME, McKee RW, Fu CS and Clemens RA (1989) Biochemical markers for assessment of niacin status in young men: urinary and blood levels of niacin metabolites. *Journal of Nutrition* 119:591–598.

Sauberlich HE, Dowdy RP and Skala JH (1974) *Laboratory Tests for the Assessment of Nutritional Status* pp 70–74. Boca Raton: CRC Press.

Swendseid ME and Jacob RA (1984) Niacin. In: Shils ME and Young VR (eds) *Modern Nutrition in Health and Disease*, 7th edn, chap. 22, pp 376–382. Philadelphia: Lea & Febiger.

Pellagra

D A Bender, University College London, UK

Pellagra is a nutritional disease caused by the combined deficiency of the vitamin niacin and the essential amino acid tryptophan. The clinical features of pellagra are dermatitis, diarrhoea and dementia. It is commonly known as the 'disease of the four Ds', since it is also fatal – the fourth 'D' is death.

The first description of pellagra was by Casal in Spain in 1735, who called it *el mal de la rosa* – the red disease. He recognized that the underlying cause was nutritional, a result of the limited diet of many people in central Spain at the time, although he did not associate it with the then recent introduction of maize from central America. The name *pellagra* was coined by Frapolli in Italy in 1771, from the Italian *pelle* for skin and *agra* for rough, thus describing the most striking feature of the disease, the roughened sunburn-like appearance of areas of the skin exposed to sunlight.

Other early studies showed that feeding additional protein, and especially the essential amino acid tryptophan, would also prevent or cure pellagra, suggesting that it was a protein deficiency disease rather than due to lack of a vitamin. It was not until 1947 that the problem was resolved, when it was shown that tryptophan is a metabolic precursor of the nicotinamide moiety of the coenzymes NAD and NADP. The coenzymes can be formed in the body either from preformed niacin or by *de novo* synthesis from tryptophan.

Aetiology and Prevalence

The cause of pellagra is an inadequate intake of both the vitamin niacin and the essential amino acid tryptophan, which acts as a precursor for the endogenous synthesis of nicotinamide, as shown in **Fig. 1**.

Although Casal described pellagra as a nutritional disease, at the beginning of the twentieth century it was generally assumed to be due to an infectious agent. The nutritional basis of the disease, and the interaction between deficiencies of both niacin and tryptophan, was established mainly by Goldberger and coworkers in the USA between 1913 and 1948. A 'pellagra-preventing factor' isolated from protein-free yeast extract was shown in 1937 to be nicotinic acid, and either nicotinic acid or its amide, nicotinamide, was shown to prevent or cure the disease in both man and experimental animals. The name *niacin* was coined when it was decided to enrich foods with the vitamin, since it was considered that nicotinic acid would be unacceptable as a food additive, because of its chemical (but not metabolic) relationship with nicotine. In the USA 'niacin' is commonly used to mean nicotinic acid, while the amide is niacinamide: elsewhere 'niacin' is used as a generic descriptor for nicotinic acid and/or nicotinamide.

The spread of pellagra largely followed the introduction of maize as a dietary staple, and by the nineteenth century it was a major problem around the Mediterranean, in the Balkans and Ukraine, as well as the southern USA and southern Africa. In South Africa pellagra became a problem following the outbreak of rinderpest in 1897, which killed most of the cattle, leading to a marked deterioration in the diet of people who had previously had ample supplies of milk and meat to supplement their maize-based diet. In the USA it was the social and economic upheaval of the Civil War which led to large numbers of subsistence farmers living on a diet based very largely on maize.

During the first half of the twentieth century, pellagra was a major problem of public health in the southern USA, with some 87 000 deaths attributed to the disease between 1900 and 1950. It is now largely eliminated in Europe, the Mediterranean and the USA, as improved living standards have permitted people to be less reliant on maize as their dietary staple. It continues to be a problem in southern and central Africa, with recent reports of outbreaks among people living on very restricted rations in refugee camps, and in parts of the Deccan plateau in India, where the dietary staple is jowar (a variety of

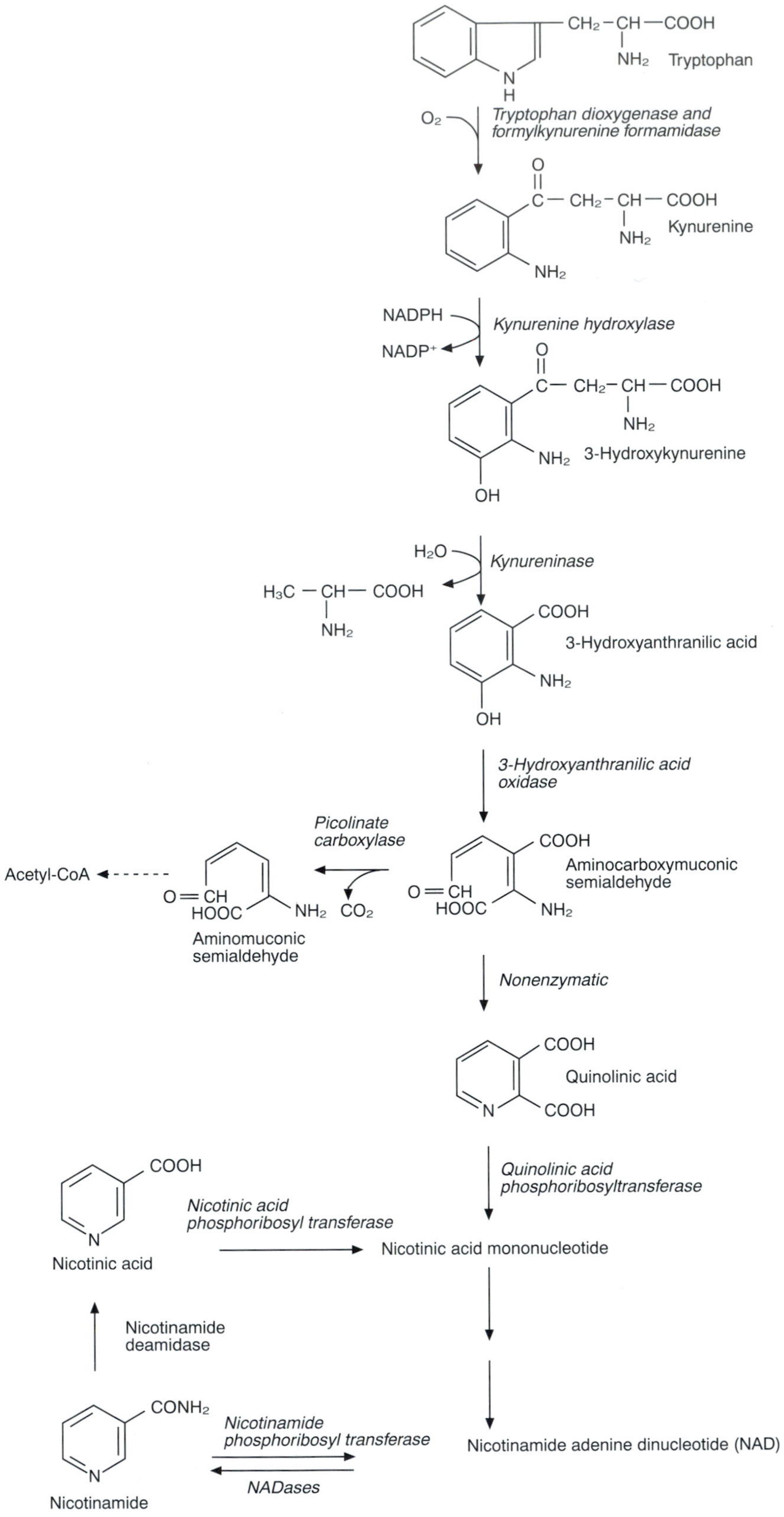

Figure 1 Tryptophan metabolism and the synthesis of NAD. Tryptophan dioxygenase EC 1.13.11.11; formylkynurenine formamidase EC 3.5.1.9; kynurenine hydroxylase EC 1.14.13.9; kynureninase EC 3.7.1.3; 3-hydroxyanthranilic acid oxidase EC 1.10.3.5; picolinate carboxylase EC 4.1.1.45; quinolinic acid phosphoribosyltransferase EC 2.4.2.19; nicotinic acid phosphoribosyltransferase EC 2.4.2.11; nicotinamide phosphoribosyltransferase EC 2.4.2.12; nicotinamide deamidase EC 3.5.1.19; NADases: NAD glycohydrolase EC 3.2.2.5; NAD pyrophosphatase EC 3.6.1.22; ADP ribosyltransferases EC 2.4.2.31 and 2.4.2.36; poly(ADP-ribose) polymerase EC 2.4.2.30.

millet, *Sorghum vulgare*), rather than maize. Rarely, pellagra occurs as a result of a disease or drug affecting the metabolism of tryptophan, despite an apparently adequate intake of tryptophan and preformed niacin.

The reason a maize-based diet predisposes to pellagra is that the proteins of maize are particularly poor in tryptophan, so that a diet in which there are few other sources of protein provides insufficient tryptophan for nicotinamide synthesis. Other cereals, such as wheat, barley, rye, rice and millet, contain enough tryptophan to meet the requirement for niacin synthesis. The problem with millet is probably one of amino acid imbalance, as discussed below.

All cereals contain preformed niacin. However, this is largely present as a variety of nicotinoyl esters, collectively known as niacytin, which are not hydrolysed by digestive enzymes to any significant extent, so that most of the niacin present in cereals is nutritionally unavailable. Interestingly, pellagra has never been a problem in central America, the original home of maize. This is because of the traditional way in which the cereal is prepared. Rather than milling the grain, it is steeped overnight in lime water (calcium hydroxide solution), then squeezed to form the dough from which tortillas are made. This alkali treatment results in hydrolysis of most of the nicotinoyl esters, so releasing free nicotinic acid, which is nutritionally available. Although maize spread to many countries following its discovery, it was generally milled like other grains rather than being treated in the traditional Mexican manner.

The Equivalence of Dietary Tryptophan and Niacin

As shown in Fig. 1, the nicotinamide ring of the coenzymes NAD and NADP can arise either from preformed dietary niacin or by *de novo* synthesis from quinolinic acid, an intermediate in the oxidative metabolism of tryptophan. For an adult in nitrogen balance, an amount of tryptophan equivalent to nearly all of the dietary intake is available for oxidative metabolism, since the utilization of tryptophan for the synthesis of protein is balanced by the catabolism of existing tissue proteins, releasing their tryptophan for metabolism.

A number of studies have shown that, under normal conditions, 60 mg of dietary tryptophan is equivalent to 1 mg of preformed dietary niacin, and it is usual to express the total niacin intake in terms of niacin equivalents – the sum of preformed niacin plus 1/60 of the tryptophan. On this basis, average Western diets, which contain about 1 g of tryptophan per day, provide more than enough niacin to meet requirements from tryptophan alone, ignoring preformed niacin.

Additional Factors in the Aetiology of Pellagra

Modern re-examination of the dietary records of pellagrins in the southern USA during the first part of the twentieth century suggests that their intake of tryptophan and preformed niacin was marginally adequate to meet requirements. It is likely that the effect of a marginal intake of tryptophan and niacin was compounded by inadequate intakes of vitamin B_6 and riboflavin (vitamin B_2). As shown in Fig. 1, these two vitamins are required for the endogenous synthesis of nicotinamide from tryptophan: riboflavin is the coenzyme for kynurenine hydroxylase (EC 1.14.13.9), and vitamin B_6 is the coenzyme for kynureninase (EC 3.7.1.3)

Mycotoxins

A number of mycotoxins cause DNA damage, and activate poly(ADP-ribose) polymerase (EC 2.4.2.30) as part of the DNA repair mechanism. This enzyme uses NAD as the source of ADP-ribose, releasing nicotinamide. While theoretically this nicotinamide could be re-used for synthesis of NAD, the enzymes involved, nicotinamide phosphoribosyltransferase (EC 2.4.2.12), nicotinamide deamidase (EC 3.5.1.19), and nicotinic acid phosphoribosyltransferase (EC 2.4.2.11) are all more or less saturated with their substrates at normal tissue concentrations. This means that the additional nicotinamide released by poly(ADP-ribose) polymerase cannot be used for NAD synthesis, but will largely be methylated to N^1-methylnicotinamide and excreted. Prolonged exposure to such mycotoxins may therefore deplete the body of nicotinamide, and be a factor in the aetiology of pellagra when intakes of tryptophan and niacin are marginal.

Dietary excess of leucine

It was noted above that although maize proteins are poor in tryptophan, the other cereal associated with pellagra, jowar, provides an apparently adequate amount of tryptophan to meet requirements. The proteins of jowar are considerably richer in leucine than most other proteins, and a diet based largely on jowar provides a considerable excess of leucine. There is a considerable body of evidence that this amino acid imbalance may be a precipitating factor in the development of pellagra when the dietary intake of preformed niacin is extremely low and the intake of tryptophan is only marginally adequate.

Leucine inhibits kynureninase, and hence reduces the rate of oxidative metabolism of tryptophan, resulting in reduced formation of quinolinic acid and NAD. In addition, leucine competes with tryptophan for tissue uptake, and thus has a further inhibitory effect on the rate of tryptophan oxidative metabolism and NAD synthesis.

Oestrogens and progestogens

Through the first half of the twentieth century, when pellagra was a major problem in the southern USA, there was a two-fold excess of women over men among those affected. In a number of reports of more recent outbreaks, there is a similar sex ratio between the menarche and menopause. There is no difference in the numbers of males and females affected among prepubertal children or adults aged over about 40 years. This suggests that oestrogens and/or progestogens may have a pellagragenic effect. Oestrogen metabolites are competitive inhibitors of kynureninase, and the administration of progesterone results in reduced activity of kynurenine hydroxylase, although *in vitro* neither progesterone nor its conjugates affects the activity of kynurenine hydroxylase. When the intake of preformed niacin is low, and that of tryptophan is marginal, the impairment of tryptophan metabolism by oestrogens and progesterone may be sufficient to precipitate pellagra more commonly in women than men.

Non-nutritional Pellagra

Pellagra can occur as a result of impairment of tryptophan metabolism owing to a variety of diseases which affect the tryptophan oxidative pathway, or as a result of drugs which inhibit one or more enzymes of the pathway, despite an apparently adequate intake of tryptophan. In most cases the condition responds well to supplements of nicotinamide.

Carcinoid syndrome

Under normal circumstances, about 1% of the daily intake of tryptophan is metabolized by way of 5-hydroxytryptamine in the central nervous system and gut, with the remainder being oxidized by way of kynurenine, and thus available for NAD synthesis. Carcinoid is a tumour of the enterochromaffin cells of the gastrointestinal tract, which form 5-hydroxytryptamine from tryptophan. The carcinoid syndrome occurs when the tumour has metastasized, usually to the liver. In extreme cases as much as 60% of the daily intake of tryptophan may be metabolized by way of 5-hydroxytryptamine. The result is a considerable reduction in the rate of oxidative metabolism through kynurenine, and hence a considerable reduction in the synthesis of NAD from tryptophan, resulting in the development of pellagra in a significant proportion of patients.

Inborn errors of tryptophan metabolism

A number of inborn errors of metabolism affecting enzymes of the tryptophan oxidative pathway have been reported, as shown in **Table 1**, all of which result in the development of pellagra. In addition, pellagra is the presenting feature of Hartnup disease, an inborn error of metabolism affecting the membrane proteins which transport the large neutral amino acids (including tryptophan). The same proteins are involved in the absorption of free tryptophan from the gastrointestinal tract into the bloodstream, from the bloodstream into tissues, and in the reabsorption of amino acids from the urine. The result of the defect is a considerable reduction in the amount of dietary tryptophan which is absorbed, as well as considerable loss in the urine. Thus, despite an apparently adequate intake, there is a deficiency of tryptophan (and other large neutral amino acids), resulting in the development of pellagra.

Drug-induced pellagra

A number of drugs can precipitate pellagra despite an apparently adequate intake of tryptophan. The best documented such drug is the antituberculosis drug isoniazid (isonicotinic acid hydrazide), although two anti-parkinsonian drugs, Benserazide and Carbidopa, are also associated with niacin depletion. These drugs have an indirect effect on tryptophan and niacin metabolism. They are hydrazine derivatives which act as carbonyl-trapping reagents and

Table 1 Conditions associated with the development of non-nutritional pellagra

Condition	Mechanism
Carcinoid syndrome	Diversion of tryptophan to serotonin synthesis
Hartnup disease	Failure of tryptophan absorption
Tryptophanuria	Tryptophan dioxygenase (EC 1.13.11.11) deficiency
Xanthurenic aciduria	Kynureninase (EC 3.7.1.3) deficiency
Kynureninuria	Kynurenine hydroxylase (EC 1.14.13.9) deficiency
Hereditary lethal pellagra	? Elevated picolinic carboxylase (EC 4.1.1.45)
Isoniazid treatment	Inhibition of kynureninase (EC 3.7.1.3)
Dopa decarboxylase inhibitors	Inhibition of kynureninase (EC 3.7.1.3)

therefore cause depletion of vitamin B_6 by forming inactive adducts with the metabolically active form of the vitamin, pyridoxal phosphate. Among other effects this results in impaired activity of kynureninase and hence a reduced rate of tryptophan oxidative metabolism and NAD synthesis. Although the pellagra responds to supplements of nicotinamide, it is more usual to give supplements of vitamin B_6 in combination with isoniazid, in order to minimize the other metabolic effects of vitamin B_6 depletion.

Clinical Features of Pellagra

The feature for which the disease was named is the severe sunburn-like dermatitis in areas of the skin exposed to modest amounts of sunlight. Mechanical pressure can cause similar lesions, especially around the wrists and ankles. The skin in the affected areas is red and slightly swollen at first, and then becomes rough, thickened, cracked and dry, with scaling, a shiny surface and brown pigmentation.

The cause of this photosensitive dermatitis in pellagra is unknown, and cannot be attributed to the known metabolic functions of either tryptophan or the nicotinamide nucleotide coenzymes. There is some evidence that there is increased metabolism of the amino acid histidine in the skin in pellagra, resulting in a lower than normal concentration of both histidine and an intermediate in its metabolism, urocanic acid, both of which are believed to have a role in absorbing ultraviolet light, and so minimizing damage to the skin from exposure to sunlight. Treatment with niacin both clears the dermatitis and also increases the concentration of histidine and urocanic acid in the dermis.

Diarrhoea is common in pellagrins, but it is not a constant feature of the disease, and indeed in some cases there may be chronic constipation. The cause of the diarrhoea is almost certainly general nutritional deficiency, resulting in atrophy of the intestinal mucosa.

The psychiatric disturbances of pellagra range from mild hallucinations with some psychomotor retardation, through confusion with increasing hallucinations, to severe dementia and anxiety psychosis, with melancholia, intermittent stupor and possibly epileptiform convulsions. In many ways this resembles schizophrenia, but the dementia of pellagra can be differentiated from schizophrenia and the organic psychoses by the sudden lucid phases which alternate with the most severe mental symptoms.

Although the cause of the psychiatric disturbance in pellagra remains to be firmly established, it is likely that it is largely due to deficiency of tryptophan, as a precursor for synthesis of the neurotransmitter serotonin (5-hydroxytryptamine), rather than a direct result of inadequate supply of the nicotinamide nucleotide coenzymes in the brain.

Chemical Pathology and Diagnosis of Pellagra

Unlike coenzymes such as those derived from other vitamins, the nicotinamide nucleotide coenzymes do not remain tightly bound to enzymes, but bind and leave, as do substrates. This means that enzyme activation assays and metabolic loading tests are not available for the assessment of niacin nutritional status. Most studies have depended on the urinary excretion of nicotinamide metabolites. Measurement of the excretion of N^1-methyl nicotinamide in depletion/repletion studies is the basis of estimates of niacin requirements and the equivalence of dietary tryptophan and preformed niacin.

Table 2 shows the ranges of urinary N^1-methyl nicotinamide and its onward metabolite, methyl pyridone carboxamide, associated with adequate, marginal and deficient niacin nutritional status. Rather than absolute amounts of metabolites excreted, the ratio of methyl pyridone carboxamide to N^1-methyl

Table 2 Urinary metabolites as indices of niacin nutritional status

	Deficient	Marginal	Adequate
N^1-methyl nicotinamide			
μmol per 24 h	<5.8	5.8–17	17–47
mg per g creatinine	<0.5	0.5–1.6	1.6–4.3
mmol per mol creatinine	<0.4	0.4–1.3	1.3–3.9
Methyl pyridone carboxamide			
μmol per 24 h	<6.4	6.4–18.9	>18.9
mg per g creatinine	<2.0	2.0–3.9	>4.0
mmol per mol creatinine	<0.44	0.44–4.3	>4.4
Ratio of methyl pyridone carboxamide : N^1-methyl nicotinamide	<1.0	1.0–1.3	1.3–4.0

nicotinamide is reported to provide a more sensitive index of status.

While urinary excretion of niacin metabolites may be useful in field studies to assess niacin nutritional status, it may not yield useful information in conditions such as carcinoid syndrome, where there can be normal excretion of metabolites, presumably arising from tissue catabolism, despite clear evidence of pellagra which responds to supplements of niacin.

The total concentration of nicotinamide nucleotides and the ratio of NAD to NADP in erythrocytes have been determined in a small number of experimental studies, but there is inadequate evidence on which to base reference ranges for use in field studies or population screening.

See also: **Amino Acids**: Chemistry and Classification; Metabolism. **Niacin**: Physiology, Dietary Sources and Requirements. **Riboflavin**: Physiology. **Vitamin B$_6$**: Physiology.

Further Reading

Bender DA (1983) Biochemistry of tryptophan in health and disease. *Molecular Aspects of Medicine* 6:101–197.

Bender DA (1992) Niacin. In *Nutritional Biochemistry of the Vitamins*, chap. 8, pp 184–222. Cambridge: Cambridge University Press.

Bender DA and Bender AE (1986) Niacin and tryptophan metabolism: the biochemical basis of niacin requirements and recommendations. *Nutrition Abstracts and Reviews (Series A)* 56:695–719.

Bender DA and Bender AE (1997) Niacin and tryptophan. In: *Nutrition: a Reference Handbook*, chap. 19, pp 305–321. Oxford: Oxford University Press.

Roe DA (1973) *A Plague of Corn: the Social History of Pellagra*. Ithaca: Cornell University Press.

Sydenstricker VP (1958) The history of pellagra, its recognition as a disease of nutrition and its conquest. *American Journal of Clinical Nutrition* 6:409–414.

Nitrogen *see* **Amino Acids**: Chemistry and Classification; Metabolism. **Protein**: Digestion and Bioavailability; Quality and Sources; Requirements and Role in Diet; Synthesis and Turnover; Deficiency.

NUCLEIC ACIDS

Physiology, Toxicology and Dietary Sources

H A Simmonds, United Medical and Dental Schools of Guy's and St Thomas's, London, UK

Physiology

Origin and properties

The nucleic acids are essential constituents of living cells and consequently are found in many foods, particularly in yeast, organ meat and seafoods. They were discovered by Miescher in 1868, the name being derived from the substance called 'nuclein' isolated from the nuclei of pus cells and spermatic fluid of Rhine salmon. The major constituents of nucleic acids were shown to be the purine and pyrimidine bases, now considered to be some of the first chemicals to emerge from the primordial soup. The chemical structure of the purine bases, including uric acid – the end product of purine metabolism in humans – was worked out also at the end of the last century by Emil Fischer and his colleagues (1884–1899), who demonstrated clearly their interrelationships and derivation from nucleic acids.

This article outlines the biosynthesis of nucleic acids, gives a brief overview of their physiological functions and concentrates on the problems resulting from the degradation of both endogenous and dietary (exogenous) nucleic acids in humans and ends with a summary of the nucleic acid content of different foods.

Structure

The nucleic acids are vital constituents of all living cells. They are composed of purine and pyrimidine bases linked as polymerized nucleotides via a pentose sugar (*nucleosides*) and esterified with phosphoric acid (*nucleotides*).

Two types of nucleic acid have been identified: deoxyribonucleic acid (DNA), where the pentose is 2'-deoxyribose (**Fig. 1**(a)) and the bases are principally adenine (A), guanine (G), cytosine (C) and thymine (T); and ribonucleic acid (RNA), where the pyrimidine uracil (U) replaces thymine and the pentose is ribose. In either case the pentose is bound by the C1 atom through a glycosidic linkage to the N9 atom of the purine group, or the N1 of the pyrimidine group.

DNA is comprised of two strands wound in the well-defined helical structure. Each nucleotide of one strand is linked by hydrogen bonding to a complementary nucleotide on the other (A–T and G–C) with the deoxyribose and phosphate groups performing structural roles. RNA is single-stranded.

Importance of nucleic acids in human metabolism

The role of DNA and RNA in the storage and transmission of genetic information is well established and the subject of many excellent reviews. Genes, the hereditary material in the nucleus of human cells, are long chains of double-helical DNA packed into 23 chromosomes. The human genome is considered to contain between 50 000 and 100 000 genes. The four bases, the purines adenine (A) and guanine (G) and the pyrimidines thymine (T) and cytosine (C), which constitute the backbone of DNA, carry the genetic information of all prokaryotic and eukaryotic organisms, the infinite variation in genetic programming being achieved by the particular sequence of these bases.

Nucleic acid biosynthesis in humans

The first step in the synthesis of DNA and RNA in humans involves the formation of the purine and pyrimidine ribomononucleotides which are derived endogenously by one of two routes. The first is the energetically expensive multistep *de novo* route (**Fig. 2**). The second is the single-step, energetically less expensive so-called 'salvage' pathway, which for purines occurs at the base level, and for pyrimidines

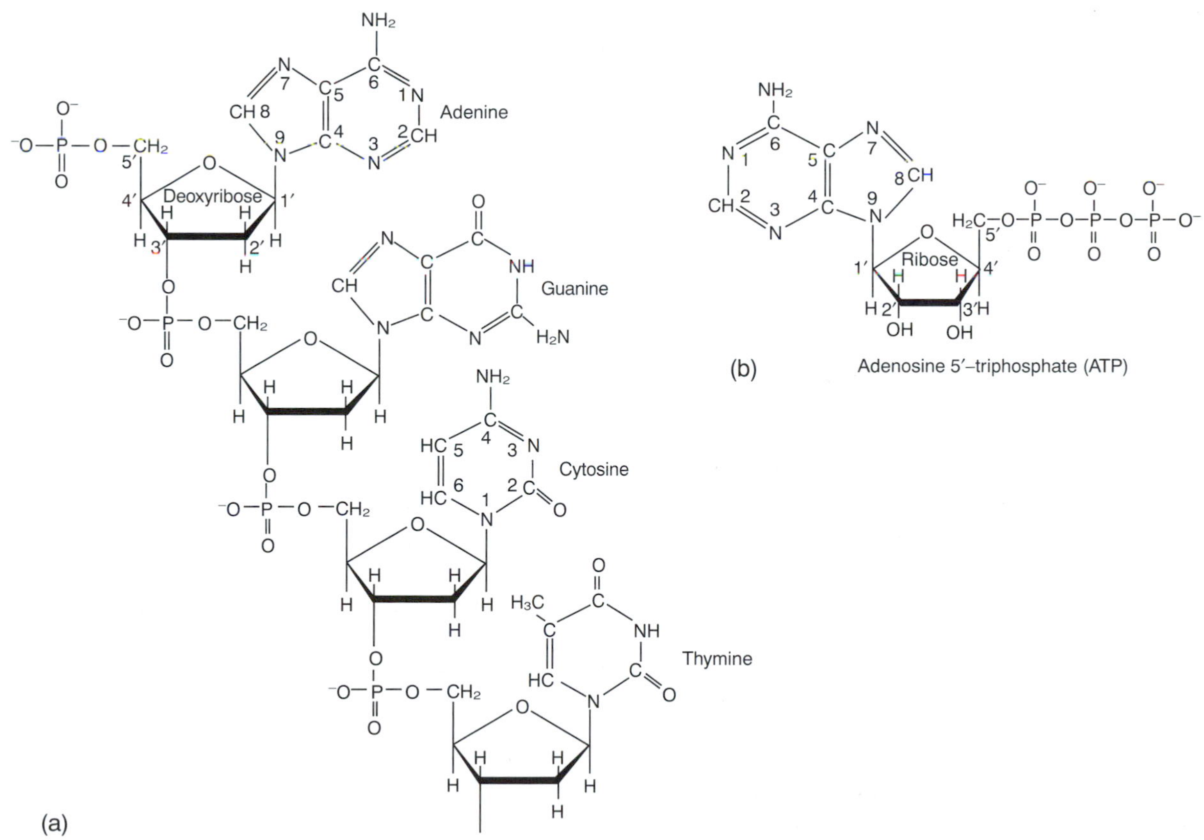

Figure 1 (a) Schematic representation of part of a DNA strand showing the structural formulae of the four constituent bases, adenine, guanine, cytosine and thymine, linked via the 3'-OH group of the deoxyribose phosphate moiety to the 5'-OH group of the next deoxyribose. Also shown is the numbering of the atoms in the deoxyribose, as well as the pyrimidine and purine rings. The latter consist of a six-membered pyrimidine ring fused to a five-membered imidazole ring. (b) Structural formula of ATP indicating that the ribose, as distinct from deoxyribose, has an OH group at the 2' position on the pentose ring.

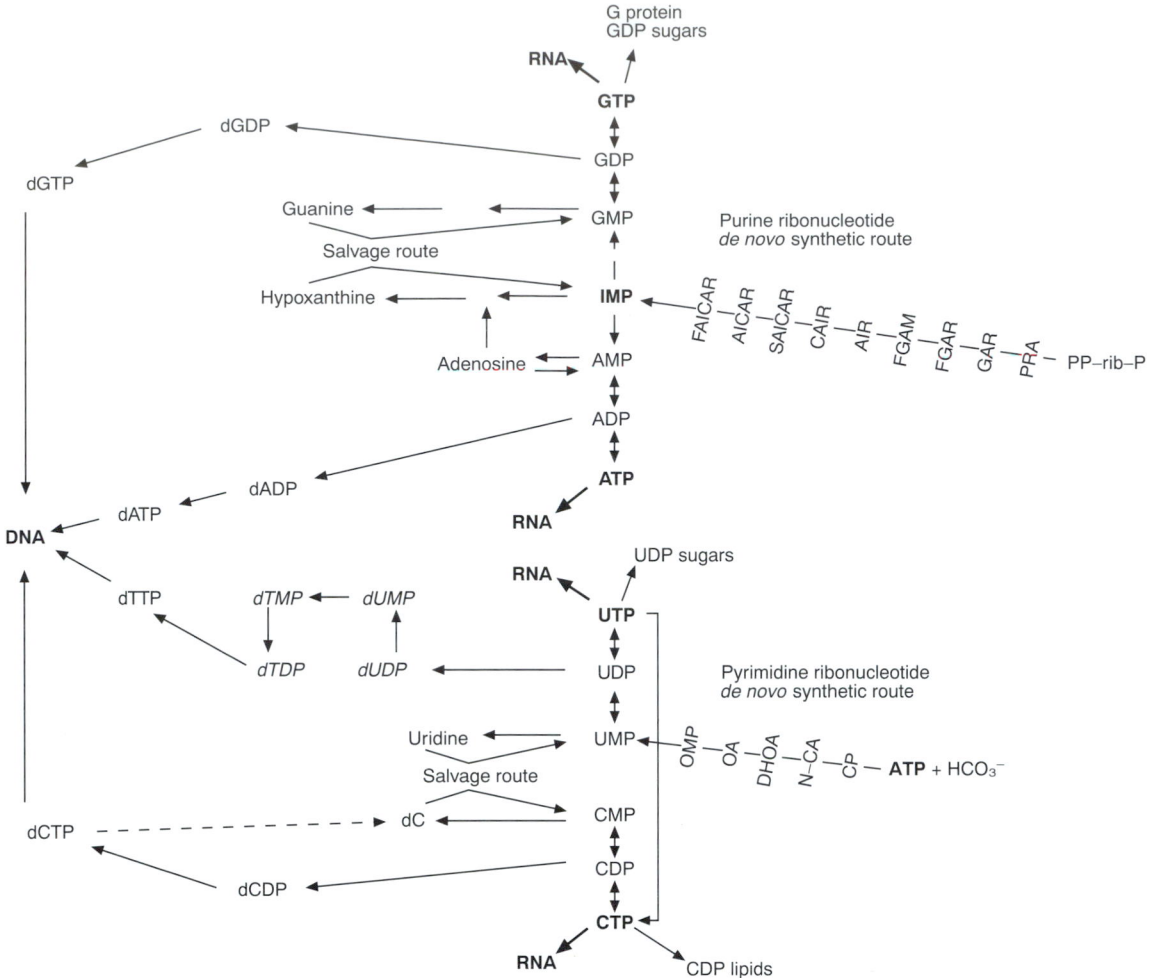

Figure 2 Metabolic pathways for the synthesis of DNA and RNA from their purine and pyrimidine ribo- and deoxyribonucleotide precursors. The dotted line from dCTP indicates the route of breakdown to deoxycytidine (dC), which can be salvaged by deoxycytidine kinase and incorporated into dCDP lipids or DNA.

Abbreviations: HCO_3^-, bicarbonate; CP, carbamolyl phosphate; N-CA, carbamoyl aspartate; DHOA, dihydroorotic acid; OA, orotic acid; OMP, orotidylic acid; PP-rib-P, 5-phosphoribosyl-1-pyrophosphate; PRA, 5-phosphoribosylamine; GAR, glycinamide ribotide; FGAR, N-formyl glycinamide ribotide; FGAM, N-formylglycinamidine ribotide; AIR, 5-aminoimidazole ribotide; CAIR, 5-aminoimidazole-4-carboxy ribotide; SAICAR, N-succino-5-aminoimidazole-4-carboxamide ribotide; AICAR, 5-aminoimidazole-4-carboxamide ribotide; FAICAR, 5-formamidoimidazole-4-carboxamide ribotide.

at the nucleoside level. 'Salvage' normally predominates over synthesis, the 5'-monophosphates so recycled exerting feedback control on the *de novo* routes.

The ribonucleotide 5'-monophosphates do not exist normally as such inside the cell, but are rapidly phosphorylated to the diphosphate. From here the diphosphates may be further phosphorylated to the triphosphate to be utilized directly in a variety of cellular processes, e.g. ATP (adenosine 5'-triphosphate), the universal energy carrier of all living organisms (Fig. 1(b)). In addition to providing energy, ATP also forms the basis of the coenzymes (NAD, NADP, FAD, etc.) and with GTP is involved in signal transduction and translation (cAMP,

cGMP, G proteins). Pyrimidines also fulfil diverse functions, either as the mononucleotides (UTP and CTP), or as the precursors of the UDP or CDP sugars and lipids which are active intermediates in the synthesis of glycogen, lipids and membranes, as well as protein glycosylation.

Alternatively, the diphosphates are reduced to the corresponding 2'-deoxyribonucleoside diphosphates in a reaction catalysed by ribonucleotide reductase. This reaction produces dADP, dGDP, dCDP and dUDP, the last being converted to dTTP to provide the four substrates essential for DNA synthesis. It was the development of this reaction which enabled evolution from the early 'RNA world' to the present 'DNA world'. DNA seemingly provides a much more stable form for storage of genetic information – a prerequisite for the development of multiple and separate species.

All RNAs are synthesized initially on a DNA template by a DNA-dependent RNA polymerase in a process called transcription and subject to a complex process of posttranscriptional modification. Like DNA, RNA is a long, unbranched macromolecule consisting of ribonucleotides joined by 3′–5′ phosphodiester bonds. In the case of RNA the molecule is single-stranded, except in some viruses. However, RNA does contain some double-helical regions resulting from the formation of the characteristic hairpin loops.

Cells contain three types of RNA, all modified after transcription to give rise to the particular functional form of RNA in question. The three kinds of RNA synthesized from DNA together play an important role in translation of the genetic message in the form of protein and thus enzyme synthesis in human cells. Most RNA is in the cytoplasm principally in the form of ribosomal RNA (rRNA: 80% of the total), the site of the growing polypetide chain in protein synthesis, while messenger RNA (mRNA: 5% of the total) provides the template for protein synthesis. The amino acids are brought to the assembly site covalently bonded to transfer RNA (tRNA: 15% of the total), their order in the growing protein being specified by the order of the bases in mRNA.

Synthesis of nucleic acids and their precursors in different human cells relates to cellular function DNA is principally found in the nucleus and is considered to be relatively stable in most cell types. Synthesis of both DNA and RNA is particularly active in cells and tissues with a high rate of turnover or metabolism (e.g. gut epithelium, skin, dividing lymphocytes, bone marrow, gonadal epithelium, etc.). The complex interplay between cells, and their ability to proliferate and differentiate depending on function is being unravelled with the assistance of advanced molecular methods. Such diversity is achieved through a tissue- and cell-specific complement of enzymes and is associated with characteristic ribonucleotide profiles. For example, nucleotide profiles in heart and muscle, as in the erythrocyte, are relatively simple, relating to the major requirement to sustain ATP. By contrast liver and intestine show a complex nucleotide pattern, supporting these organs as major sites of nucleic acid metabolism. The gut is particularly important in this respect. The nucleic acid content of intestinal mucosa is high, as is the rate of cell turnover in the luminal villi, and it has been calculated in rat that about 30 mg of endogenous nucleic acid enters the lumen daily. This means that the nucleic acid content of muscle is much lower than that of liver and intestine.

Metabolism and excretion of nucleic acids

There is a considerable turnover of endogenous nucleic acids and ribonucleotides daily during muscle work, wound healing, erythrocyte senescence, mounting an immune response, etc. However, as mentioned above, the active 'salvage' route normally ensures that only a small fraction of these vital endogenous compounds are actually degraded and lost to the body. The polynucleotides DNA and RNA must first be degraded to mononucleotides by enzymes capable of hydrolysing phosphodiester bonds – ribonucleases for RNA and deoxyribonucleases for DNA. The next step is degradation by specific 5′-nucleotidases to nucleosides or deoxynucleosides, which in turn can be deaminated and deribosylated to give the purine bases hypoxanthine, guanine or the pyrimidine bases uracil and thymine. Nucleoside/deoxyribonucleoside degradation is an essentially irreversible reaction owing to the high inorganic phosphate and low ribose/deoxyribose 1-phosphate concentrations in most tissues.

End products of endogenous nucleic acid metabolism in humans As we shall see, the potential toxicity of nucleic acids to humans relates not to the nucleic acids themselves, but to their metabolic end products, and involves primarily dietary, not endogenous nucleic acids. The pyrimidines are not a problem in either context. Catabolism of pyrimidine nucleosides not salvaged proceeds first to the bases uracil and thymine, which are then further catabolized in a series of steps to β-amino acids. All are soluble readily excreted non-ultraviolet-absorbing compounds. There is thus normally no measurable pyrimidine end product.

By contrast, in the case of purines, the bases hypoxanthine and guanine which escape salvage are catabolized via xanthine (an equally insoluble metabolic end product) by xanthine dehydrogenase (XDH) to the insoluble end product uric acid. In the case of endogenous nucleic acids this is a problem only in the rare genetic disorders described briefly below.

Metabolism of dietary nucleic acids in humans The normal human diet is rich in both DNA and RNA. The metabolism of these exogenous nucleic acids follows a similar pattern to that described above, but the first point of attack is by the bacterial flora of the intestine. This is rapid, if experiments in animals can be translated to humans. Studies in pigs demonstrated that up to 50% of radiolabelled dietary purine was degraded and lost as CO_2 within 30 min, the remaining 43% being recovered in the urine, with 5% in the faeces (**Fig. 3**).

Barrier action of the gut mucosa Humans have no apparent requirement for dietary purines, and the intestinal mucosa represents a second line of attack. It provides an effective barrier through the possession of a battery of enzymes which rapidly degrade purines derived from dietary nucleic acids (already partly processed by gut bacteria) to the non-reutilizable metabolic waste, uric acid. This may represent an important evolutionary development to protect the integrity of the human genome. Studies in humans and animals have confirmed that purine nucleotides, nucleosides and bases absorbed from the gut lumen are largely converted to uric acid during passage across the mucosa and released as such in serosal secretions.

By contrast, studies of humans with a defect in *de novo* pyrimidine synthesis at the fourth step, involving conversion of orotic acid (OA) to UMP (hereditary oroticaciduria), have confirmed that dietary pyrimidine mononucleotides, or uridine, but not the base uracil, are absorbed readily from the intestine and utilized for nucleic acid synthesis. Such patients present with severe megaloblastic anaemia, nonresponsive to the usual forms of treatment. They have been sustained for over 30 years on oral uridine, indicating that dietary pyrimidine can compensate totally for lack of *de novo* synthesis in humans. Recent studies using radiolabelled purines and pyrimidines in mice have provided further evidence for the incorporation of dietary pyrimidine nucleosides, but not purine nucleosides into hepatic RNA.

Beneficial effects of dietary nucleic acids

The above studies also suggested that provision of preformed nucleosides is of benefit to cellular proliferation in the gut. Human milk reputedly contains large quantities of nucleosides, particularly cytidine and uridine. It has been proposed that addition to infant diets of dietary pyrimidines, but not purines, might be beneficial.

Purine ribonucleotides as flavour-enhancing additives The purine 5'-nucleotide monophosphates IMP and GMP, derived from ATP, GTP and RNA degradation, have received much attention as the taste-active components in a variety of seafoods and meat. Both IMP and GMP seemingly enhance the effect of the flavour potentiator, monosodium glutamate (MSG). Studies in humans showed that the preference scores for MSG with IMP were higher than for MSG alone. Japanese research has also shown that the brothy taste of beef, pork and chicken soups could be reproduced by free amino acids plus IMP and sodium chloride. This synergistic effect with monosodium glutamate was specific for the purine 5'-nucleotides. The pyrimidines CMP and UMP exhibited practically no effect.

Toxicology

Role of nucleic acids in the pathophysiology of genetic metabolic disorders

Our knowledge of the important physiological roles played by nucleic acids and their precursor ribo- or deoxyribotide triphosphates in humans has been extended since the 1970s by the recognition of 23 different inborn errors of purine and pyrimidine metabolism. The spectrum of clinical manifestations ranges from fatal immunodeficiency syndromes, muscle weakness, severe neurological deficits, anaemia, renal failure, to gout and urolithiasis.

These 'experiments of nature' have highlighted the importance of individual steps in these pathways to a particular cell or tissue, and in particular the need

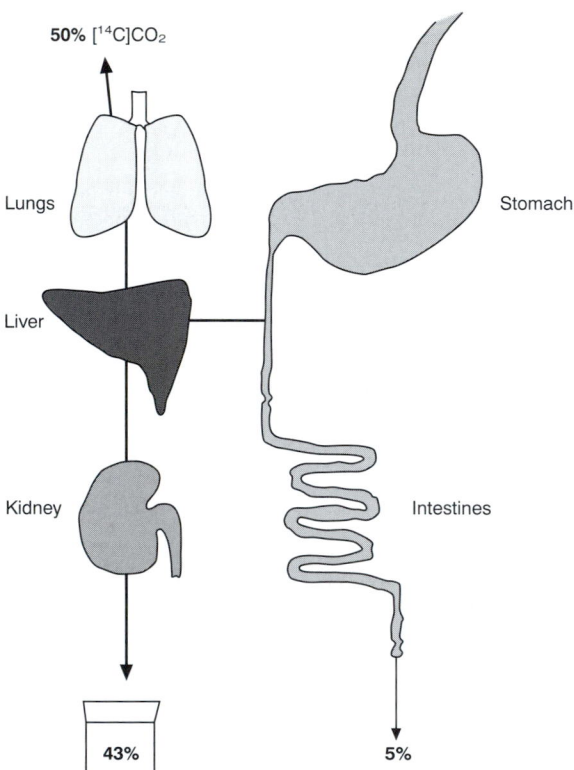

Figure 3 Diagram showing the fate of ^{14}C-labelled exogenous purine (guanine) in an animal model (pig). Radiolabel was recovered only in CO_2, urine or faeces. No incorporation into any tissues was found.

for intact pathways both for nucleic acid synthesis, as well as for their metabolism, degradation and recycling. Although DNA in most tissues is relatively stable, it is evident from the two genetic disorders associated with immunodeficiency – adenosine deaminase (ADA) and purine nucleoside phosphorylase (PNP) deficiency – that rapid turnover of cells of the haematopoietic system (e.g. extrusion of nucleus during erythrocyte maturation) normally produces significant amounts of free deoxyribonucleotides from DNA which must be degraded to the corresponding nucleobase for recycling. Absence of the two enzymes critical to this pathway, ADA and PNP, results in the accumulation of deoxy-ATP or deoxy-GTP, respectively, both of which inhibit DNA synthesis at the level of ribonucleotide reductase. The lymphospecific toxicity in these disorders results in an inability to combat infection and a potentially fatal immunodeficiency syndrome, the clinical course of which is similar to that in acquired immune deficiency syndrome (AIDS). Other rapidly dividing cells, such as those of the skin or the gut, are also affected. These disorders highlight the importance of the effective removal of waste from DNA catabolism to the normal human immune response.

Role of DNA in chemical carcinogenesis DNA normally possesses active repair systems to protect against damage by a variety of chemical and physical agents, including ionizing radiation and ultraviolet light. Ultraviolet light induces the formation of pyrimidine dimers which are recognized and cleaved by specific endonucleases. Strands may become cross-linked, bases can be altered or lost, and phosphodiester bonds may be broken.

Xeroderma pigmentosum is a rare autosomal recessive disease where the skin is sensitive to sunlight or ultraviolet light. This disease is an example of a faulty DNA repair system caused by a defect in the endonuclease which hydrolyses the DNA backbone near the pyrimidine dimer. Skin cancer usually develops and patients may die from metastases of these malignant skin tumours before the age of 30.

Toxicity of exogenous nucleic acids to humans

The potential toxicity of nucleic acids themselves to humans relates primarily to purines derived from dietary nucleic acid. This is due to a single mutational event: the fact that primates lack expression of the gene for the hepatic enzyme uricase, which degrades uric acid to the extremely soluble allantion in all other mammalian species. Although the gene appears to be present in human liver, the promoter regions are not activated. The biological value of failing to break down urate has

been debated, but it is worth noting in the context of toxicity that uric acid is considered by some to provide more than half the antioxidant activity of primate plasma.

The importance or uricase to nonmammalian species such as rodents is highlighted by the development of urate nephropathy in a genetically engineered uricase-deficient mouse. In reptiles, snakes, spiders and birds, uric acid is the total end product of nitrogen metabolism, analogous to urea in mammals. The main advantage of using this insoluble end product is that there is no obligatory water loss for its excretion, as there is for urea. Consequently, uric acid can be excreted as a slurry; an evolutionary adaptation enabling survival in arid environments.

Role of the kidney in the genesis of nucleic acid toxicity in humans The pathological changes resulting from uric acid being the exclusive end product of purine metabolism in humans derive not only from the insolubility of this metabolic waste, but also from the fact that the renal proximal tubule reabsorbs around 90% of the filtered uric acid (**Fig. 4**). Net reabsorption is higher in healthy males (92%) than in females (88%) and is lower in children of either sex (80–85%), but is much higher in 'primary gout' (95%) – predominantly middle-aged males. This difference explains the higher plasma uric acid in adult males and means that uric acid is circulating in their plasma at concentrations already close to its solubility limit. Hence the greater propensity of males to gout.

Derivation of the body uric acid pool in humans

The body pool of urate, and hence the plasma urate concentration, is the result of a balance between production, ingestion and excretion. The principal causes of increased plasma uric acid concentrations are (1) increased intake of exogenous nucleic acid (purine), and (2) overproduction of endogenous purine.

Overconsumption versus overproduction of endogenous urate The only way to establish the contribution of diet is to place the subject on a purine-free diet for a week and measure the urinary excretion of urate. Purine excretion will then equal endogenous production. In this way less than 5% of patients with gout have been found to excrete abnormally large amounts of urate (>3 mmol per day). In the majority of the latter an underlying genetic defect of purine metabolism is identified which results in the absence of the normal feedback controls. Two such disorders, both sex-linked, are hypoxanthine-guanine phosphoribosyltransferase (HPRT)

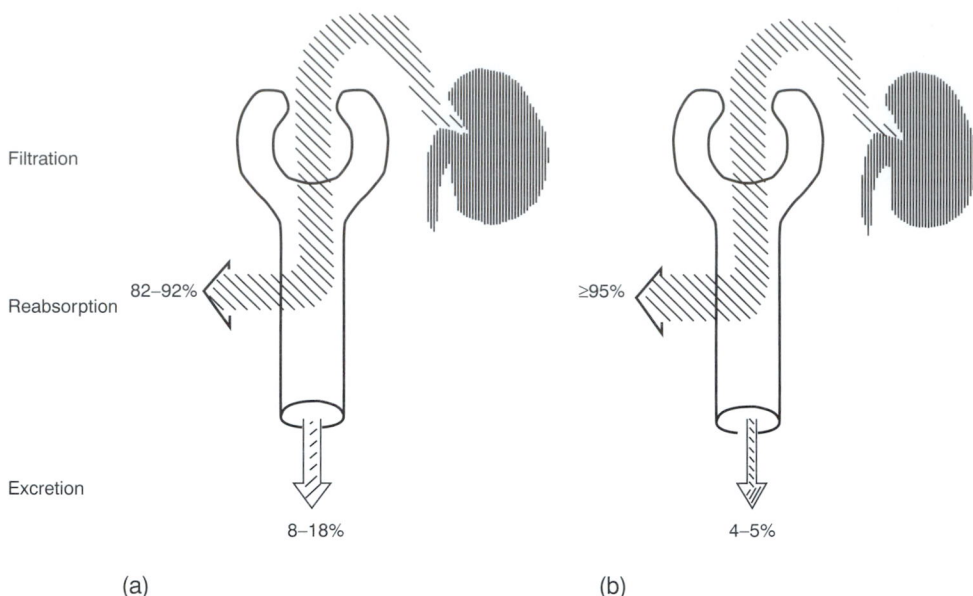

Figure 4 Schematic diagram showing the role of the kidney in influencing plasma uric acid concentration. This involves a complex interaction in the brush border membrane of the proximal tubule between reabsorption by the urate anion exchanger and secretion via a voltage-sensitive pathway. This results in a mean fractional urinary excretion of only 8–18% of the filtered load in healthy subjects and 5% or less in 'primary' gout. The net uric acid reabsorption which occurs is: (a) higher in healthy men (92%) than in women (88%) and lower in children of either sex (82%); (b) much higher in middle-aged males with primary gout (5.4%).

deficiency and phosphoribosyltransferase superactivity (PRPS), invariably presenting first in childhood or adolescence. Patients presenting in infancy usually have severe and eventually fatal neurological deficits. In patients presenting in adolescence the neurological problems are milder or absent. It is important for clinicians to be aware of this, especially when presented with a young patient with gout, or an older male with a history dating back to adolescence, particularly if siblings are involved. Treatment will differ.

Role of dietary nucleic acid in determining circulating uric acid levels in normal versus gouty humans The ingestion of food rich in nucleic acids has been noted for millennia to be high in subjects with what has been designated 'primary' gout – the gout affecting predominantly middle-aged males. The fact that gout was extremely prevalent among wealthy Englishmen for more than three centuries is not surprising. Up till World War I these affluent gentlemen habitually consumed vast nucleic acid-rich meals (**Tables 1** and **2**), frequently including many different courses and at least 16 different meats. A frugal dinner described in a seventeenth century cookery book consisted of 'a shield of brawn with mustard; a boiled capon; a chine of beef roasted; a neats tongue; a roast pig; roast goose, swan and turkey; a haunch of vension; a venison pastry; a kid with pudding in its belly; an olive pie; a couple more capons and a custard'. Beer, ale and port also played

their part, beer being particularly rich in purines derived from yeast RNA.

Both hyperuricaemia and gout are more common in Polynesians and in Australasians, traditionally high consumers of nucleic acid-rich seafood, meat

Table 1 A quick reference guide to the purine content of foods

Foods and beverages rich in nucleic acids/purines
Offal: sweetbreads, liver, kidney, heart, and paté
Seafoods: sardines, sprats, herring, bloaters, fish roe, trout or salmon; lobster, crab, prawns
Vegetables: asparagus, avocado pears, peas, spinach, mushrooms, broad beans, cauliflower
Pulses and grains: legumes, pulses and soya products
Cereals: all bran, oat, rye or wheat cereals and products; wholemeal, rye and brown breads
Other: beer and yeast extracts/tablets (Barmene™, Tastex™). Meat or vegetable extracts (Marmite™, Vegemite™, Bovril™, Oxo™)

Foods and beverages purine-free
Milk, cheese, eggs, butter, margarine, cream, ice cream
Sugar, jam, marmalade, honey and sweets
Cucumber, tomato, onions, pumpkin
Fresh, cooked or tinned fruits, nuts
Puddings, custards (milk, etc.)
Fruit juices, soft drinks

Foods low in purine
Beef, lamb, pork (steak or chops), bacon, ham, sausages, some poultry, tongue: once daily
Carrots, parsnip, potatoes, lettuce, leeks, cabbage, sprouts, marrow, courgettes: small helpings
White bread or flour, cakes, scones, biscuits, cereals
Some fish (see Table 2)

Table 2 Concentrations of purines in common foods and beverages; results are recorded relative to protein

Food	Purine (mg per 100 g)	Protein (g per 100 g)	Food	Purine (mg per 100 g)	Protein (mg per 100 g)
Meat			**Poultry**		
Beef liver	333	19.7	Chicken flesh	181	20.6
Beef kidney	285	15.4	Chicken liver	372	22.1
Beef heart	285	16.8	Chicken heart	223	18
Beef tongue	167	16.4	Duck	181	16
Beef steak	151	19.5	Goose	177	16.4
Calf liver	348	19	Turkey	239	20.1
Sweetbreads	1212	19.6			
Veal cutlet	152	19.2	**Fish, seafoods**		
Sheep kidney	312	16.8	Anchovies	411	20
Lamb chop	196	14.9	Bass	73	19.5
Pork liver	289	22	Bloaters	133	22.6
Pork cutlet	164	16.4	Bream	72	19.7
Bacon	85	9.1	Cod	62	18
Ham	136	19.5	Crab	61	19.2
Sausage (beef)	79	13.8	Clams	136	17
Sausage (pork)	66	11.5	Eel	108	18.6
Rabbit	118	20.4	Fish cakes	36	12.1
Venison	156	20	Herring	378	17
			Kippers	91	21.2
Vegetables			Lobster	100	20
Asparagus	32	2.1	Lemon sole	54	19.9
Cauliflower	32	2.4	Mackerel	246	29
Celery	20	1.1	Plaice	53	18.1
Kohlrabi	44	2.1	Salmon	250	23
Mushrooms	72	3.5	Sardines	345	23
Peas	72	6.7	Scallops	117	22.3
Spinach	96	2.2	Sprats	250	25.1
			Squid	135	15
Dried legumes			Trout	92	19.2
Split peas	195	21			
Red bean	162	20	**Canned seafoods**		
Lentils	222	28	Anchovies	321	30
Haricot beans	230	22	Herring	378	17
Lima bean	149	21	Mackerel	246	26
			Oysters	116	6
Other			Salmon	88	26
Bovril™	340	18	Sardines	399	24
Marmite™	356	2	Shrimp	231	22
Oxo™ cubes	236	10	Tuna	142	29
Yeast extracts	2257	46			

and beer. In such countries the prevalence of gout is as high as 10%, compared with 1–4% in Europe. In Europe the prevalence is higher in countries such as France where the consumption of seafoods and paté is high. The role of diet in the aetiology of 'primary' gout is confirmed by the fact that during and immediately after the two world wars this type of gout was virtually unknown. With returning affluence, or a change to Western diets of some nations such as Japan, gout, a hitherto little-known disease, is being recorded with increasing frequency.

Importance of nucleic acid type in determining toxicity   Many investigators have shown that the fate of the dietary purine moiety varies depending on whether the purine is administered in the form of DNA, RNA, mononucleotides, nucleosides or bases, some being absorbed and catabolized more readily than others. When normal subjects are fed RNA, the increase in the excretion of uric acid is dramatic when the rise in plasma urate is modest. In 'primary' gout subjects the rise in plasma urate concentration is greater and the excretion of urate less than in normals. The effect of RNA is also twice that of DNA.

Generation of urolithiasis by dietary nucleic acid
Although modest overingestion of purines by normal subjects does not precipitate gout, it can predispose to uric acid lithiasis. Uric acid stones are relatively common in the countries mentioned above where the

consumption of nucleic acid-rich beverages and food is high. Uric acid lithiasis may also occur in subjects addicted to health foods such as yeast tablets.

A number of compounds used daily such as vitamin C increase the renal clearance of uric acid and thus can precipitate urolithiasis. Perhaps not so well recognized is the uricosuric effect of a high-protein diet and the fact that purine-rich foods also predispose to calcium stone formation. A possible explanation for the latter may be that purine-rich foods such as spinach are equally rich in oxalate. About 25% of vitamin C intake is also excreted as oxalate, which can compound the problem. Diet can also produce significant alterations in urine pH. In the case of uric acid this can be important: the solubility in urine at pH 5.0 is low (around 1 mmol l^{-1}), but can be increased 12-fold at pH 8.0 by alkalinizing regimes.

Exacerbation of kidney stone formation by dietary nucleic acids in inherited purine disorders Diet can also be a precipitating factor which first draws attention to inherited genetic defects associated with overproduction of insoluble purines. This can produce urolithiasis, particularly in adults with HPRT deficiency and PRPS superactivity. Crystalluria, uric acid lithiasis or nephropathy can result, with gout developing secondarily to this. A third genetic defect leads to the accumulation of adenine, which is converted by XDH to the even more insoluble uric acid analogue 2,8-dihydroxyadenine (2,8-DHA). Undiagnosed, such subjects have progressed to renal failure, dialysis and transplantation. One child presenting in coma was from a kindred addicted to macrobiotic diets – full of pulses and grains with a particularly high adenine content. This would exacerbate stone formation and nephrotoxicity. Since this disorder is treatable with allopurinol, such nephrotoxicity can be avoided if the defect is recognized and the consumption of nucleic acid-rich foods reduced to a minimum.

Dietary Sources

Nucleic acid content of foods

What then are the nucleic acid-rich foods which should be avoided by susceptible individuals? The nucleic acid content of different foods is expressed generally in terms of purine equivalents, the data being derived from the hydrolysis of nucleic acids and free nucleotides to the constituent bases.

Foods may be classified into three groups, low, high or essentially purine-free, as indicated in Table 1. Nucleic acid-rich shellfish are probably the greatest culprits in consumers addicted to seafoods (oysters, sea-eggs, cockles, etc.) followed by the crustaceans (crayfish, crabs, etc.), with sardines and herrings equal contenders (Table 2). Organ meats rich in nucleic acids (sweetbreads, liver, paté, kidney), poultry and game (goose, turkey, pheasant, grouse) and all meat and yeast extracts are also extremely nucleic acid-rich. Amongst the vegetables are cauliflower, avocado, mushrooms as well as spinach, peas and broad beans and most pulses and grains (lentils, wheat, rye and oats).

The purine content of the principal purine-rich foods consumed daily by Europeans is listed in Table 2. The ideal diet for subjects at risk is one meat meal per day containing only the low-purine meat and vegetables indicated.

See also: **Ascorbic Acid**: Physiology, Dietary Sources and Requirements. **Gout**: Aetiology and Nutritional Management. **Renal Function and Disorders**: Nutritional Management of Renal Disorders.

Further Reading

Berthold HK, Crain PF, Gouni I, Reeds PJ and Klein PD (1995) Evidence for incorporation of intact dietary pyrimidine (but not purine) nucleosides into hepatic RNA. *Proceedings of the National Academy of Sciences, USA* 92:10123–10127.

Cameron JS and Simmonds HA (1994) Gout, purines and interstitial nephritis. In: *Oxford Textbook of Medicine*, chap. 20.10.2, pp 133–135. Oxford: Oxford University Press.

Clifford J and Story DL (1976) Levels of purines in foods and their metabolic effects in rats. *Journal of Nutrition* 106:435–442.

Diem K and Lentner C (eds) (1970) *Scientific Tables – Chemical Composition of Foodstuffs*, 7th edn, pp 230–243. Basle: Geigy.

Fuke S and Konosu S (1991) Taste-active components in some foods: a review of Japanese research. *Physiology and Behaviour* 49:863–868.

Henderson JF and Paterson ARP (1973) *Nucleotide Metabolism: An Introduction*. New York: Academic Press.

Scriver CR, Beaudet AL, Sly WS and Valle D (eds) (1995) Purines and pyrimidines. In: *The Metabolic and Molecular Basis of Inherited Disease*, 7th edn, vol. II, pp. 1655–1940. New York: McGrew-Hill.

Uauy R (1989). Dietary nucleotides and requirements in early life. In: Lebenthal E (ed.) *Textbook of Gastroenterology and Nutrition in Infancy*, pp 265–280. New York: Raven Press.

Zöllner N and Gresser U (eds) (1991) *Urate Deposition in Man and its Clinical Consequences*. Berlin: Springer-Verlag.

NUTRIENT REQUIREMENTS

International Perspectives

D A Bender, University College, London, UK

Most countries, United Nations agencies and international groupings publish tables of reference intakes of nutrients. Most of these are revised, in the light of new information, at approximately 10-year intervals. Despite the fact that the different authorities are interpreting the same body of scientific evidence, there are considerable differences between the recommendations. These may be attributed to:

1. The paucity of experimental data, so that the estimation of requirements requires the exercise of judgment.
2. Differences in the assumptions made in extrapolating from the results of controlled experiments involving purified nutrients, to eating foods, where nutrients are present in a complex mixture of chemical forms, with different biological activity and availability.
3. Differences in the basis of calculation. Energy, and nutrients related to energy intake, may be expressed in calories or joules, and considerable differences may arise in rounding off to avoid spurious precision.
4. Differences in the goals for which the recommendations are being made, and the criteria of adequacy that are considered appropriate. This will reflect national priorities; the goals are different in countries where food supplies are marginal and deficiency may be common, compared with countries where the problems are largely associated with overabundant food supplies.

Determination of Requirements

Energy requirements

The basis for estimating energy requirements for adults is measurement or calculation of energy expenditure. Direct measurement of heat output requires a thermally insulated chamber, and does not generally permit measurement for more than a relatively short time. Furthermore, only a restricted range of activities is possible in a calorimeter.

The mean energy yield of the various metabolic fuels is 20 kJ (4.8 kcal) per litre of oxygen consumed, therefore energy expenditure can be calculated from oxygen consumption. Respirometers are considerably less restricting than calorimeters, so that it is possible to determine energy expenditure in a wide variety of tasks.

Having measured energy expenditure in a given task, it is usual to express this, not in absolute units (i.e. kcal or $kJ\,min^{-1}$), but rather as a physical activity ratio (PAR) – a multiple of the basal metabolic rate (BMR). From the time spent in each type of activity and the PAR of that activity, it is possible to calculate an overall physical activity level (PAL) and use this as a basis for calculating energy requirements. A desirable PAL, in terms of cardiovascular and respiratory fitness, is $1.7 \times BMR$; the mean in the UK is $1.4 \times BMR$. This immediately introduces a problem in assessing average energy requirements for a population. Should the figures be based on desirable levels of physical activity, or on what is actually observed?

The BMR is usually calculated from a series of experimentally derived equations based on gender, age, body weight and height. This introduces a further problem in assessing energy requirements: should average BMR be calculated on the basis of actual or desirable body weights? Furthermore, there is some evidence that the equations for estimation of BMR that have been derived in temperate climates are not applicable to people living in the tropics.

An alternative approach to estimating energy requirements comes from the use of the double-isotopically labelled water technique, which provides a noninvasive way of determining total energy expenditure in free-living subjects, averaged over 2–3 weeks. Such studies permitted revision of the estimates of children's energy requirements in the 1991 UK tables, and have permitted considerable revision of estimates of the energy cost of pregnancy and lactation.

International differences in estimates of energy requirements   A review of reference intakes around the world published in 1983 quoted energy requirements published by 41 authorities. For young adult men, the average requirement was 2855 kcal, (12 MJ), with a coefficient of variation of 7.4%. The range was 2500–3200 kcal (10.5–13.4 MJ), a range of 25% around the mean.

Three factors account for these differences in estimated energy requirements:

1. *Average body weight.* Both basal metabolic rate and (more importantly) the energy cost of physical activity increase with increasing body weight, so that heavier people have a higher energy requirement. In estimating energy requirements, any national authority will have to reach a balance between considering energy requirements to maintain desirable body weight and those for the average body weight of its population.
2. *Climate.* In a cold climate more energy is expended to maintain body temperature than in tropical and subtropical areas.
3. *Average physical activity.* In countries where there is a high degree of mechanization, average energy expenditure will be considerably lower than where manual work is required for most tasks. The effect of increasing mechanization and reduced physical activity can be seen in the energy requirements published by seven European countries since the 1983 review. In all seven, the average energy requirement of young adult men fell by between 5% and 19% (mean 11%).

Protein requirements

Since 1985, estimates of protein requirements have been based on the combined report of the Food and Agriculture Organization, the World Health Organization and the United Nations University, which relied on studies of the amount of protein required to maintain nitrogen balance. Data from 23 studies were quoted, involving a total of 200 subjects. The average requirement was 600 mg protein per kg of body weight (630 mg kg^{-1} in short-term studies and 580 mg kg^{-1} in long-term studies). The report did not quote a series of studies involving a further 100 subjects (published in 1973), which showed that nitrogen balance could be maintained on intakes as low as 460 mg protein per kg body weight (range 375–590 mg kg^{-1}).

The difference between short-term and long-term studies suggests that there is adaptation to habitual protein intake. This is also shown by isotope studies of total body protein turnover. These have shown that the rate of turnover varies with intake, and several weeks are needed to adjust to changes. Higher intakes of protein than are necessary for maintenance of nitrogen balance lead to higher rates of protein turnover, but it is not known if this implies higher requirements for protein than estimates based on nitrogen balance studies.

International differences in reference intakes of protein

One approach to setting reference intakes of protein is to consider protein in its own right, and extrapolate from the average requirement to main-

tain nitrogen balance (600 mg per kg body weight), making allowance for individual variation, by adding 2 standard deviations (SD) to the mean observed requirement, to reach a figure of 750 mg kg^{-1} which is more than adequate to meet the needs of all members of the population. In the UN reports, this is termed a 'safe level of intake'; depending on estimates of average body weight, it is 40–50 g per day for adult men.

An alternative approach is to consider protein as percentage of energy intake. The safe level of intake, at average energy requirements is 7.5% of energy from protein, giving a reference intake for adult men of 50–60 g per day.

Average Western diets provide some 10–15% of energy from protein, and a number of national authorities have used this as the basis for setting reference intakes of protein, on the assumption that as energy requirement increases, it will be met by eating more of the same pattern of foods, and therefore protein intake will increase with energy requirement. The result is that what are interpreted as protein requirements increase with energy expenditure, however, there is no evidence that this is so – it is just that the reference intakes for protein are based on practical considerations rather than requirements.

Vitamin and mineral requirements

For any nutrient, there is a range of intakes between those that are clearly inadequate, leading to clinical deficiency disease, and those in excess of the body's metabolic capacity and therefore potentially toxic. Between these two extremes is the level of intake that is adequate for the maintenance of normal health and metabolic integrity. The choice of criterion of adequacy for any nutrient will both depend on which are appropriate for the nutrient in question, and also reflect national goals and priorities. The following criteria, in order of increasing adequacy of intake, may be used to estimate requirements.

Absence of clinical deficiency disease Severe deficiency leads to clinical deficiency disease, with clear anatomical, functional and metabolic lesions, possibly proving fatal. Prevention of deficiency is a minimal goal in determining requirements, and in countries where food supplies are marginal this will be the first priority. In countries where food supplies are adequate, and deficiency is more or less unknown, then simple prevention of deficiency is not an appropriate goal.

Covert deficiency At a less severe level of deficiency there are no signs of deficiency under normal conditions, but any trauma or stress reveals the precarious state of the body reserves and may precipitate clinical signs. For example, intakes of vitamin C as low as 10 mg per day will prevent or cure scurvy, but wound healing is impaired at daily intakes below 20 mg.

Biochemical deficiency At inadequate levels of intake there may be metabolic abnormalities, although there is no clinical deficiency disease. For example, thiamin deficiency results in impaired carbohydrate metabolism, with accumulation of high plasma concentrations of lactate and pyruvate; vitamin B_{12} deficiency results in excretion of methylmalonic acid; in early vitamin D deficiency there is a marked elevation of plasma alkaline phosphatase concentrations.

Covert biochemical deficiency Although the intake may be adequate for the maintenance of normal metabolic integrity, a small additional metabolic stress can reveal the inadequacy of tissue reserves, with an abnormal response to a metabolic load. Examples include the metabolism of a test dose of histidine to assess folate nutritional status, and of tryptophan or methionine for vitamin B_6 status.

Inadequate saturation of enzymes with coenzymes If total body reserves of a vitamin are inadequate there may be free apoenzyme in tissues, which is catalytically inactive in the absence of coenzyme. Measurement of the enzyme activity *in vitro* with and without added coenzyme permits determination of the degree of unsaturation of the enzyme, and hence the adequacy or otherwise of body reserves of the nutrient.

For three vitamins, there are enzymes in red blood cells that can be used in this way – transketolase for thiamin, glutathione reductase for riboflavin and one or other of the transaminases for vitamin B_6. It is not clear whether complete saturation of these enzymes with their vitamin-derived coenzymes is a desirable goal, since some degree of unsaturation (and hence some reserve of inactive, but potentially activatable, enzyme protein) may be important in metabolic regulation.

Low plasma concentrations of the nutrient Low plasma concentrations indicate that tissue reserves are not adequate to permit normal transport between tissues. The sharp increase in plasma concentration of vitamin C with increasing intake provided the basis of the (1991) UK estimates of vitamin C requirements. For some nutrients, a low plasma concentration may reflect failure to synthesize a transport protein rather than deficiency of the nutrient

itself – thus there may be a low plasma concentration of vitamin A, with functional vitamin A deficiency, in protein–energy malnutrition, despite adequate liver reserves of the vitamin, because of impairment of the synthesis of plasma retinol-binding protein.

Low excretion of the nutrient or its metabolites Low excretion reflects low intake and possibly also changes in turnover as adaptation to the inadequate intake. Early estimates of riboflavin requirements were based on the intake at which significant amounts of the vitamin were excreted; at low levels of intake there is conservation of the vitamin, and little or none is excreted. The excretion of niacin metabolites is still the only method available for assessment of niacin adequacy and requirements, and low urinary excretion of iodine is widely used to assess the adequacy or otherwise of iodine nutrition. Requirements for many minerals are estimated on the basis of balance studies.

Incomplete saturation of body reserves For some nutrients such as thiamin and vitamin C, the degree of saturation of body reserves can be assessed by giving a test dose of the vitamin and measuring the amount excreted. This is not appropriate for many minerals, or for vitamins A and D, since excessive intake may be toxic.

Optimum health Optimum health is the (possibly untestable) goal. As problems of deficiency have become less important (at least in developed countries), and levels of intake to meet the criteria of adequacy discussed above have been established, so increasing attention is being focused on the development of more sensitive indices of optimum levels of nutrient intake, such as immune responses.

Higher levels of intake There may be beneficial effects of intake of some nutrients at levels higher than are required to meet requirements. In general, these are greater than can readily be achieved from foods, and national and international authorities are, understandably, concerned about recommendations implying that normal diets may be inadequate.

At levels of intake far higher than those achieved from foods, some nutrients have pharmacological (drug-like) actions which may be useful in the treatment of diseases. Thus, nicotinic acid has a useful lipid-lowering action in hyperlipidaemic patients, and vitamin B_6 has been used to treat premenstrual syndrome (although the evidence of efficacy is weak).

Determination of requirements Minimum requirements can be estimated by measuring habitual intakes in regions where deficiency disease is common, compared with regions where deficiency is unknown. Experimental determination of requirements normally depends on depletion-repletion studies. After an appropriate criterion of adequacy has been established, volunteers are fed an otherwise adequate diet which lacks the nutrient under investigation, until there is a detectable metabolic or other abnormality. The subjects are then repleted with graded intakes of the nutrient until the abnormality is just corrected. Significant differences in apparent requirements may arise as a result of the interpretation of such studies. Thus, both the US reference intake of 60 mg of vitamin C and the Netherlands figure of 85 mg are based on the same depletion-repletion studies, but make different assumptions about the changes in vitamin C metabolism during depletion.

An alternative approach is to measure the total body pool of the nutrient and the rate at which it turns over (e.g. using isotopically labelled nutrients); the requirement is then the amount needed to replace what is lost each day, plus an allowance for digestion, absorption and metabolism. Here problems may arise in determining whether or not the total body pool determined in the studies is in fact appropriate, since the rate of turnover may well change with the size of the body pool.

Dietary Reference Values

Having established an average requirement to meet the chosen criterion of adequacy, the next problem is to convert this to a reference figure – an amount of the nutrient that is (more than) adequate to meet the requirements of all members of the population, and thus ensure that everyone achieves the chosen level of adequacy. For energy, the average requirement is used, since it is obviously not desirable to encourage intakes in excess of requirements to meet energy expenditure.

If it is assumed that individual requirements are distributed in a statistically normal fashion around the observed mean requirement, then a range of ± 2 SD around the mean will include the requirements of 95% of the population (**Fig. 1**). It is conventional to assume that requirements are normally distributed around the mean, although there is little evidence to support this assumption. Indeed, the only nutrient for which there is good evidence on the distribution of requirements is iron, which has a markedly skewed distribution, with a significant group of people having very high requirements.

A level of intake 2 SD above the mean requirement is greater than the requirements of 97.5% of the

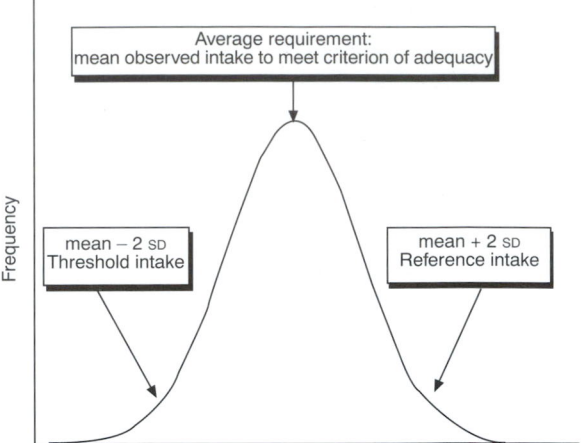

Figure 1 Determination of reference and threshold intakes from the mean observed requirement to meet the chosen criterion of adequacy. The graph shows the distribution of requirements around the mean and the reference range of ± 2 SD around the mean. The reference intake (RDA, RNI, PRI) is the mean + 2 SD; the threshold intake at or below which it is unlikely that metabolic integrity could be maintained is the mean $-$ 2 SD. From Bender DA and Bender AE (1997) *Nutrition: A Reference Handbook*. Oxford University Press, by permission of the copyright holders.

population. This level of intake is variously known as the 'recommended daily (or dietary) allowance' (or 'amount'), or the 'reference nutrient intake' (**Table 1**). An intake 2 SD below the mean requirement will be inadequate to meet the requirements of all but 2.5% of the population. In the UK tables this is termed the 'lower reference nutrient intake', implying solely that it is the lower end of the reference range; in the European Union (EU) tables it is called the 'lower threshold intake', implying that it is a level of intake at or below which it is improbable that normal metabolic integrity can be maintained.

Scaling reference intakes for different population groups

Most of the studies on which estimates of requirements are based have been performed on young people – typically college students, although there were studies on long-stay psychiatric patients and prisoners during the 1950s and 1960s. There is a problem in extrapolating to the requirements of other population groups. Most authorities extrapolate on the basis of body weight. In the absence of adequate information, this is probably appropriate for most nutrients, although it is not known whether the nutrient requirements of elderly people change in proportion to body weight and energy intake. Because evidence was available on the iron requirements of women of child-bearing age, the EU

Table 1   Terms used to describe reference intakes of nutrients

RDA	Recommended Dietary Allowances	USA 1941	The name was deliberately chosen to allow the possibility of future modification of the values and was not intended to carry any connotation of minimum or optimal requirements
RDI	Recommended Dietary Intakes	UK 1969	The term is meant to emphasize that the recommendations relate to foodstuffs as actually eaten
RDA	Recommended Daily Amounts	UK 1979	'Amounts' refers to averages for a group of people and not to amounts that individuals must meet, as implied by the term 'allowances'
	Safe levels of intake	UN agencies	Means safe and adquate, but does not imply that higher intakes are unsafe
RNI	Reference Nutrient Intakes	UK 1991	Analogous to clinical chemistry reference ranges, which encompass 95% of 'normal' values. The term emphasizes that they are not recommendations for individuals, nor are they amounts to be consumed daily
PRI	Population Reference Intakes	EU 1993	Like the RNI, but with the emphasis that these are population ranges, and not applicable to individuals
US-RDA		USA 1973	Reference intakes for labelling purposes, the highest RDA value for any population group
RDI	Reference Daily Intakes	USA 1990	Reference intakes for labelling purposes, numerically equal to US-RDA
DRV	Daily Reference Values	USA 1990	Reference values for fat, carbohydrate, sodium, potassium and protein, for labelling purposes

From Bender DA and Bender AE (1997) *Nutrition: A Reference Handbook*. Oxford University Press, by permission of the copyright holders).

committee published separate reference intakes for iron for men and women.

Pregnancy, lactation and growth   Estimates of the additional nutrient requirements of pregnancy and lactation can be made by consideration of the amount of the nutrient that must be accumulated in the fetus, or secreted in the milk. This assumes that the maternal turnover of the nutrients remains unchanged. There is, however, excellent evidence that pregnancy is associated with significant changes in the metabolism of energy, protein and some micronutrients. Older tables of reference intakes make generous allowances for additional energy and protein intake in pregnancy (and scale micronutrient requirements proportionally). More recent tables take account of the new data on energy metabolism, and make considerably lower allowances for pregnancy and lactation.

The energy and protein needs of children are reasonably well established (although use of the doubly labelled water method has resulted in changes in estimates of children's energy needs). Their requirements for micronutrients are generally less well established. Traditionally, reference intakes for children have been determined by interpolation between the two points for which there is information: young adults (on whom most of the experimental studies have been performed) and breast-fed infants, for whom it is assumed that breast milk is (more than)

adequate to meet requirements. The composition of breast milk can therefore be taken as a reference intake for suckling infants. The EU committee, however, took a different approach. Rather than interpolation between these two points, they extrapolated backwards from the data for young adults, on the basis of the established energy requirements, and assuming that the nutrient density of foods should remain constant. While there may be little more scientific justification for this extrapolation than for interpolation, it is noteworthy that the extrapolated values for breast-fed infants match those for the composition of breast milk.

Uses and limitations of tables of reference intakes

The original US tables of recommended dietary allowances (RDA) were published to provide 'standards to serve as a goal for good nutrition'. They, and all similar publications by other national and international authorities, are intended to provide reference levels of intakes for groups of the population. This is emphasized in the EU tables by use of the term 'population reference intake'. The 10th edition of the US RDA includes the important note that 'RDAs are neither minimal requirements nor necessarily optimal levels of intake ... RDAs are safe and adequate levels (incorporating margins of safety intended to be sufficiently generous to encompass the ... variability among people'.

The main use of reference intakes is in planning food supplies and diets for populations or specific groups of people, e.g. in planning institutional feeding and national food policies. Here the aim is to ensure that the requirements of all members of the population are met. National priorities will determine the criteria of adequacy that are chosen, and hence the level at which the reference intake is set. Reference intakes can also be used to assess the adequacy of intake of populations and groups of people, for example in nutritional surveys. As the number of people whose intake is below the reference intake increases, so does the risk of deficiency in the population as a whole. The third use of reference intakes is in nutritional labelling of foods, to permit consumers to compare the nutrient content of different products. For this purpose, a single labelling reference value is derived from the tables as either the average requirement or the highest reference intake of any group of the population.

A potential use of reference intakes would be in distinguishing between nutrients sold as nutritional supplements and those sold for pharmaceutical purposes (at relatively high levels of intake), when evidence of efficacy and safety may be required. A nutritional supplement providing just the reference intake, in addition to even a poor diet would be more than adequate to ensure freedom from deficiency. Unless there is evidence of toxicity, a more generous ruling would be to take some multiple of the reference intake (perhaps 5 to 10-fold) as the upper limit for products sold as nutritional supplements. Preparations with contents above this level would then have to be licensed for pharmaceutical use, rather than being freely available as nutritional supplements.

Reference intake figures are not appropriate for assessing the adequacy of an individual's intake. Because the reference intake is higher than almost every individual's requirement, an intake below the reference intake does not imply deficiency. However, it is possible to replot the frequency curve of requirements (Fig. 1) as a cumulative graph of the proportion of the experimental subjects whose requirements have been met at any given level of intake (**Fig. 2**). It is then possible to reinterpret this graph as indicating the probability that a given level of intake is adequate to meet an individual's requirements.

See also: **Adolescents**: Dietary Habits and Nutrient Requirements. **Ascorbic Acid**: Physiology, Dietary Sources and Requirements; Scurvy. **Carotenoids**: Chemistry, Sources and Physiology. **Energy**: Energy Requirements. **Iodine**: Physiology, Dietary Sources and

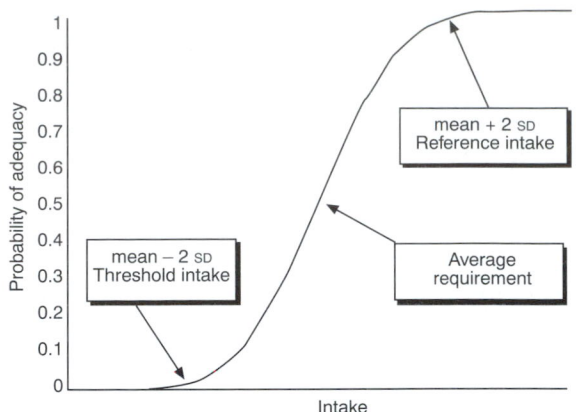

Figure 2 The same data as in Fig. 1 are plotted as the cumulative percentage of the group whose requirements have been met at any given level of intake. This can be reinterpreted as showing the probability that a given level of intake is adequate for an individual. From Bender DA and Bender AE (1997) *Nutrition: A Reference Handbook*. Oxford University Press, by permission of the copyright holders.

Requirements. **Lactation**: Dietary Requirements. **Nutritional Status**: Dietary Assessment. **Protein**: Requirements and Role in Diet. **Riboflavin**: Physiology. **Thiamin**: Physiology. **Vitamin B$_6$**: Physiology.

Further Reading

Beaton GH (1988) Nutrient requirements and population data. *Proceedings of the Nutrition Society* 47:63–78.

Department of Health (1991) *Dietary Reference Values for Food Energy and Nutrients for the United Kingdom*. Report of Health and Special Subjects 41. London: HMSO.

Food and Nutrition Board of the National Academy of Sciences (1989) *Recommended Dietary Allowances*, 10th edn. Washington: National Academy Press.

Food and Nutrition Board of the National Academy of Sciences (1997) *Dietary Reference Intakes: Calcium, Phosphorus, Magnesium, Vitamin D and Fluoride*. Washington: National Academy Press.

Harper AE (1987) Evolution of Recommended Daily Amounts – new directions? *Annual Review of Nutrition* 7:509–537.

Scientific Committee for Food (1993) *Nutrient and Energy Intakes for the European Community*. Luxembourg: Commission of the European Communities.

Trichopoulou A and Vassilakou T (1990) Recommended dietary intakes in the European Community member states: an overview. *European Journal of Clinical Nutrition* 44 (supplement 2): 51–125.

Truswell AS (1983) Recommended dietary intakes around the world. *Nutrition Abstracts and Reviews* 53:939–1119.

Turnlund JR and Schneeman BO (eds) (1996) New approaches to define nutrient requirements. *American Journal of Clinical Nutrition* 63:983s–1001s.

Nutrient-drug interactions *see* **Drugs**: Drug-Nutrient Interactions.

Nutrition claims *see* **Nutrition Labelling**: European Perspectives.

NUTRITION EDUCATION

Health Professionals

T Gill and **V Lakin**, Rowett Research Institute,
Aberdeen, UK

Copyright © 1998 Academic Press

Background

The interrelationship between nutrition, health and disease has long been recognized as fundamental to medical care. It was emphasized in the recommendations of great physicians such as Hippocrates and Galen, and in the activities of Florence Nightingale. Indeed, for a large part of the history of medical science, dietary modification was the most powerful and effective tool for the maintenance and rehabilitation of health. This concept was clearly elaborated by the Jewish scholar and physician Moses Maimonides in the twelfth century:

> The knowledge of dietetics is probably one of the most helpful things in the field of medicine because of the constant need for food, which is never ending, during health as well as illness.

Today, despite increasing dependence on advanced technology and pharmaceutical agents, the role of nutrition in the prevention and management of disease is as important as it was in the time of Maimonides. This article addresses the need for effective nutrition education and training at all stages of a health professional's career. It examines the key aims, approaches and appropriate strategies for delivering nutrition training programmes to health professionals and emphasizes the importance of comprehensive evaluation.

Why do health professionals require nutrition training?

Several studies have shown that health professionals, and in particular general medical practitioners, are trusted sources of health and dietary advice (**Table 1**).

Table 1 The ten most important sources of health information from a UK general population sample

Source	Rank	Percentage
General medical practitioner	1	48
Magazines/newspapers	2	16
Television	3	13
Friends and relatives	4	8
Practice nurse/health visitor	5	6
Pharmacist	5	6
Leaflets in GP waiting room	7	5
Other health professional	7	5
Radio	9	3

Adapted from OHE Briefing No. 30 – Health Information and the Consumer, May 1994. London: Office of Health Economics (with permission).

However, studies also show that health professionals frequently lack the skills, knowledge and confidence required to give appropriate dietary advice and to offer support with dietary changes. This is not surprising because nutrition has long been a neglected area of education for health professionals.

Which health professionals require nutrition training?

All health professionals have a role in promoting healthy eating and dietary change and all require a certain degree of nutrition training. However, it is those working within primary care who are most ideally placed to deliver dietary advice and education to the general public, and who therefore have a particular need to develop their nutrition knowledge and skills. Health professionals working in hospitals and specialist care facilities and services also have an important responsibility for maintaining the nutritional wellbeing of patients, particularly in long-stay facilities. There has been a widespread discussion of the need for improved nutrition training and education of health professions, especially for those listed in **Table 2**.

Table 2 The key health professionals requiring nutrition training

Profession	Opportunities to provide nutrition care
Nurses	
General	Nursing care involves detailed assessment and regular follow-up contact with patients/clients. Nutrition can be a direct or indirect element of this process.
Midwives Child health School health Occupational Community	Specialist nursing care is provided to specific target groups of the population from preconception through adulthood to terminal illness.
Primary care	Primary care nurses address the health concerns of all the family and often undertake active health promotion roles involving nutrition.
Medical practitioners	
Primary care physicians	General practitioners provide regular, ongoing care to individuals and their families. They are a well-respected source of health and nutrition advice. Patients regularly consult with their GP about nutrition-related illnesses and conditions where nutrition should be an integral component of the management.
Specialist physicians	Specialist physicians have enormous credibility and have the opportunity to indicate the value and importance of nutrition in disease management and prevention of illness in the whole family.
Dietitians	Dietitians are responsible for the provision of specialist nutrition advice and care and for the general promotion of nutrition in the community. They are also a major provider of nutrition training and support for other health professionals
Dentists	
Dentists	Dentists have regular, although not frequent, contact with healthy individuals. Many young children see the dentist more often than the doctor.
Dental hygienists	Hygienists have an educational role in addition to assessment and management which can address the general diet of children.
Pharmacists	Pharmacists have regular contact with patients requiring medication and their carers. They are also frequently approached by consumers seeking health advice or wanting clarification of information they have been given. A large part of pharmacy sales now includes nutrition supplements.
Other health professionals	Many other health professionals and therapists have extended contact with the public and are often approached to discuss health issues including nutrition.

Levels of education and training

Qualification and continuing practice as a health professional usually requires training at three levels: undergraduate or basic training, postgraduate or specialist training, and continuing education. Nutrition education and training should be integrated into each of these, albeit with considerable variation in content and delivery methods.

Undergraduate or basic training This leads to the basic qualification. There are usually very strict competencies set for students to achieve before they are allowed to practice. As a result, curricula are often full, established well in advance and bound by the constraints of academic requirements.

Postgraduate or specialist training This provides qualified health professionals with specific knowl-

edge and skills to carry out specialist duties. There is an academic component but the student has more opportunity to direct the learning and there is greater time and freedom to deal with issues in detail.

Continuing education Most health professions have a system of continuing education, either formal or informal, that encourages practitioners to maintain and upgrade their knowledge and skills in response to recent developments in their field. This stage usually involves more practical skills training than other stages as experienced practitioners are more concerned with the way in which they practice their profession than with the theory on which it is based.

Who provides nutrition education and training?

Undergraduate and postgraduate nutrition training is usually provided through academic institutions or professional associations, often by individuals without a specialist nutrition background. The involvement of practising nutritionists in the development and teaching of such programmes is important. Continuing nutrition education is mostly provided through local hospitals, community health care services or professional organizations, and is delivered by local dietetic departments.

Aims of Training

The main aim of nutrition training and education should be to ensure that all health professionals have a sound nutrition knowledge, as well as counselling and communication skills, necessary to support people in making dietary changes. In particular, comprehensive nutrition training should aim to:

1. develop a positive attitude among trainees towards the value and relevance of nutrition in all aspects of health care;
2. provide the basic principles of good nutrition and the rationale for dietary guidelines and food selection guides;
3. develop the skills required to identify nutrition-related problems in individuals and in the community;
4. develop the knowledge and skills necessary to give consistent and sound dietary advice to individuals and groups in an appropriate manner;
5. develop confidence in the health professional's ability to assess the validity and merit of nutritional literature and reports in the scientific and lay media.

Learning outcomes should be developed for all training programmes. These allow the effective development of the curricula, but also provide an important element in the evaluation of the programme. Learning outcomes should be related to the specific requirements of both the health profession being trained and the agency that has commissioned the training, as well as the level and purpose of training. A European workshop on nutrition training in medical education recommended a number of key learning outcomes that should be integral to basic nutrition training of all health professionals. These are set out in **Table 3**.

Analysis of Current Programmes

Despite the recognition that nutrition, health and disease are interrelated, nutrition has long been a neg-

Table 3 Some proposed nutrition learning outcomes for basic training of health professionals

Every health professional should be able to:

- appreciate the importance and relevance of nutrition for the promotion of good health and for the prevention and management of disease
- describe the scientific principles of human nutrition
- identify nutrition-related problems in individuals and the community
- provide safe and appropriate clinical nutrition support
- be able to give consistent and well-founded advice to patients and know when to refer them to specialists
- to understand and be able to promote the current dietary recommendations
- to understand the relative costs and benefits of therapeutic, preventive and public health approaches to health care and nutrition

lected area of education for health professionals. Widespread acceptance of the need for improved nutrition training is a recent development and studies on the extent and effectiveness of such training are still limited. Most attention has been focused on the training of medical doctors or primary care nurses, with a limited number of reports assessing the place of nutrition in the training of other health professionals.

Undergraduate or basic training

Nutrition rarely features as a core subject in the undergraduate curricula of health professionals. In the USA, the Association of American Medical Colleges reported that only 22% of medical schools included nutrition as a required course in 1995 and that more than 30% of medical schools excluded nutrition from the curriculum completely, failing to include nutrition either as a separate subject or as a distinct component of other subjects. In general, nutrition is only taught from a biochemical or physiological perspective.

Investigations into undergraduate medical programmes in the USA, Europe and Australia have found considerable variation in approach between schools and have generally concluded that the nutrition component is inadequate, poorly planned and poorly coordinated. As a result, positive attitudes towards the role of nutrition in health care seen in the majority of students entering medical school are essentially nonexistent by the end of the final year. Lack of established guidelines defining goals, course content, and best approaches to developing a successful medical-nutrition education programme have been identified as central to these problems.

A number of potential barriers to improving the status of nutrition in undergraduate medical curricula have been identified. These tend to relate to the medical education system and include financial pressures, time constraints in the curriculum, absence of nutrition coordinators, and the minimal coverage of nutrition issues in professional exams (see **Table 4**). However, some experts argue that these barriers can be overcome with appropriate planning and that the current situation has more to do with apathy and fear of change.

Nutrition training for nurses is generally integrated with other disciplines rather than being specified as a subject in its own right. This is despite the fact that nutrition has always been a key concern of nursing care and, before the advent of the dietetic profession, nurses were seen as the specialists in this area. However, reports have indicated that teaching of health and nutrition is increasing; use of nutrition resource materials and training packages by nurse trainers has increased, and dietitians are more involved in the basic training of nurses than of doctors. Nurse training is moving away from the traditional practical-based learning towards a more theoretical and academic framework, and specialization is occurring at the undergraduate level of training. The question remains whether nutrition should be taught in a theoretical or practical framework.

Nutrition education in the undergraduate training of health professionals other than doctors and nurses is generally limited. Nutrition rarely features in core curricula and tends to be restricted to final year elective options or as part of other speciality topics. Dentistry provides an exception, with nutrition being incorporated into the undergraduate curricula both in the basic science element and in clinical training. In addition some dental training facilities also include behavioural science, communication and counselling skills as part of clinical training.

Postgraduate or specialist training

The demand for postgraduate training of health professionals has been increasing, primarily as a result of moves towards 'specialization' in the provision of health care. Postgraduate courses tend to be provided

Table 4 Potential barriers to improving nutrition training for health professionals

- Limited funding
- Increased time spent in patient care at expense of education
- Negative perception of value of nutrition in preparing physicians for practice
- Competition from other disciplines
- Lack of nutrition specialists among teaching staff
- Absence of departments and boards for certification
- Apathy, inertia and fear of change

through training institutions for a fee, and are less heavily influenced by the major health professional bodies than was once the case.

Postgraduate nutrition courses are readily available in most regions. However, those participating in such courses tend to be looking for a change in career rather than for specialization within their own profession. In some cases, students have no training whatsoever in a health profession and seek basic nutrition training through a university postgraduate course following successful completion of a general science degree.

With the exception of the nursing profession, specialist postgraduate training in nutrition is rarely an option for health professionals. Nurses have increasing opportunities to take course in areas of special nursing responsibility such as enteral and parenteral feeding. However, this has been unpopular with many dietitians who may be concerned about the erosion of their professional role. The dietetic profession has also responded to increasing specialization within health-care services by developing specialist postgraduate training courses for dietitians.

Continuing education

The increasing prominence given to health promotion has led to increased recognition of the importance of nutrition by practising health professionals. However, there are few continuing nutrition education programmes for health professionals, and there is no formal requirement that they be undertaken.

Surveys of doctors, nurses, and other health professionals show considerable variability in nutrition knowledge between and even within professions. Knowledge associated with practical issues such as food guides, assessment and nutrition education tools is generally poor, and primary health-care teams are particularly unsure when endeavouring to translate knowledge into practical advice for individuals. This is not surprising, given the current focus of undergraduate nutrition training on nutritional biochemistry and clinical management of disease. Newer graduates tend to have a better nutrition knowledge, but this is by no means the rule. In the absence of continuing nutrition education opportunities, nutrition information is obtained from a variety of sources including medical journals, the lay media, and information sheets from food and pharmaceutical companies.

The nursing profession appears to provide the most opportunities for continuing education in nutrition. This is an indication of the large size of the profession, its central role in the health-care process, and the eagerness of nurses to attend training.

However, the resistance of nutrition trainers to extend beyond nurses and thereby reach less easily targeted and compliant professions may also be a factor. Various modes of training are available, including study days run by local dietitians, self-directed training manuals, audio and video cassettes, and courses run by professional groups. However, many are commercially funded and so editorial control by a neutral body, together with approval through validation or accreditation systems, are essential to ensure quality and consistency. Recently, the dentistry and pharmacy professions have developed distance learning programmes in nutrition that reflect their perceived growing role as nutrition educators.

Trends in training

There have been a number of attempts to address the perceived barriers to improving nutrition training. In the USA, for example, the formation of networks for developing and sharing resources among medical schools is helping to overcome shortages of qualified staff, suitable training materials, access to practical nutrition experience and appropriate examinations. Other benefits include the development of material that is of a consistent quality and format, and is directly relevant to the agreed curriculum. The approach is being adopted for the basic nutrition training of other health professionals and is gaining acceptance in the development of postgraduate nutrition courses. In the UK, a multiprofessional taskforce has produced a document which sets out the rationale and objectives of nutrition training of health professionals, and proposes a core curriculum that is applicable to all levels of training and to all health professions.

The traditional system of undergraduate medical training, with clinical practice not featuring until the later years when students have obtained a firm grounding in basic science, is currently undergoing revision in a number of training institutions. Practical problem-solving exercises are being introduced at an earlier stage of training, in parallel with large group lectures, as a means of developing theoretical knowledge and practical skills in unison. A similar shift towards problem-based learning is occurring in other professions and is expected to aid the inclusion of nutrition into the undergraduate curricula. Problem-based learning focuses on the person rather than the disease and is often taught using a multidisciplinary approach. Nutrition spans all specialities and all levels of care, and so should gain more curriculum space in this type of training approach.

A significant trend in continuing education relates to the access of accredited material and programmes over the internet. The rapid spread of computer technology into all aspects of office and domestic activities means that a large proportion of the population can access and exchange information with remote computers from home or work. Regular education bulletins, individual training units or even complete training programmes can be accessed and downloaded onto personal computers from a central server. Furthermore, the progress of learners can be assessed by the return of questionnaires, and assignments through the same media. This makes internet-based training a cost-effective and interactive educational approach that is also suitable for postgraduate level training. A number of health-care organizations have established websites that provide accredited continuing education training programmes for health-care professionals. With a huge number of people joining the web each day, the internet is destined to play a major role in training of health professionals in the future.

Developing Programmes for the Nutrition Training of Health Professionals

Nutrition should be an important component of training for health professionals during all three periods of professional learning. Given the perceived barriers and lack of enthusiasm for adding new material to already full training programmes and curricula, it may not always be appropriate for nutrition to be taught as a separate unit or subject area. The integration of a nutrition component into existing professional training is therefore also an important strategy.

Undergraduate or basic training

Undergraduate training usually consists of a number of consecutive years and so provides the opportunity to integrate nutrition into existing curricula through a variety of modes.

- Vertical integration – as a discrete theme through all years, allowing for the gradual accumulation of knowledge and skills as students progress through their basic training.
- Horizontal integration – into the teaching of specific topics for one or more years such as physiology, therapeutics, public health or health promotions.
- Elective option – in the final year of basic training

Undergraduate/basic training focuses strongly on the acquisition of knowledge and competency in basic skills (**Table 5**), but is also a period when attitudes to subject areas can be shaped. It generally

Table 5 Nutrition training strategies for different stages of health professional education

Stage	Key concepts	Teaching formats
Undergraduate or basic	Basic principles of nutrition science and clinical nutrition including: • Energy and nutrients • Physiological mechanisms that affect nutrient requirement • Nutrition through life stages • Basis of nutrition-related illness and therapeutic diets • Assessment of diet and nutritional status • Epidemiology of nutrition • Basic nutrition promotion	• Lectures • Assignments • Placements within nutrition departments • Case studies • Problem-solving exercises • Computer-aided learning programmes • Formal assessments
Postgraduate or specialist	Broader issues of clinical and public health nutrition including: • Specialist nutrition clinical care • Unusual nutrition issues • Nutritional surveillance and markers of nutritional health • Social aspects of nutrition • Public health nutrition strategies • Nutritional adaptation	• Self-completed modules • Problem-solving • Lectures • Distance learning • Dissertations and electives • Research projects • Discussion of journal articles • Internet-based programmes • Self-assessment
Continuing education	Improving the management of nutritional problems of individuals and communities including: • Revision of basic nutrition principles • Dietary assessment • Dietary management of common conditions • Achieving dietary change • Use of dietary education tools • Nutritional health of the community • Principles of public health nutrition	• Case studies • Role play • Small group discussion • Distance learning • Educational outreach • Computer-assisted learning packages • Protocol development • Internet-based programmes • Self-assessment

involves the teaching of large groups of students. This requires an approach that is economical in terms of both time and resources, but which also shapes positive attitudes towards the role of nutrition in health care and stimulates students to undertake further personal learning in the subject. Structured lectures, delivered by important opinion leaders or motivational speakers, still have an important role to play in achieving these objectives. Table 5 suggests some other suitable teaching formats for this level of training, including computer-assisted learning programmes for increased flexibility and case studies to demonstrate the relevance of course material to health-care practice. The inclusion of nutrition in formal examinations is also important.

All training should be relevant to the community in which the students will later practice. However, this level of basic nutrition training should focus more on the broader national and international nutrition issues rather than on local or regional concerns. In this way, trainers and resources can be shared between institutions on a regional or even national basis.

Undergraduate training also provides the opportunity to teach the basics of nutrition jointly to a range of health professionals. This conserves resources and ensures that there is consistency in the manner and content of training between disciplines. It also promotes a greater understanding of the complementary roles of other health professionals, a vital factor for the formation of health alliances.

Postgraduate or specialist training

Postgraduate specialist training offers greater opportunities to deal with nutrition in depth, and is more concerned with facilitation and guidance of students than with direct teaching. Teaching formats must be challenging and should not attempt to provide all required information within the prepared resources (Table 5). As with other subjects, training manuals, reading lists and research topics need to be regularly updated.

The development of discrete nutrition modules can facilitate integration of nutrition into the curricula of a wider range and number of postgraduate programmes; high-quality resources produced by one profession or institution can be utilized by others. Such an approach allows uniformity in both the content and the standard of learning achieved among different institutions and different professions, and even between different countries.

Moves towards a more self-directed mode of learning in postgraduate/specialist education require that the subject areas covered are both interesting and relevant to the particular health profession. A clear understanding of the principles of nutrition science is fundamental, but the application of acquired knowledge and skills in practice is an equally important outcome. Ideally, students will later contribute to improved understanding and practice of nutrition by their profession in general. The topic areas presented in Table 5 illustrate those most appropriate for this level of nutrition training, although they should be adapted according to the existing level of knowledge and specific nutrition concerns of each health profession.

Continuing education

Continuing education is a period when most health professionals focus on the development of practical skills relevant to their daily work. Nutrition training during this period should therefore aim to improve competence in nutrition care. This can involve correcting existing misconceptions, remedying deficits in important nutrition knowledge and skill, and reorienting attitudes towards the role of nutrition in health care. Regular advances in nutritional science and dietary management must also be disseminated to health professionals in an uncomplicated and practical format. A valuable tool for nutrition training of practising health professionals is self-assessment of current nutrition knowledge, skills and attitudes. The key issues that should be addressed at this stage of training have been outlined in Table 5.

The time available for continuing education of practising health professionals is extremely limited, usually restricted to short periods in lunch breaks or early evening. This prevents detailed analysis of issues and presents a challenge to trainers to get the important messages across with maximum efficiency. Traditional training techniques often fail in the continuing education environment. Although formal lectures still have a place within this process, there is a need to develop strategies that allow information to be delivered in short, discrete blocks. Small group discussion based on case histories is a useful and popular format for dealing with difficult health issues within such time restrictions.

Time restrictions also have important implications for course content. Thorough needs assessments are required to ensure that training is directly relevant to practice. However, it is often difficult to balance the assessed training needs of health professionals at this stage against their perceived wants, particularly if a course fee is involved. Furthermore, when nutrition education at an undergraduate and postgraduate level has been inadequate, it is often difficult to remedy the situation through continuing education.

Educational outreach, or academic detailing, is attracting increasing attention as a method for providing and reinforcing important nutrition messages and dietary practices to active health professionals. The process has been widely utilized by the pharmaceutical industry to increase awareness and provide supporting information for the uptake of new drugs by general medical doctors. It is based on a set of important principles set out in **Table 6** and usually involves a series of short sessions with individuals or groups where key messages or practices are raised and reinforced. A major advantage of the academic outreach approach is that training is delivered within the workplace and requires only a short amount of time for each visit (10–15 min). Other forms of workplace-based training have also proved popular with busy health professionals and the spread of personal computers has allowed the development of computer-based training packages that include an element of self-assessment.

There is now an increased focus on involving different health professionals who work together in the same centre into team-oriented training. The advent of evidence-based health care has led to a focus on formalized processes or protocols which are utilized by health professionals to deal with common health

Table 6 Key techniques of educational outreach

1. Conducting background assessments of health practitioner knowledge, attitudes and motivation
2. Focusing programmes on key health professionals and opinion leaders
3. Defining clear educational and behavioural objectives
4. Establishing credibility through a respected organizational identity, use of authoritative and unbiased sources of information and presenting both sides of controversial issues
5. Stimulating active participation from health professionals in education sessions
6. Using concise, graphical education material
7. Highlighting and repeating essential messages
8. Providing positive reinforcement of improved practice at regular follow-up visits

issues. Nutrition training can be made more attractive and relevant if it can provide dietary management tools which can support existing protocols or can be used as the basis for developing new protocols.

Evaluation of Nutrition Training

Although much has been written about the importance of evaluation, it remains a poorly understood and performed element of the training process. Proper evaluation is crucial for designing new programmes, improving and justifying the existence of current programmes, and eliminating ineffective programmes. It is an integral component of the training cycle (**Fig. 1**). Evaluation that is poorly designed and conducted, by contrast, can be misleading and counterproductive, and often leads to the squandering of scarce resources.

Evaluation is concerned with the collection and analysis of information to judge whether training needs have been correctly identified, and whether design and delivery are appropriate. It also measures the effectiveness and impact of the programme. Evaluation involves value judgments of the merit of training. It should not be confused with assessment, which is more to do with progress and performance of the learner. In the case of nutrition training, evaluation is usefully split into two components.

1. Formative evaluation – concerned with the inputs of the training programme (content, style, relevance and delivery) and improving the design.
2. Summative evaluation – concerned with the outcomes of the training programme (knowledge, competence, performance) and proving its worth.

In a climate of cost-effectiveness, quality control and

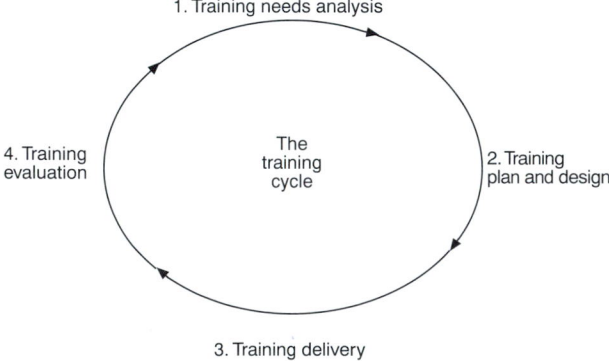

Figure 1 Evaluation is a critical component of training and assesses the effectiveness of every aspect of the training cycle. This includes evaluating whether training needs have been correctly identified, whether the training programme meets those needs and whether it was planned and delivered appropriately, as well as assessing the outcomes of the training.

accountability, both forms of evaluation must assume a high priority within the design and delivery of nutrition education and training.

Issues in planning and interpreting evaluation

Evaluation of nutrition training is associated with a number of theoretical and practical limitations, especially because of the highly subjective nature of the process. The question of who should judge the merit of the training programme – whether it is the learner, the teacher, the profession, the community or the organization that funds the training – is inevitable. Each is likely to have a different perspective and so allowing the training objectives to be driven by one party alone may give inappropriate outcomes. This is the case with most undergraduate and formal postgraduate training programmes where the learning objectives and outcomes are set almost exclusively by the training institution or professional body.

Education and training performance indicators often relate to changes in knowledge, skills and behaviour. It is important to recognize, however, that training does not occur in a vacuum; the health professional is subject to a number of external influences which may intervene during the process of learning or behaviour change (see **Fig. 2**).

The process of evaluation requires time and resources. It is important, therefore, to ensure that the procedures adopted produce valid and reliable conclusions and that they are feasible and practical. The concept of validity relates to whether the evaluation process is truly measuring what you want it to measure, while reliability relates to how consistent the results would be if the evaluation was repeated several times.

Levels of evaluation

There are numerous models on which to base the evaluation of nutrition training. Kirkpatrick, for example, has described a useful stepwise approach which breaks the evaluation process down into four logical steps and allows the development of clear and achievable goals. This approach requires specific criteria to define success but, at the same time, recognizes the many factors that may influence evaluation. The steps are defined as follows:

Step 1   Reaction – How well did the participants like the programme?

Step 2   Learning – What principles, facts and techniques were learned?

Step 3   Behaviour – What changes in behaviour resulted from the programme?

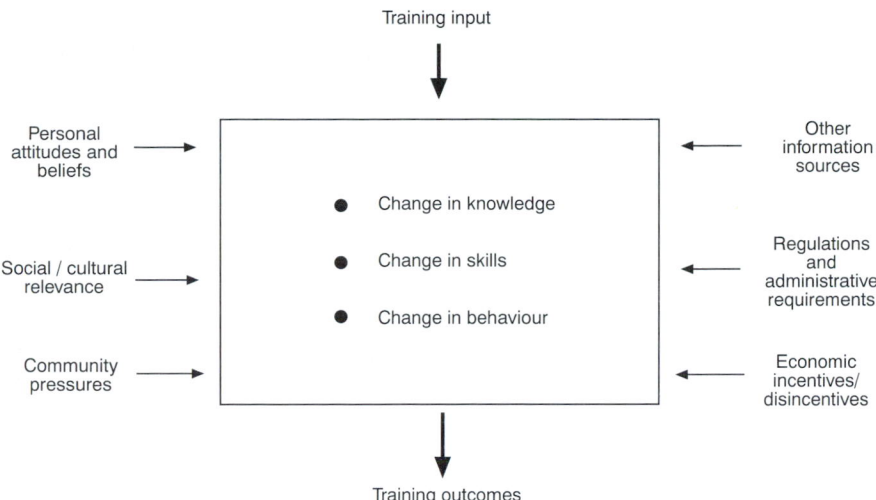

Figure 2 The outcomes of any training programme for health professionals are subject to a number of influences external to the training process. Economic and regulatory requirements, social and community pressures, media and existing attitudes and beliefs can exert powerful influences on individual participant's response to a training programme.

Step 4   Results – What are the tangible results of the programme?

Kirkpatrick presents these steps as a hierarchy of evaluation and emphasizes the need to extend the process beyond the training period. It is important to determine whether learning has been transferred into everyday practice as well as any impact on the wider community.

Table 7 presents an extended version of the Kirk-patrick hierarchy and sets out examples of appropriate evaluation measures for each level. An additional level associated with initial development of the programme precedes the first step of the Kirkpatrick approach, and the final step has been subdivided into short-, medium- and long-term outcomes. These higher levels of evaluation may face a number of complications in terms of developing valid and reliable measures and are usually inappropriate for most nutrition training programmes. However, if the

Table 7   Evaluation measures for the nutrition training of practising health professionals

Stage	Level of evaluation	Potential measures
Development of training programme	Formative	Needs assessments Piloting Uptake
Implementation of training	Reaction	Participant satisfaction Participant feedback Ongoing participation
Practitioner learning	Learning	Changes in awareness, knowledge, skills, attitudes, confidence
Change in practitioner behaviour	Behaviour change	Acceptance and use of materials Change in practice protocols Time spent in dietary management
Patient education and support	Short-term outcome (impact)	Change in patient/client satisfaction Change in patient/client awareness, knowledge, attitudes, skills, confidence, enthusiasm.
Change in patient dietary behaviour	Short/medium-term outcome	Change in patient dietary habits
Improved clinical markers	Medium-term outcome	Improved anthropometry Biochemistry Reduced clinical intervention
Improved health and reduced illness	Long-term outcome	Morbidity Mortality

true effectiveness of nutrition education and training is to be assessed, evaluation at some level of outcome is crucial. Evaluation that stops at level one is clearly inadequate, but unfortunately all too common.

See also: **Dietetics**: The Role of Dietetics in Health Care.

Further Reading

Glanz K (1992) Nutrition interventions: a behavioural and educational perspective. In: Ockene IS and Ockene JK (eds) *The Prevention of Coronary Heart Disease; A Skills-Based Approach*, pp 231–265. Boston: Little, Brown and Co.

Green LW and Kreuter MW (1991) *Health Promotion Planning; An Educational and Environmental Approach*, 2nd edn. London: Mayfield Publishing House.

Group on Nutrition Education of the Society of Teachers of Family Medicine (1995) *Physician's Curriculum in Clinical Nutrition*. Kansas City: Society of Teachers of Family Medicine.

International Union of Nutrition Sciences (IUNS) (1986) *Guidelines for the Training of Clinicians for Academic Research and Clinical Nutrition*. Report of Committee v/14. IUNS.

Kirkpatrick DL (1967) Evaluation of training. In: Craig RL and Bittel LR (eds) *Training and Development Handbook*, chap. 5, pp 87–111. New York: McGraw-Hill.

Kushner RF, Thorp FK, Edwards J, Weinser RL and Brooks CM (1990) Implementing nutrition into the medical curriculum: a user's guide. *American Journal of Clinical Nutrition* 52:401–403.

Nutrition Task Force Project Team, The Health of the Nation (1994) *Nutrition: Core Curriculum for Nutrition in the Education of Health Professionals*. London: Department of Health.

Oshaugh A, Benbouzid D and Guilbert J-J (1993) *Educational Handbook for Nutrition Trainers*. Geneva: World Health Organization.

Somerai SB and Avorn J (1990) Principles of educational outreach ('academic detailing') to improve clinical decision making. *Journal of the American Medical Association* 263(4):549–556.

Truswell AS (ed.) (1997) Nutrition attitudes and practices of primary care physicians. *American Journal of Clinical Nutrition* 65(Supplement 6S).

World Health Organization (1973) *Development of Educational Programmes for Health Professions*. Public Health Papers, no. 52. Geneva: WHO.

NUTRITION POLICIES

Contents
In Developed Countries
In Developing Countries

In Developed Countries

A Draper and **E Dowler**, London School of Hygiene and Tropical Medicine, UK

Policy is about who gets what, when, where and how, and who controls these processes. It is often seen as a process of problem definition, the setting of objectives and targets, the allocation of resources and the creation or maintenance of institutions and instruments to meet these objectives in order to produce measurable effects. Various conceptual frameworks have been developed to describe and understand the policy process and its various component parts.

Food and nutrition policies are concerned with citizens' physical and economic access to food that is nutritious, safe, reliable, reasonably priced and of good quality. In most developed free-market economies, where subsistence production is minimal and market exchange the main source of food, policies are premised on citizens being able to make informed choices about the food they purchase, prepare and consume. Food usage is essentially a personal matter: the choice of what to eat, when and with whom, reflects cultural, social and individual circumstances and desires. The role of the state in peacetime is largely indirect, in ensuring an economic and practical climate in which such choices can be expressed, and in trying to influence choice by providing information. The state does not set out to limit personal freedom either by prescribing what should be bought, or by providing a ration, although for those whose circumstances are such that they have neither the money nor opportunity to express choice – for instance, those in destitution or institutions – subsidies or rations are necessary.

By and large, nutrition policy in developed countries has largely been concerned either with redressing the adverse consequences of market failure (that is, meeting the food needs of those who are poor, for whatever reasons), or with intervention to improve human productivity (ensuring that workers are fed or that they do not become ill). Nutrition as a component of social justice or human rights seldom reaches to the policy agenda either through state machinery or the action of public health professionals. For example, the 1996 World Food Summit Rome Declaration and Plan of Action, affirmed the 'right of everyone to have access to safe and nutritious food, consistent with the right to adequate food and the fundamental right of everyone to be free from hunger'. While delegates from developed countries signed their agreement to this statement, their public responses indicated that the issues were seen as primarily concerning developing countries only. However, there are good reasons for supposing inadequate household food access will be a growing problem in developed countries. These reasons include the increasing globalization of food production and distribution with declining public sector control; the rapid economic transition that many countries (for instance, the former Soviet Union) are experiencing, leading to rising problems of social inequality and domestic food insecurity; and finally, in developed countries, the problems of rising unemployment, family breakdown and ageing populations which are producing considerable strain on national systems of social provision. Social policy sector responses will increasingly need to include nutritional needs.

The increasing globalization of the world food supply also presents a challenge to policy implementation within national contexts. A number of commentators argue that the globalization of food production, distribution and marketing means that the location of control over these processes is increasingly outside the public sector. The role of the state in influencing individuals' food consumption is also weakening. Consumers' exposure to a wide range of different cuisines and food commodities is growing, and since World War II there have been enormous changes in food habits and patterns of dietary intake in many developed countries, along with growing industrial innovation in the processed food sector. Demand for new commodities is said by some to be difficult to predict; others argue that shopping patterns and resulting diets are increasingly directed by international food retailing conglomerates.

Another postwar challenge to nutrition policies in developed countries is the need to tackle diet-related chronic diseases, such as coronary heart disease, which are increasing in incidence. In the earlier part of the twentieth century, food and nutrition policies were primarily concerned with ensuring a safe and adequate food supply and, in relation to disease, the prevention of deficiency diseases. Diet-related chronic diseases present a more complex problem: in terms of aetiology the problems were initially attributed to over- rather than underconsumption of certain foods and/or nutrients. Lately, changes in diet that have led to lower intakes of antioxidants and complex carbohydrates, perhaps below desirable levels, have been associated with increases in chronic diseases. Concepts such as the 'prudent diet' and 'optimal nutrition' have been designed to address both of these problems, although there is still scientific uncertainty about the precise formulation of these ideas in practice, and of the significance of genetic differences and individual nutrient needs.

Two international conferences on nutrition have tried to raise the profile of food and nutrition across a number of sectors in developed and developing countries: the International Conference on Nutrition (ICN), held in Rome in 1992 (**Table 1**), and the World Food Conference, held in Rome at the end of 1996. The Food and Agriculture Organization (FAO) and World Health Organization (WHO) of the UN convened the first; the FAO alone convened the second. Some are convinced that the ICN contributed to formulation of national nutrition policies in developed countries; others argue that such policies as exist would have happened anyway, although they concede the ICN strengthened the hand of national nutrition professionals in promoting nutrition's cause.

Nutrition and Agriculture Policies

The scope and objectives of nutrition policies versus food and agricultural policies

Food and nutrition policies tend to be elided in both definition and practice, but for analytical purposes it is useful to distinguish the two. The goal of food and agricultural policies is to maintain national food supply, through domestic production or imports and storage; to this end, the maintenance of an economically sound farming sector and healthy food industry, whether in the public or private sector, is a crucial objective. In contrast, a nutrition policy can be defined as one that seeks to promote healthy nutrition. The principal objective is the provision of a nutritionally satisfactory diet. This is conventionally defined in relation to recommended dietary

Table 1 Outcomes of the International Conference on Nutrition

At the UN's International Conference on Nutrition held in Rome in 1992 a World Declaration and Plan of Action for Nutrition were formulated and launched. Representatives from 159 countries attended and committed themselves to the elimination of hunger and all forms of malnutrition, and to the plan of action to achieve this. In order to achieve nutritional wellbeing for all, the Plan of Action defined nine action-oriented themes:

1. The incorporation of nutrition objectives into development plans and programmes.
2. Improvement of household food security.
3. Protection of consumers through improved food quality and safety.
4. Prevention and management of infectious diseases.
5. Promotion of breast-feeding.
6. Caring for the socioeconomically deprived and nutritionally vulnerable.
7. Prevention and control of specific micronutrient deficiencies.
8. Promotion of appropriate diets and life-styles.
9. Assessment, analysis and monitoring of nutrition situations.

The ICN also called on governments to draw up national plans of action to implement these objectives by the end of 1994. However, an audit of countries in the European region conducted by the Nurition Unit of the WHO Regional Office revealed a patchy response and variability in which themes had been adopted; the themes most commonly picked up were 3, 8 and 9.

The WHO report *Our Planet, Our Health* published in 1992 also advocated the incorporation of health goals within agricultural, nutrition and food policies.

The European Union president Jacques Santer has made a statement that health and nutrition objectives should be incorporated in reform of the Common Agricultural Policy

intakes or nutrient reference values, usually devised to avoid deficiency, but, as mentioned above, there is also now a need to incorporate the prevention of chronic disease. These two aims present a scientific and technical challenge in defining food and nutrient recommendations. They also carry implications for the agricultural, food and retail sector. For instance, the current focus on recommending increases in fruit and vegetable consumption raises several questions. If the general population responds, can developed countries produce or import sufficient commodities? What would be the implications of increased water and fertilizer usage in countries where fruit or vegetable production was markedly increased?

Few countries have an explicit nutrition policy *per se* and the extent to which nutrition policy objectives are integrated with food and/or agricultural policies is variable. This is often an area of conflict, for instance in the representation of the interests of public health and consumer protection versus the interests of agriculture and the food industry.

Food and nutrition policy is thus often a focus for struggle between competing interests. Although nutrition itself is relatively noncontentious (no-one is against good nutrition or in favour of malnutrition), it is a weak area in policy practice. Nutrition has no powerful lobby to argue its case and defend its outcome: few governments have a strong commitment to effect lasting changes in nutritional well-

being; they react to crises and pressures, whether internally generated from consumers or producers, or externally from international agencies. Where governments do adopt an explicit nutrition policy, as some European countries have done, the institutional and legislative framework for activities is seldom put in place. Most commentators on food and agricultural policies note that they seldom explicitly address nutritional objectives in practice, even though the maintenance of a healthy national diet may be a stated goal. Norway is a much-cited example of an exception (**Table 2**).

Actors in the Policy Arena

There are four main interest groups operating at national and international level on food and nutrition policy: the state decision-making and executive bodies, who by definition operate in the public sector; consumers (both individuals and households) and those who represent them; producers or suppliers, who largely operate in the private sector (producers, exporters and importers, processors, distributors, the food and retail industry); and the scientific and medical communities, which operate from academic and other public or private institutions. In addition, the media (primarily television, radio and newspapers) have an important role, either in informing consumers and enabling

Table 2 Norway's food policy

In 1975 Norway adopted a comprehensive Food and Nutrition Policy (FCP). This was designed to bring food and agricultural production in line with both national nutrition goals and also developing country needs. The FNP had four principal objectives:

1. To encourage a health-promoting diet, reduce fat consumption and in particular saturated fats, and to replace them with polyunsaturated fats, whole grains and vegetables.
2. To promote domestic food production and reduce food imports and so increase national self-sufficiency from 39% of total energy supply to 52% by 1990.
3. To promote agricultural development in less advantaged, outlying regions with regard to the preservation of the environmental resource base.
4. To contribute to world food security, promoting food production and consumption in poor countries.

Norway's FNP was unusual in taking such a broad 'farm-to-fork' approach and can be seen as the result of a complex clustering of social, economic, political and scientific factors (see Milio 1989 and 1990 for an analysis of these). In order to achieve these goals a number of policy instruments were used, which included economic measures (incentives/disincentives), regulation, information and education, and research evaluation. The goals of the FNP were met by the 1990s, although the goals that were achieved first and that had received the most funding were the food economics objectives (2 and 3).

Adapted from Tansey and Wolsey (1995).

their views to be aired publicly, or in being part of campaigning and promotion efforts by any or all of the interest groups described. Non governmental organizations, such as consumer and trade organizations and health-related charities, may also be involved in the policy formulation process. International agencies, such as WHO and FAO, may play a role in policy-making through their ability to review, research, collaborate, inform, promote and advise, but they have no power or right of intervention unless agreed or invited by national governments. Generally they are more influential in developing rather than developed countries. However, in 1993, food and agricultural commodities were included for the first time in the General Agreement on Tariffs and Trade (GATT) Uruguay round. This inclusion increased the importance of UN bodies such as the Codex Alimentarius Commission and the WHO/FAO Joint Executive Committee on Food Additives (JECFA), although their actual role is primarily confined to legislative activities, such as the setting of food standards.

State decision-making and executive bodies

It has often been pointed out that nutrition has no natural home in government and few countries have an explicit or exclusive state department or agency with responsibility for nutrition. Nutrition policy in terms of both formulation and implementation is essentially intersectoral and usually falls primarily under health or agriculture, although social and employment policies and the private sector food industry also have important roles. The constitutional arrangements that have been established in different developed countries to deal with issues related to food and nutrition vary greatly, and official agencies differ in terms of their remit and in

the demarcation of zones of responsibility and power over different components of the food chain. They also differ in how they attempt to resolve the sometimes conflicting interests of the consumer and public health, versus agriculture, industry or trade. In some countries autonomous or semiautonomous nutrition institutes have been created, often placed within ministries of health. These institutes sometimes have responsibility for negotiation with international trading and legislative bodies, such as the European Union Common Agricultural Policy, or the Codex Alimentarius Commission; sometimes this negotiation is done within the agricultural sector. In addition, food safety in relation to additives, non-adulteration, noncontamination, microbiological hazard and veterinary practices, and food product information in relation to labelling, often fall under agriculture's institutional and legislative remit. Agricultural departments are often also engaged in surveillance – of food safety, and (sometimes) of food consumption.

Many developed countries are either in the process of restructuring their state agencies for dealing with nutrition, particularly for issues relating to food safety, or have already done so. This restructuring is in response to heightened consumer sensitivity on issues of food safety, growing concern about diet and health and the need to deal with issues such as bovine spongiform encephalitis (BSE), which require a broad multisectoral approach. There is also some restructuring within the European Union (EU) of responsibilities between Directorates General which deal with nutrition, particularly in relation to food safety issues.

An example of two contrasting agencies Some agencies have a fairly narrowly defined remit and powers. One example is the semi-autonomous Australian and New Zealand Food Authority. This body is primarily concerned with the development of food standards and codes of practice to protect public health and promote fair trade, although there is consumer pressure for them to also address issues relating to food production and public health and take a broader 'farm to fork' approach to food safety. In contrast, the Swedish National Food Administration has a broader remit and powers. It is located within the Ministry of Agriculture, but takes consumer and health interests as its primary responsibility and it is independent from the Board of Agriculture. The commitment to open government means that any tensions between the interests of industry and the consumer are openly addressed.

Consumers

Consumers' nutrition interests usually cover a wide range of issues. Those actively wanting advice on how to avoid specific diseases through diet tend to be those who already have experienced heart problems or cancers themselves or in their family. Many express general health aims (such eating to be fit and strong, or having children growing well). Many are concerned about long-term safety of food production and preservation techniques (such as genetic engineering, pesticide residues, growth promoters, or potential for interspecies transfer of slow-acting prions – the BSE controversy). Others express interest in the information on food packaging (such as nutrient contents lists, or the reliability of health claims). Other recent food production concerns have been over animal welfare (animal rearing, production and transport), and the environmental sustainability of intensive agricultural and horticultural systems. Finally, there has been recent pressure for those on low incomes to have access to appropriate, healthy food. National and international consumer or voluntary sector pressure groups often focus on one or more of these consumer issues. Few, if any, national nutrition policies explicitly address all these concerns.

Scientific and medical communitites

The scientific or medical communities are the source for Expert Committees, who aim to provide consensus statements of nutrient and growth reference levels, sometimes with explicit policy targets, which are used by public sector agencies for policy formulation. In practice, the scientific nutrition arena is often one of divergence rather than consensus, particularly over reference levels and policy goals. For example, there was controversy in the USA over the setting of nutrient standards in 1985, when proposals to lower the reference values, particularly those of vitamins A and C, met with opposition from practitioners using the standards as well as from other nutritional scientists. Much of the literature about nutrition policy in developed countries is written from the perspective of public health professionals, whose current interest is largely the potential of nutritional or dietary intervention, at individual and national levels, to prevent particular diseases, such as coronary heart disease or cancers, or to contribute to increasing general or optimal levels of health and wellbeing.

The food sector

The large and diverse food sector encompasses agriculture, importers and exporters, food processors and distributors, the retail sector and caterers. Each of these has different interests in relation to policy, although ultimately all are concerned with the maximization of profits. Economically this sector is very important and it is a powerful and successful political lobbying group in many developed countries, with powerful trade organizations to represent their interests. The food industry is dominated by large multinational companies, mainly American and European, and within this there are a few who predominate, such as Unilever, Nestlé and Philip Morriss Companies Inc.

In recent years some parts of the food sector, such as supermarket chains, have begun to show considerable interest in nutrition issues, and to employ nutritional professionals for nutrition promotion as well as work on product development. The extent of industry's involvement in government is variable. In some countries, such as the UK, industry representation is included on governmental committees. In others, industry representation is excluded. For instance, in Ireland industry representation has been deliberately excluded from the newly formed Food Authority in order to create consumer confidence in its independence. In policy formation there can be conflicts of interest between the food sector and scientists working in public health. An illustration of this is the controversy in the UK over salt recommendations. In 1994 the UK government's advisory Committee on Medical Aspects of Food Policy (COMA) recommended that people should reduce their average intakes of salt from 9 g to 6 g. This provoked a fierce response from the food industry (salt is the main flavouring agent in most processed foods) and they intensively lobbied the government. When the report was launched, the Chief Medical Officer, while accepting all its other recommendations, publicly distanced himself from the one regarding salt.

Problem Definition and the Role of Surveillance

Most developed countries have some system of surveillance: regular measurement of food usage and nutritional outcomes. Problem definition is an essential step in formulating food and nutrition policies, and the task is broadly to establish who is eating what, and with what outcomes in terms of public and individual health (child growth, obesity, disease and mortality patterns). Measurement is made of food and nutrient intakes, child growth and adult body size, in many countries with validation by biological markers. These activities, which require reference standards to interpret both intakes and body dimensions, enable governments to identify who has what kind of nutrient deficiency or excess, how that might link with disease outcomes, and to monitor change with time. The problems are defined for different physiological or demographic groups (such as infants, pregnant women, and middle-aged men), and in some countries they are also defined geographically and in terms of socioeconomic conditions of the household or individual.

In some countries these quantitative data are complemented by qualitative studies of how and where people obtain and use food, and why, to establish patterns of behaviour correlated both with household sociodemographic circumstances and health outcomes.

Individuals' health is also used as the basis for monitoring national intakes of harmful substances.

The Instruments of Policy

There are a number of instruments or tools that can be used to implement the objectives or targets defined by a nutrition policy. These are mostly rather blunt and indirect in action; governments cannot force people to eat what they do not want to eat, they can only encourage and enable. Despite this, the state has considerable scope for intervention to influence individuals' nutritional wellbeing and there are various ways to do this. These vary in whether they affect the whole population or whether they are targeted at specific population groups who are deemed to be at risk, and in their mode of action. This can be direct: for instance, in setting and monitoring the implementation of standards for institutional meal provision (such as in hospitals, schools, nurseries or care centres for the elderly); or in legislating for welfare food provision for those on low incomes (such as the Women, Infant, Children supplementary feeding programmes in the USA). It can also be indirect, through improving availability and access to foods or the health impact of specific foods: for instance, promoting the construction or maintenance of retail food shops in one site rather than another; the regulation of local taxation and subsidies towards farmers' markets to influence the availability of specific food commodities; and the creation of legislation and enforcement systems to maintain food safety, purity and nutrient content. There has been little assessment of the relative efficacy of these different instruments in achieving nutrition objectives; for instance, whether nutrition education is more effective in altering food purchase and eating patterns than price subsidies.

Nutrient recommendations and dietary guidelines

Nutrient recommendations were originally recommendations for desirable population level intakes of nutrients for different age and sex groups to avoid deficiency disease and optimal growth. These recommendations were converted into food-based dietary guidelines for the purpose of nutrition education (although such population based recommendations cannot be used for individual dietary guidance). More recently, recommendations have also been set to try to address the prevention of chronic disease; initially heart disease and hypertension, followed by obesity, osteoporosis, diabetes and cancer. There has also been a move from nutrient to food-based recommendations, such as the WHO recommendation to consume 400 g of fruit and vegetables a day. The process and outcome of defining nutrient and food recommendations may be a source of controversy.

Food and nutrient recommendations are used for a number of policy-related purposes: these include monitoring and surveillance, the assessment of population food supply adequacy, the setting of toxic intake limits, and food labelling.

Education

The provision of nutrition education is based upon the notion of informed choice and that the provision of information about how to make healthy food choices will influence individual consumer choice and hence dietary intake. This is, perhaps, a questionable assumption as much social science research has shown the complexity of eating behaviour and the numerous factors that influence it.

The content of nutrition education is based on official dietary recommendations and provides advice and encouragement about how to achieve these via dietary guidelines. These may be aimed at the whole population or targeted at groups with special needs, such as pregnant or lactating women and the elderly. Education may be delivered via a number of channels: mass media (via leaflets, television and radio), schools, supermarkets, worksites, health centres, charities and so forth. In addition to state-sponsored nutrition education the retail sector is increasingly also providing dietary advice to customers. Nutrition education is sometimes given to health professionals, although many in practice receive little formal training in nutrition.

Regulatory measures

A number of regulatory measures can be used to implement policy objectives. These include the setting of food compositional standards, codes of practice, specifications for food labelling, the control of health claims on food packaging and in advertising, and planning law to influence the siting of and access to food retail outlets. Food laws are complex and until recently have been set and enforced within national contexts, but with the development of regional market groupings such as the EU, and (following the Uruguay round in 1993) the inclusion of agricultural commodities within GATT, there has been a move to base national food laws on international standards set by the *Codex Alimentarius*.

Supplementation and fortification

Both supplementation and fortification are intended to increase the intakes of specific micronutrients in either the whole population or in particular population groups. Supplementation usually refers to tablets or pills, or occasionally drops, which are consumed by the individual in addition to their usual food intake. Sometimes these are purchased by consumers 'over the counter'; sometimes they are provided by the health sector to targeted groups. In the past the use of supplements was sometimes recommended to correct measured low intakes and prevent deficiency disease, but now they may be used for other purposes, such as the prevention of neural tube defects in children via folate supplements to women. There is also controversy concerning their use; for instance, the potential of antioxidant supplements to prevent chronic diseases such as cancer.

Fortification, on the other hand, is designed to increase intakes of specific nutrients, such as iron, via their addition to specified food vehicles. The vehicle may be a staple food consumed by the whole population, or a food consumed only by certain population groups, such as infant formula. If the fortification is a government instrument, legislation is required to enforce the addition of specified micronutrients to particular food products, and to govern how much is added, at what stage, and how products should be labelled. The only choice consumers have about consuming the extra nutrient is to avoid purchasing the food used as its vehicle. For instance, in the UK the addition of iron and calcium to bread and flour has been mandatory since World War II, as has, more recently, the addition of vitamins A and D to margarine. In 1996, the USA passed the first new fortification order since 1943, which made the addition of folate to various cereal products mandatory in order to increase the folate intakes of women of child-bearing age. However, in many countries foodstuffs are fortified voluntarily by food manufacturers; the presence of the extra nutrients is often used to promote sales.

Fiscal and economic measures

Economic measures tend to be directed towards production, although fiscal measures can also be used to subsidize health-promoting foods and tax those deemed undesirable and so change the availability of these foods to the consumer. Measures such as these were used in Norway. After World War II most fiscal measures in developed countries gave subsidies and tax incentives to the production of animal-based foods, such as meat and the dairy sector.

See also: **Nutrition Policies**: In Developing Countries. **United Nations Children's Fund**: History and Role. **World Health Organization**: Role.

Further Reading

Consumers in Europe Group (1997) *The Common Agricultural Policy, Diet, Nutrition and Health*. Proceedings of a seminar, 26 February 1997. London: Consumers in Europe Group, 20 Grosvenor Gardens, London SW1W 0DH.

Gabriel Y and Lang T (1995) *The Unmanageable Consumer: Contemporary Consumption and Its Fragmentations*. London: Sage Publications.

International Congress on Nutrition (1992) *World Declaration and Plan of Action for Nutrition*. Geneva: FAO/WHO.

James WPT (1993) Policy and a prudent diet. In: Garrow JS and James WPT (eds) *Human Nutrition and Dietetics*, 9th edn. Edinburgh: Churchill Livingstone.

Leatherwood P, Horisberger M and James WPT, eds (1993) *For a Better Nutrition in the 21st Century*. Nestlé Nutrition Services. New York: Raven Press.

Lang T (1997) The public health impact of globalization of food trade. In: Shetty PS and McPherson K (eds) *Diet, Nutrition and Chronic Disease: Lessons from Contrasting Worlds*, Chap. 9. Chichester: John Wiley.

Maurer D and Sobal J, eds (1995) *Eating Agendas: Food and Nutrition as Social Problems*. New York: Aldine de Gruyter.

Milio N (1989) Nutrition and health: patterns and policy perspectives in food-rich countries. *Social Science and Medicine* 29:413–423.

Milio N (1990) *Nutrition Policy for Food-rich Countries*. Baltimore: Johns Hopkins University Press.

National Consumer Council (1992) *Your Food: Whose Choice?* London: NCC.

Pinstrup-Andersen P, ed. (1993) *The Political Economy of Food and Nutrition Policies*. Baltimore: Johns Hopkins University Press, for the International Food Policy Research Institute.

Rome Declaration on World Food Security and World Food Summit Plan of Action. World Food Summit, Rome, 13–17 November 1996. Rome: FAO.

Smith DF, ed. (1997) *Nutrition in Britain: Science, Scientists and Politics in the Twentieth Century*. London: Routledge.

Tansey G and Worsley T (1995) *The Food System: A Guide*. London: Earthscan.

Traill B and Henson S (1996) Consumption implications of agri-food policies. *Proceedings of the Nutrition Society* 55:649–659.

Walt G (1994) *Health Policy: An Introduction to Process and Power*. London: Zed Books.

WHO Nutrition Unit (1995) *Nutrition Policy in WHO European Member States: Progress Report Following the 1992 International Conference on Nutrition*. Copenhagen: WHO.

Wiseman MJ (1990) Government: where does nutrition policy come from? *Proceedings of the Nutrition Society*, 49(3):397–401.

In Developing Countries

C Geissler, Kings College London, UK

What is a Nutrition Policy?

Nutrition is the process whereby living organisms use food for maintenance of life, growth, the normal functioning of organs and tissues, and the production of energy. Human nutrition therefore encompasses food composition, food consumption, food habits, the nutritive value of foods, nutritional requirements, the relationship between diet and health, and research in all these fields. Diet in this context means the total solid and liquid foods consumed by an individual or a population group. Nutrition is therefore at the centre of a web of a number of disciplines, and so policy affecting nutrition involves many government sectors.

In the process of national development planning and policy formulation, various ministries and departments of the government (sectors) prepare development programmes for implementation during a specific plan period. These are implemented through detailed projects for which budgetary allocations are earmarked. Para-statal and private sectors such as the food industry follow a similar course of action for implementing their priority projects. Those aspects of the national policy which are specifically designed to improve the state of nutrition in a country are together defined as 'nutrition policy' or 'food and nutrition policy.'

In developing countries national policies are published for each sector in periodic National Development Plans, usually every 5 years. Nutrition does not constitute a separate sector and so aspects of nutrition policy appear under the policies of specific sectors such as agricultural, food, health, education and social welfare. These aspects are by no means comprehensive and during the stage of implementation are generally not coordinated through any official mechanism.

Policy Differences in Developing Countries

Nutrition policy preparation and implementation in developing countries differs from that in developed countries in two main respects.

1. *The types of nutrition problems addressed*. These are mainly undernutrition labelled as protein–energy malnutrition (PEM) and specific deficiency conditions, most commonly vitamin A, anaemia and goitre. Although the so-called 'diseases of affluence' often affect the richer urban sections of the population, they have not been policy priorities although they have recently become so in some Latin American and other developing countries. However some countries such as China, which are in nutritional transition between the predominance of diseases of poverty and of affluence, have to consider how to reduce remaining nutritional deficiencies but avoid the nutrition-related problems afflicting developed countries.

2. *The influence of external aid agencies*. In many developing countries governments are assisted in the formulation of nutrition policies by agencies such as the World Bank, the United Nations Children's Fund (UNICEF), the World Health Organization (WHO) and the United Nations Food and Agricultural Organization (FAO). Specific projects are often resourced by external funding, technical assistance and food aid.

National Nutrition Policies and Government Structures

Since the 1970s nutrition has been recognized as an important objective of national development and an indicator of such development. In developing countries this objective determines the goals which form the major ingredients of a national nutrition policy. A typical policy would aim to ensure a biologically safe and physically clean food supply sufficient to meet amply people's physiological, social and cultural requirements of variety of foodstuffs at commonly affordable prices. The specific programmes to implement such policies usually include a mixture of analyses of the situation and individual interventions of the types outlined in the following section. Analyses for the purpose of monitoring the nutritional situation and providing public information and recommendations may include: the periodic assessment of consumption patterns and energy and nutrient intakes; the identification of populations at risk of deprivation and excessive or imbalanced food consumption through specific studies and surveys; analysing and composing dietary patterns in terms of food groups and nutrients; defining minimum and desirable standards of the requirement of food energy and nutrients for various age groups and specific groups of the population with special needs.

As nutrition is not a sector *per se*, it usually does not have a direct budget line and in many countries the Ministry of Health is charged with improving the state of nutrition of the people, while aspects of food come under the Ministry of Agriculture. In most developing countries implementation of the nutrition policy is carried out by these Ministries or a Ministry of Planning, through autonomous or semiautonomous Councils, Commissions or Committees, which may or may not be intersectoral in their compositions. The weakness or strength of such bodies can be judged from the change in nutritional status of the people since their establishment.

Examples of government structures

In the Philippines a National Nutrition Council is attached to the Department of Agriculture with regional, provincial, city, municipal and village nutrition committees to ensure coordination at all levels. It has funds to support some sectoral and nonsectoral nutrition projects. The Governing Board consists of 10 members of the Philippines Cabinet, but despite this high-powered board the Council encounters weakness in political commitment.

In contrast in Sri Lanka the Food and Nutrition Planning Division (F&NPPD) of the Ministry of Policy, Planning and Implementation reports directly to the President of Sri Lanka and therefore has the necessary political strength to cut across sectors and override departmental barriers in order to bring about effective coordination for nutrition improvement.

In Pakistan a Nutrition Cell with authority to plan, coordinate and monitor or evaluate nutrition programmes at various levels of administration in the country is sited in the Ministry of Planning and is guided by a Nutrition Syndicate, composed of representatives of various nutrition-related sectors. Nutrition Boards and Units exist in all provinces.

In Thailand the National Food and Nutrition Committee (NFNC) works closely with the Nutrition Division of the Ministry of Public Health, and gets advice on specific subjects from *ad hoc* technical committees appointed from time to time as the need arises. This infrastructure has a distinct advantage of dealing with the food and nutrition problems as and when they arise.

Many of these and other institutions dealing with nutrition policy were established in developing countries in the early 1970s (see below), but some have a longer tradition. In Uganda, for example, a National Food and Nutrition Council was set up in 1964 to advise the Government on all food and nutrition policy strategies and has been revived in the improved political climate since 1986. It is answerable to the Cabinet and is composed of representatives of relevant ministries, institutions and NGOs, with donors involved in food and nutrition activities as observers.

Types of Programmes and Interventions

The types of interventions that form part of national nutrition policies tend to be limited to palliative measures such as vitamin supplementation, nutrition education and child feeding programmes, because many of the underlying factors that lead to malnutrition such as unemployment, low wages, land tenure arrangements, etc. involve fundamental economic and political interests that are much more difficult and contentious to address. The types of interventions that affect nutrition can be divided into general categories summarized in **Table 1.**

Historical Trends

There have been changes in emphasis in the type of programmes advocated over the decades to improve nutrition as knowledge of nutrition has grown and as governments and development agencies have experienced success or failure in various approaches.

During World War II and the postwar period of the 1940s the emphasis in developed countries was on institutional feeding such as school meals, school milk, and the distribution of concentrated vitamin sources to children and mothers. These approaches were continued in developing countries by the international agencies such as the FAO and WHO following their establishment after the war.

Table 1 Types of nutrition programmes

Explicitly nutritional
Programmes directly related to food, including those aiming to improve food availability, accessibility, quality, safety, consumption and knowledge.

1. Nutrition-oriented food policies
   1.1 gricultural production, kitchen gardens, marketing, storage, processing, safety
   1.2 Food price and distribution control: food price subsidies; taxation; food stamps; rationing
2. Feeding programmes
   2.1 Mother and child: nutrition rehabilitation centres; on site, take home
   2.2 Schools: lunch, breakfast, snack, milk
   2.3 Workers: canteens, Food for Work
   2.4 Old age: community centre; Meals on Wheels
3. Weaning foods
   3.1 Formulated, fermented, amylase-rich
4. Fortification, supplementation
   4.1 Iodine, vitamin A, iron, vitamin D, vitamin C, amino acids
5. Nutrition education

Implicitly nutritional
Programmes with indirect nutritional impact through improvement of effective food demand, food utilization and energy balance.

1. Health
   1.1 Primary health care: immunization, antiparasites, rehydration, basic medicines, prenatal care, health education, first aid
   1.2 Sanitation: water supply, water treatment, water storage, waste disposal, drainage and spraying, hygiene education
2. Economic
   2.1 Income generation
   2.2 Income maintenance: welfare benefits, unemployment benefits, child allowances, etc.
   2.3 Income substitution of subsidized basic needs
3. Labour saving
   3.1 Cereal mills, water storage and transport, child care crèches, etc.

Integrated
Combining explicit and implicit nutritional interventions: e.g. 'Applied Nutrition Programmes', 'Community Development Programmes'

As decolonization progressed a growing interest in the process of economic development and nutrition led to the recognition that individual interventions had little impact on malnutrition and that a more integrated approach was needed to improve the use of available resources. From the 1950s the international agencies therefore promoted 'Applied Nutrition Programmes': village-based programmes with components addressing several of the multiple factors of malnutrition such as income generation activities, horticulture, health care and nutrition education.

During the 1960s attention became focused on the world food supply and concern that population could outstrip production. Food and nutrition programmes were centred around the production and dissemination of high-yielding varieties of cereals, wheat, rice and maize – the 'Green Revolution' package. In the same decade the idea developed that a specific 'protein gap' existed between the amount of protein available in national food supplies and population needs. A second focus was therefore on means to increase the production and consumption of protein from a variety of novel sources.

By the 1970s, after 25 years of experience in nutrition interventions within economic development strategies, it was recognized that increased national wealth did not always result in improved welfare and nutrition as predicted by the 'trickle-down' theory of development. Nutrition was therefore proposed as a specific goal for national development, as a better nourished population would achieve more effective development. Government nutrition policy should be integrated and coordinated by a Nutrition Planning Unit in an umbrella organization such as a Ministry of Planning or a Prime Minister's Office so that the underlying causes would be simultaneously addressed by the appropriate government sector. This approach was fostered by development agencies such as FAO and USAID (United States Agency for International Development) and was adopted by several countries such as those cited above, particularly after it was endorsed at the World Food Conference in 1974.

By the 1980s attempts to apply the rational procedures advocated by this National Nutrition Planning approach for the selection of appropriate interventions had demonstrated: the paucity of data on which to decide nutritional priorities and the effectiveness of various interventions; the difficulties of placing a policy priority on nutrition; and the problems of effective intersectoral coordination. This approach was therefore subsequently abandoned. These hurdles, however, led to better evaluation of interventions, and to measurements of the functional impact of malnutrition. In the 1980s the promotion of intersectoral planning gave way to ensuring that existing sectoral interventions such as agricultural development programmes included nutrition considerations. The other main theme was the targeting of nutrition interventions to those most in need and the involvement of local communities in self-sustaining development programmes. This was brought about by the Structural Adjustment Programmes described below.

All of the approaches particularly favoured in different decades remain ongoing in the 1990s, but with various emphases. The main theme of the 1990s is micronutrient intervention, including in particular vitamin A, iron, iodine and more recently folate. There is current research interest in population trials with several micronutrients which may or may not lead to changes in nutrition policy and interventions. For example the importance of vitamin A is being investigated not only for eye lesions and blindness, but also in resistance to respiratory and diarrhoeal infections; antioxidants are being tested for their possible role in protection against cancers, heart disease and other conditions; and zinc and other micronutrients are being explored as a means to address the issue of restricted growth which is widespread in developing countries.

International Context

International promotion

Hunger and malnutrition were put on the international agenda by the League of Nations in the 1930s and the first conference of the United Nations in 1943 was devoted to food and agriculture. It remained an important focus of the UN technical agencies, the FAO, WHO and UNICEF, which were created immediately after World War II. Other international organizations have since been established including the World Food Programme (WPF), World Food Council (WFC), International Fund for Agriculture Development (IFAD) and United Nations Fund for Population Activities (UNFPA). All these organizations and other international supporting bodies have explicit objectives to eradicate human suffering caused by hunger and malnutrition, and to promote wellbeing and sound standards of health for all peoples of the world.

These organizations have played an important role in relation to nutrition policies in developing countries by:

1. providing technical assistance in the formulation and implementation of policies, programmes and activities;
2. providing programme and project funding;
3. collecting and disseminating data, such as the World Food Surveys conducted by FAO every decade since 1946 which have greatly influenced the ideas of nutritionists and development policymakers in estimating the extent and defining the causes of malnutrition, and shaped the technical assistance deemed to be appropriate;
4. organizing fora for debate on topics relevant to food and nutrition policy such as the: World Food Conference, 1974; Alma Ata Conference of Primary Health Care, 1978; World Conference on

Agrarian Reform and Rural Development, 1979; Convention on the Elimination of All Forms of Discrimination Against Women, 1979; Fourth UN Development Decade, 1990; World Summit for Children, 1990; Innocente Declaration on Protection, Promotion and Support of Breastfeeding, 1990; Montreal Policy Conference on Micronutrient Malnutrition, 1991; Rio Declaration on Environment and Development, 1992; and International Conference on Nutrition, 1992. The World Food Summit in November 1996 was set to convene two decades after the influential World Food Conference of 1974 with the objective 'to renew the commitment of the world leaders at the highest level to the eradication of hunger and malnutrition and the achievement of lasting food security for all'.

The main resolutions of some of the recent actions of the international organizations are briefly recorded below. Some are very broad and clearly unachievable, such as the nutrition goals of the Fourth United Nations Development Decade (1990s), which are to:

(a) eliminate starvation and death caused by famine;
(b) reduce malnutrition and mortality among children substantially;
(c) reduce chronic hunger tangibly;
(d) eliminate major nutritional diseases.

Others are more specific, such as those of the World Summit for Children (1990) (to be reached by the year 2000:

(a) reduction in severe, as well as moderate, malnutrition among children under 5 by half of 1990 levels;
(b) reduction in the rate of low birthweight (2.5 kg or less) to less than 10%;
(c) reduction of iron deficiency anaemia in women by 1/3 of the 1990 level;
(d) virtual elimination of iodine deficiency disorders;
(e) virtual elimination of vitamin A deficiency and its consequences, including blindness;
(f) empowerment of all women to breast-feed their children exclusively for 4–6 months and to continue breast-feeding with complementary food, well into the second year;
(g) growth promotion and its regular monitoring to be institutionalized in all countries by the end of 1990;
(h) dissemination of knowledge and supporting services to increase food production to ensure household food security.

At the International Conference on Nutrition (ICN) (1992) governments committed themselves to a Global Plan of Action for Nutrition with the aim of ensuring a safe and nutritionally adequate diet for all people through environmentally sound and socially sustainable development. They agreed to implement national plans before the end of the century with assistance from international funding agencies and bilateral aid. Major policies are to include commitment (social, economic and political) to promoting nutritional wellbeing; growth with equity; participation of NGOs and local communities including families and households; and focus on women and gender equality. Agreed strategies and actions to guide the national plans of action for nutrition included:

1. Incorporating nutritional objectives, considerations and components into development policies and programmes;
2. improving household food security, ensuring access by all people at all times to food needed for a healthy life;
3. protecting consumers through improved food quality and safety ensuring that the food supply must have an appropriate nutrient content, sufficient variety and quality, and must not endanger health of consumers through biological, chemical and other contaminants;
4. preventing and managing infectious disease;
5. promoting breast-feeding of infants;
6. caring for the socioeconomically deprived and nutritionally vulnerable;
7. preventing and controlling specific micronutrient deficiencies;
8. promoting appropriate diets and healthy lifestyles; and
9. assessing, analysing and monitoring nutrition situations.

International constraints

Since the early 1980s many developing countries have experienced severe economic crises and have had to implement a variety of 'structural adjustment policies', enforced by the international finance agencies, the International Monetary Fund (IMF) and the World Bank (IBRD), to reduce government spending and improve balance of payments. Reduced spending has resulted in cutting a variety of welfare programmes that had been effective in controlling malnutrition, such as food price subsidies. Structural adjustment conditions are rigidly imposed by the agencies to obtain new financial loans. These institutions are funded by quotas from members who have voting rights in proportion to their contri-

bution, assessed according to economic status, so that decisions are effectively in the hands of the major industrialized countries, especially the USA. This banking structure means that the policies of borrowing countries are dictated by the richer industrialized nations.

Structural adjustment frequently results in changes of particular concern to the poor, such as increased food prices and decreased expenditure on social programmes. The effects of these policies on health care, food consumption, incomes and prices appear to have led to a serious deterioration in indicators of nutrition, health status and school achievement in several countries, although it is difficult to distinguish policy effects from those of general economic decline. Efforts are now being made by UNICEF and other bodies to buffer vulnerable groups from these effects.

International Trends in Malnutrition

To what extent have nutrition policies in developing countries been effective in reducing malnutrition? Over the 20 years between the World Food Conference in 1974 and the International Nutrition Conference in 1992 there have been considerable changes in the extent of malnutrition. The percentage of underweight children has declined in all parts of the world except in Subsaharan Africa and South America, but the numbers have declined only in China, and have increased markedly in South Asia and Subsaharan Africa. Most data on nutritional status relate to preschool children as these are considered the most vulnerable, but other age groups are certainly not immune to malnutrition.

What Is the Secret of Success?

Although undernutrition is clearly related to poverty, some countries are better nourished than others at similar levels of national wealth. At the same gross national product (GNP) some countries fare much better than others, in terms of indicators of nutrition and health such as food available for consumption and infant mortality. Countries that have done best in improving nutrition in recent years are those where there is greater equity or where policies have concentrated on ensuring the satisfaction of basic needs, including adequate food. Their political ideologies range from communist China to capitalist South Korea and Taiwan. China is the classic example of a country that is still poor but has dominated malnutrition and famine through effective organization of food production and distribution. Other examples are Costa Rica, Chile, Cuba, Kerala state in India, Sri Lanka and Thailand, which have better nutrition conditions than other countries with similar GNPs. In contrast some countries have extensive chronic malnutrition, e.g. Bangladesh, despite massive aid, and Brazil despite rapid economic growth.

These improvements cannot all be ascribed to specific nutrition policies. What are the lessons that can be learned about the effectiveness of the nutrition interventions commonly used to implement nutrition policies? This is not an easy question to answer as the evaluation of effectiveness of specific interventions is theoretically simple, but practically difficult as evaluation has to take into account general economic change. An important function of international development and research agencies such as the World Bank, the International Food Policy Research Institute, FAO, UNICEF and WHO since the 1970s has been to draw together research on the impact of policies and programmes on the economic, health and nutritional status of beneficiaries, to distinguish the characteristics of success. Several features of successful large-scale nutrition interventions in relation to undernutrition have been extracted and can be summarized as follows.

The objectives must be based on a careful analysis of the real problem and be achievable in a timescale set within the programme design. Community involvement in the design and implementation is essential for self-sustaining success. The overall effectiveness depends on coverage and if interventions are targeted at specific groups there has to be a trade-off between the cost-effectiveness of targeting and wider coverage of the population. Good leadership and management are essential and the appropriate mix of components must be accompanied by effective administration. Most successful programmes included strong training and supervision. Effective implementation is helped by monitoring and evaluation of the process, with flexibility to modify the programme where necessary. The attitude of the workers is crucial in determining the potential for scaling up from a pilot project with selected staff to a large-scale operational programme which has to use existing staff. These common characteristics are a useful basis for the planning of future programmes to maximize their success.

Conclusions

A nutrition policy is easy to draw up on paper but is useless unless implemented. Many countries have adopted nutrition policies that were ineffective because they were not or could not be implemented. Some policies could not be implemented even if the political will existed, as they were too complex, such as National Nutrition Planning, or could not be scaled up successfully from pilot projects to operational programmes as they did not have funding for an equivalent level of training and supervision, such as the Applied Nutrition Programmes. Successful implementation depends on many economic and technical factors but most importantly on political will. Success in improving nutrition has been achieved in countries with a wide range of political ideologies but with a common theme of government commitment to promoting equity and to satisfying basic needs. Some types of specific intervention can be successful without such commitment, for example nutrient supplement programmes, but the criteria of success have to be clearly defined in terms of population coverage, sustainability, and to what extent the programme addresses the main nutritional problems.

See also: **Dietary Guidelines**: International Perspectives. **Famine**: Population Responses. **Food Aid**: Overview. **Food Aid Organizations**: History and Role. **Malnutrition**: Definition, Classification and Epidemiology. **Nutrient Requirements**: International Perspectives. **Nutritional Surveillance**: In Industrialized and Developing Countries. **Seasonality**: Nutritional Implications. **Socioeconomic Status**: Relationship with Diet and Nutritional Status. **Urban Nutrition**: Overview.

Acknowledgements

The author wishes to acknowledge the help given by Dr Rahmat U Qureshi, Visiting Senior Research Fellow, Kings College London, formerly Food & Policy Nutrition Officer, FAO Asia & Pacific Region, in providing references and information on food policy and nutrition, and the state of the art in some of the countries of Asia and the Pacific, and also on the impetus given to the developing countries by various international organizations.

Further Reading

ACC/SCN (1991) *Managing Successful Nutrition Programmes*, ACC/SCN State-of-the-Art Series, Nutrition Policy Discussion Paper no 7. Geneva: ACC/SCN.

ACC/SCN (1992) *Second Report on the World Nutrition Situation* (October). Geneva: ACC/SCN.

ACC/SCN (1994) *Update on the Nutrition Situation* (November). Geneva: ACC/SCN.

Berg A (1973) *The Nutrition Factor. Its Role in National Development*. Washington, DC: The Brookings Institution.

Berg A (1987) *Malnutrition. What Can Be Done? Lessons from the World Bank Experience*. Baltimore and London: Johns Hopkins University Press.

Biswas H and Pinstrup-Anderson P (eds) (1985) *Nutrition and Development*. United Nations University. Oxford: Oxford University Press.

FAO (1975) *Food and Nutrition Planning*. Nutrition Consultants Reports Series 35. Rome: FAO.

Geissler C (1993) Stature and other indicators of development: comparisons in Thailand and Philippines, Korea and Iran. In: Geissler C and Oddy DJ (eds) *Food, Diet and Economic Change Past and Present*. Leicester: Leicester University Press.

Geissler C (1995) Nutrition intervention. In: Ulijaszek SJ (ed.) *Health Intervention in Less Developed Countries*. Oxford: Oxford University Press.

Gillespie S and Mason J (1991) *Nutrition-relevant Actions: Some Experiences from the Eighties and Lessons for the Nineties*, UN Administrative Committee on Coordination, Subcommittee on Nutrition (ACC/SCN) State-of-the-Art Series, Nutrition Policy Discussion Paper no 10. Geneva: ACC/SCN.

Gittinger JP, Leslie J and Hoisington C (eds) (1987) *Food Policy: Integrating Supply, Distribution and Consumption*. Baltimore & London: Johns Hopkins University Press.

Gwatkin DR, Wilcox JR and Wray JD (1980) *Can Health and Nutrition Interventions Make a Difference*? Washington DC: Overseas Development Council Monograph 13.

Horwitz A (1987) Comparative public health: Costa Rica, Cuba, and Chile. *UNU Food and Nutrition Bulletin* 9(3):19–29.

International Conference on Nutrition (1992) *World Declaration and Plan of Action for Nutrition*. Rome: FAO/WHO.

Jolly R and Cornia GA (eds) (1984) *The Impact of World Recession on Children*, UNICEF report. New York: Pergamon Press.

NUTRITION LABELLING

European Perspectives

M A Hunt, Food and Drink Federation, London, UK

To exercise choice, modern consumers need to be well informed about the products they buy. Labelling is the usual means of providing this information; it is subject to laws which ensure that it is accurate, truthful, sufficient and not misleading. The principal purpose of food labelling is to provide information to enable consumers to select products according to their needs and to store and prepare them appropriately.

Within the EU there is a general Directive on the labelling, presentation and advertising of foodstuffs (79/112/EEC; as amended). More specific additional requirements on nutrition labelling are provided by the Directive on nutrition labelling for foodstuffs (90/496/EEC).

This article concentrates on the development, role and content of EU nutrition labelling requirements. Current UK practice is outlined, and the main aspects requiring further consideration and adaptation to progress are discussed. Finally some key analytical and enforcement aspects are identified.

Context and Role

The basic requirements of the EU Directive on food labelling (79/112/EEC) are, in general terms, to inform consumers about the nature and content of the product, shelf life and storage conditions, any necessary information about its handling and preparation, the identity of the manufacturer or distributor and the quantity being sold. Other information may be required in specific cases and further, voluntary information may be given. Labelling must not mislead the purchaser 'to a material degree'.

The Nutrition Labelling Directive (90/496/EEC) lays down rules for the provision of nutrition information on a uniform basis throughout the European Community. It concerns certain nutrient components of food and drink products, e.g. protein and fat, and not 'added ingredients'. The use of standard terms, and a standard approach to presenting nutrition information, provides consumers with information on individual products which can be readily compared with that on others. Given nutrition information on a range of products, the consumer can, if desired, select products to produce a balanced diet according to his/her requirements.

The distinction between ingredients and components is an important one. For example, the fat content of a product shown in nutrition labelling may be higher than any figure for oil/fat added if it has also to take account of fat present in other ingredients, such as egg or cocoa powder.

Historical Development

Before the adoption of the Nutrition Labelling Directive (90/496/EEC), the UK Ministry of Agriculture, Fisheries and Food (MAFF) had issued guidelines on voluntary nutrition labelling. These had been widely adopted by the UK industry which was supportive of the principle of introducing an EU Community-wide framework for the voluntary provision of nutrition labelling.

The EU Commission initially put forward, in 1988, two linked proposals, one on compulsory nutrition labelling and the other setting out the nature of that labelling. The compulsory nutrition labelling proposal provided a mechanism whereby the Commission could introduce nutrition labelling of certain nutrients for various foods, if this were deemed necessary in the light of scientific evidence, and after consideration had been given to other means of achieving the same goal. This led to substantial debate on the evidence required and on the regulatory mechanisms by which it was proposed that decisions be made. A significant factor within the UK, seen at the time as pushing the Commission proposal forward, was the UK Government's desire to introduce compulsory fat content labelling and the Commission's claim that the UK's freedom to do so was severely constrained by its Community obligations, notably those arising from the Food Labelling Directive (79/112/EEC).

The mandatory labelling proposal was formally dropped at the end of 1992, by which time the Nutrition Labelling Directive (90/496/EEC) had been adopted. Trade in complying products was permitted by 1 April 1992 and prohibition of trade in products not complying was effective from 1 October 1993.

The Commission's initial proposal for a nutrition labelling format required the declaration of energy and six nutrients, i.e. carbohydrate, protein, fat, sugars, sodium and fibre. It was of concern to interested parties that this proposal went well beyond the guidelines developed by the FAO/WHO Codex Alimentarius Commission which, as endorsed by all member governments of the European Community, acknowledged the appropriateness of providing information on a food's main nutrition profile, deeming this to be energy, protein, carbohydrate and fat.

The requirements of the Nutrition Labelling Directive (90/496/EEC) are implemented in the UK in the Food Labelling Regulations, the most recent being *The Food Labelling Regulations 1996* (SI 1996 no. 1499). The most recent MAFF *Guidance Notes on Nutrition Labelling* were issued in March 1994.

The Basic EU Rules

The following description covers the principal aspects of the Nutrition Labelling Directive (90/496/EEC) and is not a substitute for reference to the Directive itself or to national, implementing legislation. The Directive relates to foodstuffs to be delivered to the ultimate consumer. It does not apply to natural mineral waters or other waters intended for human consumption or to 'diet integrators/food supplements'. It applies without prejudice to the labelling requirements of Council Directive 89/398/EEC, on foodstuffs intended for particular nutritional purposes. This so-called PARNUTS Directive includes some basic labelling rules and provides for the development of specific Directives for identified groups of such foods, e.g. infant formulae and low-energy and energy-reduced foods intended for weight control.

Format

The provision of nutrition information is voluntary unless a nutrition claim is made, but must be given in accordance with one of two standard formats: either Group 1 (known also as the 'Big 4': energy, protein, carbohydrate and fat) or Group 2 (the 'Big 4' plus the 'Little 4': sugars, saturated fats, fibre and sodium). These must be presented in the specified order. Other, identified nutrients may also be added to these basic groups. The units to be used in declaring nutrients are specified. Quantities must be given per 100 g of food or per 100 g and per serving; 'average values' (as defined) may be used; and the information 'must be presented together in one place in tabular form, with the numbers aligned if space permits'. In addition, 'Where space does not permit, the information shall be presented in linear form'.

The amounts declared must usually be those for the food as sold. Where appropriate, however, the information may relate to the food after preparation for consumption, provided that sufficiently detailed preparation instructions are given. Some manufacturers give the information per 100 g or per 100 ml as sold and, where relevant, per serving after preparation. Examples of the latter are a fruit cordial, on the basis of a 250 ml serving diluted one part concentrate to four parts water; and a breakfast cereal, on the basis of a 40 g serving with 125 ml of semi-skimmed milk.

A resulting format of the sort most usually found on UK prepackaged products, covering Group 2, is shown in **Table 1**. The extent to which nutrition information is given, and to which the tabular format is adopted, varies considerably across the EU Member States. It is estimated that the UK currently leads the EU, approximately 80% of prepacked foodstuffs carrying nutrition labelling.

The option to make either a Group 1 or a Group 2 declaration is useful in that it recognizes the basic importance of Group 1; the potentially inverse relationship between quantity and intelligibility of information; and that some of the 'Little 4' nutrients might not be present in some products, or be present only in trace amounts. For the first 5 years after the adoption of the Directive, declaration in nutrition labelling of one of the 'Little 4', whether or not triggered by a claim, did not carry the obligation to make a Group 2 declaration. After 6 October 1995, however, it did. Views differ as to whether or not this development was in the best interests of consumer information. On the one hand, it ensures adherence to standard formats in terms of the nutrients listed. On the other hand, it may occupy label space with 'trace' and zero declarations which can only be avoided to the detriment of not giving information on those of the 'Little 4' nutrients which are present in significant amounts.

Nutrients

The definition of nutrition labelling, given in **Table 2** (Articles 1.4(a) and 4.3), identifies the nutrients which may be included in nutrition labelling, apparently excluding all others. The vitamins and minerals which may be declared, and their recommended daily allowances (RDAs), are given in the Annex to the Directive, which is shown in **Table 3**. Vitamins and minerals may only be listed if present in 'significant amounts', as defined in the Annex in terms of 15% of the RDA.

Table 1 Example of Group 2 declaration: nutrition information for canned baked beans in tomato sauce

Typical values	Amount per 100 g	Amount per serving (210 g)
Energy	232 kJ/56 kcal	487 kJ/118 kcal
Protein	4.7 g	9.9 g
Carbohydrate	8.6 g	18.1 g
(of which sugars)	(0.7 g)	(1.5 g)
Fat	0.2 g	0.4 g
(of which saturates)	(Trace)	(0.1 g)
Fibre	3.7 g	7.8 g
Sodium	0.3 g	0.6 g

Table 2 Nutrients identified in Articles 1.4(a) and 4.3 of the EU Nutrition Labelling Directive

Article 1

4. For the purposes of this Directive:
(a) 'nutrition labelling' means any information appearing on labelling and relating to:
(i) energy value;
(ii) the following nutrients:
- protein
- carbohydrate
- fat
- fibre
- sodium
- vitamins and minerals listed in the Annex and present in significant amounts as defined in that Annex.

Article 4

3. Nutrition labelling may also include the amounts of one or more of the following:
- starch
- polyols
- monounsaturates
- polyunsaturates
- cholesterol
- any of the minerals or vitamins listed in the Annex and present in significant amounts as defined in that Annex.

Table 3 Annex from EU Nutrition Labelling Directive: vitamins and minerals which may be declared and their recommended daily allowances (RDAs)

Vitamin/mineral	RDA	Vitamin/mineral	RDA
Vitamin A	800 µg	Vitamin B_{12}	1 µg
Vitamin D	5 µg	Biotin	0.15 mg
Vitamin E	10 mg	Pantothenic acid	6 mg
Vitamin C	60 mg	Calcium	800 mg
Thiamin	1.4 mg	Phosphorus	800 mg
Riboflavin	1.6 mg	Iron	14 mg
Niacin	18 mg	Magnesium	300 mg
Vitamin B_6	2 mg	Zinc	15 mg
Folacin	200 µg	Iodine	150 µg

As a rule, 15% of the recommended allowance specified in this Annex supplied by 100 g or 100 ml or per package if the package contains only a single portion should be taken into consideration in deciding what constitutes a significant amount.

Nutrition claims

A 'nutrition claim' is defined in the Directive as 'any representation and any advertising message which states, suggests or implies that a foodstuff has particular nutrition properties due to the energy (calorific value) it provides, at a reduced or increased rate or does not provide; and/or due to the nutrients it contains, in reduced or increased proportions or does not contain'. The only nutrition claims permitted are those relating to energy, to the nutrients listed in Article 1.4(a)(ii) and to substances which belong to, or which are components of, a category of those nutrients. If a claim is made for any such component, it must be quantified in the nutrition labelling.

Review date

The Directive requires that, by October 1998, the Commission shall submit to the European Parliament and to Council a report on the application of the Directive. At the same time, it shall submit to the Council any appropriate proposals for amendments. Since several of the provisions of the Directive are appropriate for review, principally to keep pace with technological developments, these are dealt with in this context in the following section.

Technical Adaptation to Progress

The Nutrition Labelling Directive (90/496/EEC) already provides the possibility for a number of amendments by means of a procedure of the Commission-chaired EU Standing Committee on Foodstuffs. Amendments may include changes to the given energy conversion factors and to the list of vitamins and minerals and the RDAs. The list of substances and energy conversion factors may be extended to enable more precise calculation of energy values. By the same procedure, it may be decided in, specific cases, whether or not a statement is a nutrition claim. It may also be decided to restrict or prohibit certain nutrition claims. Formats may be determined for the additional, graphical presentation of nutrition information. Rules may be established regarding the differences between 'average' values and those determined by 'official checks'. Rules may be adopted on the extent of information to be required with non-prepacked foods or food packed for immediate sale. So far as the writer is aware, none of these options has so far been officially pursued, other than Commission proposals to regulate claims (see below). The October 1998 review of the Nutrition Labelling Directive (90/496/EEC) provides a stimulus to decide on priorities for change.

The priorities for revision of the Nutrition Labelling Directive (90/496/EEC) have occupied discussion in both UK and EU fora and views vary substantially between EU Member States. These reflect in some measure the extent to which nutrition labelling is applied and the manner in which the Directive has been implemented into national legislation. The UK industry regards the Nutrition Labelling Directive as a generally useful piece of legislation which does not require fundamental change but to which a number of amendments are needed. Simplification

and flexibility in the operation of the Directive are sought, while ensuring consistency, and updating is needed to take account of technological developments.

Definitions and energy conversion factors

The energy conversion factors currently provided in the Directive are shown in **Table 4**. Technological developments have led to the increasing use of 'new', low-energy substances such as polydextrose and inulin. These fall within the current definition of 'carbohydrate', which requires review as this is not entirely appropriate for such lower-energy substances which are only partially metabolizable.

Similarly, the current definition of fats applies to all such substances, whether or not they are metabolizable. Pressure to reduce fat intakes for health reasons seems likely to encourage the use of fat replacers for which energy conversion factors much less than 37 kJ g^{-1} (9 kcal g^{-1}) would be appropriate. The conventional factor for fats is itself a compromise, since factors will vary around this value according to the pattern of component fatty acids.

Thus the relevant definitions need to be reviewed and provision needs to be made for the application of a wider range of energy conversion factors. If this is not addressed, non- or partially metabolizable substances, used in the interest of producing lower-energy foods, will attract an inappropriately high energy conversion factor, giving a misleadingly inaccurate result. As a proliferation of additional energy conversion factors would be impracticable, and not necessarily relevant to more than one substance, the industry has proposed that, in the case of any 'new' substance, the conversion factor recommended by the manufacturer of that substance should be adopted. The manufacturer would be responsible for substantiating this value.

A key, outstanding problem is that of the definition of 'fibre'; the Directive states that this will be defined and be measured by a method of analysis to be determined in accordance with an EU Commission Standing Committee procedure. The EU

Table 4 Energy conversion factors

Substance	Energy conversion factor	
	(kcal g⁻¹)	(kJ g⁻¹)
Carbohydrate (except polyols)	4	17
Polyols	2.4	10
Protein	4	17
Fat	9	37
Alcohol (ethanol)	7	29
Organic acid	3	13

Scientific Committee for Food reviewed dietary fibre in 1994/95 but did not make recommendations. This needs to be resolved and is addressed further below.

Admissible nutrients

The restrictive lists of nutrients do not allow for information to be given, in standard nutrition labelling, on all components of these nutrients. For example, clarification is needed in respect of some components of fats, such as stearic acid and *trans* fatty acids, which have attracted considerable consumer interest as a result of research findings. By contrast with the restrictions on nutrition labelling, it is permissible to make claims about any components of a listed nutrient, in which case nutrition information must then be given. Some manufacturers wish to provide such information without necessarily making a claim, however, and need the flexibility to respond to consumer interests and specific information requirements, which may be only transient.

Basis of declaration

Consumer research has shown a preference for information to be given per serving. Accordingly, many manufacturers would prefer provision of information per 100 g or per 100 ml to be optional and to offer nutrition information per serving instead of, rather than in addition to, the per 100 g or per 100 ml information that is currently required. Label space does not always permit both and the consumer may have difficulty in calculating the nutrition information for the amount of the product actually consumed. Unless there were generally agreed serving sizes, however, this approach may not necessarily assist consumers in comparing the nutrient value of alternative products.

Vitamin and mineral declaration

It is currently required to declare vitamins and minerals in terms of both the RDA and quantity present. Where both per 100 g or per 100 ml, and per serving declarations are made, four columns of figures are thus required. Some argue that the mg and μg units for micronutrients are of little relevance to consumers and that only the declaration of the percentage RDA amount, which is more readily understandable, should be mandatory, and be given either per serving or per 100 g or 100 ml. For enforcement purposes, the authorities can readily convert percentage RDA to weight amounts for comparison with any analytical measurements.

The '15% rule' stated at the foot of the table of vitamins and minerals (Table 3) also merits review as the current drafting relates the information provided not only to the product, but also to the size of pack in which it is sold. For example, a beverage sold in a 330 ml, single serving, may contain 15% of the RDA for vitamin C, which may thus be declared in nutrition labelling. If the footnote in the Annex is interpreted strictly, however, this would not apply if the same beverage were sold in a 1 litre bottle and did not contain 15% of the RDA per 100 ml. Similarly, calcium could not be declared for whole milk unless the milk were sold in a single serving. A possible alternative wording would be: '15% of the RDA specified in the Annex supplied by 100 g or 100 ml or per serving should be taken into consideration in deciding what constitutes a significant amount'.

The exclusive list of vitamins and minerals is restrictive in preventing declaration of other vitamins and minerals in which interest has arisen more recently, for example minerals such as selenium, chromium and molybdenum. Whilst recognizing that consistent terminology assists comprehension, it might also be argued that the use of synonyms for vitamins and minerals, rather than their biochemical name, would be more easily understandable, e.g. folic acid rather than folacin, vitamin B_1 instead of thiamin and vitamin C rather than ascorbic acid.

The EU Standing Committee on Foodstuffs has agreed in principle to adopt recommendations on revised vitamin and mineral RDAs (termed Labelling Reference Values – LRV) made by the Scientific Committee for Food in December 1992. This would create significant differences between the hitherto essentially identical EU RDAs and Codex Nutrient Reference Values (NRV), suggesting a need to review the latter in the light of more recent scientific opinion. The three sets of values are compared in **Table 5**.

Alternative presentations

The Directive provides that, in accordance with a specified procedure, 'it may be decided that the required nutrition information may also be given in graphical form according to formats to be determined'. This is taken to mean a system to enhance the comprehensibility of the standard, numerical information. The issue has been reviewed by the UK Food Advisory Committee and consumer research has been carried out by independent bodies. Here again, views differ substantially between the governments and interested parties of the EU Member States as to whether or not, and how, graphical labelling should be addressed. Any agreement must be EU-wide but, so far, no formal proposals have arisen.

UK manufacturers and retailers are exploring possibilities for highlighting specific nutrition information, within the nutrition labelling, notably energy

Table 5 Vitamin and mineral reference values for labelling

Nutrient	Unit	EU RDA	Codex NRV	SCF-proposed EU LRV
Vitamin A	μg	800	800	500
Vitamin D	μg	5	5	5
Vitamin E	mg	10	–	–
Vitamin C	mg	60	60	30
Thiamin	mg	1.4	1.4	0.8
Riboflavin	mg	1.6	1.6	1.3
Niacin	mg	18	18	15 (niacin equivalents)
Vitamin B_6	mg	2	2	1.3
Folacin	μg	200	200 (folic acid)	140 (folate)
Vitamin B_{12}	μg	1	1	1
Biotin	mg	0.15	–	–
Pantothenic acid	mg	6	–	–
Calcium	mg	800	800	550
Phosphorus	mg	800	–	–
Iron	mg	14	14	7 for men 14 for women
Magnesium	mg	300	300	–
Zinc	mg	15	15	7.5
Iodine	μg	150	150	100
Copper	mg	Value to be established	–	0.8
Selenium	μg	Value to be established	–	40

RDA, Recommended Daily Allowance; NRV, Nutrient Reference Value; SCF, Standing Committee on Foodstuffs (EU); LRV, Labelling Reference Value.

and fat, in line with the previous administration's Health of the Nation recommendations. Such presentation appears, strictly, not to be permitted under the Directive but is believed by both manufacturers and retailers to be helpful to the consumer. The UK industry would support a revision of the Directive to allow such additional presentation. Any graphical representation should be quantitative rather than qualitative, encouraging consumers to make an informed choice about the nutrition content of the foods they purchase.

It may be useful to determine whether or not the development of EU-agreed 'symbols' to denote both macro- and micro-nutrients would be an effective means of communicating information to the consumer. Manufacturers of products sold in small packs may be deterred from providing nutrition information because of lack of space, particularly if the information is multilingual. The adoption of commonly agreed symbols would require only one nutrition panel on multilingual packs, and save considerable space. Some also argue that, where words are used, it should suffice for the nutrition panel to appear in one language only, given that the words used for the nutrients are reasonably understandable in the languages of the various EU Member States and the order in which the nutrients appear is well established and familiar to consumers who use the information.

Voluntary or mandatory?

Views differ as to whether nutrition labelling should remain voluntary or become mandatory for all, or most, products. A number of factors need to be taken into account. Consumer research indicates particular interest in energy and fat. Nutrition labelling is arguably less relevant for some products than for others. There is a limit to the amount of information that can be sensibly included on some food labels, particularly if they are multilingual. All numerical data on labels attract a cost, owing to the need to establish and monitor the values declared. An estimated 80% of UK-produced, pre-packed foods now carry nutrition labelling. Increasing consumer interest indicates that attention should be given to means of providing equivalent information on non-prepacked products.

Nutrition Claims

Various attempts at developing an EU Directive on claims, including nutrition claims, have failed. The Codex Alimentarius Commission is developing Guidelines. In the UK, nonmandatory recommendations have been developed by the Food Advisory Committee, seeking to clarify the meaning of high/low (absolute) and reduced/increased (comparative) claims in respect of certain nutrients. The UK industry is generally supportive of guidance on the level of change implied by comparative claims, in order to facilitate consumer understanding, and discussions continue between interested parties. Given the overriding requirement that labelling must not be misleading, it might be argued that guidance on the meaning of relative claims is all that is needed, since a nutrition claim triggers nutrition labelling which will give a value for the absolute level of the relevant nutrient in the product.

Non-Prepackaged Foods and Catering Establishments

The Directive provides that the nutrition information to be given with non-prepacked food, and food packed at point of sale at the request of the purchaser, may be determined by each Member State until Community measures are adopted. There are currently no proposals to this end. The UK Food Labelling Regulations require that foods sold loose (non-prepacked) need not be accompanied by full nutrition labelling if a claim is made. Information must be given, however, about the subject of the claim. For example, a 'low-fat paté' sold loose from a delicatessen counter must give the amount of fat per 100 g on the display label. Other information may be given voluntarily for energy or any of the nutrients listed in the Regulations. Food which is not prepacked and which is sold at a catering establishment does not have to carry any nutrition labelling even if a claim is made. Again, however, information may be given voluntarily. It is anticipated that growing public interest in diet and health may lead to an increasing voluntary provision of information by catering and other retail outlets.

Consumer Understanding

Consumer understanding of nutrition labelling is developing slowly. It is broadly accepted that consumers who do read the label for nutrition information focus on energy and to a lesser extent on fat. Moreover, many consumers may not have a reasonable idea of how much energy (kcal/kJ) they need per day and may have little or no idea of what guideline targets mean with respect to fat. In any revision of the Directive, it would appear prudent to alter the familiar format as little as possible, in order to minimize confusion. The forthcoming review of the Nutrition Labelling Directive (90/496/EEC) could be used to simplify the provision of nutrition information and introduce more flexibility to allow manufacturers to provide information in a consumer-friendly way. It must be remembered, however, that the nutrition label itself cannot perform a complete educational function and the information provided on-pack must be supported by other materials to assist consumer understanding. The Directive appropriately states: 'Whereas the provision of nutrition labelling should assist action in the area of nutrition education for the public.' National governments have a significant role to play in providing and encouraging consumer education against the consistent background of harmonized EU nutrition labelling requirements. The UK industry is committed to specific activities to increase consumer awareness of the importance of increased physical activity and healthy eating in the avoidance of obesity.

Analytical and Enforcement Aspects

Sources and precision of data

Sources The Directive provides that 'the declared values shall, according to the individual case, be average values based on:

(a) the manufacturer's analysis of the food;
(b) a calculation from the known or actual average values of the ingredients used;
(c) a calculation from generally established and accepted data.'

Average/typical values Given the inherent variability of food raw materials and the heterogeneous nature of many products, the concept of 'average value' is important. It is defined as 'the value which best represents the amount of the nutrient which a given food contains, and reflects allowances for seasonal variability, patterns of consumption and other factors which may cause the actual value to vary'. The term 'typical value' is taken in the UK more accurately to fit this definition and is accepted for the purposes of nutrition labelling (see Table 1).

Tolerances Enforcement analysis must take account of the typical nature of the declarations which, in practice, means the acceptance of realistic tolerances. The following are a number of factors which may contribute to the uncertainty of declared quantities and of which account needs to be taken. Individual circumstances will determine the weighting to be given to each factor.

- Raw materials: composition influenced by geography, season, breed, variety, preparation.

- Process effects, e.g. attributable to heating, mixing, metering.
- Ingredient interactions.
- Product heterogeneity, e.g. multicomponent products, complete meals.
- Storage/distribution, e.g. constituent migration or degradation, separation, desiccation.
- Sampling error.
- Analytical error.

Bearing in mind that nutrition labelling concerns components of foodstuffs and not ingredients, in-factory enforcement cannot be practised as it can with the checking of recipes, at point of production or by checking inputs over a number of batches. Companies must be prepared, therefore, to justify the values which they select for nutrition declarations. A company's diligence will clearly be better demonstrated if analytical determinations over a period of time indicate that the values declared are a fair average of the results obtained.

Rounding Relevant to the accuracy of nutrition data, and to consumer understanding, is the concept of the rounding of declared values. This would both simplify presentation and avoid a misleading impression of precision.

There is no EU standard for the rounding of nutrition data. Companies may employ their own criteria. As an example, an industry/enforcement agreement in Switzerland has given rise to the following guidelines in respect of the rounding of levels for energy values, protein, fat and carbohydrate:

Less than 0.3%	= 0
From 0.3% to 0.5%	= 0.5
From 0.5% to 5.0%	= Rounded up or down to the nearest half unit
Greater than 5%	= Rounded up or down to the nearest unit.

Definitions

Agreement on definitions of nutrients and methods of analysis for their determination is a key aspect of both harmonized labelling and uniform enforcement practice.

Dietary fibre is an important case in point. In the absence of a recommendation from the EU Scientific Committee for Food, following its 1994/95 review of dietary fibre, EU-wide agreement is needed on a definition and method of analysis for 'fibre'. The UK and Irish approach has been to determine fibre by the Englyst method, which measures non-starch polysaccharides (NSP). The rest of Europe determines fibre by the method adopted by the Association of Official Analytical Chemists (AOAC) of the USA, which measures resistant starch and lignin as well as NSP. In the absence of official progress, the Confederation of Food and Drink Industries of the EU has elaborated a definition and recommended the AOAC method of analysis, supplemented as necessary by other methods to detect 'new' substances, such as polydextrose (see above), which exert a physiological effect similar to NSP fibre. The issue highlights an important consideration in respect of a number of nutrients in that their effective presence in a foodstuff is related not only to quantity, but also to physiological activity.

Further examples are clarification of the definitions of vitamins A and C, i.e. whether or not the former includes carotene and the latter includes dehydroascorbic acid.

Conclusions

Voluntary nutrition labelling, as defined by the EU Nutrition Labelling Directive, is gaining increasing application in EU Member States, accompanied by a gradual increase in consumer understanding of the information given. Experience and technological progress are showing the need for some adaptations to the Directive and several groups are considering how the presentation of nutrition information can be improved. The formal review date for the Directive, of October 1998, provides a focus for these considerations and, in the meantime, various views on needs and priorities are being debated within and between interested parties. The overall objectives are adequate flexibility, to take account of technological developments and changing consumer information requirements, while ensuring a consistent approach to nutrition labelling, and its enforcement, across the EU.

See Colour Plate 1.

See also: **Catering**: Nutritional Aspects. **Dietary Fibre (Fiber)**: Physiological Effects and Effects on Absorption. **Energy**: Energy Balance. **Food Composition Data**: Compilation, Uses and Limitations. **Nutrient Requirements**: International Perspectives.

Further Reading

Department of Health (1996) *Guidelines on Educational Materials Concerned with Nutrition*. London: HMSO.
European Communities (1990) Council Directive of 24 September 1990 on nutrition labelling for foodstuffs

(90/496/EEC). *Official Journal of the European Communities* no. L276/40–44, 6 October 1990.

Food Advisory Committee (1989) Food Advisory Committee Report and Recommendations for Controls on Certain Nutrition Claims. In: *Food Advisory Committee Report on its Review of Food Labelling and Advertising* (1990). London: HMSO.

Food and Agriculture Organization (FAO) (1992) Codex general guidelines on claims. In: *Codex Alimentarius* 2nd edn, vol. 1. Rome: FAO.

Food and Agriculture Organization (FAO) (1993) Codex guidelines on nutrition labelling. In: *Codex Alimentarius*, vol. 1, supplement 1. Rome: FAO.

Food Labelling Regulations (1996) *Statutory Instrument 1996* no. 1499. London: HMSO.

Holland B, Welch AA, Unwin ID, Buss DH, Paul AA and Southgate DAT (1991) *McCance and Widdowson's The Composition of Foods*, 5th edn. London: Royal Society of Chemistry/Ministry of Agriculture Fisheries and Food.

Institute of Grocery Distribution (1998) *Nutrition Labelling Guidelines to Benefit the Consumer*. Watford (UK): I.G.D.

Ministry of Agriculture, Fisheries and Food (MAFF) (1994) *MAFF Guidance Notes on Nutrition Labelling*. London: MAFF.

Richardson DP (1993) The role of the food industry in developing and communicating better nutrition, for a better nutrition in the 21st century. In: Leathwood P, Horisberger M and James WPT (eds) *Nestlé Nutrition Workshop Series*, vol. 27. New York: Nestec Ltd, Vevey/Raven Press.

Richardson DP and Brady MC (1997) The UK food and drink manufacturing industry: a strategy for health. *British Food Journal* 99(6):220–232.

Royal Society of Chemistry (1992) *Food Labelling Data for Manufacturers*. Cambridge: Royal Society of Chemistry.

Scientific Committee for Food (1993) *Nutrient and Energy Intakes for the European Community*, Reports of the Scientific Committee for Food, 31st series. Luxembourg: Office for Official Publications of the European Communities.

Wood JG and Insall LM (1997) Regulatory aspects of new technologies. *Proceedings of the Nutrition Society* 56, 865–877.

NUTRITIONAL STATUS

Contents
Dietary Assessment
Anthropometric Assessment
Biochemical Assessment
Clinical Examination

Dietary Assessment

Johanna T Dwyer, Tufts University School of Medicine and Nutrition, Boston, Massachusetts, USA

Dietary assessment is the process of evaluating what people eat. Specifically, it is the measurement of indicators of dietary status, which is one of several methods used to identify the possible occurrence, nature and extent of poor diet or impaired nutritional status. The reasons why dietary information is of interest vary from one investigator to another, but usually they include dietary assessment or dietary planning. The goals of dietary assessment range from simple descriptions of the intakes of different foods or food groups, to descriptions of intakes of individual dietary constituents in foods.

Usually the intake is compared against some standard that represents good nutritional health.

This article briefly reviews how dietary intake reports and food composition data can be manipulated to provide estimates of nutrient intakes. It discusses various 'gold standards' that are utilized as recommended nutrient intakes, and how these are constructed. Differences in standards and recommendations in various countries are briefly reviewed. Next, a process based on the probability approach for evaluating the nutrient intakes of individuals and populations is outlined.

General Problems in Dietary Assessment and Planning

Many problems arise in the assessment of intakes of individuals and groups. Dietary assessment tools are still crude, and human memory is fallible, so it is difficult to obtain adequate reports of what was eaten. These problems have been discussed at length elsewhere, and are only briefly summarized here.

A second set of problems involves the choice of the standards or reference values that are chosen. The values themselves vary; estimated average requirements even for the same nutrients vary from one country to another. Also, the ways in which the recommendations are stated may vary.

Discussion here is limited to recommended nutrient intake values for individuals and groups, using as an example recent standards jointly developed by the USA and Canada. The users of such standards are primarily health professionals and government or private sector decision-makers. However, recommendations for nutrient intakes can also be stated as dietary guidelines or eating plans that specify particular foods, food groups, or eating patterns. Such recommendations are more useful for laypersons in daily life.

Another group of problems involves gaps in nutrient databases. Often the chemical analytical data on foods are sparse or unrepresentative. For some nutrients in foods, only limited data may be available. Bioavailability of some nutrients also varies depending on the food source, for example for calcium, iron, zinc and folic acid. The presence or absence of inhibitors or enhancers of absorption in the digesta in the gut may further influence the net utilizable amount of nutrient that is finally absorbed. Nutrient content is often highly variable; it is best for macronutrients, and fluctuates most widely for micronutrients, especially vitamins and other substances such as dietary fibre. For many of the phytochemical and zoochemical substances thought to have beneficial effects on health that are present in foods, very few data have been compiled.

There is also the problem of nutrient availability. For usual mixed US diets, the work of Atwater and others at the beginning of the twentieth century describing net utilizable energy from protein, fat, carbohydrate and alcohol remains useful. The so-called 'Atwater factors' to correct for digestibility are already incorporated into the values that are published in food tables. However, the factors do not apply to new food ingredients, such as fats and sugars that are deliberately formulated to be poorly digestible or to provide less food energy. The problem of assessing nutrient availability is even more difficult for other nutrients than it is for food energy. This is particularly the case for the mineral elements. The composition of the digesta will largely determine the nutrient–nutrient interactions which take place and ultimately the nutrient availability. Nutrient

availability also varies between food forms of vitamins and minerals and supplements, and between organic and non-organic sources of nutrients in either vehicle. There is no general rule that applies to all situations. For example, food folates are less well absorbed than supplementary sources of folicacid, and haem iron is better absorbed than non-haem iron.

Obtaining Reports of Dietary Intake

The many different methods for obtaining information on dietary intake are described in detail elsewhere. For dietary assessment purposes, the intake must be representative of usual intakes, and must provide at least some information on levels of intake of the various nutrients. The user must keep the goals of the study and the strengths and weaknesses of each method of obtaining dietary information in mind in choosing the appropriate method for obtaining dietary reports.

The major methods for obtaining dietary information and examples of instruments available have been summarized in several recent monographs on the subject.

Retrospective methods

Retrospective methods focus on recall of intakes during some reference time period, usually in the recent past. All rely heavily on the respondent's motivation and on their ability to recall what they have eaten or their usual dietary patterns. In general, recall is best for most recent intakes, but sex, age, cognitive ability, health, weight status, the stability of the respondent's diet over time, and the complexity of the diet also influence validity of the report. The retrospective methods include the 24-hour recall, food frequency recalls, semiquantitative food frequency questionnaires and dietary histories.

Twenty-four-hour recalls   These can be obtained on a single occasion or multiple occasions. They have the advantage of providing the respondent with the opportunity to describe all of the foods, beverages, and nutrient supplements which have been consumed over the past 24 h, without suggesting responses. They provide information on intakes of all nutrients rather than only a few nutrients. A single recall cannot be used to describe habitual dietary intakes of individuals because in most Western populations food intakes vary considerably from day to day. Therefore an individual who reports a low intake on a single day may not have habitual intakes that are low, and quantitative estimates of usual intakes from a single 24-hour recall are highly suspect for describing an individual's diet. Single 24-hour recalls should not be used in surveys of groups to report the number of individuals below some cutoff point for dietary adequacy because they will overestimate those whose intakes are truly low compared with data that better reflect typical or usual intakes. A greater number of observations on a single individual gives a better estimate of usual diet. With several random 24-hour recalls, accuracy improves, and such multiple estimates can be used to provide information on usual levels of dietary intakes of individuals. However, underreporting is common; usually at least 20% for energy and most other nutrients, and the resulting data must be assessed keeping this in mind. The major disadvantage of 24-hour recalls is that they require time – at least 20–30 min, and a skilled interviewer; additional time is needed for coding the dietary information once it is obtained. Thus costs are high. Another major disadvantage of 24-hour recalls is that the completeness of the report depends not only on the respondent but on the skill of the interviewer in probing. Also, until recently computerized methods for obtaining 24-hour recalls in a standardized fashion were not available.

Food frequency questionnaires Food frequency questionnaires are useful for obtaining information on one or a few nutrients that are high in particular foods or for nutrients that are provided by only a limited number of foods in the diet. The food list that is employed usually consists of commonly eaten foods that are good sources of the nutrient or nutrients of interest. The respondent is prompted by the food list to recall whether he has eaten the food over the time period in question and if so how often. Special lists of foods high in particular food constituents such as dietary fibre or lactose can also be constructed to obtain information on these dietary constituents. Food frequency questionnaires are more straightforward and rely less on the skill of the interviewer than do 24-hour recalls, and some versions can be self-administered. The major disadvantage of food frequency questionnaires is that precise quantitative estimates of levels of nutrient intake are not usually provided, although the information may permit classification of individuals into tertiles or quartiles with respect to consumption.

A recent innovation is the semiquantitative food frequency questionnaire, which consists of a more extensive food list, often of 100 or more foods which are the major sources of the nutrients of interest in usual diets in the population group of interest. In the USA, several instruments are available which have been calibrated to data obtained from population-based surveys. Information on portion size and frequency of consumption are also queried so that rough quantitative estimates of nutrient intakes can be obtained. The questionnaires are usually self-administered and are frequently used in large studies when 24-hour recalls or other methods are not feasible and the purpose is to rank individual intakes rather than to describe absolute levels of nutrient intakes. They are inexpensive to use and computerized analysis programs are available. The disadvantages of semiquantitative food frequency questionnaires are that the food lists must be developed on the populations for which they are used for the resulting nutrient estimates to be accurate. Most food lists contain groups of foods, and the nutrient values used for these food groups are based on weighted averages or medians in the population that was used for constructing the list. If the target group being surveyed has different food consumption habits from these groups, the estimates will be inaccurate. Another disadvantage is that statistical adjustments are used to deflate intake reports since the tendency is to overreport aggregate intakes. The statistical adjustments to bring energy intakes into line may not reflect true energy intakes.

Dietary histories The dietary history involves an interview on usual diet conducted by a trained interviewer, usually a nutritionist, who queries the individual on his or her usual diet. The advantages are that it is less directive than list-based methods and that it gives a fuller picture of usual intake than does a 24-hour recall. However, the interview is time-consuming, usually close to an hour, and the results are difficult to code and process. For these reason it is not frequently used.

Prospective methods

The prospective dietary assessment methods focus on obtaining food records at the time the food is eaten or shortly thereafter.

Food records or diaries This technique involves providing the respondent with food diaries or records that they are to fill out as they eat. Most individuals are not accustomed to keeping detailed records of what they eat, and so in order to obtain satisfactory records they must be instructed on weighing or measuring methods and alerted to collect details on methods of food preparation, brand names and cooking techniques. The advantage of food records is that if they are collected to provide representative samples of usual intakes they can provide highly precise estimates of nutrient intakes that may be needed for research purposes. Weighed records are probably the most accurate, but it is difficult to obtain cooperation of respondents who are unfamiliar with weighing and measuring their foods to provide the information. A compromise to increase response rates is to use household measures, but this introduces errors since such measurements tend to be less precise than weighed records. A disadvantage of food records and diaries is that some respondents unconsciously adjust their food choices to simplify the process of weighing or measuring, and thus usual intakes may not be obtained. Also, respondent burden is considerable, and inevitably the records are incomplete or difficult to interpret for some foods, necessitating probing by a trained observer with a good knowledge of food composition and food habits. Once the food records are obtained, they must be coded and entered into a nutrient database for subsequent analysis and calculations of nutrient intakes must be obtained. This process is greatly facilitated by computerized nutrient analysis programs, but it is still time-consuming and expensive.

Collection of duplicate portions or observations of foods consumed In metabolic research very precise measures of food intake are often needed. If respondents are willing to live on a metabolic ward or under other controlled conditions where all food and drink can be provided and food consumption can be monitored, very accurate estimates of food consumption can be obtained. In the metabolic ward or in the field, if observers are permitted to observe respondents at all eating occasions and to collect duplicate portions of all food that is consumed, food composites can be analysed directly and the nutrient content can be determined chemically. These methods are very precise but also very costly, and they are not usually amenable to long-term studies. Also, the very presence of an observer or the artificial situation of the metabolic ward makes it unlikely that usual habitual food intakes similar to those that the eaters might consume in a free-living situation will be obtained.

Shortcomings of Dietary Assessment Methods

None of the dietary assessment methods in use is perfect. Prospective methods, such as food records or direct observation by an observer, may cause the eater to select different foods than he or she would normally do, so that the intake is not representative of usual consumption. Retrospective methods, such as the 24-hour recall or the semiquantitative food frequency questionnaire, are marred by forgetfulness, so that intakes are often seriously underreported.

The shortcomings of dietary reports have led some investigators to include indirect measures of dietary intake in addition to dietary record or recall information to delineate actual intakes further. Such methods include doubly labelled water to estimate energy outputs and intakes, various biochemical measures of protein catabolism that provide estimates of protein intake, and serum levels of vitamins to measure markers of habitual intake of these nutrients. When dietary assessment is being used to assess nutritional status, it is also important to include anthropometric, biochemical, and clinical information to obtain a complete picture of the nutritional status of the individual or group.

Assessment of Nutrient Intakes from Food Composition Data

The presence of nutrients in food and the chemical or other analyses that were necessary to characterize the levels present in foods became available in the first third of the twentieth century. Since then sampling techniques have improved and efforts are now made to make sure that the foods analysed are typical of those eaten by the population. Also, the analytical techniques used in food composition studies have become more precise, reliable, economical, automated and rapid. Nevertheless, there are still many problems involved in amassing and interpreting food composition data that have been dealt with in detail in several recent books. The situation is becoming even more complex. Many new food ingredients such as fat and sugar substitutes are becoming more widely available. New foods are being fortified with nutrients. Medications and other products sold over-the-counter provide substantial amounts of some nutrients, such as magnesium and fluoride, to some individuals. Also, the use of nutrient supplements is becoming common, and their content with respect to nutrients must also be ascertained. Nutrient supplement databases are generally poorly developed and these shortcomings need to be remedied. Finally, intakes of nutrients from foods and supplements need to be merged to provide overall estimates of usual nutrient intakes from all sources. In addition to considering nutrients, there is an increasing need for food tables that describe other characteristics, such as dietary fibre, the isoflavonoids and carnitine.

Usually the agricultural or health ministries of national governments are responsible for collecting and disseminating information on food composition for foods commonly eaten in the country, and for providing the food tables that are used for assessment of information collected in government-sponsored surveys. These country-specific efforts are augmented by regional and international efforts. In the 1970s and 1980s, under the auspices of the United Nations University and bilateral aid agencies the INFOODS program was launched to organize regional groups to deal with the tasks of collecting, evaluating and disseminating food composition data. These regional activities continue and are important sources of up-to-date information on nutrient data bases in different countries. Some countries actively update food composition and nutrient database information. For example, there is an annual nutrient data bank conference in the USA where such developments and new computerized dietary analysis programs are annually reviewed.

Probabilistic Approach to Evaluating Nutrient Intakes

The natural history of the development of deficiency disease is well worked out for many nutrients, and changes in biochemical and clinical parameters as well as signs and symptoms with decreasing levels of intakes are also often well documented. Studies of dietary intake levels and chronic degenerative disease risk have clarified the doses of nutrients needed for certain biochemical responses or parameters that are known to be associated with health risks, such as low-density lipoprotein (LDL) cholesterol levels. This makes it possible to relate levels of intake with functional measures. We never know with exactitude what an individual's nutrient requirements really are. Therefore, although the evaluation of intakes of individuals is an exercise in probabilities, and the exact risk of inadequacy resulting from a low intake is always unknown, we know the sequence of some of the development of disorders and the signs and symptoms that accompany getting too little of some nutrients and we can ascertain, therefore, with some certainty the nutritional status of the individual from dietary, biochemical, clinical and anthropometric indicators.

Just as we never know with certainty an individual's nutrient requirements, neither are the levels of intakes apparent at which adverse effects are likely to be present because of excessive intakes. In contrast to concerns about dietary deficiency, concerns over what the upper levels of intake that are appropriate are relatively recent for most nutrients. For large doses of many nutrients, the type, sequence and prevalence of adverse effects are still not well worked out. The upper level (UL) is the intake for which there is good assurance that intakes at or below that level will not cause adverse effects. Intakes between the recommended dietary allowances (RDA) and the UL constitute a spectrum of consumption levels that are compatible with health. Although there is no established benefit from consuming intakes above the RDA, so, too, is there little reason for concern about adverse effects developing from excess, as long as intakes remain below the UL. At present, the medical literature consists largely of anecdotal reports, which are insufficient to develop firmly grounded estimates. Until more adequate data are available, UL estimates must be considered tentative. It must be remembered that the absence of reported effects cannot be assumed to represent the true prevalence of adverse effects; in effect such an absence may only signal that little has been done to study the potential adverse effects of the nutrient in question. For some nutrients, no doubt, there are myriad possible adverse effects resulting from excessive amounts of nutrients. These need to be documented and the dose levels at which they appear quantified and clarified.

Reference Values for Nutrient Intakes
International differences

It is now recognized that in order to assess or plan dietary intakes, a variety of different reference values are needed. These have been developed by many countries and regions. The most common types of reference values are estimates of average requirements (estimated average requirements) for nutrients and estimates of intakes (reference nutrient intakes) that are thought to meet the needs of virtually all of the individuals in the population. The reference nutrient values differ in the assumptions they use, the functional end points that they focus on, the quantitative estimates they provide, the number of life stage breakouts given, and in the weights given to various types of evidence in the judgment of the expert group that is developing the standard. These differences mean that estimates, even for the same estimated average requirements of nutrients, vary by two-fold or greater. Theoretically, since human biology is the same throughout the world, the underlying assumptions for calculating estimated average requirements should be similar in all countries. The United Nations agencies and other expert groups are currently striving to harmonize approaches to developing estimated average requirements, but it is likely to take many years to complete the effort.

In contrast to the similar biological capabilities in all parts of the world, the heterogeneity of dietary intakes of foods and nutrients and other differences in environmental circumstances are apparent from country to country. Therefore population recommendations for nutrient intakes, which depend not only on the estimated average requirement but upon the variability and distribution of nutrient intakes, are likely always to differ appreciably from one country to another.

Age/life stage and gender groupings and reference weights

The rationale for age/life stage and gender groupings is that these characteristics sometimes help to explain the variability in nutrient needs and thus in the appropriate standards that should be employed, although their utility varies from nutrient to nutrient. The number of life-stage groups, the number of infant groups, and the age in childhood at which males and females are first treated separately varies from one set of nutrient standards to another. However, there are certain conventions which are employed in most of the reports. The first is that intakes from breast milk of the healthy, exclusively breast-fed infant born from a term pregnancy are often used as the basis for making recommendations for infants in the first 6 months of extrauterine life. The adequate intakes (AI) which are developed for nutrients using this model are not based on estimated average requirements (EAR) for the nutrients, and the ethics of human experimentation are such that it is not possible to determine what the EAR and potentially inadequate levels might be. While there is good evidence that such a standard permits good growth in term infants, it is less likely that breast milk nutrient content is optimal for all prematurely born babies, particularly if they are very small. Therefore other models might be more appropriate for that purpose. A second convention is that breakouts by age, sex and life stage may be important for some nutrients but not for others. In some instances, additional breakouts may be needed. A final convention is that the reference weights and heights that are selected are usually chosen to be representative of the population for which the recommendations are addressed. The reference weights are used to indicate the extent to which the reference intakes may have to be adjusted for individuals and population groups. The dietary reference intakes (DRI) are usually stated as single values, not in relationship to weight or height. Although for some nutrients such as calcium, phosphorus, magnesium, vitamin D and fluoride it might be expected that those with larger skeletal masses would have greater needs, the variability and errors from other sources in the data make it very difficult to determine how requirements vary by size. Therefore to avoid the error of implying greater precision than the data actually warrants, vitamins and minerals are not stated per unit weight.

North American perspectives

For over a half century, the Food and Nutrition Board of the National Academy of Sciences in the USA has provided recommendations on daily dietary allowances of nutrients, or recommended dietary allowances (RDA), that would minimize the risk of dietary deficiency disease in healthy individuals. These recommendations were periodically revised to incorporate new scientific developments and were used for many purposes. The Canadian government issued similar but not identical standards, calling them recommended nutrient intakes (RNI). Intakes were reformulated as described below in the early 1990s.

The DRI refers to a set of generic nutrient reference values, including EAR, RDA, AI and tolerable UL that have been developed for 12 life-stage groups by a joint US–Canadian committee. The intakes referred to are all average, mean, intakes.

Estimated average requirement (EAR) The EAR is the intake estimated to meet the specified indicator of adequacy's requirement in 50% of the life-stage and gender group being considered. The other half of individuals consuming this level of intake would not have their needs met. The indicator chosen may vary. However, the RDA had a number of limitations. They were calculated to provide enough of the nutrient to avoid deficiency, but neither the issue of minimizing chronic degenerative disease nor how best to avoid excess was addressed for nutrients other than food energy. Moreover, although the values actually applied to individuals and not to groups, they often were applied incorrectly to groups. Also, means and descriptive statistics on distributions of requirements were seldom provided, so that population recommendations were difficult to formulate. In contrast to older recommendations, in some instances the EAR may be a requirement to decrease risk of chronic degenerative disease rather than to prevent a classical nutrient deficiency. Before such a functional outcome is chosen, however, biological plausibility must be apparent. Epidemiological evidence that is supported by clinical trials and other corroborating evidence from animal and laboratory studies is also necessary. When decreases in chronic degenerative disease are chosen as the criterion on which the requirement is based, usually intermediate markers are used as proxies for the decreased risk expected. Such markers are necessary because associations with disease end points themselves may not be apparent over the short term, but only over many years. This is the case, for example, with calcium intake and osteoporosis.

Recommended dietary allowance (RDA) The RDA represents the level of intake sufficient to meet the daily nutrient needs of most individuals in a specific life-stage and gender group. It is used to provide a goal for individual intakes. The RDA is set at two standard deviations (SD) above the EAR when the variation in requirements is known and well defined. Therefore under these circumstances the RDA can be calculated from the EAR plus 2 SD of the EAR. For some nutrients, sufficient data on variation in nutrient requirements are not available or they are inconsistent. Under these circumstances a convention is used and a standard estimate of the variance is applied based on the coefficient of variation (the coefficient of variation, or CV%, is the SD divided by the mean times 100). The CV is assumed to be 10%, which is equal to one SD; this is a reasonable assumption based on protein and energy needs. Under these circumstances, then, the RDA is equal to the EAR times 1.2.

Adequate intake (AI) For some nutrients, there is not sufficient scientific evidence to calculate an EAR. When this is the case the AI, which is based on observed or experimentally determined approximations of the average nutrient intake of a defined population or subgroup that appears to sustain the desired nutritional state, is used instead. The AI is calculated when data are not sufficient to permit estimation of the EAR. Because less information is available, it must be regarded only as a provisional number. Nevertheless, when definitive data are lacking so that an EAR and RDA cannot be calculated, the AI may be used as a goal for nutrient intakes of individuals and for group intakes. However, the estimates are rough, and caution is needed. The characteristics of individuals and groups need to be examined for how well they fit the information under consideration. The desired nutrient state specified in the AI may be growth or maintenance of a specified serum level of nutrients in some cases, and in others reduction in chronic disease risk using some surrogate marker rather than the prevention of nutrient deficiency. For young infants, whom it is recommended that the sole feed be human milk until 4–6 months of age, the AI is the daily mean nutrient intake supplied by human milk for healthy term infants who are exclusively breast-fed. In most instances the AI is thought to be a value that exceeds the EAR and possibly the RDA for the specific end point chosen. The AI varies depending on the indicator of nutrient adequacy that is chosen. It also varies by other factors, including the dietary intake characteristics of the groups upon which it is based, the database, and methods that are used to estimate

it. Compared with the EAR or the RDA, the AI it is less precise. The excess of the AI compared with a true EAR differs from one nutrient to another, from one population group to another, and from one distinct sociocultural setting to another. Therefore, although it is assumed that the AI is higher than the EAR, the relationship cannot be stated mathematically.

Upper intake level (UL) The tolerable UL is the maximum level of daily nutrient intake that is unlikely to pose risks of adverse health effects to almost all individuals in the specified life-stage and gender group. The level of intake is one that can be tolerated from the biological standpoint, but it is not intended to be a recommended level of intake. That is, there is no established benefit from healthy individuals associated with nutrient intakes that are this high.

The UL can be used to assess characteristics of individuals and groups, but it should be taken as a rule of thumb rather than as a definitive judgment. Other factors, such as physiological state of the individual, length of sustained high intakes, and so on must also be considered.

Evaluating Nutrient Intakes of Individuals

Neither dietary intake nor any other single criterion is sufficient in itself for evaluating the nutritional status of the individual. However, dietary intakes can provide useful clues. For optimal health, the nutrient intakes of individuals should be adequate without being excessive. Therefore the process of evaluating nutrient intakes of individuals must address both of these issues.

Adequacy

Since we never know an individual's true requirement, estimates of nutrient needs must be based on educated guesses. The most appropriate measure to base our best guess of an individual's requirement on is the EAR. The EAR meets individual needs for half of the population, by definition. The EAR plus 2 SD is adequate for 97.5% of individuals, assuming that the distribution of requirements is normal. It is therefore assumed that such an intake is adequate. An intake below the RDA will be inadequate for a certain percentage of individuals, but for any single individual their inadequacy is not easy to determine. However, it is reasonable to conclude that the lower the intake is, the greater is the risk of inadequacy. For nutrients that have EAR, the actual probability of inadequacy can be calculated as the area under the requirement curve that is to the right of the intake. This cannot be calculated if there is only an AI for the nutrient.

For example, a correct assessment of an individual's intake would be as follows: 'Mr Smith's intake did not meet the RDA/AI for calcium, magnesium or ascorbic acid. Therefore he needs to consider eating more sources of these nutrients, which include milk and milk products, whole grain cereals, and orange juice'. An example of an incorrect dietary assessment would be this: 'From the computer printout Mr Smith's intake was only 60% of the AI for calcium, 86% of the RDA for magnesium, and 95% of the RDA for ascorbic acid, so he is deficient in all three nutrients, and especially in calcium'.

In North America, the DRI are being issued sequentially rather than in a single volume, as was the case in the past, and this has created some confusion. As a general rule, the most recent DRI should be utilized. Where revised RDA are not yet available, existing RDA should be used.

Avoiding excess

Individual assessment must also be concerned about balancing; getting enough of each nutrient without getting too much. 'Too much' is defined as amounts above the UL. The UL is defined as the maximum level of daily intake of a nutrient that is unlikely to pose risks of adverse effects to almost all individuals in a specified group, when applied to usual intakes from all sources (e.g. food, fortified food, water and supplements). For example, the UL for calcium in an adult female is 2.5 g from all sources. The UL definition is based primarily on studies in which hypercalciuria was found to be associated with both dietary and supplemental intakes of calcium. Thus for calcium food, water and supplements must all be considered. There is no known benefit from intakes that are above the RDA, and when intakes exceed the UL, there is a risk of adverse effects. A difficult issue is when a beneficial attribute is present only at levels at which other attributes are negative. For example, very large, pharmacological doses of nicotinic acid give rise to flushing, altered liver enzymes and other problems, although at the same time they have beneficial effects in decreasing serum cholesterol levels.

A current problem in assessing UL in individuals is that information on dietary supplement use, medications and water is often not obtained during the process of dietary assessment, and even when it is, there may be difficulties in integrating it with information on intakes of nutrients from foods. More comprehensive supplement databases are needed, which might include information on medications and water sources.

Planning Individual Intakes

Another reason for obtaining a dietary assessment is to plan an individual's intake. Using current usual dietary intakes, the gender and life-stage appropriate recommended dietary intake values are selected and these are used as a guide for planning the individual's food intake, taking into account food preferences, economics and other factors.

Dietary planning involves achieving the 'golden mean'; that is, achieving the appropriate RDA or AI without exceeding the safe upper level of nutrient intakes. The means of achieving such optimal intakes include nutrition education to help individuals select foods widely and the use of fortified foods or supplements. Each of these strategies has both strengths and limitations.

The use of usual foods as sources of nutrients provides the benefit that is often present from other biologically active substances such as fibre that have positive health effects and that might not be present in single sources of nutrients. Also in some instances the presence of other nutrients, such as ascorbic acid, may increase the bioavailability of another nutrient (such as iron) over what it would be if the mineral were given in a purified form. It is also true that most of the epidemiological associations between decreased incidence of certain chronic diseases and conditions and dietary intake are between intakes of foods high in specific nutrients rather than between disease and intakes of sole sources of nutrients. Finally, excess consumption of a single nutrient is rare when foods are used as nutrient sources.

Fortified foods also have their place, particularly when it is difficult to alter food habits to the extent that is likely to be necessary to bring about a desirable change in intake levels. For successful food fortification, a suitable staple food must be found which can be fortified.

For individuals at very high risk of not meeting the RDA, and for individuals in certain life-stage groups for which needs are very high, another strategy to assure dietary sufficiency is to use vitamin or mineral supplements.

Evaluating Nutrient Intakes of Populations

When the focus is on groups, for both assessing and planning, the EAR are necessary, as well as information about the distribution of intakes in the population being studied. The RDA are not helpful for planning or assessing nutrient intakes of free-living groups because such populations vary so much in their nutrient intakes. Since there are no EAR for some nutrients, such as calcium, vitamin D and fluoride, the assessment and planning of nutrient intakes is made much more complicated. More research is needed to provide the information that is necessary to obtain EAR. In addition to EAR, which provide information on the requirement, information on intake is also necessary. If the intakes are normally distributed or if they can be transformed to conform to a normal distribution, then a recommended intake for the group can be estimated based on the EAR and the variance of intake. The measure of distribution of intake that is used to calculate the mean recommended target intake is the coefficient of variation (the SD divided by the mean). This is used rather than the standard deviation, because the standard deviation usually varies in relation to the magnitude of intake. When a CV is unknown, 10% is usually assumed. If assumptions about normality of intake distributions are met, then a simplified formula can be used to calculate the recommended mean nutrient intake at which no more than 2 or 3% of the population will be two SD or more below the EAR. The formula is as follows:

$$\text{Target mean intake for a group}$$
$$= \text{EAR}/(1-[2\times \text{ CV of intake}]).$$

The target mean recommended intakes for individuals and groups vary. For example, an older woman living in an assisted living facility would have a phosphorus RDA of 800 mg, whereas the target mean recommended intake for 100 similar individuals living in the same facility would depend on their intakes. If the women all ate more or less the same diet, and the CV of intakes was 0.16, assuming that the intakes were normally distributed, the achievement of a group mean intake of 853 mg would ensure that only about 2–3% of the women would have an intake below the EAR of 580 mg. In contrast, if the women's intakes were highly variable, with a CV double this (CV = 0.32), then the target mean intake would be very much higher than this; approximately 1810 mg. Therefore the distribution of intakes in a population is critical in determining the amount of a nutrient that must be recommended.

When assessment of the intake of a group is of concern, it is important to make sure that intakes reflect usual intakes, not a single day's intake. Statistical adjustments are needed if intakes are only based on a single day's intake before the intake centiles for groups are calculated, since the distributions without adjustment will be very wide and provide unstable overestimates of the prevalence of inadequate intakes. Statistical procedures are available to adjust such intakes to account for day-to-day variance; such adjustments should be done before calculating intake centiles for groups.

Consider, for example, representative intakes of phosphorus, adjusted and unadjusted for day to day variance in intakes obtained in a recent study. The EAR for women aged 20–29 years is 580 mg phosphorus, and that for boys aged 12–19 years is 1055 mg. If only the unadjusted means were used, many more women aged 20–29 years would be judged deficient than if the adjusted means were used. Using unadjusted 1 day intakes, between 5 and 25% of women's intakes would fall below the EAR of 580 mg; with adjustments, less than 5% do so. Similarly, for boys aged 12–19 years, with an EAR of 1055 mg, almost 25% of the population using unadjusted values, but less than 5% using adjusted values would be below the EAR of 1055 mg. Unfortunately, usual intakes are not always available, and if one day of data is used the prevalence of inadequate and excessive intakes will be overestimated (since the intake distributions will be very spread out, especially when micronutrient supplements are included). Finally the variability of intakes differs from one nutrient to another. When the range of intakes is very wide, some individuals may experience excess while others will be deficient.

Methods for Estimating the Prevalence of Inadequate Intakes in Groups

The usual method of estimating the prevalence of inadequate intakes is to calculate the probability of inadequacy for each individual in the group. The group prevalence of inadequate intakes is the average of the individual probabilities. A simplified method of estimating the prevalence of inadequate intakes can be used when the variance of intakes is greater than the variance of requirements, and the requirement distribution is symmetrical. Then it is possible to determine the prevalence of inadequate intakes simply by determining the prevalence of intakes below the EAR.

Planning Recommended Intakes for Groups

Level of significance

In making recommendations for intake of groups, conventional practice among nutritionists has been to recommend levels of intake that ensure that most individuals (e.g. 97–98%) meet their nutrient requirement, and this is the degree of risk that is thought to be tolerable in planning for groups. However, under certain circumstances, more or less risk may be tolerable. For example, if the deficiency of the nutrient is associated with very serious and permanent sequellae, such as neural tube defects in the offspring of pregnant women, even a lower level of risk (e.g. 1%) might be appropriate. Conversely, when the upper level of intakes is close to the recommended level of intakes for a group but is relatively minor in its effects and rare in its occurrence, but the consequences of not achieving the EAR are severe, it may be appropriate to tolerate more risk.

Selection on the distribution of intakes for calculating requirements

Early in the process of planning the decision must be made on what distribution of intakes will be used for calculating recommendations for groups; actual or 'ideal'. It seems reasonable to use actual distributions of intakes. However, such distributions should include not only intakes from food sources, but also those from other sources (e.g. supplements, medications, etc.). A problem arises when distributions of intakes are not normally distributed or they cannot be transformed to be so. Under these circumstances other mathematical approaches must be employed. Actual distributions are seldom normally distributed. One method for dealing with this problem is to substitute ideal distributions of population intakes to calculated recommendations for groups. The advantage is that the distributions are likely to be more normally distributed, permitting easier mathematical manipulation. The disadvantage is that such 'ideal' recommendations may have little to do with the reality of what people eat, particularly in populations which are very heterogeneous.

Adjustments of intakes for day-to-day variance

Once the distribution of intakes that is to be used has been determined, it may be necessary to adjust it if it does not represent usual diets. The procedures for doing this are the same as those used for evaluating nutrient intakes of populations.

Evaluation factors increasing or decreasing risk

A final consideration in planning intakes is to take into account the many factors that may reduce or increase actual intakes of the nutrient in question in a given population. The planning of intakes does not need to accept the status quo of intakes, although it must always be based on reality. It is possible to craft interventions that will alter intakes. There are two different concerns. One is to reduce the prevalence of inadequate intakes in population subgroups. Another concern is to avoid excessive intakes that put individuals at risk of other effects. One strategy might be to increase intakes at the lower end of the intake distribution, since these are the individuals whose intakes that are the most likely to fall below the EAR. For example, if such individuals could be identified they could be given foods especially high in the nutrient needed, or meal planning could emphasize increasing intakes of the nutrient from many foods.

Use of AI

Often only the AI is available. Professionals who are used to using the AI for setting tentative recommendations for a group can do so, but should be aware of the considerable variability in these estimates. The AI is not some lower limit of the population mean intake range that is desirable for nutrient sufficiency. The World Health Organization (WHO) does specify a mean intake which is the lower limit of the population mean intake range for nutritional sufficiency.

Conclusions

Dietary assessment methods are increasingly computerized and standardized to lessen both observer and respondent burden, but they continue to have major shortcomings with respect to both validity and reliability. Therefore they alone cannot be relied upon to provide definitive evidence on nutritional status, and they are best used in combination with other methods, including anthropometric, biochemical and clinical measures. Food composition tables provide more useful information than ever before but are continuing to evolve. Sufficient new information has accumulated so that dietary reference intakes for several different purposes can be and are being formulated by expert groups in many parts of the world. In these recommendations, when sufficient data for efficacy and safety exist, the reduction in risk of chronic degenerative disease is included in selecting criteria for determining requirements. This is consonant with an emphasis on functional criteria that have meaning in terms of health and disease. Dietary reference intakes include not only recommendations about sufficiency of nutrients, but also avoidance of excess. Finally, in addition to nutrients, other food constituents that have health effects are also receiving attention in dietary assessments.

See also: **Adolescents**: Dietary Habits and Nutrient Requirements. **Ageing**: Biological Aspects. **Dietary Guidelines**: International Perspectives. **Dietary Intake**

Measurement: Methodology; Validation. **Nutritional Status**: Clinical Examination.

Further Reading

Beaton GH (1994) Criteria of an adequate diet. In: Shile RE, Olson JA and Shike M (eds) *Modern Nutrition in Health and Disease*, 8th edn, pp 1491–1505. Philadelphia: Lea & Febiger.

Beaton GH (1996) Statistical approaches to establish mineral element recommendations. *Journal of Nutrition* 126:2301S–2308S.

Bingham SA (1987) Dietary assessment of individuals: methods, accuracy, new techniques and recommendations. *Nutrition Abstracts and Reviews* 57:707–742.

Block GE and Hartman AM (1989). *Dietary Methods in Nutrition and Cancer Prevention*, pp 159–181. New York and Basel: Marcel Dekker.

Cameron ME and Van Staveren WA (eds) (1988) *Manual on Methodology for Food Consumption Studies*. Oxford: Oxford University Press.

Committee on Medical Aspects of Food Policy (1991) *Dietary Reference Values for Food Energy and Nutrients for the United Kingdom*. Report on Health and Social Subjects, no. 41. London: HMSO.

Dietary Reference Intakes (1997) In: *Dietary Reference Intakes: Calcium, Phosphorus, Magnesium, Vitamin D and Fluoride*, chap. 1. Food and Nutrition Board, Institute of Medicine. Washington, DC: National Academy Press (also published in *Nutrition Reviews* (1997) 555:319–326).

Dwyer JT (1997) Dietary assessment. In: Shils ME, Olson JA, Ross K and Shike M (eds) *Modern Nutrition in Health and Disease*. Philadelphia: Lea & Febiger.

European Community (1993) *Nutrient and Energy Intakes for the European Community*. Report of the Scientific Committee for Food, 31st sereis. Brussels: EC.

Food and Agriculture Organization of the United Nations/World Health Organization/United Nations (1985) *Energy and Protein Requirements*. Report of a joint FAO\WHO\UN consultation, Technical Report Series no. 724. Geneva: WHO.

Health Canada (1990) *Nutrition Recommendations*. Report of the Scientific Review Committee 1990. Ottawa: Canadian Government Publishing Centre.

Institute of Medicine, Food and Nutrition Board (1994) *How Should the Recommended Dietary Allowances be Revised?* Washington, DC: National Academy Press.

National Food Administration (1989) *Swedish Nutrition Recommendations*, 2nd edn. Uppsala: National Food Administration.

National Research Council (1989) *Recommended Dietary Allowances*, 10th edn. Report of the Subcommittee on the Tenth Edition of the RDA, Food and Nutrition Board, and the Commission on Life Sciences. Washington DC: National Academy Press.

Nusser SM, Carriquiry AL, Dodd KW and Fuller WA (1996) A semi-parametric transformation approach to estimating usual daily intake distributions. *Journal of the American Statistical Association* 91:1440–1449.

Pao EM and Cypel YS (1996) Estimation of dietary intake. In: Zeigler EE and Filer LJ (eds) *Present Knowledge in Nutrition*, 7th edn, chap. 50, pp 498–505. Washington, DC: International Life Sciences Institute/Nutrition Foundation.

Rand WM, Windham CT, Wyse BW and Young VR (eds) (1987) *Food Composition Data: A User's Perspective*. Tokyo: United Nations University.

Standing Nordic Committee on Food (1989) *Nordic Nutrition Recommendations*, 2nd edn (English version).

Thompson RE, Byers T and Kohlmee L (1994) Dietary assessment resource manual *Journal of Nutrition* 124(11S):2245S–2218S

Willett WH (1992) *Nutritional Epidemiology*. Oxford: Oxford University Press.

World Health Organization (1996) *Trace Elements in Human Nutrition and Health*. Prepared in Collaboration with the Food and Agricultural Organization of the United Nations and the International Atomic Energy Agency. Geneva: WHO.

Anthropometric Assessment

J Eaton–Evans, University of Ulster, Coleraine, Northern Ireland, UK

Anthropometric measurements include weight, height, length, selected skinfold thicknesses, and head, waist, hip and arm circumferences. When compared with reference values, these measurements or combinations of these measurements can provide information on body size and the proportion and distribution of body fat and lean body mass in adults; they can also be used to assess growth in children. Anthropometric measurements indirectly indicate present or past nutrition and may be markers of future ill-health.

This article reviews the uses, advantages and limitations of anthropometric measurements, discusses the technical errors of the measurements, describes the most frequently used measurements, derived nutritional indices and reference values and summarizes the laboratory methods which may validate the assessments.

Uses of Anthropometric Measurements

In adults and children, anthropometric measurements can be used to estimate body fat and lean body mass and assess their distribution and change over time. Body fat includes storage fat, found inter- and intra-muscularly, around the organs and gastrointestinal tract and subcutaneously, as well as lipids in bone marrow, central nervous tissue, mammary glands and other organs. Normal-weight men and women have about 10% and 20% body fat, respectively. Lean body or fat-free mass is mostly water and protein with relatively small amounts of glycogen and minerals. Inadequate diets are associated with low body fat stores and reduced lean body mass in adults and growth failure of children. Consumption of food greater than requirements results in excessive body fat stores in adults and children. Body fat stores that are too low or too high are associated with increased risk of morbidity and mortality. The proportion and distribution of fat and fat-free mass varies with age, sex, genetics, disease, some hormones and some drug treatments. Extensive physical exercise may be associated with increased muscle mass.

Different anthropometric measurements and combinations of measurements provide information on body composition and fat distribution and, therefore, nutritional status. The choice of measurements depends on the purpose of the assessment, the equipment available, the subjects being measured, and the skills of the observer making the measurements. Measurements can be made in laboratories, clinics and hospitals using fixed, precision equipment with a high degree of accuracy, or in the field, including peoples' homes or rural centres, with lighter, robust and portable equipment.

Advantages and Limitations of Anthropometric Measurements

Anthropometric measurements are noninvasive. Compared with other methods of assessing nutritional status, the measurements are quick and easy to make using relatively cheap and simple equipment. They can be made by relatively unskilled people.

Anthropometric measurements cannot identify protein and micronutrient deficiencies, detect small disturbances in nutritional status, nor identify small changes in the proportions of body fat to lean body mass. Some anthropometric measurements may not be socially or culturally acceptable, such as the measurement by men of womens' subscapular and supra-iliac skinfold thicknesses; some measurements may be impractical to make, such as the height in people who are unable to stand straight. Observers with limited literacy skills may not be able to read and therefore record some measurements. A single anthropometric measurement, such as weight, does not normally in itself assess growth and/or body composition and, therefore, indicate nutritional status. To interpret anthropometric measurements, single measurements or combinations of measure-

ments must be compared with reference values, by age and sex. Such reference values are not available for all population groups nor for all ages.

Errors of Anthropometric Measurements

All anthropometric measurements should be made as accurately as possible. Measurement errors may result in the misclassification of subjects' nutritional status or may lead to changes in nutritional status over time being over- or underestimated. Very precise and accurate measurements are needed for nutrition research and in some clinical situations. The same degree of precision may not be possible in nutritional screening and surveillance programmes in field studies. Errors in making measurements arise from the equipment, the physical state and age of the subjects, the time of day when the measurements are made, misreading of measurements by the observer, and as a result of rounding up or down to the nearest half or whole integer. These technical errors of measurement (TEM) vary with the age of the subjects, the measurements being made, and between (inter-) and within (intra-) observers. Values for a particular anthropometric measurement of a group of people by age and sex can be considered accurate if the inter- and intraobserver error is close to a reference value for TEM in a series of repeated measurements and if there are no biases in the measurement. For measurements of subjects outside the age range, the coefficient of variability (R) can be calculated as $R = 1 - [(\text{TEM})^2/(\text{SD})^2]$, where SD is the total intersubject variance including measurement error. It has been recommended that an R of 0.90, that is a measurement 90% error-free, is an acceptable lower limit of accuracy, although an intraobserver R of 0.95 might be more realistic in some circumstances.

TEM can be minimized by careful training of all observers, and by making measurements using appropriate equipment in triplicate and then calculating the mean. If measurements for a research study are to be made by more than one person, the interobserver measurements made must be comparable. R can be calculated for interobserver variability by making a series of measurements.

Anthropometric Measurements

Height

Height, or stature, is measured in adults and children over the age of 2 years using a stadiometer, a portable anthropometer, or a moveable headboard on a vertical measuring rod. The measuring device should be checked for accuracy using a standard 2 m steel tape. Subjects should be measured to the nearest 0.1 cm. Subjects, in minimal clothing with bare heads and feet, should stand straight, arms hanging loosely to the side, feet together and with heels, buttocks and shoulder blades in contact with the vertical surface of the stadiometer. Errors occur if subjects either do not stand straight, do not keep heels on the ground, or overstretch. Diurnal variation results in people being 0.5–1 cm shorter in the evening than in the morning.

–Height cannot be measured accurately in adults with severe kyphosis of the spine and in those who are bed- or chair-ridden. Since knee height is highly correlated with stature, height in such adults can be estimated from the measurement of knee height, using a sliding calliper. The regression equations, derived from a nonrandom sample of American people over the age of 60 years, are:

Height (cm) for men = (2.02 × knee height, cm) − (0.04 × age, years) + 64.19;

Height (cm) for women = (1.83 × knee height, cm) − (0.24 × age, years) + 84.88.

Variations in the proportion of limb length to trunk length can lead to a standard error in the estimate (SEE) of height from knee height of ± 8 cm. Demispan, which is the distance between the sternal notch of the right collar bone and the left finger root of the middle and ring finger when the subject's arm is horizontal and in line with the shoulders, can also be used to estimate height.

Length, rather than height, is measured in infants and children under the age of 3 years. Length is measured by laying a child face upwards on a measuring board with the head against the fixed headboard, and moving another board up to and resting against the child's heels with the legs straight. Small changes in length (±0.5 cm) may not be significant as it is a difficult measurement to make. Children wriggle and will not stretch out their legs. Length measurements are 1–2 cm longer than height.

Height (stature) or length indicates attained size or growth of adults and children. Long periods of inadequate food intake or increased morbidity result in a slowing of skeletal growth and individuals being short for their age, or stunted. Consecutive measurements of height every 3–6 months can be used to assess growth velocity in children and to indicate the timing of the adolescent growth spurt.

Weight

Weight is measured with digital weighing scales, using a pan, basket, sling, standing platform or chair, depending on the age and mobility of the people being measured. Weighing scales must be set on a hard, level and even surface. Scales should be accurate, sensitive and robust. They must be carefully maintained, calibrated, regularly checked for accuracy using known weights and always set at zero before use. Weight is usually measured to the nearest 0.1 kg for adults and 0.01 kg for infants.

Weight measures total body mass but does not provide information on the proportions of fat, water, protein and minerals. Weight and fat are only synonymous in very heavy people. Adults can be heavy for height if very muscular, over-fat and/or big framed. With accurate scales, small changes in weight are detectable but may not necessarily reflect change in body fat or lean body mass. In healthy persons, day-to-day variation in body weight is usually small (±0.5 kg). Consecutive measurements of weight can be used to monitor the effects of treatment such as weight loss on reduction diets or weight gain with nutritional interventions and supplementation. Weight changes are assumed to reflect changes in the amount of body fat. However, changes in body weight may also result from differences in hydration, oedema, tumour growth and trauma, as well as from factors such as the amount of food in the gastrointestinal tract and the fullness of the bladder. Weight may remain constant if the loss of muscle mass is masked by increased fat as seen in sarcopenia, the age-related loss of muscle, or by increased fluid retention.

Weight-for-height (or length) can be used to indicate body composition in adults and is an age-independent measure of body composition in children. Growth can be measured in children by consecutive measurements of weight over time (growth velocity) or by weight-for-age if the children's ages are known.

Head circumference

Head circumference is measured in infants and young children, to the nearest 0.1 cm, with a narrow flexible nonstretch tape laid over the supraorbital ridges and the part of the occiput which gives the maximum circumference. The head circumference of infants increases rapidly in the first 2 years of life. Increase in head circumference in the first 2 years of life is affected by nutritional status and non-nutritional problems including some diseases, genetic variation and cultural practices.

Mid upper arm circumference

Mid upper arm circumference (MUAC) is measured in adults and children, to the nearest 0.1 cm, using a flexible nonstretch tape laid at the midpoint between the acromion and olecranon processes on the shoulder blade and the ulna, respectively, of the left arm. MUAC is a measure of the sum of the muscle and subcutaneous fat in the upper arm. In severe malnutrition both fat and muscle are reduced in the upper arm. Oedema may increase a limb's circumference but it is not usually a problem of the upper arm. MUAC can be used as a indicator of body composition in adults and children. Since MUAC increases little between the age of 6 months and 5 years, it can be used in preschool children as an age-independent screening tool for severe malnutrition. A MUAC less than 12.5 cm suggests malnutrition. A MUAC greater than 13.5 cm is normal.

Skinfold thickness

Precision skinfold thickness callipers are used to measure the double fold of skin and subcutaneous fat to the nearest mm. The usual sites of measurement are at the triceps (TSFT), the midpoint of the back of the upper left arm; the biceps (BSFT) at the same level as the TSFT but to the front of the upper left arm; the subscapular (SSFT) just below and laterally to the left shoulder blade; and the suprailiac (SISFT) obliquely just above the left iliac crest. Skinfold thicknesses can also be measured at the mid thigh, mid calf and abdomen.

Skinfold thicknesses are difficult measurements to make with precision and accuracy: it is difficult to pick up a consistent fold of skin and subcutaneous fat; in the very obese, the skinfold may be bigger than the callipers can measure; the fold of skin and fat compresses with repeated measurements; and the careless use of the callipers causes pain, bruising and skin damage to subjects. There is, therefore, likely to be considerable inter- and intraobserver error in the measurements.

Skinfold thicknesses measure subcutaneous body fat and, therefore, indicate body composition. TSFT and SSFT indicate subcutaneous fat on the limbs and body trunk, respectively. Skinfold thickness measurements mistakenly assume that subcutaneous fat, measured at one or more selected sites, measures total body fat stores. However, subcutaneous fat at one site may not reflect fat stores at another site, and may not be positively correlated with the amount of visceral fat deposited around the internal organs of the body. Subcutaneous fat, and therefore skinfold thicknesses at the different sites, changes at varying rates with age, weight change, with diseases such as diabetes, and in women during pregnancy, postpartum and at the menopause. Skinfold thicknesses are not useful for monitoring short-term change in fat stores. If only one skinfold thickness measurement is made, TSFT is most commonly selected. TSFT correlates with estimates of total body fat in women and

children. SSFT is better than TSFT as an indicator of total body fat in men. SSFT has been shown to be a predictor of blood pressure in adults independently of age and racial group.

Waist and hip circumferences

Waist and hip circumferences are measured to the nearest 0.1 cm ' using a flexible narrow nonstretch tape in adults wearing minimal clothing, standing straight but not pulling in their stomachs. Waist circumference is measured halfway between the lower ribs and the iliac crest, while hip circumference is measured at the largest circumference around the buttocks. Measurement error occurs if the tape is pulled too tight or loose, or if subjects wear clothes with belts and/or full pockets.

With increase in waist circumference there is an increase in insulin sensitivity, while a waist circumference greater than 94 cm in men and 80 cm in women has been associated with increased risk factors for cardiovascular disease.

Elbow width

Elbow width is the width of the epicondyles of the humerus with the elbow flexed at 90°. Sliding callipers are used to measure elbow width in adults to the nearest 0.1 cm. Elbow width is a measure of bone size. Frame size can be determined by comparison with reference values either by age, or by height and sex.

Nutritional Indices

Most single anthropometric measurements do not in themselves assess nutritional status. Nutritional indices are derived by either combining two or more anthropometric measurements, shown in laboratory studies to be predictive of body composition, or by comparison of the anthropometric measurements with reference values of healthy, well-fed populations. A combination of these methods can also be used.

Body mass index

Body mass index relates weight (kg) with height (m) by a simple calculation to indicate body composition (BMI = weight/height^2). It is the most commonly used screening measurement for both obesity and underweight as very low and high BMI are associated with increased mortality and morbidity. BMI classifies adults as underweight, normal, overweight or obese (see **Table 1**). BMI and percentage body fat is only highly correlated at extremes of the distribution. BMI cannot distinguish between adults who are

Table 1 Classifications of nutritional status as a percentage of ideal body weight and body mass index

% of ideal body weight for height	Body mass index (BMI)	Nutritional status
>120	>30	Obese
110–120	25–29.9	Overweight
90–109	20–24.9	Normal
<90	<20	Underweight

heavy because of fat or heavy because of muscle, takes no account of frame size, and provides no information on body fat distribution. These limitations may result in heavy, muscled sports people being classified as overweight or obese.

In children, BMI is age-dependent. BMI increases rapidly in the first year of life and then more slowly. Children, at extremes of the distribution of reference values by age and sex, can be identified as being abnormally thin or fat for height. The BMI classification used for adults should not be used for children.

Weight-for-height

Weight-for-height is an indicator of body composition in adults. Reference values by age, sex and frame size can be used to estimate desirable body weights (% desirable body weight = (actual weight ÷ ideal body weight) × 100); which are categorized by cutoff points (Table 1).

Weight-for-height by sex is a sensitive indicator of body composition in children. It appears to be relatively independent of ethnic group in children aged 1 to 5 years and age-independent in children aged from 1 to 10 years. Children with weights less than 85% of the median reference weight-for-height are considered wasted. It is a useful screening tool for current malnutrition, especially if used with height-for-age. Oedema and obesity, however, may confound the index.

Weight-for-age

Weight-for-age can be used to monitor growth in children of known age when a series of measurements are made and compared with reference values by sex. A single measurement of weight-for-age does not discriminate between a child who is light for age because of stunting and/or wasting owing to malnutrition, and one who is small for age but healthy and well fed. Children should gain weight as a percentile of the reference values. Failure to gain weight as expected or a weight loss indicates an inadequate diet, infection and/or lack of care and should be investigated. Maintenance of weight or weight gain

may mask the loss of lean body fat and the increased oedema of kwashiorkor.

Growth velocity

Growth velocity, or change in weight or height over time, can be used to assess growth in children when compared with reference values by age and sex. Growth rates decline in the first few years of life and then increase with the pubertal growth spurt. Premature and small-for-dates children and those recovering from malnutrition and severe infections tend to have higher growth velocities (catch-up growth). Growth velocities are useful to monitor growth and assess the response to therapy including nutritional supplementation.

Head circumference-for-age

Head circumference-for-age by sex is used by paediatricians to identify children up to 2 years of age with severe chronic malnutrition pre- and postpartum and the need for further medical investigations. It is not a good indicator of children's nutritional status.

Mid upper arm circumference-for-age

Mid upper arm circumference (MUAC)-for-age indicates body composition (upper arm fat and muscle) in adults and children when used with measurements of weight and height. MUAC measurements are compared with reference values by age and sex. Since the rate of change of arm circumference is slow, it cannot be used to assess growth or monitor the response to therapy.

Mid upper arm circumference-for-height

Mid upper arm circumference-for-height (the QUAC stick) is a cheap, quick, age-independent screening tool for children with malnutrition. It is a vertical stick on which are inscribed the 80% and 85% median reference values for MUAC and height, respectively. A child is considered malnourished if the MUAC is less than 80% of the MUAC expected for height.

Skinfold thickness-for-age

Skinfold thickness measurements-for-age and sex indicates subcutaneous body fat stores in adults and children. Reference values for TSFT, SSFT, and the sum of the TSFT and SSFT, are available by age and sex.

Measurement of BMI with skinfold thicknesses can identify people who are heavy owing to excess fat or muscle mass. A high BMI and low TSFT and/or SSFT indicate a large muscle mass; a high

BMI and high TSFT and/or SSFT indicate a high subcutaneous body fat.

Mid upper arm muscle circumference and upper arm muscle area

Mid upper arm muscle circumference (MUAMC) and upper arm muscle area (AMA) are estimates of upper arm muscle and, therefore, body composition. They can be used as indicators of muscle mass and protein stores. Both MUAMC and AMA are calculated from measurements of MUAC and TSFT on the mistaken assumption that the arm is cylindrical, the subcutaneous fat is equally distributed, the bone atrophies in proportion to muscle wastage in malnutrition and the cross-sections of neurovascular tissue and bone are small. The formula, with MUAC and TSFT in mm, is:

$$MUAMC = MUAC - (\pi \times TSFT).$$

AMA can be calculated from revised formulae which take account of errors resulting from the noncircular nature of muscle and the inclusion of nonskeletal muscle with MUAC and TSFT in cm:

$$\text{For men: AMA} = \left[\frac{MUAC - (\pi \times TSFT)}{4\pi} \right]^2 - 10.0;$$

$$\text{For women: AMA} = \left[\frac{MUAC - (\pi \times TSFT)}{4\pi} \right]^2 - 6.5.$$

MUAMC and AMA can be compared with reference values by age and sex. AMA cannot be used to monitor change in muscle stores because of the problems in making this measurement. The ratio of AMA to total body muscle mass changes with age and certain diseases.

Arm fat area

Arm fat area (AFA) can be derived from measurements of MUAC and TSFT. AMA is a better indicator of total body fat but not percentage body fat, than TSFT alone. The formula used to calculate AFA (with MUAC and TSFT in mm) is:

$$AMA = \frac{TSFT \times MUAC}{2} - \frac{\pi \times (TSFT)^2}{4}.$$

AMA can be compared with reference values by age and sex. Theoretically, limb fat area can be calculated for other limbs and the body trunk, but there are no reference values available.

Total body fat

Total body fat can be estimated as a percentage of body fat by comparing the sum of TSFT, BSFT, SSFT and SISFT with reference values derived from laboratory studies by age and sex, or via the estimation of body density from regression equations with skinfold thickness measurements. There are no specific empirical equations which can be used for specific population groups. Lean body mass is calculated by difference. These calculations may overestimate body fat in lean individuals and underestimate body fat in fat adults. They should not be used in undernourished individuals or in those with diseases where the total body water content may be markedly increased.

Waist-to-hip ratio

The waist-to-hip ratio (WHR) in adults discriminates between those with upper body or intraabdominal obesity (WHR greater than 1 in men and 0.8 in women) and those with lower body or peripheral obesity. Genetics, sex and age partly determine body fat distribution. A high WHR is associated with an increased risk of premature mortality and morbidity.

Reference Values

Anthropometric assessments are interpreted by comparison with reference values by age and sex. Ideally, reference values should represent the range of 'optimum' measurements for health and longevity of a population of the same ethnic origin. Individuals should be considered at nutritional risk when above or below predetermined reference limits or cutoff points, based on functional impairment, clinical signs of deficiency or increased risk of mortality and morbidity.

In practice, reference values are derived from large sets of cross-sectional anthropometric measurements of representative samples of populations of the same ethnic origin, who are assumed to be well nourished and free from infection, parasitic disease and any other environmental factors which may affect growth and nutritional status. These data can be supplemented by data derived from direct laboratory studies of body composition. International reference values are used if local reference data are too difficult, time-consuming and expensive to obtain.

Normal, healthy, well-fed people vary in size. Therefore, reference values are usually presented as percentiles, with values less than the 5th centile or greater than the 95th centile considered outside the normal range. If international reference values are used, it may be necessary to modify the cutoff points used for identifying those at risk for particular populations. Since the rate of growth of children is age-dependent, growth charts of the most commonly used anthropometric measurements and derived indices, have been constructed. Children's growth is best monitored by plotting their sequential measurements on growth charts. A well-nourished healthy child should progress along a centile between the 5th and 95th centile for each measurement. When a child's measurements cross centiles of the growth charts, whether owing to growth faltering, failure-to-thrive or excessive growth, the cause needs to be investigated. In this way anthropometric measurements can indicate the adequacy of a child's diet, the timing of the introduction of weaning foods, the impact of illness and the response to treatment. To use growth charts such as weight-for-age, height-for-age and head circumference-for-age, it is essential to know the age of a child accurately. A child's age cannot be estimated accurately by examination. A malnourished child is smaller and looks younger and less mature than a well-fed, healthy child.

To analyse data for screening, surveillance or research programmes, measurements can be compared with the median (50th centile) of the reference data and expressed as either a percentage of the median value or as a modified statistical z-score transformation where

$$\text{SD score} = \frac{\text{individuals' measurement} - \text{median value of reference value}}{\text{standard deviation value of reference value}}.$$

SD scores are appropriate for use in areas with a high incidence of malnutrition. A high proportion of the population have measurements less than the 5th centile of reference values in these areas. A child with a SD score less than -2, irrespective of the nutritional indices used, is considered malnourished. A SD score greater than 2 suggests obesity.

The most commonly internationally used anthropometric reference values for noninstitutionalized adults aged 25–74 years, have been derived from the American NHANES I and NHANES II studies, which were undertaken during 1971–74 and 1976–80, respectively. Reference values by sex, height and frame size for desirable weights-for-height have also been derived from data on the longevity of holders of life insurance policies. These reference values are not taken from a random sample of the population, as only the more affluent in society are likely to hold life insurance; in addition, these values take no account of body composition and make no reference to the incidence of disease.

Since anthropometric measurements are quick and objective methods of monitoring children's growth and therefore nutritional status, several anthropometric reference databases are available. The Harv-ard reference data, derived from a small sample of American children in the 1930s and 1940s, has been used for the 'Road to Health' (weight-for-age) charts for monitoring growth of children in many developing countries. The American National Center for Health Statistics (NCHS) data, derived from large, cross-sectional, nationally representative samples of children aged 0 to 18 years between 1963 and 1975, were adopted by the World Health Organization as the international reference data for children's growth. The UK growth reference data were derived from mixed cross-sectional and longitudinal data of children aged 0–18 years, living in London. Other countries such as Canada, France and Australia also have their own growth reference data.

Children's growth is influenced by many factors including sex, ethnic group, breast or bottle milk feeding, their birth order, gestational age of premature children, as well as the size (height) of their parents. Growth charts do not allow for these factors. With the secular changes in height and weight, growth charts derived from anthropometric measurements of children made over 30 years ago may no longer be appropriate to monitor growth of all children today. However, they may still be relevant to disadvantaged groups in the population. Similarly, growth charts of children derived from reference data of today may not be relevant to the children of the future.

A new reference data set, derived from mostly cross-sectional studies undertaken between 1978 and 1990 of 23 000 British children aged from 0 to 20 years, has been developed by the Human Measurements Anthropometry and Growth Research Group (HUMAG). Growth charts from these data have been produced by sex for weight-for-age, height-for-age, length-for-age, head circumference-for-age and BMI-for-age.

Laboratory Assessment of Body Composition

Body fat and lean body mass can be measured by the direct chemical analysis of cadavers, or in the laboratory by various indirect methods (**Table 2**). All laboratory assessments of body composition are expensive to make in time, equipment and/or materials. Except for the chemical analysis of cadavers, they all make assumptions as to the physical properties of body fat or fat-free mass. They can be used for research, to validate anthropometric estimates of body composition and to derive regression equations for body composition from anthropometric measurements.

Table 2 Indirect methods of laboratory assessment of body composition

Method	Principle
Dual-energy X ray absorptiometry (DXA)	Measures bone and soft tissue as fatty and lean tissue components absorb energy from a photon beam at different rates
Underwater weighting to measure density	Body density depends on the proportion of body fat and lean body mass
Bioelectrical impedance with a very low electrical current and measuring electrical resistance	Electrolyte-containing tissues, found mainly in the lean body mass, conduct electricity more efficiently than body fat
Total body potassium using ^{40}K using a whole body counter	Potassium, an intracellular cation, is found mainly in fat-free mass
Total body water using an isotope dilution technique of deuterium (^2H), tritium (^3H) and oxygen (^{18}O)	Water is found in the fat-free mass
Urinary creatinine excretion	The proportion of creatinine excreted is proportional to total body creatinine; 98% of all creatinine is in muscle, provided the person is on a meat-free diet

Conclusions

Anthropometric measurements are quick and relatively easy to make. They can be used to assess body composition and fat distribution of adults and to monitor the growth of children by comparison with reference values from data of populations considered well-fed and healthy. These values may not be the optimum values for health. More data are required to determine the risk to future health of deviating from normal anthropometric reference values.

See also: **Malnutrition**: Definition, Classification and Epidemiology. **Nutritional Support**: Parenteral Nutrition; In the Home Setting. **Obesity**: Treatment. **Older People**: Nutritional Management of Geriatric Patients. **Parasitism**: Effects on Growth and Nutritional Status.

Further Reading

Freeman JV, Cole TJ, Chinn S, Jones PRM, White EM and Preece MA (1995) Cross sectional statue and weight reference curves for the UK, 1990. *Archives of Disease in Childhood* 73:17–24.

Frisancho AF (1990) *Anthropometric Standards for the Assessment of Growth and Nutritional Status*. Ann Arbor: University of Michigan Press.

Gibson RS (1990) *Principles of Nutritional Assessment*, pp 155–262. New York: Oxford University Press.

Ulijasek SJ and Mascie-Taylor CGN (eds) (1994) *Anthropometry: the Individual and the Population*. Cambridge: Cambridge University Press.

World Health Organization (1983) *Measuring Change in Nutritional Status*. Geneva: WHO.

Biochemical Assessment

F Fidanza, Institute of Nutrition and Food Science, Perugia, Italy

Biochemical methods are considered to be the most objective measures for assessment of the nutritional status of an individual. The method should be specific and sensitive to depletion of the nutrient body pool or tissue store.

The evolution of deficiency for most nutrients, and particularly vitamins, progresses in successive stages. The first stage of deficiency is when nutrient body stores begin to be depleted; at this stage nutrient urine excretion decreases, while homeostatic regulation ensures that the level of nutrient in the blood does not change. At the next stage depletion is more marked; the nutrient urinary excretion drops and its concentration in blood and other tissues is reduced.

A lowering of nutrient metabolites and/or dependent enzymes often characterizes the subsequent stage. Sometimes lower hormone concentrations and some physiological alterations are observed. At the last stages morphological and/or functional disturbances are present, at first reversible and then irreversible. Nonspecific signs and symptoms can be present; without therapeutic interventions death can be expected.

Within the framework of the evolution of nutrient deficiencies the biochemical static and functional tests most commonly used in nutritional status assessment in humans are examined.

Static Biochemical Tests

Static tests measure chemically the content of nutrients, their active or inactive metabolites or other related components, in blood or blood fractions, other tissues and urine. The choice of tissue or fluid depends on the information required (short-term or long-term status, body pool or tissue store) and on the condition of the subject.

Various confounding factors affect static biochemical tests. Some are of a general kind such as age, sex, ethnic group, physiological and hormonal status, and so cannot be eliminated; others are of a technical nature and can be reduced or eliminated by standardization; and others are biological or environmental. The most relevant confounding factors will be considered for each method; those during infection will be examined in a sub-heading.

Protein nutritional status

The *total serum protein* test is very seldom used because it is no longer considered to be a sensitive index of status.

Serum albumin, measured by an automated dye-binding method, has a rather large body pool and a long half-life, and so it is a less sensitive index of immediate nutritional status. Albumin is a negative acute-phase reactant. Confounding effects of protein-losing diseases, such as reduced protein synthesis diseases and conditions involving an increase of plasma volume or haemodilution and zinc depletion, have been reported.

Plasma transport proteins (thyroid-binding pre-albumin (PA), retinol-binding protein (RBP) and transferrin (TF)) and fibronectin (FB, an opsonic glycoprotein) have a smaller pool size and a shorter half-life than serum albumin, and so their concentrations can change more rapidly. They are therefore a more immediate indicator of protein status. Plasma transport proteins are usually measured on radial-immunodiffusion plates, or alternatively with laser nephelometry. Plasma fibronectin is measured only with laser nephelometry. Like albumin, these are negative acute-phase reactants. Confounding effects additional to those for serum albumin include pregnancy, energetic exercise and altered metabolism. RBP is sensitive to deficiencies of vitamin A and zinc and TF is affected by iron status. Insulin has also been demonstrated to interfere with plasma transport protein levels.

Urinary creatinine, usually measured with a colorimetric method (also automated), is used as a biochemical marker of muscle mass. In fact urinary creatinine is a nonenzymatic product of creatine and cannot be reutilized. Various assumptions are required for a correct urinary creatinine determination and various confounding effects have been reported (age, diet, intensive exercise, pregnancy, injury, fever and renal diseases with impaired creatinine clearance). In a clinical setting the creatinine/height index is preferred, but because of some limitations, its usefulness is not very great.

Urinary 3-methyl-histidine (3-MH) can be measured by ion-exchange chromatography or by high-performance liquid chromatography (HPLC). 3-MH is present in myofibrillar proteins and during breakdown it is excreted quantitatively because it can be neither reused nor oxidized. Accordingly it is used as an indicator of muscle protein turnover. Various confounding effects are reported (sex, age, diet, intensive exercise, stress, hormonal and catabolic states, etc.) and so the use of the urinary 3-MH test is considered to be very problematical.

Insulin-like growth factor I (IGF I), also called somatomedin C, is a regulator of anabolic properties. It has recently been proposed as a sensitive indicator of protein deficiency. It is assayed by a radioimmunoassay method which is also available in a kit. More research is needed before a correct indication on the use of this test can be provided. Confounding effects of stress, some hormonal diseases and obesity have been reported.

Plasma amino acid levels have been used in the past to diagnose protein–energy malnutrition. The ratio of free nonessential amino acid levels (glycine, serine, glutamine, taurine) to essential amino acid levels (leucine, isoleucine, valine, methionine) was proposed for the diagnosis of kwashiorkor. In children with this disease this ratio can be much higher than the normal value of 2. Plasma amino acids were previously assessed by paper chromatographic methods; automated ion exchange or HPLC techniques are now preferred. However in recent years there has been much less interest in this test.

Essential fatty acid status

A number of measures can be used to assess deficiency of essential fatty acids. In serum cholesterol esters fatty acid determination is related to recent intake, in erythrocyte membranes to intake of the previous 2–3 months, and in subcutaneous fat tissue to intake of fatty acids over a period of more than a year. Essential fatty acids are measured by gas–liquid chromatography.

Vitamin nutritional status

Vitamin A (retinol) status can be assessed in the liver and plasma. The best method is determination in the liver, but hepatic biopsy is very invasive and unsuitable in population studies. Plasma retinol is usually measured by HPLC after separation from its carrier (RBP), but its marginal values do not always reflect status because of homeostatic control and confounding effects (e.g. protein–energy malnutrition, zinc deficiency, liver disorders, infection, parasitic diseases, chronic alcoholism). Isotope dilution methods are considered satisfactory, but further investigations are needed.

In connection with vitamin A, its provitamins, the carotenoids, need some consideration. Beta-carotene and a few other carotenoids play an independent and specific role in preventing oxidation, genotoxicity and malignancy. The plasma level of most relevant carotenoids is measured by HPLC. Confounding effects of diet and season, sex and age, smoking and drinking habits are reported.

Vitamin D status is generally assessed by measurement of serum 25-hydroxycholecalciferol (25-OHD); other vitamin D metabolites are not considered reliable indicators of vitamin D status. The most prevalent test for 25-OHD in serum is by competitive protein-binding assay. The HPLC method with UV detection can be used as an alternative. Confounding effects of seasons, age, sex, drugs, liver and renal diseases are reported.

Vitamin E status can be assessed in plasma, erythrocytes, platelets and adipose tissue. The most common and practical measure is α-tocopherol in plasma by HPLC. Because α-tocopherol is bound to lipoproteins it is preferred to express plasma α-tocopherol relative to serum cholesterol (as μmol $mmol^{-1}$). The determination of α-tocopherol in adipose tissue biopsy provides information on long-term nutritional status, but this test is too invasive. Confounding effects of chronic enteropathies, protein–energy malnutrition, haemolitic anaemia, cholestatic liver disease, some drugs and heavy metals are reported.

Vitamin K status requires a multiple approach including a functional test. The determination of plasma phylloquinone by reversed-phase HPLC using postcolumn chemical reduction followed by fluorometric detection is still in use. More recently determination of the serum undercarboxylated form of protrombin (PIVKA-II) by enzyme-linked immunosorbent assay (ELISA) and urinary γ-carboxyglutamic acid (Gla) by HPLC with fluorometric detection have been proposed. Confounding effects of age, sex, malfunction of gastrointestinal tract, osteoporosis, liver diseases, antibiotics and other drugs are reported.

Thiamin status can be assessed by urinary excretion and erythrocyte thiamin pyrophosphate (TPP) tests. Thiamin urinary excretion is indicative of recent dietary intake; thiamin is detected fluorometrically after conversion to thiochrome. If 24 h urine cannot be collected, thiamin should be determined in the fasting morning urine and expressed in relation to creatinine concentration. Erythrocyte TPP is indicative of long-term nutritional status and is assessed by HPLC using fluorometric detection after precolumn derivatization to thiochrome pyrophosphate. The only limitation is TPP instability and determination should be carried out within 2 h of drawing blood. Erythrocyte TPP levels present large interindividual variation, probably as a result of con-

founding factors (age and sex, alcohol intake, smoking habits, physical activity and drugs).

Riboflavin status can be assessed by urinary excretion and whole blood FAD tests. Riboflavin urinary excretion is indicative of recent dietary intake; riboflavin is measured by HPLC using fluorometric detection. As for thiamin, if fasting morning urine is collected, riboflavin value is expressed in relation to mmol of creatinine. Confounding effects of physical activity, bed rest, chronic alcoholism, antibiotics and other drugs are reported. Whole blood FAD is considered a reliable indicator of long-term nutritional status and is assessed by reversed-phase HPLC using fluorometric detection. This test presents some advantages over the functional erythrocyte glutathione reductase activation coefficient (EGR-AC) test (see later).

Vitamin B_6 status is generally assessed by urinary 4-pyridoxic acid (4-PA) and whole blood or plasma pyridoxal-5′-phosphate (PLP) tests. The 4-PA test is indicative of recent intake but also of a deep compartment with slow elimination rate. 4-PA is measured by reversed-phase HPLC using fluorescence detection. When the completeness of 24 h collection is impossible, 4-PA is expressed in relation to mmol of creatinine. PLP in whole blood or plasma is considered to be an indicator of depletion of vitamin B_6 reserves. In whole blood PLP can be measured by reversed-phase HPLC using fluorometric detection. Plasma PLP can be measured by radioenzymatic assay, which is more sensitive than other methods of analysis. Confounding effects of age and sex, tissue injury, catabolic state, smoking habits, chronic alcoholism, pregnancy, drugs, physical exercise, organic diseases and some inborn errors of metabolism are reported.

Niacin status can be assessed by measuring the two end products N'-methylnicotinamide (N'-MN) and N'-methyl-2-pyridone-5-carboxamine (2-pyridone) in urine by HPLC. The ratio of these two urinary products is considered to be the best index of niacin nutritional status. Other major metabolites of nicotinamide have been assessed by HPLC; their value for nutritional status assessment needs further investigation.

Folate status can be assessed by serum folate, which provides information on recent intake, and erythrocyte folate, which is indicative of body folate stores and long-term nutritional status. Folate is measured by radioassay kits, sometimes simultaneously with vitamin B_{12}. Less practical, although more accurate, are microbiological assays. In a EC-Flair programme intercomparison study it was observed that radioassay tends to overestimate serum folate and presents a considerable between-kit variability; improved standardization of diagnostic kits and the provision of suitable reference material were demanded. Confounding effects of starvation, dietary folate intake, alcohol abuse, pregnancy, smoking habits and drugs are reported for serum folate; iron deficiency, age and other disease states are confounding factors for erythrocyte folate.

Vitamin B_{12} status can be assessed by measuring serum or plasma total cobalamins by competitive protein-binding assay. Kits are available to measure folate simultaneously. Microbiological assays tend to give lower results. Confounding effects of age, sex, impaired absorption by some diseases or drugs, myeloproliferative disorders, worm infestations and severe liver disease are reported. Serum holotranscobalamin II has been reported as a sensitive indicator of tissue depletion, but further investigations are needed.

Biotin status can be assessed in whole blood by microbiological assay. Radioimmunoassay tests are also available, not only for plasma but also for urine. These tests give slightly enhanced values compared with microbiological assay.

Vitamin C status can be assessed by ascorbic acid in plasma, buffy coat, erythrocytes and leucocytes. Ascorbic acid in plasma is considered to be indicative of the amount available to tissues, in buffy coat it is indicative of the intracellular content, in erythrocytes it presents great variability, and in leucocytes (particularly polymorphonuclear) it is believed to be a good indicator of tissue store. For ascorbic acid determination a dinitrophenylhydrazine assay and a more practical HPLC micromethod are available. Confounding effects of acute stress, infection, surgery, smoking habits, chronic alcoholism, sex and drugs are reported. The urinary excretion of ascorbic acid is an index of recent intake; because of instability of the collected sample the determination is limited to special cases.

Essential mineral and trace element nutritional status

Sodium and potassium in plasma have little meaning in nutritional terms; total body Na or K are measured by radioisotope dilution.

Calcium status can be assessed by measuring serum or plasma ionized calcium or indirectly by measuring bone mass and bone density. Plasma ionized calcium provides information on physiological function and is measured by a calcium-selective electrode; bone calcium content is an index of body calcium stores and is measured by neutron activation analysis or dual-photon absorptiometry. Confounding effects of venous stasis, cardiac arrest, large volumes of citrated blood infusion and high or low pH are reported for plasma ionized calcium.

Magnesium status can be assessed by measuring magnesium in serum, erythrocytes, leucocytes and urine. Serum magnesium is the method most commonly used. Confounding effects of haemolysis, energetic exercise and pregnancy are reported. Erythrocyte magnesium is indicative of long-term status. Confounding effects of age, thyroid disease and premenstrual tension are reported. Urinary magnesium is used as an indicator of magnesium deficiency after a load test. Some precautions are necessary for this test. Magnesium is measured by flame atomic absorption spectroscopy (AAS) or automated colorimetric methods.

Iron status is assessed in relation to three stages of development of iron-deficient anaemia. At the first stage, to evaluate the size of body iron stores, serum or plasma ferritin can be measured by radiometric methods, or better still using the more recent ELISA. Confounding effects of infection, liver and malignant diseases, acute leukaemia, Hodgkin's disease, rheumatoid arthritis, thalassaemia major, age and sex are reported. At the second stage, to indicate the adequacy of iron supply to the erythroid marrow, serum iron (by colorimetric or AAS methods), plasma or serum iron-binding capacity (TIBC by colorimetric or radioactive methods), erythrocyte protoporphyrin (EPP by specific haematofluorometer) and serum transferrin receptor (by ELISA developed with monoclonal antibodies) are measured. Confounding effects of infection, chronic alcoholism, deficiencies of folate and vitamins B_6, B_{12} and C, acute viral hepatitis, malignancy, shock and physical trauma are reported for serum iron; infection, protein–energy malnutrition, alcoholic cirrhosis, malignancy, nephrotic syndromes, enteropathy, pregnancy, viral hepatitis are reported for total iron-binding capacity; infection, lead poisoning and porphyrin disorders are reported for erythrocyte protoporphyrin. At the third stage, as indicators of iron-deficiency anaemia, haemoglobin (by spectrophotometry or automatically with an electronic counter), haematocrit or packed cell volume (by specially designed centrifuge or an electronic counter) and red cell indices (mean cell volume (MCV) and mean corpuscular haemoglobin (MCH), both by electronic counter) are measured. Confounding effects of chronic infection, deficiencies of folate and vitamin B_{12}, chronic diseases, haemoglobinopathies, parasitosis, sex, altitude and smoking habits are reported. All the tests of the third stage present low sensitivity and, for the confounding factors, low specificity. The measure of serum transferrin receptor seems a promising technique for the evaluation of iron deficiency or toxicity because it presents some advantages in regard to serum ferritin. The assessment of both variables is considered valuable in screening iron deficiency. Because the measure of only one variable is not enough for the assessment of a mild iron deficiency, and also to avoid other limitations, it is recommended to combine two or more independent variables.

Zinc status can be assessed by using AAS to measure zinc in plasma or serum, leucocyte and leucocyte subsets, urine, hair, nails and saliva. Plasma or serum zinc is the method most commonly used. Many precautions are required in sample collection to avoid haemolysis and contamination. There are also many pathophysiological conditions that can negatively influence specificity and sensitivity of serum zinc. Leucocyte subset zinc, and particularly monocyte zinc, is considered a useful indicator of zinc deficiency, but monocyte separation is rather difficult and quite a large blood sample must be collected. Zinc in other fluids or tissues is not considered a useful or reliable indicator of zinc deficiency.

Copper status is most frequently assessed in serum or plasma by AAS, even if this measure is of low sensitivity or specificity in the general population. Levels of copper in other tissues or fluids are difficult to assess or are not considered valid indices of copper status. Confounding effects of infection, pregnancy, leukaemia, Hodgkin's disease, some anaemias, myocardial infarction, malabsorption, ulcerative colitis, Wilson's disease, high level physical activity, age and sex are reported.

Selenium status is usually assessed measuring plasma or serum selenium by AAS with a Zeeman background correction and also by a fluorometric technique. While the plasma Se determination provides information on short-term Se status, the determination in whole blood or erythrocytes is indicative of long-term status. Confounding effects of some inborn errors of metabolism, congestive cardiomyopathy, age and some physiological conditions are reported. The determination of Se in urine presents some limitations and Se levels in hair and nails display some drawbacks.

Iodine status is generally assessed by measuring urinary iodine by a colorimetric method, which reflects iodine intake. If 24 h urine cannot be collected, iodine excretion can be expressed per g of creatinine. Better tests are the determinations of the thyroid hormones thyroxine (T_4) and $3,5,3'$-triiodothyroxine (T_3) and pituitary thyroid stimulating hormone (TSH) in serum by specific competitive radioimmunoassay methods (available in kits). In clinical settings the measurement of uptake of radioactive iodine is used.

Functional Tests

Functional tests are defined by Solomons as:

> those behavioural, physiological or biochemical functions of the organisms dependent on the adequate availability of a nutrient or responses to the regularity process to maintain body stores and harmonic internal distribution for those many nutrients that are homeostatically regulated by the organism.

The number of reliable and specific functional tests is still not very large; other simpler tests, not commonly used, lack specificity. Further studies are required on these tests because they are important for a correct assessment of nutritional status in humans.

Vitamin nutritional status

Vitamin A functional tests are the dark adaptation and the relative dose–response (RDR). The conventional dark adaptation test has been superseded by a rapid test which is more suitable for field studies. It is more specific and sensitive but of limited use in children. The relative dose–response test can provide information on liver store and is indicative of marginal status of vitamin A. It consists of the determination of plasma retinol level at baseline, administration of a small dose of retinyl acetate or retinyl palmitate, and a second determination of plasma retinol 5 h later. The response is related to the release from the liver of holo-RBP and in deficient subjects the plasma retinol will increase after 5 h. A modification of the RDR test has been proposed using an oral dose of 3,4-didehydroretinol (vitamin A_2), but its application to humans needs further investigation. Confounding effects of protein–energy malnutrition, malabsorption and liver disease are reported for RDR test.

The measurement of serum alkaline phosphatase activity can be used as a *vitamin D* functional test. The specificity is not very high and it is affected by age, sex, pregnancy and unrelated pathologies.

Vitamin E functional tests are the following peroxidative indices: erythrocyte haemolysis, erythrocyte malondialdehyde, breath pentane, susceptibility of low-density lipoprotein to oxidation and diene conjugate second derivatives. For the first two tests there are methodological limitations; for the other tests further experimentation is needed.

A *vitamin K* functional test which has been recently proposed is the serum determination of undercarboxylated osteocalcin by radioimmunoassay. This test is well correlated with static indices; further investigations are in progress.

A *thiamin* functional test which is commonly used is the erythrocyte transketolase activation coefficient (ETK-AC) test. Transketolase is a thiamin-dependent enzyme with a specific role in the glucose oxidative pathway. Transketolase activity in haemolysed erythrocytes (ETK) is measured either by disappearance of pentose or appearance of hexose by spectrophotometry. In the case of thiamin deficiency the quantity of hexose is reduced. When TPP is added to the reaction mixture the enzyme activity is enhanced in thiamin-deficient haemolysates only. The activation coefficient is given by the ratio of enhanced (with TPP addition) to basal (without TPP addition) activity. Because of some limitations, for a correct thiamin nutritional status, basal activity should be carried out together with the activation test. Automation of this test is available. Confounding effects of chronic ethanol exposure, conditions that reduce thiamin intake or absorption, uncontrolled diabetes, hyperparathyroidism, age, stress and also infections are reported. Because various methods of measurement have been proposed, in order to reach a better interpretation and comparison of results, the standardization of the procedure and the use of quality control samples on various occasions have been requested.

A *riboflavin* functional test which is commonly used is the erythrocyte glutathione reductase activation coefficient (EGR-AC) test. Glutathione reductase is a flavoenzyme with flavin adenine dinucleotide (FAD) as a prosthetic group. By measuring the EGR activity by spectrophotometry in erythrocyte haemolysate without FAD addition (basal) and with FAD addition (stimulated), the activation coefficient (that is the ratio of stimulated to basal activity) can be calculated. The higher the coefficient, the lower is the coenzyme content. Automation of this test is available. Confounding effects of glucose-6-phosphate dehydrogenase deficiency, severe uraemia, liver cirrhosis, biliary disorders, diabetes, thyroid diseases, congenital heart disease, chronic alcoholism, pyridoxine deficiency, stress and drugs are reported.

Vitamin B_6 functional tests are the erythrocyte aspartate aminotransferase activation coefficient (EAST-AC) test and the tryptophan load test. Erythrocyte aspartate aminotransferase activity is measured spectrophotometrically in erythrocyte haemolysate without PLP addition (basal) and with PLP addition (stimulated). The activation coefficient is given by the ratio of stimulated to basal activity. Automation of this test is available. Confounding effects of renal and liver diseases, cancer, coeliac disease, high protein diet, thiamin status, alcohol intake, stress and drugs are reported. The tryptophan load test was used in the past because vitamin B_6-dependent enzymes are involved in the conversion of tryptophan to niacin. After an appropriate loading

dose of tryptophan and under controlled conditions, vitamin B_6-deficient subjects excrete tryptophan metabolites (kynurenine, kynurenic acid, xanthurenic acid) in urine measured spectrophotometrically after thin-layer or ion exchange chromatography separation. Confounding effects of protein intake, exercise, pregnancy, some hormones and viral infections are reported.

Folate functional tests are the urinary formiminoglutamic acid (FIGLU), plasma homocysteine, lymphocyte deoxyuridine suppression (dU) and leucocyte lobe average tests. FIGLU acid is eliminated owing to the inhibition of the conversion of histidine to glutamic acid in folate deficiency. However the specificity of this test is low and its use limited. All the other tests are either too complex, not very specific, or require more investigation.

Vitamin B_{12} functional tests are the urinary/serum methylmalonate (MMA), lymphocyte deoxyuridine suppression (dU) and serum homocysteine tests. Methylmalonic acid increases in vitamin B_{12} deficiency; the loading with valine or isoleucine produces a marked increase in both urine and serum. Methylmalonic acid is measured by gas–liquid chromatography. The other tests are not very specific or are too complex.

Vitamin C functional tests are considered to be the lingual vitamin C and intradermal 2,6-dichlorphenolindophenol solution tests. The time to decolorize this solution is inversely correlated with plasma vitamin C levels. However in humans both methods have low precision. The Hess test, which measures capillary fragility, is not specific of vitamin C deficiency.

Zinc functional tests are serum or plasma alkaline phosphatase, taste acuity and serum thymulin tests. Alkaline phosphatase is a zinc metalloenzyme; rather than being indicative of zinc deficiency, it is considered to be of some value after zinc supplementation. Taste acuity is impaired in zinc deficiency; to measure this test, four taste qualities (salt, sweet, bitter, sour) and detection and recognition thresholds for evaluation of each taste quality are used. If the assessment is carried out carefully, this test is reliable and valid for marginal zinc deficiency. Serum thymulin activity is decreased in zinc deficiency because it needs zinc to maintain its structure. This test needs further investigation.

Copper functional tests are serum caeruloplasmin and erythrocyte superoxide dismutase (SOD) tests. The measure of serum caeruloplasmin, an acute phase reactant protein, is based on its oxidase activity on various substrates. Confounding effects of exercise, stress, pregnancy, trauma, malignancy, nephrosis, advanced liver disease and drugs are reported. Cu,Zn-superoxide dismutase is a cytosolic metalloprotein which catalyses reduction of superoxide to hydrogen peroxide and oxygen. It is considered to be a better indicator of reduced copper status than serum copper or caeruloplasmin. The determination presents analytical problems and the methods available are not uniformly standardized. Thus the results from different laboratories cannot be easily compared. Confounding effects of Down syndrome, uraemia, various anemies, Duchenne muscular dystrophy, glutathione reductase deficiency and porphyria are reported.

Selenium functional tests are plasma, erythrocyte and platelet glutathione peroxidase activity tests (GSF-px). The plasma GSH-px is a useful index only in populations with low Se intake; it responds rapidly to supplementation. Erythrocyte GSH-px presents a plateau at $1.77\ \mu mol\ l^{-1}$ above which it is independent of Se status. In addition, erythrocyte GSH-px responds slowly to depletion and supplementation. Platelet GSH-px responds rapidly to Se dietary changes and presents the maximum activity at Se levels of $1.25–1.45\ \mu mol\ l^{-1}$. Accordingly it is considered to be a sensitive indicator of changing Se status. Confounding effects of age and sex, physical activity, deficiencies of essential fatty acids, vitamin B_{12} and iron, and stress from antioxidants are reported.

Choice of Laboratory Tests

The choice of laboratory test will depend on the type of study to be carried out.

In field nutritional epidemiology studies, particularly in developing countries, the number of tests will be limited by the sample size, the suspected prevalence of deficiencies, the local laboratory possibilities, the availability of skilled personnel and economic resources. In general the following common tests can be suggested: haemoglobin, haematocrit, serum iron, total iron-binding capacity, serum ferritin, blood protoporphyrin, serum albumin, plasma transport proteins and serum zinc. For specific reasons serum retinol, other vitamins in blood or urine, some hormones (thyroxine, TSH) and minerals (urinary iodine) can be added.

In population studies to be carried out in developed countries with high-level laboratory facilities, the selection of laboratory tests depends on the purpose of the study, sample size and financial resources. The assessment of protein status is generally limited to plasma transport proteins, unless there are other specific reasons for other variables. Essential fatty acid status is assessed in lipid pattern studies; the choice of test is determined by the interest in recent intake or long-term status. In association with this test serum cholesterol, triacylglycerols and also lipoprotein fractions are measured. The selection of micronutrient tests can be determined by the suspected deficiencies from previous dietary surveys; in the absence of dietary data several tests should be conducted because preclinical deficiencies can be rather common in developed societies. A sensible selection can be found in **Table 1**.

In a hospital setting the selection of laboratory tests depends on the clinical conditions of patients at

Table 1 Summary of Flair Concerted Action No 10 recommended methods[a]

Micronutrient	Recommended method	'Best available' method	Promising method
Vitamin A		Serum retinol	RDR test
Carotenoids		Serum carotenoid profile	
Vitamin E	Lipid standardized serum α-tocopherol		
Vitamin D	Serum 25-OH-vitamin D		
Thiamin		ETK stimulation test	RBC TPP
Riboflavin	EGR stimulation test		
Vitamin B_6		Plasma PLP	
Vitamin B_{12}	Serum cobalamins		Serum MMA
Folate	RBC folate		Serum homocysteine
Vitamin C	Plasma vitamin C		
Selenium		Plasma selenium	RBC GSHPx
Iron	Serum ferritin		Transferrin receptors
Copper		Serum copper	RBC SOD
Zinc		Serum zinc	RBC metallothionein

[a]From van den Berg H, Heseker H, Lamand M, Sandstrom B and Thurnam D (1993) Flair Concerted Action No. 10 Status Papers – Introduction, Conclusions and Recommendations. *International Journal for Vitamin and Nutrition Research* **63**: 247–251, with permission.

admission and during the subsequent course of injury or illness. Because protein–energy malnutrition may be present in some cases, protein status should be assessed using laboratory tests for serum albumin, plasma transport proteins and urinary creatinine and 3-methylhistidine, as also other acute-phase proteins. Using some of the above values associated with other variables (immunological functions, anthropometric measurements), indices relating nutritional status to clinical outcome can be computed. Among hospital patients, vitamin and trace element deficiencies are also rather common; the determination of deficient variables suspected on the basis of history and physical examination is suggested.

Because on various occasions large differences in interlaboratory comparisons and ring tests have been observed, it is essential in the selection of laboratory tests to favour standardized and validated methods for which a careful collection and handling of samples is compulsory and also appropriate quality control.

Evaluation of Laboratory Indices

Reference values are, in general, population-specific; accordingly each main laboratory in homogeneous areas has to derive them from a clinically healthy reference population selected using very careful criteria. These values should preferably be given in percentiles.

Cut-off points for an appropriate interpretation of results are usually derived statistically from reference values. A current procedure for constructing cut-off point consists of determining the biochemical values which correspond to the earliest determinable physiological, metabolic, functional and morphological alterations. Such an approach has been followed only in a very few cases, and consequently most available cut-off points should be considered as tentative.

For albumin the guidelines for interpretation suggested in 1974 are still in use. For children and adults, values <28 g l^{-1} are indicative of a deficient (high-risk) status and for pregnant women this value is <30 g l^{-1}. A marginal (moderate risk) status is indicated by the following values: infants, <25 g l^{-1}; children 1–5 years, <30 g l^{-1}; children 6–17 years, <35 g l^{-1}; adults, 28–34 g l^{-1}; pregnant women at first trimester, 30–39 g l^{-1}; pregnant women at second and third trimester, 30–34 g l^{-1}. All values above the moderate risk are indicative of an acceptable (low-risk) status.

Reference values for transport proteins are provided by plate producers. Tentatively 0.10 g l^{-1} for prealbumin and 25 mg l^{-1} for retinol-binding protein are considered indicative of protein deficiency. For transferrin values below 1 g l^{-1} are considered indicative of severe protein depletion; marginal status values are between 1 and 2 g l^{-1}.

For the interpretation of serum phospholipid essential fatty acid values Holman considered the ratio $C_{20:3\ n-9} : C_{20:4\ n-6}$ above 0.2 the upper limit of 'normalcy'. For deficiency this value is grater than 0.4. Because of advanced methods of determination now available, a revision of the above criteria is compulsory.

The current cut-off points of the most widely used micronutrient tests in adults are reported in **Table 2**.

Cut-off points are different in other physiological conditions (children, pregnant and lactating women, the elderly). These values can be found in reference texts. For antioxidant vitamins and provitamins to prevent chronic diseases the following *optimal plasma levels* have been proposed: retinol, >2.5 µmol l^{-1}; β-carotene, >0.40 µmol l^{-1}; α-tocopherol, >30 µmol l^{-1}; ascorbic acid, >50 µmol l^{-1}.

Confounding Effects of Infection on Laboratory Assessment

As already indicated, many confounding effects of infection have been observed in many laboratory tests for nutritional status assessment. This problem will now be examined in more depth.

For protein status confounding effects of infection are reported for almost all laboratory tests, excluding that for total serum protein. In particular serum albumin, plasma transport protein and fibronectin levels decrease because of the increase of acute-phase proteins.

For vitamin A, severe systemic infections (e.g. pneumonia, bronchitis, diarrhoea, septicaemia, rheumatic and scarlet fever) cause a marked decrease of serum retinol level. This decrease can be due to various factors (e.g. increased retinol excretion in urine, reduced liver release of retinol and RBP to plasma). A reduction of vitamin A liver reserves assessed by the RDR test has been observed in children with chicken pox.

Tests for thiamin status can be confounded by infections that prevent normal absorption (diarrhoea, dysentery) or increase the requirement (fever).

For vitamin B_{12}, fish tapeworm or hookworm infestations give a low level of serum vitamin B_{12} because of their preferential consumption of this vitamin.

For vitamin C, acute and chronic infections can depress markedly serum ascorbic acid level owing to a decrease of vitamin C reserves.

Table 2 Cut-off points for interpretation of results of micronutrient tests in adults[a]

	Severe deficiency	Marginal deficiency	Physiological level or range
Liver retinol (μmol g^{-1})	<0.17	0.17–0.70	>0.70
P retinol (μmol l^{-1})	<0.35	0.35–0.70	>0.70
Relative dose–response (%)		>20	<20
S 25-OHD (nmol l^{-1})	<12.5		
P/S α-tocopherol (μmol l^{-1})	<11.6	11.6–16.2	>16.2
P α-tocopherol (μmol l^{-1b})	<9.25	9.25–13.9	>13.9
E TPP (nmol l^{-1})	<120	120–150	>150
U thiamin (μg per 24 h)	<27	27–65	>66
ETK-AC[c]	>1.25	1.15–1.25	1.00–1.15
E FAD (nmol l^{-1})	<200		
U riboflavin (μg per g creatinine)	<27	27–79	>80
EGR-AC[c]	>1.4	1.2–1.4	<1.2
EGR-AC[b]	>1.30	1.20–1.30	<1.20
P PLP (mmol l^{-1})	<20		20–86
U 4-PA (nmol per mmol creatinine)			128–680
EAST-AC[bc]	>1.80	1.70–1.80	<1.70
P cyanocobalamin (pmol l^{-1b})	<110	110–150	>150
S TCII (pmol l^{-1})	<15		
S methylmalonic acid (μmol l^{-1})	>1		
S homocysteine (μmol l^{-1})	>20		
P folate (nmol l^{-1b})	<5.7	5.7–11.4	>11.4
	<7		
L lobe average	>3.6		
P biotin (nmol l^{-1b})	<0.5	0.5–1.0	>1.0
P ascorbic acid (μmol l^{-1b})	<11.4	11.4–17	>17
B ascorbic acid (μmol l^{-1})	<17	17–27	>28
L ascorbic acid (nmol per 10^8 cells)		53–95	114–301
S/P ferritin (μg l^{-1})	<12	20	100
S iron (μmol l^{-1})	<10.7	20	
S TIBC (μmol l^{-1})	<71.6		
E PP (μmol l^{-1})	<1.24		
Haemoglobin (g l^{-1})			
M	<130		
F	<120		
Haematocrit (%)			
M	<40		
F	<36		
MCV	<80		
P Zn (μmol l^{-1})	<9		9–22
Mixed *L* Zn (ng per 10^6 cells)	<4.5		5–8
P/S copper (μmol l^{-1})			13–22
S caeruloplasmin (μmol l^{-1})			2–4
P Se (μmol l^{-1})	0.25–0.38	0.63–0.76	0.76–1.52
E Se (μmol l^{-1})	~0.45		1.13–2.41

Abbreviations: *P*, plasma; *S*, serum; *E*, erythrocyte; *U*, urine; *L*, leucocytes; *B*, whole blood.
[a]From van den Berg H, Heseker H, Lamand M, Sandstrom B and Thurnam D (1993) Flair Concerted Action No. 10 Status Papers. *International Journal for Vitamin and Nutrition Research* **63**: 252–316, with permission.
[b]From Benton D, Haller J and Fordy J (1997) The vitamin status of young British adults. *International Journal for Vitamin and Nutrition Research* **67**: 34–40, with permission.
[c]The percentage stimulation is now very seldom used. It can be calculated as follow: (AC $\times$ 100) $-$ 100.

For iron status tests, infection induces an increase of serum ferritin and blood protoporphyrin levels and a decrease of serum iron-binding capacity, serum iron and haemoglobin.

Zinc status tests are influenced by acute and chronic infections. A decrease of plasma zinc has been reported, owing initially to redistribution of zinc within the body tissues, and then to a negative body balance. This is due to anorexia, which reduces dietary intake, and also to increased losses via the faeces (diarrhoea), sweat and urine.

Regarding copper status tests, infection gives a rise in serum copper level because leucocytic endogenous mediator (LEM) induces an increase of serum caeruloplasmin.

Trauma, surgery, burns and inflammatory diseases

present similar confounding effects to infection on laboratory assessment.

See also: **Alcohol**: Effects of Alcohol Consumption on Diet and Nutritional Status. **Alcoholism**: Effects on Nutritional Status. **Ascorbic Acid**: Physiology, Dietary Sources and Requirements. **Biotin**: Physiology, Dietary Sources and Requirements. **Carotenoids**: Chemistry, Sources and Physiology. **Cholecalciferol and Ergocalciferol**: Physiology, Dietary Sources and Requirements. **Cobalamins**: Physiology, Dietary Sources and Requirements. **Copper**: Physiology, Dietary Sources and Requirements. **Folic Acid**: Physiology, Dietary Sources and Requirements. **Infection**: Nutritional Interactions. **Iodine**: Physiology, Dietary Sources and Requirements. **Iron**: Physiology, Dietary Sources and Requirements. **Magnesium**: Physiology, Dietary Sources and Requirements. **Niacin**: Physiology, Dietary Sources and Requirements. **Potassium**: Physiology, Dietary Sources and Requirements. **Protein**: Deficiency. **Retinol**: Physiology. **Riboflavin**: Physiology. **Selenium**: Physiology, Dietary Sources and Requirements. **Thiamin**: Physiology. **Tocopherols**: Physiology. **Vitamin B$_6$**: Physiology. **Vitamin K**: Physiology. **Zinc**: Physiology.

Further Reading

Brody T (1994) *Nutritional Biochemistry*. San Diego: Academic Press.

Christakis G (1973) Nutritional assessment in health programs. *American Journal of Public Health* 63:November supplement.

Fidanza F (1991) *Nutritional Status Assessment – A Manual for Population Studies*. London: Chapman & Hall.

Gibson RS (1990) *Principles of Nutritional Assessment*. New York: Oxford University Press.

lyengar GV (1989) *Elemental Analysis of Biological System*. Boca Raton: CRC Press.

Jelliffe DB and Jelliffe EFP (1989) *Community Nutritional Assessment – With Special Reference to Less Technically Developed Countries*. Oxford: Oxford University Press.

Jensen TG, Englert DAM and Dudrick SJ (1983) *Nutritional Assessment – A Manual for Practitioners*. Norwalk, CT: Appleton-Century-Croft.

Report of the International Nutritional Anemia Consulative Group (1985) *Measurements of Iron Status*. Washington DC: Nutrition Foundation.

Sauberlich HE, Dowdy RP and Skala JH (1974) *Laboratory Tests for the Assessment of Nutritional Status*. Cleveland: CRC Press.

Sommer A, West KR (1996) *Vitamin A Deficiency: Health, Survival and Vision*. Cary (NC): Oxford University Press.

van den Berg H, Heseker H, Lamand M, Sandstrom B and Thurnam D (1993) Flair Concerted Action No. 10 Status Papers. *International Journal for Vitamin and Nutrition Research* 63:247–316.

Wright R and Heymsfield S (1984) *Nutritional Assessment*. Boston: Blackwell Scientific.

Clinical Examination

M Meguid and **A Laviano**, SUNY Health Science Center, New York, USA

The prognosis of a primary medical disorder significantly influences the direction of the patient's clinical course. Concomitant malnutrition greatly enhances the risk of serious complication and prejudices ultimate survival. If this association is causative, the prevention or correction of nutrient depletion can minimize or eliminate malnutrition-related morbidity and mortality. Thus, the main purpose for assessing a patient's nutritional status is to:

1. identify patients who have, or are at risk of developing, protein–energy malnutrition or specific nutrient deficiencies;
2. quantify a patient's risk of developing malnutrition-related medical complications;
3. monitor the adequacy of nutritional therapy.

The problem of malnutrition in hospitalized patients and of its consequences on clinical outcome was highlighted by several publications in the 1970s. Surprisingly, after more than two decades, malnutrition in hospitalized patients is still a significant issue, adversely affecting patients' outcome.

As outlined in **Fig. 1**, malnutrition is a continuum that starts with inadequate nutrient intake, followed by a progressive series of metabolic, functional and body compositional changes. Unfortunately, defining and quantitating the degree of nutritional depletion, particularly in terms of protein–energy malnutrition diagnosis, is an unsettled topic. Indeed, the ability to use nutrition assessment to predict clinical outcome can be problematic because the interaction between malnutrition and other factors that influence outcome makes it difficult to isolate the specific contribution from malnutrition alone. Therefore, the presence of malnutrition can participate in determining a poor clinical outcome, or may simply be associated with a poor outcome if the disease *per se* affects markers of nutritional status. Moreover, as recently stated by the advisory committee appointed jointly by the National Institutes of Health, The American Society for Parenteral and Enteral Nutrition, and The American Society for Clinical Nutrition:

there is no gold standard for determining nutritional status because: a) there is no universally accepted

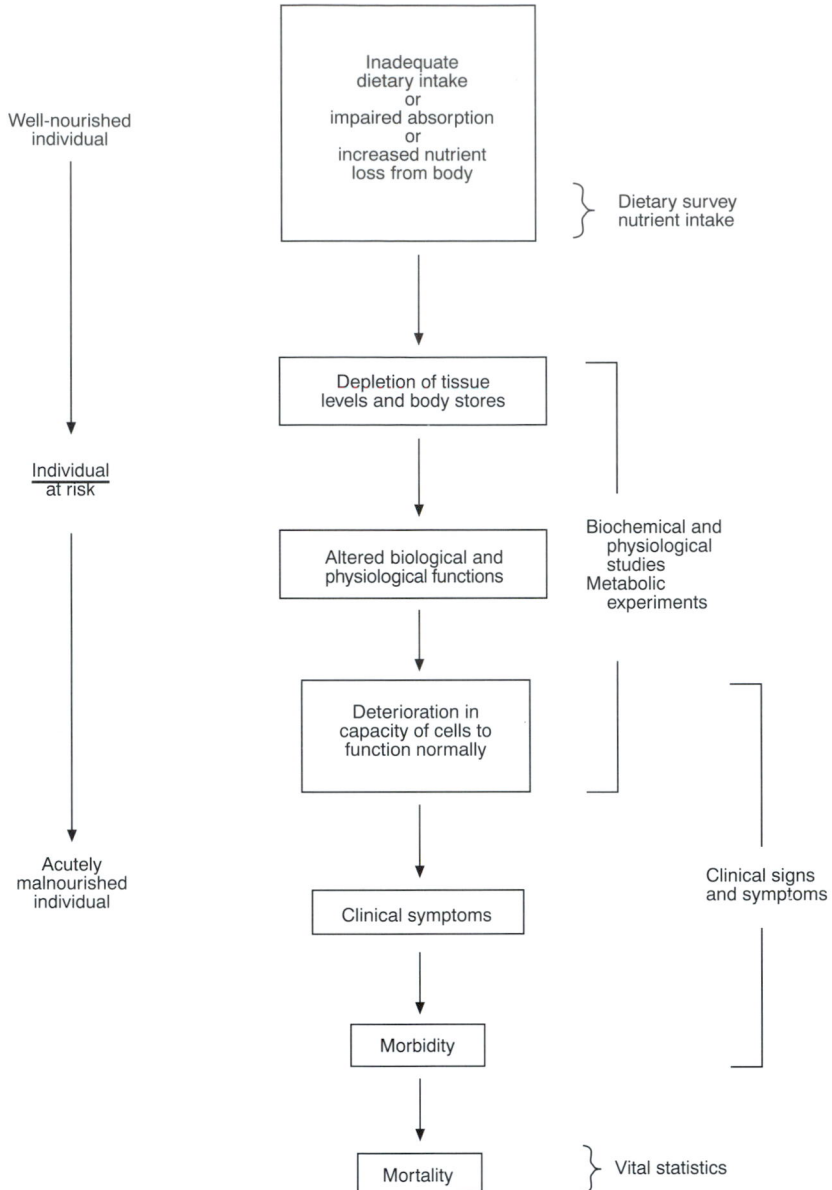

Figure 1 Sequence of events leading to the precipitation of clinically significant nutritional disease and the methods used to assess nutritional status. Modified from Beaton and Bengoa (1976) Nutrition in Preventive Medicine; Geneva: World Health Organization.

definition of malnutrition; b) all current assessment parameters are affected by illness and injury; c) it is difficult to isolate the effect of malnutrition from the influence of the disease on clinical outcome; and d) it is not clear which of the commonly used nutrition assessment techniques is the most reliable because of the paucity of comparative data.

Medical History and Physical Examination

On admission to the hospital, the patient's history is reviewed to help identify factors adversely affecting nutritional status. These include psychosocial factors (i.e. substance and/or alcohol abuse): duration, degree and severity of the current illness as it may affect appetite, food intake and physical activity; medications which a patient is taking; and a history of past operations and therapies. The clinical assessment of nutritional status requires a focused history, physical examination, and selected laboratory tests aimed at detecting specific nutrient deficiencies and patients who are at high risk for future nutritional abnormalities. Unfortunately, the ability of this approach reliably to identify patients at increased risk for medical complications has not been evaluated in clinical studies.

More data are available on the subjective global assessment (SGA). Controlled studies have suggested that SGA, based on comprehensive history, physical examination and clinical acumen, is superior to a single nutritional index in predicting the development of nutritionally associated complications. The prediction is based on: (1) past nutritional intake, disease process, operative effect on future intake of nutrients, catabolic disease (if present); and (2) the current physical state as regards weight loss, muscle wasting, functional status, oedema, skin rash and neuropathy. The findings of the history and physical examination are subjectively weighted to rank patients as being well-nourished, moderately malnourished or severely malnourished, and is used to predict their risk for medical complications. The use of SGA in evaluating hospitalized patients has been shown to give reproducible results with more than 80% agreement when two blinded observers assessed the same patient. In prospective studies, SGA has been shown to be a good predictor of complications in general surgical patients, patients undergoing liver transplantation and patients on dialysis. In one study, preoperative SGA was found to be a better predictor of postoperative infectious complications than serum albumin, serum transferrin, DCH, anthropometry, creatinine-height index and the prognostic nutritional index.

Combining SGA with some of the 'traditional' markers of nutritional status, such as serum albumin, DCH and creatinine-height index, increased (from 82% to 90%) the ability to identify patients who developed complications, but also increased (from 25% to 30%) the percentage of patients identified as 'malnourished' but who did not develop a postoperative complication. Therefore, combining nutrition assessment techniques increases sensitivity but may also increase the number of patients who might receive unnecessary nutrition support.

The physical examination is performed to seek more subtle indications of nutritional deficiency reflected in changes of the patient's skin, hair, head, eyes, mouth, abdomen and extremities, as summarized in **Table 1**.

Nutritional Assessment of the Hospital Patient

On admission to the hospital, each patient undergoes an initial nutritional screening (an example is outlined in **Table 2**). Approximately 60% of patients pass this initial screen and, therefore, do not warrant aggressive nutritional intervention. In contrast, if a patient is admitted with any one of the diagnoses associated with a high frequency of malnutrition

(**Fig. 2**) or exhibits components, behaviours or physical manifestations of the malnutrition sequelae, then a high-risk nutritional assessment should be performed (an example is given in **Table 3**). The sum of the data obtained allows the patient's nutritional status to be identified in accordance with international classification of disease (ICD) standards (i.e. quantitates the type and extent of malnutrition), provides the basis for the calculation of energy/protein requirements, and also provides for the development of a rational nutritional treatment plan.

As outlined in Table 3, the step-by-step approach to the patient's comprehensive nutritional assessment is as follows:

Section A collects relevant medical data, which is usually obtained from the patient or by reviewing the patient's medical record.

Section B involves determination of patient's nutrient intake profile with emphasis on the presence or absence of anorexia, and the adequacy of their oral intake prior to admission. The pattern and the amount of alcohol consumption are also acertained because they influence the quality and quantity of oral intake, as well as vitamin and mineral status.

In Section C are recorded the anthropometric measurements, their calculation, and standardizations based on these measurements. Section C also includes questions about any known weight change and its corresponding time frame, and the notation of the patient's biochemical data.

Prognostic Value of Nutritional Assessment Indices

Most of the methods used for nutritional assessment are directed toward providing information regarding body composition (**Fig. 3**). The available methods range from routine bedside physical measurements, body weight, anthropometric measurements, and standard biochemical and immunological tests, to highly sophisticated techniques which are at present used primarily for research purposes. The most relevant parameters measured for determining nutritional status have been extensively discussed in other articles. This article examines them in terms of their prognostic value. Their limitations are also discussed.

Height and body weight

Height and body weight are practical and simple measures of total body components, as well as of frame size. The correct procedure for their determination is as follows.

- *Height.* The patient stands without shoes to full

Table 1 Physical symptoms of nutritional deficiency

Clinical finding	Deficiency
Hair	
-easily pluckable, sparse	Protein, biotin
-straight, dull	Protein
-coiled, keratinized	Vitamin A
Skin	
-xerosis	Essential fatty acids
-petechiae	Vitamin A, vitamin C
-pigmentation/desquamation	Niacin
-follicular keratosis	Vitamin A
-'flaky-paint' dermatitis	Protein
-seborrheic dermatitis	Essential fatty acids, pyridoxine, zinc, biotin, riboflavin in infants
-dermatitis	Biotin, possibly manganese
-poor tissue turgor	Water
-purpura	Vitamin C, vitamin K
-perifollicular haemorrhage	Vitamin C
-pallor	Folacin, iron, B_{12}, copper, biotin
-ecchymoses	Vitamin C, vitamin K
-pressure sores	Protein–energy
-poor wound healing	Protein–ergy, zinc, and possibly essenttial fatty acids
-dry scaling	Nonspecific
-thickening of skin	Essential fatty acids
Eyes	
-dull (dry-xerosis), conjunctiva	Vitamin A
-blepharitis	B complex
-Bitot's spot	Vitamin A
-corneal vascularization	Riboflavin
-photophobia	Zinc
Lips and oral structures	
-angular fissures, scars, stomatitis	B complex, iron, protein, riboflavin
-cheilosis	B_6 niacin, riboflavin, protein
-ageusia, dysgeusia	Zinc
-swollen, spongy, bleeding gums	Ascorbic acid
Tongue	
-magenta	Riboflavin
-fissuring, raw	Niacin
-glossitis	Pyridoxine, folacin, iron, B_{12}
-increased size, swelling	Iodine, niacin
-fiery, red	Folacin, B_{12}
-pale	Iron, B_{12}
-atrophic lingual papillae	Riboflavin, niacin, iron
Teeth	
-tooth decay	Fluorine
-loss of dental fillings, dental caries	Vitamin C
Glands	
-parotid enlargement	Protein
-'sicca' syndrome	Ascorbic acid
-thyroid enlargement	Iodine
-hypogonadism, delayed puberty	Zinc
Nails	
-spoon-shaped (koilonychia)	Chromium, iron
-brittle, ridged, lined	Nonspecific

Table 1 Continued

Clinical finding	Deficiency
Heart	
-tachycardia, cardiomegaly, congestive heart failure	Thiamin
-decreased cardiac function	Phosphorus
-cardiac arrhythmias	Magnesium, potassium
-cardiomyopathy	Selenium
-small heart, decreased output, bradycardia	Protein–energy
-sudden failure, death	Ascorbic acid, thiamin
Abdomen	
-hepatomegaly (fatty liver)	Protein
-wasting	Energy
-enlarged spleen	Iron
Bones and joints	
-epiphyseal thickening, deformities	Vitamin D
-bone pain	Calcium
Muscle, extremities	
-wasting	Protein–energy
-pain in calves, weak thighs	Thiamin
-edema	Protein, thiamin
-muscular twitching	Pyridoxine
-muscular pains	Biotin, selenium
-muscular weakness	Sodium, potassium
-muscular cramps	Sodium, chloride
Neurological	
-ophthalmoplegia, foot-drop	Thiamin
-disorientation	Thiamin, sodium, water
-decreased position, vibratory sense, ataxia, optic neuritis	B_{12}
-weakness, paraesthesia of legs	Thiamin, pyridoxine
-hyporeflexia	Thiamin
-mental disorders	Niacin, magnesium, B_{12}
-convulsions	Pyridoxine, calcium, thiamin (infants), magnesium, phosphorus
-depression, lethargy	Biotin, folacin, vitamin C
-sleep disturbances, impaired coordination	Pantothenic acid
-nonketonic hyperosmolar syndrome	Sodium
-aphonia	Thiamin
-hyperaesthesia	Bitotin
-peripheral neuropathy	Pyridoxine
Other	
-diarrhoea	Niacin, folacin, B_{12}
-delayed wound healing and tissue repair	Vitamin C, zinc, protein–energy
-anaemia, pallor	Vitamin E, pyridoxine, B_{12}, iron, folacin, biotin, copper
-anorexia	B_{12}, chloride, sodium, thiacmin, vitamin C
-nausea	Biotin, pantothenic acid

This table was compiled from numerous sources.

height on a flat surface. If the patient is unable to stand or has kyphoscoliosis, a crown-to-heel length is measured and compared with the patient's stated height. An alternative method which can be used to estimate height is to measure the distance between the tip of one middle finger of the right hand to the tip of the other middle finger of the left hand with the patient's arms fully extended and the hands facing forward. Height should be recorded in cm.

- *Weight*. The patient stands on a scale wearing a light hospital gown, pajamas or nightgown. Bed scales should be used if patient is unable to stand. Weight is recorded in kg.

Table 2 Initial nutritional screening form

Admission date _____

Dx/CC: _____

_____

Current diet Rx: _____   Diet PTA: _____

Ht. _____cm Wt. _____kg   (Date)_____   Usual Wt. _____kg

IBW. _____kg   Wt. change _____kg   In _____ Days/Wks/Mos   Serum alb: (   )_____ mg l⁻¹

Appetite change: _____   Duration: _____

Chewing/swallowing problems: _____   Food intolerance: _____

Need for diet instruction: _____

Screening reviewed with dietitian: _____

☐ High-risk nutritional assessment by dietitian to follow.

☐ Nutritional status will be monitored.

Evaluation/Plan:

Screened by: _____   Date: _____

- *Wrist circumference to determine frame size.* This is measured with a tape just distal to styloid process of ulna and is recorded in cm.

Wrist circumference is used to determine frame size using the following calculation:

Circumference ratio (r) = height (cm)/wrist circumference (cm)

For males an r value >10.4 indicates a small frame, 10.4–9.6 a medium frame, and <9.6 a large frame. For females an r value >10.9 indicates a small frame, 10.9–9.9 a medium frame, and <9.9 a large frame.

Weight can be compared with an ideal or desirable weight. The ideal body weight range for height and frame size can be extrapolated from standardized tables developed by Metropolitan Life Insurance Company (see **Table 4**). Weight for height and frame size is related to somatic protein and/or fat stores. Interpretation of these data is as follows:

$$\frac{>100\% \text{ of lowest}}{\text{value on range}} = \frac{\text{adequate nutritional}}{\text{status}}$$

$$\frac{95–99\% \text{ of lowest}}{\text{value on range}} = \frac{\text{mild}}{\text{depletion}}$$

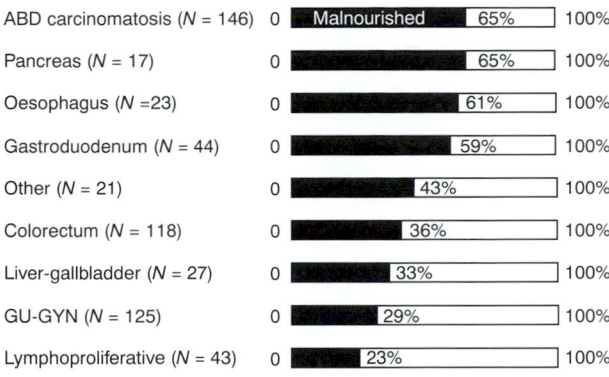

Figure 2 Incidence of malnutrition in 464 patients with benign and malignant disease. ABD, abdominal, GU-GYN, Genitourinary gynaecological. Modified from (1983) *Lancet* **2**:230–231.

$$\frac{<95\% \text{ of lowest}}{\text{value on range}} = \frac{\text{severe}}{\text{depletion}}$$

Body weight and height may also be used to assess body mass index (BMI: weight in kg/(height in m)^2), which is useful in determining both undernutrition and overnutrition. Unfortunately, the use of body weight in determining a patient's nutritional status is limited by a series of factors. Indeed, the measurement of body weight in sick patients is confounded by changes in body water resulting from dehydration, oedema and acites. The percentage of ideal body weight does not account for differences in body build (i.e. muscle mass versus fat mass). Furthermore, a person who starts at the upper end of the normal range may be classified as normal despite considerable changes in the measured value.

Weight loss

Estimation of weight loss has played a key role in the nutritional assessment of hospitalized patients since 1936, when Studley showed that a preoperative weight loss of more than 20% was associated with a 33% mortality rate, whereas a 4% mortality rate occurred in those with a weight loss of less than 20%. More than 10% loss over any time period has been taken as evidence of malnutrition, while a weight loss of more than 4.5 kg has recently been reported to be highly predictable of surgical mortality.

Reference to time frame of change is also important, as shown in **Table 5**. Unintentional weight loss greater than 10% within the previous 6 months is a reliable prognosticator of clinical outcome. However, it can be difficult to determine true weight loss because of errors in recall. When weight loss is based on patient recall up to 33% of patients with weight loss are likely to be missed and 25% of weight-stable patients would be diagnosed as having lost weight.

Another factor is that small changes in body weight can be confounded by changes in hydration status. Retention of fluid can occur during catabolism of lean body mass, therefore masking true weight loss, while diuretic therapy can confound body weight change interpretation by promoting fluid shifts.

Anthropometry

Triceps skinfold thickness provide an index of body fat, while midarm circumference and midarm muscle circumference provide a measure of muscle mass. These measurements are carried out as follows.

- *Triceps skinfold.* Measurement of triceps skinfold is made by grasping the skin and adjacent subcutaneous tissue of the patient's non-dominant arm at the midway point between the acromion process of the shoulder and the olecranon process of the elbow, using a Lange caliper. After the caliper reading diminishes, the dial can be read. Duplicate readings are made to improve validity and reliability. Observations are made and recorded in mm.
- *Midarm circumference.* Using the midpoint of the non-dominant arm, the arm circumference is measured in cm.
- *Midarm muscle circumference.* Midarm muscle circumference (MAMC) is calculated from the triceps skinfold (TSF) thickness and midarm circumference (MAC) according to the following equation:

$$\text{MAMC} = \text{MAC} - \frac{(\text{TSF} \times \pi)}{10}$$

- where MAC is measured in cm, TSF in mm, and MAMC is calculated in cm.

The two most commonly used standards for triceps skinfold thickness, midarm circumference and midarm muscle circumference are the 1966 standards based on measurements of European military men and low-income American women and the 1981 standards (see **Tables 6–8**) based on measurements of white males and females participating in the 1971–1974 US Health and Nutrition Survey. Triceps skinfold thickness, midarm circumference and midarm muscle circumference measures are compared against tables of percentiles (Tables 6–8), which allows nutritional status to be described as follows:

>10th percentile = adequate
5th–10th percentile = mild depletion
<5th percentile = severe depletion

Table 3 Nutritional assessment form

A. MEDICAL DATA

Admitting Dx/cc

Past medical Hx

Current medications

Treatment plan

Current diet order

B. ASSESSMENT OF PAST NUTRITIONAL HISTORY

Appetite evaluation

Adequacy of P.O. intake (in hospital/PTA): _____ alcohol consumption: _____

Need for diet instruction

C. NUTRITIONAL PROFILE   LABORATORY/ANTHROPOMETRIC CRITERIA

Ht (cm)	Wt (kg)	Usual wt (kg)	Wrist circum (cm)	Frame size	LB wt range kg	Weight change	% Wt loss of usual Wt
				L M S		.......kg in ...... days/wks/mos	

ITEM	Hcl	Hgb	Na	K	Cl	HCO₃	BUN	Cr	Glu	TLC	Ca	Phos	Mg	Chol	Trg
DATE															
VALUE															

PARAMETERS	PATIENT VALUES	PERCENTILES	ASSESSMENT		
			Severely Depleted	Mildly Depleted	Adequate
Wt for Ht %			<95% of lowest value on range	95–99%	>100%
Tricep skinfold arm L R			<5th percentile	5th–10th	>10th
Midarm circum.			<5th percentile	5th–10th	>10th
Midarm muscle circum.			<5th percentile	5th–10th	>10th
Albumin (Date)			<2.8 g l⁻¹	2.8–3.4 g l⁻¹	>3.5 g l⁻¹
Transferrin			<180 mmol l⁻¹	<160–179 mmol l⁻¹	>180 mmol l⁻¹
Retinol binding protein				<3 mmol l⁻¹	>3–6 μmol l⁻¹

The use of these standards to identify malnutrition in many patients is problematic because of the restricted database and the potential confounding influence of age, hydration status and physical activity. Several studies have demonstrated that 20–30% of healthy control subjects would be considered malnourished on the basis of these standards; there is also poor correlation between the two standards

Table 3 Continued

OVERALL CLASSIFICATION OF NUTRITIONAL STATUS

☐ Severe malnutrition ☐ Moderate or mild malnutrition ☐ Other (specify) ???? ☐ Normal

_____

☐ Marasmus (281) ☐ Moderate (233 ?) _____ ☐ Lacks sufficient data for classification

☐ Kwashiorker (259) ☐ Mild (293,?) _____

☐ Mixed Marasmus-Kwashiorker (252)
☐ Other Protein Ca??? Malnutrition (263.8/263.9)

D. ENERGY/PROTEIN REQUIREMENT B.E.E. based on usual wt/IBW/present wt/average of BW and present wt _____kg

Basal energy expenditure = Current protein requirement = Current energy requirement =

_____ _____ gm/kg _____ kcal/kg body wt

_____ g/day _____ kcal/day

E. SUMMARY AND RECOMMENDATIONS

ASSESSED BY: _____ **DATE:** _____

---

in classifying patients. Furthermore, interpretation of the data may be limited by inter-rater variability and the patient's hydration status. Nevertheless, markedly abnormal values (below the 5th percentile) are often associated with poor clinical outcome.

The triceps skinfold thickness provides reasonable estimates of subcutaneous fat reserves, which serve as the major energy source during prolonged starvation. Although this one site has been claimed to be representative of total body fat, the best evidence shows that at least four sites should be used, including subscapular skinfold thickness. Moreover, individuals with flabby, easily compressible tissue or with very firm tissue that is not easily deformable present a problem in obtaining valid measures of skinfold thickness.

Midarm muscle circumference gives an indication of the body's muscle mass and hence represents the main protein reserve. The assumptions inherent in the equation used to derive midarm muscle circumference, however, are that arm and muscle compartments are circular, that a concentric ring of fat covers muscle, and that bone area is a constant fraction of

muscle area, regardless of nutritional status. The recent application of computerized tomography in depleted patients demonstrates that this simplified formula underestimates muscle mass loss by 15–25% because the calculated muscle circumference includes the bone, which does not decrease proportionally in cachectic patients. Hence, there is no sound basis for classifying as malnourished those males with a midarm muscle circumference of <23 cm or those females with <21 cm, as is commonly practised.

As a whole, anthropometric measurements incorporate a wide margin of error. Sources of error include observer error, instrument error, tissue compartment changes and inaccurate application of measurements. Also, the relationship between internal and subcutaneous fat changes and fat in skinfolds is dependent on factors other than nutritional status, such as the ageing process, skin compressibility changes and total body water changes. The limited sensitivity and specificity of anthropometric measures precludes their use as absolute indicator of protein–energy malnutrition in the nutritional assessment of hospitalized patients.

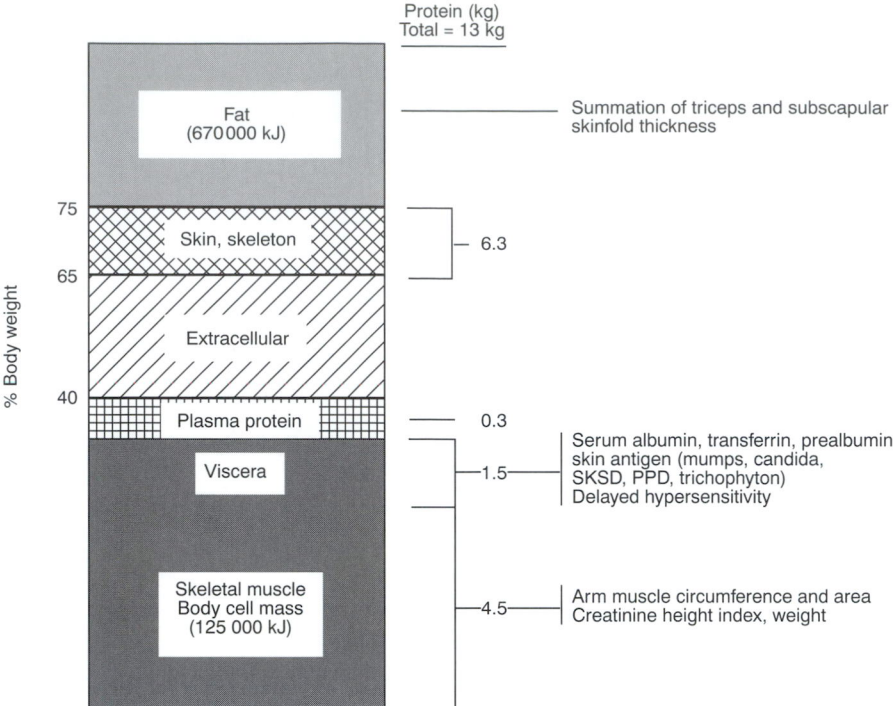

Figure 3 Current techniques for the assessment of nutritional status with corresponding components of body composition. Modified from Blackburn and Bothe (1978) *Cancer Bulletin*.

The best application of these measurements is in long-term monitoring of nutritionally stable populations in which serial measures are made by the same observer.

Serum protein concentrations

Albumin Albumin is included in the laboratory tests obtained on admission. Serum albumin's long half-life of approximately 18–20 days makes this an insensitive marker in detecting early stages of malnutrition. Although the use of albumin as a prognostic indicator of nutritional status (**Fig. 4**) has been criticized, several studies demonstrated that a low serum albumin concentration correlates with an increased incidence of medical complications.

Albumin values are used to classify nutritional status as follows:

$$\text{adequate:} \quad \geq 35 \text{ g l}^{-1}$$
$$\text{mild depletion:} \quad 28\text{–}34 \text{ g l}^{-1}$$
$$\text{severe depletion:} \quad <28 \text{ g l}^{-1}$$

Hypoalbuminaemia is associated with a variety of non-nutritional factors. Inflammatory disorders cause a decrease in albumin synthesis, an increase in albumin degradation, and an increase in albumin transcapillary losses. Gastrointestinal and some cardiac diseases increase albumin losses through the gut,

and renal diseases can cause albuminuria. In burns, peritonitis and intestinal obstruction, the vascular space is rapidly depleted of both fluid and protein. Treatment of this kind of dehydration with colloid-free fluid leads to dilutional hypoalbuminaemia. While these patients may be in an acutely negative energy balance, their overall protein stores are better than their serum albumin concentrations suggest. Furthermore, because the exchange between intravascular and extravascular albumin is so large, even small variations in the percentage of exchange can cause significant changes in plasma albumin levels. The normal rate of albumin exchange between intravascular and extravascular compartments is more than 10 times the rate of albumin synthesis or degradation. During serious illness, vascular permeability increases dramatically. Albumin losses from plasma to the extravascular space were increased two-fold in patients with cancer cachexia and three-fold in patients with septic shock. Plasma albumin levels are usually not affected by nutritional intake and will not increase in stressed patients until the inflammatory stress remits.

Serum albumin may not be a good measure of adequacy of nutrient intake. Although protein–energy malnutrition causes a decrease in the rate of albumin synthesis, this may have little impact on albumin levels because of albumin's long half-life

Table 4 1983 height and weight tables

(a) Desirable weights for women aged 25–59[a]

Height (with shoes on)		Small frame		Medium frame		Large frame	
Feet	Inches	lb	kg	lb	kg	lb	kg
4	10	102–111	46.4–50.5	109–121	49.5–55.0	118–131	53.6–59.5
4	11	103–113	46.8–51.4	111–123	50.5–55.9	120–134	54.5–60.9
5	0	104–115	47.3–52.3	113–126	51.4–57.3	122–137	55.5–62.3
5	1	106–118	48.2–53.6	115–129	52.3–58.6	125–140	56.8–63.6
5	2	108–121	49.1–55.0	118–132	53.6–60.0	128–143	58.2–65.0
5	3	111–124	50.5–56.4	121–135	55.0–61.4	131–147	59.5–66.8
5	4	114–127	51.2–57.7	124–138	56.4–62.7	134–151	60.7–68.6
5	5	117–130	53.2–59.1	127–141	57.7–64.1	137–155	62.3–70.5
5	6	120–133	54.5–60.5	130–144	59.1–65.5	140–159	63.6–72.3
5	7	123–136	55.9–61.8	133–147	60.5–66.8	143–163	65.0–74.1
5	8	126–139	57.3–63.2	136–150	61.8–68.2	146–167	66.4–75.9
5	9	139–142	58.6–64.5	139–153	63.2–69.5	149–170	67.7–77.3
5	10	132–145	60.0–65.9	142–156	64.5–70.9	152–173	69.1–78.6
5	11	135–148	61.4–67.3	145–159	65.9–72.3	155–176	70.5–80.0
6	0	138–151	62.7–68.6	148–162	67.3–73.6	158–179	71.8–81.4

Source: Metropolitan Life Insurance Company.
[a]Weights in pounds according to frame (indoor clothing weighing 3 lb, shoes with 1 in heel).

1 lb ~ 450 g; 1 in ~ 2.5 cm.

(b) Desirable weights for men aged 25–29[a]

Height (with shoes on)		Small frame		Medium frame		Large frame	
Feet	Inches	lb	kg	lb	kg	lb	kg
5	2	128–134	58.2–60.9	131–141	59.5–64.1	138–150	62.7–68.2
5	3	130–136	59.1–61.2	133–143	60.5–65.0	140–153	63.7–69.5
5	4	132–138	60.0–62.7	135–145	61.4–65.9	142–156	64.5–70.9
5	5	134–140	60.9–63.6	137–148	62.3–67.3	144–160	65.5–72.7
5	6	136–142	61.8–64.5	139–151	63.2–68.6	146–164	66.4–74.5
5	7	138–145	62.7–65.9	142–154	64.5–70.0	149–168	67.7–76.4
5	8	140–148	63.6–67.3	145–157	65.9–71.4	152–172	69.1–78.2
5	9	142–151	64.5–68.6	148–160	67.3–72.7	155–176	70.5–80.0
5	10	144–154	65.5–70.0	151–163	68.6–74.1	158–180	71.8–81.8
5	11	146–157	66.5–71.4	154–166	70.0–75.5	161–184	73.2–83.6
6	0	149–160	67.7–72.7	157–170	71.4–77.3	164–188	74.5–85.5
6	1	152–164	69.1–74.5	160–174	72.7–79.1	168–192	76.4–87.3
6	2	155–168	70.5–76.4	164–178	74.5–80.9	172–197	78.2–89.5
6	3	158–172	71.8–78.2	167–182	75.9–82.7	176–202	80.0–91.8
6	4	162–176	73.6–80.0	171–187	77.7–85.0	181–207	82.3–94.1

Source: Metropolitan Life Insurance Company.
[a]Weights in pounds according to frame (indoor clothing weighing 5 lb, shoes with 1 in. heel).

Table 5 Time frame of weight loss

Time frame	Significant weight loss	Severe weight loss
1 week	1–2%	>2%
1 month	5%	>5%
3 months	7.5%	>7.5%
6 months	10%	>10%

and large pool size. Indeed, plasma albumin concentration may actually increase during short-term fasting because of contraction of intravascular water. Even during chronic malnutrition, plasma albumin concentration is often maintained because of a compensatory decrease in albumin degradation and a transfer of extravascular albumin to the intravascular compartment. Prolonged protein–energy restriction induced experimentally in human volunteers or

Table 6 Assessment of tricep skinfold

Age group	n	Triceps skinfold percentile (mm)						
		5	10	25	50	75	90	95
Females								
1–1.9	204	6	7	8	10	12	14	16
2–2.9	208	6	8	9	10	12	15	16
3–3.9	208	7	8	9	11	12	14	15
4–4.9	208	7	8	8	10	12	14	16
5–5.9	219	6	7	8	10	12	15	18
6–6.9	118	6	6	8	10	12	14	16
7–7.9	126	6	7	9	11	13	16	18
8–8.9	118	6	8	9	12	15	18	24
9–9.9	125	8	8	10	13	16	20	22
10–10.9	152	7	8	10	12	17	23	27
11–11.9	117	7	8	10	13	18	24	28
12–12.9	129	8	9	11	14	18	23	27
13–13.9	151	8	8	12	15	21	26	30
14–14.9	141	9	10	13	16	21	26	28
15–15.9	117	8	10	12	17	21	25	32
16–16.9	142	10	12	15	18	22	26	31
17–17.9	114	10	12	13	19	24	30	37
18–18.9	109	10	12	15	18	22	26	30
19–24.9	1060	10	11	14	18	24	30	34
25–34.9	1987	10	12	16	21	27	34	37
35–44.9	1614	12	14	18	23	29	35	38
45–54.9	1047	12	16	20	25	30	36	40
55–64.9	809	12	16	20	25	31	36	38
65–74.9	1670	12	14	18	24	29	34	36
Males								
1–1.9	228	6	7	8	10	12	14	16
2–2.9	223	6	7	8	10	12	14	15
3–3.9	220	6	7	8	10	11	14	15
4–4.9	230	6	6	8	9	11	12	14
5–5.9	214	6	6	8	9	11	14	15
6–6.9	117	5	6	7	8	10	13	16
7–7.9	122	5	6	7	9	12	15	17
8–8.9	117	5	6	7	8	10	13	16
9–9.9	121	6	6	7	10	13	17	18
10–10.9	146	6	6	8	10	14	18	21
11–11.9	122	6	6	8	11	16	20	24
12–12.9	153	6	6	8	11	14	22	28
13–13.9	134	5	5	7	10	14	22	26
14–14.9	131	4	5	7	9	14	21	24
15–15.9	128	4	5	6	8	11	18	24
16–16.9	131	4	5	6	8	12	16	22
17–17.9	133	5	5	6	8	12	16	19
18–18.9	91	4	5	6	9	13	20	24
19–24.9	531	4	5	7	10	15	20	22
25–34.9	971	5	6	8	12	16	20	24
35–44.9	806	5	6	8	12	16	20	23
45–54.9	898	6	6	8	12	15	20	25
55–64.9	734	5	6	8	11	14	19	22
65–74.9	1503	4	6	8	11	14	19	22

From Frisancho AR (1981) New norms of upper limb fat and muscle areas for assessment of nutritional status. *American Journal of Clinical Nutrition* **34**: 2540–2545.

Table 7 Arm circumference standards

Age group	Arm circumference (mm)						
	5	10	25	50	75	90	95
Males							
1–1.9	142	146	150	159	170	176	183
2–2.9	141	145	153	162	170	178	185
3–3.9	150	153	160	167	175	184	190
4–4.9	149	154	162	171	180	186	192
5–5.9	153	160	167	175	185	195	204
6–6.9	155	159	177	179	188	209	228
7–7.9	162	167	166	187	201	223	230
8–8.9	162	170	177	190	202	220	245
9–9.9	175	178	187	200	217	249	257
10–10.9	181	184	196	210	231	262	274
11–11.9	186	190	202	223	244	261	280
12–12.9	193	200	214	232	254	282	303
13–13.9	194	211	228	247	263	286	301
14–14.9	220	226	237	253	283	303	322
15–15.9	222	229	244	264	284	311	320
16–16.9	244	248	262	278	303	324	343
17–17.9	246	253	267	285	308	336	347
18–18.9	245	260	276	297	321	353	379
19–24.9	262	272	288	308	331	355	372
25–34.9	271	282	300	319	342	362	375
35–44.9	278	287	305	326	345	363	374
45–54.9	267	281	301	322	342	362	376
55–64.9	258	273	296	317	336	355	369
65–74.9	248	263	285	307	325	344	355
Females							
1–1.9	138	142	148	156	164	172	177
2–2.9	142	145	152	160	167	176	184
3–3.9	143	150	158	167	175	183	189
4–4.9	149	154	160	169	177	184	191
5–5.9	153	157	165	175	185	203	211
6–6.9	156	162	170	176	187	204	211
7–7.9	164	167	174	183	199	216	231
8–8.9	168	172	183	195	214	247	261
9–9.9	178	182	194	211	224	251	260
10–10.9	174	182	193	210	228	251	265
11–11.9	185	194	208	224	248	276	303
12–12.9	194	203	216	237	256	282	294
13–13.9	202	211	223	243	271	301	338
14–14.9	214	223	237	252	272	304	322
15–15.9	208	221	239	254	279	300	322
16–16.9	218	224	241	258	283	318	334
17–17.9	220	227	241	264	295	324	350
18–18.9	222	227	241	258	281	312	325
19–24.9	221	230	247	265	290	319	345
25–34.9	233	240	256	277	304	342	368
35–44.9	241	251	257	290	317	356	378
45–54.9	242	256	274	299	328	362	384
55–64.9	243	257	280	303	335	367	385
65–74.9	240	252	274	299	326	356	373

These percentages were derived from data obtained on all white subjects in the United States Health and Nutrition Examination Survey 1. 1971–1974 (from Frisancho AR, (1981) New norms of upper limb fat and muscle areas for assessment of nutrition status. *American Journal of Clinical Nutrition* **34**: 2540–2545).

Table 8 Assessment of midarm muscle circumference

Age group	Arm muscle circumference (mm)						
	5	10	25	50	75	90	95
Females							
1–1.9	105	111	117	124	132	139	143
2–2.9	111	114	119	126	133	142	147
3–3.9	113	119	124	132	140	146	152
4–4.9	115	121	128	136	144	152	157
5–5.9	125	128	134	142	151	159	165
6–6.9	130	133	138	145	154	166	171
7–7.9	129	135	142	151	160	171	176
8–8.9	138	140	151	160	171	183	194
9–9.9	147	150	158	167	180	194	198
10–10.9	148	150	159	170	180	190	197
11–11.9	150	158	171	181	196	217	223
12–12.9	162	166	180	191	201	214	220
13–13.9	169	175	183	198	211	226	240
14–14.9	174	179	190	201	216	232	247
15–15.9	175	178	189	202	215	228	244
16–16.9	170	180	190	202	216	234	249
17–17.9	175	183	194	205	221	239	257
18–18.9	174	179	191	202	215	237	245
19–24.9	179	185	195	207	221	236	249
25–34.9	183	188	199	212	228	246	264
35–44.9	186	192	205	218	236	257	272
45–54.9	187	193	206	220	238	260	274
55–64.9	187	196	209	225	244	266	280
65–74.9	185	195	208	225	244	264	279
Males							
1–1.9	110	113	119	127	135	144	147
2–2.9	111	114	122	130	140	146	150
3–3.9	117	123	131	137	143	148	153
4–4.9	123	126	133	141	148	156	159
5–5.9	128	133	140	147	154	162	169
6–6.9	131	135	142	151	161	170	177
7–7.9	137	139	151	160	168	177	190
8–8.9	140	145	154	162	170	182	187
9–9.9	151	154	161	170	183	196	202
10–10.9	156	160	166	180	191	209	221
11–11.9	159	165	173	183	195	205	230
12–12.9	167	171	182	195	210	223	241
13–13.9	172	179	196	211	226	238	245
14–14.9	189	199	212	223	240	260	264
15–15.9	199	204	218	237	254	266	272
16–16.9	213	225	234	249	269	287	296
17–17.9	224	231	245	258	273	294	312
18–18.9	226	237	252	264	283	298	324
19–24.9	238	245	257	273	289	309	321
25–34.9	243	250	264	279	298	314	326
35–44.9	247	255	269	286	302	318	327
45–54.9	239	249	265	281	300	315	326
55–64.9	236	245	260	278	295	310	320
65–74.9	223	235	251	268	284	298	306

From Frisancho AR (1981) New norms of upper limb fat and muscle areas for assessment of nutritional status. *American Journal of Clinical Nutrition* **34**: 2540–2545.

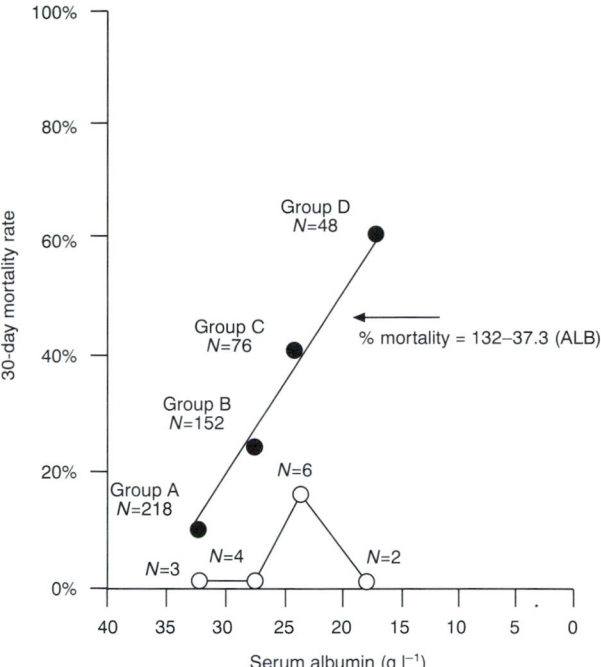

Figure 4 Relationship between lowest recorded serum albumin and 30-day mortality rate among 509 hospitalized veterans with low serum albumin levels. Mortality rate of 1551 veterans with serum albumin levels > 34 g l⁻¹ during the study period was 1.74%. ●–●, no total parenteral nutrition (TPN); ○–○, TPN. Modified from Reinhardt et al., 1980 *Journal of Parenteral and Enteral Nutrition*.

observed clinically in patients with anorexia nervosa causes marked reduction in body weight, but little change in plasma albumin concentration. A protein-deficient diet with adequate energy intake in elderly persons decreases lean body mass and muscle function without a change in plasma albumin concentration. As a consequence of its limitation, other circulating proteins are used.

Transferrin Serum transferrin may be measured directly by radioimmunodiffusion, but more commonly is derived indirectly from a measurement of the serum total iron-binding capacity as follows:

serum transferrin
= (0.8 × total iron-binding capacity) − 43

Translation of serum transferrin concentrations to nutritional status identification is as follows:

adequate: > 180 mg dl⁻¹
mild depletion: 160–179 mg dl⁻¹
severe depletion: < 160 mg dl⁻¹

Transferrin, with a half-life of approximately 8

days, responds more quickly than albumin to nutritional changes. A 2.5-fold increase in hospital mortality was observed, while a significant increased risk of sepsis and death was found in patients with serum transferrin levels below 170 mg dl^{-1}. Although transferrin can be a useful measure of nutritional status, transferrin concentrations are affected by non-nutritional factors, including iron deficiency, which leads to its increased synthesis, cirrhosis, nephrotic syndrome, and hematopoietic disorders which result in decreased circulating concentrations. For this reason other short-life serum proteins, i.e. retinol-binding protein and prealbumin, have also been used as predictors of morbidity and mortality outcome.

Retinol-binding protein This is yet another biochemically useful marker of visceral protein status. The range of normal serum concentration of retinol-binding protein is 4–5 μg dl^{-1}; a level below 3 μg dl^{-1} is suggestive of protein depletion. The very short half-life of retinol-binding protein of 10 h makes it a very rapid and sensitive indicator of nutritional status and therapeutic responsiveness. Retinol-binding protein concentrations, however, do not respond to depletion if there is a concomitant vitamin A deficiency.

Prealbumin Prealbumin is a transport protein for thyroid hormones and exists in the circulation as a retinol-binding–prealbumin complex. The tunover rate of this protein is rapid, with a half-life of 2–3 days. It is synthesized by the liver and is catabolized partly in the kidneys. Protein–energy malnutrition reduces the levels of prealbumin, while refeeding (particularly with carbohydrate) restores levels. However, prealbumin levels decrease without malnutrition in infections and in response to cytokine, hormone infusion and bone marrow transplantation for haematological malignancies. Renal failure increases, while liver failure may decrease, plasma concentrations.

Creatinine height index

Since creatinine is present almost entirely within muscle (as creatinine phosphate) and is converted to creatinine at a relatively constant rate, the excretion of creatinine in urine provides an index of lean body mass. This has been shown to be reasonably accurate in patients without renal failure, if based on multiple measurements. However, it is dependent upon an accurate and complete urine collection while the patient is consuming a meat-free diet, which can be difficult to achieve in some patient care settings. Furthermore, it has been reported that urinary creatinine

excretion correlates with the total body nitrogen, except in cancer patients; in these, creatinine excretion remained steady when total body nitrogen fell, indicating increased creatinine loss as the disease progressed. Creatinine height index has not been shown to be of value for predicting complications.

Immunological tests

Total lymphocyte count Standards have been developed for the interpretation of total lymphocyte count:

1500–1800 per mm^3 = mild depletion
900–1500 per mm^3 = moderate depletion
< 900 per mm^3 = severe depletion

Total lymphocyte count is limited to cases in which infection, cancer, metabolic stress or steroid and immunosuppressive drug use are not factors.

Immune competence Immune competence, as measured by delayed cutaneous hypersensitivity (DCH), has been shown to be associated with a poor clinical outcome

Although total lymphocyte count and DCH are affected by severe malnutrition, they are also influenced by several diseases and drugs. Infections (viral, bacterial and granulomatous), illnesses (uraemia, cirrhosis, hepatitis, trauma, burns and haemorrhage), medications (corticosteroids, immunosuppressants, cimetidine, warfarin and perhaps aspirin) and general anaesthesia and surgery alter total lymphocyte count and DHC in the absence of malnutrition. Also, simple drainage of an abscess can reverse anergy. Therefore, while potentially useful as predictors of morbidity, without the ability to separate the effects of malnutrition from those of disease, it is difficult to justify the utilization of results from such tests as reliable nutritional indicators in individual patients.

Discriminant function analysis

In attempts to predict more accurately patients' outcomes as affected by nutritional variables, mathematical equations, developed by the use of stepwise multiple regression analyses of selected nutritional parameters, have been used as an objective measure to identify patients at increased risk for medical complications. A prognostic nutritional index (PNI) has been developed based on serum albumin, triceps skinfold, serum transferrin and DHC to three recall antigens. At the University of Auckland, a new approach to nutritional assessment has been developed and tested which is based on a careful history and physical examination of a patient, and incorporates a clinical assessment of physiological functions. In 1981 a discriminate function test based on serum albumin, skin test response, presence of sepsis at the time of assessment and diagnosis of cancer was developed. Another predictive nutritional index uses only serum albumin and total lymphocyte count.

Since these indices are only mathematical manipulations of numbers derived from tests which at best are only secondarily related to actual nutritional status, they do not provide satisfactory solutions to the problems of nutritional assessment. However, only the PNI has been shown to predict clinical outcome in a prospective evaluation.

Muscle function

Muscle function tests represent the newest approach for evaluating nutritional status. They include measuring grip strength, respiratory muscle strength, and the response of specific muscles to electrical stimulation. In 120 elective gastrointestinal surgical patients, grip strength had a sensitivity of 90% in predicting postoperative complications. A technique using electrical stimulation of the ulnar nerve at the wrist has been developed; this results in contraction of the adductor pollicis muscle. It does not require the cooperation of the patient and is not affected by sepsis, drugs, trauma, surgical intervention or anaesthesia. Starvation causes specific alterations in adductor pollicis muscle response to electrical stimulation: it causes the forced muscle contraction to decrease and fatigue to develop, while similar changes occur in the diaphragm of malnourished patients. The phenomenon is not rendered abnormal by surgery, anaesthesia, steroids or sepsis, and is only temporarily altered by severe trauma (crush injuries). Our laboratory studied the effects of postoperative anorexia and reduced food intake on muscle function and plasma creatinine phosphokinase (CPK) in patients undergoing cardiac and general abdominal operations. A close correlation existed between rises in CPK and fall in force frequency and a prolongation of the relaxation rate of adductor pollicis in both groups of patients. However, when the cardiac surgical patients started to eat enough to meet daily energy requirements, muscle function and CPK levels both normalized. A similar response was observed in the abdominal surgery patients. Furthermore, changes in muscle function induced by nutritional therapy occur rapidly and before there are any changes in body nitrogen or protein content. In one study, the combination of an abnormal force–frequency curve and slow relaxation rate was more specific and sensitive than other parameters of nutritional status, such as arm muscle circumference, serum albumin and transferrin concentrations, as a preoperative predicator of postoperative complications.

Hand grip, respiratory muscle strength and relaxation rate of adductor pollicis have also been shown to be better than weight loss as a predicator of postoperative complications. It is not known whether restoring muscle function with nutritional therapy improves clinical outcome. However, in the future a more relevant and specific way of assessing nutritional status may be through further studies of muscle function.

Body Composition Analyses

The body consists of 35 components, which are organized into five levels of increasing complexity: atomic (e.g. nitrogen, potassium); molecular (e.g. water, protein); cellular (e.g. body cell mass, intracellular and extracellular fluid); tissue (e.g. skeletal muscle, adipose tissue); and whole body (e.g. weight, height). Although modern technology now allows measurements of all major body components *in vivo*, these methodologies are not readily available for clinical use. Sophisticated tools and techniques of body composition analysis, which may presently be available at institutions with metabolic wards, include: bioelectrical impedance analysis, dual energy X ray absorptiometry, electromagnetic or sound wave application, total body neutron activation systems and amino acid profile analysis. Unfortunately, no body composition measurement has been shown consistently to predict clinical outcome. These techniques are briefly summarized below.

Bioelectrical impedance analysis

The bioelectrical impedance analysis method is based on measurements of changes in the conduction of an applied electrical current through the body. Intra- and extracellular fluid are thought to act as electroconductors; cell membranes are considered to act as electrocapacitors. Since lean body tissue has a far greater electrolyte content than fat, this marked difference in ionic content permits an estimation of the lean body mass from the assessment of body electrical impedance.

Dual energy X ray absorptiometry (DEXA)

DEXA uses an X ray system that generates two energy distributions, enabling the clinician to separate body weight into three chemical components: fat, fat-free soft tissue and bone mineral.

Computerized axial tomography

This permits direct measurement of total body area as well as areas of fat, muscle and bone. Volume measurements made via computerized tomography can be extrapolated to estimate total body lean and fat mass. Two limitations of this method are the relatively high cost and the radiation exposure.

Nuclear magnetic resonance (NMR)

This approach provides information on organ volumes, tissue composition and cellular function. A second use of NMR is to obtain the spectra of certain metabolic substrates; this is termed NMR spectroscopy. NMR spectroscopy can differentiate water-bound protons from lipid protons. This facilitates differentiation between lean (rich in water and, therefore, correlated with water-bound protons) and lipid tissue. *In vivo* phosphorus NMR spectroscopy is important in body composition research owing to the significance of phosphorus compounds in cellular energy metabolism. Carbon NMR spectroscopy is not yet available. Carbon spectra from human arms have, however, shown enough resolution to identify essential fatty acids.

NMR represents a safe way to evaluate human tissue mass and composition. The high cost of instrumentation and operation, however, limits its widespread application.

Near-infrared interactance

This technique is based on the relationship between the absorptive and reflective properties, and the chemical composition of given tissue. Interactance is calculated as the ratio of energy reflected from the tissue to that reflected by a reference standard. The shape of the interactance spectrum allows for a quantitative analysis of tissue (i.e. water and fat content).

Ultrasound

This technique is based on analysis of sound wave motion. When a transmitted sound wave reaches an interface between two media of different density, the wave undergoes reflection and refraction. Differences in tissue composition as well as organ motion can thus be detected as ultrasound displays these changes in useable form.

The major advantages of ultrasound include safety, portability and reasonable cost. The disadvantages are the limited degree of structure resolution and the lack of instrumentation designed for body composition analysis.

Total body neutron activation

Total body neutron activation involves delivery of a moderated beam of fast neutrons to the subject. Capture of these neutrons by atoms of the target elements in the body creates unstable isotopes, such as calcium-49 and nitrogen-15. The isotopes revert to a stable condition by the emission of one or more γ rays of characteristic energy. These emissions are recorded in a radiospectrum. Analysis of emissions identifies energy and activity levels, which correspond with element determination and its abundance, respectively.

Applications of neutron activation analysis to assessment of body composition are the determination of total body calcium and of body nitrogen. Knowledge of the muscle and nonmuscle components from total body nitrogen, bone mineral mass from total body calcium, and body mass allows for calculation of body fat by mathematical difference.

Factors such as the high cost, the need for skilled operators, and the use of ionizing radiation generally preclude its routine application to assess human body composition.

Amino acid profile analysis

The relationship between disease state and plasma amino acid profile is being investigated. It is known that starvation and weight loss result in lowered plasma valine levels, and that sepsis increases aromatic and sulfur-containing amino acid levels. Although the physiological role of plasma amino acid alterations in various disease states is undeniably important, monitoring of amino acid levels is not yet practical.

Conclusions

In describing the techniques of nutritional assessment and in summarizing their individual as well as collective strengths and weaknesses, we have provided what seems to be an internally contradictory body of information. Most current nutrition assessment techniques are based on their ability to predict clinical outcome. However, the validity of any of these techniques truly to measure nutritional risk in hospital patients has not been proved and the effect of nutritional therapy to influence outcome in patients judged to be malnourished has not been consistent in prospective randomized clinical trials.

Thus, nutritional assessment is in a state of flux. Technical proficiency in diagnosing nutritional status is the ultimate goal, as the profound impact of nutritional status on overall bodily function/recovery in health and disease has received universal recognition by medical practitioners.

See also: **Amino Acids**: Chemistry and Classification. **Malnutrition**: Definition, Classification and Epidemiology. **Nutritional Status**: Anthropometric Assessment; Biochemical Assessment. **Protein**: Requirements and Role in Diet.

Further Reading

Antonas KN, Curtas S and Meguid MM (1987) Use of CPK-MM to monitor response to nutritional intervention in catabolic surgical patients. *Journal of Surgery Research* **42**:219.

Baker JP, Detsky AS, Wesson DE, Wolman SL, Stewart S, Whitewell J, Langer B, Jeejeebhoy KN (1982) Nutritional assessment: a comparison of clinical judgement and objective measurements. *New England Journal of Medicine* **306**:969.

Blackburn GL, Bistrian BR, Maini BS, Schlamm HT, Smith MF (1977) Nutritional and metabolic assessment of hospitalized patient. *Journal of Parenteral and Enteral Nutrition* **1**:11.

Frisancho AR (1981) New norms or upper limb fat and muscle areas for assessment of nutritional status. *American Journal of Clinical Nutrition* **34**:2540.

Giner M, Laviano A, Meguid MM and Gleason, JR (1996) In 1995 a correlation between malnutrition and poor outcome in critically ill patients still exists. *Nutrition* **12**:23.

Gray GE and Meguid MM (1990) Can total parenteral nutrition reverse hypoalbuminemia in oncology patients? *Nutrition* **6**:225.

Heymsfield SB and Casper K (1987) Anthropometric assessment of the adult hospitalized patient. *Journal of Parenteral and Enteral Nutrition* **11**:36S.

Jeejeehboy KN and Meguid MM (1986) Assessment of nutritional status in the oncologic patient. *Surgical Clinics of North America* **66**:1077.

Jelliffe DB (1966) *The Assessment of the Nutritional Status of the Community: with Special Reference to Field Surveys in Developing Regions of the World*. Geneva: World Health Organization.

Keys A, Brozek J, Henschel A, Mickelsen O, Taylor HL, Simonson E, Skinner AS, Wells SM (eds) (1950) *The Biology of Human Starvation*. Minneapolis: University of Minnesota Press.

Mughal MM and Meguid MM (1987) The effect of nutritional status on morbidity after elective surgery for benign gastrointestinal disease. *Journal of Parenteral and Enteral Nutrition* **11**:140.

Muscaritoli M, Conversano L, Cangiano C, Capria S, Laviano A, Arcese W, Fanelli FR (1995) Biochemical indices may not accurately reflect changes in nutritional status after allogenic bone marrow transplantation. *Nutrition* **11**:433.

NUTRITIONAL SUPPORT

Contents
Enteral Feeding
Parenteral Nutrition
In the Home Setting

Enteral Feeding

H D Duncan, Queen Alexandra Hospital, Portsman, UK.

David B A Silk, Central Middlesex Hospital NHS Trust, London, UK

Malnutrition amongst hospitalized patients is common and can result in an increase in morbidity and mortality as well as in increased costs. Many patients who are malnourished are not referred for full dietary assessment and remain malnourished throughout their hospital stay. This state of affairs is due to failure to recognize the importance of nutrition and the effect it may have on the patient's speed of recovery. Hospital workers may focus on the immediate problem that entailed admission to hospital, such as an acute pneumonic episode, while ignoring the malnourished state of the patient, thus potentially adversely affecting the clinical outcome.

This article is intended to give an overall view of the indications for nutritional support, the various techniques of achieving this, the types of enteral diets available and the importance of monitoring patients being enterally fed. Complications associated with enteral tube feeding from the different techniques used and as a result of refeeding are discussed.

Indications for Enteral Feeding

The need to avoid prolonged starvation is well recognized. Nonetheless, despite studies in the 1970s demonstrating the high incidence of malnutrition in medical and surgical patients, the problem of malnutrition amongst hospitalized patients remains as high today with a reported incidence of up to 40%, with as many as 10% of these being severely malnourished. Patients may be malnourished on admission or become so during their stay. Although malnutrition in hospitalized patients remains a common problem, the indications for instituting nutritional support remain controversial and ill defined, complicated by lack of training in nutrition in medical school. Indications for nutritional support depend partly on the underlying disease process, the anticipated clinical benefit and natural history of disease. Malnutrition can be difficult to diagnose and has many causes and manifestations. It comprises a group of clinical conditions that can arise from abnormal nutrient intake, digestion, absorption, metabolism and excretion. Malnutrition can cause severely abnormal structural and functional changes that affect health and survival.

The most common nutritional deficiency in hospitalized patients is protein–energy malnutrition. This type of malnutrition can develop rapidly with acute illnesses and over many months or years with chronic disease. The main manifestation of protein–energy malnutrition is depletion of tissue energy stores and loss of total body proteins with consequent morbidity and mortality. Death from malnutrition occurs within 70 days of total starvation in normal-weight adults. Total starvation in healthy adults for less than 2 to 3 days causes predominantly glycogen and water loss and minor functional consequences. After about 2 weeks of semi starvation in healthy adults, more severe functional deficits develop. Many patients are hypermetabolic and often malnourished before hospitalization, and depletion of nutrient reserves will proceed more rapidly. Weight loss is associated with increased morbidity in hospitalized patients, particularly if the weight loss is greater than 10% of the premorbid weight.

Attempts should be made not only to treat malnutrition, but also to prevent it from developing in at-risk patients. There are three main categories of patients suitable for enteral nutritional support, which are summarized in **Table 1**. The first category of patients should not be difficult to diagnose, and comprises those patients who are severely malnourished as indicated by weight loss of greater than 10% in the preceding month, a serum albumin of less than

Table 1 Indications for enteral nutritional support

1. Severe malnutrition:
- weight loss greater than 10%
- albumin less than 30 g l^{-1}
- marked muscle wasting
- oedema
- BMI < 15

2. Moderate malnutrition:
- inadequate nutritional intake for preceding 2–4 weeks
- nutritional measurements suggestive of protein–energy malnutrition
- BMI 15–19

3. Normal/near normal nutritional status:
- underlying medical or surgical disease likely to result in malnutrition if nutritional support not given

30 g l^{-1}, and muscle wasting with or without peripheral oedema. The second category of patients comprises those who are moderately malnourished and have had a reduced nutrient intake for the preceding 2–4 weeks. The third category of patients comprises those who on admission are normally or near normally nourished, but are likely to become malnourished while in hospital as a result of their disease. Patients can be clinically divided into those who have a physical obstruction to swallowing (e.g. tumour), disordered swallowing (e.g. motor neuron disease, multiple sclerosis), inability to reach and ingest food (e.g. stroke, patients on intensive care) and anorexia as a result of their underlying disease (e.g. cancer, inflammatory bowel disease, chronic lung disease). **Table 2** lists some of the disease states suitable for enteral nutrition.

Enteral nutrition is cheaper, more physiological and has fewer complications than parenteral nutrition, and should in general be used in patients with a functioning gastrointestinal tract who do not have any contraindications to this method of nutrition. It should be remembered that these two methods of feeding are not mutually exclusive, and a combination of enteral and parenteral nutrition is useful when a patient cannot tolerate full enteral nutritional support. Contraindications to enteral

Table 2 Disease states suitable for enteral nutritional support

Anorexia	Pre- and post-radiotherapy and chemotherapy
Neurological or mechanical dysphagia	Trauma
Acutely ill elderly patients	Hepatic failure
Burns	Renal failure
Sepsis	Respiratory failure
Intensive care	Distal fistulas
Pre- and post-operative	Inflammatory bowel disease
Stomatitis	Gastroparesis
HIV/AIDS	Short bowel syndrome

nutrition include intestinal obstruction, paralytic ileus, perforation, failure and major intra-abdominal sepsis.

Providing adequate nutrition to hospitalized patients is important because it reduces the incidence of malnutrition and mortality in these patients, improves respiratory function and muscle strength and general activity and can reduce disease severity. Inadequate nutrition promotes apathy, exacerbates anorexia and malnutrition and increases the risk of developing pressure sores.

The route of nutritional support needs to be individualized, but we shall only be discussing the enteral route here. Having made the decision to administer enteral nutrition, a number of considerations have to be taken into account. These include the route of access, type of enteral feeding diet to be used, gastrointestinal function, risk of aspiration and expected duration on nutritional support.

Techniques

Nasoenteric feeding tubes

The majority of patients require nutritional support for 4 weeks or less. If a patient is unable to ingest adequate nutrition using oral supplements, then enteral tube feeding is required. There are a number of different methods of enteral tube feeding, and these are listed in **Table 3**.

Nasogastric tube feeding The majority of patients require nutritional support for less than 3–4 weeks with nasogastric tube feeding being the most commonly used route of access for enteral feeding. Fine-bore nasogastric feeding tubes should be used in preference to Ryle's type of tubes which more commonly cause rhinitis, pharyngitis, oesophagitis, oesophageal erosions and strictures and gastro-oesophageal reflux. Physical complications of nasoenteric tubes are listed in **Table 4**. Fine-bore tubes with wire stylets should be inserted by trained personnel, not only to minimize the risk of misplacing the tube, but because

Table 3 Methods of tube feeding patients

Nasogastric tubes
Nasoenteric tubes
Percutaneous endoscopic gastrostomy
Percutaneous endoscopic gastrojejunostomy
Direct percutaneous endoscopic jejunostomy
Fluoroscopically inserted percutaneous gastrostomy
Surgical jejunostomy
Laparoscopic gastrostomy
Needle catheter jejunostomy
Cervical pharyngostomy
Oesophagostomy

Table 4 Complications arising from the physical presence of nasoenteric feeding tubes

Nasopharyngeal discomfort	Laryngeal ulceration
Nasal erosions and necrosis	Reflux and oesophagitis
Acute sinusitis	Oesophageal erosions and stenosis
Otitis media	Tracheo-oesophageal fistula
Hoarseness	Rupture of oesophageal varices
Intracranial passage	Duodenal perforation

only trained personnel will be sufficiently experienced to recognize that this problem may have occurred. Tube misplacement into the trachea and bronchi can cause aspiration of feed and pneumothorax, and there is a risk of oesophageal perforation. Patients most at risk from tube misplacement are those with altered swallowing or impaired gag reflex. Methods for checking the gastric position of the tube include air insufflation and auscultation of the epigastrium, and aspiration of gastric contents and testing with litmus paper. Ability to aspirate gastric contents is more successful with polyurethane tubes with a modified outlet port than with standard polyvinyl chloride tubes or polyurethane tubes with standard outlet ports. If aspiration or auscultation is unsuccessful, or if there is any doubt about tube position, then X ray confirmation is mandatory.

Other common complications include tube clogging, extubation and gastro-oesophageal reflux. Precipitation of protein of the enteral diet infused through feeding tubes at an acid pH is an important cause of tube clogging. A further important change in clinical practice has been the administration of medication via enteral feeding tubes in liquid or crushed form. Tube clogging can develop as a result of the effects of the medication on enteral diet protein precipitation, incompatibility or by means of particle occlusion. Risk of tube clogging can be reduced by flushing the tube before and after administration of medication and using modern designed feeding tubes. Inadvertent extubation may be minimized by securing the enteral feeding tube securely with tape and regular observation of the patient.

Postpyloric nasoenteral feeding tubes Patients at risk from pulmonary regurgitation and aspiration can be prescribed prokinetic drugs such as metoclopramide, cisapride or erythromycin. However, in patients at risk of aspiration (e.g. gastric atony or paresis), it would be preferable to feed the patient with a postpyloric feeding tube to reduce this hazard, although there remains a risk of aspiration in the order of 2.4%.

Placing nasoenteral feeding tubes postpylorically

can prove to be a problem. Spontaneous transpyloric passage of feeding tubes after 24 h is only in the order of 30% and is not affected by tip profile or the addition of a weight to the tip of the feeding tube. This issue is further complicated by the high incidence of spontaneous reflux of the tube back into the stomach owing to retroperistalsis and because postpyloric feeding tubes are often situated in the first and second parts of the duodenum. Metochlopramide can be tried to improve the success rate of spontaneous transpyloric passage of the tube, although in our experience the success rate is quite variable. Fluoroscopic and endoscopic techniques can be used to place postpyloric feeding tubes with variable success, but are time-consuming procedures.

Feeding by enterostomy tube

As a result of some of the difficulties encountered with nasoenteric feeding tubes, alternative routes of tube feeding have been developed. Some of these methods are particularly useful for long-term feeding.

Tube enterostomies can be placed using surgical, endoscopic or radiological methods into the gastrointestinal tract. Tube enterostomies can be either permanent or temporary, and are usually placed if it is anticipated that long-term feeding of more than 4 weeks will be required, or if nasoenteric access is compromised.

Surgical enterostomies Adjunctive tube enterostomy is usually placed at the time of surgery, when it is expected that postoperative nutrient intake will be delayed. Primary tube enterostomy is indicated for those patients requiring long-term nutritional support (**Table 5**).

Table 5 Patients suitable for tube enterostomy

Enterostomy tube inserted at time of surgery:
Head and neck surgery
Oesophagectomy
Gastrectomy
Pancreaticoduodenectomy
Pancreatectomy

Tube enterostomy for primary feeding:
Neuromuscular dysfunction
  Strokes
  Motor neuron disease
  Multiple sclerosis
  Myasthenia gravis
  Connective tissue diseases
  Head injury
Upper gastrointestinal obstruction
  Oropharyngeal cancer
  Oesophageal cancer or stricture
  Gastric or duodenal cancer
  Pancreatic cancer

Pharyngostomy This involves inserting a tube into the oropharynx and was first described in 1967. Pharyngostomy can be used in patients with congenital anomalies or trauma of the maxillofacial area, oropharyngeal tumours and following cervical or maxillofacial surgery or radiotherapy for partially obstructing oesophageal tumours. Contraindications include complete oesophageal obstruction, gastric, duodenal or jejunal obstruction, or extensive neck tumours. Complications include cellulitis, wound infections, haemorrhage, aspiration pneumonia as well as mechanical complications including injury and stricture of the oesophagus, irritation of skin and soft tissue, tubal obstruction and accidental removal of the feeding tube.

Surgical gastrostomy Surgical gastrostomy is indicated for patients in whom percutaneous endoscopic gastrostomy cannot be performed, or as adjunctive procedure at the time the patient is undergoing a surgical operation. Indications include oesophageal atresia, stricture and cancer, dysphagia due to neuromuscular disorders or following trauma. Contraindications include primary disease of the stomach, abnormal gastric and duodenal emptying, and significant oesophageal reflux, especially in those patients with a poor gag reflex. Complications of surgical gastrostomy include local irritation, haemorrhage, skin excoriation from leaking of gastric contents, wound infection, accidental tube removal, tube blockage, aspiration, gastric outlet obstruction (from tube migration), intraperitoneal leakage of gastric contents, wound dehiscence, hernia, delayed closure of the stoma, peritonitis and death.

Surgical jejunostomy Surmay created the first jejunostomy in 1878. There are three basic types of surgical jejunostomy in use: a Witzel jejunostomy, needle catheter jejunostomy and Roux-en-Y jejunostomy. The principle of the Witzel jejunostomy is to appose a loop of jejunum to the anterior abdominal wall. A small wound is created in the jejunum through which a feeding tube is inserted, and a purse string suture used to secure the feeding tube. The needle catheter jejunostomy technique involves inserting a needle obliquely through the mesenteric border of the jejunum and a Seldinger technique is used to subsequently insert the feeding tube through the jejunal wall. The external end of the feeding tube is then brought out through the anterior abdominal wall at a site distant from the laparotomy wound. A Roux-en-Y jejunostomy is used when a permanent jejunostomy is required.

Needle catheter jejunostomy and surgical jejunostomy are usually performed while the patient is undergoing major abdominal surgery, although can be formed as a separate surgical procedure. These jejunostomies are useful for both short- and long-term enteral feeding and when feeding into the stomach is contraindicated, for example following oesophageal, gastric, pancreatic or hepatobiliary surgery. Contraindications include local Crohn's disease, ascites, coagulopathies and severe immunosuppression. Complications of jejunostomy include infection, accidental removal of the feeding tube, leakage, tube blockage, volvulus and bowel obstruction, knotting of the tube and small bowel perforation. Surgical management of patients requiring long-term nutritional support is discussed in more detail (*See:* **Surgery:** Perioperative Feeding).

Percutaneous endoscopic gastrostomy and jejunostomy   Although surgical gastrostomies have been in use successfully since 1875, there are a number of problems associated with them, including wound dehiscence, infection, leakage, aspiration and bleeding. The complication rate of surgical gastrostomy varies from 2 to 75%, and mortality from 6 to 37%. This variability in morbidity and mortality is likely to relate primarily to the medical and surgical condition of the patient in whom a surgical gastrostomy is being performed. Patients are often elderly, malnourished and suffering from strokes, cancers or head injury, and many surgical gastrostomies were performed under general anaesthesia which may add to the potential morbidity.

In 1980, a method of inserting a gastrostomy tube percutaneously by endoscopy under local anaesthesia was described. Since then the percutaneous endoscopic gastrostomy (PEG) tube has become widely accepted, and their use is likely to continue increasing. PEGs are relatively simple and easy to insert, are cheaper than surgical gastrostomies, have a low morbidity and mortality, and avoid the need for a general anaesthetic. If necessary, the gastrostomy can be converted into a gastrojejunostomy using widely available commercial kits. There are two popular methods of inserting PEGs called the 'Pull – or Gauderer–Ponsky method' and the 'Push – or Sacks–Vine method'. The initial stage of both procedures is identical. An endoscope is inserted into the stomach which is distended by air insufflation. The anterior abdominal wall is transilluminated with the endoscope (or the tip of the endoscope is identified by fluoroscopy). Local anaesthesia is infiltrated into the skin following which a small wound is made with a scalpel. A large gauge needle catheter is inserted through the abdominal wall into the stomach heading towards the light from the endoscope. The stylet is removed and a wire or suture is passed through the needle into the gastric lumen. The wire or suture is grasped with forceps through the endoscope, following which the endoscope is slowly withdrawn, bringing the wire out through the mouth. The wire exiting from the mouth is held securely by an assistant and the forceps loosened to release the wire. In the Gauderer–Ponsky technique, the gastrostomy tube is tied to the wire and lubricating jelly applied. The assistant who inserted the needle into the stomach then gently pulls on the wire exiting from the abdominal wall, pulling the gastrostomy tube through the mouth, oesophagus, stomach and anterior abdominal wall, until the internal bumper is felt to catch on the stomach wall. An external fixation device is then applied. In the Sacks–Vine technique, the wire is kept taut and a tapered gastrostomy tube is inserted over the wire. The gastrostomy tube is then pushed down over the wire. After the tube tip penetrates the abdominal wall, it can be grasped and pulled through. Both techniques are equally successful with little difference in time of insertion or complications. An alternative method called the Russell technique places a J-wire into the stomach under endoscopic guidance. A dilating catheter is passed and then a feeding tube inserted using a peel-away sheath. The Russell technique has been modified to include placement of four nylon T-fasteners into the stomach at each corner of a square, which are then pulled up to appose the gastric and anterior abdominal walls. The gastrostomy tube is inserted into the middle of the square. The theory of this approach is that it avoids contamination by oral bacteria and may be useful in oesophageal obstructing tumours.

Aspiration of gastric contents may occur with PEGs and there are commercially available kits to enable conversion of PEGs into percutaneous endoscopic gastrojejunostomy (PEGJ) to try and overcome the problem of aspiration. The term percutaneous endoscopic jejunostomy (PEJ) is often to be found in the literature when describing conversion of PEGs. The term PEJ in this situation is not strictly correct, as no stoma is formed in the jejunum, and thus can cause confusion. A suitably long catheter is inserted via the gastrostomy and guided through the pylorus into the duodenum by endoscopy and forceps. The technique can be difficult and often the tip of the jejunostomy tube is little further than the first or second part of the duodenum, increasing the risk of regurgitation of the tube into the stomach. A novel wire-guided method to insert the jejunal tube via the gastrostomy further along the small bowel may prove to be more successful. PEGJs however do not appear to reduce the incidence of aspiration compared with PEGs.

The indication for a PEG is long-term feeding in a patient who cannot eat or swallow adequately or safely. Suitable patients include those with neuromuscular diseases (e.g. strokes, motor neuron disease), head and neck cancer or surgery, or oesophageal cancer. Contraindications are a completely occluding pharyngeal or oesophageal tumour, ascites, peritoneal dialysis and disorders of coagulopathy.

Complications of PEG tubes include wound infection, leakage, accidental tube removal, tube blockage, aspiration pneumonia, bleeding and death. We have recently shown a trend for fewer complications when smaller bore PEG tubes are used, and risk of complications may be further reduced by appropriate patient selection and insertion of PEGs by an experienced endoscopist and assistant.

Direct percutaneous endoscopic jejunostomy Despite the major advances in techniques of enteral gastrostomy feeding, aspiration remains a problem with PEGs and PEGJs. Infusing nutrient solutions in the small bowel distant to the ligament of Treitz can significantly reduce the risk of aspiration and placement of a feeding tube at such a distal site by direct percutaneous endoscopic jejunostomy may be useful in patients with previous gastric resection, gastric outlet obstruction and gastroparesis. The direct percutaneous endoscopic jejunostomy method essentially uses the 'pull' technique of Gauderer and Ponsky. An endoscope of 160 cm or longer is passed through the duodenum, distal to the ligament of Treitz into the jejunum. The anterior abdominal wall is transilluminated and a needle inserted at this point. The rest of the technique is as for inserting a PEG tube using the 'pull' method. Complication rates of this technique are similar to PEGs and include peristomal infections, abdominal wall abscess and colonic perforation, leakage and tube malfunction.

Fluoroscopically inserted percutaneous gastrostomy The morbidity and mortality of inserting gastrostomy tubes under fluoroscopic guidance is similar to PEG tubes, and can be used to place gastrostomies in patients with ascites or peritoneal dialysis which are relative contraindications to PEG insertion. The technique involves air insufflation of the stomach via a nasogastric tube and direct puncture of the stomach under ultrasound/fluoroscopic guidance. T-fasteners can be used as in the Russell technique.

Laparoscopic gastrostomy and jejunostomy Laparoscopy to place gastrostomy and jejunostomy tubes is a particularly useful technique in patients with complete occlusion of the oesophagus, or if previous surgery has been performed associated with adhesions. Disadvantages of this method include the need to empty the bladder by urinary catheter, a general anaesthetic is usually necessary, and the time taken to perform the procedure plus recovery time.

Enteral Diets

Although there are over 100 enteral diets available, enteral diet formulation can be classified into a few different categories (**Table 6**).

Oral dietary supplements

Oral dietary supplements are by definition not nutritionally complete and should be used to supplement dietary intake. Supplements are usually in 200–250 ml portions, are essentially lactose and gluten free and some contain a fibre source.

These supplements are usually prescribed to patients with normal or near normal gastrointestinal function, and it is important that they are palatable to the individual patient or they will not be consumed. Nitrogen is supplied as whole protein, carbohydrate as partial hydrolysate of starch, and lipid as long-chain triacylglycerols. The lipid component contains a mixture of n-3 and n-6 fatty acids. Studies have suggested that n-3 fatty acid supplementation improves survival after burns trauma, reduces post injury infectious complications and reduces immunosuppression following blood transfusion. The optimum ratio for n-6 to n-3 fatty acids is unknown, but a 5:1 ratio may be suitable, although this is not based on firm evidence from controlled clinical trials.

It has been empirically recommended that each 250 ml of oral dietary supplement should contain 25% of the recommended daily allowances of micronutrients (trace elements and vitamins) (i.e. 100% in 1 litre). Nitrogen-rich supplements have an energy density of 4.2 kJ ml^{-1} (1 kcal ml^{-1}) and the energy-rich supplements 6.3 kJ ml^{-1} (1.5 kcal ml^{-1}).

Polymeric enteral diets

There is a range of polymeric enteral diets currently available, differing in the energy, protein, fat, carbohydrate, mineral, vitamin, fibre and water content. Polymeric diets are indicated for those patients

Table 6 Categories of enteral diets

Oral dietary supplements
Polymeric enteral diets
Predigested chemically defined elemental diets
Disease-specific diets
Specialized diets

Table 7 Sources of carbohydrate in enteral feeds

Carbohydrate	Source
Starch (polysaccharides)	Pureed peas, beans, carrots Hydrolysed cereals Tapioca starch
Polysaccharides	Soya polysaccharides
Monosaccharides	Glucose Fructose
Glucose polymers	Glucose oligo- and polysaccharides Maltodextrins Corn syrup
Disaccharides	Sucrose Maltose

Table 9 Sources of fat in enteral feed

Fat	Source
Long-chain triacylglycerols	Soya bean oil Corn oil Sunflower oil Safflower oil Sesame oil Fish oil Rapeseed oil

Medium-chain
  triacylglycerols
	Hydrolysed and re-esterified
	  coconut oil

requiring enteral tube feeding who have a normal or near normal functioning gastrointestinal tract. They contain whole protein as the source of nitrogen and a mixture of carbohydrate and lipid as the energy source. Carbohydrate is derived from partial enzymatic hydrolysates of starch and constitutes 45–50% of the total energy content. The type of lipid contained in these feeds is usually either a pure long-chain triacylglycerol (LCT) source or a mixture of LCT and medium-chain triacylglycerols (MCT), and contributes 30–35% of the total energy content. Patients with normal bowel function should be able to absorb a pure LCT lipid source, but some manufacturers take the view that severely stressed patients may not be able to assimilate a pure LCT source adequately, and so add MCTs. MCTs may be more easily used as a source of energy because, unlike LCTs, they can be transported intact across the mitochondrial membrane, probably independently of carnitine. **Tables 7–9** list some of the different sources used in polymeric enteral diets.

'Standard' polymeric enteral diets contain 4.2 kJ

Table 8 Protein sources used in enteral feeds

Protein	Source
Intact protein	Soya protein Pureed beef Egg white Casein Lactalbumin Whey
Hydrolysed protein	Casein Soya protein Whey Lactalbumin
Amino acids	L-Amino acids

ml^{-1} (1 kcal ml^{-1}) of energy, 6–7 g l^{-1} of nitrogen, a nonprotein energy to nitrogen ratio of 544 kJ per g nitrogen (130 kcal per g nitrogen). The energy–nitrogen dense enteral diets contain 8–10 g l^{-1} of nitrogen, energy content 5–6.3 kJ ml^{-1} (1.2–1.5 kcal ml^{-1}), with a nonprotein energy to nitrogen ratio of 473–699 kJ (113–167 kcal per g nitrogen). Trace elements and vitamins constitute 66.7% RDA per litre. Example of the typical mineral content of standard and energy dense diets is given in **Table 10**.

There are a number of hypotonic polymeric enteral diets available. The rationale of these diets is that the incidence of gastrointestinal complications may be reduced by using 'starter regimes' whereby the load (concentration × rate) is raised slowly over a period of days. There is usually little benefit to be gained from using these diets as controlled clinical trials have shown that the incidence of gastrointestinal complications is not reduced by using 'starter regimes'.

Several polymeric enteral diets contain fibre, although currently there is little evidence to support its routine use in hospitalized patients. The interest in fibre and enteral nutrition is based on the possible effects of fibre on bowel function and morphology, generation of short-chain fatty acids and gut mucosal barrier function which have been reviewed in detail elsewhere. Constipation may be a problem in long-term enterally fed patients. Daily wet stool weights in normal subjects fed an enteral diet is approximately 80–90 g, which is not significantly increased by fibre supplementation. Enterally tube-fed patients daily mean wet stool weight is approximately 50–60 g and is not significantly altered by addition of fibre. Clinical and physiological studies have generally demonstrated how difficult it is to increase daily stool weights by supplementing enteral diets with fibre, even when a mixed rather than single fibre source has been used.

Diarrhoea remains a common problem during enteral tube feeding. Infected diets, lactose intolerance, concomitant antibiotic treatment, 'inert'

Table 10   Daily requirements and mineral content of a standard polymeric enteral diet

Minerals	Daily requirement	Units	Standard	Energy–nitrogen dense
Na	1 mmol kg^{-1} (1600 mg)	mg per 100 ml	80	80 (3.5 mmol)
K	5 mmol per g N (3500 mg)	mg per 100 ml	135	135 (3.5 mmol)
Cl		mg per 100 ml	125	125 (3.5 mmol)
Ca	700 mg	mg per 100 ml	50	57 (1.4 mmol)
P	20–30 mmol	mg per 100 ml	50	57 (1.8 mmol)
Mg	300 mg	mg per 100 ml	20	20 (0.8 mmol)
Fe	8.7–14.8 mg	mg per 100 ml	1	1
Zn	7–9.5 mg	mg per 100 ml	1	1
Cu	1.2 mg	µg per 100 ml	150	150
I	140 µg	µg per 100 ml	10	10
Se	75 µg	µg per 100 ml	4.25	4.25
Cr	>25 µg	µg per 100 ml	3.35	3.3
Mn	>1.4 µg	µg per 100 ml	300	300
Mo	50–400 µg	µg per 100 ml	5	5

carriers of medication, laxatives and hypoalbuminae-mia are all factors that may contribute towards the development of enteral feeding-associated diarrhoea. A common method of tube feeding is to use a pump to infuse enteral diet continuously. This method of feeding has been shown to promote diarrhoea in healthy subjects by suppression of colonic motor activity and causing a secretory response in the ascending colon. Likewise, high-energy loads fed by a novel bolus method of tube feeding also cause diarrhoea, although using a low-load bolus does not. The abnormal colonic responses to enteral tube feeding occurs, we believe, primarily because of the absence of a normal cephalic response to enteral tube feeding associated with failure to stimulate a normal postprandial PYY response. The secretory response can be reversed by infusing short-chain fatty acids directly into the caecum, which does provide a basis for including a fibre source in polymeric enteral diets. This positive effect of fibre may not have been demonstrated in clinical practice owing to concomitant antibiotic treatment. Short-chain fatty acids promote colonic water and electrolyte absorption, increase colonocyte proliferation and metabolic energy production, and enhance colonic blood flow. Whether fibre supplementation exerts a protective effect on gut mucosal barrier function, or whether this occurs as a result of luminal nutrition alone has not been fully elucidated. Overall, the addition of fibre in polymeric enteral diets may be beneficial, and multiple rather than single fibre sources should be used. To avoid any adverse effects on availability of trace elements for absorption, the quantity of fibre should be restricted to 15 g l^{-1} as estimated by the American Organization of Analytical Chemists (AOAC) method.

Predigested chemically defined elemental diets

There is little evidence that predigested chemically defined elemental diets are any better than polymeric enteral diets for the majority of patients. Elemental diets are useful for patients with severely impaired gastrointestinal function affecting nutrient absorption, e.g. nutritionally inadequate short bowel syndrome. In short bowel syndrome, nutrient assimilation is limited by inadequate luminal hydrolysis and brush border hydrolysis as well as by reduced functional absorptive capacity of the transport processes responsible for mediating the enterocyte uptake of the end products of luminal and brush border membrane nutrient hydrolysis. Therefore in these patients it is appropriate that nutrients should be provided in a form in which they are optimally absorbed.

The nitrogen source is derived from the partial enzymatic hydrolysis of protein, and consists of free amino acids, small peptides of 2–3 amino acid residues in chain length, and a variable proportion of longer peptide chains. The carbohydrate source consists of 'maltodextrins' derived from the partial hydrolysis of starch. The resulting composition is a heterogeneous mixture of glucose polymers with approximately 50% of the glucose content being present as polymers containing more than 10 glucose molecules. High molecular weight fractions can reduce the diet osmolality.

Steatorrhoea in the short bowel syndrome can be severe, often owing to multiple factors. This can include reduced contact time between substrate and lipase enzyme systems, reduced functional absorptive capacity, and decreased luminal bile acid concentrations resulting from interruption of the interhepatic circulation of bile salts. Assimilation of LCTs may therefore be limited, so in recognition of this most elemental diets contain LCTs predominantly in the form of linoleic acid in amounts thought to prevent essential fatty acid deficiency, as MCTs do not contain essential fatty acids. MCTs are prepared by the fractionation of coconut oil and contain predominantly octanoic (C_8) to decanoic (C_{10}) triacylglycerols. MCTs are more water-soluble than LCTs, do not require pancreatic lipase activity, and intraluminal hydolysis occurs more rapidly and more completely than with LCTs. MCTs are transported directly into the bloodstream and do not need the complex digestive and absorptive processes that LCTs require. MCTs are likely to be assimilated more efficiently than LCTs in patients with malabsorption and hence many elemental diets will also contain MCTs. If patients also have pancreatic insufficiency, then pancreatic supplements may be beneficial.

Patients with short bowel syndrome are at risk from water and electrolyte depletion, particularly when the ileum and colon have been resected. Large quantities of sodium, potassium, magnesium and zinc are lost in the jejunostomy effluent. Jejunal sodium absorption is promoted by luminal carbohydrate, bicarbonate and amino acids, but active transcellular absorption is easily overwhelmed by passive secretion down a concentration gradient via the intercellular junctions of jejunal mucosa. Perfusion studies have shown that sodium concentrations of 60–90 mmol l^{-1} are required for net sodium absorption in the jejunum, leading to the recommendation that elemental diets contain sodium in the range 80–90 mmol l^{-1} if these diets are to be used in the short bowel syndrome.

Disease-specific diets

Diets specially formulated for patients with specific diseases such as hepatic, renal and respiratory failure have been developed. Enteral diets for renal failure contain a nitrogen source consisting of all the essential amino acids plus histidine, without the nonessential amino acids. Nutritional support in renal disease is reviewed in detail (*See:* **Renal Function and Disorders**: Nutritional Management of Renal Disorders).

Patients with respiratory failure are adversely affected by diets containing high carbohydrate loads, when total energy load exceeds energy requirements. A high-fat : low-carbohydrate ratio in enteral nutrition reduces the respiratory quotient, decreases carbon dioxide production, and can reduce the length of time patients spend being ventilated.

Patients with liver disease requiring enteral nutritional support who are not encephalopathic should receive a standard polymeric or elemental diet according to clinical status. Patients who are encephalopathic, however, should probably have a nitrogen source of free amino acids containing high concentrations of branched-chain amino acids and low concentrations of methionine and the aromatic amino acids phenylalanine, tyrosine and tryptophan. As many of these patients will have cholestatic jaundice and be unable to assimilate LCTs, the energy content should predominantly be based on carbohydrate rather than lipid. Approximately 5% of the energy content needs to be presented as linoleic acid to prevent essential fatty acid deficiency. Sodium content of these diets should be low because of the underlying hyperaldosteronism and high total body sodium content.

Specialized diets

A number of enteral diets have recently been marketed supplemented with novel substrates such as n-3 fatty acids, structured lipids, short-chain fatty acids, growth factors and hormones with specific amino acids such as glutamine, arginine, cysteine, histidine, proline as well as nucleotides. In general terms the action of these novel substrates is directed towards modifying the metabolic response to trauma and sepsis, including immunomodulation, and interacting with inflammatory mediators and the gut. Examples include optimization of whole body protein synthesis by structured lipids, alteration of prostaglandin synthesis by n-3 fatty acids, the beneficial effects of arginine on hormone release, immune function, collagen synthesis and hepatic gluconeogenesis, and the roles that exogenous nucleotides may have on enhancing immune function. Arginine has immunostimulatory effects, increasing interleukin-2 production, reducing bacterial translocation and increasing survival in peritonitis, as well as improving nitrogen balance. Although glutamine has classically been considered a nonessential amino acid, recent studies suggest that it may be conditionally essential in stress and starvation. Glutamine has been shown to be beneficial in intensive care patients and following bone marrow transplantation. The role of glutamine on gut barrier function is currently unclear. It has been suggested that glutamine improves gut barrier function, although this has been disputed. Further research is required to examine more closely the role of these novel substrates in enterally fed patients.

Monitoring

General assessment

Patients receiving enteral nutrition support should be monitored closely, particularly severely malnourished patients who are at greatest risk from refeeding syndrome. It is important to take an appropriate history and examination of the patient before initiating feeding and at intervals thereafter. Formal guidelines for the assessment of patients by a nutritional risk score have recently been published by the British Association of Parenteral and Enteral Nutrition (BAPEN). Malnourished patients are apathetic, appear depressed, and may show little interest in food. These symptoms can be reversed by nutrition, but often malnourished patients must initially be persuaded to start eating to stimulate their appetite. Assessing muscle bulk and subcutaneous fat and examining for oedema will give a rough guide to the general nutritional status of the patient. Weighing the patient is a simple way of assessing if a patient is receiving adequate nutrition. However, changes in the patient's weight must be viewed with caution. It is essential that the same set of weighing scales is used, the patient must be in a similar state of dress at each weighing, and the time of weighing should be similar. The patient should have preferably emptied their bladder and bowels before being weighed. Furthermore, if the patient has gross oedema, the weight often falls with adequate nutrition as the hypoalbuminaemia is reversed and excessive fluid moves intravascularly to be excreted. A weight increase of 1–2 kg per week is suggestive of adequate nutrition to replete body mass. The body mass index (BMI) (weight (kg)/height (m)^2) can provide an approximate guide to the nutritional status of the patient. A BMI of less than 20 suggests malnutrition. However, the BMI is not ideal, as height and weight need to be accurately measured and presence of oedema may confound the true weight.

Diet charts help record exactly what the patient has received rather than what was prescribed, as the two do not always agree. Formal assessment of body fat stores can be made using skin callipers and triceps skinfold thickness (TSF), although in advanced malnutrition the correlation between TSF and total body fat stores may be poor. Patients with cirrhosis with a midarm muscle circumference and TSF below the 5th percentile of standard values however have significantly lower survival rates compared with patients above the 5th percentile. In the presence of severe fluid retention, assessment of protein–energy malnutrition by measuring midarm muscle circumference and TSF may be helpful and can identify those patients at greater risk of mortality. Isolated measurement of TSF is often of little value, but serial measurements may be more useful in assessing progress of the general nutritional status of the patient. As malnutrition is characterized by loss of skeletal protein, the assessment of muscle strength has been utilized to assess quantitatively the degree of protein depletion. Sex- and age-related hand grip strength measurements have been derived for assessing protein depletion and predicting postoperative complications. Serial measurements should be made to assess improvement in strength. To derive meaningful data from hand grip strength and TSF, the techniques need to be performed by personnel trained in using these methods.

Haematological and biochemical assessment

Basic haematological and biochemical parameters should be measured before introducing nutritional support. Initially close monitoring of potassium, phosphate, sodium and glucose is required. Patients on long-term enteral nutrition may require vitamin and trace element analysis if clinically indicated. Albumin, transferrin and thyroid-binding prealbumin may be useful in assessing response to nutrition support.

Refeeding syndrome

Refeeding malnourished patients results in a reversal in insulin, thyroid and adrenergic endocrine systems, causing an increase in basal metabolic rate and the rebuilding of lost body tissue, with glucose being the predominant energy source. This anabolic response causes intracellular movement of minerals, and serum levels may fall. These rapid changes in metabolism may cause severe cardiorespiratory and neurological problems including cardiac and respiratory failure, oedema, lethargy, confusion, coma, convulsions and death. These symptoms of the 'refeeding syndrome' have been mostly attributed to hypophosphataemia, but abnormal metabolic changes in potassium, magnesium and glucose probably also contribute. Hypokalaemia and hypomagnesaemia usually accompany the development of hypophosphataemia. Intracellular fluid increases, and extracellular fluid may decrease or increase depending on the refeeding regimen and previous fluid intake. Our standard policy on initiating refeeding is to measure urea, creatinine, sodium, potassium and glucose daily, and to test phosphate, magnesium, calcium and liver function twice weekly. The frequency of biochemical monitoring is, however, dependent on the patient's clinical and metabolic status and is adjusted accordingly.

Dehydration and refeeding oedema Dehydration is most likely to occur in patients on diuretics and who are dependent on others for their fluid intake. Additional fluid may be required during the summer months. Clinical monitoring and regular measurement of urea and electrolytes should indicate that dehydration is developing.

Refeeding may cause extracellular fluid retention. This is thought to occur as a result of refeeding with carbohydrates, which results in marked sodium and water retention. The mechanism for the antidiuretic effect of carbohydrate arises from the stimulation of endogenous insulin secretion, which enhances absorption of sodium from the renal tubules along with water.

Hyper- and hypoglycaemia Hyperglycaemia may develop owing to rapid infusion of high-carbohydrate enteral formulae, especially if the patient develops an intercurrent illness which may cause a relative insulin resistance. If hyperglycaemia is not controlled, dehydration, coma, acidosis and death may result. Rebound hypoglycaemia should not develop if nutrition is stopped abruptly unless the patient is also receiving exogenous insulin.

Potassium Potassium is primarily an intracellular cation. Insulin-induced glucose uptake by muscle and fat facilitates the intracellular movement of potassium. If inadequate potassium is supplied to meet anabolic requirements, hypokalaemia may develop. If potassium fails to rise despite adequate supplementation with potassium, magnesium levels should be checked as hypomagnesaemia often accompanies hypokalaemia. Hypokalaemia can result in muscle weakness, confusion, coma, convulsions, lethargy, and cardiac arrhythmias. Hyperkalaemia is an uncommon complication of refeeding; it may occur secondary to metabolic acidosis or renal disease and can result in cardiac arrest.

Phosphate Hypophosphataemia can develop as a result of insulin-induced uptake of phosphate by cells in the presence of glucose during refeeding. Chronic alcoholics are at high risk of developing refeeding hypophosphataemia because of existing nutritional deficiencies and depletion of whole body phosphate. Although the risk of hypophosphataemia is greater with parenteral rather than enteral feeding, the seriousness of hypophosphataemia, should it occur, warrants regular monitoring, particularly during the early stages of refeeding. Hypophosphataemia can cause muscle weakness, confusion, paraesthesia, coma, convulsions, haemolytic anaemia, cardiac arrhythmias, rhabdomyolysis and respiratory depression.

Magnesium During starvation and refeeding, magnesium levels can be low and are often accompanied by hypocalcaemia and hypokalaemia. Patients particularly at risk for hypomagnesaemia are chronic alcoholics, and those with severe malnutrition or on diuretics. During the initial stages of refeeding, magnesium should be checked twice weekly in severely malnourished patients. Symptoms of hypomagnesaemia include anorexia, nausea, depression, irritability, tremors, tetany, hyperreflexia and paraesthesia.

Calcium Hypocalcaemia may develop secondary to malabsorption causing true loss of calcium, or a relative hypocalcaemia may develop due to intercurrent critical illness. Hypocalcaemia can also develop secondary to magnesium deficiency and if the corrected calcium is low in the hypoalbuminaemic patient, magnesium should be checked and corrected if required. Hypocalcaemia can cause tetany and convulsions.

Liver function tests Changes in liver function tests may develop with enteral nutrition, but liver function usually returns to normal on discontinuing feeding. However, it is not always necessary to stop feeding. Unless liver function is severely abnormal, we continue to feed with a few hours' break each day, which usually resolves the problem.

Vitamins and trace elements Commercially produced polymeric enteral feeds contain adequate amounts of vitamins and trace elements. Supplementation may be required for some patients with severe malabsorption. Some enteral diets contain large amounts of vitamin K which may interfere with warfarin anticoagulation. If clinically indicated levels of zinc, copper, selenium, manganese, chromium and molybdenum can be quantified. A review of adult micronutrient and vitamin requirements and monitoring of these has recently been published.

Conclusions

Enteral nutrition should be viewed as a form of treatment and preventative therapy in malnourished patients. There is a range of different methods of accessing the gastrointestinal tract for enteral tube feeding, one of which should be suitable for most patients requiring enteral nutritional support. There are potential complications with tube feeding, most of which can be avoided if they are anticipated. Individualization of feeding regimens to each patient and close monitoring, both clinical and metabolic, should prevent most complications from developing.

See also: **Amino Acids**: Chemistry and Classification;

Metabolism. **Calcium**: Physiology. **Dehydration**: Physiological Effects and Management. **Dietary Fibre (Fiber)**: Physiological Effects and Effects on Absorption. **Hypoglycaemia (Hypoglycemia)**: Dietary and Metabolic Aspects. **Lipids**: Chemistry and Classification. **Liver Disorders**: Nutritional Management. **Magnesium**: Physiology, Dietary Sources and Requirements. **Malnutrition**: Definition, Classification and Epidemiology. **Phosphorus**: Physiology, Dietary Sources and Requirements. **Potassium**: Physiology, Dietary Sources and Requirements. **Renal Function and Disorders**: Nutritional Management of Renal Disorders. **Therapeutic Dietetics**: Lung Diseases.

Further Reading

Allison S (1995) Malnutrition in hospitalised patients, and assessment of nutrition support. In: Payne-James JJ, Grimble G and Silk D (eds) *Artificial Nutrition Support in Clinical Practice*, chap. 7, pp 115–126. London: Edward Arnold.

American Gastroenterological Association (1995) American Gastroenterological Association Medical Position Statement: Guidelines for the Use of Enteral Nutrition. *Gastroenterology* 108:1280–1301.

ASPEN Board of Directors (1993) Guidelines for the use of parenteral and enteral nutrition in adults and pediatric patients. *Journal of Parenteral and Enteral Nutrition.* 17(4):5SA–6SA.

Deveney KE (1990) Endoscopic gastrostomy and jejunostomy. In: Rombeau JL and Caldwell MD (eds) *Clinical Nutrition: Enteral and Tube Feeding*, vol. 2 chap. 12, pp 217–229. Philadelphia: WB Saunders.

Gottschlich MM, Shronts EP and Hutchins AM (1997) Defined formula diets. In: Rombeau JL and Rolandelli RH (eds) *Clinical Nutrition: Enteral and Tube Feeding*, vol. 2, chap. 13, pp 207–239. Philadelphia: WB Saunders.

Havala T and Shronts E (1990) Managing the complications associated with refeeding. *Nutrition in Clinical Practice* 5:23–29.

McWhirter JP and Pennington CR (1994) Incidence and recognition of malnutrition in hospital. *British Medical Journal* 308:945–948.

Payne-James JJ (1995) Enteral nutrition: tubes and techniques of delivery. In: Payne-James JJ, Grimble G and Silk D (eds) *Artificial Nutrition Support in Clinical Practice*, chap. 14, pp 197–213. London: Edward Arnold.

Rombeau JL and Palacio JC (1990) Feeding by tube enterostomy. In: Rombeau JL and Caldwell MD (eds) Clinical Nutrition: Enteral and Tube Feeding, chap. 13, pp 230–249. Philadelphia: WB Saunders.

Shenkin A (1995) Adult micronutrient requirements. In: Payne-James JJ, Grimble G and Silk D (eds) *Artificial Nutrition Support in Clinical Practice*, chap. 10, pp 151–166. London: Edward Arnold.

Silk DBA (1993) Fibre and enteral nutrition. *Clinical Nutrition* 12:S106–113.

Silk DBA (1995) Enteral diet choices and formulations. In: Payne-James JJ, Grimble G and Silk DBA (eds) *Artificial Nutrition Support in Clinical Practice*, chap. 15, pp 215–245. London: Edward Arnold.

Sizer T, Russell CA, Wood S, Irwin P, Allison S, Wheatley C and Whitney S (1996) *Standards and Guidelines for Nutritional Support of Patients in Hospitals*. Maidenhead, Berks: BAPEN.

Souba WW (1997) Drug therapy: nutritional support. *New England Journal of Medicine* 336:41–48.

Parenteral Nutrition

B Caballero, Johns Hopkins University, Baltimore, Maryland, USA

Background

Attempts to use of the intravenous route to heal and nurture humans date from the early 1800s. The first blood transfusion to a human was performed by Blundell in 1818, and in 1831 Latta reported the first successful intravenous rehydration in a patient with cholera. But progress in intravenous feeding had to wait for the developments in biochemistry and metabolism later in the nineteenth and early twentieth centuries. The identification of essential nutrients, the understanding of their biological role and metabolism, and the development of practical methods to quantify their concentration in blood and urine provided the scientific foundations for modern parenteral nutrition.

In 1949 Rhode and Vars described a technique for the continuous infusion of hypertonic solutions via a superior vena cava catheter in dogs. These investigators pioneered many of the access techniques that were later adapted for use in humans. But it was perhaps a case report by Wilmore and Dudrick in 1969 that launched parenteral nutrition as a practical clinical tool. They described the case of an infant with massive intestinal resection and severe malnutrition, who was kept on exclusive parenteral alimentation for 6 weeks. During that time, the child gained weight, length and head circumference. The dramatic success of this first application rapidly opened the field to application and research of intravenous feeding.

Another advance that greatly expanded the use of parenteral alimentation was the development of safe, nutritionally balanced solutions for intravenous use. Today, amino acid solutions, some customized for use in specific disease conditions, are widely available. The development of a lipid emulsion for intravenous use, pioneered by Wretlind in the early 1960s, facilitated the administration of energy while avoiding fluid overload. As these advances became well established, concerns for the parenteral nutrition of patients focused more on its appropriate indications and on the prevention of its potential adverse effects.

Indications

A basic principle of nutrition support is that the gut should always be the preferred route for nutrient administration. Therefore, parenteral nutrition is indicated when there is severe gastrointestinal dysfunction, usually as a result of acute injury, massive surgical resection or severe, intractable malabsorption.

The prevalence of malnutrition in the hospitalized patients is remarkably high. Although diagnostic criteria vary widely, several studies over the past decade have reported prevalences of malnutrition in large university hospitals as ranging from 30% to 70%. These high rates are likely to result from a combination of nutritional and nonnutritional factors, including severity and rate of complications of the primary disease, as well as poor nutritional screening and follow-up.

There is compelling evidence that poor nutrition impairs wound healing and tissue repair, and increases vulnerability to infection. As a consequence, malnutrition also increases the cost of hospitalization. One study compared the cost incurred by patients with high risk of malnutrition on admission with that of patients with low nutritional risk, admitted with similar diagnosis. Patients with nutritional risk had two to three times more complications during their stay, resulting in an excess cost $3000 to $6000 relative to the low-risk group. The same study estimated that nutrition support would cost the hospital $18 for enteral or $102 for parenteral nutrient administration.

The goals of nutritional support are to prevent or limit the metabolic derangements caused by acute illness, and to ensure the supply of essential nutrients to patients unable to receive regular diets. A specialized nutrition support team, which includes physicians, dietitians, nurses and pharmacists, should be responsible for assessment and monitoring of patients receiving specialized nutritional support. This support may use two major approaches for providing nutrients: enteral administration of special formulae, or intravenous infusion of solutions of amino acids, lipids and carbohydrates with micronutrients. The existence and regular function of this team, even in its most reduced form, is essential to provide adequate nutritional care and avoid iatrogenic complications associated with complex nutritional support.

Central venous access is fundamental for adequate parenteral nutrition support. Peripheral access cannot sustain full parenteral support, and is acceptable only when it is anticipated that only supplemental support for a few days will be needed (in which case the use of parenteral nutrition itself may be reconsidered). Ideally, the venous line should be used exclusively for parenteral nutrition. This can be achieved by placing multilumen lines whenever possible. Care of the line is as important as provision of nutrients, since continuing parenteral support depends on availability of venous access and avoidance of line contamination.

Requirements

Energy

The estimation of energy requirements for parenteral nutrition usually rely on predictive equations. Some of these equations, while appropriate for normal conditions, may lead to overestimates of energy needs, depending on the 'stress' factor used to account for increased energy requirements due to illness. Furthermore, energy requirements of severely ill patients tend to exhibit significant fluctuations, so even single measurements of energy expenditure by indirect calorimetry may not provide a reliable estimate of average requirements. The most common source of parenteral energy supply is glucose. Glucose is not only readily metabolized in most patients, but it also provides the obligatory need for this substrate, thus reducing gluconeogenesis and sparing endogenous protein. Most stable patients tolerate rates of 4–5 mg kg^{-1} min^{-1}, but insulin resistance in critically ill patients may lead to hyperglycaemia even at these rates. A decision on whether moderate elevations in blood glucose are acceptable should be made based on its duration, presence of glucosuria, and anticipated course of the primary illness.

Glucose in 5% solution can be safely administered via a peripheral vein, but higher concentrations require a central venous line. Twenty per cent or higher solutions may be needed to administer meaningful amounts of energy to fluid-restricted patients.

Nitrogen

Stress has a major impact on nitrogen balance. The nitrogen lost in the urine derives primarily from amino acids released by protein breakdown in response to catabolic mediators that include corticosteroid hormones, catecholamines and cytokines. Although modest increases in protein synthesis may be induced by substrate availability, this is rarely sufficient to compensate for breakdown, and attaining a positive nitrogen balance in the critically ill patients is extremely difficult. High nitrogen losses may continue for several weeks after a critical illness. Performing nitrogen balance is usually not practical in the patient care setting. At least 3–4 days of stable nitrogen intake need to be attained before performing the study. Collection of urine and faeces may be difficult, and relatively minor errors in faecal collections (usually incomplete collections) may lead to significant overestimations of net nitrogen retention. Urinary nitrogen alone is not a good index of nitrogen retention, although it can provide an estimate of the degree of protein catabolism.

Estimation of amino acid requirements is discussed elsewhere. Amino acid solutions for parenteral administration can provide all known essential amino acids (**Table 1**). Special amino acid solutions are also available containing higher levels of certain amino acids, most commonly the branched-chain amino acids (valine, leucine and isoleucine). These solutions are aimed at the management of liver diseases, sepsis and other stress conditions. Conversely, solutions containing fewer amino acids (primarily the essential ones) are available for patients with renal failure. The amino acid profile of solutions for neonatal use were developed to compensate for the immaturity of some enzymes of amino acid metabolism. For example, the rate of hydroxylation of phenylalanine to tyrosine may be insufficient to provide enough endogenous supply of this amino acid, and would increase its dietary requirement. Similar limitations have been reported for histidine and glycine synthesis in the preterm newborn. Clinical trials using growth and plasma amino acid profiles as outcome appear to support the use of these specialized solutions. The incidence of parenteral nutrition-induced cholestasis has also been reported to be lower with the use of these solutions, although the precise role of amino acid intake in the aetiology of cholestasis is still uncertain.

The concept of *organ-specific amino acid requirements* has received attention in recent years, particularly the requirement of the GI tract for the amino acid glutamine. Several studies have shown that the gut is a major nitrogen-processing organ which contributes significantly to the supply of glutamine to peripheral tissues. When this gut function is impaired, glutamine levels fall significantly. Low intracellular glutamine levels, in turn, have been correlated with impaired ability of skeletal muscle to incorporate amino acids into protein. Some clinical trials have also shown that glutamine-enriched solutions improve nitrogen balance and gut morphology. Accurate patient selection for administration of these solutions appears to be a critical factor for successful outcome.

Table 1 Examples of three amino acid solutions for parenteral use

Use	Aminosyn 10% (Abbott)	Renamine 6.5% (Clintec)	TrophAmine 5% (McGaw)
	Standard	Specialized (renal disease)	Neonatal/paediatric
Osmolarity (mOsm m^{-1})	1000	600	525
N (g per 100 ml)	1.57	1.0	0.9
Amino acids (mg per 100 per ml)			
Alanine	1280	560	320
Arginine	980	630	730
Glycine	1280	–	220
Histidine	300	420	290
Proline	860	350	410
Cysteine	–	–	<14
Serine	420	300	230
Tyrosine	44	40	140
Leucine	940	600	840
Isoleucine	720	500	490
Valine	800	820	470
Lysine	720	450	490
Methionine	400	500	200
Phenylalanine	440	490	290
Tryptophan	160	160	120
Threonine	520	380	250
Acetate (mEq per 100 ml)	14.8	6.0	56

Arginine has been added to enteral formulae. Results of clinical trials with these formulae are inconclusive, with some studies claiming positive effects on immune function and length of hospital stay. The combination of arginine with other 'immunomodulating' nutrients, such as n-3 fatty acids, has also been proposed. At this time, these approaches are primarily focused on enteral and not parenteral formulations.

Fat

Fat mobilization is a major response to stress and infection, and triacylglycerols are an important fuel source in those conditions, even when glucose availability is adequate. The development of fat emulsions for parenteral administration was a major advance in nutrition support. These emulsions can be safely administered via peripheral veins, provide essential fatty acids, and are a concentrated energy source for fluid-restricted patients (**Table 2**). Ideally, energy from fat should not exceed 40% of the total, and amounts of 2–3 g per kg per day are adequate. Patients on high-fat infusions may exhibit increased plasma triacylglycerol levels, particularly when drugs affecting lipid transport or lipoprotein lipase activity are administered concurrently.

Electrolytes

Normalization of acid–base balance is a priority and constant concern in the management of critically ill patients. Most electrolytes can be safely added to the parenteral amino acid/dextrose solution, up to a safe limit. Attempting to correct large electrolyte deficits via the parenteral mixture is not advisable, and is best done by a separate drip or bolus injection when appropriate. Even in the presence of normal serum levels, potassium and sodium administration should be carefully monitored in patients with oedema, ascites, oliguria or congestive heart failure.

Calcium salts should be added to the solution with caution. Calcium phosphate can precipitate if added in too high concentration. This is a particular risk in fluid-restricted neonates, who have relatively high calcium requirements. Concentrations of calcium salts (usually gluconate) of less than 12 mEq l^{-1} in dextrose/amino acid mixtures usually pose little risk of precipitation. However, at any given calcium concentration, increases in temperature and/or pH of the solution will increase the risk of precipitation.

Sodium bicarbonate in high concentrations will tend to generate carbon dioxide at the acidic pH of the amino acid/glucose mix. Acetate salts are preferred and can usually be used generously (always considering other concurrent sources of acetate). Acute corrections of acid–base status using sodium bicarbonate are best done by direct administration independent of the parenteral nutrition solution.

Vitamins

In the US there are two multivitamin formulations for parenteral use. One, intended for adult patients, contains 12 vitamins at levels estimated to provide daily requirements. Additional amounts can be provided separately when indicated. A paediatric formula contains 13 vitamins. Most adult vitamin formulae do not contain vitamin K, which is added according to the patient's coagulation status.

Trace minerals

These are essential component of the parenteral nutrition regimen (**Table 3**). Indeed, the discovery of the essential nature of some of these minerals was as a result of signs of deficiency developed by patients receiving total parenteral nutrition in the early days, when these substances were not added to the solutions. A multielement solution is available commercially, and can be supplemented with individual minerals. It should be noted that most trace elements may be toxic at high doses. In particular, minerals excreted via the liver, such as copper and manganese, should be used with caution in patients with liver disease or impaired biliary function. As our understanding of the essentiality and level of requirement

Table 2 Comparative composition of two common fat emulsion products

	Intralipid (Kabi-Vitrum) 10%	Liposyn II (Abbott) 10%
Lipid source	Soya bean	Soya bean, safflower
Osmolarity (mOsm l^{-1})	260	276
Phospholipids (%)	1.2	1.2
Glycerin (%)	2.25	2.5
Linoleic acid (%)	50	66
Linolenic acid (%)	9	4
Energy density (kcal ml^{-1})[a]	1.1	1.1

[a]1 kcal ~ 4.2 kJ.

Table 3 Trace mineral daily recommendations for parenteral use

Mineral	Newborns (μg kg^{-1})	Children (μg kg^{-1})	Adults (μg)
Zinc	200–300	100	2.5–4.0 mg
Selenium	2.0	2.0	40–80
Copper	20	20	0.5–1.5 mg
Manganese	1.0	1.0	60–100
Chromium	0.20	0.20	10–15

Modified from Shils et al. (1994).

of trace minerals evolves, more of them will become a required component of parenteral nutrition support.

Growth factors

Although growth factors are not recognized as required components of the usual parenteral alimentation regimen, there has been increasing interest in their use as coadjuvants in the nutrition support plan. Catabolism is a universal result of stress, sepsis and surgery, and thus it seems appropriate to attempt to counteract it with anabolic factors (usually hormones or endocrine mediators).

Insulin use as part of the parenteral regimen is relatively common. The main indication is hyperglycaemia at moderate glucose infusion rates, usually due to the insulin resistance associated with stress or to corticosteroid hormone therapy. Insulin infusion is usually effective in lowering blood glucose levels. However, kinetic studies using labelled glucose have shown that insulin administration may have little effect on endogenous hepatic glucose release and on gluconeogenesis. Thus, a high-glucose plus insulin regimen may actually increase lipogenesis and carbon dioxide production, without having a major effect on net energy balance. The decision to add insulin to the parenteral alimentation plan should be based on the overall condition and response of the patient, and monitoring accordingly.

Growth hormone (GH) and insulin-like growth factor I (IGF-I) have been the focus of several clinical trials as adjuvants to nutrition support, both enteral and parenteral. GH is an anabolic, lipolytic, insulinotropic agent that stimulates tissue protein synthesis. It has been extensively studied over the past decades as a means to revert the catabolic response to stress. From the studies of Cuthberson in the 1940s using pituitary extracts to current use of recombinant human GH, the data are consistent with a strong effect on reducing weight loss, promoting positive nitrogen balance, and mobilizing fat. More recent clinical trials have also shown its effectiveness in reversing many of the catabolic effects of corticosteroids. Other studies, however, have suggested that GH is less effective in severely injured or burnt patients. IGF-I (formerly known as somatomedin C) is released, primarily by the liver, in response to GH. Besides its role as GH mediator, it has also, as its name implies, insulin-like activity. It has been shown to be effective in enhancing protein synthesis but it lacks any significant lipolytic action. Other anabolic factors under study for possible use in nutrition support include synthetic anabolic steroids, neurotensin, epidermal growth factor and several cytokines. Further studies may eventually provide the basis for developing consistent criteria for indications of anabolic factors as part of the parenteral nutrition support plan.

Monitoring

The monitoring plan for the patient on parenteral alimentation should be customized to the specific response to intravenous therapy, as well as to the overall status of the patient. Serum electrolytes, acid–base status and blood glucose are perhaps the most important acute, short-term indicators. Once these are stable, monitoring should focus on the potential adverse effects of continuing intravenous feeding, particularly on liver function in infants and children. Monitoring of blood glucose and triacylglycerols should be done regularly when relatively high levels of these substrates are being administered. Nitrogen metabolism (plasma urea) should be regularly monitored in patients with impaired renal function receiving amino acid solutions.

Complications

The complications resulting from parenteral alimentation can be grouped in two major categories: those related to the catheter and those associated with the incorporation, metabolism and excretion of nutrients.

Catheter-related complications

The most frequent catheter-related complication is infection, which can be localized or systemic. The infection can be initially managed with appropriate antibiotic therapy, but it may require catheter removal. Other catheter-related complications include thromboembolism, pneumothorax, and vein or artery perforation.

Metabolic complications

Perhaps the most significant metabolic complication is liver toxicity, also know as parenteral nutrition cholestasis. It typically occurs in infants receiving total parenteral nutrition for weeks or months. Infants with very short gut appear to be particularly at risk. The disorder causes severe cholestatic jaundice, elevation of transaminases, and may lead to irreversible liver damage and cirrhosis. Multiple causes have been proposed, including high infusion rates of aromatic amino acids, high proportion of energy intake from glucose, and others. There is no specific treatment, other than anticholestatic therapy.

Other common metabolic complications include hyper- or hypoglycaemia, hypertriacylglycerolaemia, alterations in acid–base balance, including overproduction of carbon dioxide, and toxicity of contaminants of the parenteral solution. The lack of direct provision of nutrients to the intestinal epithelia during total parenteral nutrition is also of concern. Trophism and permeability of the GI mucosa may become altered, thus compromising any potential recovery of the patient's ability to receive nutrients enterally. Furthermore, bypassing the GI tract blunts the neurondocrine response to foods by the entero-insular axis. Studies have shown that the release of tumour necrosis factor (TNF), glucagon and catecholamines in response to endotoxin is significantly higher after parenteral than after enteral isocaloric feedings. In many circumstances it is possible to provide a minimal enteral nutrition supply to avoid or minimize this risk.

See Colour Plates 2, 3 and 4.

See also: **Amino Acids**: Chemistry and Classification; Metabolism. **Calcium**: Physiology. **Electrolytes**: Water-Electrolyte Balance; Acid-Base Balance. **Energy**: Energy Requirements. **Growth and Development**: Physiological Aspects. **Insulin Resistance**: Aetiology and Association with Disease. **Malnutrition**: Definition, Classification and Epidemiology.

Further Reading

Rombeau JL and Caldwell MD (1993) *Parenteral Nutrition*, 2nd edn. Philadelphia: WB Saunders.

American Society of Parenteral and Enteral Nutrition (ASPEN) (1993) Guidelines for the use of parenteral and enteral nutrition in adult and pediatric patients. *Journal of Parenteral and Enteral Nutrition* 17:1–52.

Brooks S and Kearns P (1996) Enteral and parenteral nutrition. In: *Present Knowledge in Nutrition*, 7th edn, pp 530–539. Washington, DC: ILSI Press.

Wilmore DW and Dudrick SJ (1968) Growth and development of an infant receiving all nutrients exclusively by vein. *Journal of the American Medical Association*. 203:860–.

Shils ME (1994) Parenteral nutrition. In: Shils ME, Olson JE and Shike M (eds) *Modern Nutrition in Health and Disease*, 8th edn, pp 1430–1458. Philadelphia: Lea & Febiger.

In the Home Setting

C Baldwin and **M Elia**, Dunn Clinical Nutrition Centre, Cambridge, UK

Patients suffering from chronic conditions often prefer to be treated in the familiar surroundings of their home, rather than in hospital. When the treatment involves sophisticated techniques, it is essential that either the patient or the carers are adequately trained and are able to distinguish between problems that can be easily dealt with at home and those that need expert advice and treatment in hospital. With the increasing pressure for hospital beds and the increasing cost of hospital stays, many techniques that were previously restricted to the hospital environment have extended into the community. These include renal dialysis, cytotoxic drug therapy and home parenteral and enteral tube feeding. Of these, home enteral tube feeding has recently grown rapidly in developed countries, so that its prevalence in countries such as Britain and the USA is greater than in hospital. In contrast, parenteral nutrition, which is a more sophisticated form of therapy, is still practised less commonly outside hospital than in hospital, and is likely to remain so in the foreseeable future. Both forms of treatment have brought into the arena health professionals specializing in nutritional support, and new problems, which range from simple day-to-day management problems to difficult ethical problems concerned with withholding or withdrawing nutritional support. Some of these problems can be appreciated by considering the origins and development of home artificial nutritional support in the context of the initiation of home artificial feeding and the organization, care and monitoring of patients.

Origins and Development

The first report of home parenteral nutrition (HPN) appeared in 1970 from North America. The numbers of people receiving HPN has grown rapidly since that time. During 1986 it was estimated that 18 000 people in North America received HPN; in 1992 this had increased to 39 000. In 1994, based on an estimated growth rate of 25%, 60 000 people were expected to receive HPN.

In Europe the development of HPN has been slower. The first reports appeared in the literature in the late 1970s. In the UK in 1994 the estimated point prevalence of HPN was 250–300 or 4–5 per million of the population. The annual prevalence is about 8–10 per million of the population. The numbers are probably similar in other Western European countries but they are much lower in Eastern European countries.

Home enteral tube feeding (HETF) is a much older technique, with the first reports appearing centuries ago. Accurate information on the numbers of people receiving HETF is difficult to obtain because HETF tends to be initiated from many centres and centralized reporting and record keeping is not fully established. **Table 1** shows the increasing annual prevalence of home artificial nutrition in North America (population ~300 million). As with HPN, HETF is less common in Europe than in North America and is practised much less in Eastern Europe, India and China than in industrialized Western countries.

The rapid growth of HETF is attributable to developments in tube technology (flexible fine bore tubes) and endoscopic procedures for placement of gastrostomy tubes (facilitating the easier initiation and management of feeding), as well as aggressive marketing associated with the development of commercial home care companies.

The difference in the prevalence of home artificial nutrition between countries and between different areas in the same country are likely to be the result of many factors. One survey in East Anglia examined the local incidence of HETF and factors influencing it. It demonstrated a 4-fold difference in the prevalence of HETF between the eight districts studied. The differences seemed to be explained by variations in expertise and support staff between districts. Districts with a high prevalence of HETF had a higher number of hospital dietitians to initiate and coordinate HETF. It is also possible that there are local differences in attitudes towards feeding disabled patients and that districts with a low prevalence of HETF may have a larger number of people in more expensive extended care facilities, although this explanation was not supported by the East Anglia study.

Globally the main influence on incidence of home artificial feeding appears to be related to health-care economics. There is a relationship between expenditure on health care, as a percentage of the Gross Domestic Product (GDP), and incidence of HPN and HETF. In India, Pakistan and Africa, where spending on health is less than 4–5% of the GDP, home artificial nutrition is uncommon. In Western Europe, where health care accounts for 6–9% of the GDP, home artificial nutrition is more common. In the USA in 1991 health care represented 11.7% of private expenditure alone, and was responsible for more home artificial nutrition than anywhere else in the world.

Indications

The main indications for HPN are Crohn's disease, ischaemic bowel disease, motility disorders of the bowel and malignant disease. The main difference in indications for use of HPN between countries concerns malignant disease. In the UK (1977–91) malignant disease accounted for only 5% of people receiving HPN. In contrast it accounted for 40% of cases in North America and 50% of cases in Italy. These differences contribute to a wide variation in age of people receiving HPN. In the UK (1977–91) less than 4% of patients were aged 55 years and over, compared with 19% in North America (1988) and 25% in Italy (1980–93). However, the figures change with time, as for example in the UK where more elderly patients with malignancy are being treated with HPN.

The indications for HETF are different in adults and in children. In adults the most common indications are neurological disorders of swallowing resulting from cerebrovascular accidents, multiple sclerosis, motor neuron disease, Parkinson's disease and obstructive lesions of the upper gastrointestinal tract. In children HETF is most usually used in conditions that lead to failure to thrive such as cerebral palsy, cystic fibrosis, congenital malformations and metabolic disorders. As with HPN, malignant disease accounts for differences in indications between countries. In North America 43% of people receiving HETF had malignant disease of all sites and in Italy malignant disease accounted for 67% of all adult HETF. A local survey in East Anglia in 1992–93 reported only 14% of adults on HETF to have malignant disease, usually of the upper gastrointestinal tract. The age distribution of people receiving HETF is once again influenced by the indications. As disorders of swallowing (strokes, motor neuron disease and other neurological conditions) and malignant disease of upper gastrointestinal tract tend to occur in older age groups, adults receiving HETF tend to be elderly. The numbers of children receiving HETF also varies between countries. In the UK they account for 30–40% of the total (and as high as 63% in one district owing predominantly to the high rate of HETF in children with cerebral palsy) compared

Table 1 Annual prevalence of home artificial nutrition in North America

Year	PN[a] at home	Enteral tube feeding[b]	
		Home	Extended care facilities
1986	18 000	22 000	20 000
1992	39 000	148 000	~150 000
1994[c]	60 000	230 000	~230 000

[a]Mainly Crohn's disease, radiation enteritis, malignancy.
[b]Mainly swallowing disorders (neurogenic/obstructive) and anorexia/failure-to-thrive.
[c]If growth rate ~25% per year in 1992 continued the extrapolated annual prevalence in 1994 is >0.1% of the population.

with 20% in the USA (1985–90) and 4% in Italy (1992–94).

Organization

In most parts of Europe home feeding has grown on an *ad hoc* basis, but without national regulation, from centres with interest and enthusiasm in the area of artificial nutritional support. The number of centres initiating and managing HPN tends to be small, partly because the number of people needing HPN is small and because a greater degree of expertise is required. HETF is managed from many more centres but with different systems of organization, resources and protocols. France is unusual within Europe in that home artificial nutrition is under the control of the Ministry of Health. HETF can be managed from any public health hospital but HPN is restricted to ministerially approved specialist centres. In 1994 there were 15 approved specialist centres for HPN, 11 for adults and 4 for children. In Italy home artificial nutrition is not nationally regulated but in 1994, 7 out of 20 regions had established regulations that were implemented by politicians. Formal applications have to be made to start home artificial feeding but there were often considerable delays in gaining approval.

In the USA the majority of HPN is managed by commercial companies. As well as being responsible for the delivery of feed and ancillary equipment, as is common in companies operating within Europe, they are also responsible for much of the management of the patients. Such companies often employ clinicians, nurses and dietitians and provide the training, support and follow-up of patients.

In the UK general practitioners are often involved in the provision and management of artificial nutritional support. They are expected to prescribe the feed for patients on HETF, although they are not able to prescribe the ancillary equipment. The costs for equipment are usually met by the hospital initiating the feeding or a community trust. For HPN neither the feed nor equipment is prescribed by the General Practitioner (GP), although until recently (1995) the GP was expected to prescribe the feed. Nevertheless the GP is expected to approve the plans for managing his or her patient, which are usually coordinated and implemented by teaching hospitals with experience in HPN.

The UK is unusual in Europe in having a well established patients' organization, Patients on Intravenous and Nasogastric Nutrition Therapy (PINNT). This organization provides support and information to people on home feeding as well as being active members of the British Association for Enteral and Parenteral Nutrition (BAPEN), through which they can influence policy and decision-making as well as advocate on behalf of their members. This organization has also been responsible for designing equipment specifically for home use.

Standards of Care

In the UK a number of problems with the provision of artificial nutrition have been reported. A survey of HETF in East Anglia reported inadequacies in training (23%) and in support and follow-up (20%). Specific problems such as lack of written instructions, lack of telephone contacts for use in emergency, lack of confidence and inadequacy of equipment for home use were also reported. They highlight the importance of facilitating follow-up at home for people who may be severely disabled and unable easily to attend hospital, and also of a multidisciplinary approach to home care. The British Association of Parenteral and Enteral Nutrition (BAPEN) further highlighted the problems that may be encountered in its 1994 report. The pressure on hospital beds means that patients may be discharged too early before training is complete. There may be a variety of people carrying out the training which may reduce the quality. Clear written instructions and contact telephone numbers were not always provided. Not all districts are able to provide a community follow-up service but may rely on GPs and district nurses. As home artificial nutritional support, especially HPN, is still relatively uncommon in the population, many practices may never have encountered a patient on this form of therapy and may be inexperienced in its management. The anomaly in the prescription of feed and equipment (see above) means that different people are providing each aspect of the care, which may not be ideal. Equipment designed for use in hospital is not always suitable for use at home. Finally, patients' needs may change throughout the course of their treatment and therefore there is a need to establish an organizational infrastructure for follow-up care. Many hospitals do not have a nutrition team nor policies that embrace the needs of people receiving artificial nutrition at home.

In 1994 a report published by the British Association for Enteral and Parenteral Nutrition (BAPEN) reviewed the role of enteral and parenteral nutrition in the community in the UK. The report examined the benefits and problems associated with the current system of organization and proposed a series of guidelines for the management of artificial nutrition in the community (**Table 2** and **Table 3**). The guidelines cover all aspects of training prior to discharge

Table 2 Standards of practice for home enteral tube feeding (HETF)

Structure	Process	Outcome
There will be a training programme for the health care professionals involved in the care of patients receiving home enteral nutrition.	Discharge planning will be performed only by professionals who have the necessary experience or who have undertaken a course of training in the topic.	The patient has confidence in the hospital team planning his/her discharge.
There will be a model of care for patients needing home enteral nutrition.	The members of the multidisciplinary team will be involved in writing the 'mission statement' on which the model is based.	The patient will know the benefits, aims and objectives of the HETF team.
There will be a relaxed, quiet area suitable for private discussion.	There will be a caring and compassionate atmosphere with adequate time for discussion.	The patient will feel able to express his/her fears and expectations.
The discharge planning documentation will include sections on domestic, family and social circumstances.	The nutrition team will evaluate, with the patient and family, how HETF will alter his/her way of life.	The patient will believe that the feeding system can be integrated into an acceptable way of life.
There will be written patient/carer learning goals for HETF.	A designated nurse or dietitian will be responsible for teaching the patient according to his/her individual capacity for learning.	The patient will be able to demonstrate the necessary skills and achieve all the learning goals.
There will be an instruction manual for HETF.	Information and procedures will be regularly updated in order to reflect developments and innovations in tube feeding, access, nutrients and delivery systems.	The patient will perform therapy based on current practice.
A relative, friend or appropriately trained health care professional will be available to deliver therapy if the patient is unable to do so.	The nurse/dietitian will help the patient identify the most appropriate carer. A community nurse will be given the opportunity to visit the patient in hospital and observe therapy before the patient is discharged.	The patient has confidence that safe care will be available at home.
Access to the gastrointestinal tract will be achieved by a tube suitable for long-term use.	The patient, nurse and doctor will choose the most appropriate tube and access site.	The patient will use a feeding tube which is acceptable and accessible.
There will be a policy for sharing care with the patient's General Practitioner.	The GP will be contacted and a shared care protocol agreed.	The patient will know the responsibility of each health care professional.
Written information describing HETF will be avaialbe for the General Practitioner.	The hospital team will provide the GP with the information before the patient is discharged, together with the discharge date and on-call telephone numbers.	The patient will have confidence in his/her GP's knowledge of HETF.
There will be written procedures for the management of feeding tubes.	The nurse/dietitian will adapt the procedures according to the patient's physical skills and domestic circumstances.	The patient's daily life will not be restricted by prolonged inappropriate procedures.
There will be a written prescription for the enteral feed (and other prescribable items)	The patient's GP will be contacted and advised on how to prescribe the feed.	The patient will have the enteral feed available at home on the day of discharge.

Table 2 Continued

Structure	Process	Outcome
There will be a list of the required equipment, e.g. syringes, connectors, administration sets, pump, drip stand, telephone.	Before discharge the patient's home health authority will be provided with the list and asked to arrange supply by making local arrangements or establishing a contract with a commercial supplier.	The patient will have all the necessary supplies in his/her home on the day of discharge.
There will be an on-call system for providing expert advice to the patient by telephone day and night.	The nurse/dietitian/doctor will explain the system to the patient and identify the professions involved.	The patient will know the names and telephone numbers of health care professionals to contact in case of emergency day or night.
Information will be available describing how the nutrient solutions and supplies will be provided following discharge.	The nurse/dietitian will explain the ordering system and discuss storage, depending on the patient's home circumstances.	The patient will know how to obtain supplies and store and dispose of unwanted material.
There will be a post-discharge monitoring protocol, established by the nutrition team.	Monitoring will be performed by a designated health professional as defined by the protocol.	The patient will know what the follow-up arrangements are.

from hospital and support from specialist trained staff once the patient is at home. In addition to the guidelines the committee proposed a system of national and local organization for the provision of parenteral and enteral feeding at home. They recommend that HPN is managed only from specialist centres that have developed an expertise in this area. HETF should operate from individual districts, but they suggest that the most effective organization of this might be to have one centre for adults and one for children within each district. Although these recommendations were intended for the British health-care system, it is clear that the basic principles also apply to many other countries.

Monitoring

The basic elements of monitoring are similar for both parenteral and enteral feeding. They include an assessment of the activity of the underlying disease, the nutritional and metabolic state of the patient, and the complications associated with nutritional support (**Table 4**). The clinical history alerts the attending health professional to the general well-being as well as the likelihood of specific problems such as dehydration, electrolyte imbalance (e.g. diarrhoea), local infection (e.g. local redness and swelling near the catheter exit site or peristomal area), blocked tubes and catheters, and so on. Catheter-related sepsis is an important complication of parenteral nutrition and aspiration pneumonia is an important complication of enteral tube feeding. The patient/carer should have written instructions about the basic procedures, which aim to reduce the com-

plication rate, how to deal with simple problems, and to how recognize problems that they cannot readily deal with. Specialist advice should be available 24 h a day.

Dietary intake should be monitored, especially in patients whose clinical status is changing. Appropriate dietary advice may facilitate return to normal oral feeding in some patients. Blood tests should be carried out at intervals to check for metabolic stability and specific nutrient deficiencies (e.g. vitamins, minerals and trace elements) and toxicities. The frequency with which they are carried out depends on the patient, e.g. whether the patient is receiving enteral or parenteral feeding, length of feeding, the extent of oral intake, and disease activity.

The frequency of complications depend at least partly on the support provided by health professionals.

Outcome

The most important predictor of outcome in patients receiving home artificial nutritional support (enteral or parenteral) is the underlying disease. Therefore, mortality statistics strongly depend on the initial indications. Nevertheless a few general conclusions can be made.

First, the complications associated with nutritional support (enteral and parenteral) are responsible for less than 3–5% of the deaths. Second, the outcome is dependent not only on the type of disease, but also on the stage of the disease, e.g. patients with advanced HIV who start HPN are only expected to survive a few months whereas patients with less

Table 3 Standards of practice for home parenteral nutrition (HPN)

Structure	Process	Outcome
There will be a training programme for health care professionals involved in the care of patients receiving home intravenous nutrition.	Discharge planning will be performed only by professionals who have the necessary experience or who have undertaken a course of training in the topic.	The patient has confidence in the hospital team planning his/her discharge.
There will be a model of care for patients needing home intravenous nutrition.	All members of the multidisciplinary team will be involved in writing the 'mission statement' on which the model is based.	The patient will know the beliefs, aims and objectives of the HPN Care Team.
There will be a relaxed, quiet area suitable for private discussion.	There will be a caring and compassionate atmosphere with adequate time for discussion.	The patient will feel able to express his/her fears and expectations.
The discharge planning documentation will include sections on domestic, family and social circumstances.	The nutrition team will evaluate with the patient and family how the HPN will alter his/her way of life.	The patient will believe that the feeding system can be integrated into an acceptable way of life.
There will be written patient/carer learning goals for HPN.	A designated nurse will be responsible for teaching the patient according to his/her capacity for learning.	The patient/carer will be able to demonstrate the necessary skills and achieve all the individual learning goals.
There will be an instruction manual for home intravenous nutrition.	Information and procedures will be regularly updated in order to reflect developments and innovations in venous access, nutrient solutions and delivery systems.	The patient will perform therapy based on current practice.
A relative, friend or appropriate health care professional will be available to deliver therapy if the patient is unable to do so (e.g. parent or guardian of a child)	The health care professional will help the patient to identify the most appropriate carer. The district nurse will be given the opportunity to visit the patient in hospital and observe therapy before the patient is discharged.	The patient has confidence that safe care will be available at home.
Venous access will be achieved by a central venous catheter suitable for long-term use.	The patient, nurse and doctor will choose the most appropriate catheter and access site.	The patient will use a central venous catheter that is acceptable and accessible.
There will be written procedures for the management of central venous catheters	The nurse will adapt the procedures according to the patient's physical skills and domestic circumstances.	The patient's daily life will not be restricted by prolonged inappropriate procedures.
There will be a policy for sharing care with the patient's general practitioner.	The GP will be contacted and a shared care protocol agreed.	The patient will know the responsibility of each health care professional.
Written information describing HPN will be available for the GP.	The hospital teams will provide the GP with the information before the patient is discharged, together with the discharge date, and on-call telephone numbers.	The patient will have confidence in his/her GP's knowledge of HPN.
There will be a written prescription for the nutrition solutions (and other prescribable items).	The patient's GP will be contacted and advised on how to prescribe the feed.	The patient will have the feeding solution available at home on the day of discharge.

Table 3 Continued

Structure	Process	Outcome
There will be a list of the required equipment, e.g. refrigerator, infusion pump, syringes, sterile gloves, telephone.	Before discharge, the patient's home health authority will be provided with the list and asked to arrange supply by making local arrangements or establishing a contract with a commercial supplier.	The patient will have all the necessary supplies at home on the day of discharge.
There will be an on-call system for providing expert advice to the patient by telephone day and night.	The nurse will explain the system to the patient and identify the professions involved.	The patient/carer will know the names and telephone numbers to contact in case of emergency by day or night.
Information will be available describing how the nutrient solutions and supplies will be provided following discharge.	The nurse will explain the chosen supply system and discuss storage depending on the patient's home circumstances.	The patient will know how to obtain supplies, store them and dispose of unwanted material.
There will be a post-discharge monitoring protocol, established by the nutrition team.	Monitoring will be supervised by the nutrition team.	The patient will know the date of the first outpatient visit and what monitoring will be performed.

Table 4 Some complications associated with parenteral and enteral nutrition

	Parenteral	Enteral
Mechanical	Catheter malposition. Insertion trauma (e.g. pneuneothorax, brachial plexus injury, cardiac arrhythmia) Catheter blockage, kinking or occlusion Catheter embolus Air embolus Clot embolus (from catheter tip) Lack of access site	Tube malposition (e.g. into lung) Inserstion trauma: drainage to stomach and bowel: peritonitis and peristomal leakage and inflammation. Tube blockage, e.g. kinking or occlusion
Feed/flow	Nutrient overload (e.g. hyperglycaemia, infusional hyperlipidaemia)	Diarrhoea or constipation Bloated adbomen/cramps Regurgitation/aspiration of feed
Infections	Catheter-related sepsis Infected feed/administration set	Infected feed administration set Infection around gastrostomy
Metabolic	Fluid and electrolyte disturbances Hyperglycaemia Deficiency syndromes, e.g. trace elements and vitamins Nutrient overload (see above) and toxicity (e.g. some trace elements)	Fluid and electrolyte disturbances Deficiency syndromes (rate with standard feeds given to typical patients) Hyper/hypoglycaemia
Organ tissue dysfunction	e.g. Abnormal liver function, intestinal atrophy, metabolic bone disease	Mainly disease related, abnormal liver function Aspiration pneumonia
Psychological	Anxiety, depression, disturbance in self-image, social isolation	Anxiety, depression, disturbance in self-image, social isolation
Financial	Economic issues vary from centre to centre and country to country	Economic issues vary from centre to centre and country to country

advanced disease are expected to survive longer. Third, outcome of a variety of conditions is available from the North American Registry. For example, in patients with AIDS and malignancy there is 80–90% mortality at 1 year. Patients with ischaemic bowel disease and motility disorders have intermediate mortalities (13% per year) with 25–30% returning to oral nutrition within 1 year. Patients with Crohn's disease often have a good prognosis (4% mortality per year) with 70% returning to full oral nutrition at 1 year.

For patients on HETF overall mortality is high: 70% mortality at 1 year for malignancy, and 45% mortality for neurological disorders of swallowing (with considerably better results in patients <25 years than >65 years). Patients receiving HETF because of impaired small bowel absorption have a 20% mortality at 1 year.

Intestinal Transplantation

Intestinal transplantation may be considered as an alternative to long-term parenteral feeding in some patients. The first intestinal transplantations in humans took place in the early 1960s. The limitations of immunosuppressive therapy at that time meant that none of the group survived beyond 76 days. From 1985–90 a series of 20 patients were given cyclosporin but only two patients were able to resume normal nutrition and most of the grafts failed. The development of a new immunosuppressive agent, tacrolimus, has revived interest in the area. An international intestinal transplant registry recently reported the results of 180 transplants carried out on 178 patients. Sixty-one per cent of the group were less than 20 years of age with 44% aged between 0 and 5 years. In 64% of cases the indication for transplantation was the short bowel syndrome. Survival at 1 and 3 years in those receiving tacrolimus was as follows; 65% and 29% for isolated small bowel transplantation; 64% and 38% for combined small bowel and liver transplantation; and 51% and 37% for multivisceral transplantation. Of the 86 survivors at 3 years 78% had stopped PN and returned to full oral nutrition and 12% were receiving PN intermittently.

Intestinal transplantation is a life-saving option for people who cannot be maintained on PN or for those who require massive abdominal evisceration of locally aggressive tumours. Transplantation is still considered too risky for children and adults successfully maintained on PN and is not appropriate for patients in whom multisystem disease is expected to progress rapidly or those who may be able to resume oral nutrition, e.g. a healing intestinal fistula or in

the short bowel syndrome where functional intestinal adaption occurs with time (up to 1–3 years).

Ethical Issues

The provision of nutritional support to people who are chronically sick or who have progressively disabling diseases or who are terminally ill raises many ethical questions. Opinions about withholding or withdrawing artificial nutritional support vary from country to country, because of different philosophical, religious and social beliefs as well as different national economies.

The legal position is not clear cut. In the USA the courts have often ruled that competent patients have the right to refuse nutritional support in the same way that they are allowed to refuse medical treatment. The situation is complicated when patients have not made their wishes known and are unable to do so because of their clinical condition. In Europe there have been fewer examples. A recently publicized report in England concerned a teenager who was in a persistent vegetative state following a crush injury at a football stadium. The local coroner ruled that withdrawing feeding would constitute an act of murder. This was overruled by the House of Lords in 1993. Feeding was withdrawn and the patient was allowed to die.

The issues raised are not easily resolved, and in some cases the distinction has to be made between withholding and withdrawing artificial nutritional support.

Conclusions

Home artificial nutritional support is an important modality of treatment which can be used to support a small group of patients with severe disabilities, which may be progressive. Without parenteral nutrition many patients with intestinal failure would die quickly and without enteral tube feeding many patients with swallowing difficulties would also die quickly. Artificial nutritional support outside hospital can also be used successfully to prevent or treat suffering associated with undernutrition and growth failure. However, the treatment itself may restrict normal lifestyle and may lead to life-threatening complications. These can be prevented or treated by establishing an adequate organizational infrastructure for training and follow-up of patients and when necessary admitting patients to hospital for more intensive therapy. Ethical difficulties about withholding or withdrawing artificial nutritional support are likely to continue and to vary with time and from country to country.

See also: **Nutritional Support**: Parenteral Nutrition.

Further Reading

Allison SP, Micklewright A, Rawlings J and Hull M (1993) Organisation and evaluation of home enteral nutrition services. *Clinical Nutrition* 12 (supplement 1):38–43.

American Dietetic Association Reports (1994) Position of the American Dietetic Association: Nutrition monitoring of the home parenteral and enteral patient. *Journal of the American Dietetic Association* 94(6):664–666.

Elia M (1994) Home enteral nutrition: some general aspects and a comparison between the USA and Britain. *Nutrition* 10:1–9.

Elia M (ed.) (1994) *Enteral and parenteral nutrition in the community*: a report by the working party of the British Association for Parenteral and Enteral Nutrition (BAPEN). Maidenhead, Berks: BAPEN.

Elia M (1995). An international perspective on artificial nutritional support in the community. *Lancet* 345:1345–1349.

Grant D (1996) Current results of intestinal transplantation. *Lancet* 347:1801–1803.

Howard L, Ament M, Fleming CR, Shike M and Steiger E (1995) Current use and clinical outcome of home parenteral and enteral nutrition therapies in the United States. *Gastroenterology* 109:355–365.

McWhirter, Hambling CE and Pennington CR (1994) The nutritional status of patients receiving home enteral feeding. *Clinical Nutrition* 13(4):207–211.

North American Home Parenteral and Enteral Nutrition Patient Registry (1993) *Annual Report with outcome profiles 1985–1991*. Albany, New York: The Oley Foundation.

Parker T, Neale G and Elia M (1995) Home enteral tube feeding in East Anglia. *European Journal of Clinical Nutrition* 49:47–53.

Parker T, Neale G, Cottee S and Elia M (1996) Management of artificial nutrition in East Anglia: a community study. *Journal of the Royal College of Physicians of London* 30:27–32.

Pennington CR (ed.) (1996) *Current perspectives on parenteral nutrition in adults*: a report by the working party of the British Association for Parenteral and Enteral Nutrition (BAPEN). Maidenhead, Berks: BAPEN.

NUTRITIONAL SURVEILLANCE

In Industrialized and Developing Countries

K F A M Hulsof and **Michiel R H Löwik**, TNO Nutrition and Food Research Institute, Zeist, The Netherlands

In Industrialized Countries

Since the 1980s, evidence has accumulated that prevailing dietary patterns have adverse health effects. Nutritional assessment has become an important topic on the health policy agenda. This article describes the aim of nutritional surveillance, the availability and usefulness of nutritional surveillance indicators (especially food consumption), and some trends, risk groups and risk areas. Nutrition-related health problems and surveillance systems differ among countries, in particular between developed and developing ones. Therefore, this article deals only with industrialized countries in Europe and Australia, Canada and the USA.

Aim of Nutritional Surveillance

As stated by a Joint FAO/UNICEF/WHO (Food and Agriculture Organization, United Nations Children's Fund, World Health Organization) Expert Committee, the objectives of nutritional surveillance are as follows: to describe the nutritional status of the population, with particular reference to groups at risk; to contribute to the analysis of causes for changes and differences; to promote decisions by governments on food and nutrition policy issues; to predict future trends and to evaluate the effects of nutritional programmes.

As illustrated in **Fig. 1**, nutritional surveillance ideally provides information on a wide range of variables, from food availability, distribution and consumption and nutrient utilization (as reflected in nutritional status) to, ultimately, health status and mortality. This results in identification of public health problems that call for specific action and lead to nutrition research priorities (both applied and more fundamental). The data can be obtained from either existing sources, including administrative data, or surveys undertaken specifically for surveillance purposes.

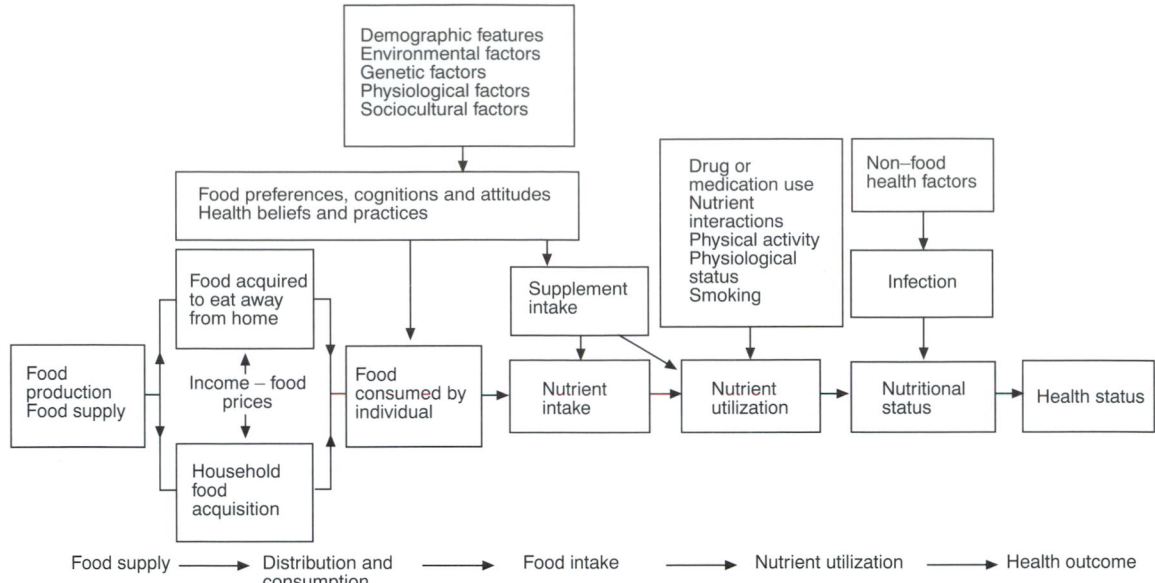

Figure 1 A conceptual model of the relationships of food to health. Source: Life Sciences Research Office, FASEB (1989).

Sources of Dietary Information

Insight into dietary patterns is a core target of nutritional surveillance since this provides a comprehensive basis for nutritional risk assessment. In principle, three different types of data can be used: food supply data, data from household consumption surveys, and data from dietary surveys among individuals. Each type of data corresponds with a different stage in the food distribution chain and is obtained by different methods.

Food supply data

Food supply data provide information on the type and amount of food available for human consumption, to the country as a whole. The supply is calculated in food balance sheets (FBSs) which are accounts, on a national level, of the annual production of food, changes in stocks, imports and exports, and agricultural and industrial use. Food supply is usually expressed per head of the population in kilograms per year, or grams per day. Per capita consumption of energy and some additional nutrients is calculated using food composition tables.

Food supply data refer to food availability, which gives only a crude impression of potential consumption. Food and nutrient losses prior to consumption, owing to processing, spoilage, trimming and waste, may not be adequately accounted for. Furthermore, these data provide no information about the distribution of food among population groups or districts.

International FBSs are prepared and published by the FAO, the Organization for Economic Cooperation and Development (OECD) and the stat-

istical office of the Commission of the European Communities (EURO-STAT). The FAO has published FBSs since 1949, also covering the period 1934–1948. Since 1949, FBSs have been compiled on an annual basis from data supplied by about 200 countries. Information is available for all European countries, Australia, Canada, Japan, New Zealand and the USA. Since 1971, the FAO has included its FBS data in the Interlinked Computer Storage and Processing System of Food and Agricultural Commodity Data (ICS). The OECD FBSs cover 23 countries, i.e. 18 European countries, Australia, Canada, Japan, New Zealand and the USA. EUROSTAT publish FBSs for its 12 member countries. Although FBSs are compiled in a similar way, they differ in coverage, food grouping and level of processing of commodities (e.g. FAO lists 300 food items classified into 17 food group categories; OECD 70 items in 13 categories) and in nutrient conversion factors. The FAO and OECD usually publish summaries of FBSs every 3–5 years, with a time-lag of 3–4 years between data collection and publication. The ICS supplies more up-to-date figures both on magnetic tape and on floppy disk (see also http://apps.fao.org/). EUROSTAT publish supply balance sheets in the Agricultural Statistical Yearbook.

In addition to the international FBSs, many countries publish national FBSs, mostly in statistical yearbooks or special statistical publications. For example, US food supply statistics are available for 1909 onwards, and in The Netherlands FBSs are available for 1950 onwards – both on a yearly basis. National FBSs tend to be more up-to-date and are normally available annually, again with a time-lag of up to 3 years. Owing to different methodologies underlying their compilation and presentation, these data can differ from the international FBSs.

Despite their limitations, FBSs are useful in that they indicate the (in)adequate aspects of food supply, provide material for planning food supply (production, imports and exports) and give crude indications of (un)desirable changes in terms of expected health impact. As a result of their long history, FBSs are especially useful for assessing trends over time. In contrast to national FBSs, the international FBSs can be used for comparative studies, provided that the FAO and OECD data sets are not mixed up. **Figure 2** illustrates the use of FBS data (FAO) for comparisons across countries and for trends over time. This figure shows the consumption of meat and meat products in five selected countries. Only in the UK has the consumption of meat and meat products remained remarkably steady since the 1960s. In the other countries the total consumption of meat has increased considerably, especially in Spain. The same tendency has been observed in other southern European countries and reflects one of the important changes in the Mediterranean diet over the past decades. Such comparisons implicitly assume that the demographic changes across the countries are similar.

Household surveys

Food available at the household level may be estimated by budget surveys and by consumption surveys. The first type of survey gives information on the purchases of food in terms of expenditure, used in economic policy. For example, weights for the construction of consumer price indices can be calculated. In household consumption surveys the amounts of foods and drinks brought into the household are also recorded. For the most part, only the expenditures of meals taken outdoors are noted. Some household surveys may even measure changes in food stocks, in addition to acquisition.

In general, household surveys do not provide information on how food is handled within the household, or on actual consumption by its members. Sometimes, the consumption data are converted to individual intake levels. The methods vary from simply dividing the total consumption by the number of people in the households, to assigning factors (consumer units) to persons weighed according to age and sex. In most countries, household surveys started in the 1940s or 1950s. Only very few countries have a continuous system, some repeat surveys every 3–4 years, others only every 5–10 years. In The Netherlands, the household budget surveys started in

1951, and since 1978 they have been conducted annually. In Europe, the best-known study is the specialized and ongoing household food consumption survey of the UK. Australia, Canada and Japan have regularly conducted household consumption surveys. In the USA, the first national household food consumption survey was conducted in 1936–1937. Between 1942 and 1965, four nationwide studies on household consumption were carried out. Since 1965, US household food consumption surveys also provide information of food intake at the individual level of household members. At present, a wide range of data on household surveys are available, as shown in the FAO Food and Nutrition Policy Papers and a recent WHO publication. However, since the dietary data are based on a variety of methods, the surveys are not very suitable for comparisons among countries. Differences exist in sampling procedures, food grouping, conversion to nutrients and period, frequency and technique of data collection. For example, sample sizes vary from less than 500 households (Switzerland) to over 30 000 (Italy), which is only partially explained by population size. Snacks, sweets, soft drinks and alcoholic beverages are excluded from some surveys. Data on the quantity of and/or expenditure on food may be collected by recordkeeping, by interviews or by both methods. Household accounts for nonfood items can cover a period of 4 weeks, but for foodstuffs 2 weeks is more usual.

In contrast to FBSs, household surveys can supply information on food (and nutrient) patterns in subgroups of households. These groups may be classified by economic, demographic and other factors, which provides the opportunity for risk group identification. The results of household surveys play an important role in nutritional surveillance within countries, particularly when surveys are carried out annually, which reveals trends in food consumption. To improve the possibilities for international comparisons of these data, an ongoing project of the European Union (DAPHNE, Data Food Networking) is now attempting to harmonize at the international level dietary exposure from household budget surveys.

Individual dietary surveys

In contrast to FBSs and household surveys, data from individual dietary surveys provide information on average food and nutrient intake and their distribution over various well-defined groups of individuals. Data more closely reflect actual consumption and can provide additional information on meal patterns, etc.

To collect dietary intake data on an individual

level, several methods can be used. Briefly, the methods can be divided into two categories: record and recall methods. Record methods collect information on current intake, keeping a record of all foods and drinks based on menu, household measures and/or weighing, over one or more days. Recall methods reflect past consumption, varying from intake over the previous day (24-hour recall) to usual food intake (dietary history or food frequency). Each form has its own strengths and weaknesses, and there is no single ideal method. Details of the available methods for assessing food consumption of individuals are given in numerous reviews and manuals.

To characterize the average intake of food and nutrients and their distribution over various groups of individuals a 24-hour recall or 1-day food record is appropriate, provided that the sample is representative of the population under study, and day-of-the-week and seasonal variations are taken into account. To determine the proportion 'at risk' of inadequate intake, the food consumption of each subject must be measured over more than one day, or retrospective information on intake over a longer period may be used (e.g. dietary history method). The appropriate period depends on the purpose of making an estimate, the precision desired, the food component(s) of interest, the intra- and interindividual variation components and the period over which an intake has to be low or high before health risks are introduced.

Most industrialized countries, if not all, have carried out small-scale dietary surveys. These surveys provide valuable information, but owing to samples of convenience and different food consumption methods their usage in national nutrition policy and nutritional surveillance is of limited value. The number of countries that have conducted individual dietary surveys within the framework of nutritional surveillance is relatively low. It appears that Australia, Canada, the USA and several European countries (Belgium, Denmark, FRG, Ireland, The Netherlands, Portugal, Sweden, UK) have performed individual nutritional surveys on a national basis. Although some surveys are planned to be repeated, until now the majority of the surveys have been conducted only once. **Table 1** presents examples of national surveys.

These surveys differ in coverage of population, methods used to collect dietary data, nutrition-related health indices, etc. In several countries dietary data were collected using a record method, but the number of record days varied from 1 to 7. A 7-day weighed record is thought to be the most accurate method of dietary assessment. However, this method has a high respondent burden, which can have consequences for the response rate and representativeness of the sample. Response rates vary widely. Some-

times, weighing factors are used to adjust for sources of nonresponse. Most surveys focus on the general population. Some subgroups (such as ethnic minorities, pregnant or lactating women) do not occur in the population in sufficient numbers to appear in the survey sample with sufficient representation to allow for reliable estimates of their diet and nutritional status. Oversampling can improve the precision of estimates in nutritional assessment in specific groups, and is used in several surveys, including those in the USA. Special (vulnerable) groups can also be examined in separate studies. For example, nationwide surveys based on a random sampling of an elderly population are conducted in Australia, The Netherlands, Sweden, the UK and the USA (not included in Table 1).

Nutritional Status and Health Indices

The assessment of nutritional status includes, in addition to dietary-intake, indicators of nutrition-related health status, such as anthropometric measurements, haematological and biochemical tests, clinical signs of deficiencies, and risk factors for diseases associated with diet (e.g. high blood pressure and overweight). Furthermore, determinants of food- and health-related behaviour, such as nutritional knowledge and attitudes, may be studied as well. These indicators can be included in the surveys or studied in separate samples. As shown in **Table 1**, most national surveys studied both dietary intake and nutrition-related health status indicators. Nutritional surveillance in the USA has a long tradition and its surveys can be considered the most comprehensive in the world. For brevity, this article reports only a part of its activities.

A major advantage of possessing comprehensive (broad oriented) information at the individual level is that interrelationships can be studied. In studying correlations between diet and nutritional status indicators, one of the characteristics of a cross-sectional study is that mostly low correlations are found. This is attributable to, among other things, intraindividual variation and inaccurate assessment of intake and status indicators. In a cross-sectional design, the observation that a particular dietary factor is positively or inversely associated with a relevant variable is meaningful, even when there is a low p value, since this provides suggestive evidence for diet–health relationships which should be studied in more detail. To establish a causal link between diet and health, both intervention and (semi)-longitudinal studies are necessary. End-points, such as morbidity and mortality data, provide very valuable additional information on the role of nutritional factors in diseases.

Table 1 Nationwide food consumption surveys with data on an individual level

Country	Year	Survey	Population Sex	Population Age	Sample size[a]	Response rate (%)	Dietary method[b]	Dietary data[c]	Other information[d]
Australia	1983	National Dietary Survey of Adults	F + M	25–64	6255	75	24h Rcl	F, N	A, BP, BC, HM, PE, PA Component of Secondary Risk Factor Prevalence Study
	1985	National Dietary Survey of school children	F + M	10–15	5224	65	1d Rcd	F, N	A, BP, BC, HM, PE, PA In conjunction with health and fitness study
Belgium	1980–1985	Nutrition and Health (BIRNH)	F + M	25–74	11 076	37	1d Rcd	F, N	A, BP, BC, MH
Canada	1970–1972	Nutrition Canada	F + M	0–65+	12 795	47	24h Rcl, FF	F, N	A, DE, HM, BC, MH, ME
Denmark	1985	Dietary Habits in Denmark	F + M	15–80	2442	NA	DH	F, N	A
	1995	Danskernes Kostvaner	F + M	1–80	3098	65	7d Rcd	F, N	NA
Former West Germany	1985–1989	National Nutrition Survey	F + M	4–65+	24 632 ind 11 141 hh	71	7d Rcd	F, N	A, BC, HM, PE($n = c.$ 2000, ≥18 years) NK, ATT, BH ($n =$ 11 141, ≥14 years)
France	1993–1994	Etude Nationale des Consommations Alimentaires	F + M	2–65+	1500	NA	7d Rcd	F, N	A
UK	1986–1987	The Dietary and Nutritional Survey of British Adults	F + M	16–64	2197 ind	70	7d Rcd	F, N	A, BP, BC (≥18 years), HM (≥18 years)
	1992–1993	National Diet and Nutrition Survey	Child	1½–4½	1675	88	4d Rcd	F, N	A, BC, DH

Continued

Table 1 Continued

| Country | Year | Survey | Population | | Sample size[a] | Response rate (%) | Dietary method[b] | Dietary data[c] | Other information[d] |
			Sex	Age					
Ireland	1990	Irish National Nutrition Survey	F + M	10–65+	1214 ind	NA	DH	F, N	NA
The Netherlands	1987–1988	The Dutch National Food Consumption Survey (DNFCS-I)	F + M	1–85	5898 ind 2203 hh	81 79	2d Rcd	F, N	A (self-reported data)
	1992	The Dutch National Food Consumption Survey (DNFCS-2)	F + M	1–92	6218 ind 2475 hh	72 72	2d Rcd	F, N	A (self-reported data)
Northern Ireland	1986–1987	Diet, Life-style and Health in Northern Ireland	F + M	16–64	616	NA	7d Rcd	F, N	A, BP, BC, HM, MH, PA
Norway	1993–1994	NORKOST	F + M	16–79	3144	63	FF	F, N	A (self-reported) PA, Att
Portugal	1980	Portuguese Food Consumption Survey	F + M	0–65+	13 000	72	1d Rcd 1d Rcl, FF	F, N	A, BP, BC, HM, MH
Sweden	1989	Household Food Survey	F + M	0–74	3000	70	7d Rcd	F, N	A, PA

Table 1 Continued

Country	Year	Survey	Population Sex	Population Age	Sample size[a]	Response rate (%)	Dietary method[b]	Dietary data[c]	Other information[d]
USA	1971–1974	National Health and Nutritional Examination Surveys (NHANES I)	F + M	1–74	20 749	74	24th Rcl, FF	F, N	A, HM, BC, PE, MH
	1976–1980	NHANES II	F + M	½–74	20 322	73	24h Rcl, FF	F, N	A, HM, BC, PE, MH
	1988–1994	NHANES III	F + M	2 months onwards	40 000 planned	NA	24h Rcl, FF	F, N	A, DE, HM, BC, PE
	1977–1978	Nationwide Food Consumption Survey (NFCS)	F + M		30 770 ind 14 930 hh	70 61	1 × 24h Rcl, + 2 d Rcd	F, N	
	1987–1988	Nationwide Food Consumption Survey (NFCS)	F + M		25 100 ind 9600 hh (target)	NA	1 × 24h Rcl, 2d Rcd	F, N	
	1985–1986	Continuing Survey of Food Intakes by Individuals (CFS II)	Child F M	1–5 19–50 19–50	996 2784 635		1–6 × 24h Rcl 1 × 24h Rcl	F, N	
	1989–1996	CSFII	F + M	all ages	NA	NA	1 × 24h Rcl + 2 d Rcd	F, N	

[a]ind, individuals; hh, household.
[b]Information other than sociodemographic and other background information: 24h Rcl, 24-hour recall; 1d Rcd, 1-day record; FF, food frequency; DH, dietary history.
[c]F, food groups; N, nutrients.
[d]A, Anthropometry; BP, blood pressure; BC, biochemical tests; HM, haematological tests; PE, physical examination; MH, medical history; DE, dental examination; PA, physical activity; NK, nutritional knowledge; Att, attitudes and behaviour; NA, not available.

Risk areas and risk groups

Nutritional assessment includes a normative evaluation of dietary intake and nutritional status indicators in order to estimate the proportion of the population at risk. Nutritional status indices can be evaluated by comparing them with reference values mostly obtained from healthy adults. Alternatively, predetermined (based on consensus reports) cutoff points can be used. In evaluating dietary intake the reference values applied in recommended dietary allowances (RDAs) or dietary guidelines are often used. However, cutoff values are prone to some misclassification owing to (biological) variation within and among individuals. Estimates of prevalence values can be adjusted for within-person variation by statistical procedures. Despite the weaknesses of cutoff points, these criteria are commonly used and very often needed to evaluate dietary intake as well as nutritional status parameters.

In most industrialized countries, the principal nutrition-related health problems are related to overconsumption of some nutrients, particularly energy, fat, saturated fatty acids, cholesterol, sodium and alcohol. Although mean intake of energy among adults is mostly lower than the recommendations, the data available from nutritional surveillance indicate a high prevalence of overweight in several countries. In many subjects, intake levels of total fat, saturated fatty acids and cholesterol are too high, leading to an increase in average serum cholesterol levels. The prevalence of hypertension, for which mineral intake and alcohol consumption may be relevant factors, is high in most adult groups. **Table 2** gives an example of the prevalence estimates of obesity, hypercholesterolaemia and hypertension, as found in some of the presented studies. Since the age-range covered in the surveys varied, comparisons were restricted to the common age-range of 25–64 years. Although **Table 2** can give only a rough impression (the periods in which the studies were conducted differed; exclusion criteria might vary, etc.), the proportion of subjects classified as overweight is relatively similar for all three countries. The exception is Australia, where there are noticeably more overweight women, but this could in part be the consequence of different criteria. The prevalence of obesity was highest in the USA; the prevalence of hypercholesterolaemia was considerably higher in the UK, and the percentages of hypertensive subjects in Australia and the USA were relatively similar. Figures for the latter were not available for the UK, since the Dietary and National Survey of British Adults only presented separate values for the systolic, diastolic and the calculated mean blood pressure, and excluded subjects receiving treatment for hypertension.

In most countries, the average intake of most minerals and vitamins appears adequate for the population. In general, iron is an exception in that many subjects have a low iron intake in comparison with RDAs. In most countries, groups with a low intake are young children, adolescents and women of childbearing age. The intakes of vitamins (e.g. vitamin A and its precursors, vitamin B_6, vitamin C, folic acid) and minerals and trace elements (e.g. calcium, magnesium, zinc, iodine, fluoride) are considered to be potentially at risk in several countries. For example,

Table 2 The prevalence of overweight, obesity, hypercholesterolaemia and hypertension in adults aged 25–64 years in Australia, the UK and the USA

Country	Sex	Age (years)	Overweight BMI[a] >25–30 (%)	Obesity BMI ≥30 (%)	Serum cholesterol[b] ≥6.5 mmol l^{-1} (%)	Hypertension[c] (%)
Australia[d]	M	25–64	43	7	19	17
	F	25–64	35[g]	7	21	13
UK[e]	M	25–64	42	9	32	NA[h]
	F	25–64	25	13	29	NA
USA[f]	M	25–64	44	13	21	18
	F	25–64	28	17	23	15

[a]Body mass index (kg m^{-2}).
[b]Serum cholesterol: 1 mmol l^{-1} = 38.7 mg dl^{-1}.
[c]Systolic blood pressure ≥160 mmHg and/or diastolic blood pressure ≥90 mmHg and/or treatment of hypertension.
[d]Risk Factor Prevalence Study, 1983.
[e]The Dietary and Nutritional Survey of British Adults, 1986–1987.
[f]Second National Health and Nutrition Examination Survey (NHANES II), 1976–1980.
[g]Overweight in women defined as BMI ≥ 24–30 kg m^{-2}.
[h]NA, not available for comparisons.

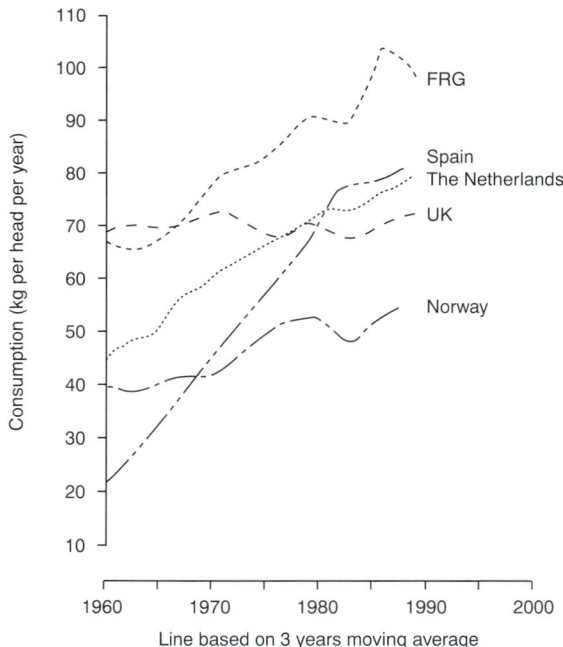

Figure 2 Available consumption of meat and meat products (kg per head per year) in five European countries. Source: (1990) *Food and Health Indicators in Europe*. Copenhagen: WHO Regional Office for Europe.

the high prevalence of low vitamin A levels in blood suggests that young children having parents with a low income are at risk in the USA; the prevalence of low plasma vitamin C levels is generally higher in groups with low socioeconomic status and in smokers (several countries). These data show that evidence for nutritional risk obtained through biochemical data is essential for the assessment of risk areas and risk groups. See individual nutrients.

Trends in Nutritional Surveillance

Biochemical and clinical measurements can be used to study trends provided that the measurements are standardized over time. For example, this is the case for some indicators (such as overweight, hypertension, elevated serum cholesterol levels) in the USA. These data indicate a recent decline in the prevalence of hypertension and hypercholesterolaemia, but no decline in the prevalence of overweight.

Concerning dietary intake, almost all industrialized countries possess information on trends in food supply over time in the national diet. An example is presented in **Fig. 2**. In several countries, data suggest that some changes in dietary patterns are in agreement with current health recommendations, but there is still a substantial difference

between the guidelines and actual consumption patterns in most countries.

Growing awareness of potential relationships between diet (as part of lifestyle) and health is accompanied by increasing demand for data at the individual level. The use of data of this type for trend analyses is hampered by the irregularity of data collection at the national level and/or by changes in survey methods over time. During the past decade, several countries (e.g. Former West Germany, The Netherlands and Sweden) have followed the example of the USA and collected individual dietary data using the framework of a household. This method of sampling and data collection has practical advantages, offers the opportunity to use the data on a household level and lowers costs. In the USA there is a tendency to collect data continuously on an individual level between larger 10-yearly surveys. For most other countries a more regular collection of data and an integration of other appropriate data from existing information systems (e.g. census data) is of primary concern.

See also: **Alcohol**: Absorption, Metabolism and Physiological Effects. **Ascorbic Acid**: Physiology, Dietary Sources and Requirements. **Calcium**: Physiology. **Cholesterol**: Sources, Absorption, Function and Metabolism; Factors Determining Blood Cholesterol Levels. **Coronary Heart Disease**: Lipid Theory of Coronary Heart Disease. **Dietary Intake Measurement**: Methodology; Validation. **Dietary Surveys**: Surveys of National Food Intake; Surveys of Food Intake in Groups and Individuals. **Folic Acid**: Physiology, Dietary Sources and Requirements. **Hypertension**: Physiology. **Iodine**: Physiology, Dietary Sources and Requirements. **Magnesium**: Physiology, Dietary Sources and Requirements. **Obesity**: Definition, Aetiology and Assessment. **Retinol**: Physiology. **Sodium**: Physiology. **Vitamin B6**: Physiology. **Vitamin K**: Physiology. **World Health Organization**: Role. **Zinc**: Physiology.

Further Reading

Becker W and Helsing E (1991) *Food and Health Data. Their Use in Nutrition-Policy Making*. WHO Regional Publications, European Series, No. 34. Copenhagen: World Health Organization.

Bingham SA (1987) The dietary assessment of individuals: methods, accuracy, new techniques and recommendations. *Nutrition Abstract Reviews* 57:705–742.

FAO (1977, 1981, 1985, 1988) *Review of Food Consumption Surveys*. Nos 1, 27, 35, 44. Rome: Food and Agriculture Organization.

Kelly A (ed.) (1987) *Nutritional Surveillance in Europe: A*

Critical Appraisal. (EURO-NUT Report No. 9). Wageningen: Stichting Nederlands Institutut voor de Voeding.

Life Sciences Research Office, FASEB (1989) *Nutrition Monitoring in the United States. An update report on nutrition monitoring.* Prepared for the US Department of Agriculture and the US Department of Health and Human Services. DHHS Publication No. (PHS) 89-1255. Hyattsville: Federation of American Societies for Experimental Biology.

WHO (1976) Methodology of nutritional surveillance. Report of a Joint FAO/UNICEF/WHO Expert Committee. *World Health Organization Technical Report Series 593.*

NUTS AND SEEDS

Nutritional Value

J Gray, Guildford, Surrey, UK

In botanical terms, the word 'nut' is used to describe a wide range of seeds, mostly from trees, with a tough, often lignified, seed coat or shell. True nuts include the chestnut, brazil nut and hazelnut. In practice, these are usually classified together with certain other so-called nuts, for example the almond, cashew and peanut, and other seeds which are all used in similar ways in the diet. Nuts and seeds come from a diverse range of different plants, so their nutritional composition is quite varied, but like most plant seeds they contain a food reserve designed to meet the needs of the developing plant embryo. In many nuts and seeds this is fat, but in others it is starch or other polysaccharides. Therefore, these foods are concentrated sources of dietary energy, as well as sources of protein, unsaturated fatty acids, various micronutrients, and fibre (nonstarch polysaccharides, NSP).

Nuts and seeds have a wide range of uses. In the typical Western omniverous diet they tend to be used either as snack items or added as minor ingredient to savoury and sweet dishes, but they have wider applications in vegetarian diets as important sources of protein and other nutrients. Certain nuts and seeds are also made into spreads, for example peanut butter and tahini (sesame seed spread).

Types

The major types of nuts and seeds grown for human consumption are shown in **Table 1**.

Nuts

Almond The almond (*Prunus amygdalis* var. *dulcis*), sometimes called the sweet almond, is one of the oldest nut crops. It is believed to have originated in South East Asia, but is now grown more widely, including in Southern Europe, Africa, Southern Australia and California. It is closely related to peaches and plums, but in the almond, in contrast to these other fruits, the 'flesh' or mesocarp becomes hard and dry as it matures, and splits open to leave the thin shell or endocarp which contains the edible almond seed or 'nut'. The nuts are eaten fresh, often in the ground form in prepared dishes, as well as roasted and salted.

Another species, *Prunus amara* or the bitter almond, is inedible, but is cultivated for its oil, which is also present in the sweet almond and in the kernels of apricots and peaches. This oil contains benzaldehyde, the essential oil, and hydrocyanic acid, from which the benzaldehyde is separated to be used in flavourings and perfumes.

Brazil nut The triangular-shaped Brazil nut (*Bertholletia excelsa*) grows in large forests in the Amazon river basin in South America. The nuts are actually hard-shelled seeds which are produced in groups of between 12 and 30 within a large, hard,

Table 1 Major types of nuts and seeds grown for human consumption

Almond	Pecan
Brazil	Pine nuts
Cashew	Pistachio
Chestnut	Walnut
Coconut	Pumpkin seeds
Hazelnut	Sesame seeds
Macadamia	Sunflower seeds
Peanut	

thick-walled woody fruit or pod. The sweet-tasting nut meat is consumed in the fresh state and brazil nut oil may be extracted for use as a lubricant.

Cashew nut The cashew (*Anacardium occidentale*) originated in Brazil but is now cultivated extensively in all tropical areas, notably in India and East Africa. The cashew fruit, which contains the seed or 'nut', hangs at the end of what is referred to as the cashew 'apple' – the edible swollen fruit stem or pedicel. The fruit itself is kidney-shaped, about the size of a large bean, and has a two-layered shell. The outer layer of this shell contains a caustic oil that must be burned off before the nut is touched. The nuts are then roasted again or boiled to remove other toxic substances and the second shell is removed. The nuts may also be used as a source of oil.

Chestnut The sweet or Spanish chestnut (*Castanea sativa*) is a native tree of Southern Europe, believed to have been introduced into Britain by the Romans. The fruit consists of two to four compartmentalized seeds or burrs, covered with numerous needle-sharp branched spines and containing the seeds or 'nuts', which are covered with a tough outer coat. The flesh of the nut is hard and inedible and is cooked, often by roasting or boiling, before being eaten. The cooking process changes the texture so that the chestnut becomes much softer than other nuts and more like a vegetable, largely as a result of its high carbohydrate content (see below).

Coconut The coconut (*Cocos nucifera*) grows on the coconut palm, which is common in tropical areas throughout the world. The native origin of the palm is uncertain, as the nuts were easily dispersed between both islands and continents by ocean currents and by early explorers. The fruits are borne on the tree in clusters of about 15 to 20, and are enclosed in a thick outer husk and covered in a mass of fibres (the mesocarp and exocarp), which is normally removed when the coconut is harvested. The familiar hard shell of the coconut is the endocarp, or inner layer, of the mature ovary of the fruit, and within the shell is the actual seed, covered with a thin brown seed coat. The white coconut 'meat', which can be eaten either fresh or desiccated, is actually part of the endosperm (storage tissue) of the seed. Coconut 'milk', which is found in the unripe nut and is drunk or used in cooking, is the liquid form of the endosperm, which solidifies as the fruit ripens. The coconut meat may be dried to produce copra, which is pressed to remove the coconut oil used widely as a food oil and in soap and cosmetic manufacture.

Hazelnut (cobnut; filbert) The most widely grown hazelnut (*Corylus avellana*) is a native of Europe, although about 10 different species of *Corylus* grow throughout Europe, North America and Asia. There is evidence that these nuts were cultivated in Ancient Greece and collected by Mesolithic peoples. The shell of the hazelnut is the matured ovary wall of the flower and the edible nut meat within this is the matured embryo.

Macadamia nut The macadamia nut (*Macadamia integrifolia*), smooth-shelled; *M. tetraphylla*, rough-shelled) is native to eastern tropical Australia, but was subsequently introduced to Hawaii, which is now the leading producer of these nuts, and also to parts of Africa and South America. It is the smooth-shelled variety that has been developed commercially. The edible kernel of the nut is the seed, consisting mostly of the cotyledons of the embryo. It is enclosed in a hard, thick, brown shell, which is itself encased in a fibrous husk that splits open when the husk dries. This occurs after the fruit falls, or when it is removed from the tree at maturity. After harvesting, the nuts are dried (to a moisture level of 1.5%), roasted (traditionally in coconut oil, or dry-roasted), and salted.

Peanut The peanut (*Arachis hypogaea*), sometimes referred to as the ground nut or monkey nut, originated in South America. Although referred to as a nut, it is in fact part of the legume family. The plant was introduced to Africa by early European explorers and to North America by the slave trade; it was also introduced to India and China. The name 'ground nut' derives from the fact that the flower withers after pollination to leave a stalk-like part of the plant, which pushes under the soil and carries the fertilized ovules in its tip. Underground, the tip continues to develop into the characteristic pod of the peanut, containing the seeds, or 'nuts'. The shape and size of the pod, and the number and colour of the seeds, is variable, depending on the peanut cultivar. On a worldwide basis, two-thirds of the peanut crop is crushed for oil (arachis oil) and peanut products are used widely in both food processing, with peanut butter as an important product, and for animal feed. The peanut itself may be eaten fresh or roasted and salted.

Pecan The pecan (*Carya illinoinensis*) is a member of the walnut family, and the tree is classified botanically as a hickory. The tree is a native of North America, grown in the southern central states. After harvesting, the nuts are air-dried to remove 10–20% of their moisture. The nut is similar to the walnut, but with a more mild and sweet flavour. The pecan nut kernel is eaten fresh and in the US it is used widely in confectionery and baked goods.

Pine nuts Pine nuts or kernels are small edible seeds which are extracted from the cones of various species of pine. The most commonly eaten variety is that from the European stone pine (*Pinus pinea*), which is native to northern Mediterranean regions. The small, oil-rich seeds are encased in a hard shell. The seeds are sometimes referred to as pignolia nuts, whereas the seeds of the pinyon pines (*Pinus edulis* and *Pinus monophylla*), which grow in the southwestern US and in northern Mexico, are known as pinon nuts.

Pistachio nut The pistachio nut is the seed of the pistachio tree (*Pistacia vera*). It is a native of central Asia, Pakistan and India, where it was cultivated 3000 years ago, and it has also been cultivated for many years in Mediterranean regions and more recently in California. The pistachio fruit is similar to a peach; the outer 'husk' (the exocarp and mesocarp of the fruit) encloses a hard but thin off-white shell (the endocarp). This splits open just before the nut matures to reveal the edible embryo, which consists mainly of two green cotyledons covered in a thin seed coat. The green nut kernels are highly prized and are eaten roasted and salted as well as in various Middle Eastern dishes.

Walnut The walnut (*Juglans* spp.) is the common name given to about 20 species of trees in this family. The most important species is *Juglans regia* – the English or Persian walnut – which is believed to have originated in Ancient Persia, later taken to Greece, and eventually distributed throughout the Roman empire. There are records of its growth in England in the sixteenth century. It was taken to America and called the English walnut to distinguish it from the native American black walnut (*Juglans nigrans*) and the butternut (*Juglans cinerea*), both of which have much thicker, less brittle shells. The walnut fruit has an outer leathery husk and an inner furrowed stone, which is the shell of the nut, within which is the edible seed.

Seeds

Pumpkin seeds The large flat seeds of the members of the pumpkin family (*Cucurbita maxima*; *C. moschata* and related species) can be dried and eaten raw, used in both sweet and savoury cooked dishes, or roasted.

Sesame seeds The sesame plant (*Sesamum indicum*), which is a native of Africa, grows in tropical and subtropical regions and is now common in Asia. The seeds are small and off-white in colour. They may be eaten whole, or used in confectionery and baked goods, and as a source of oil used in cooking. The seeds are also ground to a paste called tahini.

Sunflower seeds The sunflower (*Helianthus annus*) is a member of the Compositae or daisy family. It is believed to have originated in north America, where it was cultivated by the native Indians, and was introduced to Europe in the sixteenth century. The flat seeds may be dehusked and eaten raw or cooked, but the plant is generally cultivated for the oil they contain, which is a rich source of polyunsaturated fatty acids (see below), and is widely used for cooking and in margarine manufacture. The residual oil-cake is used for animal feed.

Macronutrient Content

Green nuts, as harvested, may contain 50% or more water, but these nuts must be cured or semidried for storage, so the moisture content of most nuts, as eaten, is low (1–6%). The exceptions are fresh coconut and chestnuts, with a moisture content of 45% and 52%, respectively. The water, macronutrient, and energy content of the nuts and seeds discussed in this article are shown in **Table 2**.

Fat

The total fat content of most nuts and seeds is high because, as the seed ripens, the fat store increases and its starch content declines. However, the amount of fat is quite variable, ranging from about 78% in the macadamia nut and 70% in the pecan to around 50–55% in nuts such as the almond, cashew, hazelnut and pistachio, and as low as 3% in chestnuts. The fat content of the edible seeds is between 45 and 60%.

The different fatty acid fractions contained in these nuts and seeds is also quite variable, as shown in **Table 3**. The vast majority of nuts and seeds are rich in monounsaturated and polyunsaturated fatty acids. However, in some nuts, such as the peanut, hazelnut and macadamia nut, monounsaturated fatty acids predominate, whereas in the walnut and in sunflower seeds, polyunsaturated fatty acids predominate. The exception is the coconut, in which saturated fatty acids constitute the major fat fraction.

Table 2 Water, macronutrient, and energy content of selected nuts and seeds (per 100 g, kernel only)

	Water (g)	Protein (g)	Fat (g)	Carbohydrate (g)	Energy (kJ)	Energy (kcal)
Almond	4.2	21.1	55.8	6.9	2534	612
Brazil	2.8	14.1	68.2	3.1	2813	682
Cashew	4.4	17.7	48.2	18.1	2374	573
Chestnut	51.7	2.0	2.7	36.6	719	170
Coconut	45.0	3.2	36.0	3.7	1446	351
Hazelnut	4.6	14.1	63.5	6.0	2685	650
Macadamia (salted)	1.3	7.9	77.6	4.8	3082	748
Peanut	6.3	25.6	46.1	12.5	2341	564
Pecan	3.7	9.2	70.1	5.8	2843	689
Pine nuts	2.7	14.0	68.6	4.0	2840	688
Pistachio (roasted, salted)	2.1	17.9	55.4	8.2	2485	601
Walnut	2.8	14.7	68.5	3.3	2837	688
Pumpkin seeds	5.6	24.4	45.6	15.2	2360	569
Sesame seeds	4.6	18.2	58.0	0.9	2470	598
Sunflower seeds	4.4	19.8	47.5	18.6	2410	581

Data from Holland *et al*. (1992).

Table 3 Total fat and fatty acid composition of selected nuts and seeds (g per 100 g, kernel only)

	Total fat	Saturated fatty acids	Monounsaturated fatty acids	Polyunsaturated fatty acids (total)	cis n-6 Polyunsaturated fatty acids	cis n-3 Polyunsaturated fatty acids
Almond	55.8	4.7	34.4	14.2	13.3	0.1
Brazil	68.2	16.4	25.8	23.0	22.9	0.1
Cashew	48.2	9.5	27.8	8.8	—[a]	—[a]
Chestnut	2.7	0.5	1.0	1.1	1.0	0.1
Coconut	36.0	31.0	2.0	0.8	0.5	0
Hazelnut	63.5	4.7	50.0	5.9	5.4	0.1
Macadamia (salted)	77.6	11.2	60.8	1.6	—[a]	—[a]
Peanut	46.1	8.2	21.1	14.3	—[a]	—[a]
Pecan	70.1	5.7	42.5	18.7	16.0	0.7
Pine nuts	68.6	4.6	19.9	41.1	—[a]	—[a]
Pistachio (roasted, salted)	55.4	7.4	27.6	17.9	—[a]	—[a]
Walnut	68.5	5.6	12.4	47.5	—[a]	—[a]
Pumpkin seeds	45.6	7.0	11.2	18.3	—[a]	—[a]
Sesame seeds	58.0	8.3	21.7	25.5	23.6	0.4
Sunflower seeds	47.5	4.5	9.8	31.0	—[a]	—[a]

Data from Holland *et al*. (1992) and The Ministry of Agriculture, Fisheries and Food.
[a]No data available.

Carbohydrate

With the exception of the starch-rich chestnut (almost 37% carbohydrate), the carbohydrate content of mosts nuts is relatively low at around 3–7%. However, peanuts, cashews, pumpkin and sunflower seeds contain more carbohydrate (13–19%). In most nuts and seeds this carbohydrate is a variable mixture of starch and sucrose, although in some there are small quantities of glucose and fructose as well, and in sunflower seeds there are some oligosaccharides.

Protein

The protein content of nuts is quite variable, but most nuts are considered to be a good source of protein. It is low (2–3%) in the chestnut and coconut, between 8 and 15% for most other nuts, but high (18–26%) in the cashew, pistachio, almond and peanut, so that the amount of protein in many nuts is about the same as in meat, fish or cheese. Pumpkin, sesame and sunflower seeds are also rich in protein.

However, the proportions of indispensable amino acids in any one particular type of nut or seed, and in fact all plant foods, differ from those needed in the human diet, with one or sometimes more 'limiting amino acids'. In most nuts and seeds, with the exception of pistachio nuts and pumpkin seeds, it is lysine that is the limiting amino acid. Thus, although the total amount of protein in nuts and seeds may be high, these foods must be complemented by other sources of plant protein, such as legumes and/or animal sources of protein (meat, fish, eggs, milk, cheese), to ensure that the overall protein quality of the diet is adequate.

Micronutrient Content

The vitamin and mineral contents of the nuts and seeds discussed in this article are shown in **Table 4** and **5**, respectively.

In general, nuts and seeds are a good source of the B vitamins, including folic acid, and of the tocopherols (vitamin E), although some, such as almonds, hazelnuts and sunflower seeds, contain much more vitamin E than others. Nuts and seeds do not contain vitamin C, and many nuts have little or no vitamin A activity.

Nuts and seeds contain quite large amounts of many minerals. In particular, many nuts, and seeds, especially sesame seeds, are good sources of calcium. They are also generally rich in potassium, magnesium and phosphorus, iron, and in trace elements such as copper, zinc, manganese and others such as chromium. Brazil nuts are particularly rich in selenium.

Fibre Content

Compositional values for the total amount of fibre (nonstarch polysaccharides, NSP), and the different fibre fractions where available, are shown in **Table 6** for the nuts and seeds discussed in this article. It can be seen that nuts and seeds contain significant amounts of fibre, similar to the amounts found in vegetables and fruit. Although nuts and seeds do contain some soluble fibre, most of the fibre in these foods is of the insoluble type, much of which is cellulose. Of the insoluble noncellulosic polysaccharides, arabinose predominates in most nuts, although the coconut contains large quantities of mannose. Most nuts and seeds are likely to contain quite large amounts of lignin, particularly those with a tough seed coat such as sesame seeds, although actual values are not available.

Toxins and Contaminants

Phytic acid

Phytic acid (*myo*-inositol hexaphosphoric acid) is present in all seeds, where it is believed to act as a store of phosphate and trace elements for the developing plant embryo. The phytate content of the commonly eaten nuts and seeds is variable. In general, the oil seeds, such as sesame and sunflower, and a number of the tree nuts, have higher phytate levels than the leguminous peanut, although the oils expressed from the seeds do not contain phytate. The

Table 4 Vitamin content of selected nuts and seeds (per 100 g, kernel only)

	Carotene (μg)	Vitamin E (mg)	Thiamin (mg)	Riboflavin (mg)	Niacin (mg)	Vitamin B_6 (mg)	Folate (μg)
Almond	0	23.96	0.21	0.75	3.1	0.15	48
Brazil	0	7.18	0.67	0.03	0.3	0.31	21
Cashew	6	0.85	0.69	0.14	1.2	0.49	67
Chestnut	0	1.20	0.14	0.02	0.5	0.34	N[a]
Coconut	0	0.73	0.04	0.01	0.5	0.05	26
Hazelnut	0	24.98	0.43	0.16	1.1	0.59	72
Macadamia (salted)	0	1.49	0.28	0.06	1.6	0.28	N
Peanut	0	10.09	1.14	0.10	13.8	0.59	110
Pecan	50	4.34	0.71	0.15	1.4	0.19	39
Pine nuts	10	13.65	0.73	0.19	3.8	N	N
Pistachio (roasted, salted)	130	4.16	0.70	0.23	1.7	N	58
Walnut	0	3.85	0.40	0.14	1.2	0.67	66
Pumpkin seeds	230[b]	N	0.23	0.32	1.7	N	N
Sesame seeds	6	2.53	0.93	0.17	5.0	0.75	97
Sunflower seeds	15	37.77	1.60	0.19	4.1	N	N

Data from Holland *et al.* (1992).
[a]Nutrient present in significant quantities but no reliable information available on the amount.
[b]Estimated value.

Table 5 Mineral and trace element content of selected nuts and seeds (per 100 g, kernel only)

	Sodium (mg)	Potassium (mg)	Calcium (mg)	Magnesium (mg)	Phosphorus (mg)	Iron (mg)	Copper (mg)	Zinc (mg)	Manganese (mg)	Selenium (µg)
Almond	14	780	240	270	550	3.0	1.00	3.2	1.7	4
Brazil	3	660	170	410	590	2.5	1.76	4.2	1.2	1530[a]
Cashew	15	710	32	270	560	6.2	2.11	5.9	1.7	29
Chestnut	11	500	46	33	74	0.9	0.23	0.5	0.5	Tr
Coconut	17	370	13	41	94	2.1	0.32	0.5	1.0	1[b]
Hazelnut	6	730	140	160	300	3.2	1.23	2.1	4.9	Tr
Macadamia (salted)	280	300	47	100	200	1.6	0.43	1.1	5.5	7
Peanut	2	670	60	210	430	2.5	1.02	3.5	2.1	3
Pecan	1	520	61	130	310	2.2	1.07	5.3	4.6	12
Pine nuts	1	780	11	270	650	5.6	1.32	6.5	7.9	N[c]
Pistachio (roasted, salted)	530	1040	110	130	420	3.0	0.83	2.2	0.9	6[b]
Walnut	7	450	94	160	380	2.9	1.34	2.7	3.4	19
Pumpkin seeds	18	820	39	270	850	10.0	1.57	6.6	N	6[b]
Sesame seed	20	570	670	370	720	10.4	1.46	5.3	1.5	N
Sunflower seeds	3	710	110	390	640	6.4	2.27	5.1	2.2	49[b]

Data from Holland et al. (1992).
[a]Range 230–5300 µg per 100 g.
[b]Estimated value.
[c]Nutrient present in significant quantities but no reliable information available on the amount.

Table 6 Total dietary fibre, as measured by the Englyst method, and fibre fractions in selected nuts and seeds (g per 100 g, kernels only)

			Fibre fractions		
			Noncellulosic polysaccharide		
	Total fibre	Cellulose	Soluble	Insoluble	Lignin
Almond	7.4[a]	1.9[a]	1.1[a]	4.4[a]	N[b]
Brazil	4.3	1.6	1.3	1.4	N
Cashew	3.2	0.6	1.6	1.0	N
Chestnut	4.1	1.1	1.3	1.7	N
Coconut	7.3	0.8	1.0	5.5	N
Hazelnut	6.5	2.2	2.5	1.8	N
Macadamia (salted)	5.3	1.4	1.9	2.0	N
Peanut	6.2	2.0	1.9	2.3	N
Pecan	4.7	1.2	1.5	2.0	N
Pine nuts	1.9	N	N	N	N
Pistachio (roasted, salted)	6.1	1.3	2.7	2.1	N
Walnut	3.5	1.1	1.5	0.9	N
Pumpkin seeds	5.3	1.1	1.7	2.5	N
Sesame seeds	7.9	N	N	N	N
Sunflower seeds	6.0	1.4	1.8	2.8	N

Data from Holland *et al.* (1992).
[a]Estimated value.
[b]Nutrient present in significant quantities but no reliable information available on the amount.

phytate content of the coconut and chestnut is particularly low.

Because of its molecular structure, phytic acid is a highly effective chelator, which forms insoluble complexes with mineral cations. Its presence in plant foods has led to concerns that it may reduce the bioavailability of various dietary minerals and trace elements, including calcium, magnesium, iron, zinc and copper. Although nuts are rich in iron, there is evidence that the addition of nuts to a meal can have a substantial inhibitory effect on iron absorption, presumably because of their phytate and polyphenol content. However, it appears that this can be overcome by the addition of a source of vitamin C to the meal, thereby underlining the need to mix different groups of foods within a meal, particularly when plant foods are the main source of nutrition.

The significance of dietary phytate intake to overall mineral nutriture is still uncertain. It is likely that in a mixed diet of animal and plant foods, dietary phytate may be of less significance than among people consuming diets where plant foods are the sole source of nutrition (vegans). Available data suggest that the trace element status of most adult vegetarians is adequate, but because of increased requirements for growth, vegetarian children may be more vulnerable to the reduced bioavailability of minerals and trace elements, notably zinc, which could be a consequence of the ingestion of large amounts of phytate-containing plant foods.

Intolerances/allergies to nuts

Intolerances to nuts, or more specifically, allergies to nut proteins, occur in a relatively small minority of people. However, there is some evidence that such adverse reactions have become more common, and the severity of the reaction that occurs in these sensitive individuals means that they must be taken very seriously. Peanuts are the most commonly cited cause of these severe reactions, estimated to affect between 0.1 and 0.2% of the population, but allergic reactions to tree nuts, incuding brazil nuts, almonds, hazelnuts and cashews, and also to sesame seeds, have been reported.

Contaminants

Nuts and seeds may be subject to mould growth during storage if the conditions are inappropriate. Certain moulds produce secondary metabolites which are toxic to humans and animals, known as the mycotoxins. Of these mycotoxins, the aflatoxins, notably aflatoxin B1, are produced by three closely related species of mould: *Aspergillus flavus*, *A. parasiticus* and *A. nomius*. These moulds may contaminate various food commodities in tropical and subtropical regions, including tree nuts, but one of the most important crops to be affected is the peanut. Aflatoxins are acutely toxic to the liver and may also be involved in the aetiology of human liver cancer in certain parts of the world. Ochratoxins, which are produced by other *Aspergillus* species, have also been found to contaminate nuts.

Some species of mould are able to proliferate within growing crops even before they are harvested, forming an endophytic relationship with the plant. This relationship has been found to exist between *Aspergillus parasiticus* and peanuts. It appears that when the plant is growing normally, no aflatoxin is produced by the mould, but when the plant is stressed, as occurs in drought conditions, then the mycotoxin may be produced. The concentrations of aflatoxins produced in this way are lower than would ensue from poor postharvest storage, but the economic consequences still may be considerable.

There are regulatory limits for the aflatoxin levels in foods. In the UK, the sale of nuts for direct consumption is prohibited if the aflatoxin content exceeds 4 µg kg^{-1} or 10 µg kg^{-1} for nuts which are to be subjected to further processing before being sold. A proportion of nuts imported into the UK, especially peanuts, are contaminated with aflatoxin. In 1994, 3% of samples examined under a European surveillance programme were found to exceed the UK limit. Nonetheless, such findings should be kept in perspective: the numbers are low and their significance in public health terms, relative to other diet related risks, is small.

Role in the Diet

Nuts and seeds can make a useful contribution to the dietary intake of macronutrients, notably protein and unsaturated fatty acids, micronutrients, dietary fibre and energy. Although these commodities play a relatively minor role in the average Western diet, they are more important in the diets of Western vegetarians, especially vegans. Even on a worldwide basis, the nutritional contribution of nuts and seeds is relatively small: plant foods are estimated to supply around 65% of edible protein, but only 8% of protein and 4% of total dietary energy is estimated to derive from pulses, oil crops and nuts (Young and Pellett (1994)).

In the UK, average weekly household consumption of nuts and their products, as recorded by the National Food Survey, is about 14 g per capita, with only 11% of households purchasing these commodities; there are no separate data for nuts eaten as out of home snacks. Data from the Dietary and Nutritional Survey of British Adults indicate that average weekly intake of people consuming unsalted nuts and nut mixes is 63 g per week, but again only 12% of the adults surveyed were consuming these commodities. Therefore, even for nutrients which are present in relatively large amounts in nuts, such as vitamin E, magnesium and copper, these foods only provide about 1% of the average daily intake in the UK.

See Colour Plate 5.

See also: **Dietary Fibre (Fiber)**: Physiological Effects and Effects on Absorption. **Fatty Acids**: Metabolism; Health Effects of Saturated Fatty Acids; Health Effects of Monounsaturated Fatty Acids; Health Effects of n-6 Polyunsaturated Fatty Acids; Health Effects of n-3 Polyunsaturated Fatty Acids; Health Effects of *trans* Fatty Acids. **Folic Acid**: Physiology, Dietary Sources and Requirements. **Food Allergies**: Aetiology. **Food Contaminants**: Mycotoxins - Occurrence and Toxic Effects. **Protein**: Quality and Sources. **Vegetarian Diets**: Nutritional Adequacy.

Further Reading

Englyst HN, Bingham SA, Runswick SA, Collinson E and Cummings JH (1988) Dietary fibre (non-starch polysaccharides) in fruit, vegetables and nuts. *Journal of Human Nutrition and Dietetics* 1:247–286.

Gibson RS (1994) Content and bioavailability of trace elements in vegetarian diets. *American Journal of Clinical Nutrition* 59(supplement):1223S–1232S.

Gregory J, Foster K, Tyler H and Wiseman M (1990) *The Dietary and Nutritional Survey of British Adults*. London: HMSO.

Harland BF and Oberleas D (1987) Phytate in foods. *World Review of Nutrition and Dietetics* 52:235–259.

Hartmann HT, Flocker WJ and Kofranek AM (1981) *Plant Science. Growth, Development, and Utilization of Cultivated Plants*. Englewood Cliffs, NJ: Prentice Hall.

Holland B, Unwin ID and Buss DH (eds) (1992) *Fruit and Nuts. The First Supplement to McCance & Widdowson's The Composition of Foods, 5th Edn*. London: The Royal Society of Chemistry.

Macfarlane BJ, Bezwoda WR, Bothwell TH, Baynes RD, Bo JE, McPhail AP, Lamparelli RD and Mayet (1988) Inhibitory effect of nuts on iron absorption. *American Journal of Clinical Nutrition* 47:270–274.

Ministry of Agriculture, Fisheries and Food (1994) *The Dietary and Nutritional Survey of British Adults – Further Analysis*. London: HMSO.

Morris ER (1993) Phytic acid. In: Macrae R, Robinson RK and Sadler MJ (eds) *Encyclopaedia of Food Science, Food Technology and Nutrition*, pp 3587–3591. London: Academic Press.

Moss MO (1996) Mycotoxins. *Mycological Research* 100:524–526.

Ryden P and Selvendran RR (1993) Phytic acid. In: Macrae R, Robinson RK and Sadler MJ (eds) *Encyclopaedia of Food Science, Food Technology and Nutrition*, pp 3582–3587. London: Academic Press.

Young VR and Pellett PL (1994) Plant proteins in relation to human protein and amino acid nutrition. *American Journal of Clinical Nutrition* 59(supplement):1203S–1212S.

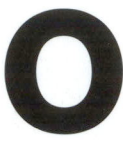

OBESITY

Contents

Definition, Aetiology and Assessment

J Garrow, Rickmansworth, Hertfordshire, UK

The total fat content of a person relates closely to their 'body mass index' (BMI), which is calculated from weight (kg) divided by height squared (m²). In adults, relative mortality rates are least among individuals in the range BMI 20–25, and health risks increase more rapidly above BMI 30. Thus people with a BMI > 25 are 'overweight', and with BMI > 30 they are 'obese'. For a given amount of fat the health risks are greater if more of the fat is intra-abdominal, rather than subcutaneous (*See:* **Obesity**; Fat Distribution).

Obesity occurs when energy intake exceeds energy expenditure over a long period, so the excess energy is deposited as fat. The abonormality in obese people is not that they have a lower than average energy expenditure, so they must have had, at some time, a higher than average energy intake from food and drink. The physiological mechanisms which regulate food intake are mainly designed to prevent undernutrition rather than overnutrition, and are easily overwhelmed by an unlimited supply of palatable food.

Obesity is commoner among women than among men, in older people than in younger people, and (in developed countries) among lower socioeconomic groups than among the more affluent. Children of obese parents, and people who have been obese, but have subsequently lost weight, are groups most liable to become obese. It appears that cognitive factors limiting weight gain are particularly important to prevent obesity.

The clinician trying to help an obese person to achieve, and maintain, a healthy weight is most concerned to assess, and if possible improve, the motivation of the patient. Substantial weight loss involves the commitment of a considerable amount of time and effort, even with the most expert guidance. Unfortunately, there are many sources of misinformation which tend to demotivate obese people.

Diagnostic Criteria

Obese people carry an excessive amount of fat, which causes a noticeable change in shape and weight. However, assessment of the amount which is 'excessive' differs in different circumstances. For example, a ballerina who is 1.7 m tall and weighs 60 kg will find employment more easily if she loses weight, although she is already well below the average weight-for-height of women in the Western world. At the other extreme it is to the advantage of a sumo wrestler to have massive fat stores, to make it difficult for his opponent to lift him off the mat. It is commonly believed that an excessively thin ideal of female beauty is a feature of modern times: certainly fashion models and beauty queens are usually unphysiologically thin. However, inspection of national art galleries will show that representations of female beauty personified as Venus, or Eve, may be thin or plump in whatever century the painting was made.

Analysis of the mortality statistics from the early part of this century gave rise to an actuarial estimate of 'ideal weight' for men and women: people who were excessively light or heavy in relation to their height tended to die young, and hence were not profitable to insure. The Metropolitan Life Insurance Company issued tables to doctors who undertook life insurance medical examinations showing the levels of weight-for-height at which an excess premium would be charged. These tables were modified in the light of increasing information, but it continued to be evident that a man or woman who was 1.7 m tall and who weighed between 60 and 75 kg was more likely to survive to normal retirement age than one who weighed more, or less, than this range.

Body mass index

The insurance weight–height tables were cumbersome to use, but the situation was greatly simplified by the use of a simple ratio which served to identify fatness in adult men and women. The Belgian astronomer Quetelet was a pioneer in systematizing measurements of people. In 1869 he reported the observation that the weight of a normal adult was proportional to the square of height: this was later used as the basis of body mass index, which is weight (kg) divided by height^2 (m^2). **Table 1** shows values of weight and height (in metric and imperial units) which correspond to a BMI of 20, 25, 30 and 40. The reasons for choosing these values will be explained later.

Relation of BMI to mortality and morbidity

The heavy continuous line in **Fig. 1** shows the relation of BMI to mortality ratio from all causes in adults, in which the minimum risk is taken to be 100. It is evident that the mortality risk increases below BMI = 20 and above BMI = 25. It increases more rapidly with increasing BMI, so the risk is approximately 125 at BMI = 30, 230 at BMI = 40, and reaches 300 at about BMI = 46. These data were derived mainly from life insurance statistics, based on many millions of insured people.

Recent studies have provided much more infor-

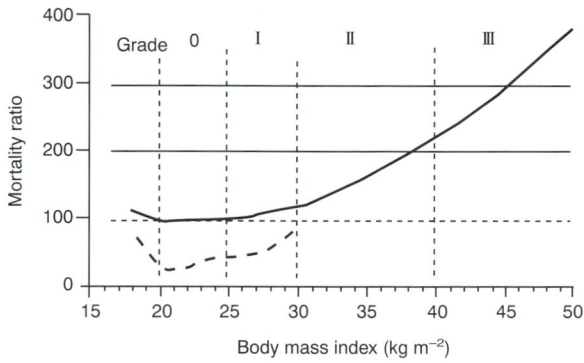

Figure 1 Relation of BMI to mortality ratio: heavy line for mixed smokers and nonsmokers, and broken line for nonsmokers only.

mation about the cause of death in different population groups. Data for healthy men and women recruited into the study at age 40–50 years, and followed for 15 years, showed that the curve of mortality ratio against BMI differs between smokers and nonsmokers; the curve for nonsmokers is indicated by the broken line in Fig. 1. The overall mortality among nonsmokers is considerably reduced relative to the smokers, and the nadir is in the range 20–22 kg m^{-2}. The relatively flat curve for mortality between BMI 20 and 30 among mixed populations of smokers and nonsmokers seems to be explained by two confounding factors: at the lower end of this range there is an increased mortality among smokers (mainly related to cancer), while at the upper end there is increased mortality among nonsmokers (mainly related to heart disease).

An empirical definition of obesity

It is evident from the above discussion that there is no threshold weight (or BMI) at which the health risks suddenly increase, but a practical compromise, which has now been adopted internationally, is to use the thresholds BMI 20, 25, 30 and 40 to define weight zones: less than 20 is underweight, 20–24.9 is desirable weight, 25–29.9 is overweight (or grade

Table 1 Variation of weight with height for adults of similar fatness indicated by body mass index (BMI)

Height		BMI = 20 Weight		BMI = 25 Weight		BMI = 30 Weight		BMI = 40 Weight	
m	ft.in	kg	st.lb	kg	st.lb	kg	st.lb	kg	st.lb
1.5	5'1''	48	7.8	60	9.6	72	11.4	96	15.2
1.60	5'3''	51	8.0	64	10.1	77	12.1	102	16.0
1.65	5'5''	54	8.7	68	10.9	83	12.12	108	17.0
1.70	5'7''	58	9.2	72	11.5	87	13.9	116	18.1
1.75	5'9''	61	9.8	77	12.1	92	14.6	122	19.2
1.80	5'11''	65	10.3	81	12.10	97	15.3	130	20.4
1.85	6'1''	68	10.10	86	13.7	103	16.2	146	21.6

I), 30–40 is obese (or grade II), and over 40 is grade III obesity.

There are two arguments against using BMI to define obesity. One is that weight-for-height is not purely determined by fatness, since heavily muscled athletes (such as boxers and weight-lifters) will have a high BMI but a relatively low fat content. Conversely, with increasing age the lean tissues of the body decrease, so old people may have a normal BMI but an excessive amount of fat. These objections are valid, but nevertheless BMI provides a reliable estimate of body fat in the great majority of adults who are not yet of retirement age and who are not body-building athletes.

The other objection to BMI is that it does not take account of the distribution of body fat, and it has been shown that the metabolic disorders associated with obesity depend much more on the amount of intra-abdominal fat than the amount of subcutaneous fat. The significance of fat distribution is discussed (*See:* **Obesity**; Fat Distribution), but we can note here that a combination of BMI and a simple measure of intra-abdominal fat (such as waist circumference) is probably the best method for defining diagnostic criteria of obesity in adults.

Mechanisms and Causes

Energy storage in the normal subject

Mammals (including man) derive energy from the protein, carbohydrate, fat and alcohol which they eat or drink. After a meal the food is digested and absorbed, mainly as amino acids, glucose and fatty acids which are then used either for biosynthesis of essential body components (such as proteins), or for fuel to provide energy for these processes and for muscular work. The metabolic processes continue over the whole 24 h cycle, so energy derived from a meal must be stored to meet demands until the next meal. The energy stores of a typical adult weighing 70 kg will contain about 12 kg fat (containing 450 MJ, or 108 000 kcal), and up to 1 kg of glycogen (containing 17 MJ, or 4000 kcal). Glycogen provides rapidly available glucose, but is an inefficient method for storing large amounts of energy. This is because 1 kg of glycogen is associated with 3 kg of water, and this 4 kg weight stores only 4000 kcal, whereas an equal weight of fat would store nine times as much energy. The energy stores of a normal adult are equivalent to about 10 weeks' requirements for sedentary living, so man can survive about 10 weeks of starvation if given adequate amounts of water.

The energy stores of small mammals (such as the laboratory rat) are relatively smaller: the rat will survive only about 10 days of starvation, so to survive the rat must match energy intake and expenditure quite accurately.

Hypothalamic feeding centres

In the early part of the twentieth century much research was done on the mechanisms by which rats achieve energy balance. Two areas of the brain were identified which seemed to be particularly important in controlling feeding behaviour: an 'appetite' centre in the lateral hypothalamus, and a 'satiety' centre in the ventromedial hypothalamus. If the former centre is destroyed the rat ceases to eat, but if the latter centre is destroyed it eats voraciously and becomes obese. Similar centres exist in the human brain, and sometimes tumours in the hypothalamus cause eating disorders in human patients. However, much research effort has failed to show any significant difference between obese and nonobese people in the functional capacity of these hypothalamic centres.

Thermoregulation and energy balance

Mammals need to maintain a constant internal body temperature of about 37°C despite changes in the ambient temperature. In part this is achieved by using a layer of fat under the skin as an insulating layer, so fat people are better able than thin ones to maintain normal core temperature when immersed in cold water. In small mammals (such as the laboratory mouse) the surface-to-weight ratio is so large that insulation alone will not protect them from hypothermia in very cold ambient conditions, so extra heat is generated in the body in specialized tissue called 'brown fat'. In a genetically obese strain of mice, designated *ob/ob*, the brown fat is defective, and these animals die of hypothermia if left in cold conditions. The energy that is used to maintain body temperature in normal mice is saved in *ob/ob* mice, and contributes to their obesity.

Attempts to apply this research to the aetiology of human obesity have been rather disappointing. The Pima Indians (like *ob/ob* mice) have a strong genetic predisposition to obesity, and also have subtle abnormalities in the sympathetic nervous system. However their energy expenditure is normal for their body composition, and since they live in the hot deserts of Arizona it is difficult to link their obesity to problems of hypothermia. Unlike *ob/ob* mice, obese human subjects have a normal thermogenic response to overfeeding, and have an increased (rather than a decreased) lean body mass.

'Cafeteria' feeding

It is rather unfortunate that so much research on

human obesity has been based on observations on small laboratory rodents which, as illustrated above, are not very applicable models of the human situation. Recently research has swung towards environmental factors which affect food intake, and this has yielded results more easily applicable to man.

If a pure-bred laboratory rat is fed a standard 'chow' diet it will gain weight in at a predictable rate. However, if it is offered a varied and palatable diet it will eat more, and become fat. Some strains of rat are particularly susceptible to overeating high-fat foods. These features all have human analogues: people in developed countries are offered a varied and palatable diet, and many of them become obese. There is some evidence that high-fat diets are particularly liable to cause obesity in susceptible people.

Measurement of energy expenditure in obese subjects

Techniques for measuring energy expenditure in free-living human subjects have improved greatly in recent years. At the beginning of the twentieth century measurements of total heat loss were made on volunteers sealed for several days into calorimeter chambers. Since then methods for measuring oxygen uptake and carbon dioxide production have become much easier and more accurate, so indirect calorimetry is practicable as a bedside procedure. The use of water labelled with stable isotopes of both hydrogen and oxygen has permitted the estimation of gas exchange in free-living subjects over periods of several weeks. The conclusions from all these studies are that the components of total energy expenditure in typical sedentary normal-weight and obese adults are as shown in **Fig. 2**. For the purpose of this illustration it is assumed that the normal subject has 58 kg fat-free mass and 12 kg of fat, while the obese subject has 66 kg fat-free mass and 34 kg of fat.

In the normal-weight subject resting or basal metabolic rate (BMR) is about 4 kJ min^{-1}, or 5.6 MJ per day (1 kcal min^{-1}, or 1400 kcal per day, and total energy expenditure is about 8 MJ per day (2000 kcal per day). Part of the nonresting component is made up of about 800 kJ (200 kcal) From the thermic effect of feeding (TEF). This is the increase in metabolic rate above resting levels which reflects the energy cost of assimilating the food, and usually amounts to about 10% of daily energy intake. The remaining 1.6 MJ per day (400 kcal per day) relates to all other forms of activity including physical activity and muscular activity to maintain posture.

In the obese subject total daily energy expenditure is increased to 10.5 MJ (2500 kcal), but the relative contributions of BMR, activity and TEF are similar to those in the normal-weight subject. BMR is

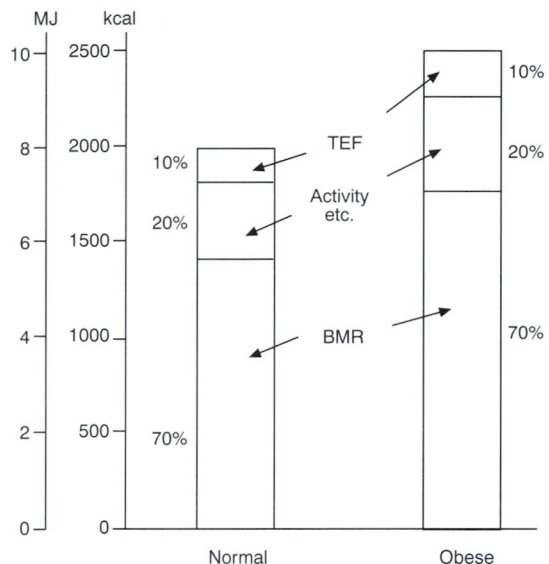

Figure 2 Components of daily energy expenditure in a typical sedentary normal-weight or obese adult. BMR, basal metabolic rate; TEF, thermic effect of feeding.

increased because the obese subject has a fat-free mass of about 66 kg instead of the 58 kg in the normal-weight subject. The daily TEF is increased from 840 to 1050 kJ (200 to 250 kcal), because a daily intake of 10.5 MJ (2500 kcal) is required to maintain energy balance in the obese person. The activity component is about 2 MJ per day (500 kcal per day) because, although the obese person may be less physically active than the lean one, the energy cost of a given activity (such as climbing stairs) will be greater on account of the greater body weight that must be moved.

Measurement of energy intake in obese subjects

The accurate measurement of habitual energy intake in obese subjects is extremely difficult. If the subject is incarcerated in a metabolic ward it is possible to measure energy intake accurately, but it is unlikely that this is the habitual intake of that individual when not incarcerated in a metabolic ward. If the subject is asked to recall food and drink taken over the previous (say) week, it is very unlikely that this recall will be accurate. It the subject is asked to record food eaten over the next few weeks both sources of error operate: the record will probably not reflect what is actually eaten, and what is actually eaten will probably differ from the habitual intake of the subject.

This scepticism about diet recording is based on the evidence obtained by biomarkers of food intake. If, for example, an adult person eats 65 g of protein daily, then, over a long period, the urinary excretion of nitrogen should be about 10 g per day, since that is the nitrogen released from the metabolism of 65 g protein. If a person makes a diet record showing that daily protein intake has been 30 g, but daily urine nitrogen is 10 g, then it is very likely that the protein intake has been underrecorded with respect to habitual protein intake. Similarly, if a person who is maintaining constant body weight is shown by calorimetry to expend 8 MJ per day (2000 kcal per day), but the diet record shows a daily intake of 4 MJ (1000 kcal), then the record cannot represent habitual intake. Unfortunately, although biomarkers can show that the record is unreliable, they cannot tell us what the true typical energy intake is – hence the difficulty in studying energy balance.

Energy balance in human subjects

At the simplest level, therefore, the cause of obesity is an energy intake which exceeds energy expenditure over a long period. Since the energy expenditure of obese subjects is on average higher than that of normal-weight persons, we must conclude that the cause is primarily a higher energy intake. Factors which predispose to this are considered below.

Epidemiology of Obesity

Association with gender, age and socioeconomic status

In the UK there were surveys in 1980, 1987 and 1991 of the heights and weights of a nationally representative sample of men and women aged 16–65 years. The prevalence of obesity (BMI > 30) found in these surveys is shown in **Fig. 3**(a) for men and Fig. 3(b) for women

The prevalence of obesity is higher in women than in men, in older people than in younger people, and in both genders and at all ages it increases in successive surveys. Similar results have been obtained in other developed countries where such serial surveys have been done. Internationally the prevalence of obesity is highest in north America and Australasia, then comes south and eastern Europe (including the former USSR), then western Europe (including the UK), with the lowest prevalence in Scandanavia and Japan.

In Third World countries subject to periodic famine the prevalence of obesity is increasing rapidly among the more affluent members of the population, but not among those who are living on a marginal diet. In developed countries there is an inverse relationship between socioeconomic status and the prevalence of obesity, for which no adequate explanation has been found. The most plausible hypothesis is that in affluent countries it is socially unaccept-

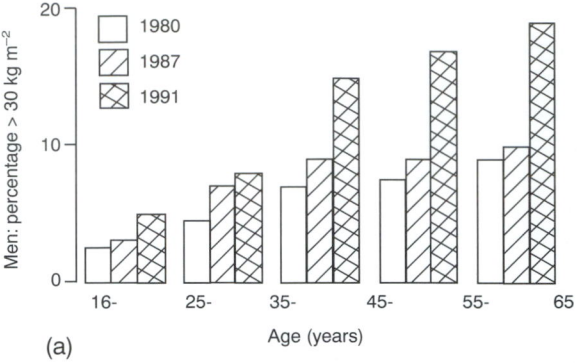

(a)

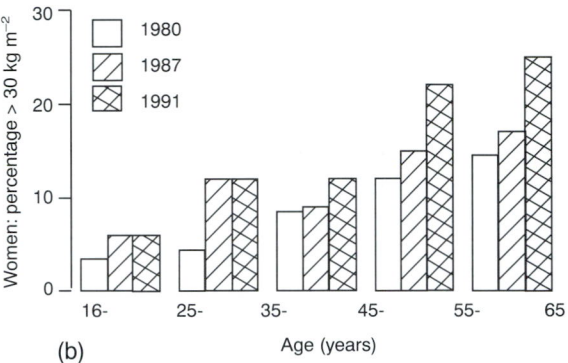

(b)

Figure 3 Prevalence of obesity in men (a) and women (b) by age in representative samples of adults in the UK in 1980, 1987 and 1991.

able to be obese, so those to whom social status is important strive to control their weight more effectively than individuals who are less concerned about their social standing.

There is also no clear reason for the relentless increase in the prevalence of obesity over the last decade. It cannot be explained on a genetic basis, since the national gene pool has not altered in the past decade. It must therefore be a result of some environmental effect, perhaps in association with certain genes which carry susceptibility to obesity. It may be that several factors are weakening the social pressures against obesity. The view that 'fat is a feminist issue' suggests that the pressure on women to be thin arises from an oppressive male stereotype, rather than a concern about health, but this does not explain the increased obesity in men. Innumerable misleading books and newspaper articles about the techniques and objectives of weight loss may have made efforts at weight control less effective.

It has been suggested that the increased proportion of energy in the diet supplied by fat, and the decreased level of physical activity in the population, are important factors in the increased prevalence of obesity. These are plausible hypotheses, but difficult to test, because it is difficult to obtain reliable data on the fat consumption, or physical activity, of those becoming obese as compared with those not becoming obese.

Pregnancy is a risk factor for obesity in some women, but overall there is no clear relationship between parity and obesity when counfounders such as age and socioeconomic group have been allowed for. For example, among better educated Finnish women there is a *reduced* chance of excessive weight gain with parity, while in less educated women the chance of excessive weight gain *increases* with parity.

Groups at Risk

It has been shown experimentally that if normal young male volunteers, with no personal or family history of obesity, are overfed substantially for 6 months, then their body weight will increase by 25%, and they will become mildly obese. Therefore everyone is at some risk of obesity, but in some people the risk is greater than in others. Two particularly high-risk groups are children of obese parents, and people who have been obese in the past, but who have reduced to normal weight.

Many life events have been identified as probable triggers for weight gain: a low level of education, chronic disease, a low level of physical activity, high alcohol consumption, getting married, and stopping smoking. However, these events do not necessarily lead to obesity, since there is another set of poorly defined characteristics which influences the ability and motivation to limit this weight gain before obesity develops.

Assessment of the Obese Person

The clinician who seeks to help a person who is obese must assess the factors which make it more, or less, likely that this person will achieve the required weight loss and maintain that weight loss indefinitely. These factors come under the general headings of motivation and technique.

Motivation to lose excess weight

A specialist who runs a hospital obesity clinic encounters a wide range of motivation among the patients whom he or she sees. The outlook is best for the patient who realizes that losing a substantial amount of weight (say 30 kg) is going to require considerable effort, but that the benefits of this weight loss outweighs the trouble involved. The benefits which a patient can realistically expect to receive on reducing from (say) 100 to 70 kg are a greatly increased exercise tolerance, improvement in blood pressure, angina, diabetes, varicose veins, pain in weight-bearing joints, and in certain disorders of reproductive function.

The outlook is worst in the patient who believes that substantial weight loss can be achieved without effort (for example by some wonder drug, or surgical operation), and that the benefits will include social success. It is true that obese patients are subject to adverse social discrimination, but it is not necessarily true that an unpopular obese person will, on losing weight, become a popular thin person.

Technique for weight loss

As explained above, the obese person carries excess fatty tissue which has an energy value of about 28 MJ kg^{-1} ($7000 \text{ kcal kg}^{-1}$). It is therefore necessary to achieve an average daily energy deficit of 4 MJ (1000 kcal) in order to achieve an average long-term weight loss of 1 kg per week. Empirically it has been found that rates of weight loss greater than 1 kg a week are associated with excessive loss of lean tissue, which is detrimental in the long run. It therefore follows that it will take *at least* 30 weeks to lose 30 kg of adipose tissue. There is absolutely no exception to this rule, and any patient is doomed to disappointment who believes that some special diet, or drug, or supplement, or exercise programme, can achieve massive, rapid, safe loss of adipose tissue.

The options for treatment of obesity are discussed (*See:* **Obesity**; Treatment), but the thermodynamic principles outlined above apply to every treatment.

Assessing the benefits to be gained by treatment

Generally speaking the younger the obese adult patient, and the greater the degree of obesity, the greater are the benefits to be gained by weight loss. Other factors concern familial disposition to the complications of obesity: in particular heart disease, hypertension and diabetes. A patient with a personal or family history of these diseases is more likely to develop them, and it is therefore more important to control the obesity than in an equally obese patient who does not have these risk factors.

See Colour Plate 6.

See also: **Body Composition**: Determination and Physiological Significance. **Energy**: Energy Balance; Measurement of Energy Intake and Expenditure. **Obesity**: Fat Distribution; Treatment.

Further Reading

Borkan GA, Sparrow D, Wisniewski C and Vokonas PS (1986) Body weight and coronary heart disease risk: patterns of risk factor change associated with long-term weight change. *American Journal of Epidemiology* **124**:410–419.

Garrow JS (1988) *Obesity and Related Diseases* pp. 329. London: Churchill Livingstone.

Garrow JS and Webster JD (1989) Effect on weight and metabolic rate of obese women of a 3.4 MJ (800 kcal) diet. *Lancet* i:1429–1431.

Han TS, van Leer EM, Seidell JC and Lean MEJ (1995) Waist circumference action levels in the identification of cardiovascular risk factors: prevalence study in a random sample. *British Medical Journal* **311**:1401–1405.

Higgins M, D'Agostino R, Kannel W and Cobb J (1993) Benefits and adverse effects of weight loss. *Annals of Internal Medicine* **119**:758–763.

Hubert HB (1984) The nature of the relationship between obesity and cardiovascular disease. *International Journal of Cardiology* **6**:268–274.

Manson JE, Colditz GA, Stamfer MJ, Wuillett WC, Rosner B, Monson RR, Speizer FE and Hennekens CH (1990) A prospective study of obesity and risk of coronary heart disease in women. *New England Journal of Medicine* **322**:822–829.

Manson JE, Willett WC, Stamfer MJ, Colditz GA, Hunter DJ, Hankinson SE, Hennekins CH and Speizer FE (1995) Body weight and mortality among women. *New England Journal of Medicine* **333**:677–685.

Rissanen AM, Heliovaara M, Knekt P, Reunanen A and Aromaa A (1991) Determinants of weight gain and overweight in adult Finns. *European Journal of Clinical Nutrition* **45**:419–430.

Seidell JC (1995) Obesity in Europe: scaling an epidemic. *International Journal of Obesity* **19** (supplement 3):S1–S4.

Sims EAH, Danforth EJr, Horton ES, Bray GA, Glennon JA and Salans LB (1973) Endocrine and metabolic effects of experimental obesity in man. *Recent Progress in Hormone Research* **29**:457–496.

Troiano RP, Frongillo EA, Sobal J and Levitsky DA (1996) The relationship between body weight and mortality: a quantitative analysis of combined information from existing studies. *International Journal of Obesity* **20**:63–75.

Webster JD, Hesp R and Garrow JS (1984) The composition of excess weight in obese women estimated by body density, total body water and total body potassium. *Human Nutrition: Clinical Nutrition* **38C**:299–306.

Early Obesity and Prognosis

B Caballero, Johns Hopkins University, Baltimore, Maryland, USA

The prevalence of childhood obesity is increasing throughout the industrialized world. In the USA, the number of children aged 6–11 years with body mass index (BMI) above the 85th percentile has increased from 15% in 1965 to 22% in 1992 (**Fig. 1**). In the same period, the prevalence of more severe obesity (BMI > 95th) has doubled, from 5.1% in 1960 to 10.2% in 1991. In a comparison of data from nine industrialized countries, in all of them there was an upward trend in the prevalence of childhood obesity. Furthermore, data from urban areas of some developing countries suggest that urbanization and socioeconomic transitions are associated with increasing prevalence of obesity in the general population.

Diagnosis of Obesity in Children

Determining whether a child is obese poses a number of problems not found in the assessment of adult obesity. Since children are constantly growing, weight gain only is of little value unless a precise measure of weight gain velocity is available. Furthermore, the use of the relationship between weight and height used commonly to define obesity, the body mass index (BMI = weight in kg/(height in m)^2) is also problematic in children. The rates of gain in weight and in height do not progress in parallel during childhood, and thus comparable BMI may be reflecting different body compositions at different ages. Ideally, the diagnosis of childhood obesity should be based on body fatness rather than body weight. Unfortunately, there is no simple, reliable means to estimate adiposity in children. The tricipital skinfold thickness has been proposed as the measure of choice, and obesity defined as a skinfold above the 85th percentile for age. Reliable measurement of skinfolds, however, is not easy, requiring proper training and constant practice. Thus, in spite of the limitations of BMI, this is still the most commonly used measure of obesity, given the large database of weight and height available for many populations. Reference data for BMI and tricipital skinfolds for

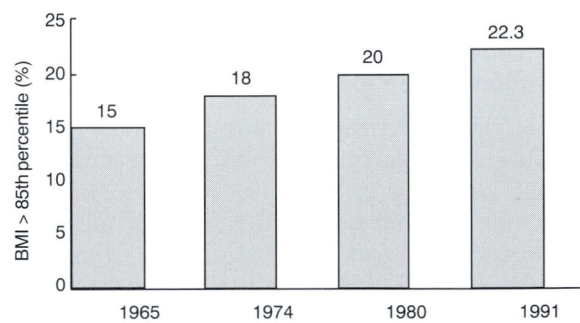

Figure 1 Trends in the prevalence of obesity in children aged 6–11 years in the USA. Data reported by Troiano *et al.* (1995) from NHES and NHANES national surveys.

the diagnosis of a paediatric obesity are available (**Table 1** and **Table 2**).

Factors Associated with Excessive Weight Gain Early in Life

Metabolic 'imprinting'

Certain metabolic changes occurring at specific periods during development appear to carry an increased risk of long-term obesity. Intrauterine malnutrition during the first trimester of pregnancy appears to increase the risk of excess weight in early adult life. It is hypothesized that a low energy supply conditions the differentiation of hypothalamic centres regulating appetite, leading to long-term patterns of energy inbalance and therefore fat accumulation. Some of the associations found between low birthweight and adult obesity may be related to these events.

Table 1 Percentiles for body mass index of children 6–19 years of age, all-race population, USA (data from Must *et al.*, 1991)

Age (years)	BMI (kg m⁻²)				
	5th	15th	50th	85th	95th
Males					
6	12.86	13.43	14.54	16.64	18.02
7	13.24	13.85	15.07	17.37	19.18
8	13.63	14.28	15.62	18.11	20.33
9	14.03	14.71	16.17	18.85	21.47
10	14.42	15.15	16.72	19.60	22.60
11	14.83	15.59	17.28	20.35	23.73
12	15.24	16.06	17.87	21.12	24.89
13	15.73	16.62	18.53	21.93	25.93
14	16.18	17.20	19.22	22.77	26.93
15	16.59	17.76	19.92	23.63	27.76
16	17.01	18.32	20.63	24.45	28.53
17	17.31	18.68	21.12	25.28	29.32
18	17.54	18.89	21.45	25.92	30.02
19	17.80	19.20	21.86	26.36	30.66
Females					
6	12.83	13.37	14.31	16.17	17.49
7	13.17	13.79	14.98	17.17	18.93
8	13.51	14.22	15.66	18.18	20.36
9	13.87	14.66	16.33	19.19	21.78
10	14.23	15.09	17.00	20.19	23.20
11	14.60	15.53	17.67	21.18	24.59
12	14.98	15.98	18.35	22.17	25.95
13	15.36	16.43	18.95	23.08	27.07
14	15.67	16.79	19.32	23.88	27.97
15	16.01	17.16	19.69	24.29	28.51
16	16.37	17.54	20.09	24.74	29.10
17	16.59	17.81	20.36	25.23	29.72
18	16.71	17.99	20.57	25.56	30.22
19	16.87	18.20	20.80	25.85	30.72

Table 2 Percentiles for triceps skinfold in children aged 6–19 years, all-race, USA (data from Must *et al.*, 1991)

Age (years)	Triceps skinfold (mm)				
	5th	15th	50th	85th	95th
Males					
6	5.04	6.19	8.36	11.10	14.12
7	5.01	6.14	8.59	12.38	15.61
8	4.96	6.08	8.79	13.66	17.18
9	4.91	6.02	8.96	14.93	18.81
10	4.84	5.95	9.10	16.02	20.68
11	4.78	5.88	9.23	16.87	22.20
12	4.69	5.79	9.35	17.26	23.25
13	4.56	5.65	9.17	17.12	23.71
14	4.47	5.60	8.93	16.35	23.46
15	4.40	5.59	8.70	15.75	22.34
16	4.33	5.55	8.45	15.75	21.53
17	4.29	5.58	8.38	15.95	21.51
18	4.25	5.63	8.53	16.59	21.83
19	4.22	5.69	8.63	17.33	22.12
Females					
6	6.00	6.76	10.01	13.44	15.57
7	6.24	7.17	10.68	14.94	17.89
8	6.47	7.58	11.36	16.41	20.18
9	6.71	8.01	12.05	17.85	22.47
10	6.95	8.44	12.74	19.01	24.38
11	7.20	8.87	13.43	20.13	26.15
12	7.45	9.31	14.13	21.25	27.98
13	7.78	9.84	14.87	22.25	29.51
14	8.15	10.37	15.47	23.27	30.86
15	8.46	10.85	16.03	24.32	32.22
16	8.78	11.34	16.62	25.12	33.22
17	9.03	11.66	17.02	25.80	33.83
18	9.21	11.79	17.24	26.51	34.26
19	9.41	11.97	17.50	27.23	34.74

Diet

During the first year of life, the ability of the child to increase total energy expenditure by increasing physical activity is quite limited. Thus, any excess energy intake will tend to be stored as body fat. Except for exclusively breast-fed babies, the level of caloric intake is usually determined by the mother or caregiver. Comparison of weight gain of healthy babies who are exclusively breast-fed with those who receive formula shows that the latter gain more weight, suggesting that excess caloric intake may be common in bottle-fed babies. Older children (2–3 years old and above) tend to share the table with the adults, and will be incorporating food preferences and eating habits accordingly. In spite of many claims on excess food consumption, most studies show no significant differences in the total dietary energy intake of normal-weight and obese children.

Reduced energy expenditure

The amount of calories the body needs to sustain physiological functions at rest, called basal metabolic rate, is quite constant when expressed by kg of lean body mass. If a child or adult is unusually efficient and requires fewer calories to sustain his or her basal metabolism, more of these calories will be available for other activities or for storage as body fat. The possibility that some individuals may have a genetically determined high energy efficiency (i.e. lower basal metabolic rates) that makes them prone to obesity has been explored in several populations. Since these differences in basal metabolic rate are quite small, they would not be expected to result in a significant accumulation of body fat in the short term, and there is no evidence of this occurring in young children. In the long term, however, it is possible that the continuing accumulation of energy 'saved' from basal metabolic rate as fat tissue may result in clinical obesity. Nevertheless, most studies show a higher energy expenditure in obese children compared with lean controls. These differences are attributed to the extra energy demands for locomotion of a larger body mass, and they disappear when the data is expressed per kg of lean mass. The finding of lower *total* energy expenditure in obese children can be usually explained by differences in physical activity levels.

Physical activity

Sedentary lifestyle is an important determinant of total energy expenditure. As the infant becomes older, the percentage of daily energy intake used for growth decreases, and voluntary activity become a major component of total energy output, besides the basal metabolic rate. Using the doubly labelled water method, significant differences in energy expenditure on physical activity have been found in infants who eventually became overweight at 12 months of age.

Levels of physical activity in school-age children vary greatly, usually determined primarily by cultural and environmental factors. Many school systems do not introduce mandatory physical education classes until middle or high school (11–14 years of age). In urban, inner city areas, opportunities for spontaneous group play after school are limited by lack of open space, street violence and limited motivation. Thus, many children of working parents remain indoors watching television after school.

Television viewing

A study examining the association between television viewing and obesity in a cross-sectional and prospective sample of over 12 000 children found that, in adolescents aged 12–17 years, the prevalence of obesity increased 2% for each additional hour spent watching television. The finding persisted when data were controlled for prior obesity, race, region, socioeconomic level, and several other family variables, and was attributed to a reduced energy expenditure and higher consumption of snack foods while watching television. In the USA, the average school-age child watches 26 h of television per week. The possible negative effect of television advertisements in shaping children's food preferences has also been of concern. In a study of television advertisements broadcast by the three major US networks during Saturday morning (a traditional children's viewing time), 71% of the commercials were for food products; of these 80% were for foods considered of low nutritional value, with candy, gum and cookies accounting for over 30%. Younger children tend to pay much more attention to the commercials than older ones. Although the impact of television advertising on children's eating habits has not been clearly assessed, there is no question that they do not favour healthy food choices, nor do they educate on the health importance of different foods.

Genetics

The heritability of adiposity has been the subject of numerous studies, yielding a wide range of results. Nevertheless, based on large cohort studies such as the Framingham Heart Study (USA), the Nord-Trondelag Study (Norway) and several others, experts concluded that heritability of body fatness is not higher than 40%, and is likely to be much lower than this figure. For example, the Framingham study, involving 74 994 people, showed a familial correlation of BMI of only 19%.

Prognosis: Tracking of childhood body weight into adulthood

The persistence of obesity from childhood into adulthood is dependent on the age of onset and the degree of excess weight. In general, only a relatively minor proportion of obese children remain obese when entering adulthood, but these tend to be those suffering from the most severe forms of obesity. In a 36-year follow-up of a cohort of 5362 children from England, Wales and Scotland, only 21% of those who were obese at age 36 years were also obese at age 11 years. The predictive value of childhood adiposity for adult adiposity also varies for different measures of fatness, possibly related to gender differences in body fat amount and distribution.

The body fat content of a child does not increase linearly with body weight, but rather undergoes periods of rapid accumulation at different stages. It has

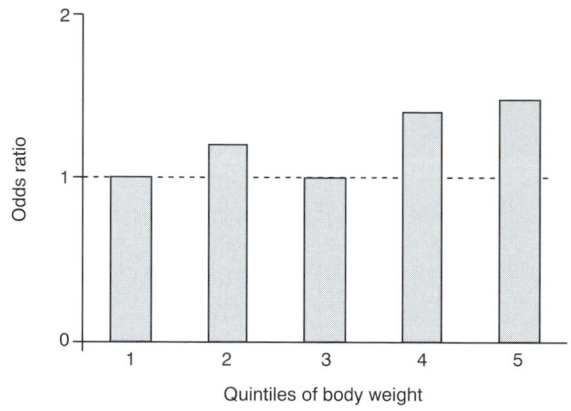

Figure 2 Prepubertal body weight and mortality risk. Data from both sexes, with mortality odds ratios adjusted for matching variables: sex, year of birth, and availability of pre- and post-pubertal body weight data. From Nieto *et al.* (1992).

been suggested that excess fat accumulation at these critical periods is more likely to persist into adulthood. The tracking of excess weight before 4–5 years of age is relatively poor, but tends to improve above 7 years of age. Regardless of time of onset, the longer a child has been obese, the higher the risk of continuing into adult obesity.

The long-term prognosis for treated obesity in children, although also dependent on age of onset and duration of the disease prior to initiation of therapy, is usually poor. Although many children are able to lose weight during the initial phase of treatment, the recurrence of excess weight at 5-year follow-up is close to 100%. Treatments that include family therapy fare better than treatments focusing only on the child.

Early Obesity and Long-term Risk of Disease

It is well established that obesity in adults is associated with increased morbidity and mortality. It has also been shown that adults who become overweight in childhood or adolescence tend to have more severe forms of the disease than those that become obese in adulthood. A different question is whether being obese during childhood increases mortality or morbidity independent of adult weight, e.g. even when weight goes back to normal after adolescence. Data from the Harvard Growth Study of 1922–35 showed that excess weight during adolescence was associated with increased risk for all-cause mortality and coronary heart disease, independent of postadolescence weight. In another study using a cohort database of 13 146 persons followed between 1930 and 1980, a significant association was found between weight at

ages 5–18 years and all-cause mortality, with odds ratios increasing linearly with prepubertal weight (**Fig. 2**). These results suggest that obesity during childhood and adolescence may have a sustained negative impact on adult health, which appears to be independent of the persistence of excess weight itself.

All this evidence, plus the great difficulty in treating obesity once established, underlines the importance of prevention. Introducing healthy dietary habits and promoting physical activity may be the two most relevant components of an obesity prevention programme for childhood.

See also: **Adolescents**: Nutritional Problems. **Energy**: Energy Requirements; Energy Balance; Measurement of Energy Intake and Expenditure. **Exercise**: Diet and Exercise; Beneficial Effects. **Infants**: Low-birthweight and Preterm Infants. **Obesity**: Treatment; Prevention.

Further Reading

Bray GA (1997) Progress in understanding the genetics of obesity. *Journal of Nutrition* **127**:940S–942S.

Caballero B (1993) Obesity. In: Avery ME and First L (eds) *Textbook of Pediatric Medicine*. Baltimore: Williams & Wilkins.

Dietz WH Jr and Gortmaker SL (1985) Do we fatten our children at the television set? Obesity and television viewing in children and adolescents. *Pediatrics* **75**:807–812.

Epstein LH, Wing RR, Koeske R and Valoski A (1987) Long-term effects of family-based treatment of childhood obesity. *Journal of Consulting and Clinical Psychology* **55**(1):91–95.

Goran MI, Figueroa R, McGloin A, Nguyen V, Treuth MS and Nagy TR (1995) Obesity in children: recent advances in energy metabolism and body composition. *Obesity Research* **3**(3):277–289.

Must A, Dallal GE, Dietz WH (1991) Reference data for obesity: 85th and 95th percentiles of body mass index (wt/ht²) and triceps skinfold thickness. *American Journal of Clinical Nutrition* **53**:839–846.

Must A, Jacques PF, Dallal GE, Bajema CJ and Dietz WH (1992) Long-term morbidity and mortality of overweight adolescents: a follow-up of the Harvard Growth Study of 1922 to 1935. *New England Journal of Medicine* **327**:1350–1355.

Nieto FJ, Szklo M and Comstock GW (1992) Childhood weight and growth rate as predictors of adult mortality. *American Journal of Epidemiology* **136**(2):201–213.

Okamoto E, Davidson LL and Conner DR (1993) High prevalence of overweight in inner-city schoolchildren. *American Journal of Diseases of Children* **147**:155–159.

Poskitt EME (1993) Which children are at risk of obesity? *Nutrition Res* **13**(1):S83–S93.

Ravelli G-P, Stein ZA and Susser MW (1976) Obesity in young men after famine exposure *in utero* and early infancy. *New England Journal of Medicine* 295:349–353.

Ravussin E, Lillioja S, Knowler WC, Christin L, Freymond D, Abbott WGH, Howard BV and Bogardus C (1988) Reduced rate of energy expenditure as a risk factor for body-weight gain. *New England Journal of Medicine* 318:467–472.

Robert SB, Savage J, Coward WA, Chew B and Lucas A (1988) Energy expenditure and intake in infants born to lean and overweight mothers. *New England Journal of Medicine* 318:461–466.

Troiano RP, Flegal KM, Kuczmarski RJ, Campbell SM and Johnson CL (1995). Overweight prevalence and trends for children and adolescents. *Archives of Pediatric and Adolescent Medicine* 149:1085–1091.

Fat Distribution

M Harris and **June Stevens**, University of North Carolina at Chapel Hill, North Carolina, USA

It has now been clearly demonstrated that the location, as well as the amount, of adipose tissue on the body has important implications for health and disease. While the relative importance of total adiposity vs. type of adiposity continues to be debated, the notion that an 'apple-shaped' (or android) body is associated with greater obesity-related health risks than a 'pear-shaped' (or gynoid) body is well accepted (**Fig. 1**). The increased risk associated with the apple shape is generally attributed to a larger amount of visceral (or intra-abdominal) fat.

Measurement of Fat Distribution

Fat patterning, the distribution of fat, is measured using either imaging or anthropometric techniques. Imaging techniques have the advantage of providing separate measurements of subcutaneous and visceral fat, but they remain too expensive for use in most epidemiological work and are generally used only in clinical studies. Anthropometric measurements cannot provide a direct assessment of visceral fat, but they are quick, inexpensive, and noninvasive.

Imaging techniques

Imaging techniques currently in use to measure fat patterning include computerized tomography, dual photon absorptiometry (DPA), dual energy X ray absorptiometry (DEXA), magnetic resonance imaging (MRI) and ultrasound. Computerized tomography and MRI are considered the most reliable methods for measuring body fat distribution. MRI, however, has the advantage of not exposing subjects to radiation. DPA and DEXA are usually used to measure bone mineral content but have also been used to measure soft tissue. These techniques are not recommended for use in fat distribution studies since they do not discriminate well between visceral and subcutaneous fat and can overestimate fat tissue in subjects with low mineral bone density. Ultrasound measurement has potential for use in studies of relatively large populations, although the ability of the technique to measure intra-abdominal fat is currently limited because it does not distinguish between different fat layers well. It may be more useful for measuring the thickness of subcutaneous layers rather than actual intra-abdominal fat.

Fig. 2 shows two different cross-sectional images of the abdomen obtained by magnetic resonance imaging. The MRI is constructed of 256 × 256 pixels which vary from white to black with different shades of grey. Each pixel represents 2.4 mm². The fat regions are depicted as the lighter portions of the images. The subcutaneous fat area delineates the perimeter of the abdomen while the visceral area is contained within the subcutaneous area. Figure 2(a) represents a cross-section of an abdomen with a relatively small subcutaneous fat area in comparison with an enlarged visceral fat area. Figure 2(b) shows a participant with a small visceral fat to subcutaneous fat depot ratio.

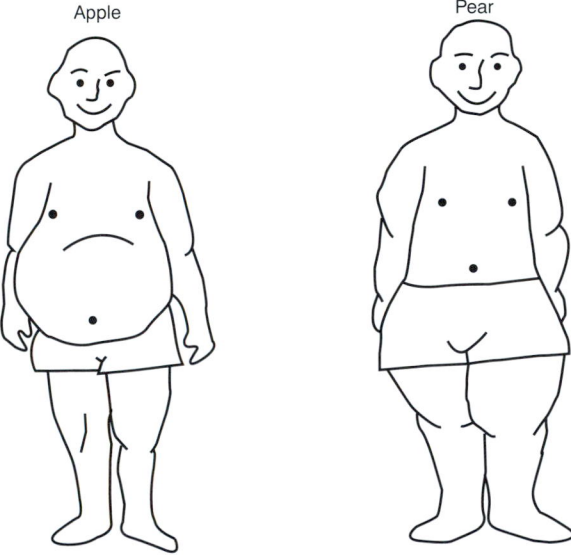

Figure 1 The apple (android) and pear (gynoid) body shapes.

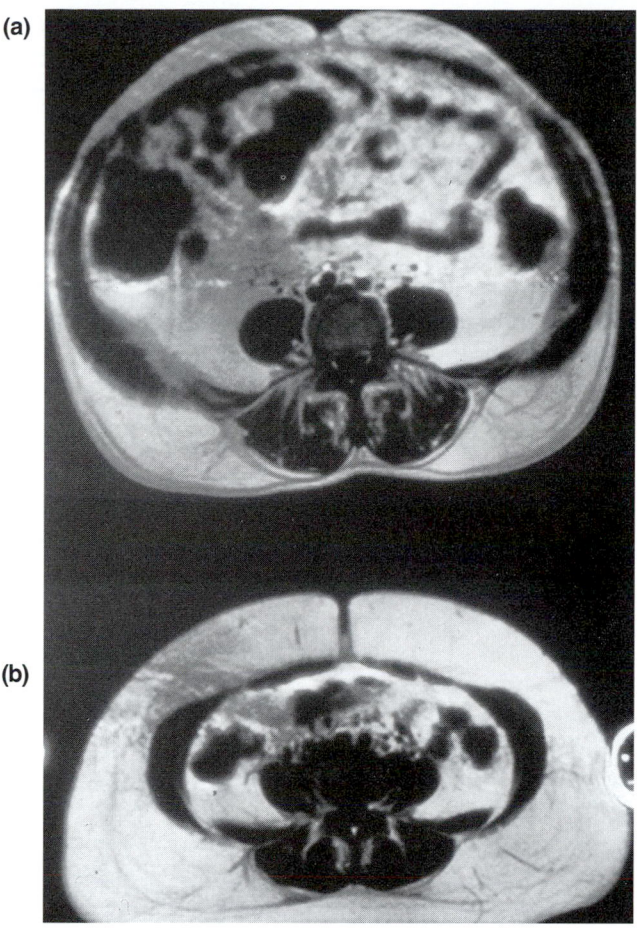

Figure 2 Cross-sectional images of the abdomen obtained by MRI. (a) Small subcutaneous fat area and enlarged visceral fat area. (b) Small visceral fat area in comparison with subcutaneous fat depot.

Anthropometric techniques

Anthropometric indices used to measure fat patterning include skinfold thicknesses, circumferences, and ratios such as waist-to-hip ratio, subscapular/triceps skinfolds, waist/thigh, abdominal circumference/height, and waist/height. Linear equations which predict the amount of visceral fat have also been derived. Sagittal diameter, the height of the abdomen measured with the subject in the supine position, is sometimes used and can be measured anthropometrically or by imaging. **Fig. 3** shows a technique for the anthropometric measurement of sagittal diameter using a caliper. Measurement is usually taken between the fourth and fifth lumbar vertebrae.

Skinfold thicknesses and skinfold ratios have not been found to be well correlated with metabolic measurements or with visceral fat and are not recommended for use as indicators of fat patterning. Combinations of anthropometric measurements in linear equations to predict the amount of visceral fat

have, thus far, not offered substantial improvement over the simpler measurements of waist or waist-to-hip ratio and an accurate equation has yet to be developed.

The waist-to-hip ratio is the most popular anthropometric method used to measure fat distribution in both clinical and epidemiological studies. One problem with this anthropometric measurement, however, is that it does not specifically measure visceral fat, although it is correlated with visceral fat.

Another problem with the waist-to-hip ratio is that there is no standardized method of measuring the waist or the hips (see **Table 1**). One reason why there is no single anthropometric measurement consistently better correlated with visceral fat is that there is no uniform method of defining the location at which the waist and hip measurement should be assessed. For instance some measure the waist at the level of the umbilicus, while others measure it at the minimal abdominal circumference. Some researchers have recently compared waist and hip circumference

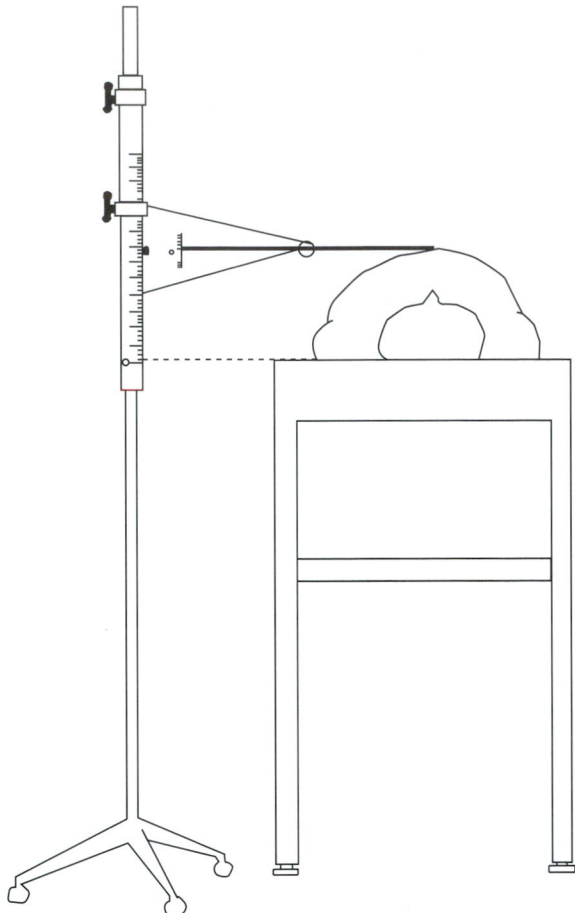

Figure 3 Sagittal diameter measured anthropometrically using callipers.

measurements, where the measurements were taken at several different locations, and examined correlations with cardiovascular risk factors. The best correlations were obtained when waist-to-hip ratio was calculated as the waist measured at the point midway between the lower rib margin and iliac crest (about 1 inch, ~2.5 cm, above umbilicus) or when the waist was measured at the umbilicus, and hips measured at the widest point of the buttocks. Although the waist-to-hip ratio using both waist measurements correlated significantly with metabolic parameters (P

< 0.001), the use of the landmark measurement (versus the umbilicus) was recommended since the umbilicus may shift positions when an individual gains or loses weight. Waist and hip measurements are also affected by body size. The more obese an individual, the more difficult it is to measure the waist and hip circumferences and the higher the measurement error. These sources of variability will contribute to the attenuation of risk estimates and error.

Sagittal diameter and waist circumferences may be better indicators of visceral fat than the waist-to-hip ratio. These techniques have been examined as predictors of visceral fat, and yielded higher correlations with visceral fat than the waist-to-hip ratio in some, but not all, studies. It is important to note that many studies measure sagittal diameter using imaging techniques. Measured anthropometrically, the sagittal diameter produces correlations with visceral fat as low as $r = 0.51$ and as high as $r = 0.87$.

Although the waist circumference tends to be more highly correlated with visceral fat than the waist-to-hip ratio, it is difficult to ascertain from the available studies the most accurate predictor of visceral fat since studies vary by the site used for waist and hip measurements and the subjects examined represent a wide range of age and total body adiposity (see below). One advantage of the use of the waist circumference versus waist-to-hip ratio as an indicator of fat patterning or visceral fat is that it consists of only one measurement instead of two, and therefore introduces less measurement error. The use of the waist measurement alone may also avoid population specific trends in hip size, that may be unrelated to the amount of visceral fat and bias waist-to-hip ratio measurements across populations. However, the waist circumference is more dependent on total adiposity than the waist-to-hip ratio and is more difficult to assess in ageing subjects. If an index of body shape is desired, independent of total body fatness, the waist-to-hip ratio may be preferred because it is less highly correlated with total adiposity than the waist.

Table 1   Anatomical locations used to measure waist and hips

Waist	Hip
One-third between the xiphoid process and umbilicus	Largest horizontal circumference around the buttocks
Narrowest part of torso	Level of iliac crest
Midway between exiphoid process and umbilicus	Maximal circumference between superior border of iliac crest
Midway between lower rib and iliac crest	and thigh region 4 cm below superior iliac crest
Level of ⅓ of distance between xiphoid process and umbilicus	
One inch (~ 2·5 cm) above umbilicus	
Level of umbilicus	
Level of iliac crest	

There is still a need for an anthropometric measurement which can accurately estimate the amount of visceral fat. Although the waist-to-hip ratio is problematic, it is a widely accepted form of fat patterning measurement. It is a good predictor of disease and metabolic disorders – generally an increasing waist-to-hip ratio indicates increasing risk. Cutpoints for elevated waist-to-hip ratio which represent an elevated risk for disease development have been defined as between 0.90–0.95 for men and 0.80–0.85 for women.

Metabolic Characteristics of Visceral and Subcutaneous Fat

The main function of adipose tissue is to store and break down fat based on energy excess or need, respectively. The storage of fat is regulated by the enzyme lipoprotein lipase (LPL). This enzyme hydrolyses triacylglycerols into free fatty acids which can then be transported into the adipocyte and rehydrolysed for storage. Greater LPL activity is associated with greater accumulation of fat. In premenopausal women, its activity is higher in the gluteal-femoral adipose areas than in the abdominal areas. The opposite is true in men where LPL activity is the same or higher in the abdominal adipose areas than in the gluteal-femoral regions.

The breakdown of fat is regulated by the enzyme hormone-sensitive lipase (HSL). This enzyme releases free fatty acids into the bloodstream for energy use (lipolysis). The rate of basal lipolysis is higher in gluteal-femoral fat tissue than abdominal tissue in both men and women. This may be due to greater cell size in that region. In the abdominal area, basal lipolysis is higher in subcutaneous fat than in visceral fat. However, when stimulated hormonally, rates of lipolysis may differ between men and women. Lipolytic rates have been shown to be higher in the visceral region compared with those in the subcutaneous region in men while the opposite trend is seen in women.

Regulators of lipolysis and fat storage

The processes of lipolysis and fat storage are regulated by hormonal factors which either enhance or suppress the activities of HSL and LPL. Through the action of glucocorticoid receptors, glucocorticoids enhance LPL activity and promote abdominal deposition of fat. The density of glucocorticoid receptors is greater in the visceral abdominal depot than the subcutaneous abdominal depot. Therefore, an increase in glucocorticoid secretion is associated with increases in abdominal fat deposition compared with other fat depots.

Insulin favours fat storage by increasing LPL and decreasing HSL activity. Insulin has stronger anti-lipolytic effects in adipose located in the abdominal region compared with the femoral regions in both men and women. Paradoxically, insulin binding is stronger in the gluteal-femoral region than the abdominal region. Therefore, it has been hypothesized that insulin regulates lypolysis at the postreceptor level.

Catecholamines regulate lipolysis through α_2- and β-adrenoreceptors. The β-adrenoreceptor increases lipolysis while the α_2-adrenoreceptor inhibits it. Although both the α_2- and the β-adrenoreceptors coexist in adipose tissue, they are regionally specific such that there may be an excess of one type of receptor relative to the other in various adipose regions. The lipolytic effect of catecholamines is 10–20 times greater in the abdominal region than the gluteal-femoral region, as marked by a 2-fold increase in the number of β-adrenoreceptors in both sexes. The lipolytic action of catecholamines is more pronounced intra-abdominally than in the abdominal subcutaneous tissue. Sex differences are displayed with the α-adrenoreceptor. Although the number of receptors is similar in both sexes, the sensitivity of the receptors in females is reduced by a factor of 10–15 in the abdominal compared with the gluteal-femoral region.

Sex hormones, such as oestrogen, testosterone and progesterone, also affect the balance of fat accumulation/mobilization, although their effects vary in men and women and the mechanisms are not clearly understood. It has been shown that testosterone stimulates lipolysis by increasing the number of β-adrenoreceptors. Oestrogen and progesterone, on the other hand, stimulate fat storage and inhibit lipolysis, preferentially in the gluteal-femoral area compared with the abdominal area.

An increased androgenic hormone profile is associated with upper body fat accumulation in women, but studies in men are conflicting. Significant inverse associations between fat distribution and testosterone have been found in population studies in men. Reduced visceral fat has also been observed when testosterone treatment was administered to men. These findings challenge the hypothesis that an androgenic hormone profile contributes to a more 'male type' of fat pattern and the associated metabolic sequelae.

The controversy over the effect of sex hormones on fat distribution is complicated by the metabolism of sex hormones. Sex hormone binding globulin (SHBG) binds circulating testosterone and oestrogen. Decreased SHBG concentration may be associated with an android shape. Therefore, studies need to distinguish between total circulating and unbound sex hormones and SHBG.

Sequelae of altered metabolism in visceral fat

Intra-abdominal adipose tissue has metabolic characteristics that are different from that of adipose tissue from other sites. These differences seem to be most pronounced in the regions that are drained by the portal circulation. These 'portal adipose tissues' have a sensitive system for the mobilization of free fatty acids due to a preponderance of β-adrenergic receptors and little α-adrenergic inhibition.

The hypothesis has been advanced that the heightened responsiveness of intraabdominal fat to lipolytic agents results in increased lipolysis with venous drainage of the released free fatty acids directly to the liver. These fatty acids may contribute to increases in triacylglycerol synthesis and hyperinsulinaemia secondary to decrements in insulin degradation. The hyperinsulinaemia could eventually produce non-insulin-dependent dependent diabetes in susceptible individuals. It has been proposed that the hyperinsulinaemia could also lead to increased blood pressure through increased sympathetic stimulation of the vessels, heart and kidneys.

In addition, insulin resistance combined with a relative increase in androgenic activity could lead to an unfavourable lipid profile. In addition to the effects of free fatty acids on insulin and glucose, an increased visceral depot decreases the activity of LPL. This causes an increase of very low-density lipoprotein (VLDL) secretion and a decrease in its catabolism. The production of high-density lipoprotein (HDL) therefore decreases, the transfer of lipids (i.e. VLDL to LDL and HDL) increases and an enrichment of triacylglycerols results.

Correlates and Possible Determinants of Fat Distribution

A large number of studies have examined correlations between fat distribution and genetic, behavioural and physiological variables. Many factors including heredity, age, gender, overall fatness, alcohol consumption, smoking and physical activity are associated with either an android or gynoid shape. The underlying reason for the observed associations between these variables and fat patterning remain to be elucidated. Some studies have found a more androgenic hormone profile in cigarette smokers, although this finding has been inconsistent. Increased cortisol secretion, an endocrine response to stressors associated with upper body fat deposition, may explain some of the association between smoking, alcohol consumption and fat distribution. Correlates

of fat distribution are important to understand since they may confound relationships between fat patterning and physiological outcomes or morbidity or mortality outcomes.

There is evidence that body shape and amount of visceral fat is partially determined by genetics. After eliminating effects of age and overall fatness, studies have shown that heritable factors can account for as much as 20–50% of the variability in waist-to-hip ratio.

Fat distribution has long been known to vary by gender. Men have a higher waist-to-hip ratio and significantly more intra-abdominal adipose tissue than women. During weight gain in normal-weight men, fat is initially deposited abdominally in the subcutaneous and visceral regions – proportionately more in the upper compared with the lower abdomen. In these men little fat is deposited in the gluteal-femoral regions until they become obese. In contrast when women gain weight, subcutaneous fat is deposited uniformly. Visceral fat begins to accumulate only after obesity has been reached.

Ageing is accompanied by changes in both weight and fat distribution. Weight tends to be gained until about 55 years of age, after which it begins to decline. Independent of the weight gained, however, fat tends to be accumulated centrally in both men and women. This increase tends to be most pronounced between young and middle age in men, and between middle age and old age in women (a function of menopausal status).

Although cigarette smokers tend to be leaner than nonsmokers, they have increased central adiposity (as indicated by higher waist and waist-to-hip ratios) compared with nonsmokers, even after the effects of age and BMI have been eliminated. Furthermore, waist-to-hip ratio increases progressively with an increase in the number of cigarettes smoked daily. The waist-to-hip ratio increases with increasing 24 h cotinine excretion, indicating that central fat accumulation is dependent on the dose of smoke inhaled.

Physical activity is negatively correlated with fat distribution in both men and women. Negative associations exist between waist-to-hip ratio and various sports and exercise indices after controlling for the effects of BMI, smoking, and education. There is some evidence that activity may be associated with a preferential mobilization of abdominal fat.

While alcohol consumption has been postulated to be correlated with fat distribution, studies have been inconclusive. Differing measurements for alcohol consumption among studies and the difficulty in obtaining reliable measurements of consumption may contribute to inconsistent findings. One recent study distinguished alcohol consumption in terms of alcohol, beer and spirits, and found that increased centralized fat accumulates with increasing consumption of beer or spirits. Interestingly, any increase in the daily consumption of wine tended to decrease the waist-to-hip ratio.

The prevalence of obesity is higher in many ethnic groups than in white Americans. African Americans, Hispanic Americans, American Indians and Polynesians are more overweight than whites, and these differences are generally more marked in women than in men. Asians appear to be different from other minority groups studied in the US as they have been shown to have the same or lower total body adiposity than reference white populations.

Since body weight is highly correlated with the waist-to-hip ratio, it is not surprising that greater abdominal fat accumulations are seen in ethnic groups which tend to be heavier than whites. The issue of whether fat distribution is different among ethnic groups after controlling for differences in overall fatness is less well studied. African American women may have lower waist-to-hip ratios than white women after the effects of total adiposity are eliminated.

Fat Distribution and Disease Risk

Numerous studies have examined associations between fat patterning and morbidity. Since fat distribution is correlated with age as well as with other risk factors for disease such as smoking, alcohol consumption, physical activity, and menopause in women, it is important to eliminate the effects of these variables in order to obtain an estimate of the independent effect of central obesity on morbidity. Few studies of the relationship of fat distribution to disease have adjusted for these factors. Admittedly, the impact of some of these correlates of fat distribution may be subtle and unlikely to seriously distort relationships between fat patterning and disease. However, age, the ultimate risk factor for disease and death, is sufficiently highly associated with fat distribution to result in substantial distortion. Similarly, cigarette smoking is related adequately strongly to fat patterning and to various diseases and outcomes to make analyses which do not adjust for smoking difficult to interpret.

The large correlation between fat patterning and overall adiposity ($r \sim 0.7$) also influences the interpretation of results, making it difficult to differentiate between the two effects. Some authors compare the size of the correlation between fat distribution (usually measured as waist-to-hip ratio) and total adiposity (usually measured as body mass index, BMI) in an attempt to show the relative importance of each. Other authors examine effects within (for example) tertiles of BMI and waist-to-hip ratio simultaneously or test for an independent effect of waist-to-hip ratio or BMI in multiple regression models that include both variables. In the latter type of analysis, the associations of both waist-to-hip ratio and BMI with an outcome can be greatly reduced or even disappear because of collinearity between the two measures.

Correlations between insulin and glucose

Visceral fat measured using imaging techniques and waist-to-hip ratio is inversely correlated with insulin sensitivity as measured by the oral glucose tolerance test (OGTT). Fat distribution as measured by waist-to-hip ratio is also correlated with fasting levels of insulin and glucose. Correlations, unadjusted for age or other covariates, are about $r = 0.4$ (range 0.1–0.7). In the few studies that do adjust for age and BMI, the correlation between insulin and waist-to-hip ratio attenuates to about $r = 0.1$.

Correlations with plasma lipids

Of the various blood lipid parameters routinely studied, plasma triacylglycerol levels are most consistently associated with the waist-to-hip ratio, with the size of unadjusted correlations approximately $r = 0.4$. After adjusting for age and BMI, triacylglycerol levels remain significantly correlated with the waist-to-hip ratio, although attenuated to about $r = 0.2$.

A handful of studies have examined VLDL levels and fat distribution. Unadjusted associations between VLDL and waist-to-hip ratio range from $r = 0.15$ to $r = 0.49$. Studies of correlations between waist-to-hip ratio and LDL and total cholesterol have not been consistent. In contrast, HDL shows a consistent negative association with waist-to-hip ratio. While unadjusted r values range from about $r = -0.2$ to $r = -0.7$, the average correlation is about $r = -0.4$. After adjustment for age and BMI, HDL continues to be significantly negatively associated with the waist-to-hip ratio, with an average correlation of about $r = -0.1$.

Correlations with blood pressure

The association between blood pressure and waist-to-hip ratio varies among studies, although it tends to be stronger than that of total cholesterol (unadjusted $r \sim 0.3$). Many studies do not eliminate nor control for subjects taking antihypertensive medication, which makes adjusted correlations difficult to identify.

Fat patterning and non-insulin-dependent diabetes

There is strong evidence to link waist-to-hip ratio with the risk of developing non-insulin-dependent diabetes, even after eliminating effects of age, smoking, BMI and other important correlates. An individual who is obese (> 150% ideal body weight) and has an elevated waist-to-hip ratio (>0.8) may have as much as a 10-fold increased risk for developing non-insulin-dependent diabetes compared with an individual who is of normal weight (< 120% ideal body weight) and has a low waist-to-hip ratio (<0.72).

Fat patterning and cardiovascular disease

Elevated waist-to-hip ratio has been positively associated with cardiovascular disease in population studies, although not as consistently as with diabetes. Cardiovascular disease risk increases with an increasing waist-to-hip ratio; however in most studies the effects of other factors such as age and BMI were not eliminated. More recent studies which did control for these factors found an independent effect of waist-to-hip ratio on CVD.

Conclusions

The relationship of body fat distribution to metabolic abnormalities and disease has now been well recognized. Individuals with a more android than gynoid body shape tend to have a more adverse metabolic profile and an increased risk for non-insulin-dependent diabetes and cardiovascular disease. Of the many plasma parameters examined, triacylglycerols and HDL have the strongest and most consistent associations with the waist-to-hip ratio after adjusting for the effects of age and total adiposity.

While much has been learned about fat distribution since the early 1980s, there are several issues that need further exploration. The question of whether body type can be changed through behaviour needs to be more fully addressed. Standardized anthropometric measurements need to be established, and differences in fat distribution among ethnic groups need to be elucidated. Finally, more research is needed to identify mechanisms of action. An increased abdominal depot may not necessarily be the cause of metabolic disturbances but an effect of underlying genetic and endocrine abnormalities.

See Colour Plate 9.

See also: **Diabetes Mellitus**: Classification and Chemical Pathology; Aetiology and Epidemiology. **Hyperlipidaemia (Hyperlipidemia)**: Overview; Nutritional Management. **Lipids**: Chemistry and Classification.

Further Reading

Abate N and Garg A (1995) Heterogeneity in adipose tissue metabolism: causes, implications and management of regional adiposity. *Progress in Lipid Research* **34**:53–70.

Björntorp P (1991) Metabolic implications of body fat distribution. *Diabetes Care* **14**:1132–1143.

Björntorp P (1993) Visceral obesity: a 'civilization syndrome'. *Obesity Research* **1**:206–222.

Björntorp P (1996) The regulation of adipose tissue distribution in humans. *International Journal of Obesity* **20**:291–302.

Bouchard C, Despres JP and Mauriege P (1993) Genetic and nongenetic determinants of regional fat distribution. *Endocrine Reviews* **14**:72–93.

Despres JP, Moorjani S, Lupien PJ, Tremblay A, Nadeau A and Bouchard C (1990) Regional distribution of body fat, plasma lipoproteins, and cardiovascular disease. *Arteriosclerosis* **10**:497–511.

Emery EM, Schmid TL, Kahn HS and Filozof PP (1993) A review of the association between abdominal fat distribution, health outcome measures, and modifiable risk factors. *American Journal of Health Promotion* **7**:342–353.

Jakicic JM, Donnelly JE, Jawad AF, Jacobsen DJ, Gunderson SC and Pascale R (1993) Association between blood lipids and different measures of body fat distribution: effects of BMI and age. *International Journal of Obesity* **17**:131–137.

Kissebah AH and Krakower GR (1994) Regional adiposity and morbidity. *Physiological Reviews* **74**:761–811.

Kumanyika K (1993) Special issues regarding obesity in minority populations. *Annals of Internal Medicine* **119**:650–654.

Schreiner PJ, Terry JG, Evans GW, Hinson, WH, Crouse JR III and Heiss G (1996) Sex-specific associations of magnetic resonance imaging-derived intra-abdominal and subcutaneous fat areas with conventional anthropometric indices. *American Journal of Epidemiology* **144**:335–345.

Shimokata H, Tobin JD, Muller DC, Elahi D, Coon PJ and Andres R (1989) Studies in the distribution of body fat: I Effects of age, sex, and obesity. *Journal of Gerontology* **44**:M66–73.

Shimokata H, Andres R, Coon PJ, Elahi D, Muller DC and Tobin JD (1989) Studies in the distribution of body fat. II Longitudinal effects of change in weight. *International Journal of Obesity* **13**:455–464.

Stevens J (1995) Obesity, fat patterning and cardiovascular risk. In: Longnecker JB (ed.) *Nutrition and Biotechnology in Heart Disease and Cancer*, pp 21–27. New York: Plenum Press.

van der Kooy K and Seidell JC (1993) Techniques for the measurement of visceral fat: a practical guide. *International Journal of Obesity* **17**:187–196.

Treatment

L Albon and **P Kopelman**, St Bartholomew's and The Royal London School of Medicine and Dentistry, London, UK

Introduction

Any treatment programme for obesity should address not only the problem of weight reduction, but also include measures to help with the maintenance of the lowered weight. The primary aim for a programme is a reduction in body fat with the assumption that this will reduce risk from comorbid conditions. Nevertheless, a successful programme should also lead to an improvement in the quality of life, self-esteem, social functioning, anxiety and depression. Obesity is a condition which may not respond to conventional methods of treatment: its management requires an approach tailored to specific needs.

The ability of a treatment to maintain long-term weight reduction is as important as its ability to cause the initial weight loss. In many instances obesity results not from an inability to lose weight, but from a considerable difficulty in maintaining a lowered weight.

Long-term strategies including weight maintenance

Obesity and overweight are chronic conditions. Short-term programmes are likely to be ineffective, with rapid weight regain once treatment is stopped. Treatment programmes must be for the longer term and include measures to prevent relapse. A better understanding of those particularly at risk from obesity is needed to ensure an appropriate use of resources. Those at risk will include moderately overweight subjects with a body mass index (BMI) of 27 to 30 $kg\,m^{-2}$, who have upper body obesity. Additionally important treatment areas include weight gain in infancy, adolescence and pregnancy. A family history of obesity or associated diseases, fat distribution and risk factors for coronary heart disease are individually important factors that may influence the treatment mode.

Associated diseases

Short-term weight loss corrects or ameliorates many of the metabolic abnormalities associated with overweight including insulin resistance, diabetes mellitus, hypertension, dyslipidaemia and blood coagulation abnormalities as well as obesity-related physical impairments. Moreover, weight loss in obese persons consistently improves negative emotions such as depression and anxiety. It also improves psychosocial functioning, mood and quality of life in the obese, but these beneficial effects may be transitory, and sometimes are offset by the adverse psychological and psychosocial consequences of subsequent weight regain.

Realistic weight goals

The success or failure of any treatment programme may be judged by an arbitrarily chosen weight or percentage weight loss. Ideal weight tables are not applicable to overweight patients and weight goals should be tailored to the individual. A weight loss of between 5 and 10% of the initial body weight is associated with clinically useful improvements in terms of blood pressure, plasma cholesterol and triacylglycerols and high-density lipoprotein (HDL) cholesterol, and a significant improvement in diabetic control. Goals for older patients will be different from those for younger ones – data suggests that a population becomes heavier with age whereas the risk from obesity does not increase proportionately. In some older patients, prevention of further weight gain may be more appropriate.

Dietary Treatment of Obesity

The modern approach to obesity treatment must focus on a healthy diet in terms of the prevention of hypertension and ischaemic heart disease and in line with the general recommendations for the population as a whole. Long-term changes in food choices, eating behaviour and lifestyle are necessary, rather than a temporary restriction of specific foods.

Low-calorie diets

There are many types of low-calorie diets (**Table 1**).

Table 1 Types of low-energy diets

- *Balanced diets* – a balanced ratio of protein, carbohydrate and fat but in reduced quantities

- *One-food diets* – single foods are eaten at each meal in the hope that an aversion to these foods will develop

- *Diets eliminating one or more nutrients* – one or more energy sources are eliminated or reduced (usually carbohydrate or fat)

- *High-fibre diets* – high-fibre diets are said to reduce calorie density, increase eating time and displace other high-calorie foods

- *Formula diets* – generally balanced diets that are low in calories and that serve to replace whole meals. These are usually in liquid or powder form and have a novelty value coupled with an ease of use

They generally involve a daily intake of between 3300 and 6300 kJ (800–1500 kcal). The efficacy of any diet is entirely dependent upon patient adherence. For long-term success the most important characteristics of dietary modification is that it is achievable and sustainable – this can only be accomplished by a balanced eating programme.

Very low-calorie diets

Very low-calorie diets (VLCDs) were introduced in the 1970s in an attempt to emulate the impressive weight loss achieved by starvation therapy. Such diets consist of a daily energy intake of below 3300 kJ (800 kcal) consumed in a liquid form. They were initially rendered unsafe by inadequate nutrient content, inappropriate selection of patients and poor supervision. However, modern VLCD regimen are relatively safe when used under professional supervision for the treatment of more severe degrees of obesity. High initial weight losses of >3 kg per week can be achieved with VLCDs, but these losses include considerable amounts of fluid and lean body tissue. VLCDs should only be used for short periods in those patients who are refractory to more moderate dietary interventions and their wider use cannot be condoned (**Table 2**). To reduce potential risks from loss of lean body tissue, such preparations must provide a daily minimum of 1600 kJ (400 kcal) for women and 2000 kJ (500 kcal) for men, accompanied by 40 and 50 g per day, respectively, of high biological value protein.

An alternative form of low-calorie liquid diet is the milk diet. It consists of 1.8 l (3 pints) of whole cow's milk which provides 4900 kJ (1170 kcal) and 59 g of high biological quality protein. It is, however, deficient in iron, fibre and vitamins, but these can be supplemented by the addition of methyl cellulose, a multivitamin capsule and ferrous sulfate (200 mg per day). Patient adherence to the milk diet is dependent upon whether the patient is able to tolerate such a volume of milk.

Table 2 Indications and contraindications for VLCD treatment

Indications	Contraindications
BMI >35 kg m^{-2}	Age <12 or >65 years
One or more complications associated with obesity	Recent myocardial infarct
	Congestive heart disease
Failure of conventional dietary restriction	Unstable angina or arrhythmias
	Pregnancy or lactation
	Significant psychiatric disease or eating disorder

Commercial slimming organizations

Such organizations are profit-making ventures. They have been shown to be economical, practical and an effective means of providing care for a large number of moderately obese people in the community. Weekly meetings serve to encourage and reinforce active participation by members, who learn through the exchange of ideas within the group. Weight losses achieved by commercial groups are comparable to those seen in general practice or hospital outpatient clinics. When behavioural techniques are added to the basic programme of balanced diet, the results are further improved.

Efficacy of dietary therapy

Published reports suggest that dietary therapy is most effective in patients over 40 years of age with a BMI of under 35, and a medical consequence of obesity which is likely to improve with weight loss. The main limitation of dietary therapy is that most weight is regained within a year to 18 months of the cessation of therapy: a weight regain of 30% is reported after ceasing to attend a slimming club for 2 years. A review of five randomized control trials of VLCD treatment suggests 37–52% of lost weight is regained after 2 years and less than 5% of the patients maintain significant weight loss by 5 years.

Behaviour Modification

All dietary regimens should ideally be linked with some form of behaviour therapy. Behaviour modification is an important technique in the management of obesity and has been incorporated into many self-help groups. Behaviour modification serves to identify the unproductive habits developed over many years and helps to unlearn them by replacing them with adaptive patterns of behaviour. The main features which behavioural programmes have in common are an agreement to keep records of food intake and weight change, an attempt to restrict cues which cause eating and to eat more slowly, and various systems for rewarding these changes in behaviour. In behavioural weight-control programmes, the focus is on behaviours related to body weight, namely food intake and physical activity. The key difference between behavioural methods and other forms of treatment for obesity is that individuals must take personal responsibility for initiating and maintaining treatment rather than relying on external forces alone. There are at least three behavioural approaches to the management of obesity (**Table 3**).

Table 3 Behavioural approaches to the management of obesity

- *Increased emphasis on low-fat intake and exercise* – In the past behaviour change programmes focused on overall calorie intake, more recently the emphasis has shifted onto low-fat diets with patients being asked to record the fat content of the foods they consume as well as the total calories

- *Direct intervention on behavioural antecedents and consequences* – To intervene more directly on environmental cues controlling eating, subjects are provided with the food they should eat; to intervene more directly on the consequences, investigators pay subjects to lose weight and maintain it

  Inclusion of low-calorie diets in the treatment programme – These programmes aim to achieve substantial initial weight loss from the use of VLCD and improve subsequent weight maintenance through behavioural techniques

- *Combination of behaviour therapy and exercise programmes* – The addition of exercise to the behavioural and dietary components seems to be beneficial in terms of weight and maintained weight

Efficacy of behaviour treatment

In most studies, behaviour therapy produces consistent weight loss for the short-term. Recent studies suggest that that programmes which focus on both calorie restriction and reduced fat are more successful than those which consider calorie intake alone. Studies which have examined cue avoidance are inconclusive whereas those which included the provision of food may be of value. Evidence suggests that lengthening treatment programmes improves the long-term outcome in relation to weight maintenance. Although controlled trials confirm that continued contact with a therapist is beneficial, the nature of this contact may be less important.

Family Therapy

Eating patterns and behaviours are, to a great extent, acquired by learning, and for this reason there has been much interest in modifying the behaviour within the family setting. Obese children are at great risk of becoming obese adults. One-third of preschool-age obese children and 50% of older children will become obese adults. The risk of adult obesity is at least twice as high for obese children compared with nonobese children.

Efficacy of family therapy

Behavioural therapy seems to be effective in arresting this process in some children. A randomized controlled study of the effects of 1 year's family therapy for obese children matched with two groups, one of which received dietary and exercise counselling alone, and another in which patients were simply weighed, showed that the increase in BMI was significantly less in the family therapy group compared with the conventionally treated or control groups. Moreover, fewer children in the family therapy group had a BMI greater than 30 kg m^{-2} at 1 year.

A review of treatment outcomes in four randomized treatment studies demonstrates that after 10 years, one-third of the treated children had decreased their degree of overweight by 20% or more, and 30% were no longer obese. Significantly greater benefits are observed when both parents and children are targeted and when exercise is included in the treatment regimen. A limitation of this type of approach is that it is time-consuming and consequently expensive.

Exercise and Physical Activity

Exercise produces fat loss in obese and normal-weight subjects, although losses rarely exceed 5% of body weight. The weight loss through exercise, although generally small, exceeds that predicted if direct energy expenditure calculations are performed. It is likely that exercise has complex effects on the body which are not fully explained by energy expenditure. It has been proposed that the two processes most likely to be affected by exercise are appetite and basal metabolism.

The effect of physical activity on appetite is far from clear. It is agreed that appetite is diminished immediately after vigorous exercise but the longer-term effects and the effects of moderate exercise on appetite are unknown. Exercise increases the resting metabolic rate (RMR) while calorie restriction, particularly sudden restriction, causes a reduction in RMR. Exercise may oppose the effect of reduced calorie intake on RMR. There may be other beneficial effects of exercise that are independent of its effect on body weight. Regular exercise reduces blood pressure and improves insulin sensitivity, both in association with or independently of weight loss. A reduction in triacylglycerols and low-density lipoprotein cholesterol and elevation of high-density lipoprotein cholesterol have also been reported with exercise and physical training in obese patients. However, persuading an obese person to take part in exercise programmes and to maintain exercise as part of daily routine is not easy. It is not necessary to increase maximal oxygen uptake in the obese to derive benefit from exercise: metabolic evidence of fitness is achieved with less vigorous exercise. The risks from exercise are not great providing it is introduced gradually and other complications such as osteoarthritis and ischaemic heart disease are taken into account.

Efficacy of exercise as therapy

The evidence that exercise alone is of benefit is lacking; any weight loss is modest. A review of 55 studies indicates that, on average, only 1.16% of body fat was lost. By contrast, other studies suggest exercise may lead to around 0.105 kg per week weight loss, depending on the degree of obesity.

Exercise and weight maintenance

A study of moderately overweight men eating hypocaloric diets, with and without an exercise programme, revealed no statistical difference in the amount of weight lost by those in the exercise or diet alone groups. Differences were observed in the type of weight loss, with the nonexercise group showing a striking reduction in lean body mass while the exercise group preserved their lean tissue and lost more body fat. Follow-up at 6 and 18 months after completion of the trial showed that many of the exercisers had maintained this weight loss whereas those in the nonexercise group had regained 92% of the lost weight by 18 months. Another study of patients 3 years after completing a multidisciplinary weight loss programme found that those performing $2\frac{1}{2}$ h aerobic exercise per week had regained 49% of the original weight lost compared with a 75% regain in the nonexercisers.

Pharmacotherapy

The complexity of obesity requires that any pharmacological agent will need to increase energy output or decrease energy intake whilst being safe and non-addictive. Currently available therapeutic agents are centrally acting (e.g. appetite suppressants), peripherally acting (e.g. thermogenic agents), or those which act on the gastrointestinal tract (e.g. bulk agents, cimetidine or pancreatic lipase inhibitors).

Indications for use of pharmacotherapy

Pharmacotherapy must be regarded as an adjunct, and not an alternative, to dietary treatment. Many physicians reserve the use of antiobesity drugs for those with severe obesity (BMI > 35 kg m^{-2}), or for those with one or more medical or metabolic consequences (e.g. hypertension, hyperglycaemia, severe hyperlipidaemia or obstructive sleep apnoea). However, they may also be indicated for patients with a BMI between 28 and 34 kg m^{-2} with upper body obesity and patients with strong family history of early death from coronary heart disease.

Centrally acting drugs

Appetite suppressants are the agents which are most widely used. The action of these drugs fall into four categories:

- those acting via catecholamine pathways;
- those acting via serotoninergic (5HT) pathways;
- a combination of catecholamine and serotoninergic actions;
- other agents, e.g. opiate receptor blockers (naloxone), serotonin precursors (trytophan) and amino acids.

The first substance shown to have an anorexic effect was dexamphetamine, which acts by releasing the catecholamine neurotransmitters noradrenaline and dopamine from presynaptic neurons. Dexamphetamine-induced anorexia is mediated via noradrenergic pathways while euphoriant and stimulant activities are mediated via dopaminergic pathways. Dexamphetamine cannot be regarded as a treatment for obesity given the potential for abuse resulting from its euphoriant activity. Fenfluramine, which is a phenylethylamine derivative chemically similar to amphetamine but with a different clinical profile, was introduced in the early 1970s. This substance does not cause catecholamine release but acts along serotoninergic pathways. It consequently produces neither stimulant nor euphoric symptoms. Fenfluramine is a racemic mixture of dextro- and laevorotatory stereoisomers. Dexfenfluramine, which is the serotoninergic d isomer, was isolated from racemic fenfluramine. Dexfenfluramine has little effect on the dopaminergic system but increases presynaptic output of serotonin and decreases postsynaptic uptake of this neurotransmitter. This not only reduces unwanted side effects, but also increases the anorexic activity of the drug to twice that of the racemic mixture, thereby allowing the dose to be half that of the racemic mixture.[1]

Efficacy of centrally acting drugs Studies of 3 month's duration comparing dietary restriction combined with placebo or dexfenfluramine confirm that most subjects lose weight on active treatment. An open multicentre study in Italy showed that 32% of patients treated with dexfenfluramine lost between 0 and 5% of their initial body weight while 44% lost between 5 and 10%. A 1 year, placebo-controlled, multicentre, European trial of dexfenfluramine in 800 obese patients found that patients receiving

---

[1] The US manufacturer of dexfenfluramine recently withdrew the drug from the market following reports of cardiac valve disease in users.

either dexfenfluramine or placebo experienced significant weight loss during the first 6 months. However, in the group receiving active treatment, weight reduction was maintained during the second 6 months while weight was usually regained in patients receiving placebo. If a 10% weight loss is taken as an end point at 1 year, twice as many patients taking dexfenfluramine achieved this compared with those taking placebo. Overall, 36% patients treated with dexfenfluramine achieved a weight loss in excess of 10% of their initial weight at 4 months and 30% of these maintained this at 12 months. The percentage of placebo group maintaining this at 12 months was 2%. An evaluation of the time course of weight loss revealed that this had stabilized at 6 months, suggesting a role for dexfenfluramine in weight maintenance.

Other serotoninergic drugs include fluoxetine and sertraline.

Combined noradrenergic and serotoninergic agents

Sibutramine is a combined serotonin and noradrenergic re-uptake inhibitor which is currently under investigation. It appears to exert a centrally mediated decrease in appetite (via noradrenergic and 5HT receptors) and a peripheral catecholamine-induced increase in resting metabolic rate. Preliminary studies suggest sibutramine to be at least as effective as dexfenfluramine in inducing weight loss. This drug has recently been granted a license in the USA.

Peripherally acting compounds

Thermogenic agents Several drugs cause a transient increase in metabolic rate. The most effective are thyroid hormones, but toxicity is common at the dosage required to achieve significant weight loss. Furthermore, lean tissue rather than fat tissue tends to be lost. Thyroxine is only indicated for use in obesity where a patient requires thyroid replacement treatment as a consequence of biochemically proven hypothyroidism.

Compounds with β_2 agonist properties have been shown to increase the basal metabolic rate by 10% at rest. Recent Danish studies have demonstrated a synergy between ephedrine and caffeine with significant weight loss being achieved in obese subjects taking a combination of the two drugs compared with patients taking a placebo. Neither drug is licensed for the treatment of obesity in the UK. Novel atypical β-adrenoreceptor agonists have been developed which increase metabolic rate in obese rodents and cause weight reduction by decreasing body lipid content. These compounds appear to act on a β-receptor (β_3) which is independent of β_1- and β_2-receptors and selectively induce thermogenesis. Preliminary

studies of one such agent (BRL 26830A) confirmed it to be effective in inducing weight loss but unacceptable side effects have halted development. One of the many disadvantages of obesity is a decrease in exercise tolerance: at rest, an obese individual has a lower cardiac reserve than a normal-weight person. Any drug which further increases resting metabolism in an obese person might further decrease this reserve, which will negate any potential benefits.

Tetrahydrolipstatin Tetrahydrolipstatin (THL), which is a chemically synthesized derivative of lipstatin, a substance produced by *Streptomyces toxytricini*, is a potent inhibitor of gastric, pancreatic and carboxylester lipase. Pancreatic lipase splits free fatty acids from the glycerol backbone and is the main enzyme responsible for the digestion of dietary triacylglycerols. Selective inhibition of pancreatic lipase leads to decreased absorption of cholesterol and triacylglycerol. Initial trials with THL have demonstrated moderate, but significant, weight loss compared with patients receiving placebo. Theoretically, inhibition of absorption of nutrients from the small intestine is a sound principle in weight reduction and THL could be seen as a useful adjunct to more conventional forms of therapy. Preliminary results from a 1 year multicentre study confirm its effectiveness in reducing weight and weight maintenance. Adverse effects experienced by some patients include loose stools, steatorrhoea, oily spotting of underwear and abdominal pain. Other possible adverse consequences of longer-term use include reduced absorption of fat-soluble vitamins (A, D and E).

Other compounds Opiate antagonists, amino acids, bulk-forming agents and human chorionic gonadotrophin do not have a role to play in the treatment of obesity. A preliminary report suggesting cimetidine to be efficacious as treatment for obesity has not been confirmed by subsequent studies.

Surgical Treatment for Obesity

At least 30 surgical techniques have been developed for the treatment of obesity. These methods can be categorized on the basis of their mode of action.

- Mechanical – removal of adipose tissue, restriction of intake.
- Malabsorptive – surgical bypass of portions of the gastrointestinal tract.

Superficial cosmetic removal of excess adipose tissue, which includes liposuction, will not be considered because it has no lasting benefit.

Internal mandibulo–maxillary fixation (dental splintage)

The rationale behind dental splintage is that the construction of a barrier will make it more difficult for patients to consume large quantities of food. The long-term results (> 12 months) from such treatment are disappointing with most patients experiencing a rapid regain of weight once the splints are removed, despite close supervision, behavioural treatment and the application of a waist cord. As a result, this form of treatment has been abandoned by most centres.

Gastric restriction techniques

Gastroplasty techniques involve the fashioning of a proximal pouch of the stomach by vertical stapling, thereby restricting the gastric volume to approximately 15 ml. The opening of the pouch may be reinforced externally by a nylon mesh, fascia or teflon. Gastric banding involves the external 'pinching off' of the upper part of the stomach with a band, usually made of dacron.

Malabsorption techniques

Intestinal bypass operations in the form of jejuno-ileostomy, with either end-to-end or end-to-side anastomoses, have now largely been abandoned for the treatment of obesity owing to long-term side effects. However, gastric bypass combined with a gastroplasty has gained popularity and is the most commonly employed surgical procedure in many centres. The procedure involves fashioning a pouch of up to 30 ml volume by stapling across the stomach and bringing up a limb of small intestine as a conduit for food, thus bypassing the distal stomach, duodenum and proximal jejunum.

Indications for surgical treatment of obesity

It is important that patients are carefully selected for surgical treatment with the following criteria being taken into account:

- those with BMI > 40 kg m^{-2};
- those with metabolic complications of obesity;
- those who have shown repeated failure to control weight with either diet or behavioural therapy;
- those who have no evidence of psychiatric disease or maladaptive eating behaviours.

Efficacy of surgical treatments for obesity

Weight loss Both types of surgery (gastroplasty and gastric bypass) successfully reduce weight (**Table 4**). Substantial weight loss generally occurs during the first 18 months postoperatively followed by a nadir in the weight. Some degree of weight regain is common by 2–5 years after operation.

Psychosocial effects Many patients report improvement in mood and other aspects of psychosocial functioning following such operative procedures. The degree to which this is sustained is unknown.

Risks of surgery

An assessment of the risks involved in the surgical treatment of obesity includes the evaluation of both perioperative and long-term complications. Published series report that the immediate operative mortality rate for both vertical banded gastroplasty and gastric bypass is low. On the other hand, morbidity in the early postoperative period may be as high as 10%. In the later postoperative period other problems may arise which require re-operation. In the long term micronutrient deficiencies, particularly of vitamin B_{12}, folate and iron, are common after gastric bypass and require continuous monitoring.

Professionals Involved

Published evidence confirms that patients do better, whatever the treatment, when seen more frequently and for a greater length of time. Moreover, strategies which involve expertise incorporating dietetic, behavioural and exercise experts as well as

Table 4 Mean weight loss achieved with gastric restriction and malabsorption techniques

Date of study	No. of patients	Technique	Mean weight loss
1986	1463	SRG	37% of preoperative weight at 5 years
1987	307	Gastric bypass	28% of preoperative weight over 12- to 84-month period
1989	139	VBG	27% of preoperative weight at 6 years
1995	1000	SRG and ASGB	30% of preoperative weight at 5 years
1995	1150	Gastric bypass and VBG	25–33% of preoperative weight

Abbreviations: SRG, silastic ring; VBG, vertical banding gastroplasty; ASGB, adjustable stoma silicone gastric banding.

Table 5 Relative success rates for various treatment strategies for obesity

Treatment	Success	Maintenance	Limitations	Conclusions
Dietary	Variable depending on diet used; VLCD can achieve up to 3 kg per week initially	Generally poor with most trials showing almost complete weight regain within a 1–5 year period	VLCD potentially dangerous if used unsupervised and for the longer-term. Concern about the detrimental effects of 'weight cycling'. Can prove expensive. Of limited use for severely overweight	Must be considered the basis for all forms of obesity treatment. Easy to implement. Weight regain very common
Commercial slimming organizations	Very variable loss between 0 and 11 kg per patient	Moderate with mean weight regain of 30% at 2 years		
Behaviour modification	About 0.5 kg per week	Weight loss maintained to a greater extent than any other nonsurgical treatment	Limited weight loss when used alone. Better results if longer-term contact with therapist and combined with exercise	Best therapy (other than surgery) for maintaining weight loss
Exercise	Variable weight loss depending on type of exercise: 10–18 kg per year	Good if exercise is maintained	Time-consuming – very fat may be reluctant to participate. Amount of exercise disproportionate to actual weight loss	Of undoubted benefit to overall health and most beneficial when used in combination with other strategies. Appears particularly effective for overweight children
Drugs	10 kg per 6 months in INDEX study of dexfenfluramine[1]	30% of patients lose 10% or greater of initial body weight and maintain this on treatment for 12 months	Side effects may limit use. Dexfenfluramine licensed currently for 12-week course only. Potential adverse effects of drug treatment for long-term prescribing (>12 months) uncertain	Possibly the most effective strategy for inducing and maintaining weight loss other than surgery. Concerns remain about long-term treatment and its cost
Surgery Dental splintage	Good short-term loss (>25 kg)	Almost 100% of patients regain within 12 months of removal	Expensive. Does not appear to modify eating habits for longer-term even if combined with behaviour therapy	Low success rate for longer-term makes it difficult to justify as treatment
Surgical procedures – gastroplasty/gastric bypass	Most patients lose >30% of preoperative weight	Good in about 40% of patients (dependent on type of operation)	Expensive. Operative risk significant if severely overweight. Possible longer-term adverse effects uncertain – probably patients require life-long follow-up	Probably most effective treatment for obesity. However, patients must be carefully selected – probably limit to those with BMI >40 or those between 35 and 40 at high risk from comorbid conditions

[1]Recently withdrawn from the market by US manufacturer. See footnote on p. 1450.

physicians and surgeons are also more successful in sustaining weight loss. This underlines the importance of a multidisciplinary approach. Strategies for weight control need to be well publicized and include opportunistic screening of both individuals and their families – treatment of obese children must be in the context of the whole family. Treatment programmes must include a system of regular audit and the provision for change as a result of the findings.

Evaluation of Efficacy and Effectiveness of Treatment Programmes for Obesity

Limited estimates of the cost-effectiveness of treatment programmes have been published. These depend entirely on predicted rather than real costs and speculate on the development and cost of related complications. Beneficial factors for the short term will include improved quality of life, reduced sick leave, fewer days off work due to disability, reduced number of visits to doctors or other health care professionals, and fewer days in hospital. For the longer term, beneficial factors are reduced mortality (from all causes) and improved control (or reversal) of associated diseases such as hypertension and diabetes.

Data on the long-term consequences of weight loss on health are presently scanty. A review of the evidence for reduced mortality rates in persons who have lost weight is inconclusive owing to methodological problems. However, the initial findings from a Swedish study, which is assessing the longer-term benefits from obesity surgery (SOS), confirm that substantial weight loss (approximately 30 kg) is associated at 2 years with 60% reduction in plasma insulin, 25% decrease in glucose and trcacylglycerols and a 10% reduction in blood pressure. Furthermore, this degree of weight loss result in a 14-fold reduction in risk of developing diabetes and a 3- to 4-fold risk reduction for the development of hypertension, hypertriglyceridaemia and low HDL cholesterol levels. These preliminary findings suggest that considerable financial savings are possible from effective measures for weight loss and subsequent weight maintenance. A summary of the success rates of curent treatment options is given in **Table 5**.

See also: **Adolescents**: Nutritional Problems. **Appetite**: Physiological and Neurobiological Aspects; Psychobiological and Behavioural Aspects. **Carbohydrates**: Requirements and Dietary Importance. **Children**: Nutritional Problems of Preschool Children; Nutritional Problems of School Children. **Coronary Heart Disease**: Prevention. **Diabetes Mellitus**: Dietary Management. **Drugs**: Drug-Nutrient Interactions. **Energy**: Energy Balance. **Exercise**: Diet and Exercise; Beneficial Effects. **Hunger**: Overview. **Hyperlipidaemia (Hyperlipidemia)**: Overview. **Insulin Resistance**: Aetiology and Association with Disease. **Meal Size and Frequency**: Effect on Absorption and Metabolism. **Nutrition Education**: Health Professionals. **Obesity**: Definition, Aetiology and Assessment; Early Obesity and Prognosis; Fat Distribution; Prevention; Complications of Obesity. **Protein**: Requirements and Role in Diet. **Smoking**: Effects on Diet and Nutritional Status. **Sucrose**: Dietary Sucrose and Disease. **Weight Management**: Approaches; Weight Maintenance; Weight Cycling.

Further Reading

Bjorntorp P and Brodoff BM (eds) (19XX) *Obesity.* New York: JB Lippincott.

Blackburn GL and Saunders BS (eds) (1994) *Obesity, Pathophysiology, Psychology and Treatment.* New York: Chapman and Hall.

Bray GA, Bouchard C and James WPT (eds) (1988) *Handbook of Obesity.* New York: Marcel Dekker.

Finer N (ed.) (1997) *British Medical Bulletin: Obesity,* Vol. 53, No. 2.

Garrow JS (1988) *Obesity and Related Diseases.* New York: Churchill Livingstone.

Guy-Grand B, Apfelbaum M, Crepaldi G *et al* (1989) International trial of long term dexfenfluramine in obesity. *Lancet* 2:1142–1145.

NIH Consensus Development Conference Draft Statement on Gastrointestinal Surgery For Severe Obesity (1991) *Obesity Surgery* 1:257–265.

Sjostrom L, Narbro K and Sjostrom D (1995) Cost and benefits when treating obesity. *International Journal of Obesity* 19:S9–S12.

Prevention

Samuel Chan and **George L Blackburn**, Center for the Study of Nutrition Medicine, Harvard Medical School, Boston, Massachusetts, USA

Obesity is a complex, refractory disease of multifactorial origins, strongly influenced by the interplay between genetic, environmental, social and cultural variables. In current medical practice, the most promising role for prevention appears to lie in primary prevention, i.e. in changing the personal health behaviours of patients long before clinical disease develops.

Risk Factors for Adult Obesity

Obesity is the result of interactions among dozens of factors from the social, behavioural, environmental, physiological, metabolic, cellular and molecular domains. Its consequence is an energy imbalance that results when the intake of energy-dense food exceeds energy output. Many variables have the potential to create this positive energy balance over long periods of time, including a high-fat diet and a low thermogenesis and resting metabolic rate for a certain body mass. A variety of risk factors for adult obesity have been identified.

Body mass index (BMI) ≥ 27

BMI, which takes height and weight into account, is found by dividing a person's weight in kilograms by the square of the height in metres. The upper 15th percentile, i.e. a BMI of more than 27.8 for a man or more than 27.3 for a woman, is considered overweight. A BMI in the range 20 to 25 is considered normal weight. A BMI of greater than 25 but less than 27 is described as overweight. The degree of obesity ranges from mild obesity at a BMI near 27, moderate obesity at 30, severe obesity at 35, to very severe or morbid obesity at 40 or greater (see **Table 1**). Estimates of excess body fat can be made by calculating differences from ideal body weight, measuring skinfold thickness, or performing bioelectric impedance analysis (BIA).

Table 1 Classification of obesity

Grade	BMI (kg m^{-2})	Classfication	% IBW (males)	% IBW (females)
0	20–25	No obesity	100	100
I	25–30	Overweight	110	120
II	30–35	Obesity	135	145
III	35–40	Medically significant obesity	160	170
IV	40–45	Severe obesity	180	195
V	45–50	Super obesity	200	220
VI	>50	Supermorbid obesity	225	245

Adapted, with permission, from Kanders BS, Forse RA and Blackburn GL (1991) Methods of obesity. In: Rakel RE (ed.) *Conn's Current Therapy*, pp 524–531, Philadelphia: WB Saunders.
BMI, body mass index; IBW, ideal body weight.

Visceral body fat

Fat that collects above the waist rather than around the hips or buttocks, i.e. upper body weight, is associated with increased health risks. For the same degree of obesity (BMI), the presence of visceral body fat signals a need for early intervention. Independent of BMI, a waist measurement of 100 cm or more in a man, or 90 cm or more in a woman, indicates a heightened risk of hypertension, heart disease, diabetes and other obesity-related conditions. A waist-to-hip ratio (circumference of the waist divided by circumference of the hips) greater than 1.0 in men, or greater than 0.8 in women, can also be a biomarker of obesity risk.

Sedentary lifestyle

Technological advances, including the development of television, have led to a marked reduction in the amount of human energy expended in earning a living, completing personal chores or engaging in other aspects of daily life. Data indicate a prevalence of obesity more than four times greater among individuals who watch 21 or more hours of television per week compared with those who watch less than 7 h. Data also show that in the US, more than 60% of adults in each state fail to achieve a recommended 30 min of daily physical activity, and in half the states at least 73% of adults are insufficiently active.

Personal and family history

Family history may provide information to alert parents, schools and health-care providers to monitor excess body weight per height in childhood. According to twin, adoptee and large cohort studies of nuclear families, similarities in fat, fat-free mass and fat distribution increase with the degree of genetic similarity. Evidence also indicates that the risk of obesity in adulthood is influenced by both childhood and parental obesity.

Gene–environment interactions Recent genomic discoveries link more than 20 candidate genes to the aetiology of obesity; in and of themselves, however, none appear to be a major cause of human obesity (i.e. pathogenesis requires interaction between environmental and genetic factors). Twin studies suggest that genetics can account for between 40% and 80% of variance in BMI or skinfold thickness. Similarly, there is a strong association between the BMIs of adoptees and their biological parents. Human obesity and its comorbidities are the results of multiple autosomal recessive genes. The major effect is most likely related to impaired thermogenesis and muscle energy expenditure.

Childhood obesity Children at risk for obesity, or in the process of developing it, are a high-priority target for intervention. Early onset of obesity, together with parental obesity, is responsible for a disproportionate share of adult cases; the risk is 40% with one obese parent, 80% with two. Some 51% of obese children with obese parents suffer from adult obesity compared with 20% of obese children with normal weight parents. Other risk factors include lower socioeconomic status and time spent watching television. Given that the relative risk of obesity rises with the obese child's age, careful attention to excess rates of weight gain in the offspring of obese parents will help identify those for whom early alterations in diet or activity should be promoted.

Environmental factors

Environmental factors include an overabundance of high-energy, dense, processed food choices; decreased opportunities and motivation for physical activity; and restaurant portions that far exceed recommended serving sizes. For example, the US Department of Agriculture standard serving for meat is 60–80 g (2–3 oz), but many cookery book and restaurant portions start at 200 g (7 oz) and go as high as 1000 g (38 oz) for one person.

Psychological variables

Depression and other psychological factors may influence eating habits. Many people also eat in response to negative emotions such as boredom, sadness or anger. Among those who seek treatment for serious weight problems, about 30% either have difficulties with binge eating, or suffer from binge eating disorder. Obesity is an infrequent antecedent or cause of depression.

Others

Secondary causes of obesity are rare. Hyperthyroidism and Cushing's syndrome may lead to excessive weight gain or obesity, as may drug treatment involving corticosteroids and some antidepressants. Such factors, however, account for only an estimated 1% of all obesity cases.

Prevention Strategies

Strategies for preventing obesity and its comorbidities focus on controllable risk factors, i.e. diet and activity levels. Data show that regular physical activity, combined with healthy eating habits, is the most efficient and healthy way to control weight. Preventive service guidelines include periodic diet and exercise assessment and counselling.

Physical activity

Physical activity maintains health and reduces risk for heart disease, colon cancer, diabetes and high blood pressure. The relationship between health and physical fitness can be used to motivate compliance to exercise guidelines of 30 min on most, if not all, days. Physical activity also helps to control weight, contributes to the development and maintenance of healthy bones, muscles and joints, and reduces symptoms of anxiety and depression. Conversely, habitually low levels of physical activity and physical fitness are associated with a marked increase in all-cause mortality.

Studies show that weight is regulated by the balance between daily energy intake and expenditure. Physical activity helps control weight by using excess energy that would otherwise be stored as fat. It also helps reduce body fat by building or preserving muscle mass, and improving the body's ability to use energy.

Physical activity need not be strenuous to achieve health benefits, but it must be regular. Many of the gains from endurance and resistance exercise diminish within 2 weeks if physical activity is substantially reduced, and disappear within 2–8 months if physical activity is not resumed. Thus, when a lapse occurs, it is important to resume the exercise routines as soon as possible.

The 1997 studies carried out in the United States have drawn the following conclusions.

1. People of all ages, male and female, receive substantial health benefits from moderate intensity physical activity; for example 30 min of brisk walking at 5–6 km h^{-1} (3–4 mph).
2. For most people, a modest increase in daily activity – an expenditure of (150–200 cal) per day – can improve both health and quality of life.
3. Additional benefits can be gained by increasing the duration or intensity of activity.
4. Benefits can be achieved through intermittent bouts of activity, as short as 8–10 min, with a total of 30 min or more on most days.

For adults, the addition of strength-developing exercises two or more times per week can improve musculoskeletal health, reducing the risk of falls and helping to maintain independence in performing the activities of daily life.

Research on physical activity continues to evolve, with growing interest in finding ways to differentiate the characteristics of physical activity that improve health; likewise efforts are being made to determine how the interrelated characteristics of amount, intensity, duration, frequency, type and pattern of physical activity are related to specific health or disease outcomes. Studies on the health effects of moderate versus high-intensity activity and intermittent versus continuous activity are also needed.

Determinants of activity

Research on understanding and promoting physical activity is at an early stage, and more studies are needed to determine the most effective ways to motivate a majority of the population to participate in a level of physical activity that can benefit health and wellbeing. Some successful interventions, however, have been evaluated.

School-based programmes are particularly promising. Data show that physical activity sharply declines during adolescence. Childhood and adolescence may thus be pivotal times for preventing sedentary behaviour among adults by maintaining the habit of physical activity throughout the school years. Interventions targeting physical education in primary schools have led to substantial increases in activity levels during physical education classes, prompting calls for compulsory daily physical education throughout the school years and greater promotion of activities that can be enjoyed throughout life.

Communities can facilitate increased physical activity by providing environmental inducements, such as pavements with curb cuts, and safe, accessible and attractive trails for walking and bicycling. They can also open schools for community recreation; form neighbourhood watch groups to enhance safety; encourage malls and other indoor/protected places to provide safe places for walking; ask employers to offer opportunities for employees to incorporate moderate physical activity into their daily lives; and provide child-care arrangements and community-based programmes that meet the needs of racial and ethnic minorities, and older, disabled and low-income women.

Among young people and adults, consistent influences on physical activity patterns include confidence in one's ability to engage in regular physical activity (i.e. self-sufficiency), enjoyment of physical activity, support from others, positive beliefs concerning the benefits of physical activity, and a lack of perceived barriers.

Physicians can also help induce behaviour change in patients through the use of certain principles/strategies. These include: developing a therapeutic alliance; counselling all patients; ensuring that patients understand the relationship between behaviour and health; working with them to assess barriers to behaviour change; involving patients in the choice of which risk factor(s) to tackle first; designing a behaviour modification plan; monitoring progress through follow-up contact; and serving as a role model. Most physicians rely on a combination of strategies, including individual counselling, group classes, audiovisual aids and community resources. They also involve members of their office staff.

Dietary guidelines

Nutritional habits are linked to some of the same aspects of health as physical activity; they may even be related lifestyle characteristics. The 1995 Dietary Guidelines for Americans, the basis for all US government nutrition-related programmes, called for 30 min or more of daily, moderate-intensity physical exercise to maintain or improve weight. The latest guidelines also ranked a recommended diet high in whole grains, fruits and vegetables ahead of one that is low in fat, saturated fat and cholesterol, and stressed the importance of lifetime weight maintenance.

Adults who are at a healthy weight, have gained less than 4.5 kg (10 lb) since reaching full height, and are otherwise healthy, are advised to maintain body weight by balancing energy consumed with physical activity. Prevention of weight gain in children is addressed through education, i.e. restricting food choices to healthy foods only (grain products; vegetables and fruits; low-fat milk products or other calcium-rich foods; beans, lean meat, poultry, fish or other protein-rich foods); limiting television time; and encouraging participation in vigorous physical activity. The food guide pyramid, **Fig. 1**, shows the types and amounts of foods most Americans need for a healthy diet, while **Table 2** lists the amounts of the various foods in one serving.

The food supply

Food suppliers and manufacturers are being encouraged to reduce the availability of high-density, high-energy snacks and foods, and to increase the availability of good-tasting, nutrient-rich, low-energy products. Other prevention strategies include reducing the number of high-energy food advertisements targeted at children and limiting the distribution of high-density foods, especially in schools.

Public policy

Individuals in the US and other developed nations are exposed to a toxic food environment that provides access to, and relentlessly encourages consumption of, a high-fat high-senergy diet. Legislation and regulation aimed at the price structure of foods, opportunities and incentives for physical activity, and control of exposure to messages that promote unhealthy eating might have a considerable impact on public health.

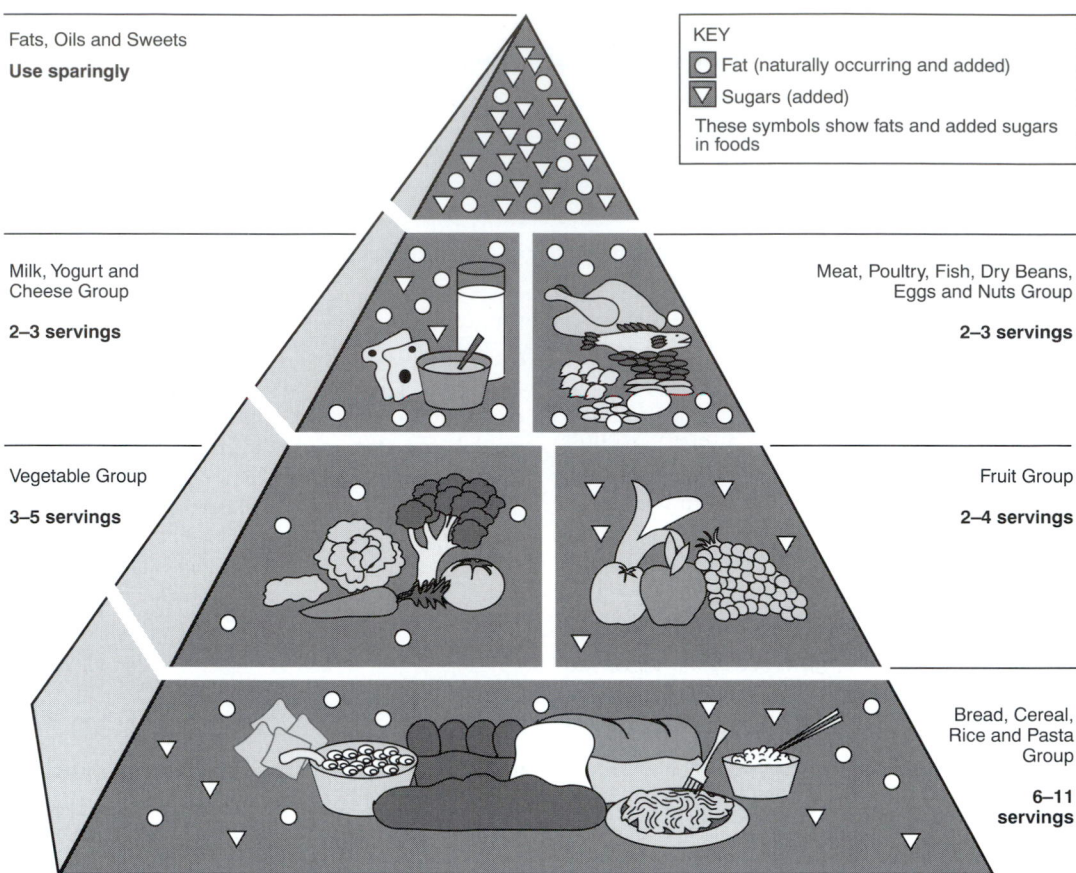

Figure 1 Food guide pyramid – a guide to daily food choices. From US Department of Agriculture/US Department of Health and Human Services.

Strategic changes, designed to encourage the intake of healthy foods and decrease the consumption of unhealthy foods, could include: (1) subsidies for healthy foods to lower prices and increase per capita consumption; (2) taxes on unhealthy foods to raise prices and decrease per capita consumption; and (3) regulation of advertising for sweets, soft drinks, fast foods and sugared cereals aimed at children.

Goals of Prevention

The goals of obesity prevention, like those of treatment, are shifting from a single focus on body weight to a broader, health management perspective. This is defined as the adoption of healthy and sustainable eating and exercise behaviours that can be followed every day. Improved feelings of energy and wellbeing are the priorities.

Studies indicate that all weight management/obesity prevention programmes should include at least the following goals:

1. a healthy eating style, with increased intake of whole grains, fruits, and vegetables;
2. a nonrestrictive approach to eating based on internal regulation of hunger and satiety; and
3. a least 30 min a day of enjoyable physical activity.

Conclusions

Prevention of obesity is an appealing concept given the prevalence, growth rate, treatment resistance, morbidity, disability and early mortality of the disease. Nevertheless, prevention has attracted far fewer resources than treatment, leaving the field with an unfortunate lack of information on, or commitment to, public health approaches. Prevention programmes for obesity, now at the earliest stages of development, have yet to develop adequate conceptual models, identify the most likely intervention targets, or even confirm that the prevention of obesity is possible in the current environment.

The pandemic of obesity is a problem of major public health significance. Despite growing

Table 2 What counts as one serving?

Food group	Amount in 1 serving[a]
Breads, cereals, rice, pasta	1 slice of bread ½ cup of cooked rice or pasta ½ cup of cooked cereal 1 oz of ready-to-eat cereal
Milk, yogurt and cheese	1 cup of milk or yogurt 1½–2 oz of cheese
Meat, poultry, fish, dry beans, eggs and nuts	2½–3 oz of cooked lean meat, poultry, or fish Count ½ cup of cooked beans, or 1 egg, or 2 tablespoons of peanut butter as 1 oz of lean meat (about ⅓ of a serving)
Vegetables	½ cup of chopped raw or cooked vegetables 1 cup of leafy raw vegetables
Fruits	1 piece of fruit or melon wedge ¾ cup of juice ½ cup of canned fruit ¼ cup of dried fruit
Fats, oils and sweets	Limit energy from these (especially if you need to lose weight)

Source: US Department of Agriculture/US Department of Health and Human Services.
The amount you eat may be more than one serving. For example, a dinner portion of spaghetti would count as two or three servings of pasta.
[a]1 oz ~ 28 g; 1 cup ~ 240 ml; 1 tablespoon (tbsp) = 15 ml.

knowledge about the relationship between nutrition and exercise, prevailing treatments have done little to stem a sharp rise in incidence rates. A current shift from a medical to a public health model is focusing attention on prevention and public policy, prompting a call for a re-examination of the paradigms on which treatment and prevention programmes are based. Research on prevention is still in its infancy, and even less is known about the impact of potential policy changes. Environmental factors, however, appear to be driving the increase in obesity, and many believe that this critical knowledge must inform a wider public health approach to the problem.

See also: **Dietary Guidelines**: International Perspectives. **Exercise**: Diet and Exercise; Beneficial Effects. **Obesity**: Early Obesity and Prognosis.

Further Reading

American College of Sports Medicine (1991) *Guidelines for Exercise Testing and Prescription*, 4th edn. Philadelphia: Lea & Febiger.

Battle EK and Brownell KD (1996) Confronting a rising tide of eating disorders and obesity: treatment vs. prevention and policy. *Addictive Behaviors* 21(6):755–765.

Blackburn GL and Kanders BS (1994) *Obesity: Pathophysiology, Psychology and Treatment*. London: Chapman & Hall.

Centers for Disease Control (1992) *Project PACE: Physician's Manual. Physician-Based Assessment and Counseling for Exercise*. Atlanta: Centers for Disease Control.

Centers for Disease Control and Prevention and the American College of Sports Medicine (1995) Physical activity and public health. A recommendation from the Centers for Disease Control Prevention and the American College of Sports Medicine. *Journal of the American Medical Association* 273(5):402–407.

Foster GD, Wadden TA and Brownell KD (1985) Peer-led program for the treatment and prevention of obesity in the schools. *Journal of Consulting and Clinical Psychology* 53:538–540.

Institute of Medicine (1995) *Weighing the Options. Criteria for Evaluating Weight Management Programs*, p 139. Washington, DC: National Academy Press.

Jackson YM, Proulx JM and Pelican S (1991) Obesity prevention. *American Journal of Clinical Nutrition* 1625S–1630S.

National Institutes of Health (1985) *Health Implications of Obesity*. NIH Consens Statement Online. 1985. Feb 11–13 [cited 1998, Jan 13]; 5(9):1–7.

US Department of Agriculture and US. Department of Health and Human Services (1995) *Nutrition and Your Health: Dietary Guidelines for Americans*. Home and Garden Bulletin no 232. Washington, DC: Department of Health and Human Services.

US Department of Health and Human Services (1988) *The Surgeon General's Report on Nutrition and Health*. Publication no. DHHS (PHS) 88–50210. Washington, DC: US Government Printing Office.

US Department of Health and Human Services (1991) *Healthy People 2000: National Health Promotion and Disease Prevention Objectives*. DHHS publication PHS 91–50212. Washington, DC: US Government Printing Office.

US Department of Health and Human Services (1995) *Physical Activity and Health: A Report of the Surgeon General*. Washington, DC: US Government Printing Office.

Wolf, AM and Colditz, GA (1996) Social and economic effects of body weight in the United States. *American Journal of Clinical Nutrition* 63(supplement):466S–469S.

Complications of Obesity

Nikhil V Dhurandhar and **Richard L Atkinson**,
University of Wisconsin at Madison, Wisconsin, USA

Obesity is a serious chronic disease associated with numerous complications and comorbidities that involve most systems of the body. The common factor in all obese people is the presence of excess adipose tissue stores and an increased percentage of body fat. Even in the absence of complications and comorbidities, obesity increases the risk of early mortality. In association with complications such as hypertension, dyslipidaemia, sleep apnoea and the glucose intolerance–insulin resistance syndrome, the risk of early mortality may be markedly elevated. It has been estimated that there are 300,000 obesity-related excess deaths in the USA each year. In addition to the medical complications, obesity is associated with psychological and social problems that may overshadow the medical problems in the quality of life for many obese people. The complications of obesity are summarized in **Table 1**.

Role of Distribution of Body Fat in the Complications of Obesity

The distribution of excess adipose tissue contributes to the complications of obesity. Obese individuals may be divided into those whose excess fat is deposited in the upper body, and those with increased lower body obesity. Upper body obesity may be localized to the subcutaneous space versus the intraabdominal space (visceral fat). Waist circumference and the ratio of waist to hip circumferences correlate with the morbidity and mortality of obesity. Individuals with increased visceral fat, as measured by the cross-sectional area on computed tomography (CT) or magnetic resonance imaging (MRI), are at greater risk for systemic complications of obesity compared with people with fat localized to abdominal subcutaneous depots or to the lower body. The mechanisms of these differences are not clear, but research has shown that visceral fat has a higher triacylglycerol turnover rate and releases greater amounts of fatty acids into the circulation than do other adipose tissue depots. Since blood vessels from the visceral fat drain into the portal vein, some investigators postulate that exposure of the liver to high levels of free fatty acids produces insulin resistance, which is known to be correlated with many of the complications of obesity described below.

Leptin is another factor that may affect the metab-

Table 1 Complications of obesity

Metabolic complications
Non-insulin-dependent diabetes mellitus
Insulin resistance, hyperinsulinaemia
Dyslipidaemia
Gout
Abnormalities of growth hormone secretion

Diseases of organ systems
Atherosclerotic and arteriosclerotic vascular diseases
    Coronary heart disease
    Hypertension
    Congestive heart failure
    Cerebrovascular disease
Respiratory system abnormalities
    Obesity–hypoventilation syndrome
    Sleep apnoea
Reproductive system abnormalities
Nervous system
    Pseudotumour cerebri
    Adiposis dolorosa
Immune system dysfunction
Digestive system abnormalities
    Gall bladder disease
    Hepatic disease
Skin diseases
Cancers
    Breast
    Uterus
    Gall bladder
    Colon
    Prostate

Mechanical complications of obesity
Increased intraabdominal pressure
Arthritis

Surgical complications
Perioperative risks: anaesthesia, wound complications, infections
Incisional hernias

Psychosocial complications
Social stigma: job and career discrimination, marriageability
Poor self-esteem
Poor body image

olism of different fat depots. Leptin is the product of the *ob* gene and is made predominantly in adipose tissue. Leptin receptors are present in the hypothalamus and it was postulated that leptin is a signal from adipose tissue to the brain that regulated fat stores. Obese mice (*ob/ob*) have a defect in leptin production and obese-diabetic mice (*db/db*) and Zucker fatty rats have a defect in the leptin receptor. When injections of leptin are given to *ob/ob* mice, they decrease food intake and lose weight and adipose tissue. Leptin injections do not affect *db/db* mice nor Zucker fatty rats, as would be expected.

Because leptin injections reduced body weight, it

was surprising to learn that serum leptin levels correlate positively with body fat stores in both animals and humans. These data required revision of the hypothesis that leptin was a signal that regulated fat stores. It now appears that leptin plays a role in signalling, but may not be the prime factor regulating fat stores. The increasing serum leptin levels with increasing obesity appear similar to the situation of insulin with obesity. Thus, obesity may produce resistance to the action of leptin.

Leptin levels are higher in females than males, but this association does not appear to be due to oestrogen levels. Leptin is found in greater concentrations in abdominal subcutaneous fat than in visceral fat. The mechanisms for these differences are not known, but it is possible that they may play some role in the differential metabolic responses of subcutaneous and visceral fat.

Metabolic Complications of Obesity

Non-insulin-dependent diabetes mellitus (NIDDM)

A strong association of obesity with the prevalence of non-insulin-dependent diabetes mellitus (NIDDM) is well documented. The risk of developing NIDDM increases with the degree and duration of obesity, to as much as 20-fold with severe obesity. The US National Diabetes Commission reported that the risk of diabetes doubles for every 20% of excess body weight. The risk of NIDDM is greater with visceral obesity. Non-insulin-dependent diabetes mellitus is frequently associated with other complications such as hypertension and dyslipidaemia, thus increasing the risk for atherosclerosis and cardiovascular disease. Poor glycaemic control in NIDDM may lead to severe microvascular complications including nephropathy, retinopathy and neuropathy. Weight loss is a very effective treatment for NIDDM and can prevent the onset of NIDDM in susceptible individuals.

Insulin resistance and hyperinsulinaemia

Insulin resistance refers to the phenomenon of insensitivity of the cells of the body to insulin's actions. Different tissues may have different insulin sensitivities. For example, adipose tissue may be more sensitive to insulin than muscle tissue, thus favouring the deposition of fatty acids in adipose tissue and diminished fatty acid oxidation in muscle. Obesity is the most common reason for insulin resistance. Several investigators have described the 'insulin resistance syndrome', which includes obesity, NIDDM, hypertension, hyperinsulinaemia and dyslipidaemia. This syndrome is associated with marked increases in morbidity and mortality.

Insulin resistance is usually associated with hyperinsulinaemia. Hyperinsulinaemia is an independent marker to predict the development of atherosclerosis. A causal relationship between hypertension and hyperinsulinaemia has not yet been well established. Hypertension associated with hyperinsulinaemia could be due to increased renal sodium retention, increased intracellular free calcium, increased sympathetic nervous system activity, or increased intraabdominal pressure due to increased visceral fat deposition.

The mechanism of insulin resistance is not clearly understood. Basal insulin levels increase with the degree of overweight, perhaps due to increased insulin secretion and/or reduced clearance by the liver. A reduced receptor number and/or post-receptor defects may lead to insulin resistance. Both basal hyperinsulinaemia and insulin resistance decrease with weight reduction.

Dyslipidaemia

Obesity is associated with high serum cholesterol, triacylglycerol and very low-density lipoprotein (VLDL) concentrations, and reduced levels of high-density lipoprotein (HDL) cholesterol. Every 10% increase in relative body weight is associated with a 0.3 mmol l^{-1}(12 mg dl^{-1}) increase in cholesterol concentration. The correlation of serum cholesterol with body mass index (BMI) is greater for men than women. (The body mass index is calculated by dividing the weight in kg by the height in metres squared.) Increased concentrations of serum triacylglycerol with weight gain may be due to increased intake of fats or to impaired removal of triacylglycerols into tissues because of low levels of lipoprotein lipase activity. Insulin resistance promotes lipolysis and increased circulating free fatty acids, which enhance the formation of VLDL in the liver. Dyslipidaemia contributes to increased atherosclerosis in obesity. Weight reduction usually reduces levels of serum cholesterol and triacylglycerols, increases HDL cholesterol, and may reduce atherosclerosis.

Gout

Serum uric acid and the prevalence of gout correlate positively with BMI. High serum uric acid levels correlate with insulin resistance and an increased risk of atherosclerotic cardiovascular disease in obesity. Serum uric acid levels may temporarily increase with acute weight loss, but usually decrease with large amounts of weight loss. The lower uric acid levels are maintained with continued weight loss.

Abnormalities of growth hormone release

Growth hormone (GH) is released by the anterior pituitary gland and affects lipid, carbohydrate, and protein metabolism. It also controls the rate of skeletal and visceral growth. Growth hormone is lipolytic in adipose tissue. Animal studies show enhanced catecholamine-induced lipolysis and increased numbers of β-adrenoreceptors in adipocytes of GH-treated animals. In obese people GH release is impaired, and the rises in levels of GH after meals, with sleep and in response to secretagogues such as arginine or levodopa are blunted. The defective release of GH can be reversed by weight reduction.

Diseases of Organ Systems

Atherosclerotic and arteriosclerotic vascular diseases

Diseases of the vascular system make the greatest contribution to the increased mortality associated with obesity. In both sexes, the excess mortality due to vascular disease increases linearly with BMIs greater than 25. The vascular complications of obesity can be categorized into four major groups:

1. coronary heart disease;
2. hypertension;
3. congestive heart failure;
4. cerebrovascular disease.

Coronary heart disease   Longitudinal studies show a positive correlation of BMI with coronary heart disease (CHD), and obesity is an independent predictor of CHD. However, in the presence of other risk factors such as hypertension, high serum cholesterol and triacylglycerol levels, low serum HDL cholesterol levels and insulin resistance, all of which are increased by obesity, the risk of atherosclerotic CHD increases dramatically. Weight loss reduces all of these risk factors associated with cardiovascular disease, but because long-term reductions in body weight have been so difficult to achieve, there are few long-term studies of changes in cardiovascular mortality due to weight loss. A very low-fat diet (10% of total energy as fat) has been shown to reduce the size of atherosclerotic plaques in coronary arteries. Such low-fat diets almost invariably produce weight loss.

Hypertension   The prevalence of hypertension among overweight adults in the USA is 2.9 times higher than that in nonoverweight individuals. Every 10 kg increase in body weight is associated with an increase of 3 mmHg in systolic blood pressure and 2 mmHg in diastolic blood pressure. Persistent hypertension can contribute to the development of left ventricular hypertrophy, coronary ischaemia, and stroke.

The aetiology of the association between hypertension and obesity is unclear. Some of the mechanisms offered to explain the association of obesity and hypertension are:

- hyperinsulinaemia due to insulin resistance leading to increased renal reabsorption of sodium;
- sodium retention due to a decreased renal filtration rate, increased intraabdominal pressure and/or increased plasma renin activity;
- increased sympathetic nervous system activity.

Except in long-standing cases, weight reduction is usually accompanied by a decrease in blood pressure. The reductions in blood pressure with weight loss are not dependent on decreases in salt intake. Many studies have shown that even modest weight losses, in the range of 5–10% of initial body weight, may produce reductions or even normalization of blood pressure in obese individuals. Certainly some of the reductions in blood pressure are due to energy restriction, but a few studies have shown that blood pressure remains low with modest weight loss despite a return of energy intake towards baseline levels.

Congestive heart failure   Total blood volume increases with excess body weight. Higher oxygen consumption in obesity and increased blood flow to the splanchnic bed and adipose tissue increase cardiac output. Also, the transverse diameter of heart, thickness of the posterior wall, and thickness of the interventricular septum increase with body weight. Left ventricular mass is a stronger predictor of morbidity and mortality than blood pressure. A combination of these factors may result in the congestive heart failure seen in severely obese people. The heart rate, stroke volume, blood volume, cardiac output and left ventricular work return towards normal with weight reduction. One study that compared weight loss by dieting to treatment with antihypertensive drugs demonstrated a greater improvement in cardiac hypertrophy with weight loss, despite similar reductions in blood pressure.

Cerebrovascular disease   Obesity-related atherosclerosis and arteriosclerosis increase the risk of cerebrovascular disease and strokes. Obesity is an independent risk factor for strokes, even in the absence of other comorbidities.

Respiratory system

Obesity is associated with reduced lung volume, altered respiratory patterns, and an overall reduction in the compliance of the respiratory system including a diminished vital capacity and total lung capacity. More severe obesity is associated with the 'obesity–hypoventilation syndrome', which is characterized by excessive daytime sleepiness and hypoventilation. The increased work required to move the chest wall, a decrease in arterial oxygenation in the lungs and a diminished sensitivity of the respiratory centre to the stimulatory effect of carbon dioxide are postulated to contribute to the obesity–hypoventilation syndrome.

The obesity–hypoventilation syndrome may be associated with or exacerbated by obstructive sleep apnoea, which is characterized by repeated collapse of the upper airway and cessation of breathing with sleep. Obstructive sleep apnoea occurs when the tongue obstructs the glottis and prevents entry of air into the trachea. As many as 25% of all obese people have sleep apnoea. Weight reduction usually reduces the severity of sleep apnoea, and massive weight reduction – such as that after gastric bypass surgery – eliminates the disease in most patients.

Digestive system

Gall bladder disease The risk of gall bladder disease, particularly gallstone formation, is increased in obesity, and the disorder occurs with greater frequency in women. The prevalence of gall bladder disease in obese individuals increases with age, body weight and parity (in women). The aetiology of the increased gall bladder disease is not clear, but genetic factors play a role. Increased cholesterol production, which leads to increased excretion of cholesterol in bile, is known to occur in obesity and correlates with increases in body weight. Many obese people skip meals, particularly breakfast, and the reduced number of meals may result in less frequent emptying of the gall bladder. The resulting bile stasis may contribute to gallstone formation. Although long-term weight loss and maintenance may reduce the occurrence of gall bladder disease, the risk of gallstone formation actually increases during the active weight loss phase. The aetiology of this increase is thought to be the mobilization of cholesterol from adipose tissue during rapid weight loss. This increased load of cholesterol in the circulation produces supersaturation of the bile, leading to gall bladder sludge in about 25% of patients and to symptomatic disease in about 1–3%. Treatment with ursodeoxycholic acid reduces or eliminates the risk of gallstone formation during weight loss.

Hepatic disease Abnormalities in hepatic function are commonly reported in obese people. Fatty liver, due to increased concentrations of fatty acids, diacylglycerols and triacylglycerols in hepatocytes, is reported in obese people; the frequency of fatty liver has been reported to be as high as 68% to 94% in very obese subjects. A small number of very obese subjects will develop micronodular cirrhosis. Abnormal liver enzymes on laboratory screening are common in obese people and do not require further evaluation unless they are markedly elevated. Weight loss results in disappearance of the excess fat and normalization of the liver function tests.

Reproductive system

Hormonal complications in males Obese men have elevated levels of plasma oestrone and oestradiol that correlate with the degree of obesity. Plasma total testosterone and free testosterone (the biologically active moiety) are reduced in obese men, and the reductions correlate negatively with the degree of obesity. The reduced levels of free and total testosterone are not generally accompanied by hypogonadism or a decrease in libido, potency or sperm count in obese men. Free and total plasma testosterone levels normalize upon significant weight reduction. Also, oestrogen levels are normalized if the individuals attain normal weight, but not if the weight loss is modest and significant obesity persists.

Hormonal complications in females Obese women have normal levels of total plasma oestradiol and oestrone but reduced levels of sex hormone binding globulins (SHBG). Thus, free oestradiol (the biological active moiety) is significantly elevated. The high levels of free oestradiol are postulated to increase the risks of endometrial and breast cancer and to reduce fertility. Obesity in women is associated with the polycystic ovary (PCO) syndrome, characterized by hyperoestrogenism, hyperandrogenism, polycystic ovaries, oligomenorrhoea or amenorrhoea, hirsutism and infertility. Weight loss usually normalizes SHBG and oestradiol levels for individuals with simple obesity, but weight loss may not restore fertility to patients with severe PCO syndrome.

Obstetric complications Obesity increases the risk of complications during pregnancy and childbirth. Increased body weight, hypertension and fluid retention during pregnancy can lead to toxaemia of pregnancy. Heavier women have a longer duration of labour and a greater frequency of abnormal labour and caesarean sections.

Nervous system

Pseudotumour cerebri This syndrome is characterized by increased intracranial pressure, headaches, blurred vision or loss of vision, and papilloedema. It is most common in massively obese individuals and may be seen in association with sleep apnoea or with the obesity–hypoventilation syndrome. It may be associated with retinal haemorrhage or loss of vision from severe papilloedema. Some investigators believe that increased intraabdominal pressure with massive obesity is an aetiologic factor for pseudotumour cerebri. Major weight loss, particularly after obesity surgery, results in dramatic improvement.

Adiposis dolorosa This is a syndrome of unknown aetiology characterized by painful deposits of adipose tissue occurring over multiple areas of the body. Adiposis dolorosa occurs predominantly in postmenopausal women (female to male ratio of about 30 : 1) and is associated with weakness, fatigue and emotional disturbances. Obesity is present initially but patients may lose weight and become asthenic as the syndrome progresses. The painful areas of fat may occur as subcutaneous lumps, with a 'bag of worms' or a 'caked breast' feeling on physical examination, or may even be diffused in a localized or generalized pattern. Painful areas of fat have been described over all areas of the body but the knees are the most commonly involved site. The disease usually begins gradually with mild pain and tenderness of the area involved, but may progress to severe pain, particularly with movement. Burning, numbness, tingling or crawling sensations of the skin may be noted. Intravenous infusions of lignocaine (lidocaine) are reported to relieve pain from 2–12 months after each infusion. The mechanism involved in the relief of pain by this drug is uncertain.

Immune system

Animal studies have shown an increased rate of infection and mortality in obese dogs compared with lean animals experimentally infected with canine distemper virus. Cell-mediated immune response is impaired in obese individuals. Maturation of monocytes into macrophages after incubation *in vitro* is significantly less for obese compared with lean subjects. Impaired cell-mediated immune response in children was demonstrated to be due to subclinical deficiencies of zinc and copper. The impairment in the immune response was reversed after 4 weeks of zinc and copper supplements.

Skin

Obese people may have several disorders of the skin. The most common is stasis changes of the skin of the lower legs in massively obese people. The aetiology of this finding is venous stasis, oedema and breakdown of the skin.

Fragilitas cutis inguinalis This condition of fragile skin in the inguinal area of obese people is diagnosed by stretching the skin of the inguinal area. A linear tear appears at right angles to an applied force that is insufficient to tear the skin of a normal person. This condition is unrelated to the sex and age of the person.

Acanthosis nigricans Seen occasionally in obesity, acanthosis nigricans is characterized by darkening of the skin in the creases of the neck, axillary regions and over the knuckles. An association between acanthosis nigricans and insulin resistance is reported in persons who have circulating antibodies to the insulin receptors. Since acanthosis nigricans also may be associated with highly malignant cancers such as intraabdominal adenocarcinoma, physicians should be alert to this possibility and not attribute the condition simply to the presence of obesity.

Cancer

Obese women have significantly greater mortality rates for endometrial, cervical, ovarian, breast, uterine and gall bladder cancers. Obese men have significantly greater mortality ratios for colorectal and prostate cancer. Some investigators postulate that the increased risk of cancer in obesity may be due to the increased production of oestrogen in fat tissue. Promotion of tumour growth by this excess oestrogen also is thought to play a role in the poorer prognosis of breast cancer. Some investigators have questioned if obesity is a primary factor in the increased prevalence of cancer in obese people, or if life-style factors may play a role. For example, obese people tend to eat a higher-fat, lower-fibre diet than lean people. Dietary fat has been implicated as a potential independent risk factor for cancer, particularly colon cancer. Conversely, dietary fibre has been thought to protect against colon cancer. Finally, exercise has been shown to reduce the prevalence of cancer, and it is well known that obese people are less active than lean people. Much additional work needs to be done to elucidate the role of obesity in the production of cancer.

Mechanical Complications of Obesity

Arthritis

Increased body weight leads to trauma of the weight-bearing joints and speeds the development of osteoarthritis in obesity. Patients with osteoarthritis have a greater mean body weight than controls without this disease. Knee and hip joints are particularly affected. Flattening of the arc of the plantar surface of the feet (flat feet) may be congenital or acquired, but flat feet occur more frequently in obese people, presumably due to the stress of carrying excess body weight. Flat feet may lead to unsteady gait and aches and pains after walking. Increased fat deposition particularly in the abdominal region can change the natural curvature of the spine, causing lordosis and resulting in backache in obese people.

Intraabdominal pressure

Central obesity is thought to increase intraabdominal pressure owing to mechanical pressure from the excess visceral fat in severely obese people. Research in animals has shown that experimentally induced acute increases in intraabdominal pressure to the levels seen in the abdomens of very obese people cause increases in pleural pressure, intracranial pressure and central venous pressure. The investigators postulated that in humans, increased intraabdominal pressure may contribute to hypertension, insulin resistance and NIDDM, obesity–hypoventilation syndrome, pseudotumour cerebri, incisional hernia and urinary incontinence. Massive weight loss following obesity surgery normalizes the increased intraabdominal pressure and reduces or eliminates all the symptoms listed above.

Surgical Complications

Obese patients are at increased risk of surgical and perisurgical complications. These risks include an increased risk of complications and death from anaesthesia, longer operating times, delayed wound healing, increased postoperative wound infections and pneumonia, and a higher frequency of incisional hernias after surgeries involving the abdominal wall. Many surgeons recommend weight reduction before elective surgery, but there are few studies to document that acute weight reduction improves the outcome of surgery.

Psychosocial Complications

Social complications

Obesity carries a social stigma that dramatically affects the quality of life for obese individuals. Physical attractiveness is highly valued in US society. A lean figure is particularly valued in women, and obese children and adults are considered unattractive by many in society, including other obese people. Other factors contributing to the social bias against the obese are beliefs that obesity is due merely to overeating and therefore obese people must lack willpower. Many members of the general public, and even health professionals, ignore the evidence for the genetic contribution to obesity, believe that obese people are responsible for their own plight, and believe that they do not deserve sympathy for their disability.

Obesity and intelligence (as judged by IQ values and the Scholastic Aptitude Test scores) are not correlated. Obese and lean high school students were found to be equally interested in attending high-ranking colleges, but a significantly lower number of obese females were admitted compared with non-obese females. The choice of mates is adversely affected by obesity, and obese individuals tend to marry mates with less education and from a lower socioeconomic class. It is more difficult for an obese person to find a job or to be promoted once hired, so lower earnings and a lower socioeconomic status are correlated with obesity. Obese employees are viewed as less competent, less productive, inactive, disorganized and less successful by employers. The bias against obesity has been shown to begin in early childhood, so the low self-esteem noted in obese people in many studies is not surprising.

Psychological complications

Severely obese persons do not have different personality types or more psychopathological disorders than lean controls. However, obesity is associated with negative emotions, low self-esteem, decreased marital satisfaction and body image disparagement. All of these conditions and beliefs show improvement with weight reduction.

Repeated cycles of intentional weight loss followed by weight gain (weight cycling) are common for obese people. Weight cycling is associated with lower levels of life satisfaction in females. However, in the initial period after weight loss, self-esteem and mood improve.

Dieting efforts correlate positively with the prevalence of eating disorders, particularly binge eating. A correlation of eating disorders with abuse of drugs and alcohol has been shown. In strictly dieting female college freshmen who were not alcohol abusers at baseline, the frequency of alcohol abuse was reported to increase after 1 year.

See also: **Arthritis**: Dietary Aspects of Aetiology and Nutritional Management. **Cancer**: Epidemiology and Associations Between Diet and Cancer. **Cholesterol**: Sources, Absorption, Function and Metabolism; Factors Determining Blood Cholesterol Levels. **Coronary Heart Disease**: Lipid Theory of Coronary Heart Disease; Aetiology; Prevention. **Diabetes Mellitus**: Classification and Chemical Pathology; Aetiology and Epidemiology; Dietary Management; Secondary Complications and Their Prevention. **Fertility**: Body Fat, Menarche and Fertility. **Gall Bladder Disease**: Nutritional Therapy. **Gout**: Aetiology and Nutritional Management. **Hypertension**: Physiology; Nutritional Management. **Insulin Resistance**: Aetiology and Association with Disease. **Lipoproteins**: Physiology. **Liver Disorders**: Nutritional Management. **Obesity**: Fat Distribution; Treatment. **Pregnancy**: Appropriate Maternal Weight Gain.

Further Reading

Atkinson RL (1982) Intravenous lidocaine for the treatment of intractable pain of adiposis dolorosa. *International Jownal of Obesity*, 6:351–357.

Bray GA (1986) Effects of obesity on health and happiness. In: Brownell KD and Foreyt JP (eds) *Handbook of Eating Disorders*, New York: Basic Books. pp 3–44.

Bjorntorp P (1993) Visceral obesity: a 'civilization syndrome'. *Obesity Research* 1:206–222.

Grundy SM and Barnett JP (1990) Metabolic and health complications of obesity. *Disease-a-Month* 36(12): 641–731.

Horton ES (1995) NIDDM – the devastating disease. *Diabetes Research and Clincas Practice* 28(supplement 1):S3–11.

Kuczmarski RJ, Flegal KM, Campbell SM and Johnson CL (1994) Increasing prevalence of overweight among US adults. *Journal of the American Medical Association* 272:205–211.

Pi-Sunyer FX (1993). Medical hazards of obesity. *Annals of Internal Medicine* 119:655–660.

Reaven GM (1991) Insulin resistance, hyperinsulinemia, hypertriglyceridemia, and hypertension. Parallels between human disease and rodent models. *Diabetes Care* 14:195–202.

Stern J, Chair *et al.* (1995) In: Thomas PR (ed.) *Weighing the Options: Criteria for Evaluating Weight-Management Programs*, p 4. Washington: National Academy Press.

Stunkard AJ and Wadden TA (1992) Psychological aspects of severe obesity. *American Jownal of Clinical Nutrition* 55:524S–532S.

Sugerman HJ, Felton WL, Salvant JB, Sismanis A and Kellum JM (1995) Effects of surgically induced weight loss on idiopathic intracranial hypertension in morbid obesity. *Neurology* 45:1655–1659.

Zumoff B and Strain GW (1994) A perspective on the hormonal abnormalities of obesity: are they cause or effect? *Obesity Research* 2:56–67.

Oils *see* **Fats and Oils**: Nutritional Value.

OLDER PEOPLE

Contents
Nutritional Requirements
Physiological Changes
Nutritionally Related Problems
Nutritional Management of Geriatric Patients

Nutritional Requirements

S B Roberts and **N P Hays**, Tufts University, Boston, Massachusetts, USA.

Life expectancy at birth in the USA is now 75.4 years, compared with about 47 years at the beginning of the twentieth century. Consequently, the proportion of the population that is elderly, as well as the mean age of the population, has increased. A continuation of these trends is anticipated through the beginning of the twenty-first century. One of the consequences of this profound demographic shift is an increased awareness that nutritional influences on health should be optimized for the older population.

Old age is a time when maintaining a good nutritional status is a critical determinant of health – but at the same time is often more challenging than it is earlier in life. As described below, the body's need for some nutrients is actually increased relative to that in earlier adult life, while the body's subconscious ability to regulate food and nutrient intakes diminishes. For these reasons, the elderly are a group particularly vulnerable to inadequate dietary intakes. The consequences of excessive nutrient intakes, particularly of energy, are also more severe in older adults. Obese elderly persons are much more likely to suffer disabling comorbidities associated with obesity such as heart disease, osteoarthritis and reduced mobility, which in turn can lead to a downward spiral of disability and frailty. Thus, it is important to know the nutritional requirements of elderly persons, and the food choices that can ensure adequate nutrition.

Determining accurate recommended dietary allowances (RDAs) for any age group is challenging. Historically, RDAs have been focused towards preventing nutrient deficiencies, whereas there is now increasing recognition that increased or lower intakes of some nutrients may also have protective functions against late-life chronic diseases such as coronary heart disease and some cancers. The newest update of the RDAs, now called Dietary Reference Intakes (DRIs), does in fact consider these protective functions as a factor in setting nutrient recommendations. (At the time of preparation of this manuscript, 1997 DRIs are available for calcium, magnesium, phosphorus, fluoride, and vitamin D. Recommendations for all other nutrients remain based on the 1989 RDAs.) In some cases, the increased intakes that appear to prevent late-life chronic disease are unfeasible without resorting to pharmacological nutrient interventions through fortification or other types of programmes. Despite increased recommendations for several nutrients in the new DRIs, the question of whether DRIs should recommend levels of nutrients compatible with what can be consumed through foods, or whether in some cases pharmacological supplementation may be appropriate, is an ongoing debate. Of particular relevance to this issue is the fact that, in epidemiological studies linking diet to disease, it is the consumption of foods rather than nutrients that is actually measured. Metabolically active 'phytochemicals' in such foods as fruits and vegetables may play important roles in disease prevention and are not at the present time understood well enough to be used as supplements.

The determination of accurate and meaningful DRIs is particularly difficult in the elderly population. Whereas the majority of young adults are healthy, the majority of elderly persons have one or more chronic diseases or disabilities that affect nutrient uptake and utilization (see Older People (b) Physiological Changes), and at the same time use multiple medications to treat chronic diseases. If nutritional recommendations are to be made not only for healthy elderly persons, but also for subgroups with different health limitations, this vastly increases the complexity of formulating accurate recommendations. Moreover, the objective of DRIs may change with adult age, with increasing focus on maintaining current health rather than preventing deficiency or future disease. For example, a recommendation to consume a low-fat diet to prevent later coronary heart disease may be inappropriate for 85-year-old men and women, who often find it hard to consume enough food to maintain weight. Finally, the 'elderly' are not one group. Currently, DRIs provide specific recommendations for individuals aged 51–70 and >70 years, which assumes that all individuals over the age of 70 years are metabolically equivalent with regard to their nutrient needs. This is certainly not the case for several nutrients and individuals in the age range 70–80 years should certainly be judged differently from those aged 80–90 years.

With these considerations in mind, we have focused this article on the effects of age on the body's ability to use different nutrients. When an increase in the intake of a particular nutrient is needed to achieve the same circulating level of the nutrient in the body or the same level of adequacy as judged by a particular enzymatic activity, this is taken as evidence of an increase in requirements. A more advanced treatment of nutritional requirements in the elderly must await the collection of data more sophisticated than is currently available.

Energy Requirements

Current recommendations on dietary energy intake define expected average amounts of dietary energy required for sustaining normal metabolic processes, together with desirable or expected levels of physical activity in healthy individuals. In weight-stable adults, energy requirements are equal to total energy expenditure because body energy stores remain approximately constant. Current RDAs also note that not more than 30% of dietary energy should be supplied by fat, and only 10% or less from saturated fat. This recommendation applies to adults of all ages. A further general consideration concerning energy requirements is that body weight should

Table 1 Estimated energy requirements by physical activity level

Physical activity level	PAL units[a]	Energy needs at 65 years (kJ per day)[b]	
		Man (75 kg)	Woman (60 kg)
Light activity	1.50	10 615	8025
Moderate activity	1.65	11 678	8828
Heavy activity	2.00	14 154	10 698

[a]Physical activity level (PAL) = Basal metabolic rate (BMR) multiplied by activity factor.
Estimated BMR of men (kJ per day)
    Age 18–30 BMR = (64.0 × weight in kg) + 2841
        30–60 BMR = (48.5 × weight in kg) + 3678
          >60 BMR = (56.5 × weight in kg) + 2038

Estimated BMR of women (kJ per day)
    Age 18–30 BMR = (61.5 × weight in kg) + 2075
        30–60 BMR = (36.4 × weight in kg) + 3469
          >60 BMR = (43.9 × weight in kg) + 2494
[b]1 kJ ≈ 0.239 kcal.

ideally be maintained within the Body Mass Index (weight in kilograms divided by square of height in metres) range of 20 to 25–28 kg m^{-2}. The question of whether an upper limit for desirable BMI is 25 or 28 remains controversial, especially for women.

Age, body weight and the level of physical activity are the primary determinants of energy requirements for body weight maintenance in adults of all ages. Concerning the effects of age, the older the person the lower the energy requirements. For body mass, the larger the body mass the greater the energy needs of the body. Height is an important determinant of body mass since taller persons tend to weigh more than shorter ones. Physical activity is also an important determinant of energy requirements. **Table 1** shows the recommended energy requirements of adult men and women of typical weight expressed as 'PAL' (physical activity level) units, which are energy requirements divided by the estimated 'basal meta-

bolic rate' (the minimum expenditure of the body when lying supine at rest at least 12 h after the last meal). PAL units are given for light, moderate and heavy levels of activity and basal metabolic rate can be calculated using the equations at the bottom of Table 1.

As predicted by the USA National Academy of Sciences recommendation, elderly adults typically have substantially decreased energy requirements relative to young adults by 1255–2510 kJ per day (300–600 kcal per day) (**Table 2**). This is thought to be for two main reasons: (1) basal metabolism decreases with age owing to a reduced amount of lean tissue (the actively metabolizing component of the body) as well as a decrease in the amount of metabolic activity per unit of lean tissue; (2) although not inevitable, the capacity for physical activity is typically decreased in older persons in concert with increased body fat mass.

The estimated energy needs given in Tables 1 and 2 have been challenged recently as being somewhat inaccurate. This is because, based on recent research using doubly-labelled water to measure energy requirements, they appear to underestimate the usual energy needs of healthy men and perhaps women also. The underestimation has been suggested to be due to an underestimate of the energy expenditure associated with normal daily living. In a summary of recent energy requirement studies in elderly persons, the measured PAL value of older men and women averaged 1.65, compared with the suggested recommendation of 1.51. This change would mean that the daily energy requirements of older men and women with typical body weights would average 10 539 kJ (2519 kcal) and 8828 kJ (2110 kcal), respectively. Like the recommended dietary

Table 2 Effects of age on estimated energy requirements

Age group (years)	Body weight (kg)	PAL units[a]	Estimated energy needs (kJ per day)[b]
Men			
19–24	72	1.67	12 134
25–50	79	1.60	12 134
51+	77	1.50	9 623
Women			
19–24	58	1.60	9 205
25–50	63	1.55	9 205
51+	65	1.50	7 950

[a]Physical activity level (PAL) = basal metabolic rate (BMR) multiplied by activity factor.
[b]1 kJ ≈ 0.239 kcal.

allowances, however, the new research confirms a substantial decrease in caloric requirements with age.

Protein Requirements

The 1985 FAO/WHO Committee on Energy and Protein requirements defines the protein requirements of an adult as 'the lowest level of dietary protein intake that will balance losses of nitrogen (N) from the body in persons maintaining energy balance at modest levels of physical activity'. Nitrogen balance is determined in metabolic studies as the difference between measured nitrogen intake (from dietary protein which is about 16% nitrogen by weight) and nitrogen losses. The major routes of nitrogen loss – in urine and faeces – are measured and miscellaneous nitrogen losses, including those in hair, skin, sweat, and breath ammonia, are assumed to be 8 mg per kg body weight. Based on this nitrogen balance methodology, it is estimated that the mean requirement for good quality protein in adults is 0.6 g per kg body weight, and the recommended safe protein intake (to cover individual variability in requirements) is 0.75 to 0.80 g per kg body weight.

No change in protein requirements with age is currently recommended, because of the limited and conflicting information in the literature at the time the most recent recommendations were developed. However, it was recognized in the recommendations that values of 0.75 and 0.80 g per kg body weight provide for higher intakes of protein per unit of lean tissue in older individuals, because of the reduced amount of lean tissue in this group. Thus, even if elderly persons have an increased requirement for protein relative to their amount of lean tissue, this may be accommodated already within the current RDAs.

Recent studies have raised the question of whether the current recommendations may underestimate usual protein needs in elderly persons. In a review and reanalysis of previous studies, protein requirements of elderly persons appeared to be increased to > 1.0 g per kg body weight per day. However, this tentative observation was based on potentially inaccurate assumptions including that miscellaneous nitrogen losses from the body are the same in young and elderly subjects (when they are probably lower in the elderly), and that an equilibration period of only 5 days is sufficient to bring elderly persons into nitrogen balance when the protein intake is adequate. Another recent study found that protein requirements were unchanged in healthy elderly women compared with younger women and reduced in elderly men. This controversy over whether the need for dietary protein is increased or decreased in the elderly cannot be resolved without further investigation.

Vitamin Requirements

RDAs and DRIs for vitamins in adults are shown in **Table 3**. Different approaches were taken to determine these estimated vitamin requirements in adults, including depletion–repletion studies conducted in a metabolic ward, measurement of intakes required to maintain constant body stores, and the activity of enzymes requiring vitamins as cofactors. In studies used to determine 1989 RDAs, there was a consistent emphasis on the prevention of clinical or biochemical

Table 3 Recommended daily vitamin needs (1989 RDAs except as indicated)

Vitamin	Younger adults		Older adults		Probable bias in older subjects
	Male	Female	Male	Female	
Vitamin A (μgRE)	1000	800	1000	800	Too high
Vitamin D (μg)[a]	5	5	10–15	10–15	Probably OK
Vitamin E (μg-αTE)	10	8	10	8	Probably OK
Vitamin K (μg)	80	65	80	65	?
Vitamin C (mg)	60	60	60	60	Too low
Thiamin (mg)	1.5	1.1	1.2	1.0	Probably OK
Riboflavin (mg)	1.7	1.3	1.4	1.2	Too low
Niacin (mg)	19	15	15	13	?
Vitamin B_6 (mg)	2.0	1.6	2.0	1.6	Too low
Folate (μg)	200	180	200	180	Too low
Vitamin B_{12} (μg)	2	2	2	2	Too low
Biotin (μg)	30–100	30–100	30–100	30–100	?
Pantothenic acid (mg)	4–7	4–7	4–7	4–7	?

[a]1997 DRI (Dietary Reference Intake) range for older adults: lower value is DRI for 51–70 years; higher value is DRI for >70 years.

deficiency as well as consideration of usual dietary intakes, rather than long-term prevention of chronic disease. The 1997 DRIs, on the other hand, were set at levels designed to reduce the risk of chronic disease. The RDA values listed are the best estimate of the same intake for the whole adult population – i.e. the mean intake plus two standard deviations (SD). The DRI value for vitamin D, however, is based simply on the observed mean vitamin D intake that appears to sustain a population's normal nutritional status.

The recommendations given in Table 3 are, for the most part, the same for young and older adults – again defined as less than and greater than 51 years of age for the RDAs, and as less than 51, 51–70, and greater than 70 years of age for DRIs. The exceptions are thiamin, riboflavin and niacin requirements, which were predicted (but not tested experimentally) to be lower in older persons. These predictions were made on the grounds that derivatives of thiamin, riboflavin and niacin function as cofactors in pathways of energy production and release. Because older adults consume and expend less energy, they can be expected to need less of the vitamins used to transform food into metabolic energy.

Recently, however, there has been increasing recognition that current RDAs for vitamins may not be correct for elderly individuals. In particular, and as summarized in Table 3, there is increasing evidence that RDAs for vitamins B_6 and B_{12} may be too low and that the RDA for vitamin A may be too high. There is also preliminary evidence that the RDAs for riboflavin and vitamin C may be inappropriately low as well.

Vitamin B_6

Vitamin B_6 is a cofactor for a large number of enzymes used in the metabolism of amino acids and related compounds. A vitamin B_6 depletion–repletion study showed that vitamin intakes equivalent to a mean of 1.96 mg per day for elderly men and 1.90 mg per day for elderly women were needed to return urinary xanthurenic acid excretion to normal following a tryptophan load (one test for B_6 deficiency), thus indicating that current RDAs may be too low for this age group. This evidence was also consistent with the previous observation that many elderly persons show evidence of biochemical vitamin B_6 deficiency.

Vitamin B_{12}

Vitamin B_{12} is used in the body as a cofactor for several essential enzymatic reactions including methionine synthase and methylmalonyl-CoA mutase. Vitamin B_{12} requirements have been suggested to be increased in elderly persons, on the grounds that 25–40% of individuals over 60 years of age have atrophic gastritis (a degenerative condition of the stomach. This condition results in impaired acid and pepsin secretion by the stomach, which in turn indirectly reduces absorption of vitamin B_{12} from the diet. Vitamin B_{12} deficiency may be the one major undetected vitamin deficiency in the elderly population and has been suggested as being responsible for a proportion of the dementia cases among the elderly population. Monthly B_{12} injections or use of a B_{12} nasal gel, both of which bypass the gastrointestinal tract, are usually most effective in restoring vitamin B_{12} levels to normal. In addition, weekly ingestion of megadose B_{12} supplements ($300 \times$ RDA) allow absorption by passive diffusion and are another means of normalizing B_{12} status.

Folate

Folate functions as a cofactor for enzymes involved in amino acid metabolism and nucleic acid synthesis. Recently, folate has received attention for its role in homocysteine metabolism and cardiovascular disease (CVD) risk. Excess levels of homocysteine in the blood have been implicated as a CVD risk factor; folate, along with vitamins B_6 and B_{12}, is involved in converting homocysteine to methionine, a harmless metabolite. In the elderly, studies have shown that folate intakes less than 400 µg per day correlate with elevated blood homocysteine levels. Unfortunately, many elderly do not consume the currently recommended 200 µg per day. Further research will be needed to determine if fortification of grain products with folate, scheduled to begin in January 1998, will bring older adult's intake up to the desired level.

Vitamin C and riboflavin

Recent research has provided preliminary evidence that elderly persons may need more of the antioxidant vitamin C and more riboflavin than previously thought. For the same vitamin C intake, elderly persons have lower circulating levels compared with young adults, perhaps because of either impaired absorption of vitamin C from the gut or impaired reabsorption from the kidney.

Elderly persons have also been reported to need the same amount of riboflavin as young adults, not less as suggested in the 1989 RDAs. Riboflavin functions primarily as a component of two flavin coenzymes, flavin mononucleotide (FMN) and flavin adenine dinucleotide (FAD), which catalyse oxidation–reduction reactions. A further observation of relevance to riboflavin requirements in the elderly is that riboflavin requirements may be increased during consumption of low-fat diets.

Vitamin A

Vitamin A is required for a wide range of metabolic reactions in the body and in particular is used in the differentiation of epithelial cells, support of reproduction and maintenance of the visual system. Concerning the possibility that the RDA for vitamin A may be too high and should be reduced, recent studies have indicated that elderly persons have decreased clearance of vitamin A by hepatic and other peripheral tissues. This finding helps to explain the observations that elderly persons have normal liver storage of vitamin A despite decreased vitamin A intakes, and that the use of vitamin A supplements by elderly persons is associated with increased circulating toxic indicators (high circulating retinyl esters).

Mineral Requirements

RDAs and DRIs for minerals in adults are shown in **Table 4**. As with the vitamin recommendations, different approaches were taken to determine these estimated mineral requirements in adults, including balance studies and summation of expected mineral needs based on metabolic demands and rates of absorption. The RDA values listed are best estimates of the safe intake for the whole adult population – i.e. the mean requirement plus 2 SD; the DRI values for phosphorus and magnesium are estimated in a similar fashion. The DRIs for calcium and fluoride, however, are based simply on an approximated mean requirement. The recommendations given in Table 4 are the same for young and older adults with the exception of iron requirements in older women, which are proposed to be lower on the grounds that iron losses are reduced following menopause, and calcium requirements in older men and women, which are higher on the grounds that higher intakes

ensure a maximal skeletal calcium retention. Evidence suggests that the DRI for calcium may be too low, and possibly that the RDA for chromium may be higher than necessary.

Calcium

Based on increased recognition that the 1989 RDA for calcium may be too low, the 1997 DRI was set at at 1200 mg per day for men and women 51 years and older. This value may still be too low for optimal calcium retention in individuals older than 65 years of age, but there are also issues of nutrient–nutrient interactions when considering an amount greater than 1200 mg per day. Calcium is the primary mineral in bone and teeth and is extremely important for the elderly, because the age-associated bone demineralization that occurs commonly in elderly persons is accelerated when calcium intake is low and leads to increased risks of bone fracture and tooth loss. Ageing is associated with an decreased ability to absorb dietary calcium and also a decreased ability to increase the fractional rate of absorption when calcium intake is low. Calcium supplementation (for example using calcium citrate malate) has been shown to prevent age-associated bone loss both in women with initially low calcium intakes and perhaps also in those with intakes in the normal range.

Chromium

Chromium mediates the hormonal effects of insulin and so is needed for a wide range of metabolic functions including maintaining glucose and lipid status. Chromium requirements for older persons are difficult to determine, owing to the scarcity of accurate measures of both chromium status and the chromium content of foods. Based on available intake data, it has been estimated that approximately

Table 4 Recommended daily mineral needs (1989 RDAs except as indicated)

Mineral	Younger adults		Older adults		Probable bias in older subjects
	Male	Female	Male	Female	
Calcium (mg)[a]	1000	1000	1200	1200	Too low?
Phosphorus (mg)[a]	800	800	800	800	?
Magnesium (mg)[a]	420	320	420	320	Probably OK
Iron (mg)	10	15	10	10	Probably OK
Zinc (mg)	15	12	15	12	Probably OK
Iodine (μg)	150	150	150	150	?
Selenium (μg)	70	55	70	55	Probably OK
Copper (mg)	1.5–3.0	1.5–3.0	1.5–3.0	1.5–3.0	Probably OK
Manganese (mg)	2–5	2–5	2–5	2–5	?
Fluoride (mg)[a]	3.8	3.1	3.8	3.1	?
Chromium (μg)	50–200	50–200	50–200	50–200	Too high?
Molybdenum (μg)	75–250	75–250	75–250	75–250	?

[a]1997 DRI (Dietary Reference Intake).

12.5 MJ (3000 kcal) of a typical diet would have to be eaten to obtain the minimum suggested amount of chromium of 50 µg. Such an intake is rare in elderly persons, and at the same time balance studies have shown that chromium balance can be achieved with dietary intakes less than 50 µg. These findings, coupled with the observation that chromium deficiency is extremely rare in adults of any age, suggests that the current suggested intake may be unnecessarily high for elderly adults.

Fluid Requirements

Water is by far the largest constituent of the body, accounting for between 50% and 80% of the body mass. It is needed for a variety of essential purposes including regulation of cell volume, nutrient transport, waste removal and temperature regulation. Water is lost from the body in urine, faeces and 'insensibly', i.e. in sweat and transepidermal routes, and so must be replaced. To replace essential water losses, water needs to be consumed at an estimated rate of 0.24–0.36 ml kJ^{-1} (1–1.5 ml kcal^{-1}) of energy expended. Thus, an elderly person with an energy requirement of 9200 kJ per day (2200 kcal per day) will need 2.2–3.3 l per day of water. As shown in **Fig. 1**, approximately half of this water intake usually comes from consumed liquids and the remainder will come from water contained in food and the metabolic water derived from the oxidation of macronutrients in the body.

Water intake is a particular concern in elderly persons. This is not because water requirements are higher in this group – they are not – but because the ability to sense a need for water appears to be blunted in older individuals, with the consequence that they do not feel thirsty when they should and so are at risk of dehydration from inadequate fluid intake. This is particularly true when water requirements are increased – for example in hot, dry weather and when body temperature is increased during a fever. For this reason, elderly persons should be given the advice that they should not rely on thirst to determine when they drink but instead should have a meal and snack plan that routinely incorporates one or more drinks.

Appropriate Food Choices for the Elderly

Elderly persons have substantially inadequate intakes of many of the micronutrients as judged by the adequacy of reported dietary intake in a number of national surveys. This finding may be due, in part, to the inaccuracy of many types of dietary records,

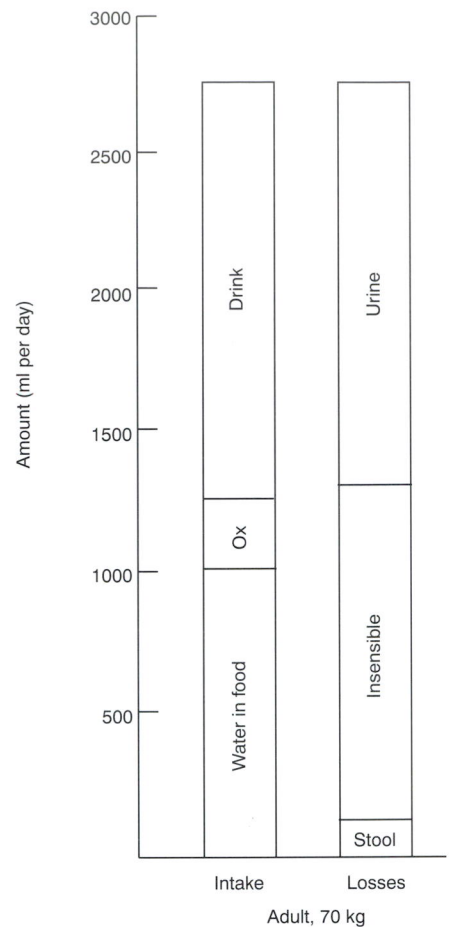

Figure 1 Routes and approximate magnitude of water intake and losses without sweating. Ox is water of oxidation. Adapted with permission from *Recommended Dietary Allowances*, 10th edn. Copyright 1989 by the National Academy of Sciences. Courtesy of the National Academy Press, Washington, DC.

especially in elderly persons. However, corroborating evidence from studies of circulating nutrient levels and enzymatic tests of biochemical deficiency suggests that micronutrient inadequacies are widespread in the elderly population. Decreased energy requirements, a reduced ability to regulate food intake accurately, and social factors all contribute to the poor dietary intake of elderly persons. This, coupled with an equivalent or even increased requirement for micronutrients, necessitates a very different dietary pattern in elderly persons with increased emphasis on consumption of fruits, vegetables, legumes, fish, lean meat and low-fat dairy products and whole grains, and decreased intake of highly processed foods with a relative deficiency of micronutrients. While dietary supplements remain a viable alternative to the provision of micronutrients to the elderly population, this should not be a preferred option because supplements do not yet replace the wide range of biologically active food constituents, many of which will probably come to be recognized as playing important roles in the prevention of chronic diseases.

Acknowledgements

This work was supported in part with NIA grants AG12829 and T32AG00209.

See also: **Calcium**: Physiology. **Chromium**: Physiology, Dietary Sources and Requirements. **Electrolytes**: Water-Electrolyte Balance. **Energy**: Energy Requirements. **Folic Acid**: Physiology, Dietary Sources and Requirements. **Older People**: Physiological Changes. **Protein**: Requirements and Role in Diet. **Retinol**: Physiology. **Riboflavin**: Physiology. **Vitamin B$_6$**: Physiology.

Further Reading

Blumberg JB and Meydani M (1995) The relationship between nutrition and exercise in older adults. In: Gisolfi CV, Lamb DR and Nadel E. (eds) *Exercise in Older Adults*, pp 353–394. New York: Cooper Publishing Group.

Boisvert WA, Mendoza I, Castaneda C, De Portocarrero L, Solomons NW, Gershoff SN and Russell RM (1993) Riboflavin requirement of healthy elderly humans and its relationship to the macronutrient composition of the diet. *Journal of Nutrition* **123**:915–925.

Brody T (1994) *Nutritional Biochemistry*. San Diego: Academic Press.

Chernoff R (1994) Thirst and fluid requirements. *Nutrition Reviews* 52 (supplement 2):S3–S5.

FAO, WHO and UNU (1985) *Energy and Protein Requirements*. Report of a joint FAO/WHO/UNU expert consultation. Technical Report Series 724. Geneva: World Health Organization.

Fereday A, Gibson NR, Cox M, Pacy PJ and Millward DJ (1997) Protein requirements and ageing: metabolic demand and effeciency of utilization. *British Journal of Nutrition* **77**:685–702.

Garry PJ and Vellas BJ (1996) Aging and nutrition. In: Ziegler EE and LJ Filer (eds) *Present Knowledge in Nutrition*, pp 414–419. Washington, DC: ILSI Press.

Heseker H and Schneider R (1994) Requirement and supply of vitamin C, E and β-carotene for elderly men and women. *European Journal of Clinical Nutrition* 48:118–127.

Institute of Medicine, Food and Nutrition Board (1997) *Dietary Reference Intakes: Calcium, Phosphorus, Magnesium, Vitamin D and Fluoride*. Washington, DC: National Academy Press.

National Research Council (1989) *Recommended Dietary Allowances*, 10th edn. Washington, DC: National Academy Press.

Poehlman ET (1993) Regulation of energy expenditure in aging humans. *Journal of the American Geriatrics Society* **41**:552–559.

Roberts SB, Fuss P, Heyman MB, Evans WJ, Tsay R, Rasmussen H, Fiatarone M, Cortiella J, Dallal GE and Young VR (1994) Control of food intake in older men. *Journal of the American Medical Association* **272**:1601–1606.

Rosenberg IR (1994) Keys to a longer, healthier, more vital life. *Nutrition Reviews* 52:S50–S51.

Russell RM and Suter PM (1993) Vitamin requirements of elderly people: an update. *American Journal of Clinical Nutrition* 58:4–14.

Russell RM (1997) New views on the RDAs for older adults. *Journal of the American Dietetic Association* 97:515–518.

Ryan AS, Craig LD and Finn SC (1992) Nutrient intakes and dietary patterns of older Americans: a national survey. *Journal of Gerontology* 47:M145–M150.

Scrimshaw NS, Waterlow JC and Schurch B (eds) (1996) Energy and protein requirements. *European Journal of Clinical Nutrition* 50 (supplement 1):S1–S197.

Wood RJ, Suter PM and Russell RM (1995) Mineral requirements of elderly people. *American Journal of Clinical Nutrition* 62:493–505.

Physiological Changes

M Wahlqvist, A Kouris-Blazos and **G S Savige**, Monash Medical Centre, Victoria, Australia

Physiological changes in the elderly generally represent a decline in reserve capacity. They may be age-related without being an obligatory part of the ageing process. Nutritional factors may minimize these changes. These changes may, however, decrease nutritional tolerance for excesses or restrictions. These include decreased appetite, less taste appreciation and diminished handling of food in the gut, with alterations in motility and digestion. The hormonal responses to food, hormonal-like properties of foods themselves (such as phyto-oestrogens) and hormonal determinants of nutritional status (such as body composition), as well as body composition itself, are all valuable in the nutritional assessment and monitoring of the aged.

Body Composition

Body composition is dynamic throughout the life span. The changes that occur with ageing include a loss of height, muscle mass, bone mass and body water, while there is an increase in and redistribution of fat mass.

Body compartments

Body composition can be broadly classified into two sections: fat mass (FM) and fat-free mass (FFM). Fat mass incorporates all body lipids, while the fat-free mass includes all body constituents other than lipids such as minerals, proteins and water. Lean body mass (LBM) is similar to the FFM compartment except that it also includes essential lipids such as phospholipids. Finally, total body water (TBW), which accounts for most of the body's weight, includes both intracellular and extracellular water.

Physiological changes that occur with ageing

In both men and women height decreases with age. Alterations in posture, vertebral collapse, osteoporosis, loss of muscle tone and reductions in disc space all contribute to this loss of height. The rate of loss after maturity has been estimated to be between 0.5 and 2.0 cm per decade, with the loss being greater in older age.

Most literature indicates that peak bone density is achieved in the middle of the third decade, although it has been suggested that this may occur towards the end of adolescence. Involutional bone loss usually begins between the ages of 35 and 40 years, with the rate of bone loss varying according to the type of bone and the skeletal site. Overall women can lose at least half of their trabecular bone mass and about one-third of their cortical bone mass during their lifetime. For men this overall loss is less and represents about two-thirds of the loss experienced by women. Bone loss in accelerated in women at the menopause, but this rate slows about 5–10 years later.

There is decrease in FFM with ageing owing to a loss in muscle mass, bone mass and body organ mass. The extent of these losses depends on age itself, activity levels, gender (men lose lean body mass at a faster rate than women) and hormonal changes. By the seventh decade LBM has decreased by an average of 5 kg in women and 12 kg in men and skeletal muscle size has declined by as much as 40%. The kidney, liver and lungs become smaller with the ageing process. It has been estimated that the weight of the kidney is reduced by 9%, the liver by as much as 18% and the lungs by 11%.

As lean body mass decreases with advancing age, the percentage of body fat increases. There is a redistribution of subcutaneous fat from the limbs to the trunk and intra-abdominal fat increases. Total body water (TBW) in healthy elderly subjects also declines with age. This decline seems to parallel the decline in lean body mass, but whether the source of loss is from intracellular water or extracellular water remains unclear.

Measurements in the elderly

Change in body weight over time (in the absence of fluid imbalances) is one of the best indicators of changes in body composition. Limb length, unlike stature, is not altered by ageing and is therefore a useful surrogate for estimating original height. Two such measures include arm span and knee height. Estimating original height and comparing it with actual height may be a useful indicator of nutritional status, because the preservation of height may be looked upon as a positive sign in nutritional terms.

Skinfold thickness measurements of subcutaneous fat can be used to predict body fat content. In elderly subjects this method becomes less reliable because increased body fat is stored intra-abdominally and intramuscularly. The reliability of these measurements is further complicated by the decline in elasticity and compressibility of subcutaneous adipose in the elderly. Despite these limitations, serial skinfold measures are still useful in assessing changes in body composition.

Abdominal circumference is a useful indicator of abdominal obesity, although decreases in trunk length owing to conditions like osteoporosis may reflect some of the increase seen in abdominal circumference with ageing. Calf circumference is recognized by the World Health Organization to be the most sensitive measure of muscle mass in elderly.

Consequences of change

The change in body composition seen with ageing can be minimized with adequate exercise and nutrient intake, producing a more favourable outcome in terms of health. It has been shown the rate and degree of loss in LBM is an important predictor of length of survival and in some studies a higher body mass index has been associated with lower mortality in the elderly.

A reduction in muscle mass impacts on mobility, increases the risk of falls, and can adversely affect the functional capacity of other muscles such as the diaphragm. Loss of muscle mass also indicates a loss of protein reserves, which are drawn upon during episodes of illness. These losses increase the risk of malnutrition and immune dysfunction, conditions more prevalent among the aged.

Osteoporosis, a metabolic bone disease in which bone mass is reduced (either by decreased bone formation or by increased bone resorption, or both) causes fragility fractures. It accounts for a considerable proportion of the morbidity and mortality seen in ageing populations, for example the expected rate of survival in those sustaining a hip fracture is reduced by 12% or more.

The Gastrointestinal Tract

The mouth

Insofar as nutritional physiology is concerned the mouth and related structures contribute to taste and release of smells for the adjacent olfactory apparatus, mastication, a limited amount of starch digestion (by way of salivary amylase) and the initial phase of deglutination (swallowing).

Mastication may be impaired in the aged because of a reduction in masseter and medial pterygoid muscle mass with age, together with poorer movement control. Additionally the edentulous mouth may contribute to masticatory impairment, although retention of teeth to older age is improving and the need for associated dental and gingival care growing (osteoporosis of mandible and maxilla may contribute to gingival disease). Although dental health may influence food choice, nutritional status need not suffer if nutritious alternatives are sought. Salivary flow may be decreased in the aged, but in general it does not appear to be an inevitable accompaniment of ageing. More work is required on salivary composition in relation to age given its lubricating, buffering, remineralization, antimicrobial and digestive functions.

Oesophagus

Before a swallow reaches the oesophagus, its transit through the pharynx may be longer by up to 10% in over 65-year-olds. In the oesophagus itself, amplitude of contraction, extent of relaxation and smoothness of peristalsis may be reduced in the aged. Oesophageal motility disorders may be sufficient to be regarded as disease states like achalasia (absence of peristalsis) or diffuse oesophageal spasm. The term 'presbyoesophagus' is sometimes applied to oesophageal motility disorders in the aged. Although degenerative changes may occur as a consequence of ageing, these changes should not be accepted as part of the normal ageing process without further investigation. For instance, underlying conditions which may be responsible for motility changes include diabetes, strictures or malignant disease.

Stomach and duodenum

Decreased gastric function may supervene when gastritis affects the stomach, as in 'atrophic gastritis', in which a reduction in acid and also intrinsic factor (necessary for vitamin B_{12} absorption further down the gastrointestinal tract in the distal ileum) occurs, although this is usually not complete. It may have an autoimmune basis (usually in the gastric fundus, for example pernicious anaemia), but more commonly is attributable to long-standing infestation with *Helicobacter pylori* (usually in the gastric antrum), which can be eradicated. Crystalline vitamin B_{12} can be absorbed in elderly subjects with 'atrophic gastritis'.

While not a physiological process, the use of NSAIDS (nonsteroidal anti-inflammatory drugs) in the elderly can contribute to significant gastric and duodenal pathophysiology, notably haemorrhage and ulceration. At the same time, there is evidence that aspirin (acetyl salicylic acid, an NSAID) may protect against gastrointestinal cancers, raising interest that this may apply to salicylates occurring naturally in foods.

Pancreas

Pancreatic size decreases in later life, with duct dilation and parenchymal fibrosis. In the aged, volume, bicarbonate and enzyme output from the pancreas generally decline, and adaptation to dietary change is less adequate.

Small intestine

The absorption of carbohydrate, fat and protein appears to be less well tolerated in elderly people when loads are high. For instance, faecal fat and nitrogen excretion have been shown to increase more among aged adults compared with young adults when these nutrient loads are increased. Higher breath hydrogen excretion in elderly adults has also occurred in response to meals high in carbohydrate. Atrophic gastritis (mentioned above) produces a pH-dependent folic acid malabsorption in the jejunum in the aged and it can also contribute to calcium, iron and vitamin B_{12} malabsorption.

The bacterial microflora of the small bowel can also change and increase with age and contribute to malabsorption.

Liver

Liver mass and blood flow decrease in the aged, in part related to decline in lean body mass – but it may not be inevitable. Kupffer cells (liver reticuloendothelial cells) accumulate lipofuscin pigment. Protein synthesis generally declines and the responsiveness or regulation of albumin synthesis is less appropriate. Drug handling may diminish with implications for dosage.

Large bowel

Colon dysmotility and disordered defaecation contribute to constipation. Diverticula develop. Some of these alterations may reflect changes in diet, for example declining intakes of energy are often associated a reduced intake of dietary fibre and resistant starch.

The faecal microflora changes with a decrease in bifido-bacterium and increases in *Escherichia coli*, streptococcus, lactobacillus and *Clostridium perfringens*. Probiotics, like oligosaccharides and resistant starch, and probiotics (ingested live organisms), may have a place in minimizing these age-related changes.

Endocrine Function

There are several alterations in circulating hormone levels and action with advancing age; diseases often present in the elderly account for these changes, while other changes are due to ageing *per se*. There is an increased propensity for the aged to develop endocrine deficiency diseases (e.g. diabetes mellitus, hypothyroidism, hypogonadism) owing to a loss of functional reserve in many endocrine organs. The classic nonspecific presentation of endocrine disease in the aged is weight loss.

Insulin

Elderly people tend to have an impaired glucose tolerance compared with their younger counterparts owing to reduced insulin secretion and insulin sensitivity (cells lose their ability to respond to insulin because of defects in insulin receptors). The hyperglycaemia of ageing is more closely correlated with the increasing level of body fat and physical inactivity with advancing years than to the ageing process *per se*. Chromium has been suggested to have a role in normal glucose homeostasis because it forms part of the 'glucose tolerance factor' which promotes efficient insulin function. Chromium deficiency may take many years to develop and is more likely to occur in the elderly and has thus been implicated in the glucose intolerance of ageing. The main sources of chromium include brewer's yeast, blackstrap molasses, egg yolk, cheese, liver and wholegrain products.

Growth hormone and prolactin

Growth hormone levels also decline with advancing age and thus may explain a number of normal changes seen with ageing. These include the diminished nitrogen retention, the decrease in lean body mass, the increase in adipose tissue, and some of the osteopenia characteristically associated with ageing. The hormone prolactin (involved in lactation) also increases with age, and helps to maintain body fat in the elderly (and in breast-feeding mothers).

Thyroid hormones

There is a decreased production of thyroid hormones with ageing that is counterbalanced by a decreased thyroid hormone degradation. The prevalence of hypothyroidism and hyperthyroidism rises significantly in people aged over 60 years. Major changes in circulating thyroid hormones are mainly seen in the elderly when illness supervenes (e.g. euthyroid sick syndrome). These changes can mimic the changes seen with hypothyroidism. Malnourished elderly often present with the euthyroid sick syndrome. Hyperthyroidism is characterized by the hyperkinetic state, thyromegaly and eye signs, but in the elderly these signs are often replaced by heart failure, fatigue, depression, dementia and unexplained weight loss.

Aldosterone and dehydroepiandrosterone (DHEA)

The levels of aldosterone tend to fall with advancing age and thus tend to increase the propensity of older people to develop hyperkalaemia. Dehydroepiandrosterone (DHEA), a product made in the body during the synthesis of steroid hormones, declines dramatically with advancing age. Diminished levels of DHEA are associated with hypercholesterolaemia, hypertension and death from cardiovascular diseases in men. DHEA administration in animals prolongs life span, which may be related to its ability to reduce weight. DHEA deficiency results in reduced levels of nicotinamide adenine dinucleotide phosphate (NADP) and stimulation of lipogenesis, which has the potential to promote atherosclerosis. DHEA as a prescription drug is currently under investigation as it may have potential in reducing fat synthesis and enhancing fat utilization.

Testosterone and oestrogen

In the majority of older men there is a marked decrease in testosterone levels and a compensatory increase in luteinizing hormone (LH) and follicle-stimulating hormone (FSH) levels. In a number of elderly men, the hypothalamus fails to detect the decrease in testosterone adequately, resulting in the development of hypothalamic hypogonadism. Apart from the role of testosterone in maintaining normal sexual function, it also promotes nitrogen retention, maintains muscle mass, protects bone from excessive calcium loss and produces a feeling of wellbeing. The median age for the cessation of the menstrual cycle is 51 years (among women in the US) and is due to the failure of the ovaries to produce oestrogens and progesterone. As a consequence, the pituitary gland becomes more active and produces FSH and LH in greater quantity. Some ovarian secretion of oestrogen generally continues but gradually diminishes until it is inadequate to maintain the oestrogen-dependent tissues: the breasts and genital organs gradually atrophy; the decrease in protein anabolism causes thinning of the skin and bones (oesteoporosis). Even after cessation of ovarian secretion of oestrogen, some oestrogen is found in plasma due to conversion of adrenally secreted androgens into oestrogen by nonovarian tissues. Androgens in the ageing female are responsible for hirsutism (e.g. hair on upper lip and chin) and abdominal fatness which in turn increases the risk of cardiovascular diseases and diabetes. Oestrogen favourably affects plasma low-density lipoprotein (LDL) cholesterol/high-density lipoprotein (HDL) cholesterol ratios, and this may explain why women have much less atherosclerosis than men until after the menopause, when the incidence becomes similar in both sexes. Consumption of naturally occurring oestrogens (phytoestrogens) in plant foods (especially legumes) have been shown to play a role in controlling menopausal symptoms and possibly in reducing the risk of breast and ovarian cancer by blocking oestrogen activity in cells, and by inhibiting endothelial cell proliferation and *in vitro* angiogenesis. The recognition that such foods (phytoestrogens) are effective indicates they may partially substitute for hormone replacement therapy (HRT).

Angiotensin and vasopressin

Elderly people are at increased risk of dehydration. This failure to develop an appropriate thirst response may be secondary to an impaired or inappropriate secretion of angiotensin and antidiuretic hormones, which may lead to hyponatraemia. Decreased free water clearance in response to vasopressin has also been noted, predominantly due to the age-related fall in glomerular filtration rate.

Activity Patterns

A moderate amount of physical activity (e.g. 30 min walk daily) throughout the life span is protective against early mortality, coronary heart disease, diabetes, stroke and osteoporosis. Exercise appears to affect the risk of death even more than heredity, smoking, hypertension or extremes in body weight. In addition to extending longevity, physical activity supports independence and mobility in later life by reducing the risks of falls and minimizing the risk of injury should a fall occur. Muscle mass and strength tend to decline with age, making older people vulnerable to falls and immobility. However, older adults who are active have less fat mass and more muscle mass, greater flexibility and better balance than those who are inactive.

Immobility

Stiffness, pain and declining mobility are unfortunately still perceived as stereotyped characteristics of 'normal ageing' rather than as being caused by potentially treatable conditions, e.g. adverse drug reactions, neurological, musculoskeletal and cardiovascular disorders or inappropriate bed rest. For example, phenothiazines are often prescribed for nonspecific 'dizziness' which is usually an undiagnosed gait disorder. These drugs can cause significant immobility by causing an extrapyramidal (parkinsonian) syndrome, postural hypotension and cognitive impairment. One dose is enough to cause immobility for weeks. Carers may unwittingly reinforce disability by discouraging activity, especially because of the fear of falls (**Table 1**). Once immobility is established ('bed and chair existence'), this will result in muscle weakness and wasting, poor balance, loss of endurance, loss of confidence, dependency and secondary complications of immobility (**Table 2**).

Physical activity

Adult energy needs decline by an estimated 5% per decade; basal metabolic rate is reduced in the aged by about 10–20% compared with their younger counterparts. This decline in metabolic rate reflects, by and large, the reduced lean body mass, which in

Table 1 Causes of gait disorder and falls in the aged which may ultimately lead to immobility

Neurological	Musculoskeletal
Stroke	Arthritis
Alzheimer's disease	Fractures
Parkinson's disease	Podiatric problems
Alcohol	Polymyalgia
Other cerebellar degenerations	Myopathy
Adverse drug reactions	**Cardiovascular**
Phenothiazines	Postural hypotension
Tricyclic antidepressants	Heart failure
Benzodiazepines	Angina
Antihypertensives	Claudication
Antiparkinson drugs	
Sensory	**Environmental**
Visions	Stairs
Hearing	Rugs
Fear of falling	Bathing, toileting
	Housework, shopping

Other
Intercurrent illness
Enforced dependency/bed rest
Depression
Pain
Malnutrition

Table 2 Some secondary complications of immobility

Venous thrombosis
Pulmonary embolism
Aspiration pneumonia
Orthostatic hypotension
Leg oedema
Impaired glucose tolerance
Constipation
Urinary incontinence
Increased bone fracture risk
Pressure sores/ulcers

turn requires that older adults eat less food energy to maintain their weight. It has been suggested that activities of growth hormone and testosterone, which promote lean tissue growth, are reduced with ageing; this may contribute to the shift in balance from lean to adipose tissue with age. A decreased capacity for muscle fibre regeneration and a decreased trophic effect of the autonomic nervous system on muscle may also be partly responsible. However, regular exercise not only impedes this loss of lean body mass, but also increases energy expenditure and energy intake, thereby enhancing nutrient intakes. Age-related conditions such as cardiovascular disease, musculoskeletal disease, osteopenia, obesity and others can result in a decline in physical activity. There is also a decline in physical working capacity (Vo_2max), amounting to about 10% per decade between ages 25 and 65 years. This means that the same physical tasks require a greater physical effort in the aged. Physical training can correct these age-related changes in physical working capacity by as much as 50%.

Appetite and Taste

Taste

The sensation of taste is perceived by taste buds located on the tongue, roof of the mouth, pharynx, larynx and the upper third of the oesophagus. Taste buds are situated in small protrusions on the surface of the tongue called papillae. Each taste bud is innervated by three cranial nerves and consists of a number of sensory receptor cells surrounded by supporting cells. These cells are renewed every 10–10.5 days. Chemical substances pass through a pore at the surface of the taste bud to reach the taste receptors. Finally, interpretation of taste occurs in the taste centre of the cerebral cortex.

Losses in taste sensitivity (hypogeusia) occurs in most elderly people. This loss was initially thought to be due to a reduced number of taste buds, but recent data indicate that a decline in the number of receptors may be responsible. The ability to detect a taste (threshold) is elevated in the aged, but the threshold varies with different substances. Taste thresholds on average tend to be 2–2.5 times higher in elderly adults when compared with young adults. For some substances, however, the threshold may be more than 20 times higher in the elderly.

Smell

The sense of taste is closely related to the sense of smell. In order to smell a chemical substance it must come into contact with olfactory receptors that are located within the olfactory mucosa at the roof of the nasal cavity. These olfactory receptors are bipolar sensory neurons that possess cilia at one end and axons at the other end. The cilia which arise from the end of the neuron facing the surface of the nasal cavity are thought to be stimulated by chemical substances. The axons of these bipolar neurons unite to form bundles which pass through a small bone known as the cribriform plate to reach the olfactory bulbs. The olfactory bulbs that are situated in the anterior section of the brain contain groups of cells called glomeruli. With ageing many of these cells degenerate. The axons of the bipolar neurons (which reach the olfactory bulbs) synapse with the dendrites of other neurons. The axons from these neurons form the olfactory tract which conveys impulses to the 'old brain' for processing.

Olfaction usually begins to decline during the sixth decade and deteriorates further after the seventh decade. The threshold for the sense of smell is higher and the ability to discriminate between different odours is diminished in the elderly. This diminished sense of smell may result, in part, from the degeneration of cells in the olfactory bulbs or in the neurons found in the 'old brain'. Neurons found in the 'old brain' (which consists of the hippocampus, amygdala and the prepyriform cortex) are the first neurons to show signs of degeneration with ageing.

Appetite

Factors which control food intake are complex and not fully understood. Salivation, gastric secretions and hormonal stimulation can arise from the sight, smell, taste and thought of food. There are 10 gastrointestinal hormones which have been shown to inhibit food intake. These include cholecystokinin, bombesin, gastrin, secretin, glucagon, insulin, somatostatin, neurotensin, substance P and pancreatic peptide. Neurotransmitters such as serotonin, norepinephrine and the opiates are known to influence food choice, however the exact mechanisms by which these operate is not clear. Changes that occur to these hormones or neurotransmitters and their effect on appetite in the elderly need further investigation.

The homeostatic mechanisms that control appetite may be impaired in the elderly. Several studies have shown elderly men less capable of regulating their energy intakes after dietary manipulations compared with younger adults. Other studies report a drop in energy intakes with ageing. This reduction can be explained, in part, by the age-related drop in basal metabolic rate. However, the decline in physical activity (and presumably appetite) that accompanies ageing appears to be the major contributor to the fall in energy intakes.

See also: **Cancer**: Epidemiology of Breast Cancer. **Dehydration**: Physiological Effects and Management. **Exercise**: Beneficial Effects. **Gastrointestinal Tract**: Structure and Function of the Stomach; Structure and Function of the Small Intestine; Structure and Function of the Colon. **Osteoporosis**: Aetiology.

Further Reading

Anderson HG (1994) Regulation of food intake. In: Shils ME, Olson JA and Shike M (eds) *Modern Health in Health and Disease*, 8th edn, vol. 1, chap. 35, pp 524–536. Philadelphia: Lea & Febiger.

Bowman BA, Rosenberg IH and Johnson MA (1992) Gastrointestinal function in the elderly. In: Munro H and Schlierf G (eds) *Nutrition of the Elderly*, Nestlé Nutrition Workshop Series, vol. 29, pp 43–50. New York: Vevey/Raven Press.

Cashman MD (1991) The ageing gut. In: Chernoff R (ed.) *Geriatric Nutrition: The Health Professional's Handbook*, pp 183–227. Gaithersburg: Aspen Publishers.

Fogt EJ, Bell ST and Blackburn GL (1995) Nutrition assessment of the elderly. In: Morley JE, Glick Z and Rubenstein LZ (eds) *Geriatric Nutrition: A Comprehensive Review*, 2nd edn, chap. 5, pp 51–62. New York: Raven Press.

Forbes GB and Reina JC (1970) Adult lean body mass declines with age: some longitudinal observations. *Metabolism* 9:653–663.

Greenberg RE and Holt PR. (1986) Influence of aging upon pancreatic digestive enzymes. *Digestive Diseases and Sciences* 31(9):970–977.

Hazzard WR, Andres R, Bierman EL and Blass JP (eds) (1990). *Principles of Geriatric Medicine and Gerontology*, 2nd edn. New York: McGraw-Hill Information Services Co.

Lipski P (1992) Immobility: causes and consequences. In: *Update in Geriatric Medicine: An Overview of Current Knowledge*, part 1, pp 1–9. Edgecliff, Australia: Excerpta Medica.

Lipski PS and James FW (1992) Small intestine. In: Evans JG and Williams TF (eds) *Oxford Textbook of Geriatric Medicine*, pp 226–236. Oxford: Oxford University Press.

Mitsuoka T (1996) Intestinal flora and human health. *Asia Pacific Journal of Clinical Nutrition* 5(1):2–9.

Morley JE and Glick Z (1991). Endocrine aspects of nutrition and aging. In: Chernoff R (ed.) *Geriatric Nutrition: The Health Professional's Handbook*, chap. 12, pp 311–335. Gaithersburg: Aspen Publishers.

Nelson JB and Costeli DO (1988) Effects of aging on gastrointestinal physiology. *Proceedings of Gastroenterology* 12:28–35.

Riggs L and Melton III LJ (1992) Involutional osteoporosis. In: Evans JG and Williams TF (eds) *Oxford Textbook of Geriatric Medicine*, section 14.1, pp 405–415. New York: Oxford University Press.

Rolls BJ, Dimeo KA and Shide DJ (1995) Age-impairments in the regulation of food intake. *American Journal of Clinical Nutrition* 62:923–931.

Russell RM (1990) Gastrointestinal function and aging. In: Morley JE, Glick Z and Rubenstein LZ (eds) *Geriatric Nutrition, A Comprehensive Review*, chap. 17, pp 231–237. New York: Vevey/Raven Press.

Russell RM, Krasinski SD, Samloff IM, Jacob RA, Hartz SC and Brovender SR (1986) Folic acid malabsorption in atrophic gastritis. *Gastroenterology* 91:1476–1492.

Schiffman SS (1993) Food acceptability and nutritional status: considerations for the aging population in the 21st century. In: Leatherwood P, Horisberger M and James WPT (eds) *For a Better Nutrition in the 21st Century*, Nestlé Nutrition Workshop Series, vol. 27, pp 149–162. New York: Vevey/Raven Press.

Steen B (1988) Body composition and aging. *Nutrition Reviews* 46:45–51.

Wahlqvist ML, Hsu Hage BB-H, Kouris Blazos A and Lukito W (1995) *Food Habits in Later Life*. Tokyo and Melbourne: United Nations University Press and Asia Pacific Journal of Clinical Nutrition.

Walls AWG (1992) The ageing mouth. In: Evans JG and Williams TF (eds) *Oxford Textbook of Geriatric Medicine*, pp 179–195. New York: Oxford University Press.

Werner I and Hambraeus L (1972) The digestive capacity of elderly people. In: Carlson LA (ed.) *Nutrition in Old Age*, pp 55–60. Uppsala: Almqvist and Wilksell.

World Health Organization (1995) Adults 60 years and older. In: *WHO Expert Committee on Physical Status: The Use and Interpretation of Anthropometry*, WHO Technical Report Series 854, chap. 9, pp 375–407. Geneva: World Health Organization.

Nutritionally Related Problems

C P G M de Groot and **W A van Staveren**, Wageningen Agricultural University, Wageningen, The Netherlands

The population over the age of 55 years is increasing rapidly all over the world. In industrialized countries the proportion of elderly people will increase by about 1% per year; in developing countries an increment of about 3% per year is expected. The nutritional needs of this population will require more and more attention from professionals working in the food industry as well as in health care.

There exists an interrelationship between ageing and nutrition. Ageing is defined as all physiological changes that occur from conception until old age and the ultimate death. In this article the term is restricted to changes that occur in adulthood, when growth has stopped.

On the one hand, nutrition is considered as one of the key determinants in the process of ageing. On the other hand, age-related changes take place in bodily appearance, in the functional capacity of the body and in the body's capacity to adapt to physical stress, which affect the nutritional needs.

It is hard to distinguish between changes due to old age *per se* and changes that are the consequences of disease. **Table 1** shows factors affecting the ageing process. In this article the effects of ageing on body composition, including energy needs and problems of over- and underweight, bone mass and the water balance are discussed. Physiological functions of the digestive system, malabsorption, nutrient drug interactions and consequences for nutritional requirements are described, together with risk micronutrients and early warning signals for malnourishment.

Changes in Body Composition and Energy Needs

Fat-free mass and energy needs

Regardless of wide differences between individuals, ageing changes in body composition with time are universal, including changes in lean tissue and fat mass, body water and bone mass. Throughout middle age, body mass tends to increase owing to an accumulation of fat, preferentially intraabdominally. Thereafter – usually from the age of 65–70 years – it declines in association with loss of lean tissue. Diminution of physical activity enhances the changes in body composition occurring with ageing, which in turn affect physical function. Ultimately these processes result in a lower requirement for energy.

The total demand for energy is dominated by the energy needed per day to maintain vital functions, the basal metabolic rate (BMR), representing 60–70% of total energy expenditure. Most of the remainder (approximately 25%) is needed to cover the costs of physical activities. The BMR declines with age by up to 5% per decade. It is the fall in lean tissue with age that determines this decline. One of the most important preventive measures in this process is the maintenance of physical activity. This helps to maintain lean body mass, physical fitness and the requirement for energy.

Partly as a response to reduced energy needs, the energy intakes of affluent populations decline with age. This places an increasing number of elderly people at risk of malnutrition, as the opportunities for providing an adequate dietary nutrient intake are very limited when total food consumption becomes low (**Fig. 1**), e.g. below 6.3 MJ (1500 kcal). Current recommendations for daily energy intake are 9–11 MJ for men and 8–10 MJ for women. Institutionalized elderly people or the elderly sick are especially likely to fail to achieve such intakes. Their energy intakes should therefore be derived from a diet containing a variety of nutrient-dense foods, even though their appetite may wane. Efforts are needed to optimize food choice and the provision of nutrient-dense foods for the most vulnerable elderly people, so that they eat similar foods to those in the diets of more successful ageing people.

Table 1   Effect of ageing on nutritional outcome variables

Genetic variables	Programmed ageing	Environmental variables
Premature ageing	Structural changes and functional deficits	Diet
Disease risk		Smoking
Intelligence	Coping skills	Education
Pharmacogenetics	Adaptive responses	Drugs
Skin colour and type	Capacity of skin to synthesize vitamin D	UV exposure

Ageing diseases:
heart disease, cancer, diabetes, dementia, others

Nutritional outcome including:
nutritional requirements, nutritional
  status, requirement for special diet,
  need for food assistance

Adapted from Roe (1990).

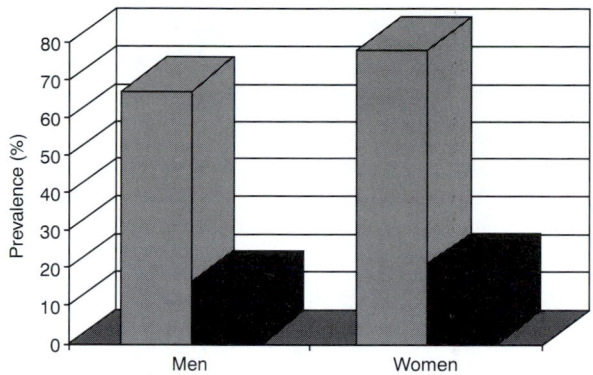

Figure 1 Prevalence of inadequate intakes of at least one nutrient among elderly people whose daily energy intake is below 6.3 MJ (shaded bar) and for those whose intake exceeds 7 MJ (solid bar). From De Groot *et al.* (1996), with permission from Macmillan Press Limited.

For health reasons it is important that elderly people avoid becoming underweight. Though losing weight may be favourable at younger ages and being overweight is a known health risk in adults, there is evidence that low body weight and loss of body weight in the elderly are more strongly associated with risk of mortality (**Fig. 2**). It is even more important to be slightly overweight than underweight for people over the age of 70 years. Therefore, except for those who are obese, elderly people should be encouraged to maintain an adequate energy intake. According to a longitudinal study among relatively healthy Europeans, 20–25% fail to do so: about 8% lost and 16% gained at least 5 kg of body weight over a period of 4 years. When appetite is reduced an increase of meal frequency may not only help to promote energy intakes but also prevents blood glucose levels from declining steeply.

Body water, dehydration and medication

As lean tissue is abundant in water there is a decrease in total body water – especially extracellular water – with advancing age, from 80% at birth to 60–70% after age 70 years. In addition, older people experience diminished sensation of thirst, and urinary concentrating ability declines as a function of age. Thus old people incur an increased risk of dehydration, particularly when diuretic or laxative medicines are used or in the presence of some diseases common in old age, such as diarrhoea, renal disease and infection with fever. As water is essential to all biological functions, fluid intakes in old age should be at least 1700 ml per day. In the body, water acts as a diluent for water-soluble drugs. Given the decrease of body water with age, old people may need lower dosages of water-soluble drugs than younger adults to achieve the desired therapeutic effect and to avoid drug toxicity.

Bone mass and nutritional factors

Throughout life bone mass changes, with a maximum (peak bone mass) achieved by age 25–30 years and bone loss occurring after the fourth decade. Higher calcium intakes in childhood and early adulthood result in a 3–8% greater bone mass later in life, thereby improving the key factor in the osteoporotic process and the age-associated risk of fractures. In women there is a perimenopausal increase in the rate of bone loss which persists after the menopause following a decline in oestrogen production (**Fig. 3**).

Factors other than age and sex that are associated with low bone mass include low body weight, smoking, alcohol consumption, reduced physical activity, low calcium absorption and secondary risk factors

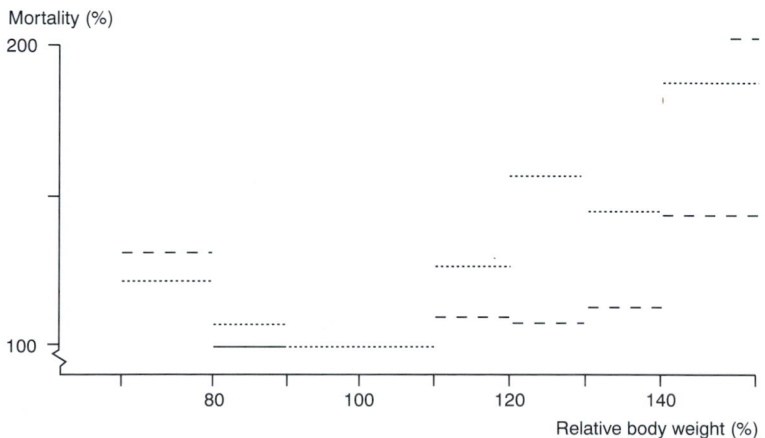

Figure 2 Mortality in relation to relative body weight in different age categories: age 30–49 years (dotted line) and age 70–89 years (dashed line). American Cancer Society Study data, from van Staveren and Deurenberg (1994).

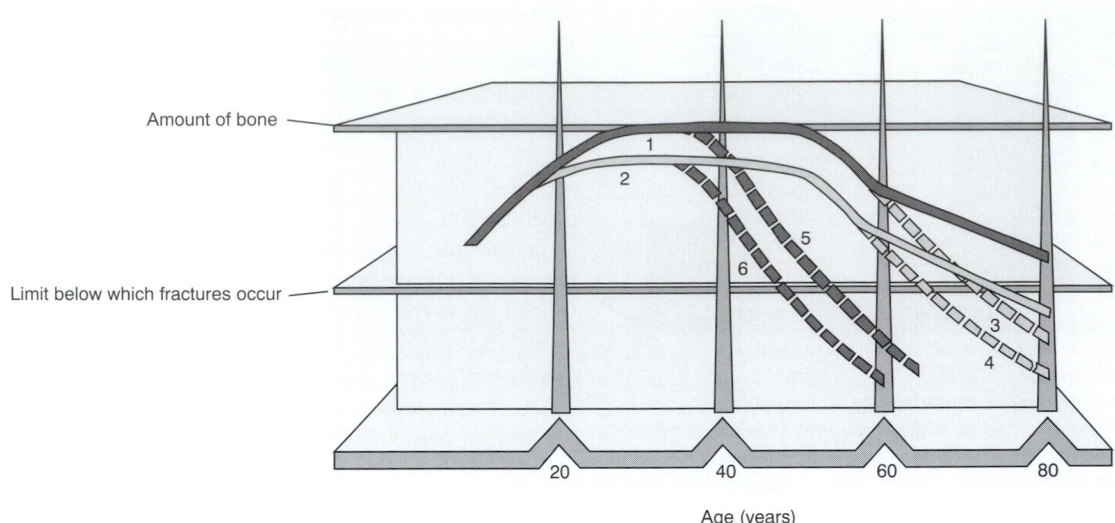

Figure 3 Rate of bone loss: 1, bone mass change in women with a high initial amount of bone and an average loss after menopause; 2, bone mass change in women with a low initial amount of bone and an average loss after menopause; 3, 4, bone mass change in women with high losses after the menopause; 5, 6, bone mass change in women with an early menopause or after surgical removal of the ovaries. First fractures occur approximately 10 years after the menopause.

such as the use of steroids. Though there is still uncertainty about the quantitative role of nutritional factors in the pathogenesis of osteoporosis, preventive measures include adequate calcium intakes (probably even in old age), and exposure to sunlight to ensure vitamin D adequacy and/or dietary supplementation with vitamin D. Restricted sunlight exposure, reduced capacity of the skin to produce vitamin D and low vitamin D intake make elderly people prone to vitamin D deficiency.

Nutritionally Related Problems and the Digestive System

The number of taste buds varies widely from person to person, but does not decline with age. Taste perception and the perceived flavour of foods decrease, but this is effected by many factors including diminishing smell, age-related changes in the olfactory system, the integration of the central nervous system, medication, oral hygiene and nutrition (**Fig. 4**).

Inadequate intakes of zinc, copper, nickel and some vitamins have been associated with decreased perception of flavour of food.

Small intestine

Transit time is not changed in the elderly; however, reduced motility of the gut in the elderly may cause stasis, with bacterial overgrowth and malabsorption. The latter also may be caused by a reduced mucosal surface due to poor oxygenation of the tips of the villi as a result of a decreased blood supply from a

low cardiac output. Decreased absorption is most frequently observed for electrolytes, lactose, vitamin D and calcium. Absorption of digested food takes place by diffusion and by active transport across membranes. Adequate fluid must be available for absorption to proceed. The dehydrated state of the aged can reduce the capacity of the gut to absorb digested food.

Colon

The mucosal and muscle layers of the colon may atrophy, resulting in weakening of the muscle wall. Reduced motility of the colon allows prolonged exposure of faeces to water absorption and drying. Reduced bulk results in further reduction of the stimulus to muscle contraction and will lead to constipation. This may be enhanced by a diet lacking dietary fibre, little physical activity and poor tone of abdominal muscles.

Liver

Liver reserves of vitamins A, D and B_{12} are unlikely to be diminished. Protein synthesis and especially the synthesis of vitamin K dependent factors are reduced. It is, however, not clear if this affects vitamin K requirements.

Nutrient and Drug Interactions

Many elderly people use drugs. In Europe, even 83% of 'apparently healthy' people aged 74–79 years use an average of two types of drugs, with antihyperten-

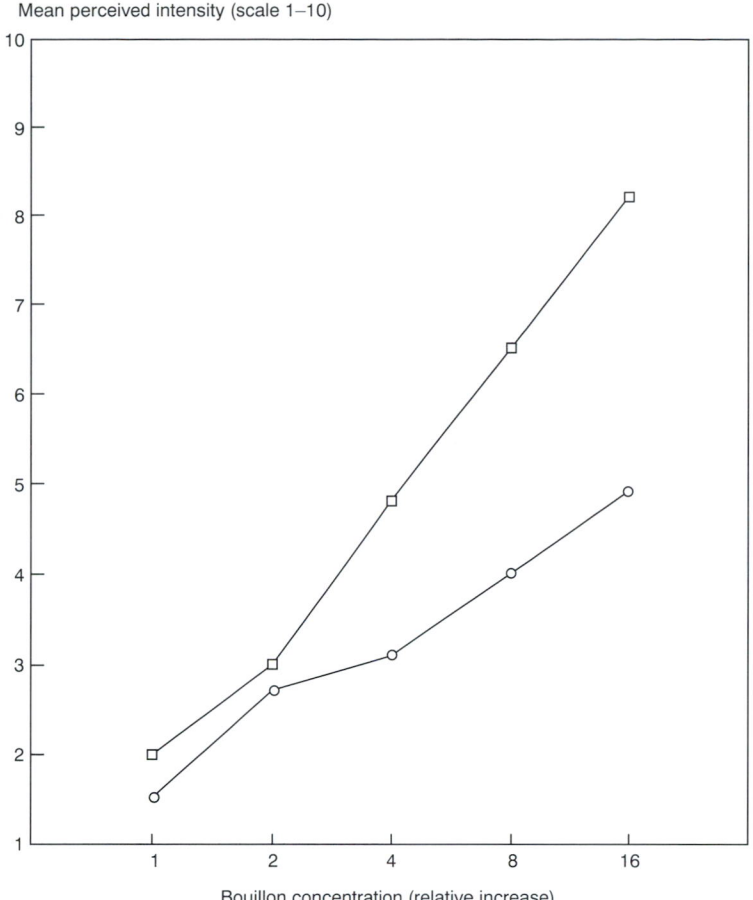

Mean perceived intensity (scale 1–10)

Bouillon concentration (relative increase)

Figure 4 Mean responses of perceived intensity of bouillon flavour, judged by a group of 23 elderly subjects (circles) and 32 young subjects (squares). From Graaf C, Polet P and van Staveren WA (1994) Sensory perception and pleasantness of food flavors in elderly subjects. *Journal of Gerontology: Psychological Sciences* 49:P93–P99.

sives (33%), analgesics (31%), diuretics (24%), sleeping pills (18%) and psychotropic drugs (17%) being taken most often. Many drugs taken by the elderly can interfere with nutritional status. The possible effects include amongst others suppression or stimulation of appetite and impaired nutrient absorption and metabolism; for example, Lis-diuretics can have adverse effects on calcium metabolism, salicylates can increase the need for vitamin C and some types of antihypertensives act as antagonists of vitamin B_6. Negative consequences of laxatives often taken by the elderly include interference with nutrient absorption. Dietary interventions may help to reduce the intake of drugs. There is evidence that moderate sodium restriction prevents or delays the development of hypertension. Also limiting alcohol intake provides protection, as about 10% of hypertension in men has been attributed to alcohol. Culinary skills become important to ensure that elderly people continue to find eating enjoyable, especially because increases in olfactory and taste thresholds occur with ageing (Fig. 4).

Risks for Malnutrition

The elderly people most at risk of developing malnutrition are those who are small eaters: because of poverty, because of disability resulting from chronic geriatric disease, or because of a combination of these factors. Malnutrition is found in elderly people living in their own homes if they are indigent, isolated or homebound because of their own disability or the serious illness of their partner. Ten main risks for noninstitutionalized elderly can easily be identified and acted upon by nonmedical personnel (**Table 2**). It must be understood that each risk mentioned in this table is only a potential danger sign; each has to be considered in relation to others. It should be stressed, however, that malnutrition is much more common in the elderly in long-term care, especially those who are unable to feed themselves.

Nutritional requirements and risk nutrients in the elderly

Nutritional requirements of the elderly and very old

Table 2 Early warning signals for malnourishment

Recent unintended weight change of about 5% or more in the preceding month

Physical disability affecting food shopping, preparation or intake

Lack of sunlight

Bereavement and/or observed depression or loneliness

Mental confusion affecting eating

High alcohol consumption

Polypharmacy or long-term medication

Poor subjective health

Missed meals, snacks or fluids

Low budget for food

Poor nutritional knowledge

may be set with different objectives. The values may serve either diagnostic or prescriptive purposes, but the ultimate goal will always be to improve the quality of life. The heterogeneity of the target population relative to needs and goals is as such that so far the nutritional requirements are largely extrapolated from those of younger populations taking age-related changes into account. Most countries do have their own set of requirements and age specificity may differ. In some countries (amongst others the Nordic countries and the Netherlands) two elderly age groups are distinguished: younger elderly people (65–75 years of age) and the older elderly (> 75 years of age). Because of ageing, environmental and life-style factors, elderly people may be at risk for an insufficient supply of a number of nutrients (**Table 3**). The values in Table 3 should be accepted cautiously, with the proviso that change may be desirable:

- when new information on nutritional needs of the elderly becomes available;
- for elderly patients who belong to particular disease groups, including mental diseases;
- for elderly people using specific drugs;
- for elderly people using specific diets that may reduce the absorption of some nutrients.

Dietary Guidelines

Dietary surveys do not indicate that dietary guidelines in the elderly should be totally different from those for younger adults. Accents in the programme, however, should be different. Nutrition education programmes for the elderly should give priority to drinking habits and to promoting the consumption

Table 3 Recommended daily allowance (RDA) and observed problems for selected food components

Component	RDA[a]	Problems
Energy (MJ)		
men	9–11	Low energy intake (<6.3 MJ per day) is highly correlated with an insufficient micronutrient supply. Immobility decreases energy requirement
women	8–10	
Protein (g kg^{-1})	0.8–1	Protein turnover may be lower than in young adults, which indicates lower requirement. However, the efficiency of protein synthesis is decreased, which increases the requirement
Vitamin A (mg RE)	0.8–1	Risk of toxicity from megadoses of vitamin A in supplements
Vitamin D (μg)		
65–75 years	2.5	Requirement increased in the oldest owing to insufficient subcutaneous synthesis with little or no exposure to UV light
>75 years	7.5–10	
Thiamin (mg)	1.1–1.4	Special attention in small eaters and elderly with alcohol addiction
Riboflavin (mg)	1.3–1.6	Those consuming few animal products may be at risk
Vitamin B$_6$ (mg)	0.9–1.1	Requirement may be higher, when using the antihypertensive drug hydralazine
Folate (μg)	200–300	Extra attention for patients with atrophic gastritis and patients using a number of medicines
Vitamin B$_{12}$ (μg)	2–2.5	Vegans and patients with atrophic gastritis have a high risk of deficiency; some drugs may interact
Vitamin C (mg)	60–70	Increased requirement for patients using salicylates. Be alert for low vitamin C supply via cooked meals from catering agencies
Calcium (mg)	800–1000	High-risk groups include elderly people using little or no milk or milk products, and patients using lisdiuretica

Table 3 Continued

Component	RDA[a]	Problems
Iron (mg)	8–10	With reduction in lean body mass, iron requirement may be decreased. However, occult blood loss (caused, for example, by salicylate intake) may increase requirement
Iodine (μg)	150–300	Supply often inadequate; in some places enriched products (salt) should be used
Water (ml)	1500–2000	Attention to fluid intake is necessary

RDA, recommended daily allowance; RE, retinol equivalent.
[a]Values recommended in the Netherlands, Scandinavia and the UK.

of foods that are good sources of calcium, zinc, magnesium, potassium, folate and vitamin B_6. Thus recommendations should focus on the importance of daily consumption of (green) vegetables, fruit, wholegrain products, milk and milk products, and should emphasize the nutritional value of lean meat, fish and legumes. As greater variety is associated with higher nutrient intakes in the elderly, the recommendation to eat a wide variety of foods is also important.

The use of dietary supplements

The few studies so far available of dietary supplementation among elderly people suggest that – as in younger adults – those elderly who need supplements do not use them, while the elderly consuming a diet with a high nutrient density do use supplements, as well. Food supplements include specially formulated preparations containing vitamins, minerals and protein, or a combination of these and other ingredients. Unnecessary use of supplements should be discouraged, because consumption of megadose levels (amounts exceeding 10 times the recommended daily allowance) of various nutrients may cause adverse health effects. There are, however, situations in which supplements have a role to play. For example, vitamin D would be indicated for the housebound elderly, and vitamin B_{12}, folate, potassium or other nutrients may be a necessary supplement in disease conditions or when certain drugs are used that influence nutrient absorption, utilization or excretion. In addition, suitable supplementation provides a means for improving the nutritional status of malnourished elderly or preventing nutritional deficiencies in people who are at risk.

See also: **Body Composition**: Determination and Physiological Significance. **Bone**: Composition, Metabolism and Bone Growth. **Colonic Diseases and Disorders**: Nutritional Management. **Dental Disease**: Aetiology and Epidemiology. **Dietary Guidelines**: International Perspectives. **Drugs**: Drug-Nutrient Interactions. **Energy**: Energy Balance. **Liver Disorders**: Nutritional Management. **Malabsorption Syndromes**: Nutritional Management. **Older People**: Nutritional Requirements; Physiological Changes; Nutritional Management of Geriatric Patients.

Further Reading

De Groot CPGM, van Staveren WA, Dirren H and Hautvast JGAJ, eds (1996) SENECA, nutrition and the elderly in Europe. Follow-up study and longitudinal analysis. *European Journal of Clinical Nutrition* 50(supplement 2):127.

Department of Health (1992) *The Nutrition of Elderly People*. Report on Health and Social Subjects 43. London: HMSO.

Expert Group Nutrition and the Elderly (1995) *Nutrition of the Elderly*. The Hague: Netherlands Food and Nutrition Council.

Hazzard WR, Bierman EL, Blass JP, Ettinger WH and Halter JB (1994) *Principles of Geriatric Medicine and Gerontology*, 2nd edn. New York: McGraw-Hill.

Horwitz A, MacFayden DM, Steen B and Williams TF (1989). *Nutrition in the Elderly*. Oxford University Press.

Roe DA (1990) Overview of effects of aging on nutrition. *Clinics in Geriatric Medicine* 6:319–334.

Sandström B, Antti A, Becker W, Lyhne N, Pedersen JI and Porsdottir I (1996) Nordiska närings-rekommedationer 1996. Nordic Council of Ministers Nord 1996: 28.

Staveren WA van and Deurenberg P (1994) Management of obesity in adult men and women in later life. In: Hills AP and Wahlqvist ML (eds) *Exercise and Obesity*, pp 195–205. London: Smith-Gordon.

Nutritional Management of Geriatric Patients

M-M G Wilson and **John E Morley**, Saint Louis University Health Sciences Center, St Louis, USA

Undernutrition

Overwhelming evidence identifies nutritional status as a prime index of disease outcomes and a major predictor of morbidity and mortality in the older population. Undernourished older persons admitted to acute care facilities have a longer duration of hospital stay. Furthermore, following discharge, early emergent readmission occurs all too frequently. Added complications of undernutrition include immune dysfunction, delayed wound healing and decreased cognitive function. Free-living older persons with suboptimal nutritional status are at increased risk of becoming dependent on care-givers as a result of compromised activities of daily living. Evidence also exists linking myopathy resulting from undernutrition with an increased incidence of gait instability and hip fractures. Yet, despite the significant negative impact of undernutrition on the functional status and quality of life of older persons, nutritional assessment and dietary management are often overlooked when health professionals evaluate the geriatric patient.

Demographic considerations emphasize the magnitude of the problem of undernutrition within the geriatric population. Reported prevalence rates in the USA of undernutrition in the older population range from 11% to 30%. Within the community-dwelling older population, which constitutes over 90% of older persons, studies have shown a prevalence of undernutrition exceeding 30%. However, data exist to show that clinical detection and appropriate intervention occur in less than one-tenth of undernourished older persons. Physicians and health professionals involved in geriatric care must remain cognizant of the fact that preservation of maximal health and function in the older person mandates routine and efficient nutritional evaluation, surveillance and management.

Diagnosis and evaluation of undernutrition

Anthropometry The clinical diagnosis of undernutrition in older persons is based solely on anthropometric indices. Diagnostic criteria are as follows:

- body weight less than 80% of the ideal body weight for height and age, *or*
- weight loss exceeding 10% of baseline weight in the preceding 6 months, *or*
- Body mass index less than 17.

The anthropometric index most frequently used in nutritional assessment is body weight. However, within the older population the usefulness of this index is hampered by the lack of age-adjusted reference values. Reference values applicable in younger adults are not suitable for use in older persons as age-related sarcopenia and a disproportionate increase in subcutaneous body fat in older adults may variably affect such norms. Using data derived from the

National Health and Nutrition Examination Survey, Frisancho established body weight norms for persons up to the age of 74 years. The use of this and other similar age-adjusted tables is mandatory to ensure accurate interpretation of weight values in older persons. Within the older population, intentional weight loss resulting from dietary restriction should not discourage comprehensive nutritional assessment, as recent evidence indicates that both voluntary and involuntary weight losses in older persons possess similar adverse health outcomes.

Calculation of the body mass index (BMI) is considered to be one of the most objective anthropometric indices, as it permits correction of body weight for height. The BMI, calculated by dividing the weight in kilograms by the height in metres squared, is based on the proven premise that weight in the younger adult increases proportionately with height squared. This concept is false in older persons as height is significantly affected by age-related changes. Loss of height with ageing occurs secondary to shortening of the axial skeleton due to age-related osteoporosis, degenerative disc changes, vertebral thinning and kyphoscoliosis. Furthermore, using height as an anthropometric index may be impractical in nonambulant and bedbound persons. Nevertheless, clinical use of the BMI in the older population has been preserved by the development of adapted nomograms. Such nomograms are based on the determination of BMI using surrogate parameters of height adopted from the appendicular skeleton, which is relatively unaffected by age-related osseous changes. These parameters include supine total arm length, arm span, erect forearm length and knee to floor height.

Skinfold thickness measurements are used as anthropometric indices of total body fat in younger adults. However, the precise relationship between skinfold thickness and total body fat remains to be determined, as does the response of subcutaneous fat to undernutrition. Furthermore, in the older adult, the accuracy of this technique is hampered by unpredictable age-related qualitative and quantitative changes in body fat. Altered compressibility of body fat has also been shown to occur with ageing, rendering skinfold thickness measurements unreliable for use in older adults. Measurement of mid-arm circumference is another frequently used anthropometric index. However, several factors influence muscle bulk including exercise, disease and genetic factors. In the older person this index is of doubtful clinical utility.

It is evident that several factors confound the use of anthropometric indices, underscoring the importance of serial measurements. These allow for quantification of response to intervention and also enhance accuracy of data interpretation by utilizing intrasubject comparison. More accurate methods of body composition analysis are available but are unlikely to be suitable for routine clinical use. These include computerized tomography, bioelectrical impedance, nuclear magnetic resonance imaging, *in vivo* neutron activation analysis and dual energy X ray absorptiometry (DEXA). Because of alterations in body water with ageing, the value of bioelectrical impedance is questionable. The DEXA technique is excellent but the migration of body fat to the abdomen with ageing has been suggested to result in an underestimation of body fat in older persons. Currently, these methods are used almost exclusively for research purposes; in both cross-sectional and longitudinal studies they have shown an increase in body fat by 40–60 years of age with a decline in body fat in those aged over 70 years.

Biochemistry Hypoalbuminaemia is often considered indicative of undernutrition in older persons. However, the diagnostic specificity of this index is poor. Serum albumin levels are determined by the interplay between nutritional intake, total body albumin distribution and several pathological changes which alter the biosynthetic and catabolic rates of albumin. In the acutely ill or stressed older person, cytokine release has been shown to suppress the synthesis of albumin and prealbumin. Additionally, the release of counterregulatory hormones in stressful situations reduces serum albumin levels by suppressing albumin synthesis and increasing catabolism. Direct downregulation of albumin gene expression has also been shown to occur in situations of acute stress. Paradoxically, undernutrition itself may result in a compensatory reduction in albumin catabolism, yielding inappropriately high albumin levels. Although these multiple confounding factors detract from the predictive value of albumin as a diagnostic index, sufficient evidence exists in support of the negative impact of hypoalbuminaemia on the health status of the older person. In free-living older persons studies have identified a positive correlation between serum albumin levels and functional status. Convincing evidence also exists linking hypoalbuminaemia to increased morbidity and mortality in community-dwelling and institutionalized older persons. In the light of current evidence, hypoalbuminaemia is best utilized as a marker that identifies a high-risk subset of older persons in whom early and aggressive nutritional intervention is crucial.

Several other biochemical indices can be used as nutritional markers. Major disadvantages of most of these indices, including serum albumin, include poor diagnostic specificity and relatively long half-lives which limit their use in the diagnosis and serial evaluation of undernutrition. Insulin-like growth factor I is considered to have the greatest positive predictive value as it has been shown to correlate well with nutritional status even during periods of acute stress. Added advantages of this index are a relatively short half-life of 2–6 h and a rapid response to fasting and refeeding. However, routine use of this assay in the evaluation of undernutrition will probably be precluded by cost. Serum albumin assays are undoubtedly the most cost-effective and readily accessible investigation. It is doubtful that the use of other biochemical markers will be of added benefit.

Haematology Normochromic, normocytic anaemia resulting directly from undernutrition is a recognized clinical entity. Studies have identified reduced erythropoiesis and alterations of erythrocyte function in undernourished persons which respond to nutritional repletion. Iron and folate deficiency anaemias may also result from inadequate micronutrient intake in undernourished persons.

Measurement of the total lymphocyte count (TLC) is helpful in the diagnosis and stratification of undernutrition according to severity. A TLC less than 1200×10^6 l^{-1} indicates mild undernutrition while counts less than 800×10^6 l^{-1} are usually found in severely undernourished persons.

Recognizing causative factors of undernutrition

Physiological anorexia of ageing, a well-documented clinical occurrence, predisposes the older person to undernutrition. Several factors have been implicated in the genesis of this phenomenon. Evidence suggests that the decrease in lean body mass, energy expenditure and metabolic rate that occur with advancing age may partially account for the reduction of food intake in healthy older persons. The reduction in the sensitivity of olfactory and gustatory receptors with ageing may compromise the hedonic qualities of meals, further reducing the desire to eat. Age-related alterations in hormonal and neurotransmitter-mediated function may also play a role in suppressing food intake. Animal studies suggest that ageing results in a reduction in the opioid feeding drive and an increase in the satiating effect of cholecystokinin. This may lead to the ingestion of smaller meals and prolonged periods of satiety between meals.

The occurrence of a variety of pathological factors superimposed on the background of age-related physiological changes may further compromise nutritional status in the older adult (**Table 1**). Existing data suggest that as many as one-third of

Table 1 Common and uncommon causes of undernutrition in older persons

Reduced food intake
Ill-fitting dentures
Periodontal disease
Oropharyngeal disease
Orofacial dyskinesias

Psychosocial factors
Depression
Eating disorders
Bereavement
Social isolation
Low financial income

Physical/mental disability
Persistent tremors
Dyskinesia/dyspraxia
Arthritides
Parkinsonism
Cerebrovascular disease
Dementia
Behavioural disorders

Increased nutrient metabolism
Hyperthyroidism
Phaeochromocytoma
Wandering, agitation
Movement disorders
Hemiballismus

Reduced nutrient utilization
Malabsorption syndrome
Chronic inflammatory bowel disease
Gluten enteropathy

Gastrooesophageal disease
Inflammatory
Neoplastic
Dysmotility

Multifactorial
Chronic bronchitis, emphysema
Cardiac failure
Malignant disease
Substance abuse

undernourished older persons suffer from untreated depression. The predominance of neurovegetative symptoms in depressed older persons often results in anorexia, social withdrawal, reduced motivation and decreased activity, all of which can compromise nutritional intake. The use of appropriate antidepressants very often reverses these symptoms, resulting in an increase in food intake and restoration of adequate nutritional status. Nonetheless, the choice of antidepressants is crucial in the management of depressed, older undernourished persons. The popularity of selective serotonin reuptake inhibitors in younger persons has led to their increasing use in the older population. However, in older persons the efficacy of such agents in improving mood may be marred by adverse gastrointestinal effects and weight loss which subsequently compromise nutritional status. Thus, where such agents are used, careful monitoring of nutritional status is mandatory. Electroconvulsive therapy is a viable option in anorexic depressed persons, as evidence exists in support of the efficacy of this treatment in restoring appetite following failure of pharmacological agents.

Minor dysphoric changes may also adversely affect nutritional status and necessitate intervention. Over 30% of older community-dwelling persons live alone, usually as a result of bereavement or migration of younger family members. Meals are often eaten alone and the lack of social interaction during meal preparation and consumption can compromise the social, recreational and hedonic aspects of dining. Consequently, this reduces the motivation to prepare and eat meals. Thus, particular attention should be paid to the recreational aspects of mealtimes, and older persons should be encouraged to socialize during meals. This can be accomplished in a variety of ways. Participation in dining clubs, where available, should be encouraged. Arrangements can also be made for older persons to attend and partake in meals at senior citizens' centres. Ambulant senior citizens should be encouraged to dine out, if this is preferred.

Effective nutritional intervention mandates due consideration of financial and socioeconomic factors. Approximately one-third of the older population live below the poverty line and may experience difficulty with the purchase of food items necessary to ensure a balanced diet. Inadequate transportation, limited mobility and poorly accessible shopping facilities may be added limiting factors. The services of social and community agencies should be employed where such considerations are relevant, and an attempt should be made to provide appropriate assistance.

A wide variety of prescribed drugs can cause anorexia, nausea and other symptoms of gastrointestinal distress in older persons, rendering medication review an important component of nutritional management. Digoxin, theophylline and nonsteroidal antiinflammatory agents are frequent culprits in this regard. Enquiry must also be made into the use and tolerance of self-prescribed medication. Offending drugs, once identified, must be discontinued. Iatrogenesis also contributes to undernutrition by way of therapeutic diets. Low-cholesterol and low-salt diets are often prescribed to older persons on the basis of data extrapolated from younger persons. There is currently little evidence to suggest that these diets are of any benefit to older persons when used as primary prevention strategies. The use of such diets in older persons should be discouraged, as they often reduce palatability and consequently discourage food intake. Health professionals should also enquire regarding self-prescribed diets. Studies indicate that the older population is more susceptible to food fads and advertised commercial diets that are often unbalanced and of dubious benefit. Prolonged ingestion of such diets can result in marked undernutrition.

A wide variety of medical illnesses require focused therapeutic intervention in order to maintain or restore adequate nutritional status. Degenerative and neurological disease can significantly impair mobility and physical function. The use of adapted appliances and cutlery in such situations may serve to improve manual dexterity and preserve the ability to self-feed. In older persons with severely impaired function, who are unable to cook, meal delivery services ('meals on wheels') may be an acceptable alternative to home-cooked meals. Tooth loss is a well-recognized risk factor for undernutrition. Periodontal disease and edentulism are highly prevalent among the geriatric population and can impair masticatory ability. Older persons who have lost teeth, experience pain on mastication or receive inadequate dental care should be carefully screened and offered appropriate therapy. The use of dentures may improve food intake. However, where dentures are poorly tolerated, alteration in the consistency of meals is helpful. Dysphagia occurs commonly in older persons with degenerative and vascular neurological conditions such as dementia, parkinsonism and cerebrovascular disease. A bedside swallowing evaluation should be an integral component of nutritional evaluation, followed by a modified barium swallow with fluoroscopy in cases where significant dysphagia is identified. In most cases oral food intake will remain possible, with appropriate modifications regarding swallowing technique, feeding precautions and food consistency.

Health professionals often wrongly assume that older persons possess adequate knowledge of basic dietetic practice and nutritional attitudes. There is evidence to suggest that the nutritional attitudes and knowledge of undernourished older persons may be inadequate, particularly with regard to food preparation. Dietary education and counselling are crucial components of nutritional intervention in undernourished older persons who retain the responsibility for preparing their own meals. Such counselling should be targeted towards identifying deficits in basic dietary knowledge and the correction of poor nutritional practices.

Nutritional assessment tools

An array of nutritional screening tools have been developed to facilitate the identification of older persons at risk for undernutrition. The Nutrition Screening Initiative (NSI) in the USA stemmed from a collaborative effort between family physicians, dietitians and the National Council of Aging. This is a three-tiered tool formulated to assist in the detection of older persons at risk for nutritional compromise and subsequent direction of such persons toward the appropriate level of care. The first level of screening is designed to be initiated by the patient or primary care-giver. Persons identified to have an increased risk of undernutrition are then referred for evaluation by health-care or social services personnel. This constitutes the second level of screening. The identification of factors that may warrant medical intervention will prompt referral to a physician for further evaluation. The NSI is of proven value as an epidemiological tool and serves to increase the awareness of patients and care-givers to undernutrition. However, its usefulness within orthodox settings may be hampered by the number of personnel and services required, which may constitute a significant drain on available resources. Added drawbacks to the use of this tool for the individual patient are the lack of professional supervision at initiation and reliance on patient compliance in adhering to the specified clinical pathway protocol.

The Mini Nutritional Assessment (MNA) is a comprehensive and simple tool designed to evaluate the nutritional status of older persons. This is the first well-validated nutritional screening instrument and is recommended for use in people aged over 75 years. Cross-validation indicates that nutritional assessment using this tool will accurately evaluate and categorize nutritional status in about 75% of older persons without the need for further biochemical tests or clinical assessment. The MNA scoring system permits the stratification of older adults into three categories: well-nourished, at risk of undernutrition, and undernourished. An advantage of the MNA is that it can easily be used by a wide range of health professionals, in a variety of clinical settings which cater for both free-living and institutionalized older persons. Several other tools are of practical value in the clinical setting. Morley has developed a useful screening tool known by the acronym SCALES (**Table 2**). This uses basic biochemical and anthropometric indices to identify older adults at risk of undernutrition, and can be readily incorporated into serial evaluation of the older person in different clinical settings. The simple mnemonic 'MEALS ON WHEELS', also devised by Morley, may prove useful in prompting consideration of the risk factors and common causes of nutritional compromise (**Table 3**).

Table 2 SCALES: screening tool for the early detection of patients at risk of protein–energy undernutrition. Patients scoring over 3 are at risk

Parameter	Score 1 point	Score 2 points
Sadness	GDS 10–15	GDS > 15
Cholesterol	<4.65 mmol l^{-1} (180 mg dl^{-1})	<4.14 mmol l^{-1} (160 mg dl^{-1})
Albumin	<40 g l^{-1} (4 g dl^{-1})	<35 g l^{-1} (3.5 g dl^{-1})
Loss of weight	<1 kg (2 lb) in 1 month	>2.7 kg (6 lb) in 6 months
Eating problems	Cognitive impairment or physical limitations	Cognitive impairment and physical limitations
Shopping problems	Inability to shop or prepare a meal	

GDS, geriatric depression score.

Table 3 MEALS ON WHEELS: common causes of undernutrition in older persons

Medication (e.g. digoxin, theophylline, psychotropic drugs)
Emotional (depression)
Anorexia, alcoholism
Late-life paranoia
Swallowing disorders

Oral and dental disease
No money (absolute or relative poverty)

Wandering (dementia, behavioural disorders)
Hyperthryoidism, hyperparathyroidism
Entry problems (malabsorption)
Eating problems
Low-salt or low-cholesterol diets
Shopping and food preparation problems

Oral nutritional repletion

Appropriate treatment of the underlying causes of undernutrition should be accompanied by oral nutritional supplementation in persons who are able to eat. Objective quantitative baseline assessment of food intake is mandatory. This is best achieved by the maintenance of a food diary, in which the patient records all food items consumed as meals or snacks over a 72 h period. Review of the food diary also permits evaluation of food preferences and eating patterns. The goal of nutritional supplementation should be the consumption of the recommended daily allowance of macronutrients and micronutrients. Several predictive equations have been derived for the purpose of determining the optimal energy intake for each individual. However, it remains unclear as to what extent corrections have been made for age-related physiological changes in nutritional requirements and energy expenditure. The Benedict–Harris equation is perhaps the best known and most frequently applied. Using this equation, the required daily energy intake in kcal is derived as follows:

- Men: $66 + 13.7W + 5H - 6.8A$
- Women: $665 + 9.6W + 1.8H - 4.7A$

where W is the weight in kg, H is the height in cm and A is the age in years. Upward adjustment is required by factors ranging from 1 to 1.5, to compensate for increased activity or pathologically stressful conditions.

For practical clinical purposes, a total daily energy intake of 147 kJ kg^{-1} (35 kcal kg^{-1}) achieves efficient nutritional repletion. It is recommended that carbohydrates constitute 50–60% of the total energy intake. Dietary fat should be limited to less than 30% of the total energy intake, with saturated fat constituting less than 10%. The current recommended daily allowance for protein is at least 1 g kg^{-1} body weight. Acutely stressful or hypercatabolic conditions necessitate an increase in protein intake to about 1.5 g kg^{-1}. Generally, compliance with these dietary guidelines achieves the dual purpose of ensuring optimal macronutrient and micronutrient intake. This obviates the need for the routine prescription of pharmacological multivitamin preparations in undernourished persons, unless specific signs of vitamin deficiency are clinically evident.

Nutritional supplementation with regular or fortified natural food items is the preferred mode of nutritional repletion. This possesses the advantages of familiarity, palatability and cost-effectiveness. Where the patient is reluctant or unable to consume the required total energy intake in natural food items, commercially formulated nutritional supplements are a reasonable alternative. The choice of preparation can be based on palatability and patient preference unless underlying medical conditions such as lactose or gluten intolerance have to be considered. Patients with malabsorption syndromes should be given hydrolysed preparations to enhance nutrient absorption. Regardless of the preparation used, an attempt should be made to vary flavours, as age-related sensory specific satiety may limit intake if only one flavour is used. The optimal timing for the administration of nutritional supplements remains to be firmly established. Such supplements are often administered with meals, but evidence suggests that liquid supplements administered at least 1 h before meals serve to enhance subsequent energy intake. When such supplements are administered with meals, a suppressant effect on food consumption is evident. Ultimately, in persons with severe undernutrition, the focus should be on energy intake and patient food preference, not on optimal proportions of macronutrient and micronutrient intake. Frequently, efforts to ensure a balanced diet necessitate the use of food items which may compromise palatability and result in a counterproductive reduction in food intake.

Enteral tube feeding

Enteral or parenteral modes of nutrient delivery may be needed in people who are unable to eat or swallow. However, in the presence of a functioning gastrointestinal tract, enteral tube feeding is preferred as it is associated with a lower incidence of complications, more efficient nutrient utilization, increased cost-effectiveness and greater ease of administration. Additionally, small bowel hypoplasia and alterations in gastrointestinal secretions have been shown to result from prolonged parenteral nutrition. Nasogastric and nasoenteric tubes are best reserved for short-term support in persons who may be able to resume oral feeding within 14 days, in order to avoid the significant morbidity associated with the use of nasal tubes. In persons in whom prolonged enteral intake is anticipated, gastrostomy or jejunostomy tubes are indicated.

In patients who retain normal gastrointestinal absorptive function, regular meals may be puréed and delivered through large-bore feeding tubes. A variety of polymeric enteral feeding formulae are also available; these are of relatively low viscosity, rendering them particularly suitable for delivery through small-bore tubes, which are usually more comfortable and aesthetically pleasing. In persons with malabsorption, hydrolysed predigested formulae are available. Specific formulations also exist for people with special nutritional requirements owing to underlying disease such as diabetes mellitus or renal or respiratory failure.

In older people, bolus tube feedings are associated with an increased risk of aspiration. Thus, where possible, continuous infusions of feeds are preferred. In order to further reduce the risk of aspiration pneumonia, it is recommended that the patient is positioned in a 30° head-up incline during feedings. Feeds may be infused over a 24 h period or over 14–18 h with a nocturnal break. The latter infusion schedule is often advocated on the grounds that it mimics normal eating patterns more closely. In addition, the absence of a nocturnal feed-free period

has been shown to obliterate the physiological diurnal variation in insulin, cortisol and glucagon secretion. Maximal nutrient utilization is also encouraged by daytime feed infusions as gastric emptying occurs more rapidly during the day. Continuous infusion of enteral tube feeds should be initiated at a rate of 30 ml h^{-1} using half-strength feeds. If tolerated, full-strength feeds may then be introduced at the same rate and increased by 25 ml h^{-1} every 8–12 h until the recommended daily energy intake is achieved.

Parenteral nutritional repletion

In the older person with a nonfunctioning gastrointestinal tract, parenteral nutrition may be unavoidable. All patients receiving parenteral nutrition must be monitored closely for adverse effects. For short-term intravenous nutritional repletion, peripheral parenteral nutrition may be employed. Low osmolality nutritional preparations, with a low risk of toxicity to soft tissue, are best suited for this purpose. There is a paucity of data regarding the safety and efficacy of most peripheral parenteral nutritional products for periods exceeding 14 days. Thus, where longer periods of intravenous feeding are required, total parenteral nutrition through a large central vein is indicated. Standard total parenteral formulations comprising 25% dextrose, 5% amino acids, electrolytes and trace elements in optimal amounts are suitable for use in most patients. During prolonged parenteral nutrition, lipid emulsion supplements should be added to prevent deficiency of essential fatty acids.

Pharmacological management of undernutrition

A number of anabolic growth factors are currently being investigated as possible pharmacological adjuncts in the management of undernutrition. Age-related anorexia, sarcopenia and osteopenia have been linked with growth hormone deficiency. The administration of human growth hormone to healthy older adults has been shown to increase muscle bulk. However, significant side effects such as carpal tunnel syndrome, gynaecomastia and hypoglycaemia were noted; furthermore, the increase in muscle bulk failed to produce a parallel increase in muscle strength. However, evidence suggests that when growth hormone is administered to older people with severe undernutrition over a short period there may be a significant increase in weight and appetite without notable adverse effects. Nonetheless, the lack of data regarding the safety and efficacy of growth hormone administration precludes routine clinical use. The role of IGF-I in the management of undernutrition is currently under investigation.

Available studies suggest that exogenously administered IGF-I may enhance nitrogen retention, gluconeogenesis and maintenance of normal gastro-intestinal function.

There is a profusion of studies regarding the role of anabolic steroids in the management of undernu-trition. However, the clinical applicability, efficacy and risk–benefit profile of anabolic steroids in the treatment of undernourished older people remains poorly defined. The use of testosterone in hypogona-dal undernourished men seems reasonable, and oxandrolone has proved useful in some women with anorexia, when used for short periods. Several other drugs are available, although these are often reserved for the treatment of undernourished younger adults with chronic wasting illnesses; they include cortico-steroids, cannabinoids, cyproheptadine, and meges-trol acetate. As a general rule, the use of pharmaco-logical agents in the management of undernutrition in older persons is actively discouraged, as currently the therapeutic efficacy and safety of most of these agents in older persons remains unclear.

Managing undernutrition in the community setting

With the increasing emphasis on home health care, there will be an inevitable rise in the number of com-munity-dwelling persons requiring alternative modes of feeding. Special consideration and appropriate modification of therapeutic regimens may be required in such cases to ease the care-giver or per-sonal burden.

If enteral tube feeding is provided at home, con-tinuous infusion may limit the patient's mobility and functional independence. This method also has the disadvantage of requiring immediate access to tech-nical support, in the event of mechanical failure of the infusion pump. Thus, care-givers and patients may find intermittent bolus feeding a more con-venient and less daunting task. To minimize the aspiration risk, intermittent bolus feeds should be administered, where possible, with the patient in a seated position. Patients should also be encouraged to remain seated for at least 1 h after feeds. Some active older people may resent the social incon-venience and embarrassment of tube feeding during daytime hours, and may prefer overnight enteral infusions of hypercaloric feeds. Hypercaloric feeds contain twice the amount of equal volumes of reg-ular enteral feeds, thereby permitting the provision of adequate nutritional support over shorter periods.

Parenteral nutrition within the home is fraught with all the hazards of intravenous therapy. The availability of skilled services to monitor such ther-apy is crucial. Additionally, adequate care-giver and social support is mandatory for candidates for this mode of nutritional repletion at home.

Physicians and health-care professionals involved in home delivery of enteral and parenteral nutritional therapy will need to develop and implement compre-hensive therapeutic programmes incorporating skilled nursing and dietary services to ensure safe and effective treatment.

Managing undernutrition in long-term care institutions

Therapeutic strategies for managing undernourished institutionalized older adults are similar to those used within the community, although owing to read-ily available medical supervision, enteral and par-enteral modes of feeding are used more often. The comparatively formal structure of the nursing home environment has the added advantage of encour-aging closer supervision of therapy and stricter nutritional surveillance.

A major drawback to oral nutritional repletion in institutionalized older persons is the restricted var-iety of meals. This can usually be circumvented by involving the residents in menu development and, where feasible, granting permission for meals of the residents' choice to be supplied by family or friends. Residents of nursing homes are often less functional than their peers and thus may be more dependent on assistance for their basic activities of daily living. When the ability to self-feed is compromised, it is imperative that all meals are supervised and assist-ance with feeding rendered where necessary. Many residents are persistent wanderers, and may expend a considerable amount of energy in this exercise. In such patients an appropriate increase in their daily energy intake is required to prevent weight loss. Simi-lar adjustments may be required for residents with persistent involuntary movements or severe agi-tation.

It is essential for institutions to preserve the social and recreational aspects of meals; all too often, meal-times are reduced to clinical, sanitized and isolated events. Within the nursing home environment meal-times are best managed as a component of rec-reational therapy. Socialization and the preservation of each resident's dignity should be encouraged dur-ing meals. Nursing facilities should also attempt to mimic community resources by making food items available outside scheduled mealtimes, from vending machines and snack carts.

Nutritional surveillance programmes are crucial to the success of established intervention strategies within nursing homes. Quality indicators, preferably employing anthropometric indices, should be defined and used to monitor the success of intervention strategies. Continuous quality improvement and total quality management programmes must also be implemented as critical components of effective nutritional intervention strategies. Finally, the development of nutrition focus groups and the use of interdisciplinary intervention strategies directed at increasing nutritional intake and preventing undernutrition should be encouraged.

Micronutrient Deficiency

In older people at risk of nutritional compromise, micronutrient supplementation deserves special attention, in order to forestall the development of micronutrient deficiency (**Table 4**). The clinical features of established vitamin deficiency are well recognized. The first recourse in the management of micronutrient deficiency states should be the provision of a well-balanced diet. In the presence of a functioning gastrointestinal tract, an adequate diet containing the recommended daily allowance of each micronutrient effectively prevents and corrects deficiency states. However, the failure to consume the required amount of food may warrant the use of oral pharmacological micronutrient supplements. Vitamin B_{12} deficiency may be considered unique in this regard as, traditionally, replacement therapy has been administered parenterally. Most cases of vitamin B_{12} deficiency occur as a complication of atrophic gastritis, which may reduce the secretion of intrinsic factor, acid and pepsin, and may encourage bacterial overgrowth in the proximal small intestine. However, studies indicate that in many cases ileal function is maintained and intrinsic factor may be present in normal quantities. Thus, it is likely that in some persons repletion may be adequately achieved by oral vitamin B_{12} replacement therapy. The simul-

taneous administration of acid-pepsin preparations and tetracycline preparations to combat bacterial overgrowth, where appropriate, may enhance repletion. Up to 5% of persons aged 80 years or older have vitamin B_{12} deficiency, and it is more common in persons with Alzheimer's disease.

There is a rising trend toward dietary supplementation with pharmaceutical preparations containing large doses of vitamins and minerals, based on conclusions drawn from the results of several studies. Evidence derived from human and animal studies indicates that antioxidant micronutrients, mainly vitamins A, C and E, play a role in boosting immunity and preventing or retarding the progression of several degenerative diseases. The reduction in the incidence of malignant neoplastic disease and atherosclerosis has received significant attention. Vitamins E and C have also been shown to reduce low-density lipoprotein (LDL) cholesterol levels and increase high-density lipoprotein (HDL) levels, in addition to lowering fasting plasma insulin levels and improving insulin efficiency. Two eye diseases in older persons – age-related macular degeneration and cataracts – are believed to be amenable to nutrient manipulation. Epidemiological studies have suggested a protective role for antioxidants such as vitamin C, vitamin E, β-carotene and glutathione in macular degeneration. Zinc supplementation may retard the rate of progression of age-related macular degeneration. Cataracts are less common in persons who eat 3.5 or more servings of fruits or vegetables a day. Dietary intake of vitamin E, vitamin C, riboflavin and carotene are also associated with reduced cataract formation. One study found that the risk of cataracts was lowest in spinach consumers (carotene) and those consuming rich animal sources of vitamin A, but not in those consuming vitamin supplements. In the older adult,

Table 4   Vitamins: recommended daily allowances (RDA) and clinical features of deficiency states

	RDA	Deficiency states
Vitamin A	600–700 μg	Decreased immunity to infections, xerophthalmia, night blindness
Niacin	12–16 mg	Pellagra (dermatitis, dementia, diarrhoea), glossitis, cheilosis
Pyridoxine	1.6–2 mg	Dermatitis, delirium, peripheral neuropathy, glossitis
Riboflavin	1.1–1.3 mg	Glossitis, cheilosis, normochromic anaemia
Thiamin	0.8–0.9 mg	Beriberi, Wernicke's encephalopathy, Korsakoff's psychosis
Cyanocobalamin	5 μg	Megaloblastic anaemia, optic atrophy, peripheral neuropathy, subacute combined degeneration of the cord, dementia
Ascorbic acid	40 mg	Hyperkeratosis, petechial haemorrhages, mucosal bleeding, lethargy
Vitamin D	10 μg	Osteomalacia, osteoporosis
Vitamin E	8–10 mg	Peripheral neuropathy, ataxia, haemolytic anaemia
Folate	200 μg	Megaloblastic anaemia, cognitive dysfunction
Vitamin K	65–80 mg	Spontaneous haemorrhage, hypothrombinaemia

NE, niacin equivalent; RE, retinol equivalent.

reduced cutaneous synthesis and enteric absorption of vitamin D increase the risk of vitamin D deficiency. Decreased renal responsiveness to parathormone is an added risk factor. It has been demonstrated that at least 500 per day of vitamin D are required to prevent significant osteoporosis in postmenopausal women. This assumes greater significance in institutionalized patients who may have reduced exposure to sunlight and consequently a marked reduction in vitamin D cutaneous synthesis. The role of calcium supplementation in the retardation of osteoporosis is also well recognized. There is also some evidence to suggest that inadequate dietary calcium consumption may play a role in the genesis of colorectal cancer and hypertension.

Currently, the safety of large pharmacological doses of micronutrient supplements in humans remain to be established. In spite of this, a considerable proportion of the older population consume large doses of these supplements as a primary preventive health measure. The risk of long-term supplementation with high doses of micronutrients, particularly in the presence of age-related changes, cannot be ignored, and few studies have addressed this issue specifically. Due caution must be exercised, even with the use of micronutrients such as vitamin D and calcium where clinical benefits have been clearly established. The complications of overenthusiastic calcium and vitamin D supplementation include hypercalcaemia, nephrocalcinosis, milk-alkali syndrome, ectopic calcification and rebound gastric acidity. Calcium supplementation may also chelate iron compounds and precipitate iron deficiency. With regard to vitamin A, available data have identified an increase in absorption and reduced peripheral clearance of this vitamin in older adults, therapy increasing the risk of vitamin A toxicity. Similarly, older persons on long-term iron therapy, particularly in the absence of proven iron deficiency, are at increased risk for the development of secondary haemochromatosis.

On the basis of existing evidence, the use of pharmacological doses of vitamin and mineral supplements is probably best restricted to low-potency supplements and reserved for persons with established micronutrient deficiency who are unable to eat an adequate diet. Close monitoring of such patients for adverse effects is mandatory.

Obesity

Men aged 60–69 years have the highest prevalence of overweight for males in the USA (42.2%). Prevalence of overweight then declines to 18% in those over 80 years of age. In women, the peak age for being overweight is 50–59 years (52%) with a progressive decline in being overweight over the next three decades to 26.2% in those over 80 years of age. In men over 60 years of age, Mexican-Americans have the highest prevalence of obesity, while in women African-American women have a higher prevalence of obesity. From 1960 to 1991 the prevalence of overweight increased in men over 60 years from 23% to 60.9% while women over 60 years showed a slight decline from 45.6% to 41.3%.

With ageing there is increasing upper and central body fat distribution. This trend is accelerated in women following menopause. In women aged 55–69 years central obesity has been demonstrated to be correlated with greater coronary artery disease mortality as well as total mortality. Even with weight loss, the waist to hip ratio remained an important predictor of mortality in old women.

Leptin is a hormone produced by fat cells. In women, leptin levels rise in middle age in concert with the increase in fat mass and then fall in late old age as fat mass declines. In men, leptin levels increase progressively from 65 years onwards. This is related to the fall in testosterone levels that occurs with ageing. In old men testosterone therapy decreased leptin levels.

As food intake declines with ageing, obesity in old age must be predominantly due to other factors. All three components of energy output – resting metabolic rate, thermic energy of feeding and physical activity – decline with ageing; thus the pathogenesis of obesity in old age appears to be predominantly due to altered energy output rather than to increased food intake.

While moderate degrees of overweight appear to confer minimal increased mortality in the older population, those above 130% of average body weight have an increased risk of death even at extreme ages. Most of the complications of obesity in older persons are similar to those seen in younger persons. Certain effects of obesity appear more commonly in older persons; for instance, functional decline is more common compared with younger persons. This is often associated with a 'fear of falling'. This syndrome is particularly common in older African-American women. The prevalence of diabetes mellitus increases with age, due in part to the increased fat mass in middle age onwards. Obesity markedly increases the prevalence of sleep apnoea in older persons. Overweight increases the rate of progression of osteoarthritis and its effects on function. In nursing homes obesity has been associated with an increase in pressure ulcers. Increasing weight decreases claudication distance in older persons with peripheral vascular disease.

Management of obesity in older persons usually should not be aggressive; surgery for obesity is not appropriate, and the use of thermogenic and anorexic agents should be avoided. A combination of exercise, diet and behaviour modification is the cornerstone of therapy, as is the case in younger persons. Old people need to be carefully monitored for the development of hypoalbuminaemia, and in all cases it is prudent to prescribe a multivitamin supplement.

See also: **Antioxidants**: Diet and Antioxidant Defence. **Body Composition**: Determination and Physiological Significance. **Nutritional Status**: Anthropometric Assessment. **Nutritional Support**: Enteral Feeding; Parenteral Nutrition. **Obesity**: Definition, Aetiology and Assessment.

Further Reading

Ciocon JO (1988) Tube feeding in elderly patients: indications, benefits and complications. *Archives of Internal Medicine* 148:429–433.

Dwyer JT, Gallo JJ and Reichel W (1993) Assessing nutritional status in elderly patients. *Am Fam Physician* 47:613.

Fleck A (1989) Clinical and nutritional aspects of changes in acute phase proteins during inflammation. Proceedings of the Nutrition Society. *Nutrition* 48(3):347–354.

Frisancho AR (1984) New standards of weight and body composition by frame size and height for assessment of nutritional status of adults and the elderly. *American Journal of Clinical Nutrition* 40(4):808–819.

Guigoz Y, Vellas B and Garry PJ (1994) Mini Nutritional Assessment: a practical assessment tool for grading the nutritional state of elderly patients. *Facts and Research in Gerontology* (supplement 2):15–59.

Heymsfield SB, Tighe A and Wang Z (1994) Nutritional assessment by anthropometric and biochemical methods. In: Shils ME, Olson JA and Shike M (eds) *Modern Nutrition in Health and Disease*, pp 812–841. Philadelphia: Lea & Febiger.

Kudsk KA and Minard G (1994) Enteral nutrition. In: Zaloga GP (ed.) *Nutrition in Critical Care*, pp 331–360. St Louis: Mosby Yearbook.

Lindpainter K (1995) Finding an obesity gene: a tale of mice and men. *New England Journal of Medicine* 332:679.

National Research Council (1989) *Recommended Dietary Allowances*, 10th edn. Washington, DC: National Academy of Sciences.

Posner BM, Jeffe AM, Smith KW and Miller DR (1993) Nutrition and health risks in the elderly: the Nutrition Screening Initiative. *American Journal of Public Health* 83(7):972–978.

Wilson MMG and Morley JE (1995) The diagnosis and management of protein energy undernutrition in older persons. *Annual Review of Gerontology and Geriatrics* 15:111–142.

Osteomalacia *see* **Cholecalciferol and Ergocalciferol**: Rickets and Osteomalacia.

OSTEOPOROSIS

Contents
Aetiology
Treatment and Prevention

Aetiology

N Minaur, Royal National Hospital for Rheumatic Diseases, Bath, UK

Osteoporosis is characterized by loss of bone and fractures that occur with little or no trauma. The bone which remains is normal. It is a major health problem throughout the Western world owing to the morbidity, mortality and cost of care which are a consequence of the fractures. Until recently, osteoporosis was considered part of the ageing process, with little scope for its treatment or prevention. This nihilistic attitude is fortunately changing, largely in response to prospective studies showing that therapeutic intervention leading to a reduction in fractures is possible. This article will discuss the definition of osteoporosis and its prevalence, risk factors, detection and clinical consequences. Finally, the role of hormones, diet and peak bone mass will be considered. Although much progress has been made in identifying groups at risk of osteoporosis and measuring bone mass, the precise aetiology of this important disorder remains unknown. The prevention and nutritional management of osteoporosis are discussed in the following article.

Definition

In 1948, Albright and Reifenstein described osteoporosis as being a condition in which there is 'too little bone, but what bone there is, is normal'. This helps distinguish osteoporosis from other bone diseases such as osteomalacia, in which fractures may also occur, but where there is a mineralization defect and abnormal bone.

The definition was refined by a group of experts at a consensus conference in 1993 to 'a systemic skeletal disease characterized by low bone mass and microarchitectural deterioration of bone tissue, with a consequent increase in bone fragility and susceptibility to fracture'. An advantage of this statement is that it allows the diagnosis to be made before a fracture has occurred, enabling preventative treatment to be instituted. Also, the important clinical consequence of osteoporosis, namely fracture, is emphasized. There is no reference to the cause of the reduced bone mass, and thus the definition holds for age-related, postmenopausal and also secondary forms of the disease, for example, steroid-induced osteoporosis.

The World Health Organization (WHO) has suggested that adult females may be classified as osteoporotic or osteopenic on the basis of their bone mass measurement (**Fig. 1**). An individual's bone mineral density is related to the young, healthy mean for that population, and expressed as a T score. A T score of

−1 means the bone density is one standard deviation below the average young, healthy mean. The WHO definition of osteopenia is a T score of between −1 and −2.5, while osteoporosis is a T score of lower than −2.5. Established or severe osteoporosis is present if a fragility fracture has occurred. Using this definition, it has been estimated by Melton that 23% of White women over age 50 and 70% of 80-year-old White women are osteoporotic.

In women, the menopause is associated with accelerated bone loss for approximately 7 years after oestrogen levels fall. Evidence from studies of postmenopausal women suggests that there is an increase in bone turnover, with both resorption and formation increased. However, resorption is increased more than formation, which leads to thinning and then perforation of the trabecular bone, resulting in fracture susceptibility. Bone biopsies from postmenopausal women have shown a reduction in the number of osteoblasts (bone-forming cells) in osteoporosis, resulting in incremental bone loss over years, as the number of bone-resorbing cells (osteoclasts) is unaffected. In the healthy adult skeleton, with normal bone turnover, the amount of bone resorbed is replaced exactly, and bone formation and resorption are said to be 'coupled' (**Fig. 2**). Uncoupling of formation and resorption may lead to net bone loss and, ultimately, osteoporosis.

Osteoporosis can be classified as age-related, post menopausal or secondary, but in an individual patient many factors may combine to produce the end result of low bone mass and increased fracture risk (**Table 1**).

Prevalence and Groups at Risk

Osteoporosis is the most common metabolic bone disease in Western countries. Using the WHO diagnostic criteria above, Melton has estimated that 54% of postmenopausal White women in the USA fulfil

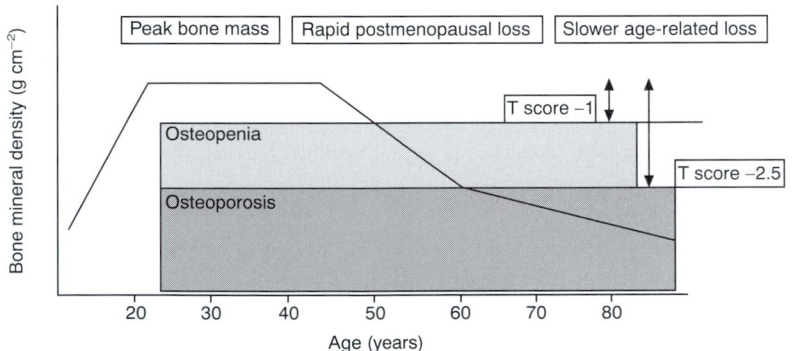

Figure 1 Schematic diagram of WHO criteria for diagnosis of osteoporosis and osteopenia. The mean bone mineral density for a female population is shown.

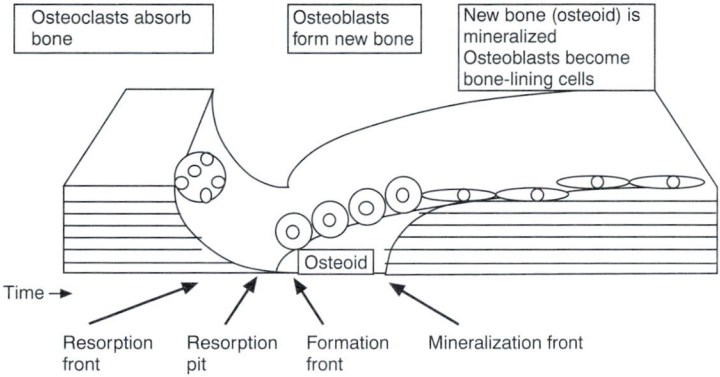

Figure 2 Bone remodelling. Adapted with permission from Eriksen EF, Axelrod DW and Melsen F (1994) *Bone Histomorphometry*, pp 3–12. New York: Raven Press.

Table 1 Classification of osteoporosis

Primary	Postmenopausal (type I)
	Age-related (type II)
Idiopathic	
Juvenile	
Secondary	Endocrine, e.g. Cushing's syndrome, thyrotoxicosis
	Associated with inflammatory diseases, e.g. rheumatoid arthritis
	Associated with drugs, e.g. corticosteroids, heparin, anticonvulsants
	Haematopoietic, e.g. multiple myeloma, lymphoma, mastocytosis
	Immobilization
	Osteoporosis of pregnancy
Congenital	Osteogenesis imperfecta

the conditions for osteopenia, and another 30% have osteoporosis (**Fig. 3**). This is a significant proportion of the population, suggesting that 26 million White women in the USA are at risk of fracture. This does not include non-White women and men, for whom there is much less data. Epidemiological studies have usually focused on fracture data, rather than bone

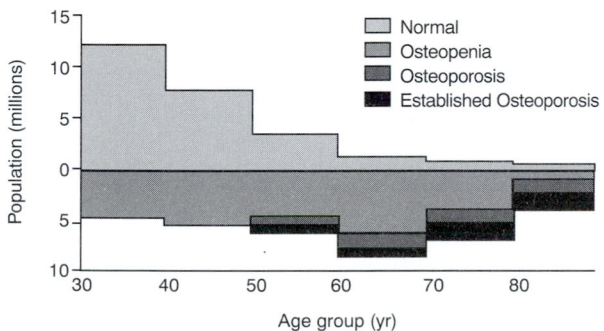

Figure 3 With permission from Melton LJ III (1995) How many women have osteoporosis now? *Journal of Bone and Mineral Research* **10**:175–177.

mineral density, for practical reasons. The data generated by such work underestimates the numbers affected as those who fulfil the criteria for osteoporosis but who have not sustained a fracture are not represented. The *fracture prevalence* refers to the number of people in a population who have already suffered a fragility or osteoporotic fracture, whereas *fracture incidence* refers to the number of new fractures which occur in the population over a given time, usually a year. Fracture prevalence varies according to the population studied. Hip fracture rates are similar in White women of northern European extraction whether they live in North America, South Africa, Scandinavia or New Zealand. By contrast, hip fracture rates are much lower in Maori (New Zealand), or Bantu (South Africa) peoples. In general, fracture rates are much lower in Black populations and there is less difference between the sexes. In Caucasians, female fracture rates usually exceed male.

It has been estimated that a 50-year-old White woman has a greater than 50% risk of sustaining an osteoporotic fracture in her remaining life, with the risk being approximately 16% for each of the three main fractures: hip, wrist and vertebral. **Fig. 4** shows that the three main osteoporotic fractures have different incidence rates and different sex ratios, depending on the stage of life studied.

The forearm (Colles') fracture incidence starts to rise in women at around the time of the menopause (there is no comparable rise in men). This is the time when women become more likely to trip and fracture the wrist of their outstretched hand.

In contrast, hip fracture incidence starts to rise in an exponential fashion after the age of 60, some 15 years after the rise of forearm fractures. People of this age have slower reaction times and are less able to reduce the fall impact on their hip with an outstretched hand.

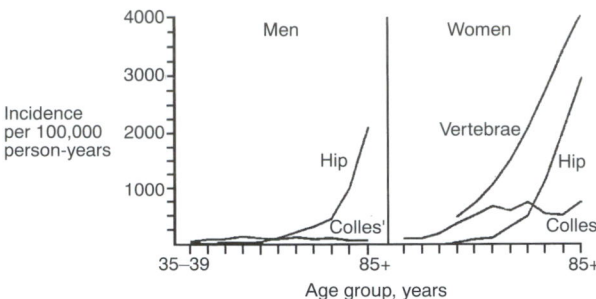

Figure 4 Incidence rates for the three common osteoporotic fractures in men and women, plotted as a function of age at the time of fracture. With permission from Riggs BL and Melton LJ III (1986) Involutional osteoporosis. *New England Journal of Medicine* **314**:1676–1686.

The prevalence of vertebral fractures has been less readily ascertained as the majority of vertebral fractures go unreported and are clinically silent, while episodes of back pain even in someone known to be at risk of osteoporosis may not be due to fracture. Furthermore, vertebral fractures are assumed to be present if certain vertebral deformities are seen on radiographs in population studies, when they may be due to other conditions such as osteoarthritis. The European Vertebral Osteoporosis Study (EVOS) compared vertebral deformity on standard radiographs in 36 European countries and found a fairly constant 10–15% prevalence in men between the ages of 50 and 70. In the case of women, however, the prevalence was lower than men at the age of 50, but increased with age to exceed the male prevalence at the age 65–69 (**Fig. 5**). The higher rate in middle-aged men was related to heavy physical work in early life. There were marked differences in prevalence

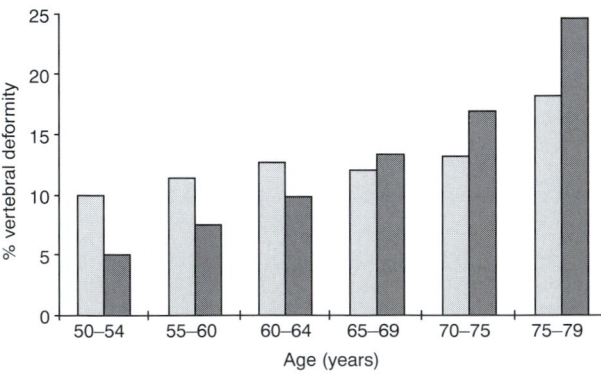

Figure 5 Prevalence of vertebral osteoporosis in European men and women. Dark shading, women; light, shading, men. Adapted from data with permission from O'Neil TW, Felsenberg D, Varlow J, Cooper C, Kanis JA, Silman AJ and the European Vertebral Osteoporosis Study Group (1996) The prevalence of vertebral deformity in European men and women: the European vertebral osteoporosis study. *Journal of Bone and Mineral Research* **11**:1010–1018.

between countries in the EVOS study, and even within countries, suggesting effects of both social and environmental factors. Generally, there were increased rates in northern European countries, possibly related to reduced sunshine exposure and consequently a state of relative vitamin D deficiency.

The incidence of hip fractures is rising. This is partly due to demographic changes and increased life expectancy. Worldwide, it has been estimated that the number of hip fractures will rise from the 1.66 million in 1990 (estimated) to 6.26 million by 2050. Although there will be more hip fractures in countries such as the UK, over 70% of these fractures will occur in Africa, the Middle East, Latin America or Asia. These projections have major cost implications.

Risk Factors

There are many risk factors which can contribute to a low bone mass (**Table 2**).

Age

Bone mass measured at any age is determined by the peak bone mass attained and rate of bone loss subsequently. The peak bone mass is reached at the end of growth, during the third or fourth decade. In premenopausal women, bone loss occurs at approximately 1% per annum. As women reach the menopause, bone loss accelerates with annual reductions in bone mineral density of up to 5–15%. Bone loss in men up to the age of 50 has been estimated as 5–10% per decade; there is an increase after the age of 50, although much less than that seen in women.

Genetics

Many groups are investigating genetic factors as a family history of osteoporosis is a risk factor and there are great geographical and racial differences in the prevalence of osteoporosis, as outlined above. Genetic factors may affect the peak bone mass attained by an individual, the rate of age-related bone loss, and the rate of bone loss in response to other stresses such as the oestrogen deficiency of the menopause or bone-wasting drugs such as corticosteroids. In addition, our genes play a part in determining other features such as our height, weight and size of our bones, although these are modified by environmental factors such as diet and exercise. The age at menarche and menopause is also largely under genetic control. Twin studies measuring bone mineral density in monozygotic (identical) and dizygotic (nonidentical) twins have suggested that more than half the variability of bone mineral density at any age is genetically determined. Research is continuing into possible relationships between polymor-

Table 2 Risk factors

Age	Longevity
Genetic	Family history
	Caucasian/Asian > Black/ Polynesian
	Vitamin D receptor, oestrogen receptor
	Negatively correlated with osteoarthritis
Related to sex hormones	Female > male
	Late menarche
	Early menopause
	Amenorrhea – including exercise-induced
	Nulliparity
	Anorexia nervosa
	Hypogonadism
Habitus	Slim
	Short
	Long femoral neck length
Diet	Low dietary calcium
	Excess protein, sodium
	Excess phosphate, e.g. in soft drinks
Lifestyle	Little weight-bearing exercise
	Smoking
	Alcohol
Concurrent illnesses	
Endocrine (other than sex hormones)	Insulin-dependent diabetes mellitus
	Thyrotoxicosis
	Hyperparathyroidism
	Hypopituitarism
Haematopoietic	Multiple myeloma
	Lymphoma, leukaemia
	Mastocytosis
Other	Previous osteoporotic fracture
	Any cause of immobilization
	Idiopathic hypercalciuria
	Gastrectomy and other bowel disease (coeliac disease)
	Osteoporosis of pregnancy
	Little or no sunlight exposure
Drugs	Corticosteroids
	Excess thyroxine replacement in hypothyroidism
	Heparin
	Anticonvulsants
	Methotrexate
	Cyclosporin A

phisms of receptors for hormones such as oestrogen and vitamin D and bone mineral density. It was thought that a vitamin D receptor polymorphism was a major genetic determinant of bone mineral density when an Australian group published their findings in *Nature* in 1995. However, other groups have failed to confirm their findings and a retraction has since been issued. A recent study in the Framingham cohort suggests that certain vitamin D polymorphisms may have an effect on bone mineral density when subjects are stratified according to calcium intake.

Also, as osteoarthritis (predominately thought of as a disease of cartilage) seems to be protective for osteoporosis, collagen genes are being studied.

Habitus

A typical sufferer of osteoporosis is a slim, White, elderly women of short stature. Shorter people have smaller bones and lower bone mass and thus lower bone density. This apparent disadvantage may be offset by the fact that shorter people are less likely to sustain a fracture if they fall. Although studies have shown that bone mineral density values are similar in Japanese and Caucasian populations, the incidence of hip fracture is much lower in the Orientals. This is thought to be due in part to the shorter hip axis length in Asian people. If two people have similar bone mineral density values of the hip, the taller one is more likely to fracture a hip following a similar fall owing to the action of forces on the femoral neck.

Detection

Osteoporosis is often diagnosed following a fracture, as there are no symptoms associated with low bone mass. In subjects at risk, however, timely (prefracture) diagnosis enables preventative treatment to be instituted.

Noninvasive measures of bone density

Osteoporosis cannot be diagnosed from plain radiographs (X rays) unless a typical fracture is seen, but the radiologist may comment that the bones are osteopenic, with apparent rarefaction of the bony substance and fewer characteristic markings than normal. The mainstay of detection is measurement of the bone mineral density (BMD). This is derived usually from a measure of bone mineral content (BMC). BMD is the most important factor in determining bone strength and has been shown to be associated strongly with future fracture risk. Each standard deviation reduction in BMD is associated with a 2- to 3-fold increase in risk of future fracture and BMD accounts for 75–85% of the variance in bone strength. There are several ways to measure BMD with good accuracy and excellent precision (**Table 3**). Radiographic absorptiometry was an early development in quantitative bone mineral measurement. Its use is limited to the appendicular skeleton,

Table 3 Bone densitometry techniques

Technique	Site	Precision error (%)	Accuracy error (%)	Radiation dose (μSv)
SPA	Radius	1–2	4–6	<1
	Calcaneus	1–2	4–6	<1
DPA	Spine	2–4	5–10	5
	Femur	3–5	5–10	3
	Total body	2–3	1–2	3
DXA	AP-spine	1–2	4–8	1
	Lat-spine	2–3	5–10	3
	Femur	1–2	4–8	1
	Whole body	<1	1–2	3
QCT	Single energy	2–4	5–15	50
	Dual energy	4–6	3–6	100
QUS	Calcaneus	2–4	2–4	0

Adapted with permission from Hagiwara S, Yang S-O, Glüer CC, Bendavid E and Genant HK (1994) Noninvasive bone mineral density measurement in the evaluation of osteoporosis. *Rheumatic Clinics of North America* **20**, 651–669.
SPA, single photon absorptiometry; DPA, dual photon absorptiometry; DXA, dual-energy X ray absorptiometry; QCT, quantitative computed tomography; QUS, quantitative ultrasound; AP-spine, antero-posterior lumbar spine; Lat-spine, lateral lumbar spine.

such as small bones in the hands, and it has been largely superseded by other techniques.

Single-photon absorptiometry (SPA) is performed at the wrist and calcaneus (heel) and may be predictive of future fractures elsewhere in the skeleton. These sites are used as they have little variation in the associated soft tissue. Dual-photon absorptiometry (DPA) uses a radionuclide source with emissions at two different energy levels (usually [153]gadolinium) which enables sites with variable amounts of soft tissues to be scanned, including the axial skeleton. Because the radioactive source has to be changed every 12–18 months, leading to difficulties with quality control, and scan times are very long (up to 40 min for lumbar spine or hip), most centres use one of the following three methods.

A major advantage of using DXA (dual-energy X-ray absorptiometry) to estimate the BMD is that the sites most prone to fracture can be studied directly (hip and lumbar spine as well as forearm). This is important as the best predictor of future fracture at a particular site is the BMD of that site. Recent improvements mean that subjects with replacement joints or other surgical instrumentation (metal) can be assessed by DXA. Also, the bone loss from the hand bones in early arthritis can be ascertained, but this is currently confined to research rather than clinical practice. DXA measures bone mineral content (BMC, g or g cm^{-1}), which is then converted into an areal (two-dimensional) density (BMD, g cm^{-2}) using the size of the bone measured. Quantitative computed tomography (QCT) is the only method available which can estimate the contribution of cortical and trabecular bone to the BMD. QCT provides a true three-dimensional measurement (rather than the two-dimensional areal density of DXA), which is particularly useful in the spine, avoiding the need for lateral spine views. However, QCT uses much more radiation than DXA and accuracy is reduced if bone marrow fat content is increased. Dual energy QCT can provide a more accurate BMD estimate regardless of bone marrow fat content, but at the cost of precision and radiation exposure.

The portability of ultrasound (QUS, quantitative ultrasound) and the fact that it uses no radiation are advantages over other methods. QUS utilizes an emitting transducer which transmits broadband ultrasound waves through the heel, with the foot placed in water. A receiving transducer measures the speed of sound (SOS, m s^{-1}) and broadband ultrasound attenuation (BUA, dB MHz^{-1}). However, relating QUS measures to bone strength is difficult as stiffness of the bone and microarchitectural factors affect readings and most experts feel unable at the present time to recommend this over other established techniques. In addition, QUS is used at the os calcis (calcaneus), and as noted above, this is less predictive of future hip or vertebral fractures than DXA of the relevant area.

There has been much debate about the wisdom of screening a population for low BMD, in the same way that mammograms and cervical smears are offered to women at different stages in their lives. The current position is that screening has been advocated for the following categories of patients.

- Oestrogen deficiency – especially premature menopause, amenorrhoea or if acceptance of hormone replacement therapy depends on result.
- Fragility fracture or radiological evidence such as osteopenia and vertebral fracture in order to confirm diagnosis.
- Long-term corticosteroid therapy.
- Conditions predisposing to secondary osteoporosis, for example, anorexia nervosa, hypogonadism and malabsorption syndromes.

However, in practice there are not enough densitometers in the UK to enable this to occur.

Invasive measurement of bone density by bone biopsy

Measurement of bone density by the above techniques provides information about a single time point, but gives no clue as to the rate of bone loss up to that point. If an individual is given tetracycline (an antibiotic which binds avidly to bone and teeth and which fluoresces) at two known time points (usually 2 weeks apart), a biopsy of their bone some 3–5 days later will reveal two lines on microscopy in recently formed bone. These relate to the doses of tetracycline and allow the rate of formation of bone in that site to be determined. Disadvantages of the technique are that it is invasive, with accompanying stitches and discomfort. Also, the site biopsied is usually the iliac crest, which is not a typical site for osteoporotic fracture. For these reasons, bone biopsy is often a research tool, although it has a place in the diagnosis of osteomalacia, osteoporosis secondary to mastocytosis and renal bone disease.

Markers of bone turnover

It is possible to assess the rate of bone turnover by invasive (bone biopsy) or noninvasive methods. Biochemical markers of bone turnover refer to the measurement of compounds in either serum or urine which are related to bone resorption and formation. As osteoporosis occurs in the setting of an imbalance (uncoupling) of formation and resorption, these markers may have clinical usefulness. An advantage over bone density measurements is that markers change much more quickly in response to therapy. Owing to the errors associated with BMD measurement, there is no point in repeating BMD estimation before a year when looking for a response to treatment. However, changes in markers of bone turnover can be seen within weeks, allowing nonresponders or those with poor compliance to be identified early. The markers of bone formation are serum alkaline phosphatase (the bone specific isoenzyme), serum osteocalcin (also called bone gla-protein) and procol-

lagen I extension peptides. Markers of resorption include fasting urinary calcium, hydroxyproline and hydroxylysine glycosides, plasma tartrate-resistant acid phosphatase and urinary collagen pyridinium cross-links. Convenient specific immunoassays are being developed for these compounds. Workers in this field have categorized subjects into fast and slow losers of bone, based on bone turnover markers. A prospective French study (the EPIDOS study) over 2 years found that two urinary markers of bone resorption, C-telopeptide and free deoxypyridinoline, were predictive of hip fracture risk, independent of BMD. The hope is that a combination of baseline BMD measurement together with marker(s) of bone turnover will enable treatment of osteoporosis to be better targeted to those at greatest risk of future fracture.

Clinical Consequences

Low bone mass without fracture causes no symptoms and osteoporosis has been called the silent epidemic. The consequences are all related to the fractures which may occur. The fractures are typically fragility in type. This means they occur with minimal trauma, for example a simple fall from standing height only resulting in a hip fracture. The three most common fractures are a Colles' fracture of the forearm, hip fracture and vertebral body fracture. Apart from the pain of the fracture itself, considerable morbidity and even mortality may result. Osteoporotic bone does not take longer to heal after fracture than normal bone, but a surgeon may have difficulty in finding enough bone stock for successful instrumentation (for example, pin and plate fixing of a fractured hip) and bone grafts are sometimes necessary.

Forearm fractures cause least problems, and do not necessarily result in admission to hospital. However, if the person lives alone, they may need help with activities of daily living. Occurring as they do some years before the incidence of vertebral and hip fractures starts to rise, Colles' fractures should be a reminder to consider osteoporosis prophylaxis in a woman around the time of the menopause.

Vertebral fractures cause pain, loss of height and change in body shape, the so-called dowager's hump. If multiple vertebral fractures have occurred, the lowest ribs may rest on the iliac crest, with abdominal protrusion which may be confused with obesity. Apart from the discomfort this causes, respiration may be impaired and the abdominal contents compressed. Many vertebral fractures are silent, or are not brought to medical attention, as they may be painless or simply attributed to 'backache'. Often, though, a sudden severe pain is felt over the fracture site, which may radiate around the thorax to the midline anteriorly. This pain is worse on taking a deep breath or moving, and usually settles after 4–6 weeks. It is important to consider underlying causes of vertebral fracture, such as multiple myeloma and metastatic disease. Only 10–15% of vertebral fractures occur on falling: the remainder are spontaneous. Vertebral fractures in the same bone may progress (**Fig. 6**). Thus, a single endplate fracture can progress to a wedge or even compression fracture.

The most serious fractures are hip fractures. These are also the most accurately recorded, as medical attention is always sought. There is significant mortality associated with hip fractures as several studies have demonstrated 10–40% excess mortality over the subsequent year. The majority of deaths occur in the first 6 months after the fracture and it has been suggested that at least some of these deaths may be the result of coexisting serious diseases, which may or may not have contributed to the fall. Estimates of deaths directly due to the fracture vary from 15 to 40%. Even for survivors of hip fracture, many have serious continuing disability and require long-term nursing care.

Other fractures may occur in osteoporosis. Rib fractures are said to be particularly common in patients on long-term glucocorticoid therapy, per-

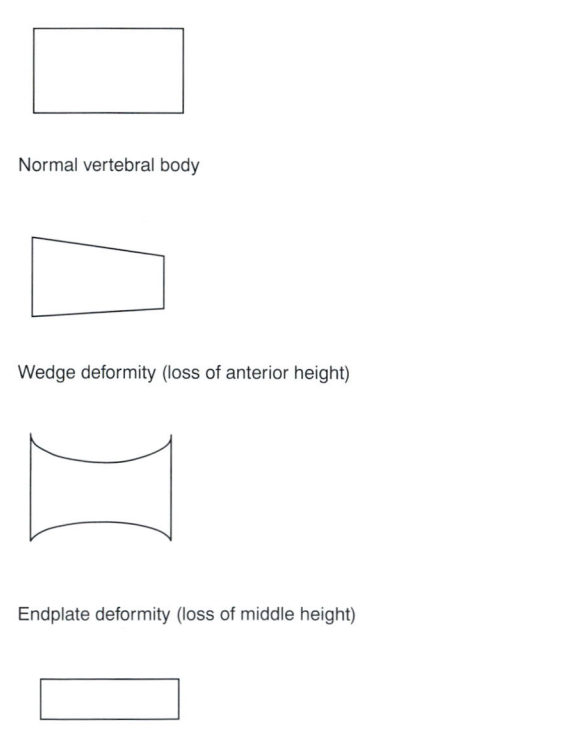

Normal vertebral body

Wedge deformity (loss of anterior height)

Endplate deformity (loss of middle height)

Compression deformity (loss of anterior, posterior and middle height)

Figure 6 Schematic representation of the alteration of vertebral body shape with osteoporotic fractures.

haps related to chronic coughing in those with airway limitation disease. Fractures of the humerus, tibia and pelvis are not unusual.

Role of Hormones

Hormones play a critical part in skeletal homeostasis, both in the growing child and adult. Bone is a target organ for parathormone, vitamin D, glucocorticoids and the sex hormones oestrogen and testosterone. Parathormone is released from the parathyroid gland in response to a low serum calcium. The principle actions of the hormone are: (1) to stimulate release of calcium and phosphate from bone; (2) to stimulate reabsorption of calcium and inhibit reabsorption of phosphate in the kidney; and (3) to stimulate the renal synthesis of 1,25-dihydroxyvitamin D_3. All these actions serve to raise serum calcium and lower serum phosphate. Osteoblasts have PTH receptors and, similar to thyroid hormone, PTH acts indirectly on the osteoclast. The effect of PTH is to increase osteoclast numbers and activity, resulting in bone resorption, through more resorption (activation) sites. The activity of osteoblasts is also increased and whether net bone loss or formation results depends on the levels of PTH over time. Continuous high levels of PTH cause bone loss, but the pulsed administration of low doses can cause bone formation in laboratory animals and man.

In both men and women, normal levels of the sex hormones are important for bone health. Women who have a short reproductive period (late menarche and early menopause) are at increased risk of osteoporosis. Menopause may be induced artificially early if the woman undergoes hysterectomy and removal of the ovaries. Amenorrhoea in female athletes, ballet dancers and sufferers of anorexia nervosa predisposes to osteoporosis. One of the major consequences of oestrogen loss is thought to be the altered production of cytokines and growth factors by resident cells in the bone marrow microenvironment. These include the 'pro-resorptive' cytokines tumour necrosis factor (TNF-α), and the interleukins IL-1 and IL-6, which are all increased. Meanwhile, the 'pro-formative' factors tumour growth factor (TGF-β) and insulin-like growth factors I and II are reduced and the net effect of these changes is to shift the balance in favour of increased bone resorption, and hence bone loss.

Osteoporosis in men is sometimes associated with hypogonadism (low testosterone levels) which may be secondary to alcohol excess. Until recently, very little research had been done on male osteoporosis and it was assumed that all cases were secondary in nature. Primary male osteoporosis is being increasingly recognized and work is continuing into similarities to and differences from the condition in females. Elevated levels of thyroid hormone, whether due to thyrotoxicosis or excess replacement therapy in hypothyroidism, increase bone remodelling by action on osteoblasts, which have specific thyroid hormone receptors. The thyroid hormone acts on osteoclasts indirectly, through the osteoblast, and bone resorption exceeds bone formation, resulting in bone loss. The normal bone remodelling cycle in trabecular (cancellous) bone lasts for approximately 200 days. Histomorphometry has shown that in thyrotoxicosis the cycle is shortened to about 110 days. Cushing's syndrome of excess glucocorticoids, either exogenous or endogenous, is associated with rapid bone loss. Glucocorticoids have multiple effects on bone, both locally and systemically. They inhibit gastrointestinal absorption of calcium and increase its renal excretion. This stimulates release of parathormone (PTH) which increases the number of bone remodelling sites. Glucocorticoids also inhibit the synthesis of new bone by osteoblasts.

Role of Diet and Peak Bone Mass

Peak bone mass is the maximum bone mass attained and has a major effect on the bone mass at each subsequent stage of life. Bone mass increases during growth, plateaus during the 20s and starts to decline after the age of about 30 (Fig. 1). The peak bone mass an individual can reach is determined partly by genetic influence and by mechanical loading (exercise) during growth, but adequate calcium during growth is also essential. A study published in 1979 from the former Yugoslavia of two villages found a lower incidence of hip fractures in the village which had a higher intake of calcium. Many other subsequent studies have failed to show such clear relationships between calcium intake and bone density or fracture incidence.

Calcium supplementation seems to most benefit those with the lowest previous intake. A consensus conference at the National Institutes of Health in 1994 has suggested optimal daily calcium intakes of 800–1000 mg for children up to age 12, 1200–1500 mg from age 12 to 24, and 1000 mg from age 25 to age 65 or the menopause (whichever comes first). After the age of 65 or postmenopausally, 1500 mg per day is recommended. These intakes are specific for the USA, but probably hold for any country where there is high intake of protein and sodium in the daily diet, each of which cause renal wasting of calcium. Recently concern has been expressed that adolescent girls are at risk of failing to attain their peak bone mass through a variety of lifestyle choices;

restricting dairy products and smoking as part of weight control and drinking carbonated drinks which contain phosphate and result in loss of calcium via the kidneys. Weight-bearing exercise is now also less often compulsory in schools. All these may increase the epidemic of osteoporosis which has been predicted for the next century.

Acknowledgments

I would like to thank Dr JN Beresford, Senior Lecturer, School of Pharmacy and Pharmacology, University of Bath, for advice in preparation of this article. NM is a Clinical Research Fellow supported by the Arthritis and Rheumatism Council, UK.

See Colour Plate 10.

See also: **Ageing**: Biological Aspects. **Bone**: Composition, Metabolism and Bone Growth. **Cholecalciferol and Ergocalciferol**: Physiology, Dietary Sources and Requirements.

Further Reading

Center J and Eisman J (1997) The epidemiology and pathogenesis of osteoporosis. In: Reid IR (ed.) *Baillière's Clinical Endocrinology and Metabolism: Metabolic Bone Disease*, pp 23–62. London: Baillière Tindall.

Consensus Development Conference (1993) Diagnosis, prophylaxis and treatment of osteoporosis. *American Journal of Medicine* 94:646–650.

Cummings SR, Kelsey JL, Nevitt MC and O'Dowd KJ (1985) Epidemiology of osteoporosis and osteoporotic fractures. *Epidemiologic Reviews* 7:178–208.

Dequeker J, Raspe H-H and Sambrook P (1994) Osteoporosis. In: Klippel JH and Dieppe PA (eds) *Rheumatology*, pp 7 32.1–7 32.10 St Louis: CV Mosby.

Genant HK, Engelke K, Fuerst T, Gluer C-C, Grampp S, Harris ST, Jergas M, Lang T, Lu Y, Majumdar S, Mathur A and Takada M (1996) Noninvasive assessment of bone mineral and structure: state of the art. *Journal of Bone and Mineral Research* 11:707–723.

Hagiwara S, Yang S-O, Gluer CC, Bendavid E and Genant HK (1994) Noninvasive bone mineral density measurement in the evaluation of osteoporosis. *Rheumatic Disease Clinics of North America* 20:651–669.

Kanis JA and Pitt FA (1992) Epidemiology of osteoporosis. *Bone* 13:S7–S15.

Kleerekoper M and Nelson DA (1997) Which bone density measurement? Editorial, *Journal of Bone and Mineral Research* 12:712–714.

Melton LJ III (1995) Perspectives: how many women have osteoporosis now? *Journal of Bone and Mineral Research* 10:175–177.

Miller PD, Bonnick SL and Rosen CJ (1996) Consensus of an international panel on the clinical utility of bone mass measurements in the detection of low bone mass in the adult population. *Calcified Tissue International* 58:207–214.

Taylor AK, Lueken SA, Libanti C and Baylink DJ (1994) Biochemical markers of bone turnover for the clinical assessment of bone metabolism. *Rheumatic Disease Clinics of North America* 20:589–607.

Wasnich RD (1996) Epidemiology of osteoporosis. In: Favus MJ (ed.) *Primer on the Metabolic Bone Diseases and Disorders of Mineral Metabolism*, 3rd edn, pp 249–251. Philadelphia: Lippincott-Raven.

Treatment and Prevention

K O'Brien, Johns Hopkins University, Baltimore, Maryland, USA.

Osteoporosis and osteopenia are currently substantial public health problems. Recent estimates suggest that 6–7 million women over the age of 50 years in the USA have osteoporosis, and 12–17 million have osteopenia and are at an increased risk of developing this disease. Once bone has lost a substantial amount of its mineral and matrix it is more susceptible to fracture. The increasing impact of low bone mass on public health can be demonstrated by the large increase in the age-specific rate of hip fractures since the 1970s.

The most unfortunate aspect of the bone loss that occurs in osteoporosis is that once the structural framework of bone is lost it cannot be restored. Because of the nonreversible aspect of this process, the most effective strategies for treating osteoporosis should focus on prevention, maintenance of existing bone mass and reduction of variables that increase the likelihood of traumas which could lead to fracture.

Prevention

Calcium intake

Calcium comprises approximately 38% of bone mineral and is the most abundant mineral found in bone. Owing to the importance of calcium in the structural integrity of bone, deficiencies or inadequate intakes of calcium will have a strong impact on bone mass. It is generally well accepted that calcium is crucial during the pubertal growth spurt in order for the attainment of maximal peak bone mass to be achieved. However, it is also essential that optimal calcium intake be consumed throughout the life cycle to meet the daily intrinsic requirements of calcium required to offset urinary, dermal and endogenous faecal calcium losses. Because serum calcium is very

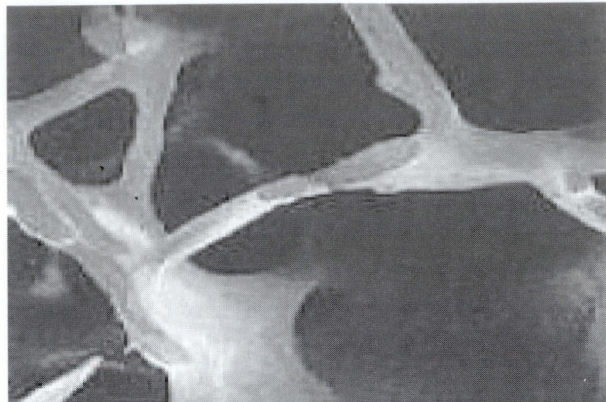

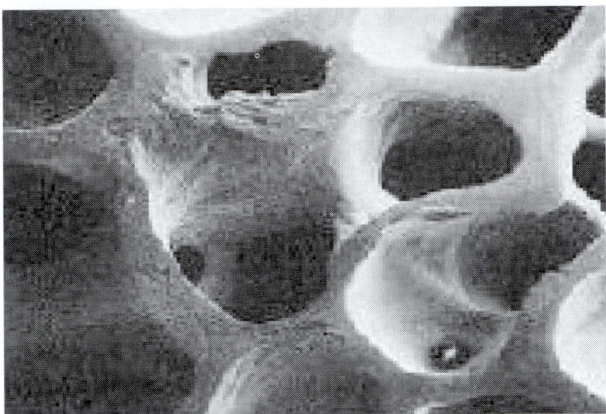

Figure 1 A scanning electron micrograph of healthy bone is shown in the top panel. In contrast, bone in the lower panel has lost a substantial amount of mineral and matrix compromising its structural integrity and increasing the risk of fracture. From Favus MJ (Ed.) Primer on the Metabolic Bone Diseases and Disorders of Mineral Metabolism (2nd Edn), Lippencott-Raven Publishers, PA, 1993.

tightly regulated, if net calcium absorption is not capable of compensating for these losses, serum calcium needs will be met by increased bone calcium resorption. Over time, imbalances between the rates of bone calcium resorption and deposition will lead to a reduction in bone mineral density.

The importance of calcium in bone mineral acquisition and maintenance has been demonstrated in several epidemiological studies in which significant relationships between an individual's lifelong intake of calcium and both bone mass and fracture risk have been identified. Many of these studies, however, have been difficult to interpret because of the difficulty in separating the impact of calcium intake from other nutritional and environmental variables which may also be influencing bone mass. Furthermore, a women's menopausal status must be taken into consideration when examining these relationships, as the rapid bone loss that occurs in the early postmenopausal period is largely refractory to calcium supplementation.

The impact of calcium supplementation on bone mass may be most evident in women whose habitual dietary calcium intakes are below 400 mg per day. Furthermore, owing to the prevalence of vitamin D deficiency in the elderly, oral vitamin D supplements up to 800 iu per day may also be required in order for calcium to be absorbed and for calcium supplementation to be efficacious.

The importance of calcium intake on bone mass was recognized by the Institute of Medicine which recommended that the daily adequate intake of calcium of women aged 31–50 years be increased to 1000 mg. The daily adequate intake of calcium recommended for all men and women aged 51 years and older was increased to 1200 mg per day (**Table 1**).

The current dietary intakes of calcium in adult women are well below these recommended levels. It is often difficult to increase consumption of dairy products in older populations because of lactose intolerance, weight reduction or low-cholesterol diets, or decreased appetite and food consumption. Many of these problems can be avoided by using lactose-free dairy products, lactase pills and the numerous fat-free products which are available for individuals who are dieting. Nonfat milk powder can also be added to a number of recipes to increase the calcium content of the food without adversely affecting taste. Increasing calcium intake from dairy products has been found to increase the intake of a number of other nutrients, including protein, magnesium, zinc, phosphorus, thiamin and riboflavin. For this reason, increasing calcium intake through dietary methods is preferable to the use of calcium supplements alone. Despite these benefits, unless marked changes are made in the current dietary habits of adult and elderly individuals, it may be necessary to obtain the recommended calcium intakes from increased use of calcium supplements or fortified food products.

Several forms of calcium supplements are commercially available, including calcium carbonate, calcium citrate and tricalcium phosphate. Although these forms may differ slightly with respect to their calcium content per tablet and their absorbability, the small differences observed between products may not be biologically significant.

Several variables will influence the optimal way in which these calcium supplements are consumed. If the calcium supplement is taken before bedtime this will counteract the nocturnal increase in the rate of bone resorption. However, gastric acid secretion may be impaired in some elderly individuals, and taking these supplements with a meal will facilitate absorption in this group. The percent of calcium that is absorbed from the gastrointestinal tract is inversely related to calcium intake: as higher calcium intakes are ingested the intestinal efficiency of calcium absorption decreases. For this reason, smaller calcium doses (<500 mg) should be taken with each meal of the day, instead of taking one large calcium supplement.

Other dietary considerations in preventing osteoporosis

In addition to calcium, a number of other minerals and dietary components are essential for optimal bone health. Vitamin D is required for active calcium absorption in the gut, and it also facilitates bone calcium resorption. Vitamin K is also important in maintaining bone health because several bone matrix proteins require vitamin K for γ-carboxylation, needed for optimal binding of these proteins to hydroxyapatite. The collagen crosslinking of bone is also dependent on vitamin C, and deficiency of this vitamin can lead to bone abnormalities.

Phosphorus and magnesium also are present in bone. Bone contains 85% of the phosphorus found in the body. Magnesium is important in calcium metabolism and bone health because it is required both for parathyroid hormone secretion and for the enzyme that converts 25-hydroxyvitamin D into the biologically active form of vitamin D.

Zinc, manganese and copper are also related to bone health. These minerals are cofactors for various enzymes required in the posttranslational modification or synthesis of bone matrix constituents. It is possible that deficiencies or inadequate intakes of these nutrients can adversely affect bone quality.

Other dietary constituents are known to influence either urinary calcium excretion or intestinal absorption. Sodium is one of the strongest predictors of urinary calcium excretion and a high dietary sodium

Table 1 Calcium requirements

Group	Adequate daily intake of calcium (mg)
Infant	
Birth–6 months	210
6 months–1 year	270
Children	
1–3 years	500
4–8 years	800
Adolescents/young adults	
9–18 years	1300
Men/women	
19–50 years	1000
51–70 years	1200
Over 70 years	1200

Source: Institute of Medicine, 1997.

intake will increase urinary calcium losses. High intakes of animal protein also increase urinary calcium excretion and may alter bone calcium turnover. Individuals with excessive alcohol intake are also at an increased risk of low bone mass due to a decreased intake of other nutrients and an increase in urinary calcium excretion. Alcohol may also directly impair osteoblast function.

Treatment

Pharmacological treatment

Several pharmacological agents are available for the management of established osteoporosis (**Table 2**). These therapeutic agents work either by primarily inhibiting the resorption of bone (antiresorptive agents) or by promoting bone mineralization (proformative agents). Antiresorptive agents include bisphosphonates, oestrogen or hormonal replacement therapy, oestrogen agonists, oral calcium and/or vitamin D supplementation and calcitonin. Proformative agents include anabolic steroids, sodium fluoride and several growth factors such as

insulin-like growth factor I (IGF-I) and transforming growth factor β (TGF-β).

Fluoride Fluoride has been administered orally at dosages ranging from 30 mg to 75 mg per day to treat individuals with low bone mass. This compound is well absorbed, binds avidly to bone and has been demonstrated to result in increased trabecular bone mass and lumbar spine bone mineral density. However, the impact of fluoride supplementation on fracture rates is less certain. Furthermore, there is also some degree of uncertainty regarding both the quality of the newly formed bone and the appropriate dosage to administer such that bone density is improved without adversely affecting bone quality. More controlled clinical studies are needed to address the dosage and efficacy issues pertaining to the use of fluoride in maintenance of bone mass.

Bisphosphonates Bisphosphonates are pyrophosphate analogues that are not metabolized by the body. They are capable of binding to bone and work primarily by inhibiting bone resorption. Because

Table 2 Osteoporosis treatment in postmenopausal women

Treatment	Primary mode of action	Typical dosage	Benefits/risks
Calcitonin	Inhibits osteoclast activity and decreases bone resorption	50–100 iu (subcutaneous or intramuscular injection) 100–200 iu (nasal spray)	May have analgesic benefits comparable to NSAIDs
Bisphosphonates (alendronate)	Inhibit bone remodelling, particularly resorption	10 mg per day	Alendronate may preferentially inhibit resorption without inhibiting bone formation; slight increases in bone mass have been observed for up to 3 years after initiation of treatment
Sodium fluoride	Stimulates bone formation	40–60 mg per day	The quality of newly formed bone may be suboptimal. Fluoride may influence the crystalline structure of bone and increase its fragility
Oestrogen	Inhibits bone resorption	Conjugated equine oestrogens 0.625 mg per day	Oestrogen replacement therapy reduces fracture and cardiovascular risk. Some studies have indicated that it may increase the risk of breast cancer
Calcium	Inhibits bone resorption	1200 mg per day	Increased calcium intake may have the most impact on fracture rates in women with habitually low calcium intakes (<400 mg per day)
Vitamin D	Decreases bone resorption	Doses of 10–20 μg per day (400–800 iu) may be required in postmenopausal women with inadequate sun exposure or vitamin D intakes	Vitamin D supplementation may limit bone loss by reducing secondary hyperparathyroidism and improving intestinal calcium absorption

NSAIDs, nonsteroidal antiinflammatory drugs.

these drugs are poorly absorbed (typically less than 1%), it is recommended that they be consumed on an empty stomach and food should be avoided for a minimum of 30 min after this medication is consumed. One side effect of this, however, is an increased likelihood of gastrointestinal upset and nausea.

A number of different bisphosphonates are currently available to treat low bone mass; these include etidronate, pamidronate, clodronate, risedronate and tiludronate. These bisphosphonates are comprised of a P—C—P backbone with varying side-chain moieties. The phosphate core of the bisphosphonate is responsible for the binding of the drug to the bone crystals, while the side chain confers the antiresorptive properties. Although bisphosphonates inhibit bone resorption, they may also decrease the magnitude of bone formation as measured using indirect markers of bone formation (urinary N-telopeptide and deoxypyridinoline). A second-generation bisphosphonate, alendronate, has been approved for use in the treatment (and the prevention) of osteoporosis. This drug may be more efficacious than earlier bisphosphonates because the dose that inhibits bone resorption is much lower than that required to affect bone formation. Studies have found that this drug increases bone mineral density, and increases bone mass over at least a 3-year period. The potential for this drug to increase bone mass over a longer period has yet to be addressed.

Thiazides   Individuals with elevated urinary calcium excretion may have an increased risk of developing low bone mass owing to excessive urinary calcium losses. Thiazide diuretics have been used in hypercalciuric individuals to reduce urinary calcium excretion. Decreasing the net losses of calcium from the body will indirectly lead to a reduction in bone resorption which will help to maintain existing bone mass. There is little information about the usage of this medication in individuals without abnormally high urinary calcium excretion, and the impact of thiazide diuretics on fracture rates has not been thoroughly investigated.

Calcitonin   Salmon calcitonin is approved for use in the treatment (not prevention) of osteoporosis. This medication can be administered either parenterally or intranasally. Little evidence of the efficacy of nasal calcitonin with respect to fracture risk is available. One benefit associated with the use of calcitonin is that it may be the only therapy that also alleviates symptoms, owing to its analgesic effect. Furthermore, calcitonin may have the fewest adverse side effects of any of the currently available treatments.

Reported side effects associated with the use of this medication are minor and include nasal irritation, flushing and nausea. Over time, the efficacy of this product may decrease, perhaps as a result of the formation of antibodies, to this medication.

Calcitriol   Calcitriol, $1,25(OH)_2D_3$, is the active form of vitamin D. Studies have demonstrated that this metabolite is efficacious in increasing both calcium absorption and bone mineral density and in decreasing fracture rates. Analogues of this metabolite such as $1\alpha\text{-OHD}_3$ or $1\alpha\text{-OHD}_2$ may also be beneficial in increasing bone mineral density and decreasing fracture rates. High-dose supplementation with these metabolites can result in hypercalcaemia, hypercalciuria and nephrocalcinosis. However, calcitriol at a dose of $0.5-1$ µg per day does not appear to influence renal function adversely. Research into the development of new analogues of calcitriol is in progress. It is hoped that these analogues will have selective effects on osteoblast function without altering renal function.

Oestrogen and hormonal replacement therapy   Oestrogen has several effects on calcium and bone homeostasis. It has positive effects on the synthesis of the active form of vitamin D, urinary calcium reabsorption and intestinal calcium absorption. The cells responsible for bone formation (osteoblasts) have receptors for oestrogen, and oestrogen may also regulate or influence the production of TGF-β, interleukin 1 (IL-1) and IGF-I. For these reasons, alterations in circulating oestrogen levels will have a substantial impact on bone remodelling. Following the loss of oestrogen in the perimenopausal period, bone undergoes a period of rapid alterations in turnover resulting in a substantial amount of bone loss. Up to 5% of bone mass may be lost each year for the first few years following menopause, and a total loss in bone mass of roughly 15% occurs during this time. During the period of rapid bone turnover in early menopause, calcium supplementation does not seem to have an effect on maintenance of bone mass. After this rapid turnover period, a new threshold in bone turnover is achieved and the annual rate of bone loss slows to approximately 1%.

In women who enter menopause with optimal bone mass the magnitude of bone loss over the menopausal period should not jeopardize bone mass. However, if inadequate peak bone mass or excessive losses of bone mineral have already occurred prior to menopause, net bone loss during the menopausal period may decrease a woman's bone mineral density such that it enters the fracture threshold.

It is often a difficult decision for women as to

whether oestrogen replacement therapy should be initiated. In women with a strong family history of osteoporosis or with other conditions that may have jeopardized bone mineral density, or who are unsure if they should take oestrogen, it may be helpful to recommend a bone density scan. This will serve as a baseline reference value to establish risk and bone density prior to menopause, and will enable the magnitude and rate of bone loss to be determined in the early postmenopausal period.

Oestrogen replacement therapy has been found to be effective at slowing the rate of bone loss in women even if initiated at the age of 70 years. However, this treatment may need to be continued for a 10-year period until a significant decrease in the risk of hip fracture is obtained. Once oestrogen replacement therapy is stopped, bone loss will continue at the rate that occurs immediately following menopause. Oestrogen replacement therapy may therefore be most efficacious if started earlier in the menopausal period so that bone mass will be maintained at a higher level until a later age. Both the oral and transdermal routes of oestrogen replacement therapy appear to confer the same degree of protection. Furthermore, equine oestrogen, oestradiol and oestrone sulfate all have comparable effects on reducing the rates of skeletal turnover.

There are both benefits and risks associated with the use of oestrogen replacement therapy. In some studies, oestrogen replacement has been found to slightly increase the risk of developing breast cancer and if oestrogen is given unopposed (without progestins) the risk of endometrial hyperplasia and carcinoma may also be increased. However, oestrogen is strongly protective with respect to the risk of coronary heart disease and alters the serum lipid profile to increase high-density lipoprotein levels and decrease low-density lipoprotein levels. Oestrogen therapy may reduce the risk of thrombotic stroke and may also decrease the risk of Alzheimer's disease.

Women with an intact uterus can be placed on hormonal replacement therapy in which progestins are added to the oestrogen replacement on either a cyclical or a continuous basis. The long-term impact of this form of treatment on endometrial cancer has yet to be thoroughly evaluated. Moreover, there are fewer data on the long-term efficacy of hormonal replacement therapy with respect to hip fracture in comparison with oestrogen replacement therapy.

In addition to hormonal and oestrogen replacement therapy, certain oestrogen agonist drugs are being investigated for their ability to maintain bone mass. It is hoped that these drugs will have comparable effects on the skeleton and fracture reduction without many of the adverse side effects associated with hormonal replacement therapy. Tamoxifen is one example of an oestrogen agonist that has been found to reduce bone loss in patients with breast cancer. To avoid the adverse effects of tamoxifen on both endometrial and mammary tissue proliferation; a newer modification of this drug, raloxifene, has been developed and approved for use in the prevention of osteoporosis.

Anabolic steroids Administration of synthetic derivatives of the androgen testosterone to both women and men can increase bone mass. One benefit of this treatment is that there may be a positive impact on both muscle and bone mass. However, the side effects associated with this treatment in women are generally unacceptable. Reported side effects of androgen use in women include increased hair growth and voice changes as well as adverse effects on lipoprotein metabolism. These medications are used for osteoporosis treatment in some countries but they are not approved in the USA.

Additive effects of pharmacological treatments There is a strong possibility that combinations of current treatments may eventually prove to be more efficacious than single treatment alone. To date, calcium has been used in combination with a number of the current therapies. It is possible that future studies will find that oestrogen and alendronate, or other combination therapies, may have additive effects on decreasing bone turnover and/or maintaining or increasing bone mass. The impact of potential multitherapy combinations on bone mass has not yet been fully established.

Nonpharmacological treatment

Although bone mass cannot be restored to normal once the bone matrix has been destroyed, there are several nonpharmacological approaches that can be used to minimize fracture risk in established osteoporosis. The majority of hip fractures occur as a result of a fall. By decreasing the likelihood of falls the adverse effect of these fractures on mortality and quality of life can be reduced. Several strategies have been recommended to assist in the prevention of falls, to protect vulnerable body areas from trauma associated with a fall, and to improve overall muscle coordination and muscle strength.

Preventing falls A number of environmental factors within the home can influence the risk of falling. To decrease the likelihood of falls or accidents, the following approaches can be recommended to osteoporotic individuals:

- Throw rugs or other floor coverings which are not firmly adhered should be avoided, and slippery floors should be carpeted.
- Poor lighting within and around the home should be corrected to improve visibility.
- Loose cords around the home should be removed, and placement of additional telephones in the home may help to minimize the risk of falls.
- Furniture should be arranged to provide a clear traffic path.
- Ambulatory devices may be helpful in individuals with impaired mobility.
- Eyeglass prescriptions should be kept up to date to insure optimal vision.
- In the bathtub or shower, protective railings can be installed to assist with mobility.
- Shoewear should be selected for comfort, stability and cushioned support.
- Medications that may impair balance, mobility, vision or neurologic function should be closely monitored.

Exercise is known to positively influence bone mass. During exercise the strain and small changes in the shape of the bone will stimulate local bone responses to positively influence the balance in bone remodelling. Many studies have reported positive associations between exercise and bone mass at a number of sites, especially the hip and the spine. The impact of exercise on bone mass is related to the intensity of the exercise, with aerobic and strength training exercises having the greatest effect on bone mass. However, the calcium intake of the individual is also important, and exercise in postmenopausal and elderly women may only increase bone mass if calcium intake is optimal.

What may not be generally appreciated is the positive impact of exercise not only on bone mass but also on muscle strength, muscle mass, balance and coordination. Improvements in muscle strength may assist with proper posture, balance, flexibility, coordination and gait stability. Although weightbearing exercises may be best in the maintenance of musculoskeletal strength, the type of exercise selected should be consistent with the physical status of the individual.

Protecting vulnerable areas   One of the most vulnerable areas from a fall is the hip. The relative impact of the fall on fracture risk will be related to both the bone quality and the ability of the subcutaneous padding to protect against the force of the impact. Lean women may have less padding over bony prominences and may be more susceptible to fracture. External hip protectors may assist in reducing the magnitude of the impact. These protectors deflect the energy from the force of the fall to the surrounding muscles and soft tissue. Studies have found that the use of hip protectors in populations at risk is capable of decreasing the fracture rate in these groups.

Targeting Groups at Risk

A number of nondietary factors are related to the risk of low bone mass. Individuals with a small body frame have a smaller bone reserve on which to draw and therefore have a higher risk of osteoporosis. Asian and white women are at increased risk in comparison with men and non-Hispanic black individuals because of a lower peak bone mineral density. Cigarette smoking has adverse effects on bone mass. Smokers may be leaner, and female smokers may experience an earlier menopause and have lower postmenopausal oestrogen levels. Women who have had an early menopause or surgical removal of the ovaries at a young age are also at an increased risk of low bone mass.

A number of illnesses that alter calcium and/or vitamin D homeostasis or bone turnover can increase the risk of developing osteoporosis. Examples of illnesses that can have negative effects on bone mass include hyperthyroidism, hyperparathyroidism, intestinal malabsorption syndromes, gonadal insufficiency, gastrointestinal diseases, paralysis or hemiplegia, hypercortisolism, thyroid disease, and insulin-dependent diabetes. Medications known to have a negative impact on bone mass include steroids, thyroid hormone, anticonvulsant therapy (phenytoin), aluminium, and glucocorticoid therapy.

One of the most crucial periods in bone acquisition occurs during the pubertal growth spurt. At this time a substantial proportion of adult bone mass is accumulated. Bone mineral acquisition curves can be viewed not only as indicators of bone growth, but also as peak periods to target optimal dietary calcium intake so that maximal bone mineralization can be achieved. Calcium is the most abundant mineral in bone, and nutritional emphasis has been placed on optimal intake of this nutrient during the adolescent growth spurt. Calcium supplementation has been found to increase bone mass, an effect which may be most apparent when implemented during the prepubertal period. It is not yet known if the additional calcium intake during the pubertal growth spurt will increase peak bone mass or if the predetermined peak bone mass is being obtained at an earlier age. Nevertheless, the importance of optimal calcium intake during childhood and early adolescence has been recognized by the Institute of Medicine, which recommended that adequate daily intakes of calcium be increased to 1300 mg per day in children and adolescents between the ages of 9–18 years (see Table 1).

Despite the importance of calcium in bone mineral acquisition, the median calcium intake of adult and adolescent females is substantially below the recommended dietary allowance. If the current calcium intake recommendation is used, an even greater proportion of the adolescent and adult population would be consuming diets which are not optimal with respect to calcium intake. Ensuring optimal calcium intakes during the pubertal growth spurt may be one of the easiest ways of helping to ensure that peak bone mass is achieved.

Although optimal nutrition is required to provide the available substrate for bone mass, it is not the only variable required for healthy bones. A substantial amount of bone mineral acquisition is believed to be due to genetic rather than environmental factors. Further research into the genetic control of bone mineral acquisition and loss will be invaluable in targeting groups at risk for low bone mass.

It is currently known that a family history of osteoporosis is a risk factor for the development of this disease. In addition, the heritability of bone mass has been examined in several familial resemblance studies in siblings, mono- or dizygotic twins, and parent–offspring pairs. These studies have demonstrated that the majority of bone mass (up to 80%) is due to genetic and not environmental causes.

Several lines of new research are attempting to identify genotypes which are predictive of low bone mass. A number of allelic variations in several receptors and binding sites have recently been implicated in the control of bone mineral acquisition. These include the vitamin D receptor, parathyroid hormone receptor, oestrogen receptor and the binding site of the type 1 α 1 collagen gene (the major protein in bone). The relative contributions of these genotypes to the control of bone mineral acquisition are still controversial, and not all reports examining these relationships have found comparable relationships. However, with further research into this area, it is hoped that individuals at risk for this disease can be identified and targeted for intervention prior to the development of osteoporosis.

See also: **Bone**: Composition, Metabolism and Bone Growth. **Calcium**: Physiology. **Cholecalciferol and Ergocalciferol**: Rickets and Osteomalacia. **Exercise**: Beneficial Effects. **Magnesium**: Physiology, Dietary Sources and Requirements. **Older People**: Nutritional Requirements; Nutritionally Related Problems. **Phosphorus**: Physiology, Dietary Sources and Requirements. **Smoking**: Effects on Diet and Nutritional Status. **Vitamin K**: Physiology. **Zinc**: Physiology.

Further Reading

Christiansen C (1992) Prevention and treatment of osteoporosis: a review of current modalities. *Bone* 13:S35–39.

Heaney RP (1996) Bone mass, nutrition, and other lifestyle factors. *Nutrition Reviews* 54(4):S3–S10.

Institute of Medicine, Food and Nutrition Board (1997) *Dietary reference intakes: calcium, magnesium, phosphorus, vitamin D and fluoride.* Washington, DC: National Academy Press.

Lips P (1996) Prevention of hip fractures: drug therapy. *Bone* 18(3):159S–163S.

Marcus R (1989) Understanding and preventing osteoporosis. *Hospital Practice* 24(4):189–218.

Marcus R (1991) Understanding osteoporosis. *Western Journal of Medicine* 155:53–60.

Myers AH, Young Y and Langlois JA (1996) Prevention of falls in the elderly. *Bone* 18(1):87S–101S.

Nordin BEC, Need AG, Horowitz M and Morris HA (1994) Treatment of osteoporosis in the elderly. *Clinics in Geriatric Medicine* 10(4):625–646.

Prestwood KM, Pilbeam CC and Raisz LG (1995) Treatment of osteoporosis. *Annual Review of Medicine*, 46:249–256.

Recker RR (1993) Prevention of osteoporosis: calcium nutrition. *Osteoporosis International* supplement 1:S163–S165.

Recker RR (1993) Current therapy for osteoporosis. *Journal of Clinical Endocrinology and Metabolism* 76(1):14–16.

Riggs BL (1991) Overview of osteoporosis. *Western Journal of Medicine* 154:63–77.

Oxidant damage *see* **Antioxidants**: Diet and Antioxidant Defence; Observational Epidemiology; Intervention Studies.

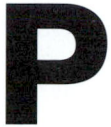

PANTOTHENIC ACID

Physiology, Dietary Sources and Requirements

C J Bates, MRC Dunn Nutrition Unit, Cambridge, UK

Absorption, Transport and Storage

A considerable proportion of the pantothenic acid that is present in food eaten by animals or humans exists as derivatives such as coenzyme A (CoA) and acyl carrier protein (ACP). The pantothenic acid in these derivatives is largely released as free pantothenic acid by pancreatic enzymes, and is then absorbed, along the entire length of the small intestine by a combination of active transport and passive diffusion, of which the active transport process seems to predominate at physiological intakes. This active transport process is dependent on sodium, energy and pH and is saturable: the K_m is c. 17 μM and V_{max} is c. 1000 pmol cm^{-2} h^{-1}, with minor variations among species.

In mice, it was found that usual dietary pantothenate levels did not affect the rate of absorption of a standard pantothenate dose, i.e. there was no evidence for feedback adaptation of the absorption pathway to low or high intakes, and it is assumed that the same is true in other species, including humans. However, there is some evidence from rat studies that the extent of secretion of enzymes degrading CoA into the gut lumen may partially limit the availability of pantothenic acid from CoA.

In humans, studies of urinary excretion of pantothenic acid after oral intakes of either free pantothenic acid or of the pantothenic acid present in food have indicated a relative availability of c. 50% from the food-borne vitamin. Urinary excretion of pantothenate was c. 0.8 mg per day, when a pantothenate-deficient diet was eaten, rising to 40–60 mg per day at a high daily intake of 100 mg. At intermediate intakes, in the range 2.8–12.8 mg per day, the daily urinary excretion rate varied between c. 4 and 6 mg.

Urinary excretion rates reflect recent intakes perhaps more closely than most other biochemical indices.

The contribution of the gut flora to the available pantothenate for humans is unknown, but there is some evidence that bacterial synthesis of the vitamin may be important in animals, especially ruminants, since severe deficiency can only be achieved by using antibiotics.

Clinical conditions such as ulcers or colitis can adversely affect pantothenate status and excretion rates, and dietary fibre may affect its absorption.

After a dose of ^{14}C-labelled pantothenate, about 40% of the dose appears in muscle tissue and about 10% in the liver, with smaller amounts occurring elsewhere. The differential affinities of the various different tissues determines their individual contents of the coenzyme derivatives, CoA and ACP, since there is no other major store of the vitamin anywhere in the body. Most organs, including placenta, exhibit evidence of a unidirectional active transport process for the intracellular accumulation of pantothenate which is dependent on sodium, energy and pH. In placenta (and probably elsewhere) this transport process is also shared by biotin and by some of its analogues, which can exhibit competitive inhibition. The only tissues which have been shown to differ with respect to transport mechanisms are red cells and the central nervous system.

In the central nervous system there is a saturable, bidirectional facilitated diffusion, but no evidence for active transport. In rabbits, for instance, pantothenate is converted only slowly to CoA in the brain. Similarly, the uptake and efflux of pantothenate into and out of red blood cells is nonsaturable and is unaffected by sodium, energy or pH. Red cells contain pantothenate, 4-phosphopantothenate and pantotheine, but *not* CoA (since they do not contain mitochondria, nor carry out CoA-dependent processes). The function of the pantothenate derivatives found in red cells is unknown, but their formation clearly results in higher concentrations of total pantothenate in red cells than in plasma, and red cell (or whole blood) total pantothenate is considered a better status index, and is more predictably related to intake, than is serum or plasma pantothenate. The latter appears to be a very short-term marker.

Unlike several other B vitamin precursors of cofactors, pantothenate is not entirely converted to coenzyme forms inside the cell, and metabolic 'trapping' is therefore less dominant than it is for some other B vitamins. There is some evidence that the free pantothenate in tissues is more closely related to dietary pantothenate than the coenzyme forms are; the latter are relatively protected during periods of dietary deficiency or of low intakes. Uptake of pantothenate from plasma into most tissues is proportional to the plasma concentration because the active transport process is nowhere nearly saturated at typical plasma concentrations of $c.$ 10^{-6} M.

Metabolism and Excretion

The primary role of pantothenic acid is in acyl group activation for lipid metabolism, involving thiol acylation of CoA or of ACP, both of which contain 4-phosphopantotheine, the active group of which is β-mercaptoethylamine. Coenzyme A is essential for oxidation of fatty acids, of pyruvate and of α-oxoglutarate, for metabolism of sterols, and for acetylation of other molecules, so as to modulate their transport characteristics or functions. Acyl carrier protein, which is synthesized from apo-ACP and coenzyme A, is involved specifically in fatty acid synthesis. Its role is to activate acetyl, malonyl and intermediate-chain fatty acyl groups during their anabolism by the biotin-dependent fatty acid synthase complex (i.e. acyl-CoA: malonyl-CoA-acyl transferase (decarboxylating, oxoacyl and enoyl-reducing and thioester-hydrolysing), EC 2.3.1.85).

The organ with the highest concentration of pantothenate is liver, followed by adrenal cortex, because of the requirement of steroid hormone metabolism there. A total of 95% of the CoA within each tissue is found in the mitochondria. However, the initial stages of activation of pantothenate and conversion to CoA occur in the cytosol. It was originally believed that the final stages of CoA synthesis must occur within the mitochondria, but later evidence indicated that transport across the mitochondrial membrane is, after all, possible. Beta-oxidation within the peroxisomes is also CoA-dependent, and is downregulated by pantothenate deficiency.

The rate of CoA synthesis is under close metabolic control by energy-yielding substrates, such as glucose and free fatty acids, at the initial activation step, catalysed by pantothenate kinase (ATP: pantothenate 4-phosphotransferase, EC 2.7.1.33). This feedback control is thought to be a mechanism for conservation of cofactor requirements. There are also direct and indirect effects of insulin, corticosteroids and glucagon, which result in important changes in tissue distribution, uptake, etc. in diabetics. The mechanisms involved here are complex and not yet fully understood.

Fasting results in a reduction of fatty acid synthase activity with loss of the coenzyme of ACP, which thus achieves the desired objective of a shift away from fatty acid synthesis, towards breakdown. This interconversion of apo-ACP and holo-ACP is thus a very important process for the short-term regulation of fatty acid synthesis.

Deficiency of sulfur amino acids can result in reduced CoA synthesis; likewise copper overload can (by interfering with sulfur amino acid function) also reduce CoA synthesis.

Excretion of free pantothenate in the urine is the primary excretion route in humans; in other mammals the glucuronide or glucoside may be excreted. There is little evidence of degradation to simpler products, and pantothenic acid appears to be very efficiently conserved in animals. Some bacteria can cleave it to yield pantoic acid and β-alanine. A potentially useful breakdown product of CoA is taurine, formed via cysteamine. This amino acid is an essential nutrient for some carnivorous animals such as cats.

In adult humans, a typical urinary excretion for pantothenate is around 4 mg per day, and excretion rates of less than 1 mg per day, are considered to be 'low'. When dietary intakes are low, the majority of the circulating vitamin, which is filtered in the kidney tubules, is resorbed by the same type of sodium-dependent active transport process that also occurs at most other sites in the body. Retention of a test dose of pantothenate is, as expected, greater in partially depleted subjects, than in saturated ones. Secretion into breast milk is proportional to intake and to blood levels of the vitamin; therefore dietary supplements to the lactating mother generally increase the breast milk content of the vitamin.

Metabolic Function and Essentiality

As noted above, the biochemical functions, and hence the basis for the dietary requirement of pantothenic acid, arise entirely from its occurrence as an essential component of CoA and of ACP, which cannot be synthesized *de novo* in mammals from simpler precursors.

In addition to the now well-established roles of CoA in the degradation and synthesis of fatty acids, of sterols and of other compounds synthesized from isoprenoid precursors, there are also a number of acetylation and long-chain fatty acylation processes which seem to require CoA as part of their essential biological catalytic sites, and which are still being explored and unravelled today. The acetylation of amino sugars and some other basic reactions of acetyl-CoA and succinyl-CoA in intermediary metabolism have been known since the 1980s. However, the addition of acetyl or fatty acyl groups to certain proteins in order to modify and control their specific and essential properties is a more recent discovery. The first category of these modifications comprises the acetylation of the N terminal amino acid in certain proteins, which actually occurs in at least half of all the known proteins that are found in higher organisms. The specific amino acids that are recipients of these acetyl groups are most commonly methionine, alanine or serine. The purposes of this terminal acetylation process are not entirely clear and may be multiple, including modifications of function (e.g. of hormone function), of binding and site recognition, of tertiary peptide structure, and of eventual susceptibility to degradation. Another possible site of protein acetylation is the side chain of certain internal lysine residues, whose side chain ε-amino group may become acetylated in some proteins, notably the basic histone proteins of the cell nucleus, and the α-tubulin proteins of the cytoplasmic microtubules, which help to determine cell shape and motility.

Proteins can also be modified by acylation with certain long-chain fatty acids, notably the 16-carbon saturated fatty acid, palmitic acid, and the 14-carbon saturated fatty acid, myristic acid. Although structurally very similar to each other, these two fatty acids seek entirely different protein locations for acylation and also have quite different functions. They have recently been explored with particular emphasis on viral and yeast proteins, although proteins in higher animals, in organs such as lung and brain, can also become acylated with palmitoyl moieties. Palmitoyl-CoA is also required for the transport of residues through the Golgi apparatus during protein secretion. It is believed that these protein acylations may enable and control specific protein interactions, especially in relation to cell membranes, and proteins which are palmitoylated are generally also found to be associated with the plasma membrane. Signal transduction (e.g. of the human $β_2$-adrenergic receptor) is one process which appears to be controlled by palmitoylation, and other palmitoylated proteins possess some structural importance, for example in the case of the protein–lipid complex of brain myelin. Clearly these subtle protein modifications, all of which depend on CoA and hence on

pantothenic acid, have a wide-ranging significance for many biological processes which is still being actively explored.

Pantothenic acid is essential for all mammalian species so far studied, namely humans, bovines, pigs, dogs, cats and rodents, as well as for poultry and fish. Pantothenate deficiency signs in animals are relatively nonspecific and vary between species. Deficiency in young animals results in impaired growth and requirement estimates based on maximum growth rates are between 8 and 15 mg kg^{-1} diet. Rats that are maintained on a diet low in pantothenate exhibit reduced growth, scaly dermatitis, alopecia, hair discoloration and loss, porphyrin-caked whiskers, sex organ disruption, congenital malformations and adrenal necrosis. Deficient chicks are affected by abnormal feather development, locomotor and thymus involution, neurological symptoms including convulsions, and hypoglycaemia. Pigs exhibit intestinal problems and abnormalities of dorsal root ganglion cells, and several species suffer nerve demyelination. Fish exhibit fused gill lamellae, clumping of mitochondria and kidney lesions. Signs specific for pantothenate depletion are not well characterized for humans. A syndrome which included 'burning feet' has been described in tropical prisoner-of-war camps during world War II, and it was said to respond to pantothenic acid supplements; however this was likely to have been a more complex deficiency. A competitive analogue of pantothenate, ω-methyl pantothenate, interferes with the activation of pantothenic acid; it also produces burning feet symptoms, Reye-like syndrome, cardiac instability, gastrointestinal disturbance, dizziness, paraesthesia, depression, fatigue, insomnia, muscular weakness, loss of immune (antibody) function, insensitivity to adrenocorticotrophic hormone and increased sensitivity to insulin. Large doses of pantothenate can reverse these changes. One of the earliest functional changes observed in mildly deficient rats was an increase in serum triacylglycerols and free fatty acids, presumably resulting from the impairment in β-oxidation. Paradoxically, CoA levels are relatively resistant to dietary pantothenate deficiency; however, there are some interorgan shifts in pantothenate in certain metabolic states.

As noted above, CoA is required for Golgi function, involved in protein transport; pantothenate deficiency can therefore cause reductions in the amounts of some secreted proteins. Other metabolic responses to deficiency include a reduction in urinary 17-ketosteroids, a reduction in serum cholesterol, a reduction in drug acetylation, a general reduction in immune response and an increase in upper respiratory tract infection.

Recently, some studies of wound healing and fibroblast growth have indicated that both pantothenic acid and ascorbic acid are involved in trace element distribution in the skin and scars of experimental animals, and that pantothenic acid can improve skin and colon wound healing in rabbits. It is not yet known, whether these observations are relevant to wound healing in humans.

Requirements

In the UK, National Food Survey records showed that in 1979 and 1986 mean adult daily pantothenate intakes were 5.1 and 6.07 mg per day, respectively. Since there is little evidence for the magnitude of minimum requirements in humans, the UK committee responsible for the revision of dietary reference values in 1991 suggested that daily intakes in the range 3–7 mg can be considered as adequate (although no specific values for the Reference Nutrient Intake, Estimated Average Requirement or Lower Reference Nutrient Intake for pantothenate were set). The US National Research Council, Food and Nutrition Board have likewise suggested 'safe and adequate' intakes of pantothenic acid at 4–7 mg per day for adults.

There are few studies in communities where intakes are likely to be low; indeed, pantothenic acid is so widely distributed in human foods that it is unlikely that any natural diets with a very low content will be encountered. Some variations in status between communities has been described, but these do not define requirements. In a group of adolescents in the USA, daily pantothenate intakes were around 4 mg; total blood pantothenate was in the 'normal' range of $c.$ 350–400 ng ml^{-1}, and intakes were correlated with red cell pantothenate ($r = 0.38$) and with urinary pantothenate ($r = 0.60$), both $P < 0.001$. In adults, these correlations were less strong.

Although expert committees have not recommended increased pantothenate intakes during pregnancy and lactation, there is some evidence that requirements may increase. As for most water-soluble vitamins, maternal blood levels do decrease significantly on normal diets during pregnancy, and the mean daily output of the vitamin in breast milk in the US is of the order of 2–6 mg, i.e. close to the mean daily maternal intake. It has been suggested that infant formulae should contain at least 2 mg pantothenate per litre.

Dietary Sources and High Intakes

Pantothenate is widely distributed in food; rich sources include animal tissues, especially liver and

Table 1 Pantothenate content of selected foods

Food	mg per 100 g wet wt	mg per MJ
Meat offal and fish		
Stewed minced beef	0.8	0.84
Grilled pork chop	1.0	0.72
Calf liver, fried	8.8	8.40
Lamb's kidney, fried	5.1	7.90
Cod, grilled	0.25	0.62
Dairy products		
Cow's milk, full cream	0.35	1.27
Cheese, cheddar	0.36	0.22
Yogurt (whole milk, plain)	0.5	1.50
Boiled chicken's egg	1.3	2.10
Human milk	0.25	0.86
Fruits		
Apples, eating, flesh and skin	trace	trace
Oranges, flesh	0.37	0.24
Pears, flesh and skin	0.07	0.41
Strawberries, raw	0.34	3.10
Dried mixed fruit	0.09	0.10
Vegetables		
Potatoes, boiled, new	0.38	1.20
Carrots, boiled, young	0.18	1.40
Brussel sprouts, boiled	0.28	1.90
Cauliflower, boiled	0.42	3.60
Onions, fried	0.12	0.17
Grains, grain products, nuts		
White bread	0.3	0.30
Wholemeal bread	0.6	0.67
Rice, boiled, white	0.1	0.17
Cornflakes	0.3	0.19
Baked beans in tomato sauce	0.18	0.50
Peanuts, plain	2.66	1.10

Compiled from Holland B *et al., McCance and Widdowson's The Composition of Foods*, (1991) 5th edn. London: Royal Society of Chemistry and MAFF. (With the permission of the Controller of Her Majesty's Stationery Office.)

yeast, with moderate amounts occurring in whole grain cereals and legumes (see **Table 1**). It is fairly stable during cooking and storage, although some destruction occurs at high temperatures and at pH values below 5 or above 7. Highly processed foods have lower contents than fresh foods.

Synthesis by gut flora in humans is suspected but not yet proven; the rarity of diet-induced deficiency has been attributed to contributions from gut flora sources.

There is little or no evidence for any toxicity at high intakes: at daily intakes around 10 g there may be mild diarrhoea and gastrointestinal disturbance, but no other symptoms have been described. Pantothenate has been prescribed for various chronic disorders, but is not known to be useful in high doses.

See also: **Amino Acids**: Chemistry and Classification; Metabolism. **Energy Metabolism**: Tricarboxylic Acid Cycle and Oxidative Phosphorylation. **Fatty Acids**: Metabolism. **Lactation**: Dietary Requirements. **Lipids**: Chemistry and Classification.

Further Reading

Bender DA (1992) Pantothenic acid. In: *Nutritional Biochemistry of the Vitamins*, chap. 12, pp 341–359. Cambridge: CUP.
Fox HM (1984) Pantothenic acid. In: Machlin L (ed.) *Handbook of Vitamins: Nutritional, Biochemical and Clinical Aspects*, pp 437–457. New York: Marcel Dekker.
McCormick DB (1988). Pantothenic acid. In: Shils ME and Young VR (eds) *Modern Nutrition in Health and Disease*, 7th edn, pp 383–387. Philadelphia: Lea & Febiger.
Plesofsky-Vig N and Brambl R (1988) Pantothenic acid and coenzyme A in cellular modification of proteins. *Annual Review of Nutrition* 8:461–482.
Robinson FA (1966) Pantothenic acid. In: *The Vitamin Co-factors of Enzyme Systems*, chap. 6, pp 406–475. Oxford: Pergamon Press.
Smith CM and Song WO (1996) Comparative nutrition of pantothenic acid. *Journal of Nutritional Biochemistry* 7:312–321.
Tahiliani AG and Beinlich CJ (1991) Pantothenic acid in health and disease. *Vitamins and Hormones* 46:165–227.

PARASITISM

Effects on Growth and Nutritional Status

P G Lunn, Dunn Nutrition Laboratory, Cambridge, UK

In common with all other animals, human beings are susceptible to a range of parasitic organisms. The most important and common of these have been with humans for countless years and have become so well adapted that in most cases the human is their major if not their only host. Although parasitic infections occur throughout the world, it is in the wet tropics and subtropics where they are found at their greatest prevalence and intensity. Most developing countries are also located in these areas and the consequent poverty, poor hygiene and inadequate sanitation augment the favourable environmental conditions to enhance proliferation of the organisms.

Parasitic infections are among the most common diseases in the world (**Table 1**) and in many developing countries there seems to have been little improvement in prevalence rates for many years. Their association with poverty ensures that these diseases occur in areas where poor child growth and malnutrition are the most important and persistent health problems. While there is no doubt that heavy infections of any parasite can result in severe illness or even death of the host, such cases are rare even in areas of high prevalence, and the norm is low to moderate parasite numbers which result in few (if any) overt clinical symptoms. Nevertheless, by causing subtle reductions in appetite, digestion and absorption, and by increasing chronic inflammation and nutrient loss particularly of iron and protein, it is believed that such low-level but long-term infections contribute to the persistently poor nutritional state of many – especially children – in the developing world.

Table 1 Estimated world prevalence of parasites important to human nutrition

	Prevalence (millions per year)
Helminth parasites	
Ascaris lumbricoides (roundworm)	800–1000
Necator americanus and *Ancylostoma duodenale* (hookworms)	700–900
Trichuris trichiura (whipworm)	500
Schistosoma haematobium, S. japonicum and *S. mansoni*	200
Strongyloides stercoralis and *S. fülleborni*	50–100
Protozoal parasites	
Giardia intestinalis	200
Entamoeba histolytica	400
Cryptosporidium parvum	?

Data from Pawlowski (1984) and Grove (1984).

The most important parasites in humans are from two main groups, the helminth worms and protozoans. Although several hundred different species have been described, the vast majority of infections are caused by only a few. Only those that are known to interfere with host nutrition are discussed below.

Epidemiology and Life Cycles

Helminth parasites

Ascaris lumbricoides, **roundworm** About 73% of all roundworm infections are estimated to occur in Asia, with many countries having prevalence rates greater than 50%. In some rural areas over 90% of children harbour the infection. It is less prevalent in Africa (about 12% of all cases) and in Central and South America (about 8% of all cases). It is uncommon but still present in some rural areas of Europe and southeastern parts of the USA.

The adults of *A. lumbricoides* live in the lumen of the jejunum, the upper part of the small intestine. The worms live for some 12–20 months and females grow to 20–35 cm in length and 3–6 mm in diameter. An adult female discharges 200 000 to 240 000 eggs per day into the lumen and these pass out of the body in the faeces. The eggs embryonate, i.e. an infective larva develops within the egg, in 3–4 weeks. Infection occurs by oral ingestion of embryonated eggs in faecally contaminated food, water, hands, kitchen utensils or playthings. Eggs hatch in the small intestine. The larvae burrow into the mucosal blood vessels and are carried first to the liver, then to the lungs where they enter the alveoli. They migrate to the pharynx (often assisted by coughing), where they are swallowed and return to the small intestine to grow into adults.

Both the prevalence and intensity of infection with *A. lumbricoides* increase rapidly during early childhood, and although prevalence often remains high throughout life, intensity of infection tends to peak in the 5–15 year age range.

Hookworms Although 13 different human hookworm parasites have been listed, only two species, *Necator americanus* and *Ancylostoma duodenale,* are responsible for virtually all cases of hookworm disease in humans. The two worms are similar in appearance, feeding pattern and life history and most clinical reports do not differentiate between the species. Humans are their only known host.

Necator americanus is the only species seen in North America and it predominates in Central and South America, Central Africa, southern India, Indonesia and the South Pacific. *Ancylostoma duodenale* is found in Mediterranean Europe, the Middle East, North Africa, Pakistan, Iran and northern India. Both species occur in parts of Brazil, India and Africa, throughout Southeast Asia, Indonesia and the Pacific islands.

Adult worms live in the upper part of the small intestine and eggs are discharged into the lumen. Up to 10 000 (*N. americanus*) or 25 000 (*A. duodenale*) eggs per day can be produced and are passed out in the faeces. Eggs hatch within 48 h and the larvae are free-living for 2–3 weeks, but then must reach a host or die. They generally enter the body by skin penetration, usually through the feet or hands. Having entered a blood vessel, they are transported to the lungs where they migrate into the alveoli and eventually reach the pharynx from where they are swallowed, finally reaching the small intestine. Infection with *A. duodenale* can also occur orally and transplacentally. Egg production starts 40–100 days after infection. Female adults of *A. duodenale* are 10–13 mm in length, *N. americanus* 9–11 mm, and the males about 2 mm shorter. *Necator americanus* can live for up to 5 years.

Both prevalence and intensity of infection increase with age in childhood up to the age of about 10–15 years, then remain constant during adulthood. High prevalence is associated with inadequate or unhygienic disposal of faeces which contaminates the soil. Lack of footwear, a common state in developing countries, allows feet to come in contact with infective larvae. Untreated human excreta is still used as a fertilizer in some countries and this may explain the heavier parasite loads frequently seen in individuals doing agricultural work.

Schistosomes The three most common species responsible for schistosomal disease are *Schistosoma haematobium, S. mansoni* and *S. japonica,* with some individuals in Africa harbouring two species. Urinary schistosomiasis, found mainly in Africa and some eastern Mediterranean countries, is caused by *S. haematobium.* Infection with either *S. mansoni* (found in Africa, the Middle East, parts of South America and the Caribbean) or *S. japonica* (occurs in China, Philippines and Indonesia) results in intestinal schistosomiasis. These worms live in blood vessels – *S. haematobium* in the vesical venules of the urinary bladder, with the other two species infecting the mesenteric veins adjacent to the intestines. Adults live in male-female pairs, and damage is caused by passage of eggs through the tissues into either the bladder (*S. haematobium*) or the gut lumen. Eggs leave the body in the urine or faeces. If they reach fresh water, they hatch to produce miracidia which must find a suitable snail host. After entering the snail, the parasites multiply by asexual reproduction, eventually producing free-swimming cercariae which are infective to humans. Infection is by skin penetration during contact with fresh water containing cercariae. Egg production starts some 2–3 weeks after infection. The parasite lives for 3–8 years.

The prevalence of this parasite in many developing countries is increasing as irrigation schemes allow the intermediary snail hosts to extend their range.

Trichuris trichiura, **whipworm** The whipworm is widespread throughout the tropics and subtropics. Most cases of infection (63% of the worldwide total) occur in Asia, with 11% in Africa and 14% in the Americas; a few cases are still seen in the USA, western Europe and Japan.

Humans are the principal host of the parasite which lives in the caecum, and the ascending and transverse colon of the large intestine. Adults are 3–5 cm in length and are whip-shaped; the long, thin anterior end is embedded in the mucosa, with the thicker posterior end in the lumen. Worms feed on mucosal cells but may also ingest red and white blood cells.

Eggs leave the host in faeces and embryonate in the soil. After reingestion, they hatch in the small intestine and larvae develop in the villi before moving down to the large intestine. Egg production starts 30–90 days after ingestion.

In some rural areas the prevalence can exceed 90%, and although prevalence remains high throughout life, peak intensity usually occurs between the ages of 5 years and 15 years. Infection occurs by oral ingestion of embryonated eggs on faecally contaminated food, hands or utensils.

Strongyloides stercoralis This worm has a worldwide distribution but is found predominantly in the tropics. Prevalence rates are uncertain as detection of the larvae by direct faecal examination (the method usually employed) gives a considerable underestimate. Prevalence rates of up to 85% have been reported but are uncommon. In parts of Africa, a closely related worm *Strongyloides fülleborni* is often more common than *S. stercoralis*.

The life cycle is unusual in that both free-living adults and larval forms exist. Adult parasites are all female, about 2.7 mm in length, and produce eggs parthenogenetically. They are usually found in the duodenum and upper jejunum. Eggs are passed into the lumen but most hatch while still in the intestinal tract. Although the majority of larvae are passed out in the faeces, some penetrate the wall of the intestine and reinfect the host, a situation known as autoinfection.

Larvae passed with the faeces live in the soil and grow into adults of both sexes. Eggs are laid and larvae hatch within 1–2 weeks. They metamorphose to an infective stage, when they must either locate a host or die. Infection is usually by skin penetration. Larvae are carried by the blood to the lungs where they burrow into the alveoli, travel up the trachea and are swallowed, so reaching the small intestine where they mature in approximately 2 weeks. Because of the autoinfection process, infection with this parasite can last indefinitely and severe disease can suddenly appear many years after an individual has left an endemic area.

Special features of helminth parasites Helminth infections all exhibit certain characteristic features by which they differ from most other infective organisms.

1. Intensity of infection shows an overdisperse distribution; it is usual for 20% of an infected population to harbour 80% of the parasites. Thus a large majority of individuals will have only light infections and show few if any symptoms.
2. Some individuals appear to be predisposed to have heavy worm burdens; they quickly reacquire a heavy load after eradication of their original infection. It is not known whether this is a genetic trait or due to the individual living under particularly unhygienic conditions.
3. Infection by several different parasites at the same time (polyparasitism) is extremely common in many areas.
4. Reinfection following deworming occurs very quickly because of considerable contamination of the environment by the large numbers of eggs produced by the parasites. In a study in Myanmar, the preinfection prevalence of *A. lumbricoides* was reached only 6–8 months after deworming.

Protozoal parasites

Giardia intestinalis (= *lamblia*) This organism is a common parasite of the human gastrointestinal tract and is found in all parts of the world. Although its prevalence is greatest in developing countries where hygiene facilities are poor, outbreaks of giardiasis continue to occur in many developed countries.

It has a simple life history. The trophozoite (the active form in the intestine) lives in the duodenum and jejunum of the host where it attaches to the enterocytes by means of a ventral disc. It reproduces rapidly by mitotic division and in heavy infections can cover large areas of the mucosa. Some trophozoites encyst; a protective wall forms around the organism and the cysts pass out in the faeces. Cysts are directly infective and after ingestion by a new host, the organisms emerge to establish a new infection. Disease can follow the ingestion of as few as 10 cysts which, given moist conditions, are viable for several months.

In developed countries, most infections can be traced to contaminated water, but direct person-to-person transmission has also been documented in nurseries, schools and other child institutions. In developing countries, poverty-related unsanitary conditions and inadequate disposal of faeces promote orofaecal spread of the parasite, but contaminated water is also likely to be important. The large number of cyst-producing individuals with asymptomatic infection constitute a reservoir of *G. intestinalis*. In addition, some animals are known to harbour *Giardia* and may be a source of human giardiasis.

Entamoeba histolytica This amoeba has a very wide distribution but is most commonly found in developing countries where lack of hygienic facilities exacerbate orofaecal contamination of water, food and hands. These parasites generally infect the large intestine where they frequently invade mucosal tissues.

The life cycle is simple: trophozoites reproduce asexually forming substantial colonies and in some cases cause ulcerative lesions in the mucosa. Some organisms encyst and pass out with the faeces. Following ingestion of the cysts by another host, the amoebae emerge when the cyst reaches the large bowel. The organism can also invade other organs, notably the liver, resulting in a life-threatening illness.

Cryptosporidium parvum This organism has only been recognized as a human parasite since 1976. It has a worldwide distribution, but in developed countries it generally causes a self-limiting disease which occurs most commonly in child institutions and in people working with animals. However, water-borne outbreaks have occurred in which large numbers of people have become infected. It is much more prevalent in developing countries where it is mainly a disease of children. The parasites live in the upper part of the small intestine, attached to the mucosal cells from which they feed.

Both sexual and asexual reproduction occur in the host and cysts are produced, most of which pass out in the faeces. Some however, do excyst while passing through the gastrointestinal tract, resulting in auto-infection which can prolong the disease long after the original source of infection has been eliminated. Infection is by ingestion of cysts in food or water, or

from unhygienic contact with infected persons. Continued exposure is facilitated by the many infected individuals who remain asymptomatic while passing cysts. The organism can also be transmitted to humans from infected animals.

Pathophysiology

Mechanisms of parasite–host nutrition interactions

Gastrointestinal parasites interfere with the nutrition of their host by one or more of the following mechanisms (**Fig. 1**).

Loss of appetite, anorexia Loss of appetite is a common feature in many illnesses, not only those involving the gastrointestinal tract. It is now thought that much of the appetite loss in disease is mediated by one or more cytokines (e.g. interleukin 1 and tumour necrosis factor), which are released by lymphocytes as part of the body's response to tissue damage or invasion. Additionally, however, parasitized individuals often complain of symptoms such as nausea, abdominal pain, flatulence, distension and discomfort, while some infections are associated with vomiting, diarrhoea or dysentery, all of which can be expected to reduce appetite.

Maldigestion and malabsorption Gastrointestinal parasites are well placed to interfere with digestion and absorption, so it is not surprising that maldigestion and malabsorption of fat, protein and carbohydrate as well as many of the micronutrients have been reported during infection. Structural damage to the mucosa of the intestine, such as the flattening or thickening of villi or villous atrophy, will reduce the absorptive surface area. Damage to the cells diminishes their absorptive properties and limits active transport processes, while accelerated replacement of damaged cells may result in immature mucosal cells with reduced transport capacity. Food that is not fully digested and absorbed in the small intestine will enter the large bowel where excessive colonic fermentation may result in diarrhoea.

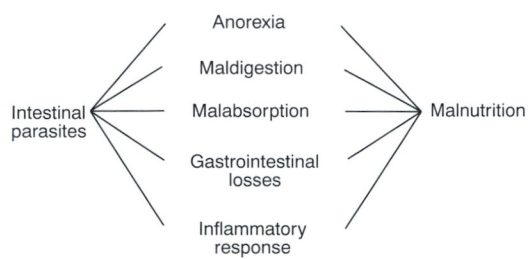

Figure 1   Mechanisms of parasite–host nutrition interactions.

Nutrient losses Accelerated loss of nutrients from the body is probably the most important mechanism by which parasitic infections compromise the nutritional status of their host. Nutrient loss can arise both directly and indirectly.

Direct losses occur during the feeding of the blood-sucking and tissue-invading parasites. Blood and tissue ingested by the worms form part of the loss, but the lesions caused by feeding and burrowing activity continue to ooze blood and tissue fluids after the parasites have moved on. Similarly, the passage of schistosome eggs through the tissues of the bladder or intestine is often accompanied tissue damage and blood loss. Increased turnover and accelerated shedding of parasite-damaged enterocytes into the lumen of the gut is another mechanism of increased nutrient loss. Even though some of the nutrients lost into the lumen will be reabsorbed, the process is far from complete. Vomiting or diarrhoea causes loss of electrolytes and trace elements.

Indirect losses arise from stimulation of the host's immunologic and inflammatory mechanisms which are mobilized to combat the infection and repair tissue damage. Localized inflammation at the site of the parasite activity, often accompanied by leucocytic infiltration of tissues, causes further damage to the mucosa, augmenting maldigestion, malabsorption and nutrient losses as more damaged cells are shed. Activation of the systemic inflammatory system, i.e. the acute-phase response, is a general reaction of the body to pathogen invasion or tissue damage. It results in a widespread cytokine-mediated catabolic response. Muscle tissue is broken down to provide substrates for gluconeogenesis and the repair of damaged cells and a negative nitrogen balance ensues. Anorexia occurs and there are increased losses of amino acids, minerals and vitamins in the urine and faeces.

Competition for nutrients Competition for nutrients is generally unlikely owing to the considerable difference in biomass of the host and parasite. However, the tapeworm *Diphyllobothrium latum* does compete for vitamin B_{12} taken in the diet. The worm concentrates large amounts of this vitamin in its own tissues, depriving the host and in some cases leading to megaloblastic anaemia.

Impact of parasites on host nutrition

Clinical studies Much of our knowledge of the impact of parasitism on host nutrition (**Table 2**) comes from hospital studies of heavily parasitized patients. Irrespective of the organism involved, nutritional status and anthropometric indices of such severely ill patients are invariably poor on admission but quickly improve following successful treatment. Such data must, however, be interpreted with caution. In developing countries, malnourished individuals admitted to hospital rarely suffer from a single infection; viral and bacterial pathogens and other parasitoses are frequently present, as are frank dietary deficiencies. Patients are routinely dosed with wide-range antibiotics and anthelmintics and given high-quality rehabilitation diets, so in general neither the cause of their symptoms nor the basis for recovery can be established with certainty. Both synergistic and antagonistic interactions between different pathogens may also occur.

Ascaris lumbricoides Despite the large size of these worms, mild to moderate infections are generally well tolerated with few, if any, overt symptoms. Clinical studies give contradictory results. Although anorexia, abnormal mucosal histology, decreased absorption of fat and carbohydrate, reduced lactase activity, decreased transit time, reduced nitrogen retention, reduced vitamin A absorption and lower vitamin A status have all been reported, they are not present in all cases. These abnormalities are in keeping with a stimulation of the host's immune and inflammatory mechanisms and it seems likely that occurrence of these symptoms depends on whether such mechanisms have been initiated. Why the immune and inflammatory response should be initiated in some cases of *A. lumbricoides* infection but not others is not known.

Hookworm Loss of blood, particularly of its iron content, is the most important pathological feature of hookworm infection. Iron deficiency anaemia is one of the most common deficiency diseases in the world and there is no doubt that hookworms contribute significantly to the estimated 1.3 billion individuals who suffer from this problem. Through its feeding activity, each *Necator americanus* worm causes the loss of about 0.03 ml of blood per day, while the larger *Ancylostoma duodenale* accounts for approximately 0.15 ml per day. Part of this loss is blood ingested by the worm, but each time the worm moves to a new site, perhaps up to six times per day, the lesions continue to ooze blood into the lumen.

Daily blood loss from an individual passing 2000 eggs per gram of faeces has been estimated at 4.3 ml (containing 2.0 mg of iron) and 8.9 ml (4.2 mg of iron) for *N. americanus* and *A. duodenale* respectively. Although approximately 35% of this iron will be reabsorbed by the intestine, daily losses will be 1.3 mg and 2.7 mg of iron, respectively. Assuming that only 10% of dietary iron is absorbed, an increased dietary intake of 13 mg and 27 mg

Table 2 Parasite interference with host nutrition

Parasite	Symptom	Nutritional effect
Ascaris lumbricoides	Anorexia and abdominal pain	Growth retardation, weight loss
	Malabsorption syndrome	Reduced fat and nitrogen uptake
		Reduced vitamin A status
	Lactose intolerance	Growth retardation, weight loss
	Acute-phase response	Growth retardation, weight loss
Hookworm	Anorexia and abdominal pain	Growth retardation, weight loss
	Diarrhoea	Growth retardation, weight loss
	Blood loss	Iron deficiency, anaemia
	Protein-losing enteropathy	Hypoalbuminaemia, oedema
Schistosoma sp.	Anorexia	Growth retardation, weight loss
	Diarrhoea	Growth retardation, weight loss
	Blood loss	Iron deficiency, anaemia
		Hypoalbuminaemia
	Acute-phase response	Growth retardation, weight loss
Trichuris trichiura	Anorexia	Growth retardation, weight loss
	Abdominal pain and vomiting	Growth retardation, weight loss
	Diarrhoea and dysentery	Loss of trace elements, e.g. zinc
		Growth retardation, weight loss
	Blood loss	Iron deficiency, anaemia
	Protein loss	Hypoalbuminaemia, oedema
	Acute-phase response	Growth retardation, weight loss
Strongyloides sp.	Anorexia	Growth retardation, weight loss
	Abdominal pain and vomiting	Growth retardation, weight loss
	Malabsorption syndrome	Reduced fat absorption
	Protein-losing enteropathy	Hypoalbuminaemia, oedema
	Acute-phase response	Growth retardation, weight loss
Giardia intestinalis	Anorexia	Growth retardation, weight loss
	Diarrhoea	Loss of trace elements
	Malabsorption syndrome	Reduced fat absorption
		Reduced vitamin A status
	Mucosal disruption	Lowered disaccharidase activity
		General maldigestion
	Acute-phase reaction	Growth retardation, weight loss
Entamoeba histolytica	Diarrhoea and dysentery	Fluid and electrolyte loss
		Electrolyte imbalance
		Loss of trace elements
	Acute-phase response	Growth retardation, weight loss
Cryptosporidium parvum	Anorexia	Growth retardation, weight loss
	Abdominal pain and vomiting	Growth retardation, weight loss
	Diarrhoea	Growth retardation, weight loss
	Mucosal disruption	Lowered disaccharidase activity
		General malabsorption
	Acute-phase response	Growth retardation, weight loss

respectively is required to make good these losses. As most diets contain only 15–20 mg of iron per day and some 10–15 mg of this is needed to cover daily metabolic requirements, intake would need to at least double to replace the loss from even this moderate hookworm load. In developing countries this is rarely possible, so without iron supplements, iron stores are soon depleted and iron deficiency anaemia ensues. Blood haemoglobin concentrations fall with increasing faecal egg counts above 2000 eggs per gram. Heavy infections of over 1500 worms with blood losses of over 100 ml per day are associated with severe anaemia and risk of death. In lighter infections, subclinical iron deficiency is shown by low plasma ferritin and iron concentrations; low transferrin saturation and elevated erythrocyte protoporphyrin content.

Protein is also lost through into the lumen of the small intestine during hookworm disease. Estimates of plasma loss vary considerably and values over 100 ml (containing 6–7 g of protein) per day have been recorded, although much of this may be reabsorbed. Nevertheless, moderate to heavy hookworm infections are associated with hypoalbuminaemia, hypoproteinaemia and oedema, especially in areas where the protein content of the diet is low.

Despite the invasive nature of hookworms, there appears to be little or no activation of the host immune or inflammatory mechanisms in most cases. Mucosal abnormalities, maldigestion and malabsorption have been described but are not common.

Schistosome species Iron deficiency anaemia associated with blood loss occurs in both urinary and intestinal schistosomiasis. Although blood loss can be severe in heavy *Schistosoma haematobium* infection, in a study of nonhospitalized children with low to moderate infection, iron losses ranged from 120 µg to 500 µg per day, increasing with rising egg count. This is less than losses due to hookworm, but dietary iron consumption would need to increase by about a third to compensate. In areas where iron status is poor, the extra burden due to *S. haematobium* will undoubtedly contribute to the onset of anaemia. Intestinal schistosomiasis caused by *S. mansoni* can also result in iron deficiency but it is generally less severe than that seen in hookworm disease. Little data is available for *S. japonicum* infection, but its effect appears to be similar to *S. mansoni*.

The poor nutritional status of infected individuals may be related to anorexia, diarrhoea and activation of the inflammatory mechanisms of the host. Blood cytokine concentrations are raised in schistosomiasis and fall with effective treatment.

Trichuris trichiura This helminth also causes loss of blood and iron from the large intestine of its host by its burrowing and feeding activities. Blood loss per worm has been estimated to be 0.005 ml, thus a moderate to heavy infection of 200 worms would cause the daily loss of 1 ml of blood containing about 400 µg of iron. Daily iron intake would need to increase by approximately 4 mg to compensate. More than 3000 worms have been found in heavy *T. trichiuris* infection and such cases do have marked iron deficiency anaemia. However, in the majority, where worm counts rarely exceed 100, the infection is usually asymptomatic. Plasma protein loss can also

be substantial in heavy infections, but although plasma albumin values are frequently reduced, hypoproteinaemic oedema is rare.

Heavy infections are characterized by persistent dysentery, abdominal pain, nausea, vomiting and tenesmus leading to rectal prolapse. Appetite is reduced and raised plasma cytokine and acute-phase protein concentrations indicate activation of host immune and inflammatory mechanisms. Loss of nutrients including zinc and other trace elements in the persistent dysentery and vomiting may further lower nutritional status.

Strongyloides stercoralis The impact of this worm on nutritional status has not been clearly defined. Most information comes from case studies of heavily infected individuals and there have been no community studies. Heavily infected subjects have a severe small intestinal illness with anorexia, abdominal pain, nausea, diarrhoea and vomiting. There is some evidence for a malabsorption syndrome; steatorrhoea is often present, but it does not occur in all cases. A substantial protein-losing enteropathy can occur, resulting in severe hypoalbuminaemia and kwashiorkor-like oedema. Protein loss arises from a combination of the burrowing activity of the worms and a local inflammatory reaction from the host. The little information on *S. fülleborni* infection suggests it has a similar impact on host nutrition.

Giardia intestinalis Infection with *G. intestinalis* can be associated with a wide range of symptoms, from mild, self-limiting watery diarrhoea to a persistent foul-smelling diarrhoea with vomiting, abdominal pain and distension, and a severe malabsorption syndrome. However, many infected individuals 20–84% of infected cases) remain asymptomatic. It is not clear why the parasite can cause such a range of degrees of illness.

The nutritional impact varies with both the severity and duration of the symptoms. In the early stages, anorexia is of major importance, but if the disease persists, intestinal aspects compound the situation. In at least 50% of symptomatic patients there is malabsorption of fat, carbohydrates, protein and micronutrients (particularly vitamin A) associated with structural and functional abnormalities in the small intestine. Damage to the mucosa can range from normal to subtotal villous atrophy, but most subjects have mild villus shortening and increased crypt depth. The abnormalities are associated with a reduction in disaccharidases, notably lactase activity, and in lowered intraluminal concentrations of the hydrolytic enzymes trypsin, chymotrypsin and lipase.

Little is known about the nutritional effects of non-symptomatic giardiasis.

Entamoeba histolytica Although *E. histolytica* can cause life-threatening diarrhoea and dysentery in some, most infected individuals remain free of symptoms. In others, persistent diarrhoea can continue for months, interspersed with periods of apparently normal bowel function. As the parasite is most commonly found in the large intestine, there is little interference with food digestion and absorption and its main effect on nutrition seems to be due to loss of trace elements and electrolytes in watery stools. In more severe cases, blood is also lost in this way but amounts are small. Infection is associated with inflammation of the large bowel (colitis) indicating that host immune and inflammatory mechanisms have been stimulated, and this may account for reports of hypoalbuminaemia. No study has assessed the impact of this disease on nutritional status in the community.

Cryptosporidium parvum Most individuals infected with *C. parvum* remain asymptomatic, but in others, acute or chronic diarrhoea associated with vomiting, abdominal pain, dehydration and fever can occur. Immunocompromised and previously malnourished cases tend to have more severe and prolonged disease. In developing countries, the disease is most frequently seen in young children.

The nutritional impact of the infection depends on the severity and duration of the infection, but growth retardation and lowered nutritional indices occur in asymptomatic cases as well as those with symptoms. Structural damage to the mucosa of the small intestine is seen in severe cases and the resulting maldigestion, malabsorption and stimulation of the host immune and inflammatory mechanisms are likely to account for the adverse nutritional effects. It is believed that the nutritional status of asymptomatic individuals is compromised by less extreme expression of these same mechanisms.

Community and intervention studies

Iron deficiency and iron deficiency anaemia A close relationship between the level of hookworm infection and severity of anaemia has been observed in many cross-sectional field studies. Similar though generally less severe levels of anaemia have been associated with intensity of *Schistosoma* sp. and *Trichuris trichiura* disease. The cause and effect relationship suggested by these data has been confirmed by longitudinal investigations of iron status following anthelmintic administration. Community studies in Kenya, India and Papua New Guinea have recorded substantial increases (up to 6 g l^{-1}) in haemoglobin concentration 4–8 weeks after treatment. These marked improvements were seen even when parasite loads were not completely eliminated. Effective treatment of *Schistosoma* sp. and *T. trichiura* infections also results in much improved iron status.

Growth and protein–energy malnutrition Although clinical studies confirm that parasites have the potential to interfere with growth and nutritional status, evidence that they are a major cause of the widespread stunting and protein–energy malnutrition seen in developing countries is not as conclusive as may be expected. This may be because most infected individuals in a community will have only low to moderate parasite loads, and whether a particular disease is important in precipitating malnutrition on a community or public health scale will depend on the nutritional impact of such low-level infections. Information has come from two types of study: (a) cross-sectional surveys, and (b) longitudinal, placebo-controlled intervention studies in which nutritional improvements are sought following the use of antiparasitic drugs.

A large number of cross-sectional community studies have associated parasitic infection with growth deficits and poor anthropometric indices. Schistosomiasis has long been associated with poor growth, and an extreme condition, schistosomiasis dwarfism, in which physical and sexual development were severely retarded, was reported to be quite common in China until the 1950s. Most recent studies of mild to moderate infection with all three *Schistosoma* species confirm an association with poor nutritional status which is more marked in girls, but the degree of impairment is variable between different regions and at best can only explain a small part of the total nutritional deficit of the subjects. Hookworm infection is similarly associated with poor appetite, slower growth and lowered nutritional indices, with the severity of these related to the severity of iron deficiency anaemia. Iron supplementation of hookworm-infected children has been reported to improve appetite and growth performance as well as iron status, suggesting that the lowered nutritional status may be secondary to iron deficiency rather than a direct effect of the parasite. Growth retardation seen in moderate to heavy *T. trichiura* infection may be similarly explained, although heavier burdens of this worm frequently cause dysentery, a symptom invariably related to poor nutritional status. The few community studies performed suggest that giardiasis is also associated with poorer child growth and anthropometric indices, but the overall impact does not appear to be great compared with the underlying level of malnutrition in the areas studied.

The results of these cross-sectional studies have been reinforced by longitudinal community-wide studies of nutritional improvement following reduction or eradication of parasite burden. Over an 8-month study, Kenyan children given praziquantel to treat their schistosomiasis gained more weight and had higher skinfold measurements than counterparts given a placebo. However, the 1.2 kg weight gain only increased the percentage weight for age from 72.9% to 74.9%, while children given the placebo showed a 1.3% fall. A similar study in the Philippines also found improved skinfold thickness, but no improvement in weight. Albendazole treatment of heavily polyparasitized Kenyan children harbouring hookworm, A. lumbricoides and T. trichiura also resulted in improvements in weight, arm circumference and skinfold thickness associated with increased appetite and fitness. Statistical analysis implicated hookworm as being the most important in compromising nutritional status. Weight gain above placebo-treated counterparts averaged 1.3 kg per 6 months, adding about 3% to a weight for age of approximately 80%. Whether A. lumbricoides infection retards growth is in dispute. Although several studies report small improvements following effective deworming (the largest being a 1.2 cm increase in height over 2 years) but a roughly equal number found that worm eradication had no effect on growth.

Overall, community and intervention studies suggest that elimination of gastrointestinal parasites would improve growth and anthropometric status of children in developing countries, but that such improvement is limited. This contrasts with the substantial improvement in iron status and iron deficiency anaemia following effective parasite treatment.

Treatment and Prognosis

Table 3 shows the drugs most commonly used in treatment of parasitic infections. Anthelmintic drugs have improved dramatically and are now highly effective; in most cases a single course of treatment will result in parasite eradication. However, immunocompromised hosts (including malnourished children) may require more extensive courses of therapy for complete elimination of the infection. This is particularly the case in the treatment of cryptosporidiosis. Iron supplements are usually provided where blood loss has resulted in iron deficiency anaemia.

Recovery from infection is usually complete and

Table 3 Drugs of choice for parasitic infections

Infection	Drug
Ascariasis	Mebendazole, albendazole, pyrantel
Hookworm infection	Mebendazole, albendazole
Schistosomiasis	Praziquantel, metrifonate, niridazole, oltipraz
Trichuriasis	Mebendazole, albendazole
Strongyloidiosis	Thiobendazole, ivermectin
Giardiasis	Metronidazole, quinacrine, furazolidone
Amoebiasis	Metronidazole, paromomycin
Cryptosporidiosis	Spiramycin, clindamycin

rapid as most parasites do not cause lasting damage to their host. Schistosomiasis is the exception and can result in granuloma formation in several tissues, particularly the liver and spleen, which may become life threatening.

Prevention

Although drugs are now available to eradicate infections, unless the home environment changes, most individuals will soon become reinfected. The transmission of all the parasites discussed occurs through close contact between the host and infected human faeces, either orally or by skin penetration. The basic requirements for prevention are an efficient and hygienic mode of disposal of faeces, improved facilities in the home (for example clean running water and a concrete floor) plus a knowledge of basic hygiene. Use of footwear and avoidance of contact with water likely to contain schistosome cercariae would help. For the foreseeable future, however, such control measures are unrealistic in most developing countries and the alternative may be the large-scale, nationwide use of anthelmintics to regularly deworm all individuals in endemic areas. Safe, effective and relatively cheap drugs are now available and their use in this way could substantially reduce the level of intestinal parasitic disease throughout the developing world. Such programmes can be expected to result in a marked reduction in the prevalence and severity of iron deficiency anaemia, but in most situations will have a lesser impact on child growth and incidence of protein–energy malnutrition.

See also: **Anaemia (Anemia)**: Iron-Deficiency Anaemia. **Cytokines**: Nutritional Aspects. **Diarrhoeal (Diarrheal) Diseases**: Nutritional Factors. **Infection**: Nutritional Interactions. **Iron**: Physiology, Dietary Sources and Requirements.

Further Reading

Bundy DAP and Cooper ES (1989) *Trichuris* and trichuriasis in human. *Advances in Parasitology* 28:107–173.

Cooper ES, Whyte-Alleng CAM, Finzi-Smith JS and MacDonald TT (1992) Intestinal nematode infections in children: the physiological price paid. *Parasitology* 104:S91–S103.

Crompton DWT (1986) Nutritional aspects of infection. *Transactions of the Royal Society of Tropical Medicine and Hygiene* 80:697–705.

Crompton DWT (1987) Human helminthic populations. *Baillière's Clinical Tropical Medicine and Communicable Diseases* 2:489–510.

Diamond LS (1982) Amebiasis: nutritional implications. *Reviews in Infectious Diseases* 4:843–850.

Grove DI (1984) Strongylodiosis. In: Warren KS and Mahmoud AAF (eds) *Tropical and Geographic Medicine*, pp 373–379. New York: McGraw-Hill.

Lunn PG and Northrop-Clewes CA (1993) The impact of gastrointestinal parasites on protein-energy malnutrition in man. *Proceedings of the Nutrition Society* 52:101–111.

Meyer EA (1990) *Giardiasis*. Amsterdam: Elsevier.

Moqbal R and MacDonald AJ (1990) Immunological and inflammatory responses in the small intestine associated with helminth infections. In: Behnke JM (ed.) *Parasites, Immunity and Pathology*, pp. 249–282. London: Taylor & Francis.

O'Donoghue PY (1995) Cryptosporidium and cryptosporidiosis in man and animals. *International Journal for Parasitology* 25:139–195.

Pawlowski ZS (1984) Implications of parasite-nutrition interactions from a world perspective. *Federation Proceedings* 43:256–260.

Solomons NW (1993) Pathways to the impairment of human nutritional status by gastrointestinal pathogens. *Parasitology* 107:S19–S35.

Stephensen LS (1987) *The Impact of Helminth Infections on Human Nutrition*. London: Taylor & Francis.

Stephensen L (1993) The impact of schistosomiasis on human nutrition. *Parasitology* 107:S107–S123.

Thein-Hlaing (1993) Ascariasis and childhood malnutrition. *Parasitology* 107:S125–S136.

Pathogens *see* **Infection**: Nutritional Interactions; Nutritional Management; Nutritional Management of Measles and Human Immunodeficiency Virus in Children.

Pellagra *see* **Niacin**: Pellagra.

Pesticides *see* **Food Contaminants**: Pesticides.

Phenylketonuria *see* **Inborn Errors of Metabolism**: Nutritional Management of Phenylketonuria.

Phosphate *see* **Phosphorus**: Physiology, Dietary Sources and Requirements.

PHOSPHORUS

Physiology, Dietary Sources and Requirements

J J B Anderson, University of North Carolina, Chapel Hill, North Carolina, USA

Phosphorus is found in foods as phosphate salts or phosphate groups that are part of organic molecules. Elemental phosphorus is toxic and therefore not consumed as such. The abbreviations P_i and P_o stand for inorganic phosphate and organic phosphate, respectively; these are the natural forms of the element in foods and in body tissues and fluids. (The general term 'phosphate' is used in this review, and 'P' refers to both P_i and P_o.) The P_i concentration in blood is under hormonal regulation, primarily through actions of the calcium-regulating hormones, but insulin and other hormones also influence P_i distribution and uptake by cells. This review of phosphorus focuses more on the inorganic anionic form than on the diverse organic molecules that incorporate the anion into their structures for various functions in the body. Most of the topics reviewed herein are covered in depth in other sources listed in the bibliography.

Functional Uses of Phosphates

Cellular uses of phosphates in intermediary metabolism are extensive. Typically P_i ions are converted to various organic phosphates (P_o). Practically all energetic steps utilize high-energy phosphate bonds (adenosine triphosphate or ATP) for the synthesis of organic molecules, to drive transport systems across cell membranes, to make muscles contract, to allow nerves to conduct impulses and transfer information, to convey genetic information, to provide skeletal support and protection, for teeth, and for other mechanisms. In addition, phosphates circulating in blood have buffering activity. Clearly, P_i ions have multiple uses within and without cells.

Mineralized bone serves as an important store of P_i ions that can be retrieved from hydroxyapatite crystals through the action of parathyroid hormone on bone cells. Therefore, hypophosphataemia and phosphate deficiency are rare events in adults without other major complications, because of the large reservoir of P_i ions in the bone fluid compartment and in the mineral phase of bone.

Physiology of Phosphates

Inorganic phosphate ions are the primary form of phosphorus absorbed from the external environment via the small intestine, dissolved in the blood and extracellular fluids, distributed to tissues throughout the body, and excreted via the kidneys and intestinal tract. In addition, P_i ions and P_o in organic molecules are secreted in sweat, lost in the exfoliation of epithelial cells, and secreted in milk by lactating women. Typically, total P is measured because organic P_o groups are cleaved in the chemical analytic steps used to determine P.

Intestinal absorption

Inorganic phosphate ions are efficiently absorbed across the small intestine. In adults the efficiency is approximately 70%, and in children it can be as high as 90%. These efficiencies are considerably greater than those for calcium ions, which are 28–30% in adults and 50% or higher in children. The net effect is that P_i ions are absorbed approximately twice as efficiently as calcium ions. For example, for every 1000 moles of P_i, approximately 700 moles are absorbed (net), compared with only 300 moles (net) of calcium from 1000 moles in the diet. Therefore, the excretory mechanisms have to work more efficiently to eliminate the extra P_i absorbed following meals.

The absorption efficiency of P_i declines later in life so that the net absorption of phosphorus from foods is somewhat reduced; probably this occurs in a similar fashion as calcium absorptive efficiency declines with age, especially after age 65 years in women.

Inorganic phosphate ions are absorbed across all three parts of the small intestine, but the rapid entry to blood of radioactively labelled phosphates suggests that duodenal absorption occurs both efficiently and at a high transfer rate. Therefore, the bulk of P_i ions absorbed are transported across this segment, lesser amounts across the jejunum, and still lesser amounts across the ileum. If the hormonal form of vitamin D, calcitriol or 1,25-dihydroxyvitamin D, is elevated, P_i absorption can be even further enhanced in all segments of the small intestine.

Distribution in blood and homeostatic regulation

Phosphates exist in three fractions in human blood plasma: 54% free or ionized as HPO_4^{2-} and $H_2PO_4^-$, 34% complexed as the ions to small organic molecules; and 12% bound to circulating proteins. The ultrafiltrable fractions (ionic and complexed P_i) that are readily available for uptake by cells or by the extracellular bone fluid compartment (BFC) represent approximately 88% of the total P_i in blood plasma.

Parathyroid hormone (PTH) is considered to be the major hormone regulating P_i homeostasis because of its powerful role in enhancing renal and possibly intestinal P_i losses, while at the same time conserving calcium ions. When PTH is elevated, renal P_i reabsorption is largely inhibited, and similarly the secretion of P_i ions by intestinal mechanisms is enhanced (although understanding of this route of P_i loss is less established). Parathyroid hormone also acts on bone tissue to increase transfer of calcium ions from the BFC and from the resorption of mineralized bone tissue to the blood plasma to restore the calcium ion concentration. By these same actions of PTH, P_i ions are also indirectly transferred from the BFC and bone to the blood.

Calcitonin and the hormonal form of vitamin D, calcitriol, also have roles in phosphate homeostasis (see below). Other hormones can also influence the utilization of P_i within cells.

Uptake by tissues

The uptake of P_i ions by cells requires carrier mechanisms or cotransport systems because of the electrical charge and water-solubility properties of these anions. Typically P_i ions cotransport with glucose in postprandial periods, but their charge must be neutralized by cations, normally not calcium ions. Also after meals, P_i ions enter the bone fluid compartment, but in this case typically with calcium ions. Calcitonin has been considered to be primarily responsible for the uptake of these two ionic species by bone tissue following food ingestion and the intestinal absorption of these ions. Within cells the P_i ions are almost immediately used to phosphorylate glucose or other molecules, and a small fraction of these ions are stored as organic molecules or inorganic salts within cellular organelles.

Some P_i ions that enter bone may enter bone cells, especially osteoblasts or lining cells, whereas other ions bypass the cells and go directly to the BFC, an extension of the blood-extracellular continuum. In the BFC, P_i ions in solution increase the P_i concentration (activity) which permits these ions to combine with calcium ions in excess of their solubility product (K_{sp}) and form mineral salts (precipitate) in bone extracellular tissue. The formation of hydroxyapatite crystals, i.e. mineralization, is essential for structural support and protection of internal organs from environmental trauma. The P_i ions are, therefore, essential for the formation of endoskeletons typical of most vertebrates except cartilaginous fish.

Secretion into breast milk

Human breast milk contains approximately 140 mg l^{-1} of phosphate, compared with almost 340 mg l^{-1} of calcium. These large quantities of ions typically cannot be entirely provided by absorbed P_i and calcium, and therefore the skeletal reservoir of mineral becomes a significant contributor to the P_i of milk during an extended lactation. Lactating mothers need adequate amounts of P_i and calcium to support the secretion of these ions in milk and subsequently to restore bone mineral lost during the peak period of a full lactation (6 months or longer).

Excretion by the kidneys and small intestine

Approximately 60–70% of the P_i ions are cleared by the kidneys each day by healthy individuals. If PTH concentration is elevated, P_i excretion is enhanced even more, so that P_i losses are further increased. Under the same conditions of elevated PTH, the secretion of P_i by the gut may also be increased, but little is known about the regulation of endogenous P_i secretion via this route. The endogenous faecal secretion of phosphates is the second major route of loss that the body uses to maintain P_i ion homeostasis.

Phosphate balance

Phosphate balance means that the intake of phosphate from foods equals its losses in urine and faeces (and other sources such as sweat and skin, which are seldom measured). In effect, P_i ions that are absorbed are accounted for by losses from the body. Under zero balance conditions, no net gain or loss of P_i ions occurs. This balance state probably only exists during adulthood (roughly 20–60 years of age). During growth and pregnancy, but not during lactation, positive balance states tend to predominate, whereas in late life P_i retention may increase and become a major health problem for individuals with declining renal function. Phosphate retention (positive balance) late in life results in part from the declining effectiveness of PTH in enhancing renal excretion of P_i ions with decreasing renal function.

A typical phosphate balance in an adult man is illustrated in **Fig. 1**. A man typically consumes 1200–1400 mg P_i + P_o a day, whereas a woman consumes 900–1000 mg per day, according to the median intakes of the US Department of Agriculture's Continuing Survey of Food Intake of Individuals (CSFII) in 1991. These estimated intakes of total phosphate by gender do not include phosphate additives in foods.

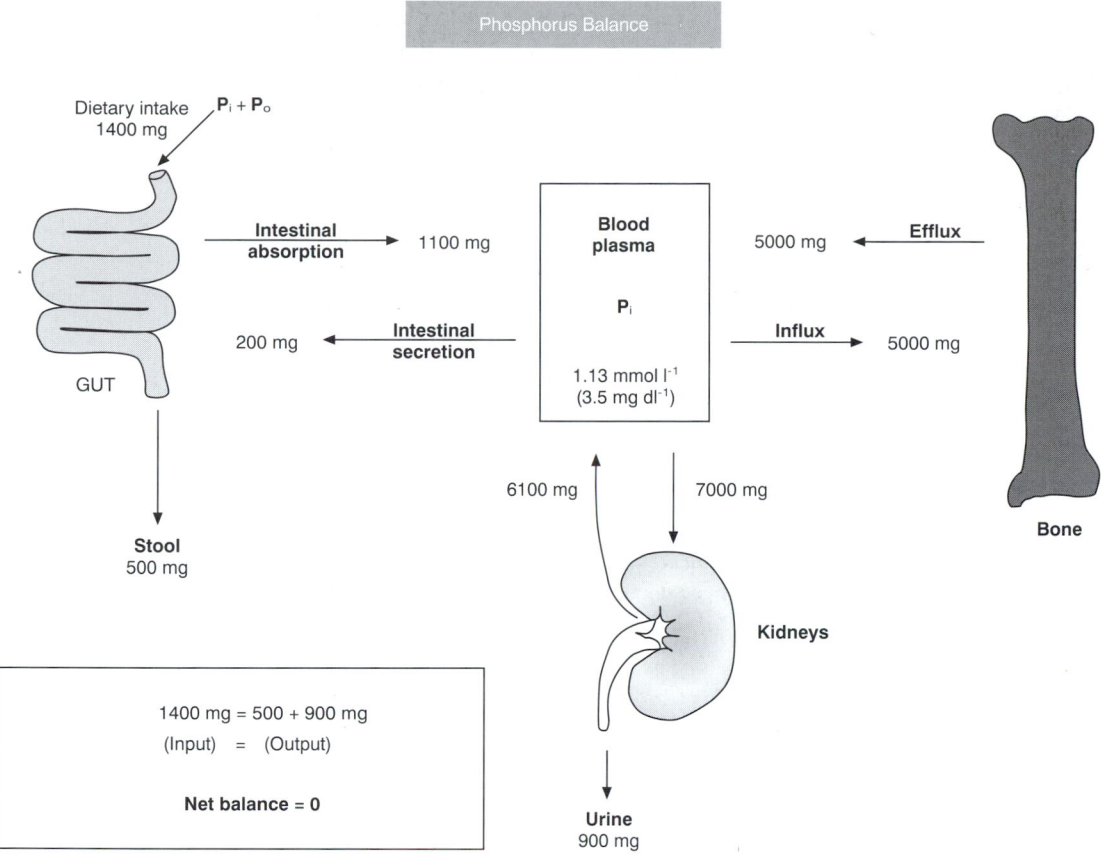

Figure 1   Phosphorus balance of an adult male. P_i = inorganic phosphate, P_o = organic phosphate.

Skeletal Tissue

Bone contains approximately 85% of all phosphates in the body; soft tissues contain about 10%, and blood and other extracellular fluids almost 1%. The 5% or so of P_i in teeth is fixed and nonretrievable. The phosphates in bone tissue exist almost exclusively in the mineral phase, i.e. hydroxyapatite. The P_i ions in the bone crystals serve as an important reservoir for transferring ions to the blood compartment via PTH. Although the regulation of serum calcium is directly linked primarily to the secretion of PTH, both calcium and P_i ions are resorbed together under the action of PTH on bone and these ions released to the blood. If excessive resorption of bone tissue occurs, then the excess P_i ions that accumulate in blood need to be removed through the renal and intestinal routes. The persistent action of PTH on bone, therefore, may have adverse effects on bone by gradually reducing its mass and its strength as described below.

Dietary Sources of Phosphates

A human dietary deficiency of phosphate is virtually impossible to develop, with the possible exceptions noted below. The reason for this encompassing statement is that almost all foods contain phosphate groups in organic (P_o) and/or inorganic (P_i) forms, and many of the foods commonly consumed are rich in P. For example, the polyphosphate phytic acid (inositol hexaphosphate) contains six P_o groups per molecule that become P_i groups when phytates are digested within the lumen of the gastrointestinal tract by phytase enzymes. (Phytates, however, are incompletely digested by humans, i.e. perhaps 50% or even less of the P_o groups.) Food composition tables should be consulted for the phosphate (total P or combined P_o and P_i) content of specific foods.

The approximate percentage distribution of foods (by food group) that provide dietary P in the USA is as follows: milk and dairy products 30%; meat, poultry and fish 27%; cereal grains and grain products 20%; legumes, nuts and seeds 8%; vegetables 7%; and other (miscellaneous) foods, including fruits, 8%. It is presumed, though accurate data are lacking, that these percentages are similar for the nations of the European Union and other Western nations. For populations that consume little or no dairy foods, the percentages would greatly increase for grains, legumes, vegetables, and fruits, depending on the food traditionally available. Vegetarians of all types, but especially vegans, have lower P intakes than do omnivores who consume several servings a day of dairy foods and meats. Intakes by vegans could be insufficient in P, but deficiency symptoms are very unlikely.

Plant foods

Cereal grains and most vegetables contain fair amounts of phosphates, compared with animal sources. Except for highly processed wheat flours and polished rice, cereal grains have much of their P_o bound in phytates that are not digested completely within the gastrointestinal tract and, therefore, the total amount of P in grains is not available for absorption. Legumes, including soya flour and peanuts, are good sources of P. Very few other plant foods are good sources of P except for nuts, such as almonds. Fruits, fruit juices and vegetable oils contain negligible amounts of phosphorus.

Animal foods

Animal foods are especially rich in phosphorus. Meats, fish, invertebrate seafoods, poultry and dairy products contain large amounts of this element. Liver, cheeses, and eggs (yolks) are highest in P, followed by meats, fish, and poultry, and then by milks (of any fat content). Mixed dishes that contain cheese or milk also contain large amounts of P.

Food additives

Processed foods currently being used by North Americans are often significantly increased in their P content through the intentional addition of one or more phosphate salts by the food industry. Phosphate additives have several functions in foods, notably as acids, as buffers and as anticaking agents. For individuals who consume many processed foods, especially those with cheese in them, it is estimated that total P intake per day can be increased by 10–15%. Therefore, P intakes from foods, both natural and processed, can tip the balance with respect to calcium to an unhealthy status (see below). The fortification of foods with P is not warranted because the diet is ample in phosphates.

Supplements

Because practically all foods contain phosphates naturally, and many processed foods have phosphates added to them, no need for supplements exists in healthy individuals with normal renal function. Except for the very rare clinical cases of the renal phosphate wasting condition and phosphate deficiency in newborns or premature babies, it is difficult to conceive of a situation requiring phosphate supplements. Therefore, phosphate supplements are not recommended for human consumption.

Requirements of Phosphorus as Phosphates

Phosphorus is an essential nutrient because it is needed for both organic molecules and the mineralized tissues, bones and teeth. Calcium phosphate salts have been speculated to have been the substratum for the synthetic steps that resulted in the origin of life in the liquid medium during the early history of the planet Earth.

Phosphorus requirements

The amounts of P needed in the diet each day depend on several variables, such as stage of development in the life cycle, gender, body size and usual physical activity. Mean requirements of dietary P are not precisely known for either sex during adulthood, but daily intakes (roughly between the 10th and 90th percentiles) of P in the USA are estimated to be approximately 1600–2400 mg for men and 1200–1600 mg for women according to data generated by the US Department of Agriculture's Continuing Survey of Food Intakes by Individuals (CSFII) in 1991.

Requirements of P may be as low as 600–800 mg a day for women and 800–1000 mg for men, but these are educated guesses only, assuming adequate consumption patterns of calcium. Excess P_i that is absorbed is excreted in a highly linear relationship to P intake in individuals with healthy kidneys. In late life and in individuals who have declining renal function, some phosphate ions may be harboured (not truly stored) in mineralized atheromatous deposits in arteries and in the skin. Phosphate balance assessment methods have been historically helpful in arriving at estimates of P requirements, but they typically have low precision of measurements in faeces and are therefore not so reliable.

Phosphorus allowances

In the USA the recommended dietary allowances for P have been established since the 1940s and they have been kept identical to those for calcium over this period. Phosphorus allowances, however, seem to be superfluous because of the widespread availability of this element from foods. The current adult US recommended dietary allowance of P for adult males and females is 800 mg per day.

Relationship to calcium and calcium : phosphorus ratio

The problem with adequate or excessive dietary phosphate intakes is the potential imbalance between calcium and phosphorus that results from typically low dietary calcium consumption patterns. Since practically all foods contain phosphates, but only a few foods have much calcium, eating behaviours that exclude calcium-rich foods, mainly milk and related dairy foods, may contribute to a condition known as nutritional secondary hyperparathyroidism. This condition may be exacerbated in individuals who consume diets rich in foods processed with phosphate additives and cola drinks with phosphoric acid, which can add considerably to the total dietary intake of P.

The high intake of total P *per se* is not such a problem, but the behaviours that lead to avoidance of the calcium-rich foods become the major problem because of the lowering of the Ca : P ratio and the development of a persistent elevation of (PTH). A diet containing adequate amounts of calcium can overcome these adverse effects of P.

Long-term prospective human studies of high-phosphate diets have not been published, so that data from short-term and cross-sectional investigations must be used to assess any adverse effects of habitual low-Ca, high-P intakes on bone status, the important end point of such studies. Only a few reports have examined this issue of the dietary Ca : P ratio. A 4-week investigation of young women consuming a Ca : P ratio of 0.25 : 1 demonstrated a persistent rise in PTH which is undesirable. Another report of cross-sectional data of healthy young adult females suggested that too much P relative to calcium in the usual diet has a negative effect on bone mineral content and density.

The mean Ca : P ratio of US adults approximates 0.5 : 1. Healthy ratios of intakes of the two elements range from 0.70 to 0.75 when the recommended numbers of servings from all food groups are consumed each day. It is very difficult to achieve a ratio of 1 : 1, the ratio recommended in the US RDAs, without taking calcium supplements. Therefore, a healthy eating pattern should contain a ratio within the range 0.7 : 1 to 1 : 1. Intake ratios at or below

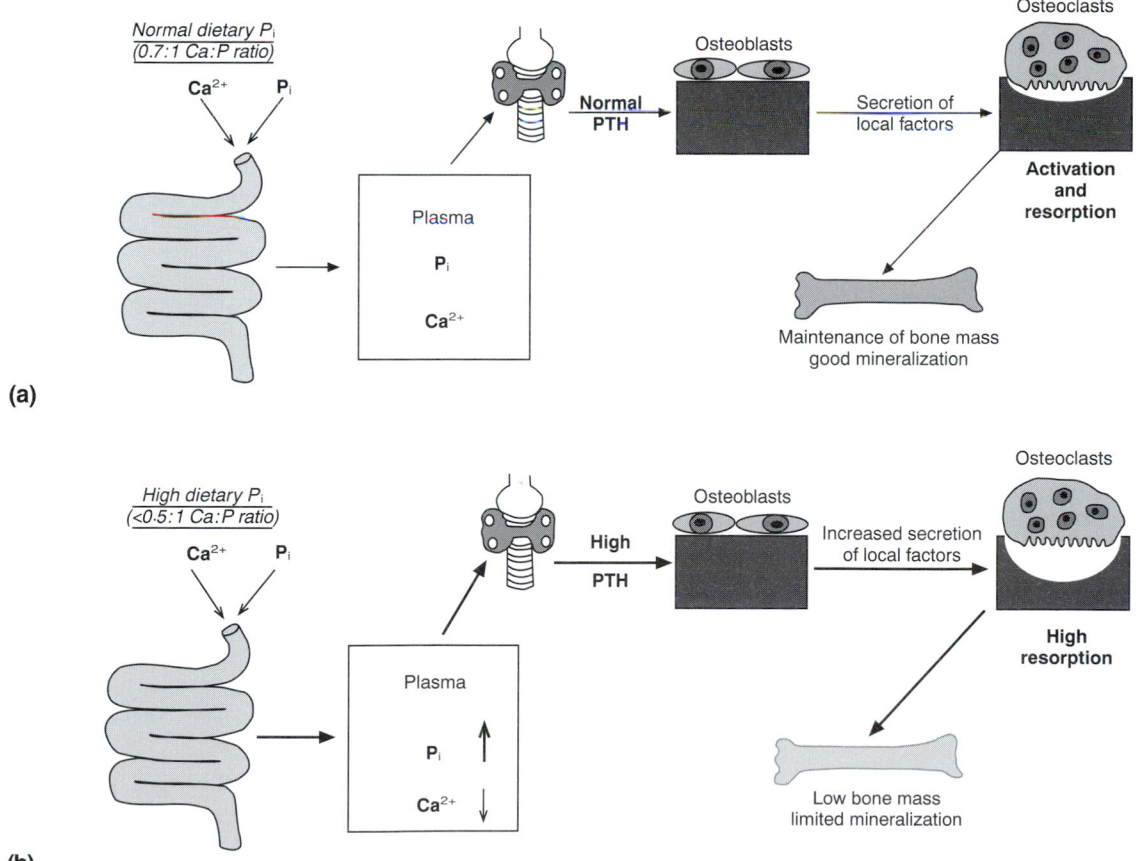

Figure 2   Comparison of parathyroid hormone (PTH) responses of (A) normal and (B) high dietary P_i intakes, and effects of PTH on bone mass.

0.5 : 1 are of concern because of the likelihood of persistently elevated PTH concentrations and the potential loss of bone mass which could lead to fragility fractures.

Fig. 2 illustrates the potential changes in bone mass and mineralization of the skeleton in individuals who typically consume diets with low Ca : P ratios compared with those who have normal intake ratios. The persistently elevated PTH is responsible for the limited bone mineralization and loss of bone mass.

Human Diseases of Phosphate Deficiency and Excess

Conditions of phosphate deficiency are extremely rare in humans because of the wide availability of dietary sources of these ions. A renal phosphate wasting condition of unknown aetiology has been reported. In addition, P_i deficiency has been reported in isolated cases of individuals with renal disease or home total parenteral nutrition who have taken excessive amounts of intestinal phosphate binders, such as aluminium and magnesium hydroxides (antacids), to reduce their P_i absorption.

On the other hand, dietary P excess is considered to be commonplace in the USA, especially among women who greatly limit their consumption of dairy products. These individuals have persistently elevated serum PTH concentrations that effectively reduce their bone mass over long periods. An increased risk of skeletal fractures is likely in individuals with diets that contain excessive amounts of P relative to limited amounts of calcium.

Conclusions

Phosphates participate in diverse roles in the human body, both intracellularly and extracellularly as P_i and P_o groups. Dietary deficiency of this element during practically the entire life cycle is highly unlikely, but high intakes are common because of the widespread availability of phosphates in foods. Phosphate additives in processed foods are increasing contributors to high consumption patterns of phosphorus. When a chronic pattern of low calcium consumption is coupled with high intakes of dietary phosphates (both P_o and P_i), parathyroid hormone becomes persistently elevated as a result of the inappropriate dietary Ca : P ratio. The potential outcome of this deleterious ratio is low bone mass and an increased risk of skeletal fractures, especially late in life but in reality at any age.

See also: **Bone**: Composition, Metabolism and Bone Growth. **Calcium**: Physiology. **Cereal Grains**: Dietary Significance and Nutritional Value. **Cholecalciferol and Ergocalciferol**: Physiology, Dietary Sources and Requirements; Rickets and Osteomalacia. **Dairy Products**: Nutritional Value. **Fruits and Vegetables**: Nutritional Value. **Legumes**: Types and Nutritional Value. **Nuts and Seeds**: Nutritional Value. **Osteoporosis**: Aetiology; Treatment and Prevention.

Further Reading

Allen LH and Wood RJ (1994) Calcium and phosphorus. In: Shils ME, Olson JA and Shike M (eds) *Modern Nutrition in Health and Disease*, 8th edn, pp 144–163. Philadelphia: Lea & Febiger.

Anderson JJB (1991) Nutritional biochemistry of calcium and phosphorus. *Journal of Nutritional Biochemistry* 2:300–309.

Anderson JJB (1996) Calcium, phosphorus and human bone development. *Journal of Nutrition* 126:1153S–1158S.

Anderson JJB and Garner SC, eds (1996) *Calcium and Phosphorus in Health and Disease*. Boca Raton: CRC Press.

Barger-Lux MJ and Heaney RP (1993) Effects of calcium restriction on metabolic characteristics of premenopausal women. *Journal of Clinical Endocrinology and Metabolism* 70:264–270.

Calvo MS (1993) Dietary phosphorus, calcium metabolism, and bone. *Journal of Nutrition* 123:1627–1633.

Calvo MS and Park YK (1996) Changing phosphorus content of the US diet: potential for adverse effects on bone. *Journal of Nutrition* 126:1168S–1180S.

Calvo MS, Kumar R and Heath H (1990) Persistently elevated parathyroid hormone secretion and action in young women after four weeks of ingesting high phosphorus, low calcium diets. *Journal of Clinical Endocrinology and Metabolism* 70:1340–1344.

Metz J, Anderson JJB and Gallagher PN (1993) Intakes of calcium, phosphorus, protein and level of physical activity are related to radial bone mass in young adult women. *American Journal of Clinical Nutrition* 58:537–542.

Nordin BEC, ed. (1976) *Calcium, Phosphorus, and Magnesium*. Edinburgh: Churchill Livingstone.

Subcommittee on Dietary Allowances, Food and Nutrition Board, National Research Council (1989) *Recommended Dietary Allowances*, 10th edn. Washington: National Academy Press.

Talmage RV, Cooper CW and Toverud SU (1983) The physiologic significance of calcitonin. In: Peck WA (ed.) *Bone and Mineral Research Annual*, vol. 1, pp 74–143. Amsterdam: Excerpta Medica.

US Department of Agriculture (1994) *Continuing Survey of Food Intakes of Individuals (CSFII): Diet and Health Knowledge Survey 1991*. Springfield: US Department of Commerce, National Technical Information Service.

Physical activity *see* **Exercise**: Physiology of Muscle; Diet and Exercise; Beneficial Effects.

PHYSICAL HANDICAP

Nutritional Management of Cerebral Palsy

Jackie Krick, Patricia Murphy-Miller and **Sally Savidge**, Kennedy-Krieger Institute, Baltimore, Maryland, USA

This article focuses on cerebral palsy and its nutritional implications. The first section will define cerebral palsy and describe its causes, rate of prevalence and classification types. Associated deficits related to cerebral palsy will also be explored. The topic of nutritional assessment of children with cerebral palsy will include sections on growth, body composition and energy, protein, fluid and nutrient needs. Feeding and swallowing problems and the influences of muscle tone on the ability to eat safely will be discussed extensively, as well as alternative feeding routes. The interdisciplinary approach is emphasized throughout as the ideal model to provide services to persons with cerebral palsy in order to assure quality of life in the community.

Definition and Aetiology

Cerebral palsy is a term that refers to a number of nonprogressive disorders of movement and posture that result from an injury to the central nervous system during early brain development.

Causes

Many diseases and conditions can affect the developing brain and result in cerebral palsy. However, up to 25% of cerebral palsy cases have no apparent aetiology. **Table 1** lists the most common causes of cerebral palsy.

Prevalence

Studies in several developed countries indicates a prevalence of cerebral palsy in 1.2–2.5 per 1000 children of early school age. In industrialized countries,

Table 1 Causes of cerebral palsy

	Causes	Percentage of cases
Perinatal		44
1st trimester	Teratogens	
	Genetic syndromes	
	Chromosomal abnormalities	
	Brain malformations	
2nd–3rd trimester	Intrauterine infections	
	Problems in fetal/placental functioning	
Labour and delivery	Pre-eclampsia	
	Complications of labour and delivery	19
Perinatal	Sepsis/central nervous system infection	
	Asphyxia	
	Prematurity	8
Childhood	Meningitis	
	Traumatic brain injury	
	Toxins	5
Not obvious		24

Adapted from Hagberg B and Hagberg G (1984) Prenatal and perinatal risk factors in a survey of 681 Swedish cases. In: Stanley F and Alberman E (eds) *The Epidemiology of the Cerebral Palsied*, pp 116–134. Philadelphia: JB Lippincott.

approximately 12–20% of persons with cerebral palsy acquired their disability after the first month of life.

Classification

There are several different classifications of cerebral palsy in the literature. The three most predominant types include pyramidal, extrapyramidal and mixed-type. The type of cerebral palsy and the degree of involvement play an important part in nutritional assessment and treatment.

Pyramidal (spastic) cerebral palsy Children with spastic cerebral palsy have increased muscle tone with a clasped-knife quality. In spastic quadriplegia (30% of pyramidal cerebral palsy) all four extremities are involved. In spastic diplegia (25%) both lower extremities are spastic with minimal upper extremity involvement. Hemiplegia (45%) implies involvement on only one side of the body, with the upper extremity usually more affected than the lower.

Extrapyramidal cerebral palsy Choreoathetosis involves the presence of abrupt, involuntary movements of the upper and lower extremities. This condition can greatly increase energy expenditure and will be explored further in the energy needs section.

Mixed-type cerebral palsy Mixed-type cerebral palsy includes characteristics of both the pyramidal and extrapyramidal types. For example, a child may have rigidity in the upper extremities and spasticity in the lower extremities.

Associated disabilities/deficits

Associated deficits of cerebral palsy are important to note since they impact on nutritional status. Cognitive impairments are quite common. Mental retardation occurs in 60% of cerebral palsy cases with the remainder at high risk for some type of learning disability. Sensory deficits are prevalent, including those in the visual and auditory modalities. Seizures occur in 20–30% of cases with the highest proportion in the spastic type. Feeding, behavioural or emotional problems are also frequently noted.

Nutritional Assessment

The goal for nutritional assessment and intervention is to have healthy, alert, interactive individuals who are able to take advantage of all the environment has to offer. Each person must be able to participate to her/his capacity in the learning and therapeutic

habilitative processes and in social, community and leisure activities.

Growth

The literature describes children with cerebral palsy who are shorter and lighter than the reference standard. This may be the result of several factors. Individuals with cerebral palsy have alterations in muscle tone affecting their limbs and torso, depending on the level of severity and topography. They often exhibit muscle contractures, depending on the type of cerebral palsy; muscle spasticity itself may retard bone growth. Limited physical activity may impede growth. Immobilization may be required after orthopaedic surgery. Immobilization inhibits bone formation and longitudinal growth and results in suppression of certain growth-stimulating hormones. It has been suggested that dysregulation of growth hormone secretion may be another factor affecting growth.

Recently a growth reference for children with spastic quadriplegia was developed to facilitate uniformity in clinical appraisal as well as to simplify comparative interpretation of growth data. These growth curves can be seen in **Figs 1–6**. It is important to view the velocity of rate of growth from one measurement to another to aid clinical management. The rate of growth in children with cerebral palsy is slower, so

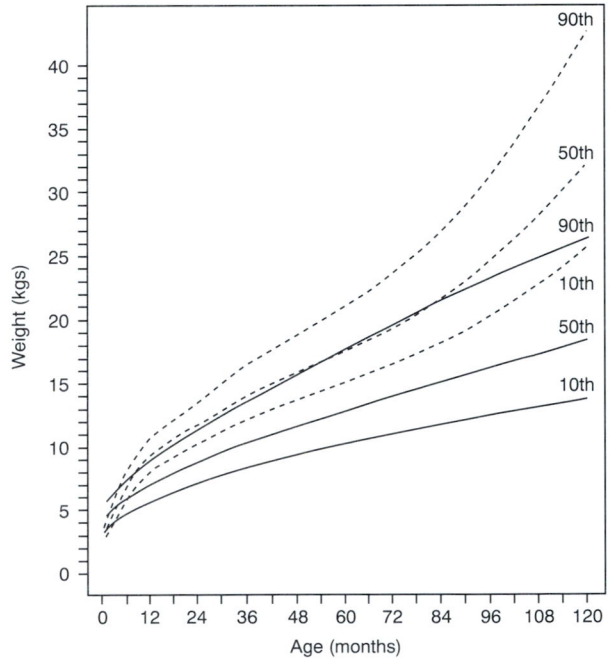

Figure 1 Weight for age for girls aged 0 to 120 months. The solid line represents girls with quadriplegic cerebral palsy and the dotted line represents the National Center for Health Statistics standard curve for 10th, 50th and 90th percentiles. (From Krick *et al* JADA **96**).

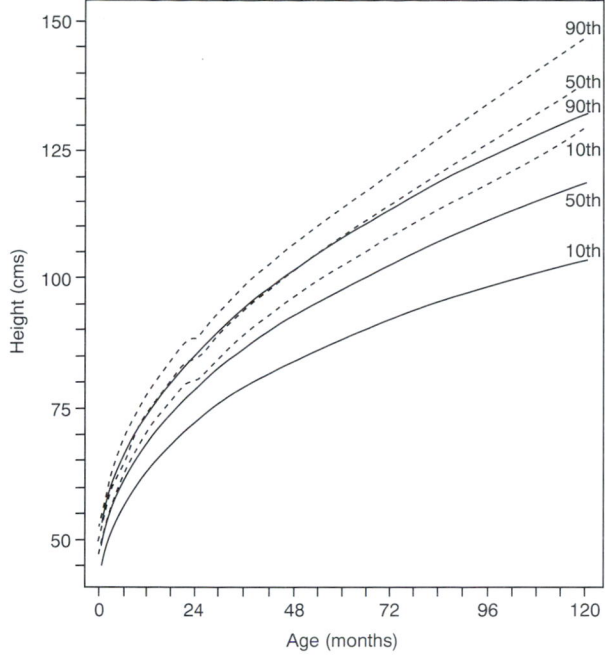

Figure 2 Length for age for girls aged 0 to 120 months. The solid line represents girls with quadriplegic cerebral palsy and the dotted line represents the National Center for Health Statistics standard curve for 10th, 50th and 90th percentiles.

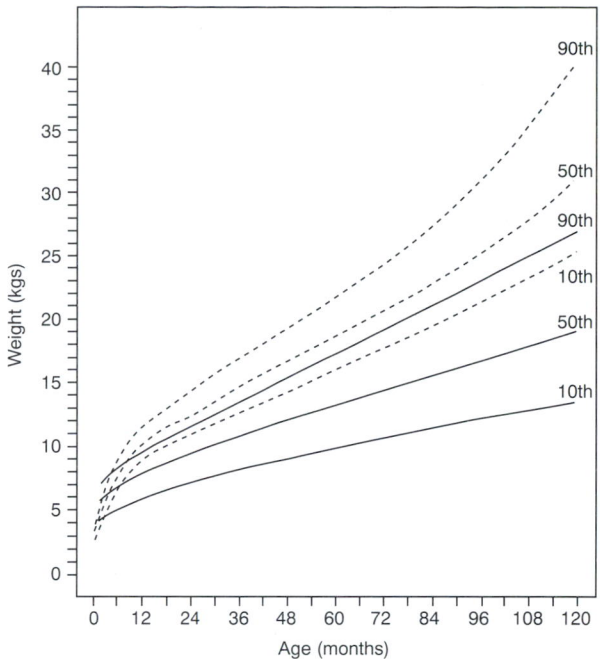

Figure 4 Weight for age for boys aged 0 to 120 months. The solid line represents boys with quadriplegic cerebral palsy and the dotted line represents the National Center for Health Statistics standard curve for 10th, 50th and 90th percentiles.

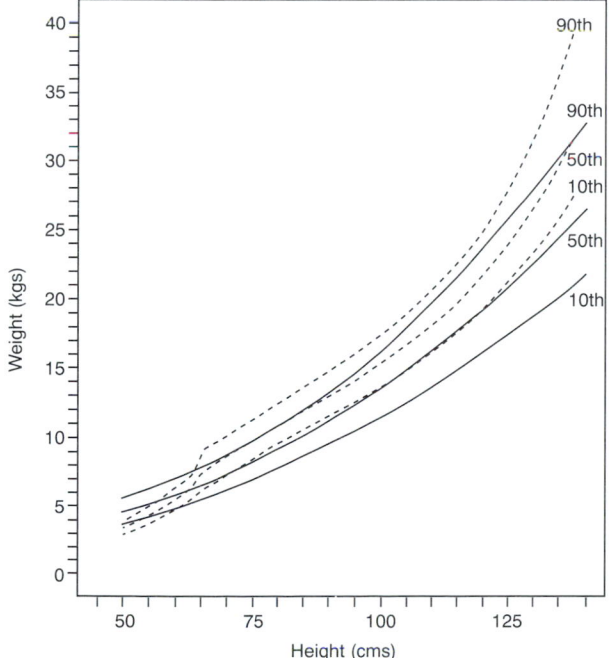

Figure 3 Weight for length for girls aged 0 to 120 months. The solid line represents girls with quadriplegic cerebral palsy and the dotted line represents the National Center for Health Statistics standard curve for 10th, 50th and 90th percentiles.

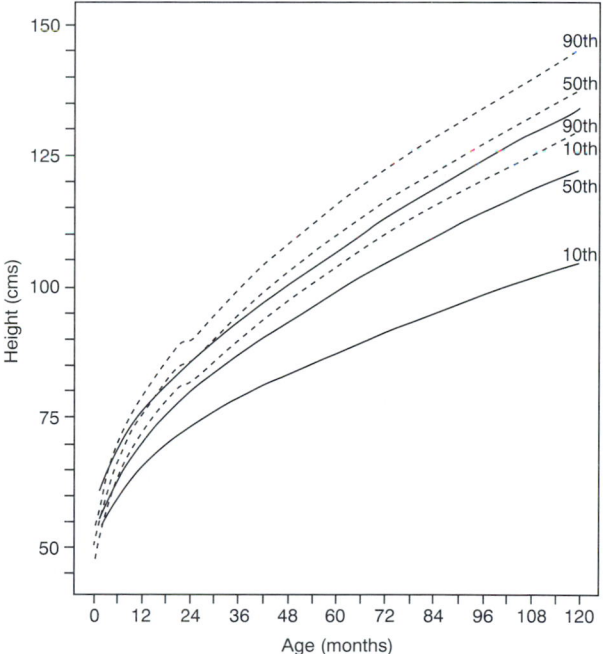

Figure 5 Length for age for boys aged 0 to 120 months. The solid line represents boys with quadriplegic cerebral palsy and the dotted line represents the National Center for Health Statistics standard curve for 10th, 50th and 90th percentiles.

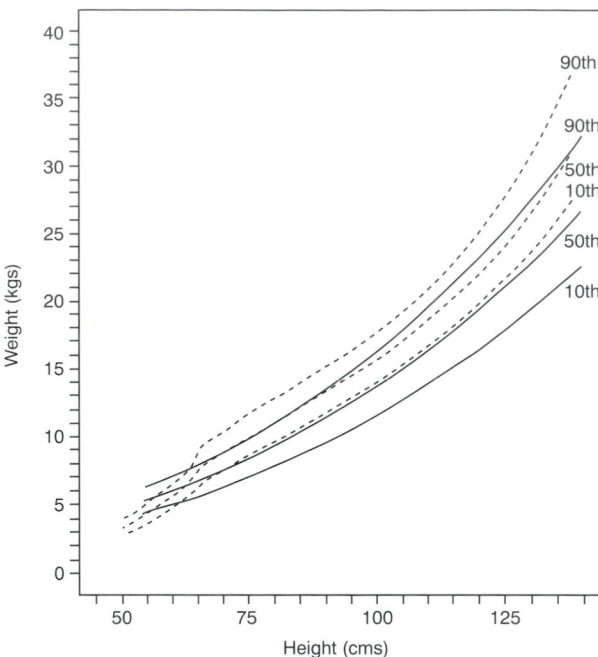

Figure 6 Weight for length for boys aged 0 to 120 months. The solid line represents boys with quadriplegic cerebral palsy and the dotted line represents the National Center for Health Statistics standard curve for 10th, 50th and 90th percentiles.

that as they get older the difference from the standard becomes greater.

The use of Z scores for length-for-age, weight-for-age, and weight-for-length promotes an accurate evaluation of discrete changes from one measurement date to another. Percentile tables describe ranges, and consequently detection of movement within the range is difficult to describe. The Z score denotes standard deviation units from the median and allows the practicing clinician and investigator to pinpoint precisely any given measurement.

Measurement of length or height for individuals with cerebral palsy may require techniques and standards using arm span, lower leg length or segmental measurements because of the difficulties encountered with joint contractures and/or scoliosis. The use of height age, rather than chronological age, is a commonly used technique and is defined as the age at which the child's height crosses the 50th percentile on the National Center for Health Statistics (NCHS) chart.

Ideal body weight

The estimate of ideal body weight (IBW) is also in part determined by the severity of the cerebral palsy. The IBW should be aimed at maintaining adequate fat and muscle stores to endure repeated surgeries or a common virus while facilitating daily physical care and management. Weight-for-length is a good indi-

cator of nutritional status because it obscures the issue of chronological age and addresses whether the individual is proportionate. Therefore, IBW should be expressed as this ratio. Those with cerebral palsy should attain and maintain an IBW that takes into account their age, the level of physical ability and their independence. Measurement of arm anthropometry will provide a description of body composition and support clinical judgements related to IBW. For example, children with spastic quadriplegia are the most dependent and the 10th percentile weight-for-length would be designated as the IBW. However, this assignment is done in tandem with assessment and monitoring of body composition and if either the arm fat or arm muscle area were less than the 5th percentile, then the IBW would be adjusted upward.

Body composition

Since the 1970s researchers reviewing body composition have noted reduced lean body mass in children with cerebral palsy. Recent work looking at adults with cerebral palsy and their age-matched controls found no difference in lean body mass or percentage of body fat.

Energy needs

Equations that are frequently used to predict energy requirements were developed using healthy children and adults in usual environmental and physical activity conditions and do not provide an accurate assessment of the needs of those with cerebral palsy. From a nutrition perspective, wide-ranging studies demonstrate underreporting of energy needs on food records, which at best provide a qualitative measure of intake. Therefore clinicians have turned to the use of more sophisticated technology such as doubly labeled water and indirect calorimetry to assess the energy needs of this population. Additionally, the energy cost of movement, whether it be wheelchair propulsion, crutch ambulation or the involuntary movements of the individual with athetosis, must be considered. Those with cerebral palsy may undergo repeated orthopaedic surgery that insults nutritional status, resulting in increased nutrient and energy demands. It has also been hypothesized that whole body metabolic rate might be related to differences in skeletal muscle fibre proportions and/or differences in enzymatic activity. Persons with cerebral palsy have abnormal variation in the size of muscle fibres and altered distribution of fibre types.

Altered energy needs are common among those with cerebral palsy and differ widely from the norm. Clinicians use a variety of approaches to estimate energy needs such as the recommended dietary allowances (RDA) for chronological age, the RDA for height age, and the World Health Organization (WHO) equation. When estimating energy needs, information related to muscle tone, activity level and needs for growth or catch-up growth must be added to the estimate for resting energy expenditure (REE).

One equation designed specifically for this population is:

REE × muscle tone factor × activity factor
+ growth factor(s) = kcal per day.

The REE can be determined using indirect calorimetry or can be derived from estimating body surface area × standard metabolic rate × 24 h. Body surface area (m^2) is calculated from length and weight, using the nomogram derived from the formula of DuBois and DuBois and the standard metabolic rate (kcal per m^2 per h) is identified using height age and sex, applying Fleisch data. The modifying factors are applied as follows:

- *muscle tone factors*: multiply by 10% for high tone (hypertonicity) and decrease by 10% for low tone (hypotonicity), no adjustment for normal tone;
- *activity factors*: multiply by 15% for bedridden state, 20% for wheelchair and 30% for ambulation;
- *Growth factors*: add 5 kcal (20.92 kJ) per g of desired growth, expected growth and catch-up.

Energy needs must be viewed on an individual basis assimilating the concepts noted above. The use of any approach is regarded as a guidepost and requires careful monitoring of body weight. Modifications to the diet should be based on clinical observation and measurement. There is a subpopulation of individuals who are obese and require less than any estimate for REE. Care should be exercised to provide adequate nutrients, protein and fluid.

Nutrient and fluid needs

Nutrient and protein needs are based on the RDAs similar to the population without cerebral palsy. Height age is often used in these determinations.

Table 2 Fluid needs based on body weight

Body weight (kg)	Fluid need (cm³ kg⁻¹)
≤10	100
11–20	+50
≥21	+25

Suggest monitoring urine specific gravities when available, quantity, colour and odour of urine, and adjust for periods of stress and temperature.
Example: 28 kg child
100 ml × 10 kg = 1000 ml
  50 ml × 10 kg =   500 ml
  25 ml × 8 kg =   200 ml
Total need = 1700 ml.

Nutrient deficiencies, drug–nutrient interactions, inability to bear weight and immobilization may lead to osteoporosis which increases the risk for bone fracture.

Fluid needs are based on body size rather than calorie intake. **Table 2** demonstrates how to calculate fluid needs. Constipation is a chronic problem for most children with cerebral palsy and is related to muscle tone, loss of sensation, limited physical activity, medications side effects and inadequate dietary fibre and/or fluid intake. Oral motor dysfunction results in diminished intake as well as in food and fluid loss. Modified food and fluid textures result in less free water and fibre in the diet. Discomfort associated with constipation may decrease appetite and increase gastrooesophageal reflux. Dietary intervention may therefore be limited and medical management may be necessary.

Assessment of Feeding Skills and Safety

Eating skills are acquired in a sequential pattern so that a developmental history will be helpful in evaluating present function and planning treatment options. Factors affecting feeding performance are shown in **Table 3**.

Table 3 General factors affecting feeding performance

Neuromotor performance	Constipation
Perceptual deficits	Amount of physical and verbal assistance required
Cognition and communication skills	Physiological support
Vision and hearing	Oral motor skills and swallowing status
Behaviour/interaction	Medications
Growth	Dental and gum disease
Dietary adequacy	Multiple orthopaedic procedures
GER and other GI-related issues	Family/psychosocial stressors

Oral motor evaluation

Feeding and swallowing problems are common in the child with cerebral palsy, depending on the type of muscle tone, presence of primitive reflexes, movement patterns and the integrity of the sensory system. Clinical indicators of feeding and swallowing dysfunction are shown in **Table 4**. Problems often include poor intake, inefficient and lengthy mealtimes, abnormal oral motor patterns, inappropriate progression of feeding skills, and/or physiological compromise with feeding. Sensory, cognitive and language deficits may also complicate the feeding process. An interdisciplinary team evaluation is essential for the assessment, development of appropriate goals and facilitation of a treatment plan which respects the developmental progression. A clinical assessment of the feeding process should include observance of facial muscle tone, oral reflex activity, functional oral motor skills, structural abnormalities, sensory responses, behaviour and interaction during feeding, respiratory and phonatory status, and posture and positioning.

Radiographic and ultrasound studies can provide more detailed information about the oral structures and the competency of the oral, pharyngeal and oesophageal phases, including the detection of aspiration. Cervical auscultation can also be helpful in evaluating the pharyngeal phase of swallowing. In addition, these techniques can assist in determining the suitable solid and liquid texture and appropriate head and neck positioning. Hypertonicity leads to abnormal movements of the tongue, lip and jaw. These abnormal movements can be manifested as tongue retraction, tongue tip elevation, tongue thrust, tonic biting, jaw thrust, jaw instability, lip retraction, and lip/cheek instability. An abnormally strong gag reflex, tactile hypersensitivity in the oral area and drooling can also complicate feeding. Individuals with cerebral palsy are also at risk for dental problems owing to poor oral hygiene, teeth grinding, hypersensitivity in the oral area and hyperplasia of the gums from long-term use of phenytoin, a medicine commonly prescribed for seizure management.

Aspiration and gastro-oesophageal reflux

Clinical signs of aspiration may include coughing, choking, gagging, inability to handle oral secretions, wet upper airway sounds with poor vocal quality, apnoea, food refusal, frequent upper respiratory infections, and/or aspiration pneumonia. Aspiration of food may occur without physical evidence if the protective cough or gag is not functioning, sensory deficits exist, and/or the swallowing mechanism is dysfunctional. This results in what is termed silent aspiration. While aspiration from solid food can be detected, the possibility of aspiration from gastro-oesophageal reflux (GER) may also need to be considered. The regurgitation of gastric contents from the stomach into the oesophagus can lead to irritability during or after feeding, arching, oesophagitis and ultimately food refusal. Other symptoms of GER include respiratory compromise, apnoea and/or drooling. Treatment for GER includes the use of antacids, H_2 blockers, medications to increase gut motility, reduction in feeding rate, positioning, thickening of foods or liquids, or surgical intervention. Small, frequent, feedings help to decrease the volume in the stomach at one time.

Fatigue may occur in the child who is not able to sustain the work involved with feeding and may be expressed by an increase in respiratory rate, diaphoresis or increased work of breathing. The causes may be muscular, respiratory or cardiac, and may increase the risk of aspiration or hypoxia. The work required to eat a meal is accomplished at a higher physiological cost to the child, thereby increasing caloric needs.

Muscle tone and positioning

It is important to understand the influences of muscle tone and proper positioning on the ability to eat safely and efficiently in this population. Increased or decreased muscle tone contributes to: difficulty preserving a patent airway, compromised self-feeding skills, poor rib cage expansion and oesophageal motility, and difficulty in maintaining a stable supported base for seating. Fluctuating muscle tone

Table 4 Clinical indicators of feeding and swallowing dysfunction

Facial weakness	Apraxia
Decreased sensation	Pain with swallowing
Congestion	Difficulty managing secretions
Noisy 'wet' sounds	History of upper respiratory infections
Multiple swallows to clear bolus	Apnoea during feeding
Unexplained fevers; unexplained irritability	Failure-to-thrive, failure to maintain weight
Coughing/choking/gagging before, during, or after swallow	
Food refusal	

leads to involuntary movements and limited postural stability. Despite the type of muscle tone, optimal positioning is crucial for feeding and swallowing. The proper feeding position includes neutral alignment of head and neck, midline orientation, symmetrical trunk position, 90 degree pelvic/femoral alignment, and symmetrical arm position with neutral shoulders. An example of proper positioning can be seen in **Fig. 7**. Consultations with orthopaedists and/or rehabilitation physicians to address present and potential musculoskeletal problems, physical and occupational therapists for functional assessment, orthotists for deformity management, and durable medical equipment specialists to customize standard wheelchair components, are valuable.

Superior mesenteric artery syndrome (SMA)

SMA syndrome is a condition in which the third portion of the duodenum is intermittently compressed by the overlying superior mesenteric artery, resulting in gastrointestinal obstruction. Symptoms include recurrent vomiting, abdominal distension, weight loss and postprandial distress. Persons with cerebral palsy are at high risk for several of the reported causes of SMA syndrome. These include body cast compression, severe weight loss, prolonged supine positioning and scoliosis surgery. Consequently, it is important to recognize the symptoms and know the appropriate treatments for this syndrome. Most persons can be treated nonsurgically with gastric aspiration, and nasojejunal or gastrojejunal feedings distal to the obstruction. One study also found that turning to the left from a supine position displaces the SMA from the right to the left side of the aorta in scoliosis cases. Thus, positioning can help alleviate symptoms and special considerations may be indicated in light of the limitations imposed by the cerebral palsy.

Behaviours around mealtime

Parent–child interactions can also influence feedings. Ineffective communication, lack of bonding, absence of social interaction or poor interactive skills, family dysfunction and decreased environmental stimuli can exacerbate feeding difficulties, or lead to frustration and anxiety with subsequent food refusal or parental withdrawal. Aversion to oral feeds can also be an outcome of medical complications such as oesophagitis and GER or lack of feeding experience at critical milestones secondary to prolonged tube feedings. Behavioural treatment should only be undertaken after thorough medical, nutritional and neurodevelopmental assessments are completed.

Feeding Issues

The feeding plan should be safe, promote growth or weight maintenance without excessive energy expenditure in order to obtain the required calories, and meet the needs of the family. It should reflect their resources in time and skill, and should address their concerns and expectations. The goals for treatment once feeding and swallowing problems are identified are to prevent aspiration and thereby respiratory compromise, to provide adequate calories, protein, vitamins, minerals and fluid, and to educate caregivers regarding nutritional requirements.

Oral motor considerations

Management strategies for daily mealtime feeding include positioning, modification of the sensory properties of the food, oral motor facilitation techniques and equipment adaptations. For those individuals with increased energy needs, the nutrient density of their meals may need to be maximized. **Table 5** lists commonly used calorie boosters. It is important to acknowledge the inability to change the underlying feeding problem, while providing a method of circumventing the problem to allow adequate nutrition and growth. For example, facilitative techniques to minimize excessive jaw movement may entail: the feeder providing physical jaw

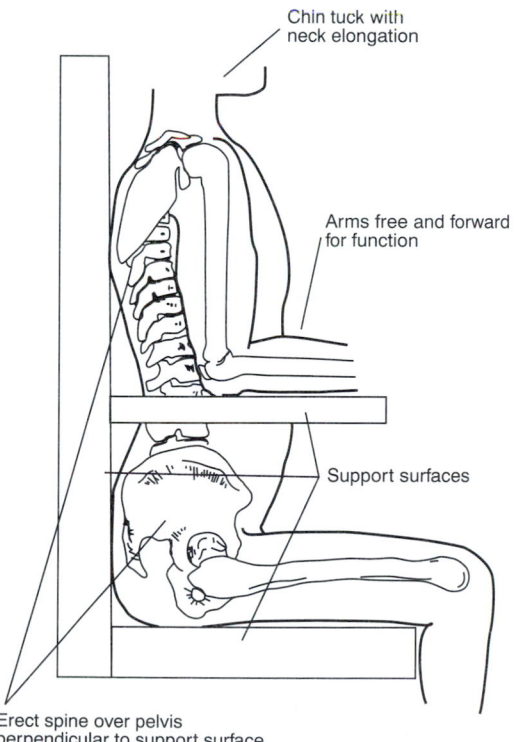

Chin tuck with neck elongation

Arms free and forward for function

Support surfaces

Erect spine over pelvis perpendicular to support surface

Figure 7 Proper seating position. Reproduced with permission from: *The Handbook of Assistive Technology*. Singular Publishing Group, Inc.

Table 5 Calorie boosters

Instant breakfast	Margarine, butter, oils, gravy
Powdered, evaporated milk	Sugar, honey, syrup
Whole milk cheeses	Cream cheese
Peanut butter	Sour cream
Wheat germ	Concentrate juices
Yogurt, pudding, custards	Breading or cracker meal
Milkshakes, eggnog	Fruit canned in heavy syrup
Supplements – such as Polycose, Promod, Microlipid, Pediasure® and Ensure®, etc.	

control/support; a change in the food consistency, texture, temperature or taste to improve the ability to propel a bolus through the oropharynx; the careful selection of adaptive feeding equipment to assist with self-feeding and/or increased intake; and an appropriate seating system. Proper positioning also allows the feeder use of both hands.

Alternative feeding routes

Many children with cerebral palsy are not able to meet some or all of their calorie needs by mouth owing to one or more of the following conditions: oral motor dysfunction, excessive energy needs, recurrent infections, illnesses, and orthopaedic surgical interventions. Consequently, if the gastrointestinal tract is functioning, supplemental or total tube feedings may be indicated. Early intervention with enteral nutrition may prevent protein–energy malnutrition and its complications. Studies have shown improvements in weight gain (fat mass as opposed to fat-free mass) with supplemental tube feedings, which better enables individuals to endure short-term medical insults.

Enteral nutrition may be delivered by nasogastric, nasojejunal, gastrostomy and jejunostomy tubes. The degree of GER and risk of aspiration determine where the tube is placed, whereas the length of time needed for tube feedings determines whether a naso-enteral or surgically placed tube is required. The decision of continuous, intermittent or combination tube feeds is dependent upon the individual needs of the patient.

Tube feedings should be considered a tool to improve nutritional status, rather than failure of the childs' ability to eat. Based on the medical diagnosis and developmental stage of the child, the prognosis for return to oral feeding varies, and the length of time to achieve this goal is extremely variable. For some children, the goal of returning to full or partial oral feeding is not realistic. Oral motor therapy should focus on maintaining existing oral motor skills, encouraging pleasurable oral experiences and tolerance of oral hygiene practices. Non-nutritive

oral stimulation must be performed when tube feedings are employed as the route of nutrition. The benefits are listed in **Table 6**. Improvement in nutritional status can result in positive changes in oral feeding.

Parenteral nutrition should only be used when the gastrointestinal tract is dysfunctional. When initiating feedings in patients with major weight loss or failure-to-thrive, whether enteral or parenteral nutrition is used, it is important to be aware of the 'refeeding syndrome'. This syndrome refers to phosphorus depletion and alterations in potassium, magnesium and glucose metabolism, resulting in severe metabolic and physiological complications. It is imperative to increase calorie delivery slowly with close laboratory monitoring.

Medications

Medication treatment options offer challenges to nutrition. These include attention to drug–nutrient interactions. For instance, diazepam, often used to decrease spasticity, increases the potential for drooling. This raises concerns of fluid loss/balance as well as loss of the protective effect of saliva on oesophageal mucosa. Additionally, attention must be paid to tone reduction in the trunk and oral structures that would compromise safety of feeding skills. Tone-lowering drugs potentially reduce energy expenditure and as a result require increased vigilance to avert excessive weight gain.

Coordinated services

The provision of nutrition services and prevention of further disabling conditions can be done in a variety

Table 6 Benefits of non-nutritive oral stimulation

Maintains oral sensation and tolerance

Facilitates saliva production, swallowing, and other oral motor patterns

Maintains or develops coordination of respiration and swallowing

Facilitates parent–child interactions

of health-care, school, vocational, home and community settings. It is the responsibility of the family in concert with the health-care team to promote nutrition care planning in these settings. More than 90% of children with cerebral palsy live to adulthood; however, their life expectancy is less than that of the general population. The chronicity of nutrition problems for individuals with cerebral palsy is recognized and has in part created a need for care coordination and integrated service planning to provide meaningful and cost-effective services.

See also: **Energy**: Measurement of Energy Intake and Expenditure. **Nutritional Support**: Enteral Feeding.

Further Reading

Capute A and Acardo PJ (eds) (1996) *Developmental Disabilities in Infancy and Childhood*, 2nd edn, vol. II: The Spectrum of Developmental Disabilities. Baltimore: Paul H Brookes.

Case-Smith J (ed.) (1993) *Pediatric Occupational Therapy and Early Intervention*. Stoneham: Butterworth-Heinemann.

Cherney L (1994) *Clinical Management of Dysphagia in Adults and Children*. Gaithersburg: Aspen Publishers.

DuBois D and Dubois EF (1916) A formula to estimate the approximate surface area if height and weight be known. *Archives of Internal Medicine* 17:863–871.

Eicher PS and Batshaw ML (1993) Cerebral palsy. In: Batshaw ML (ed.) *The Pediatric Clinics of North America. The Child with Developmental Disabilities*, vol. 40: pp 537–551. Philadelphia: WB Saunders.

Ekvall SW (ed.) (1993) *Pediatric Nutrition in Chronic Diseases and Developmental Disorders*: Prevention, Assessment and Treatment. New York: Oxford University Press.

Fleishe A (1951) Le metabolism basal standard et sa determination au moyen du 'metabolcalculator'. *Helvetica Medica Acta* 18:23–44.

Klein M and Delaney T (1994) *Feeding and Nutrition for the Child with Special Needs*. Tucson: Therapy Skill Builders.

Krick J, Murphy P, Markham J and Shapiro B (1992) A proposed formula for calculating energy needs of children with cerebral palsy. *Developmental Medicine and Child Neurology* 34:481–487.

Krick J, Murphy-Miller P, Zeger S and Wright E (1996) Pattern of growth in children with cerebral palsy. *Journal of the American Dietetic Association* 96:680–685.

Kurtz LA (1992) Cerebral palsy. In: Batshaw ML and Perret YM (eds) *Children with Disabilities. A Medical Primer*, chap. 24. Baltimore: Paul H Brookes.

PHYTOCHEMICALS

Contents
Classification and Occurrence
Epidemiological Factors

Classification and Occurrence

M Rhodes and **K R Price**, Institute of Food Research, Norwich, UK

Plants produce a wide range of low molecular weight compounds termed secondary metabolites or phytochemicals. Phytochemicals include many different chemical classes such as alkaloids, phenolic acids, flavonoids and terpenoids. There are many variations of derivatives within each class and these often show high degrees of stereochemical selectivity. Over 12 000 phytochemicals have so far been described in unprocessed food plants. A particular feature of plant secondary metabolism is that many of the products are toxic to the plant itself and a number of mechanisms have been evolved by plants to sequester these compounds, either within the plant cell or outside the cytoplasm on the plant surface or into the cell wall. An important feature of many groups of intracellular compounds is the formation of conjugates of the phytochemicals, usually with sugars, and their sequestration of these polar compounds in the plant cell vacuole. Thus, a general feature of plant secondary metabolites is the accumulation of glycosides, which can involve many different sugars and often acylation of the sugars with organic acids.

These phytochemicals play a number of roles in the plant, principally to provide a defence against attack by predators and pathogens, but they are also important in the interaction of the plant with its environment and as pigments and attractants promoting flower pollination and seed dispersal. Nearly all wild plants are either unpalatable or are toxic to phytophagous animals. An important factor in the unpalatability of plants to animals is the presence of high levels of a class of polyphenolic compounds, the tannins, which, because of their ability to bind tightly to proteins in the mouth, give an adverse reaction of high astringency. Among phytochemicals are many important pharmacologically active compounds including alkaloids and steroidal glycosides. Indeed, plants remain important sources of drugs still in current use.

However, of the vast number of available plant species, only a few hundred are regularly eaten by humans as food. Among these species, there has been considerable selection and breeding for plant species and varieties which are low in toxicants. Such plant improvement has led to the retention of those secondary metabolites which provide positive organoleptic or visual characteristics such as flavour compounds and pigments, and the reduction of those with adverse acceptability properties such as the tannins. However, low levels of tannins giving a limited degree of astringency is a desirable feature in some fruits. As a consequence of such crop improvements, current food plant varieties tend to have somewhat reduced endogenous defences against pathogens and predators and have to be defended in the field by pesticides and agrochemicals. Nevertheless, food plants retain significant levels of phytochemicals. With any diet in which plant foods form a significant element, a diverse range of plant secondary metabolites is ingested, among which are compounds having either beneficial or detrimental effects in humans. They may be taken up via the intestine into the bloodstream, metabolized by human gut or liver cells, and they or their metabolites may reach target cells within the body and influence the physiology of these cells.

These effects may be to cause cellular toxicity; indeed, some phytochemicals are potential natural toxicants to man. These include glycoalkaloids in potatoes and green tomatoes, and cyanogens (cyanogenic glycosides) in cassava. However, the balance of epidemiological evidence shows that diets rich in fruit and vegetables are correlated with low incidences of a whole range of degenerative diseases such as cancers. There is evidence that high intakes of particular classes of phytochemicals, such as the flavonols, is correlated with a low incidence of the degenerative disease, coronary heart disease. The beneficial effects of high intakes of fruit and vegetables in protecting against a range of these diseases can be ascribed to their content of particular phytochemicals. The significance of phytochemicals as protective factors is far from being understood at present and much current research is aimed at gaining an understanding of their possible role in nutrition.

Classification of Phytochemicals

Several classes of phytochemicals have been implicated as having effects in nutrition. These include potential toxicants such as glycoalkaloids, furanocoumarins and cyanogenic glycosides, and compounds such as phenolic acids, flavonoids, isoflavonoids, glucosinolates and the alk(en)yl cysteine sulfoxides, for which there is some evidence of a protective role. Among these potential protective factors a distinction may be drawn between those compounds in which the active species is an endogenous compound found in the food, and those in which the active species is not in itself an endogenous food component but is derived from a food component by the action of enzymes during preparation or during digestion. Phenolic acids and flavonoids are examples of the first group of protective factors, while glucosinolates and the alk(en)yl cysteine sulfoxides are examples of the second. Glucosinolates are sulfur-containing glucosides with a general formula of $R—C(=NOSO_3)—S—$glucose, where the function R can be an alkyl-, aryl-, indole- or sulfur-containing group. They are found in brassica vegetables where they are compartmentalized in the plant from a hydrolytic enzyme, myrosinase, which is housed in specialized cells (myrosin cells). On cell rupture, the enzyme and substrate can mix and interact to release glucose and a series of breakdown products (see **Fig. 1**) including isothiocyanates, thiocyanates, nitriles and indole derivatives, depending on the type of glucosinolate substrate, the pH and the presence of metal ions.

It is these breakdown products, principally the isothiocyanates and the indole-3-carbinol (which is formed from indole glucosinolates), which may have putative protective ability. In the alliums, the protective factors arise from the alk(en)yl cysteine sulfoxides by the action of the enzyme alliinase (see **Fig. 2**), which yields pyruvic acid and ammonia in addition to alk(en)yl sulfenic acids; these are unstable and give rise to compounds such as allicin (diallyl thiosulfinate) and alk(en)yl mono-, di- and trisulfides.

The chemical structures of typical examples of nutritionally important phytochemicals are shown in **Fig. 3**.

This distinction between natural toxicants and protective factors is not always clear cut. Compounds within the same chemical class may have

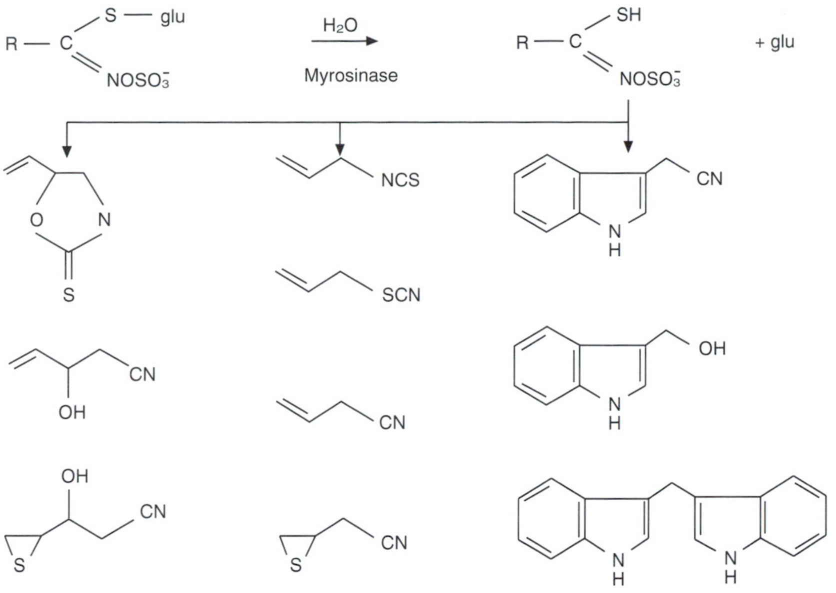

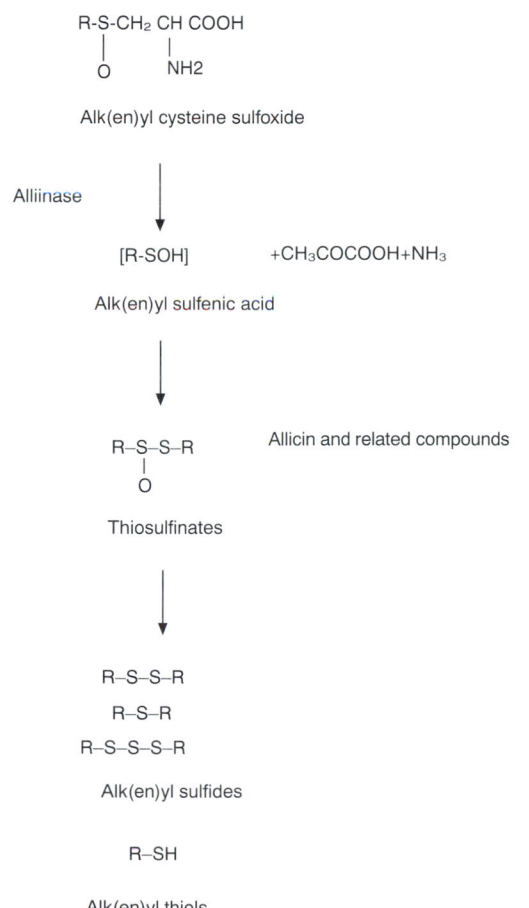

Figure 1 The breakdown of glucosinolates in brassica vegetables under the action of myrosinase.

both positive and negative effects on metabolism. For instance some glucosinolates, such as progoitrin, are known to have goitrogenic activity, while others, such as glucoiberin, may be protective as inducers of enzyme systems thought to detoxify carcinogens. In other cases a compound may be toxic at high dose and yet be protective at lower physiologically relevant doses. Thus glucobrassicin is mutagenic at high doses, yet at levels found in a normal diet appears to have a protective effect. In this article emphasis will be given to compounds which have potential protective effects and they will be classified on the basis of their physiological activity. **Table 1** lists some of these potential biological activities and some of the compounds which have been shown to exhibit them.

Evidence for potential protective effects is generally based on experiments demonstrating a biological activity in a relevant *in vitro* bioassay or in experiments using animal models. In some cases, this is supported by both epidemiological studies and by a limited number of intervention experiments in humans. The experimental evidence from work on animals does not lead to conclusions which are directly applicable to humans and often the evidence is conflicting. For instance, epidemiological evidence correlates high intakes of flavonol derivatives (principally derivatives of quercetin) with a low incidence of coronary vascular disease, but not with cancer. Experiments showing that quercetin can protect low-density lipoprotein (LDL) against oxidation both *in vitro* and *in vivo*, a process associated with the aetiology of atherosclerosis, is in agreement with the epidemiological evidence. However, experi-

R-S-CH$_2$ CH COOH
| |
O   NH2

Alk(en)yl cysteine sulfoxide

Alliinase

[R-SOH]   +CH$_3$COCOOH+NH$_3$

Alk(en)yl sulfenic acid

R–S–S–R   Allicin and related compounds
|
O

Thiosulfinates

R–S–S–R
R–S–R
R–S–S–S–R

Alk(en)yl sulfides

R–SH

Alk(en)yl thiols

Figure 2 The breakdown of alkenyl cysteine sulfoxides by the enzyme alliinase in allium vegetables. R = 2-propenyl-, allyl-, propyl-, or methyl-.

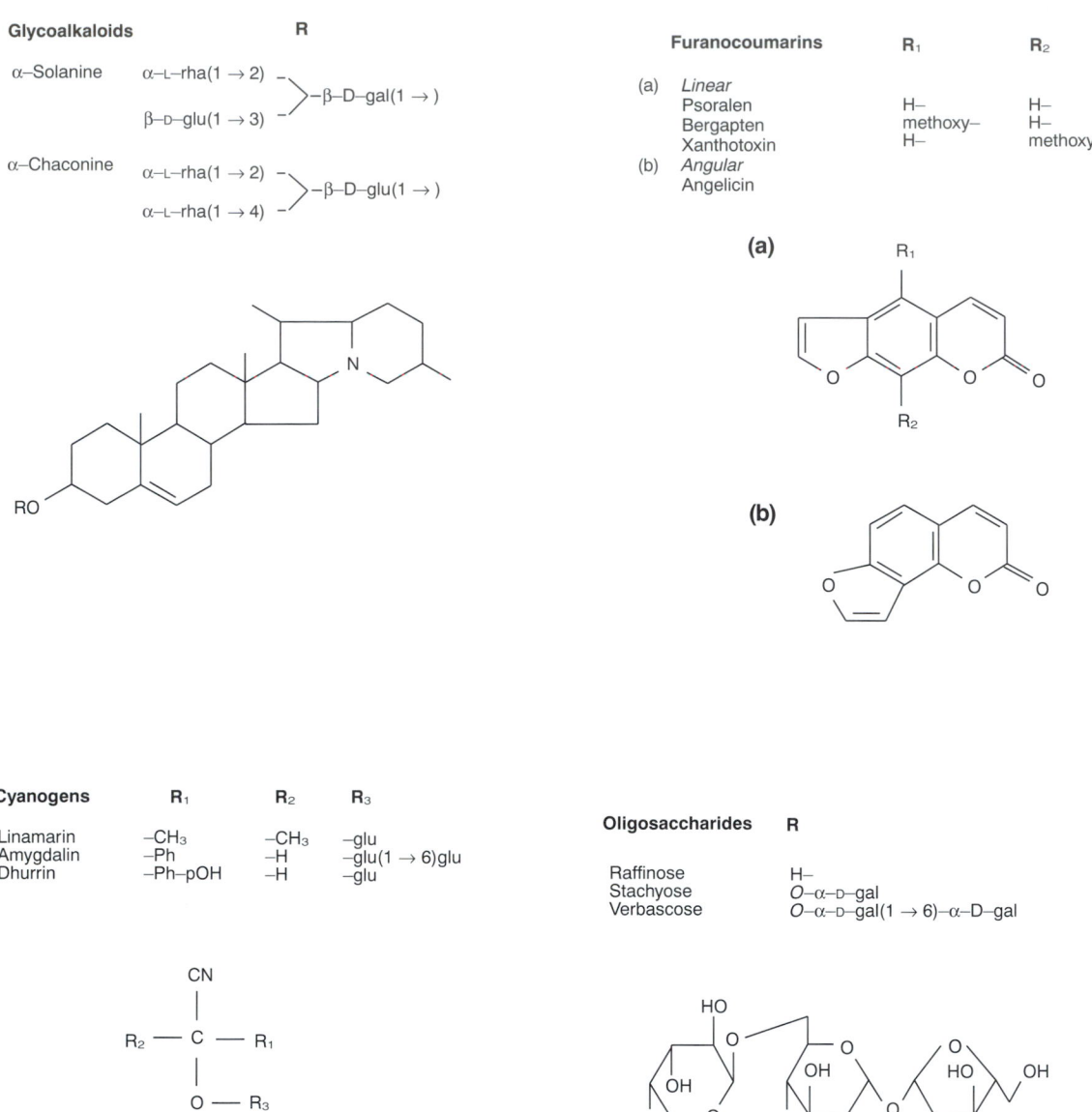

Figure 3 The chemical structures of representatives of each of the major classes of phytochemicals found in plant foods.

mental evidence in rodents suggests that quercetin and related compounds can protect against chemically induced cancers, and this clearly conflicts with the epidemiological findings in humans.

Antioxidants

Some dietary phytochemicals – the phenolic acids and flavonoids – are significantly more active as antioxidants than antioxidant vitamins such as ascorbate and tocopherol. The flavonoids can be 4- to 5-fold more active than ascorbate in *in vitro* assays designed to measure antioxidant activity. Detailed structural analysis of the requirements for this activity shows the presence of 3′,4′-dihydroxyl groups on the B ring and the presence of a 2,3 double bond in the C ring are the main requirements for high antioxidant activity. These antioxidants may promote protective effects by inhibiting the peroxidation of fatty acids in lipids and the oxidation of LDL, and by scavenging reactive oxygen species. The presence of *o*-dihydroxyl groups in the aromatic ring of cinnamic acids such as in caffeic acid or chlorogenic acid promotes antioxidant activity but significant activity is also found in cinnamic acids with a single hydroxyl group such as *p*-coumaric and ferulic acids.

Saponins	R_1	R_2
Soyasaponin A$_1$	β–D–glu(1 → 2)β–D–gal (1→2)–β–D–gluA(1 →)–	β–D–glu(1 → 3)α–L–ara(1→)–
Soyasaponin A$_2$	β–D–gal(1 → 2)β–D–gluA (1 →)–	β–D–glu(1 → 3)α–L–ara(1→)–
Soyasaponin I	α–L–rha(1 → 2)β–D–gal (1→2)–β–D–gluA (1 →)–	H–
Soyasaponin II	α–L–rha(1 → 2)α–L–ara (1 → 2)–gluA(1 →)–	H–
Soyasaponin III	β–D–gal (1 → 2)gluA (1 →)–	H–

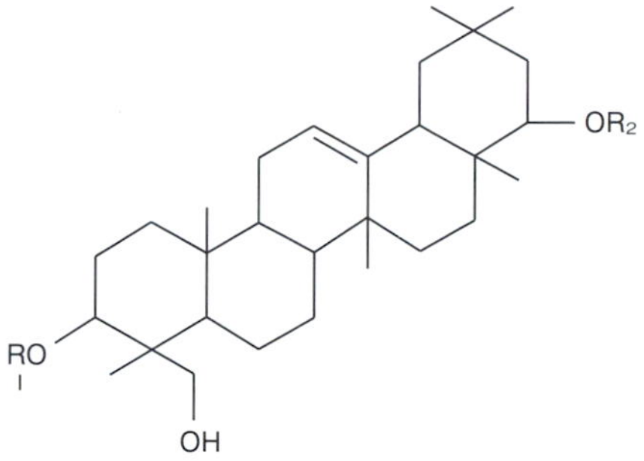

Isoflavones R

Daidzin	β–D–glu(1 →)–
Genistin	β–D–glu(1 →)–
Daidzein	H–
Genistein	H–

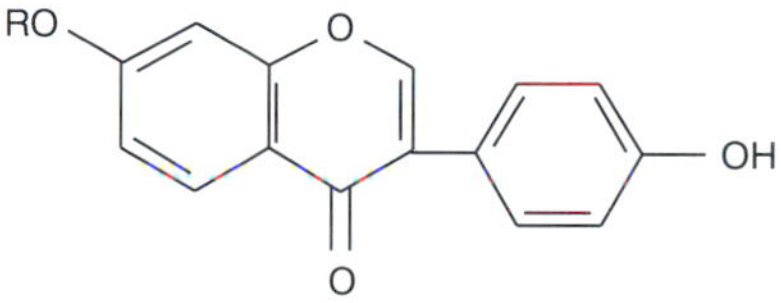

Hydroxycinnamic acids	R	R_1	R_2	R_3
Cinnamic acid	–H	–H	–H	–H
p-Coumaric acid	–H	–OH	–H	–H
Ferulic acid	–OCH$_3$	–OH	–H	–H
Caffeic acid	–OH	–OH	–H	–H
Chlorogenic acid	–OH	–OH	–H	–quinic acid

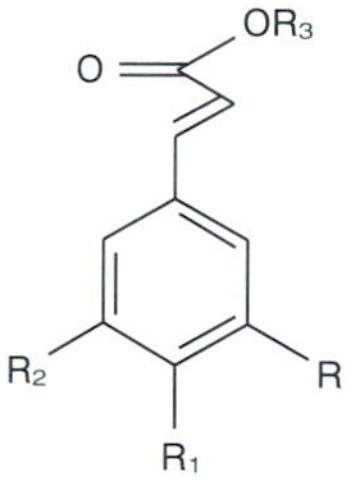

Xanthines R

Theobromine	H–
Caffeine	methyl–

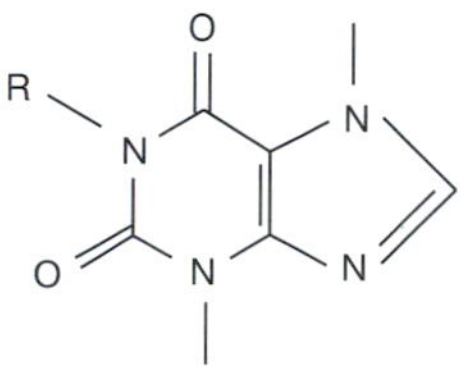

Figure 3 Continued.

Influences on Hormone Metabolism

Isoflavones found in high concentrations in some legumes and the lignans, which are found in many plants but principally in cereals, both show weak estrogenic activity. Isoflavones in the diet can protect against hormone-dependent disease including breast cancer and cardiovascular disease. More recent studies

Glucosinolates   **R**

Sinigrin	prop-2-enyl
Gluconapin	but-3-enyl
Progoitrin	2-hydroxybut-3-enyl
Glucoiberin	3-methysulphinylpropyl-
Glucoraphanin	4-methylsulphinylbutyl-
Glucobrassicin	indol-3-ylmethyl-
Neobrassicin	1-methoxyindol-3-ylmethyl-
4-Methoxyglucobrassicin	4-methoxyindol-3-ylmethyl-
4-Hydroxyglucobrassicin	1-hydroxyindol-3-ylmethyl-

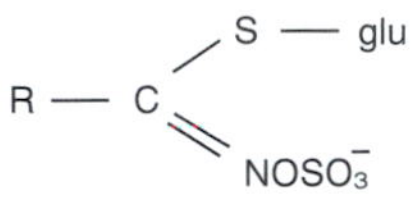

Anthocyanins   **R₁**   **R₂**   **R₃**

	R_1	R_2	R_3
Cyanidin 3-glucoside	−OH	−OH	−H
Delphinidin 3-glucoside	−OH	−OH	−OH
Malvidin 3-glucoside	−OCH₃	−OCH₃	−OCH₃
Peonidin 3-glucoside	−OCH₃	−OH	−H

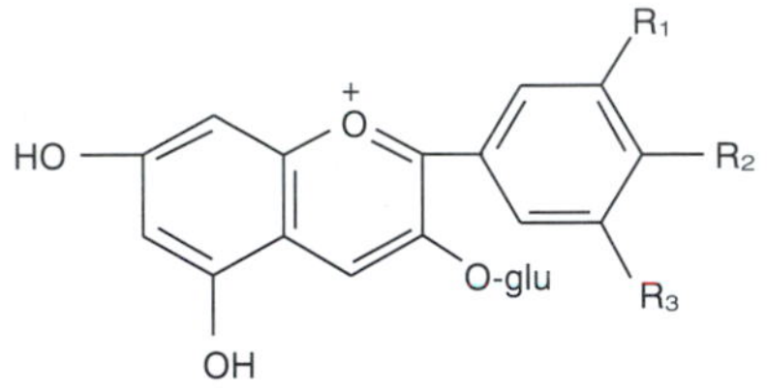

Sulfoxides   **R**

S-Methyl cysteine sulfoxide	methyl-
S-Propen-1-yl cysteine sulfoxide	prop-1-enyl
S-Propyl cysteine sulfoxide	propyl-
S-Propen-2-yl cysteine sulfoxide	prop-2-enyl

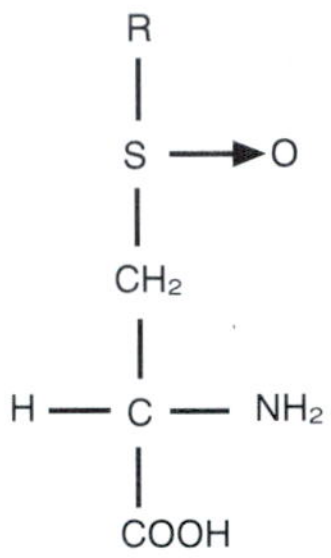

(+) − Catechin

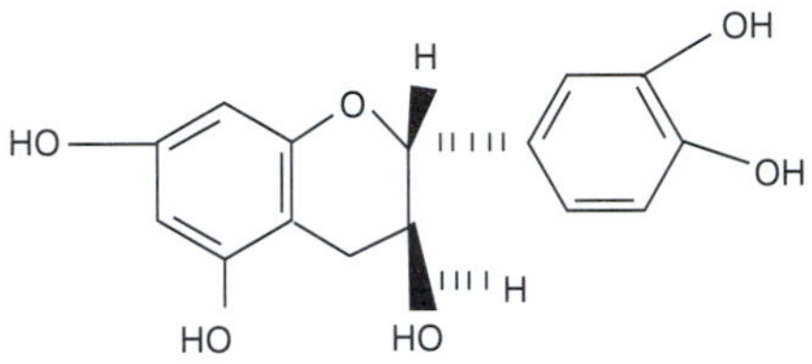

(−)-Epicatechin is an isomer of catechin.
Procyanidins are dimers of catechin and epicatechin

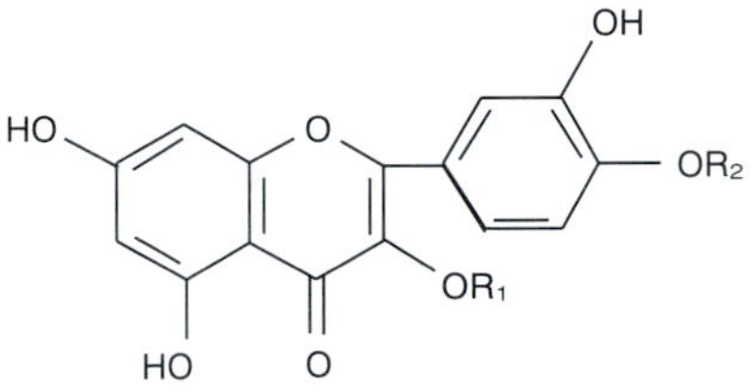

Lignans

Matairesinol

Flavonols   **R₁**   **R₂**

	R_1	R_2
Quercetin 4′-monoglucoside	H−	β−D−glu(1 →)−
Quercetin 3,4′-diglucoside	β−D−glu(1 →)−	β−D−glu(1 →)−

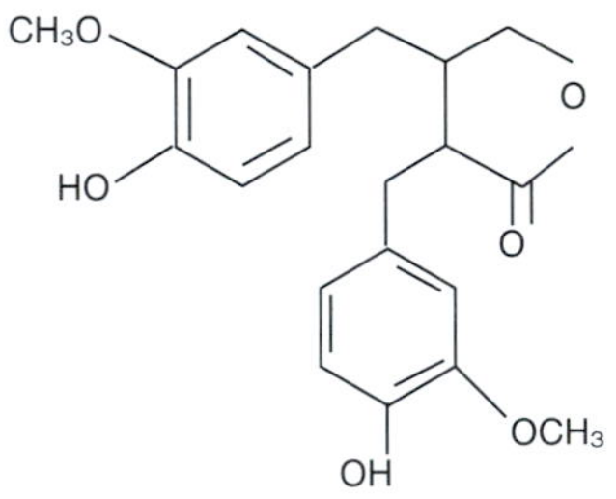

Figure 3 Continued.

have shown that they have anticancer activity in a number of animal carcinogenesis model experiments. They can inhibit growth *in vitro* of many human cancer cell lines and recent experiments have shown that feeding soya bean isoflavones to premenopausal women can potentially reduce the risk of breast cancer by increasing the length of the menstrual cycle.

Isoflavones, such as genistein and daidzein, can bind to the estrogen receptor, but such binding is weak compared with that of the natural steroidal hormones. For instance, genistein has only 1% of the estrogenic activity of diethylstilbestrol. Isoflavones have other biological activities, such as antioxidant properties, and one compound, genistein, is a potent

Table 1 Potential biological activities

Mode of action	Examples
Antioxidants	Flavonols, catechins
Protection against hormone-dependent cancers	Isoflavones, lignans
Hypocholesterolaemic effects	Saponins
Blocking agents	Isothiocyanates (glucosinolates), indoles, allium sulfur compounds
Suppressing agents	Benzylisothiocyanate
Inducers of DNA repair	Vanillin, cinnamaldehyde, coumarin, anisaldehyde
Antimetastatic agents	Tangeretin, catechin, retinoside
Inhibitors of cell proliferation	Quercetin, kaempferol, genistein, daidzein

inhibitor of tyrosine kinases involved in signal transduction in the cell. It is probable that the physiological effects of isoflavones cannot be simply ascribed to their influence on hormone metabolism.

A number of other compounds representing diverse chemical classes have been implicated as having phytoestrogenic effects. These include testrone from palm kernel, anethole from anise oil and coumestrol from alfalfa, but there have been few detailed studies of their mode of action.

Modulation of the Processes of Carcinogenesis

The process of carcinogenesis is thought to involve an 'initiation' stage in which somatic mutations occur, resulting either from DNA adduct formation with genotoxic compounds or from the oxidative modification of DNA from reactions with free radicals. If such damage is not repaired or if such repair is incomplete, then a clonal population of mutated initiated cells will develop. Such cells have high growth rates and reduced sensitivity to factors which regulate cell growth and differentiation. Such initiated cells have to undergo a further process of 'promotion' before they enter the fully transformed condition and subsequently the invasive state (metastasis), giving rise to secondary tumours at distant sites. There is potential for each of these stages in carcinogenesis to be influenced by dietary components.

Role as blocking agents

Blocking agents are defined as chemicals which offer protection against cancer formation when given in animal experiments immediately before or during treatment with the carcinogen. Phytochemicals may act as blocking agents by preventing the activation

of procarcinogens to carcinogens or by promoting their detoxification. Animal and human liver tissues detoxify xenobiotic compounds in a two-step process by which the xenobiotic is first oxidized by so-called 'phase I' enzymes, which are typically cytochrome P-450-based mixed-function oxidases, to produce electrophilic intermediates. These are then converted into a conjugated form with either uronic acids or glutathione by phase II enzymes (such as glutathione S-transferase (GST), UDP-glucuronate : glucuronyltransferase (GT) and quinone reductase (QR)) to form hydrophilic products which can be either excreted directly, or excreted after being further metabolized. In some cases, the action of phase I enzymes may be to activate procarcinogens to carcinogens and factors which can either inhibit the activity or induction of phase I enzymes or induce phase II enzymes can influence the balance of phase I to phase II activity. Altering the balance towards phase II activity would favour the detoxification of the carcinogen and protect the cell from carcinogen-induced damage to DNA, and ultimately from neoplasia and the cancerous state. Among the most active inducers of phase II enzymes are the breakdown products of the glucosinolates, the isothiocyanates. A recent hypothesis proposed that the anticancer properties of isothiocyanates are mediated by two related mechanisms. First, they suppress procarcinogen activation by downregulating the expression of the relevant P-450 enzyme and by direct inhibition of its enzyme activity. Second, they induce expression of phase II enzymes including GST and QR, and thus promote detoxification of electrophilic intermediates. Other phytochemicals including flavonols are inducers of phase II enzymes such as QR, but are less potent than the isothiocyanates.

Role as suppressing agents

Suppressing agents will inhibit the appearance of tumours in animal experiments when given after the chemical treatment used to initiate the neoplasia. The classic example of a compound having suppressing activity is the benzyl isothiocyanate which arises from the enzymic breakdown of glucotropaeolin, a glucosinolate present in cabbage and water cress. The mechanism by which suppressing agents act is unclear but a number of mechanisms by which suppression might occur have been suggested. These include selective inhibition of cellular proliferation of transformed cells, which could potentially be via the pathway of programmed cell death, apoptosis. There has, however, been little work to show whether food components can influence apoptotic effects on cells entering the cancerous state. One study showed that isothiocyanates were more toxic to cells initiated into the cancerous state than in untransformed normal cells, but the extent to which an effect on apoptosis is involved in this is, as yet, unclear.

Inducers of DNA repair

One point at which protective factors could mitigate against the development of cancers is through stimulating endogenous systems to repair damage caused by interactions between genotoxic compounds and DNA. The best characterized of the dietary components which are thought to influence DNA repair processes is vanillin (4-hydroxy-3-methoxybenzaldehyde), a flavour compound. Vanillin can protect Chinese hamster ovary (CHO) cells from the mutagenic effects of ultraviolet light and X rays. It is proposed that it promotes DNA repair via DNA nucleotidyltransferase. Other components which are thought to promote excision repair activity are tea tannins such as epigallocatechin gallate.

Role as antimetastatic agents

Factors which influence the metastatic spread of fully transformed cells from the primary tumour via the blood and lymph system to form secondary tumours can at least slow the carcinogenic process. There is some evidence from model *in vitro* experiments that flavonoids such as tangeretin and (+)-catechin can delay the spread of cancer cells. These effects have not been demonstrated in animals and their relevance to the human situation is questionable.

Inhibitors of cell proliferation

The high rate and disorganized growth of undifferentiated transformed cells is a characteristic of carcinogenesis. Such hyperproliferating cells are more prone to DNA damage than are normal cells. Factors which slow the rate of proliferation of such cells can potentially decrease the risk by allowing the endogenous surveillance systems to operate and for endogenous repair to function. The processes of cell proliferation are complex and there are many points at which protective factors might be able to influence cell growth. These include effects on expression of oncogenes such as *ras* protooncogenes and ornithine decarboxylase (ODC), effects on polyamines which control growth rate in many systems, and effects on inter- and intracellular signalling. Expression of the *ras* proteins may be influenced by limonene, a monoterpene which is a component of citrus oils. The ability of limonene to inhibit mammary tumour promotion in rats following treatment with the carcinogen 7,12-dimethylbenz[*a*]anthracene has been proposed to be due to its ability to inhibit farnesylation of the p21^{ras} protein. Both apigenin, a flavonoid, and curcumin,

a phenylpropanoid which is the yellow pigment of turmeric, are thought to act in their protective role as inhibitors of ODC. Signals within and between cells operating through a complex system of membrane-bound receptors and signal transduction pathways play important roles in regulating cell proliferation. These pathways involve sequences of events including receptor binding, hydrolysis of inositol polyphosphates, mobilization of cellular calcium, activation of protein kinases and induction of enzymes such as ODC. Dietary compounds which can influence such pathways include glycyrrhetic acid, a degradation product of glycyrrhizin, found in liquorice, which is an inhibitor of the protein kinase C and also has antitumour properties.

Occurrence and Levels of Phytochemicals in Food

Table 2 lists the main classes of phytochemicals and the foods in which they occur as major components. Some classes, the glucosinolates and the glycoalkaloids, for example, occur in only a relatively small number of forms and are very limited in their distribution in the plant kingdom, being found in only one or two families. Yet they are important since they occur in commodities such as brassica vegetables and potatoes respectively, which are major components of many diets. In contrast, flavonoids occur in many forms such as flavonols in onions, flavonones in citrus fruit, catechins and tannins in tea and pome fruits, and the red/blue pigmented anthocyanins in berry fruit. This situation is confounded since in all these classes, except the catechin and tannins, the various flavonoid aglycones exist in a diversity of conjugated forms with sugars and organic acids which often reach high levels of complexity. Flavonoids are found in almost all plant families and occur in nearly all plant foods, but the level varies considerably between plant foods.

Onion is a major dietary source of flavonols (up to 29% of the total dietary intake of flavonols in the Netherlands comes from onions), containing up to 1.5 g flavonol per kg edible material. Over 85% of this content is due to two components, quercetin 4'-O-monoglucoside and quercetin 3,4'-O-diglucoside. Most other flavonol sources contain less than one-tenth of the content of onions. Brussels sprouts are a major source of glucosinolates with sinigrin, progoitrin and glucoiberin as the major components. The content of phytochemicals can reach very high levels in some food plants. For instance, the overall level of raffinose oligosaccharides in peas can reach over 50 g kg^{-1} and the level of caffeine in coffee may exceed over 18 g kg^{-1}. The wide range of total

Table 2 The main classes of phytochemicals and the foods in which they occur as major components

Compound	Chemical form	Plant family	Major food source
Glycoalkaloids	Glycoside	Solanaceae	Potato, tomato, aubergine
Cyanogens	Glucoside	Leguminosae	Cassava, lima bean
Furanocoumarins	Aglycone	Umbelliferae	Parsnip, parsley
Oligosaccharides	Galactoside	Leguminosae	Soya bean, pea, bean
Saponins	Glycoside	Leguminosae	Soya bean, pea, bean
Isoflavones	Glucoside (acylated)	Leguminosae	Soya bean, chickpea, alfalfa
Xanthine alkaloids	Aglycone	Wide distribution	Coffee, tea
Glucosinolates	Glucoside	Cruciferae	Cabbage, brussels sprout, broccoli, turnip, swede
Alkenyl cysteine sulfoxides	–	Liliaceae	Onion, leek, garlic
Phenolic acids	Esters	Wide distribution	All fruit and vegetables
Flavonols	Glycoside	Wide distribution	Onion, tea, wine, apple, broccoli, kale
Anthocyanins	Glycoside	Wide distribution	Blackberry, strawberry, radish
Catechins	Aglycone	Wide distribution	Apple, tea
Tannins			
Condensed	Aglycone	Wide distribution	Blueberry
Ellagitannin	Glucoside		Grape
Gallotannin	Glucoside		Beans, tea
Lignans	Glycoside Acylated	Wide distribution	Cereals, linseed

concentrations of phytochemicals within a single commodity as shown in **Table 3** reflects the variations in content between plant varieties and the influence of environmental and agronomic practices on the levels of these phytochemicals.

Bioavailability

In spite of this increasing knowledge of the content of protective factors in foods, their known activity in a range of bioassays and in feeding trials with both animals and humans, there remains great uncertainty as to the form and quantity of these compounds that enter the human body. Most classes of nutritionally important phytochemicals (see Tables 2 and 3) are present as glycosides, but it is not clear to what extent this conjugation is lost during processing. Isoflavones, which are largely present in soya bean seeds as malonated glucosides of genistein and daidzein, suffer significant decarboxylation to form acetyl conjugates and lose the entire malonyl group during thermal processing. In many fermented soya products considerable degradation of isoflavones can occur and the aglycones become major components. In contrast, the flavonol glucosides of onion (Q4'-G and Q3,4'-DG) are very resistant to breakdown during normal processing operations.

The degree to which the phytochemicals are subsequently modified by metabolism or conjugation in the human cells is an important factor in their bioavailability. For nearly all classes of phytochemicals there is a lack of knowledge on their absorption in the intestine. For flavonols it has been suggested that they pass through the small bowel into the large intestine unaltered, where they are degraded by microbial enzymes, largely to the aglycone and that uptake is via the aglycone in the large intestine. Recently, however, studies have concluded that the glycosides are more bioavailable than the aglycone, and that their uptake takes place in the small intestine. It is clear from all these studies that absorption of the phytochemicals in the intestine is far from understood. The site and extent of uptake of relatively well-studied compounds such as flavonol derivatives remain uncertain, and this is even more true for compounds such as the breakdown products of glucosinolates and the allium sulfur compounds, where the nature as well as the concentration of the biologically active species are matters of dispute. With a normal diet, the gut cells are exposed to a great diversity of compounds and the possibility of interaction between phytochemicals must be considered. For instance, it has been shown that certain glycoalkaloids and saponins (see Tables 2 and 3, Fig. 3) can cause a depolarization of the potential difference across the gut wall as a result of the action of the glucose/sodium ion transport system. They also cause pores to form in the gut membrane, making the gut more permeable. Under these circumstances, glycoalkaloids and saponins may facilitate the transport of other dietary compounds into the bloodstream.

Table 3 Concentrations of phytochemicals in different foods

| Phytochemical | Food | Level (mg per kg fresh weight) | |
		Total	Individual
Glycoalkaloids	Potato	8–665	
α-Chaconine			60
α-Solanine			35
Cyanogens	Cassava	16–1100	–
Linamarin			
Furanocoumarins	Parsnip	8–105	
Psoralen			7
Angelicin			18
Bergapten			4
Xanthotoxin			26
Oligosaccharides	Peas	37 300–63 000	
Raffinose			9050
Stachyose			22 000
Verbascose			19 100
Saponins	Soya bean	1980–6500	
Soyasaponin A_1			550
Soyasaponin A_2			250
Soyasaponin I			1270
Soyasaponin II + III			370
Isoflavones	Soya bean	678–3886	
Daidzin			406
Genistin			954
Daidzein			27
Genistein			24
Xanthines	Coffee	6500–28 000	
Theobromine			175
Caffeine			18 400
Glucosinolates	Brussels sprout	900–5020	
Sinigrin			473
Gluconapin			178
Glucoiberin			305
Glucobrassicin			183
Progoitrin			341
Neoglucobrassicin			141
Glucophanin			156
Sulfoxides	Onion	46	
Methyl cysteine sulfoxide			7
1-Propenyl cysteine sulfoxide			36
Propyl cysteine sulfoxide			3
Phenolic acids	Apple	56–618	
Caffeoylquinic acid			49–518
p-Coumaroylquinic			5–62
Feruloylquinic acid			2–4
Caffeic acid glucoside			0–6
p-Coumaric acid glucoside			0–19
Ferulic acid glucoside			0–9
Flavonols	Onion	1533	
Quercetin diglucoside			1181
Quercetin monoglucoside			352
Anthocyanins	Redcurrant	159	
Cyanidin-3-glucoside			6
Cyanidin-3-rutinoside			13
Cyanidin-3-sambubioside			18
Cyanidin-3-sophoroside			4
Cyanidin-3-xylosylrutinoside			47
Cyanidin-3-glucosylrutinoside			11
Catechins/tannins	Grape skin	64	
Catechin/epicatechin			13
Procyanidins			50
Lignans	Sunflower seed	11	–
Matairesinol			

Conclusions

Humans have developed elaborate biochemical mechanisms to deal with the wide range of phytochemicals to which they are exposed when eating a diet containing a variety of plant foods. It appears that humans receive a net benefit in terms of protection from degenerative diseases on such a diet, in spite of the fact that many plant foods are known to contain a number of potentially toxic compounds. The hypothesis that the beneficial value of plant foods is due to their content of phytochemicals has centred on a few classes of compound, including flavonoids and phenolic acids, isothiocyanates and indole carbinols from brassicas, and sulfur compounds such as diallyl disulfide from onions and garlic. Before the nutritional significance of these compounds can be resolved, it is important to understand the levels of these compounds to which cells in the body are exposed. This will require a detailed knowledge of the bioavailability of these compounds. If the nature of the compounds responsible for the beneficial effects of plant foods can be defined, the developments in plant molecular biology over the past decade offer the possibility of developing new varieties of crop plants with increased nutritional value.

See also: **Antioxidants**: Diet and Antioxidant Defence. **Bioavailability**: Definition and General Aspects. **Cancer**: Epidemiology and Associations Between Diet and Cancer. **Cereal Grains**: Dietary Significance and Nutritional Value. **Fruits and Vegetables**: Nutritional Value. **Legumes**: Types and Nutritional Value. **Phytochemicals**: Epidemiological Factors.

Further Reading

Original papers

Barnes S (1995) Effect of genistein on in vitro and in vivo models of cancer. *Journal of Nutrition* 125:777S–783S.

Block G, Patterson B and Subar A (1992) Fruit, vegetables and cancer prevention. A review of the epidemiological evidence. *Nutrition and Cancer* 18:1–29.

Formica JV and Regelson W (1995) Review of the biology of quercetin and related bioflavonoids. *Food and Chemical Toxicology* 33(12):1061–1080.

Herman C, Adlercreutz T, Goldin BR, Gorbach SL, Höckerstedt KAV, Watanabe S, Hämäläinen EK, Markkanen MH, Mäkelä TH, Wähälä KT, Hase TA and Fotsis T (1995) Soybean phytoestrogen intake and cancer risk. *Journal of Nutrition* 125:757S–770S.

Hertog MLG, Feskens EJM, Hollman PCH, Katan MB and Kromout D (1993) Dietary antioxidant flavonoids and risk of coronary heart disease: the Zutphen Elderly study. *Lancet* 342:1007–1011.

Hertog MGL, Feskens EJM, Hollman PCH, Katan MB and Kromhout D (1994) Dietary flavonoids and cancer risk in the Zutphen Elderly study. *Nutrition and Cancer* 22:175–184.

Johnson IT, Williamson G and Musk SRR (1994) Anticarcinogenic factors in plant food: a new class of nutrients. *Nutritional Research Reviews* 7:175–204.

Prochska HJ and Santamaria AB (1988) Direct measurement of NAD(P)H: Quinone reductase from cells cultured in microtiter wells: a screening assay for anticarcinogenic enzyme inducers. *Analytical Biochemistry* 169:328–336.

Rice-Evans C, Miller NJ, Bolwell PG, Bramley PM and Pridham JB (1994) The relative antioxidant activities of plant derived polyphenolic flavonoids. *Free Radical Research* 22(4):375–383.

Zang Y and Talalay P (1994) Anticarcinogenic activities of organic isothiocyanates: chemistry and mechanisms. *Cancer Research* 54:1976S–1981S.

Books

Committee on Comparative Toxicity of Naturally Occurring Carcinogens (1996) *Carcinogens and Anticarcinogens in the Human Diet*, Report of the Committee on Comparative Toxicity of Naturally Occurring Carcinogens, National Academy of Sciences, USA. Washington DC: National Academy Press.

Huang MT, Ho CT and Lee CY (eds) (1992) *Phenolic Compounds in Food and their Effects on Health*. Washington, DC: American Chemical Society.

Huang MT, Osawa T, Ho CT and Rosen RT (eds) (1994) *Food Phytochemicals for Cancer Prevention*. Washington, DC: American Chemical Society.

Waldren KW, Johnson IT and Fenwick GR (eds) (1993) *Food and Cancer Prevention: Chemical and Biological Aspects*. Cambridge: The Royal Society of Chemistry.

Epidemiological Factors

H Wiseman, King's College, London, UK

Epidemiological Sources of Evidence Indicating Potential Health Benefits of Phytochemicals

Flavonoids

Epidemiological evidence suggests that dietary flavonoids, such as the quercetin, kaempferol, myricetin, apigenin and luteolin found in tea, apples, onions and red wine (usually as glycoside derivatives of the parent aglycones), may help to protect against coronary heart disease (CHD). The main epidemiological evidence comes from the Zutphen Elderly study and the Seven Countries Study. In the Zutphen Elderly study (805 men aged 65–84 years), the mean baseline flavonoid intake was 25.9 mg daily and the major sources of intake were tea (61%), onions (13%) and apples (10%). Flavonoid intake, which was analysed in tertiles, was significantly inversely associated with mortality from CHD; the relative risk of CHD in the highest versus lowest tertile of flavonoid intake ($\geq$ 28.6 mg per day versus <18.3 mg per day) was 0.42 (95% confidence interval 0.20–0.88).

The Zutphen Elderly study thus suggests that regular flavonoid consumption, as part of the food matrix, may reduce the risk of death from CHD in elderly men. This study also provides evidence for flavonoid-mediated protection against stroke. Dietary flavonoids (in particular quercetin) were inversely associated with stroke incidence. The relative risk of the highest versus the lowest quartile of flavonoid was 0.27 (95% confidence interval 0.11–0.70). Black tea contributed around 70% to flavonoid intake and the relative risk for a daily consumption of 4.7 cups or more of tea versus less than 2.6 cups of tea was 0.31 (95% confidence interval 0.12–0.84). Increased consumption of green tea (especially more than 10 cups per day) in 1371 Japanese men aged over 40 years increased the proportion of HDL (high-density lipoprotein) cholesterol ('good' cholesterol), and a decreased proportion of LDL (low-density lipoprotein) cholesterol ('bad' cholesterol), and this may be another cardioprotective effect of the flavonoids and other polyphenols in tea.

In 16 cohorts of the Seven Countries Study, the average long-term intake of flavonoids was inversely associated with mortality from CHD (**Table 1**) Flavonoid intake, surprisingly, did not appear to be an important determinant of cancer mortality in this study. This is in contrast to the anticarcinogenic effects observed in animal models and in human cancer cells *in vitro* (see below). An inverse association between tea consumption and the incidence of some cancers has been reported in a prospective cohort study of 35 369 postmenopausal women. Inverse associations with increasing frequency of tea drinking were seen for cancers of the digestive tract and the urinary tract. The relative risk for women who reported drinking $\geq$2 cups (474 ml) of tea per day compared with those who never or only occasionally drank tea was 0.68 (95% confidence interval 0.47–0.98) for digestive tract cancers and 0.4 (95% confidence interval 0.16–0.98) for urinary tract cancers. Another epidemiological study has reported a reduced risk of gastric cancer from drinking 10 cups or more daily of green tea. Tea, and especially green tea, is particularly rich in catechin-type flavonoids such as ($-$)-epigallocatechin and ($-$)-epicatechin, in addition to flavonol-type flavonoids such as quercetin, and an assessment of catechin intake may not have been made in other epidemiological studies.

Phytoestrogens

Phytoestrogens are phytochemicals found in a number of edible plants. The highest levels of dietary intakes of phytoestrogens are found in countries with low incidence of hormone-dependent cancers. The main phytoestrogens in the human diet are the isoflavonoids and the lignans. Isoflavonoid-type phytoestrogens such as the isoflavones genistein and daidzein occur mainly (as glycosides of the parent aglycone) in soya beans (*Glycine max*), a wide range of soya products (**Table 2**), and to a lesser extent in other legumes. The main source of plant lignans are various seeds such as linseed (secoisolariciresinol), sesame seed (matairesinol) and various grains (matairesinol and secisolariciresinol). The incidence of breast and prostate cancer is much greater in

Table 1 Data from the Seven Countries Study: flavonoid (flavonol and flavone) intakes of middle-aged men in various countries around 1960 and contribution of different foods to total flavonoid intake

Country	Flavonol and flavone intake (mg per day)	Quercetin intake (mg per day)	Tea (%)	Fruit and vegetables (%)	Red wine (%)
The Netherlands	33	13	64	36	0
Japan	64	31	90	10	0
USA	13	11	20	80	0
Finland	6	6	0	100	0
Croatia	49	30	0	82	18
Serbia	12	10	0	98	2
Greece	16	15	0	97	3
Italy	27	21	0	54	46

Adapted from Hertog and Hollman (1996) Potential health effects of the dietary flavonol quercetin. *European Journal of Clinical Nutrition* **50**:63–71.

Table 2 Overview of epidemiological data relating to the role of soya bean products in breast cancer risk

Study	Soya bean product	Findings	Estimate of relative risk
Case–control[a]	Soya bean protein	↓ risk	0.43
	Soya bean: total protein	↓ risk	0.29
Case–control	Soya bean	Not significant	[b]
Prospective	Miso soup	↓ risk	0.46
Prospective	Miso soup	↓ risk[c]	[b]
	Tofu	↓ risk[c]	[b]

Adapted from Messina *et al.* (1994b) Soy intake and cancer risk: a review of the *in vitro* and *in vivo* data. *Nutrition and Cancer* **21**:113–131.
[a]Premenopausal women only.
[b]Could not be calculated.
[c]Decreased risk was only found to be significant for the baseline period 1971–75.

Western countries than in Far Eastern ones, where there is an abundance of dietary phytoestrogens.

Urinary excretion of phytoestrogens can be used as a measure of intake and thus possible exposure and possible protection against cancer. A very low urinary excretion of lignans and equol (isoflavan metabolite of the isoflavone daidzein) in postmenopausal breast cancer patients compared with vegetarians has been observed. In humans, omniverous subjects usually have quite low levels of isoflavonoid excretion. The Japanese (males and females) have the highest levels of isoflavonoid excretion followed by subjects following macrobiotic, vegan and lactovegetarian diets. Urinary lignan excretion is higher in Finland compared with that in the USA and Japan. In assessing exposure to the protective effects of phytoestrogens, urinary excretion rates should be considered in combination with actual plasma levels. In some Japanese men the plasma biologically active sulfate + free lignan fraction was similar to or even higher than that in the Finnish men.

Japanese women and women of Japanese origin living in Hawaii but who consume a diet similar to the traditional Japanese diet (rich in soya products) have a low breast cancer incidence and mortality. Women in the Far East who have low rates of breast cancer are thought to consume around 30–50 times more soya products than women in the USA. A case-control study in Singapore found that premenopausal women who consumed 55 g of soya per day had a 50% reduced risk of breast cancer compared with women who infrequently consumed soya foods. A high intake of miso soup has been associated with a reduced risk of breast cancer in Japanese women. In prospective trials a trend towards an inverse association between intake of tofu and subsequent risk of breast cancer has been found, as well as an inverse association between intake of miso soup and development of breast cancer.

A trend towards protective effects against prostate cancer of tofu but not miso has been shown in a large group (around 8000) men of Japanese ancestry in Hawaii followed for 20 years. The latency period for prostate cancer appears to be lengthened in men of Japanese origin in Hawaii who have a low mortality from prostate cancer. The incidence of *in situ* prostate cancer in autopsy studies is similar, however, to that of men in Western countries. The consumption of soya isoflavones by these men may be responsible for this long latency period. This probably means that they die of other causes including old age before the prostate cancer can develop to a life-threatening stage.

Phytoestrogens may also protect against colon cancer by preventing the conversion of procarcinogens to carcinogens or by removing locally generated carcinogenic free radicals (see below). Lignan excretion is high in Finnish subjects living in regions with a low colon cancer risk and lower incidence of colon cancer has been observed in areas with high tofu consumption. There is also growing evidence for cardioprotective effects and antiosteoporotic effects of phytoestrogens; these are currently under investigation.

Brassica glucosinolates and their derivatives

Glucosinolates (previously known as thioglucosides) are sulfur-containing phytochemicals found in cruciferous or brassica vegetables, such as broccoli, cabbage, kale, cauliflower and Brussels sprouts (**Table 3**). Although around 100 different glucosinolates are found in the plant kingdom, only around 10 are found in brassica vegetables. They are also found in other plant foods in addition to brassica vegetables. Degradation products of glucosinolates include other organosulfur compounds such as the isothiocyanates and dithiothiols. Glucosinolate degradation products also include indoles.

Epidemiological data suggest that the relatively

Table 3 Case–control studies of stomach, colon and rectal cancer showing inverse, null or positive associations for the consumption of different types of phytochemical-rich fruit and vegetables

Fruit or vegetable type	Stomach cancer[a] (no. of studies)			Colon cancer[b] (no. of studies)			Rectal cancer[c] (no. of studies)		
	Inverse	Null	Positive	Inverse	Null	Positive	Inverse	Null	Positive
Fruit	14	3	0	5	2	1	3	0	1
Citrus fruit	11	1	0	2	1	3	4	1	0
Tomatoes	9	1	1	4	0	2	3	2	1
Vegetables	11	0	0	8	0	1	2	0	2
Raw vegetables	10	0	0	3	0	1	–	–	–
Allium vegetables	9	1	1	4	1	1	2	0	1
Cruciferous vegetables	–	–	–	8	3	1	5	0	0
Green vegetables	8	0	0	4	1	0	–	–	–
Legumes	7	0	2	1	2	2	–	–	–
Carrots	7	1	1	–	–	–	4	0	1

Adapted from Steinmetz and Potter (1996) Vegetables, fruit and cancer prevention: a review. *Journal of the American Dietetic Association* **96**:1027–1039.
[a]Data summarize the results from 31 studies (both statistically significant and nonsignificant results included).
[b]Data summarize the results from 21 studies (both statistically significant and nonsignificant results included).
[c]Data summarize the results from 13 studies (both statistically significant and nonsignificant results included).

high content of glucosinolates and related compounds may be responsible for the observed protective effects of brassica vegetables in the majority of the 87 case–control studies and seven cohort studies that have been carried out on the association between brassica consumption and cancer risk. In the case–control studies, 67% of studies showed an inverse association between consumption of brassica vegetables and risk of cancer at various sites. If individual brassica vegetables are considered, then the values for the number of studies that showed an inverse association between consumption of brassica vegetables and risk of cancer at various sites are: broccoli, 56%; Brussel sprouts, 29%; cabbage, 70%; and cauliflower, 67%. The cohort studies showed

inverse associations between broccoli consumption and the risk of all types of cancer taken together; between the consumption of brassicas and risk of stomach cancer and occurrence of second primary cancers; and between the consumption of cabbage, cauliflower and broccoli and the risk of lung cancer. Overall it appears that a high consumption of brassica vegetables is associated with a decreased risk of cancer (**Table 4**). The associations were most consistent for stomach, lung, rectal and colon cancer and least consistent for the hormonal cancers including prostatic, ovarian and endometrial cancer. However, further epidemiological research is required to separate the cancer protective effects of brassica vegetables from that of vegetables in general.

Table 4 Case–control studies of lung, breast and pancreatic cancer showing inverse, null or positive associations for the consumption of different types of phytochemical-rich fruit and vegetables

Fruit or vegetable type	Lung cancer[a] (no. of studies)			Breast cancer[b] (no. of studies)			Pancreatic cancer[c] (no. of studies)		
	Inverse	Null	Positive	Inverse	Null	Positive	Inverse	Null	Positive
Fruit	8	0	0	3	0	1	6	1	0
Citrus fruit	–	–	–	1	0	2	1	2	0
Tomatoes	4	0	0	–	–	–	–	–	–
Vegetables	7	0	0	–	–	–	5	1	0
Raw vegetables	–	–	–	–	–	–	2	1	0
Green vegetables	9	0	0	5	1	0	–	–	–

Adapted from Steinmetz and Potter (1996) Vegetables, fruit and cancer prevention. *Journal of the American Dietetic Association* **96**:1027–1039.
[a]Data summarize the results from 13 studies (both statistically significant and nonsignificant results included).
[b]Data summarize the results from 13 studies (both statistically significant and nonsignificant results included).
[c]Data summarize the results from 9 studies (both statistically significant and nonsignificant results included).

Allium organosulfur compounds

There is growing epidemiological evidence that other organosulfur compounds in addition to those derived from glucosinolates can protect against cancer. Allium species such as garlic (*Allium sativum*) and onions (*Allium cepa*) are a rich source of organosulfur compounds such as the diallyl sulfides. There is epidemiological evidence from the Netherlands Cohort Study (120 852 men and women 55–69 years in age) for a strong inverse association between onion consumption and incidence of stomach carcinoma (**Table 5**). However, the consumption of leeks and the use of garlic supplements were not associated with stomach carcinoma risk. The relative risk for stomach carcinoma in the highest onion consumption category ($\geq$ 0.5 onions per day) was 0.50 (95% confidence interval 0.26–0.95) compared with the lowest consumption category (no onions per day). However, this study did not support an inverse association between the consumption of onions and leeks and the use of garlic supplements and the incidence of male and female colon and rectal carcinoma. There is currently only limited epidemiological evidence concerning the beneficial influence of garlic organosulfur compounds on cardiovascular disease.

Potential Importance of Flavonoids to Human Health: Molecular Mechanisms of Action

Flavonoid-containing preparations have been used for many years in efforts to treat a wide range of human diseases. Their potential importance to human health and the molecular mechanisms by which they may act will now be examined. Flavonoids possess a broad spectrum of biological actions ranging from anticarcinogenic, anti-inflammatory, cardioprotective, immune-modulatory to antiviral. The mechanisms by which flavonoids cause these effects may include induction of the activity of some important enzymes, while inhibiting the activity of others (**Fig. 1**). Modulation of membrane function, including the activity of membrane-bound enzymes, through a protective membrane antioxidant action is likely to be of prime importance (see below).

The extent to which dietary flavonoids are actually absorbed is largely unknown and is a key question in assessing the likely importance of these compounds to human health. Originally, only aglycones (free flavonoids without sugar molecules attached)

Table 5 Cohort and case–control studies of all types of cancer showing inverse, null or positive associations for the consumption of different types of phytochemical-rich fruit and vegetables

Fruit or vegetable type	All types of cancer[a] (no. of studies)		
	Inverse	Null	Positive
Fruit	29	12	5
Citrus fruit	26	8	6
Tomatoes	35	5	10
Vegetables	55	4	9
Raw vegetables	33	4	2
Allium vegetables	27	3	4
Cruciferous vegetables	38	8	8
Green vegetables	61	5	13
Legumes	14	6	16
Carrots	50	7	7

Adapted from Steinmetz and Potter (1996) Vegetables, fruit and cancer prevention. *Journal of the American Dietetic Association* **96**:1027–1039.

[a]Data summarize the results from 194 studies (both statistically significant and nonsignificant results included).

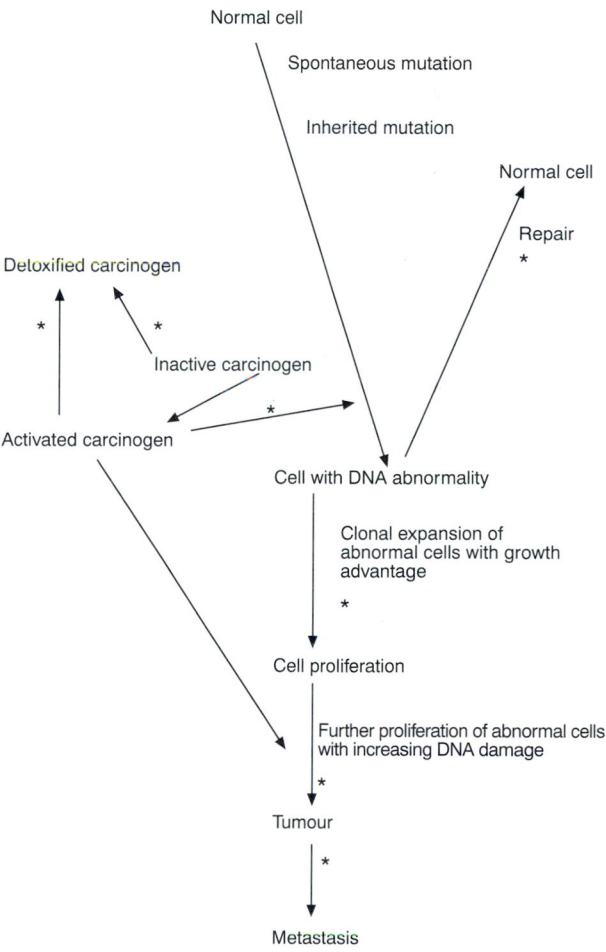

Figure 1 Overview of cancer and locations on the pathway (*) where phytochemicals may be able to block the cancer process. Adapted from Steinmetz and Potter (1996) Vegetables, fruit and cancer prevention. *Journal of the American Dietetic Association*, **96**:1027–1039.

were thought to be absorbed: no enzymes that can remove these sugar groups are present in the intestinal wall. Recent studies with ileostomy patients appear to show that humans can absorb significant amounts of quercetin. Most importantly, absorption of quercetin glucosides was 50% and absorption of pure quercetin and quercetin rutinoside was only 20–30%, suggesting utilization of an intestinal glucose transport mechanism.

Membrane function is now understood to be of vital importance to many cellular processes. These include the role of membrane enzymes and receptors in cell growth and signalling. Membrane function may be influenced by dietary components directly by altering membrane fluidity or indirectly by protection against the free radical-mediated process of membrane lipid peroxidation. This can arise from oxidative stress and result in oxidative membrane damage. Flavonoids such as quercetin and myricetin have been widely found to inhibit membrane lipid peroxidation. Flavonoids inhibit lipid peroxidation *in vitro* by acting as chain-breaking antioxidants: they donate a hydrogen atom to lipid radicals, thus terminating the chain reaction of lipid peroxidation. Additionally, flavonoids can act as metal chelating agents (see below). Furthermore, kaempferol-3-O-galactoside protected mice against bromobenzene-induced hepatic lipid peroxidation. The relative potencies of flavonoids as antioxidants is governed by a set of structure–function relationships: in general optimum antioxidant activity is associated with multiple phenolic groups, a double bond in C2–C3 of the C ring, a carbonyl group at C4 of the C ring and free C3 (C ring) and C5 (A ring) hydroxy groups. It is of related interest that consumption of 300 ml of either black or green tea greatly increased plasma antioxidant capacity in 10 volunteers. This suggests that normal levels of tea consumption could provide sufficient flavonoids to achieve a potentially health protective effect.

There is growing evidence for the role of free radicals in the oxidative DNA damage implicated in carcinogenesis (**Fig. 2**). The ability of flavonoids to act as antioxidants may contribute to the anticancer effects observed in animal models and human cells in culture *in vitro*, which could potentially be important to human health despite the present lack of epidemiological evidence (see above). Quercetin has been shown to have growth inhibitory effects *in vitro* on breast cancer cells, colon cancer cells, squamous cell carcinoma cell lines, acute lymphoid and myeloid leukaemia cell lines and a lymphoblastoid cell line. These effects appear to be mediated via binding to cellular type II oestrogen-binding sites. Furthermore, when the ability of two citrus flavonoids, hesperetin

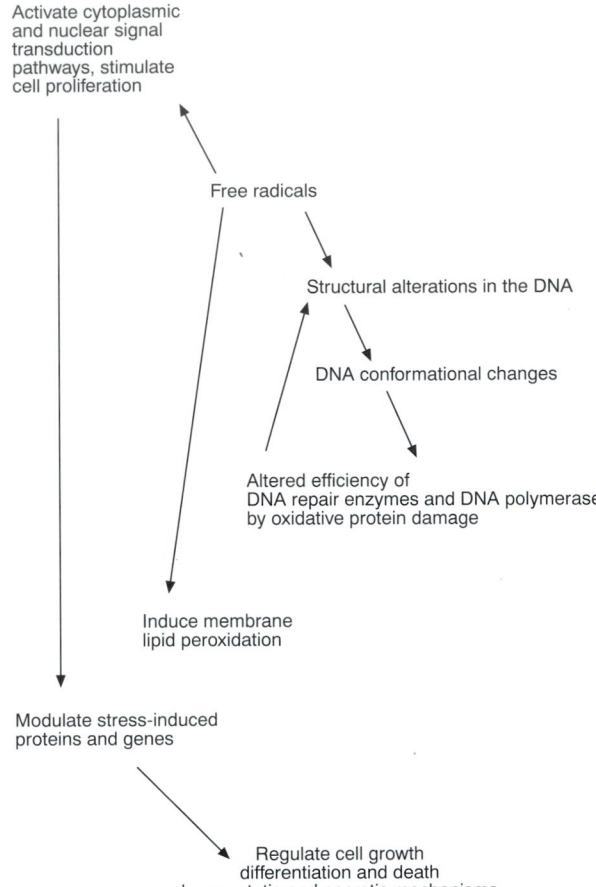

Figure 2 Overview of the role of free radicals in the cancer process. Adapted from Wiseman and Halliwell (1996) Damage to DNA by reactive oxygen and nitrogen species: role in inflammatory disease and progression to cancer. *Biochemical Journal* **313**:17–29.

and naringenin (found in grapefruit mainly as its glycosylated form naringin), and three noncitrus flavonoids to inhibit the proliferation and growth of a human breast cancer cell line was investigated, the concentrations required to achieve 50% inhibition ranged from 5.9 to 56 μg ml^{-1}. The effectiveness of the citrus flavonoids was enhanced by using them in combination with quercetin, which is widely distributed in other foods. Quercetin fed to rats in the diet at levels of 2% or 5% inhibited the incidence and multiplicity of chemical carcinogen-induced mammary tumours. Mammary tumorigenesis in rats was delayed in the groups given orange juice (rich in citrus flavonoids together with other phytochemicals and nutrients) or fed the naringin-supplemented diet compared with the other groups. A number of the phenolic compounds of green tea including the catechins have been shown to inhibit tumour formation in rats induced by N-methyl-N'-nitro-N-nitrosoguanidine and also mutation induced by aflatoxin and benzo[a]pyrene.

Quercetin has been shown to inhibit the activity of two enzymes which play an important role in mammary cell growth and development: it inhibits tyrosine protein kinase activity and phosphoinositide phosphorylation, and also inhibits protein kinase C, vital in the regulation of cellular proliferation. Furthermore, inhibition of tumour growth through cell cycle arrest and induction of apoptosis by quercetin are both thought to be functionally related to activation of the tumour supressor protein p53.

A number of mechanisms have been proposed for the protection by flavonoids against CHD, one of which is antioxidant activity. Oxidative damage to LDL (particularly to the apoprotein B molecule) is considered to be an important stage in the development of atherosclerosis: it is a prerequisite for macrophage uptake and cellular accumulation of cholesterol leading to the formation of the atheromal fatty streak (**Fig. 3**). Flavonoids such as quercetin are effective inhibitors of *in vitro* oxidative modification of LDL by macrophages or copper ions and flavonoids in red wine have been reported to protect LDL against oxidative damage. The antioxidant properties of flavonoids may contribute to the reduced risk of CHD in wine drinkers, the so-called French paradox. Resveratrol, another phenolic phytochemical found in wine, has been shown to protect LDL against oxidative damage and appears to protect against cancer in animal models. Further studies on this interesting compound are clearly warranted.

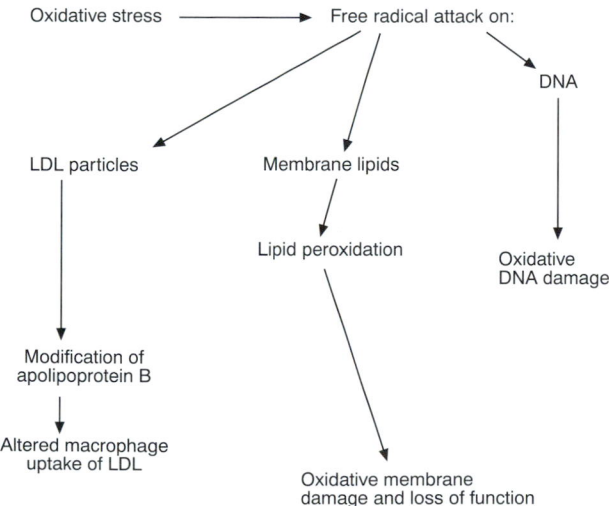

Figure 3 Overview of the role of free radicals in the oxidative damage to cellular targets likely to be harmful to human health: many phytochemicals have protective antioxidant actions. Adapted from Wiseman (1996b) Dietary influence on membrane function: importance in protection against oxidative damage and disease. *Journal of Nutritional Biochemistry* **7**:2–15. (With permission from Elsevier Science.)

Quercetin also displays potent antithrombotic effects: it inhibits thrombin and ADP-induced platelet aggregation *in vitro* and this may be through inhibition of phospholipase C activity rather than through inhibition of thromboxane synthesis. In addition, flavonoid binding to platelet membranes may inhibit the interaction of activated platelets with vascular endothelium. The antioxidant activity of flavonoids may also prevent the damaging action of lipid peroxides generated by activated platelets on endothelial nitric oxide and prostacyclin, which both inhibit platelet aggregation and have vasodilatory activity. The activity of flavonoids as inhibitors of the viral enzyme reverse transcriptase also suggests that they may be beneficial in the control of retroviral infections such as acquired immunodeficiency syndrome (AIDS).

Possible adverse effects on human health should also be considered. Quercetin was reported to induce bladder cancer in rats when administered in the diet at a levels of 2%. These results were not confirmed in another study, however, which used quercetin at levels reaching 10%. It should be noted that under certain *in vitro* conditions flavonoids and other phenols can act as pro-oxidants and cause DNA damage. However, phenols have complex pro- and antioxidant effects *in vitro*, depending on the assay system used, and it is often difficult to predict their net effect *in vivo*. For example, many synthetic and dietary polyphenols (including quercetin, catechin, gallic acid ester and caffeic acid ester) can protect mammalian cells from the cytotoxicity induced by peroxides such as hydrogen peroxide. Although tea is a good source of flavonoids, phenolic compounds including tannins and also polyphenols and phenol monomers are also good inhibitors of iron absorption, which could contribute to the nutritional problem of iron deficiency. In general it is unlikely that sufficiently toxic quantities of any particular flavonoid could be consumed from the diet, which contains many diverse varieties of flavonoids in varying quantities.

Potential Importance of Phytoestrogens to Human Health: Molecular Mechanisms of Action

Populations in the Far East have been consuming soya bean for centuries. In contrast, Western cultures and diets have only started to adopt soya foods much more recently. Western-style soya foods are produced by modern processing techniques in large soya bean processing plants. Traditional soya foods, made from soya beans, include both nonfermented and fermented foods. The nonfermented soya foods include soya milk and the soya milk product tofu, as well as whole-fat soya flour, soya nuts, whole dry beans and fresh green soya beans. Traditional fermented soya foods include soy sauce, tempeh, natto, miso and fermented tofu and soya milk products. Soya milk is the name given to the aqueous extract derived from whole soya beans. A cup of soya milk is thought to contain around 40 mg of isoflavones. In soya beans, textured vegetable protein (TVP) and tofu (soya bean curd) there are high levels of the conjugated isoflavones called daidzin and genistin. In contrast, in fermented soya bean products such as miso, nearly all the isoflavones are present in their unconjugated forms called genistein and daidzein.

The metabolism of phytoestrogens is of great importance to their ability to exert health-protective effects. Following ingestion daidzin and genistin are hydrolysed in the large intestine by the action of bacteria to release genistein and daidzein. When daidzein is ingested it is metabolized by the bacteria in the large intestine to form equol or O-desmethylangolensin, whereas genistein is metabolized to p-ethyl phenol. The lignan precursors in grain (matairesinol and secisolariciresinol) are converted to the two main mammalian lignans enterolactone and enterodiol by gut bacteria. Matairesinol undergoes dehydroxylation and demethylation directly to enterolactone, whereas secisolariciresinol is converted to enterodiol, which can then be converted to enterolactone.

Phytoestrogens, which act as weak oestrogens, can antagonize the growth-promoting effects of oestrogen in breast cells and imitate the protective action of oestrogen on the cardiovascular system and on bone. This action may contribute to their reported protective ability against heart disease and osteoporosis and may be particularly important for postmenopausal women. It also suggests their use as a natural supplement, as an alternative to hormone replacement therapy (HRT) in women. The weak oestrogenic activity of genistein may be the reason why Japanese women suffer from fewer menopausal symptoms such as hot flushes compared with women in Western countries. Indeed, it is likely that there is sufficient oestrogenic activity in soya to compensate for the lack of oestrogen production by the ovaries in postmenopausal women.

Phytoestrogens block the growth-promoting action of oestrogen (and androgens) on cancer cells, and this action may protect against hormonal-dependent cancers such as breast and prostate cancer. Genistein and daidzein appear structurally similar to the female sex hormone oestrogen. In order for oestrogen to stimulate the growth of breast cancer cells it first needs to bind to its nuclear receptor, the oestrogen receptor. Isoflavones can also bind to this receptor because of their structural mimicry, but do not produce the same effect on cell division because they are weak oestrogens. In women who produce considerable amounts of oestrogen the soya isoflavones can act as antioestrogens. They can be considered to be acting in a similar way to tamoxifen. Tamoxifen is an antioestrogen drug widely used in the treatment of breast cancer, it is currently being assessed for the prevention of breast cancer.

The phosphorylation state of oestrogen and progesterone receptors may also influence receptor activity, thus the inhibitory action of genistein on tyrosine kinase may be associated with its influences on cancer. Daidzein competes with oestradiol for binding to the rat uterine type II oestrogen-binding site (known as the bioflavonoid receptor), thus it may inhibit cancer cell growth in a similar manner to some flavonoids (see above), by competing with oestradiol for this binding site. Nuclear type II oestrogen-binding sites occur in breast, prostate and other cancer cells. Some lignans can also bind to nuclear type II oestrogen-binding sites and block the proliferative action of oestrogen.

In in vitro cancer models, genistein inhibited the proliferation of human cancer cells in culture. Genistein is a specific inhibitor of tyrosine kinases, which are involved in a signalling cascade that ultimately leads to cell division. Genistein was shown to be equally effective as an inhibitor of the growth of oestrogen-dependent MCF-7 and oestrogen-independent MDA-468 breast cancer cells. Furthermore, genistein has been found to inhibit MCF-7 growth by blocking the cell cycle at important check points and by inducing apoptosis; this probably occurs from impairment of the signal transduction pathway from the tyrosine kinase receptor. In cell cultures enterolactone at physiological concentrations can block the growth-promoting effects of oestradiol.

Enterolactone is also an inhibitor of the enzyme aromatase and genistein and coumestrol inhibit 17β-hydroxysteroid dehydrogenase type I. Aromatase inhibition and prevention of the conversion of oestrone to oestradiol in malignant cells by these compounds could inhibit the promotional phase of oestrogen-dependent cancer. The lignan enterolactone and its direct plant precursor matairesinol inhibit prostate cancer cell growth in vitro.

In order for cancer cells to spread, new blood vessels need to grow by a process called angiogenesis. Genistein appears to be a potent inhibitor of angiogenesis and thus may potentially be useful in the treatment of cancer as well as in its prevention.

Phytoestrogens are antioxidants, and the antioxidant properties of genistein may contribute to the protective effects against cancer of diets rich in soya foods. Early studies showed soya beans, soya flour, soya protein concentrates and soya protein isolates to have a marked antioxidant activity. In a model membrane system genistein can inhibit lipid peroxidation at high concentrations, although it is much less potent than flavonoids such as quercetin.

The results from 26 animal studies of experimental carcinogenesis, in which diets containing soya or isolated and purified soya bean isoflavonoids were used, show that in 17 of these studies (65%) protective effects were reported: the risk of cancer (incidence, latency or tumour number) was greatly reduced, and no studies reported that soya intake increased tumour development. Furthermore, in rats treated neonatally with 7,12-dimethylbenz[a]anthracene, genistein was found to delay the appearance of mammary tumours in association with increased cell differentiation in the mammary tissue.

Animal studies have demonstrated the antitumorigenic effect of the mammalian lignan precursor secoisolairiciresinol diglycoside. Ingestion of purified secoisolairiciresinol diglycoside by rats at 1.5 mg day^{-1} for 20 weeks commencing 1 week after treatment with the carcinogen dimethylbenzanthracene, achieved a 37% reduction in the number of mammary tumours per rat and a 46% reduction in the number of tumours per number of rats in each group. Urinary mammalian lignan excretion increased, indicating conversion of secoisolairiciresinol diglycoside to mammalian lignans. Furthermore, the secoisolairiciresinol diglycoside component of flaxseed was found to be particularly beneficial in inhibiting the promotional phase of carcinogeninduced mammary tumorigenesis in rats. The colon cancer protective effect of flaxseed in rats may be related to the secoisolairiciresinol diglycosidemediated increase in caecal β-glucoronidase activity.

Alterations in the menstrual cycle have been shown with consumption of 60 g of soya protein (45 mg of conjugated isoflavones). Overall the length of the cycles increased, so that over a lifetime there would be fewer cycles, and hence less exposure to oestrogen. This could potentially mean a lowered risk for breast cancer. The menstrual cycle is under the influence of oestrogen, which in turn is controlled by the levels of pituitary hormones. Levels of pituitary hormones were lowered in a similar manner to that observed with tamoxifen, again suggesting beneficial cancer-preventing properties of these compounds.

Lower incidence of heart disease has also been reported in populations consuming large amounts of soya products, although good epidemiological data are still awaited. Nevertheless, protection against heart disease may be another potential health benefit

of phytoestrogens. Soya protein incorporated into a low-fat diet can reduce cholesterol and LDL and raise HDL and the oestrogenic isoflavones present are likely to contribute to this effect. Indeed, removal of phytoestrogens from soya reduces its protective properties. In postmenopausal hypercholesterolaemic women 40 g per day of soya protein at an isoflavone level of 1.39 mg or 2.25 mg isoflavones per g protein increased HDL cholesterol concentrations and decreased non-HDL cholesterol and the ratio of total cholesterol/HDL cholesterol, compared with the casein/nonfat dry milk control. In a preliminary study on normolipidaemic men the majority response to soya protein was a favourable effect on both protective and harmful lipoproteins. The antioxidant action of oestrogens may also contribute to their cardioprotective properties, and although oestrogenic isoflavones can protect LDL (**Fig. 4**) against oxidative modification *in vitro* (the isoflavan metabolite equol was particularly potent), their effects *in vivo* are as yet unclear. Genistein can also inhibit cell adhesion, alter growth factor activity and inhibit the cell proliferation involved in atherosclerotic lesion formation.

Osteoporosis is a chronic disease in which the bones become brittle and break more easily. Soya bean phytoestrogens may protect against postmenopausal bone loss and osteoporosis. Again, this is because isoflavones are weak oestrogens: genistein can act in a similar way to the conjugated equine oestrogens utilized in HRT to maintain bone mass in rats. Soya protein calcium is absorbed to a similar extent to that from dairy milk, but soya protein does not increase urinary calcium excretion to the extent

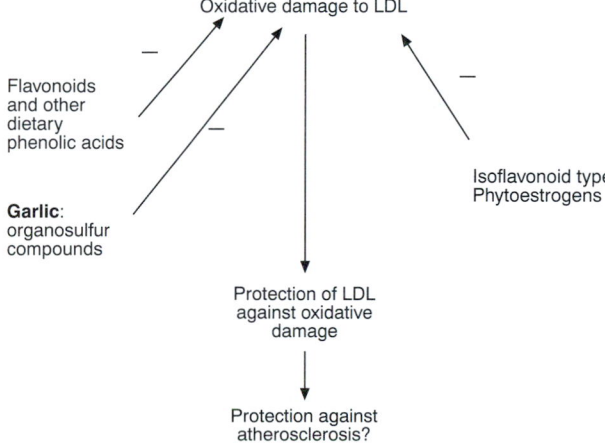

Figure 4 Overview of the role of antioxidant phytochemicals in protecting against the oxidative damage to LDL implicated in atherosclerosis. Adapted from Wiseman (1996b) Dietary influence on membrane function: importance in protection against oxidative damage and disease. *Journal of Nutritional Biochemistry* 7:2–15. (With permission from Elsevier Science.)

of animal proteins despite being of equal protein quality. Protection against osteoporosis is yet another possible health benefit of phytoestrogens.

However, there are concerns about possible adverse effects of phytoestrogens arising from their oestrogenic properties. Phytoestrogens may act like the oestrogens used in HRT and the oral contraceptive pill, and therefore may potentially adversely influence levels of blood-clotting factors, possibly increasing the risk of deep vein thrombosis (formation of blood clots). Phytoestrogens have been reported to cause infertility in some animals and there is some concern over their consumption by human infants, particularly in relation to the sexual development of male infants. The coumestan phytoestrogen coumesterol found in clover and alfalfa sprouts (not a major part of the human diet) is particularly known to cause infertility in sheep. When fed at relatively high doses phytoestrogens, including isoflavones, have been shown in some rodent studies to cause changes to the immature reproductive tract that result in developmental abnormalities. A study in peripubertal monkeys, however, showed no adverse effects. Furthermore, no reproductive abnormalities have been found in people living in countries where soya consumption is high. Indeed, dietary isoflavones are excreted into breast milk by soya-consuming mothers, which suggests that in cultures where consumption of soya products is the norm, breast-fed infants are exposed to high levels, again without any adverse effects. Furthermore, isoflavone exposure shortly after birth through breast-feeding at a critical developmental period may protect against cancer. In fact this could be a more important factor in the observation of lower cancer rates in populations in the Far East than adult dietary exposure to isoflavones.

Potential Importance of Glucosinolate Derivatives and Related Compounds to Human Health: Molecular Mechanisms of Action

There may be some important health-protective effects of glucosinolate derivatives and related compounds. The hydrolytic products of some glucosinolates have been shown to display anticancer properties. A metabolite of glucobrassicin (3-indoylmethylglucosinolate), indole-3-carbinol, has been shown to inhibit the growth of human tumours of the breast and ovary. Furthermore, indole-3-carbinol may modulate the oestrogen hydroxylation pathway such that a less potent form of oestradiol is produced, thus conferring protection against oestrogen-related cancers.

Consumption of glucosinolate-containing Brussels sprouts (300 g per day of cooked sprouts) for 1 week has been shown to increase rectal glutathione S-transferase-α and -π isoenzyme levels. Enhanced levels of these detoxification enzymes may partly explain the epidemiological association between a high intake of glucosinolates in cruciferous vegetables and a decreased risk of colorectal cancer.

Glucosinolate-derived isothiocyanates can prevent the formation of chemical carcinogen-induced tumours of the liver, lung, mammary gland, stomach and oesophagus in animal models. The anticarcinogenic effects of isothiocyanates may be mediated by a combination of mechanisms including inhibition of carcinogen activation by cytochromes P-450: this could be achieved by both direct inhibition of enzyme catalytic activity and downregulation of enzyme levels and induction of phase II enzymes such as glutathione transferases and NAD(P)H:quinone reductase (these detoxify any remaining DNA-attacking electrophilic metabolites generated by phase enzymes). Dietary glucosinolates and their breakdown products have been tested as anticarcinogens in terms of their ability to induce the anticarcinogenic phase II enzyme marker quinone reductase in murine Hep a1c1c7 cells. The relative activities observed were found to be dependent on the nature of the side chain of the parent glucosinolate. Furthermore, the ability of glucosinolates and derivatives to induce cytochrome P-450 1A1 in Hep G2 cells has been assessed.

Phenethyl isothiocyanate protects mice against nitrosoamine-induced lung tumorigenesis. It also modulates the activity of phase I and phase II xenobiotic-metabolizing enzymes (see above), resulting in the inhibition of the oxidative activation of a number of chemical carcinogens. The isothiocyanate sulforophane is a particularly potent inducer of detoxification enzymes.

Undesirable goitrogenic effects have been identified for isothiocyanates and other hydrolytic products of glucosinolates. Furthermore, in contrast to the anticancer effects of brassica vegetables discussed above, a number of genotoxic effects have also been demonstrated in bacterial and mammalian cells. In bacterial assays (induction of point mutations in *Salmonella* TA98 and TA100 and repairable DNA damage in *Escherichia coli* K-12), juices from eight brassica vegetables tested caused genotoxic effects in the absence of metabolic activation. The order of potency was: Brussels sprouts > white cabbage > cauliflower > green cabbage > kohlrabi > broccoli > turnip > black raddish. In mammalian cells, structural chromosome aberrations were observed with some of the juices; the most potent were Brussels sprouts and white cabbage, and genotoxic effects were accompanied by decreased cell viability. The fraction of these brassica juices containing isothiocyanates (and other breakdown products of glucosinolates) was found to contain 70–80% of the total genotoxic activity of the juices. The fraction containing flavonoids and other phenolics had a much weaker effect. In related studies two isothiocyanates – allyl isothiocyanate and phenethyl isothiocyanate – were found to be > 1000-fold more cytotoxic in a Chinese hamster ovary cell line than their parent glucosinolates (sinigrin and gluconasturtiin, respectively). Phenethyl isothiocyanate also induced genotoxic effects (chromosome aberrations and sister chromatid exchanges).

More evidence is therefore required before an overall recommendation can be made regarding the likely beneficial or otherwise influences of glucosinolates (and their derivatives) on human health.

S-Methyl cysteine sulfoxide

S-Methyl cysteine sulfoxide is another sulfur-containing phytochemical found in all brassica vegetables, in addition to glucosinolates (see above). Both S-methyl cysteine sulfoxide and methyl methane thiosulfinate (its main metabolite) can block chemical-induced genotoxicity in mice. S-Methyl cysteine sulfoxide is thus likely to contribute to the observed ability to brassica vegetables to protect against cancer in both human and animal studies. It is of interest that a hydrolytic product of S-methyl cysteine sulfoxide was linked in the 1960s to the severe haemolytic anaemia or Kale poisoning observed in cattle in Europe in the 1930s.

Potential Importance of Other Phytochemicals to Human Health: Molecular Mechanisms of Action

Allium organosulfur compounds

Allium organosulfur compounds may be phytochemicals of importance to human health by acting as antioxidants, thus protecting against free radical-mediated damage to important cellular targets such as DNA and membranes implicated in cancer and neurodegenerative diseases and ageing (see above). Protection against oxidative damage to LDL and cellular membranes could protect against cardiovascular disease. Aged garlic extract inhibited lipid peroxidation in rat liver microsomal membranes and investigation of the major organosulfur compounds found in aged garlic extract showed S-allylcysteine and S-allylmercaptocysteine to have free radical scavenging activity.

Organosulfur compounds such as diallyl sulfide may also protect against cancer by modulation of carcinogen metabolism. This may involve altered ratios of phase I and phase II drug-metabolizing enzymes. Various garlic preparations including aged garlic extract have been shown to inhibit the formation of nitrosamine-type carcinogens in the stomach, enhance the excretion of carcinogen metabolites and inhibit the activation of polyarene carcinogens. Inhibitory effects of organosulfur compounds on the growth of cancer cells in vitro, including human breast cancer cells and melanoma cells, have been observed. Modulation of cancer cell surface antigens, associated with cancer cell invasiveness, has been observed and in some cases cancer cell differentiation can be induced. Aged garlic extract can reduce the appearance of mammary tumours in rats treated with the powerful carcinogen dimethyl benz[a]anthracene (DMBA). Cytochromes P-450 activates this carcinogen by oxidizing it to the DNA-binding form, DMBA diol epoxide, which causes DNA lesions and cancer initiation. The antibacterial activity of these allium compounds may also prevent bacterial conversion of nitrate to nitrite in the stomach. This may reduce the amount of nitrite available for reacting with secondary amines to form the nitrosamines likely to be carcinogenic, particularly in the stomach.

Allium organosulfur compounds appear to possess a range of potentially cardioprotective effects. In one small study 432 cardiac patients were divided into a control group (210) and a garlic-supplemented group (222). Garlic feeding was found to reduce the mortality by 50% in the second year and by about 66% in the third year. Furthermore, the rate of re-infarction was reduced by 30% and 60% in the second and third years, respectively. It should be noted that only a small number of patients in both groups experienced the end event of death or myocardial infarction and a much larger-scale study is needed. Aged garlic extract lowers cholesterol and triacylglycerols in laboratory animals and can reduce blood-clotting tendencies. It has been suggested that garlic supplementation at a level of 10–15 g of cooked garlic daily could lower serum cholesterol by 5–8% in hypercholesterolaemic individuals. There may, however, be more important cardioprotective effects of garlic. In animal studies aged garlic extract suppressed the levels of plasma thromboxane B_2 and platelet factor levels, which are important factors in platelet aggregation and thrombosis. In rats frequent low doses (50 mg kg^{-1}) of aqueous extracts of garlic or onions (onion was less potent) produced significant antithrombotic activity (lowering of thromboxane B_2) without toxic side effects.

Aqueous extracts of raw garlic also inhibited cyclooxygenase activity in rabbit platelets, again contributing to an antithrombotic effect. In addition, aged garlic extract and S-allyl cysteine and S-allyl mercaptocysteine have antiplatelet adhesion effects (platelet adhesion to the endothelial surface is involved in atherosclerosis initiation). Furthermore, S-allyl mercaptocysteine inhibits the proliferation of rat aortal smooth muscle cells, another important atherosclerotic process. Indeed, this antiproliferative effect on smooth muscle cells may be indicative of a possible antiangiogenic ability in relation to the prevention of tumour growth and metastasis.

Saponins

Saponins are another steroidal phytochemical of interest that may, in addition to isoflavonoid-type phytoestrogens (see above), contribute to the health-protective effects of soya products. Soya beans have a high saponin content and soya bean saponins have been shown to have a growth inhibitory effect on human carcinoma cells *in vitro*, probably by interacting with the cell membrane and increasing membrane permeability. The proposed anticarcinogenic mechanisms of saponins include normalization of carcinogen-induced cell proliferation, direct cytotoxicity, bile acid binding and immune-modulating effects. Of particular interest is the finding that saponins actively interact with cell membrane components: they possess surface active characteristics because of the amphiphilic nature of their chemical structure. Thus they can act to alter cell membrane permeability and cellular function. Soya bean saponins have been reported to inhibit hydrogen peroxide damage to mouse fibroblast cells and thus may protect human health through antioxidant-mediated mechanisms.

Saponins from ginseng root (*Panax ginseng* C.A. Mey) may also be important. Antioxidant effects have been reported for total ginseng saponins as well as for the individual saponins (ginsenosides Rb1, Rb2, Rc and Rd; others include Re and Rg1). Furthermore, ginsenosides Rb1 and Rb2 protected cultured rat myocardiocytes against superoxide radicals; the mechanism for this may involve induction of genes responsible for antioxidant defences rather than radical scavenging. Ginsenosides stimulate endogenous production of nitric oxide in rat kidney. This may contribute to the observed antinephritic action of these compounds and may suggest a protective role in the kidney. It has also been suggested that the observed cardioprotective effects of ginsenosides in animal models may be mediated by nitric oxide release. In addition, ginsenoside-enhanced release of nitric oxide from endothelial cells, particularly from perivascular nitric oxidergic nerves in the corpus cavernosum of animal models, may partly account for the reported aphrodisiac effects of ginseng.

Other phytochemicals of interest

Additionally, a wide range of other phytochemicals may have important beneficial effects on human health if consumed in sufficient amount to be efficacious. In many cases their full spectrum of molecular actions remains to be elucidated. Netherless, the following phytochemicals and their main botanical sources are deemed worthy of a brief mention.

The phytochemicals dihydrophthalic acid, ligustilide, butylidene, phthalide and n-valerophenone-O-carboxylic acid have been isolated from angelica root (*Angelica sinensis*). They are likely to contribute to the observed effects of angelica root in modulating the circulation including increasing coronary flow, modulation of myocardial muscular contraction and antithrombotic effects.

Phytochemicals extracted from liquorice (*Glycyrrhiza glabra* L.) include glycyrrhetic acid, glycyrrhizic acid (the sweet principle of liquorice) and an active saponin glycyrrhizin (a 3-O-diglucuronide of glycyrrhetic acid). In rats, dietary supplementation with 3% liquorice elevated liver glutathione transferase activity. This suggests a potential detoxification and anticancer effect of these phytochemicals because glutathione transferase catalyses the formation of glutathione conjugates of toxic substances for elimination from the body. Antibacterial, antiviral, antioxidant and anti-inflammatory effects have also been reported for these compounds.

Phytochemicals found in ginkgo (*Ginkgo biloba*) leaves include ginkgolic acid, hydroginkgolic acid, ginkgol, bilobol, ginon, ginkgotoxin, ginkgolides (A,B and C) and a number of flavonoids common to other plants such as kaempferol, quercetin and rutin (see above). These phytochemicals are currently attracting attention for their possible effects on the circulation, in particular cerebral circulation, including improvement in mental function. A number of studies have reported that extracts of ginkgo leaves enhanced brain circulation, increased the tolerance of the brain to hypoxia and improved cerebral haemodynamics. It has been suggested that these effects are mediated via calcium ion flux over smooth cell membranes and via stimulation of catecholamine release. In addition, protection against free radical-mediated retinal injury has been reported and thus other possible antioxidant-mediated protective effects on human health are also possible. Damage to mitochondrial DNA could play a role in neurodegenerative diseases such as Alzheimer's disease and Parkinson's disease. There is limited evidence for significant improvements in CHD patients following treatment with a daily dose equivalent to 12 mg total ginkgetin.

See also: **Caffeine**: Chemistry and Physiological Effects. **Cancer**: Epidemiology and Associations Between Diet and Cancer; Epidemiology of Breast Cancer; Epidemiology of Colorectal Cancer; Epidemiology of Lung Cancer; Epidemiology of Gastrointestinal Cancers Other Than Colorectal Cancers; Diet in Cancer Treatment. **Coronary Heart Disease**: Prevention. **Fruits and Vegetables**: Nutritional Value. **Lipids**: Chemistry and Classification. **Osteoporosis**: Aetiology; Treatment and Prevention. **Phytochemicals**: Classification and Occurrence.

Further Reading

Adlercreutz CHT, Goldin BR, Gorbach SL, Hockerstedt KAV, Watanabe S, Hamalainen EK, Markkanen MH, Makela TH, Wahala KT, Hase TA and Fotsis T (1995) Soybean phytoestrogen intake and cancer risk. *Journal of Nutrition* **125**:757S–770S.

Adlercreutz H (1996) Lignans and isoflavonoids: epidemiology and possible role in prevention of cancer. In: Kumpulainen JT and Salonen JT (eds) *Natural Antioxidants and Food Quality in Atherosclerosis and Cancer Prevention*. Cambridge: Royal Society of Chemistry.

Cook NC and Samman S (1996) Flavonoids: chemistry, metabolism, cardioprotective effects and dietary sources. *Journal of Nutritional Biochemistry* **7**:66–76.

Formica JV and Regelson W (1995) Review of the biology of quercetin and related bioflavonoids. *Food and Chemical Toxicology* **33**:1061–1080.

Hertog MGL and Hollman PCH (1996) Potential health effects of the dietary flavonol quercetin. *European Journal of Clinical Nutrition* **50**:63–71.

Lea MA (1996) Organosulphur compounds and cancer. *Advances in Experimental Medicine and Biology* **401**:147–154.

Lin RI-S (1994) Phytochemicals and antioxidants. In: Goldberg I (ed.) *Functional Foods: Designer Foods, Pharmafoods and Nutraceuticals*. New York: Chapman & Hall.

Messina M, Messina V and Setchell KDR (1994a) *The Simple Soybean and Your Health*. New York: Avery Press.

Messina MJ, Persky V, Setchell KDR and Barnes S (1994b) Soy intake and cancer risk: a review of the *in vitro* and *in vivo* data. *Nutrition and Cancer* **21**:113–131.

Rao AV and Sung MK (1995) Saponins as anticarcinogens. *Journal of Nutrition* **125**:717S–724S.

Steinmetz KA and Potter JD (1996) Vegetables, fruit and cancer prevention: a review. *Journal of the American Dietetic Association* **96**:1027–1039.

Stoewsand GS (1995) Bioactive organosulfur phytochemicals in *Brassica oleracea* vegeatables. *Food and Chemical Toxicology* **33**:537–543.

Wiseman H (1996a) Role of dietary phytoestrogens in the protection against cancer and heart disease. *Biochemical Society Transactions* **24**:795–800.

Wiseman H (1996b) Dietary influences on membrane function: importance in protection against oxidative damage and disease. *Journal of Nutritional Biochemistry* **7**:2–15.

Wiseman H and Halliwell B (1996) Damage to DNA by reactive oxygen and nitrogen species: role in inflammatory disease and progression to cancer. *Biochemical Journal* **313**:17–29.

Zhang Y and Talalay P (1994) Anticarcinogenic activities of organic isothiocyanates: Chemistry and mechanisms. *Cancer Research* **54**:1976S–1981S.

Phyto-oestrogens *see* **Phytochemicals**: Classification and Occurrence; Epidemiological Factors.

Polyunsaturated fat *see* **Fatty Acids**: Health Effects of n-6 Polyunsaturated Fatty Acids; Health Effects of n-3 Polyunsaturated Fatty Acids.

POPULATION, DEVELOPMENT AND NUTRITION

Overview

Barry M Popkin, Carolina Population Center, University of North Carolina, Chapel Hill, North Carolina, USA

Biomedical and social scientists have long recognized the importance of the demographic and epidemiological transitions in higher-income countries and have more recently understood that similar sets of broadly based changes are occurring in lower-income countries. Researchers have been slow to recognize that these same changes in economic and social development have profound effects on nutrition. This entry provides a brief overview of the transition countries are undergoing. It provides some background on critical underlying shifts in economic, demographic and related forces that affect diet and activity and body composition trends.

Human diet and nutritional status have undergone a sequence of major shifts among characteristic states, defined as broad patterns of food use and corresponding nutrition-related disease. Since the seventeenth century, and more particularly in the last few decades of the twentieth century, the pace of dietary change appears to have accelerated by varying degrees in different regions of the world. The concept of the nutrition transition focuses on large shifts in diet, especially its structure and overall composition. The same underlying socioeconomic and demographic changes associated with dietary change are also leading to shifts in activity patterns. The combination of these dietary and activity changes is reflected in nutritional outcomes, such as changes in average stature and body composition. Furthermore, dietary changes are paralleled by major changes in health status, as well as by major demographic and socioeconomic changes.

Two extant theories of change address key factors that affect and are affected by nutritional change. One relates to the demographic transition – the shift from a pattern of high fertility and high mortality to one of low fertility and low mortality (typical of modern industrialized nations). Even more directly relevant is the concept of the epidemiological transition, first described by Abdel Omran in 1971. The epidemiological transition describes the shift from a pattern of high prevalence of infectious diseases and malnutrition, resulting from pestilence, famine and poor environmental sanitation, to a pattern of high prevalence of chronic and degenerative diseases strongly associated with lifestyle. The concepts of demographic and epidemiological transition share a focus on the ways in which populations move from one pattern to the next. The framework developed here mirrors these concepts of demographic and epidemiological change shown in **Fig. 1**.

It is useful to consider briefly the nutrition transition within its detailed historical context. The nutrition transition has followed five broad patterns: (1) hunting and gathering food; (2) famine; (3) receding famine; (4) degenerative disease; and (5) behavioural change. The major features of each pattern are summarized in **Table 1**. These patterns are not restricted to particular periods of human history. For convenience, the patterns are described in the past tense as historical developments; however, 'earlier' patterns are not restricted to the periods in which they first arose, but continue to characterize certain geographic and socioeconomic subpopulations. The economic and demographic changes associated with shifts in the structure of income and work and also those associated with population distribution are those components of development that are addressed in most detail in the next section.

The theory of the nutrition transition relates shifts among major nutritional patterns to the complex interplay of changing patterns of socioeconomic, demographic and health factors. Understanding the nutrition transition will require broad-based examination of critical components of development. Propositions related to the nutrition transition and development are summarized here.

Background Forces

Proposition 1

Major shifts in population growth, age structure, and spatial distribution are closely associated with nutritional trends and dietary change.

This proposition is not addressed directly here, but one of the most powerful sets of shifts linked with demographic change – rapid urbanization – receives attention in some detail.

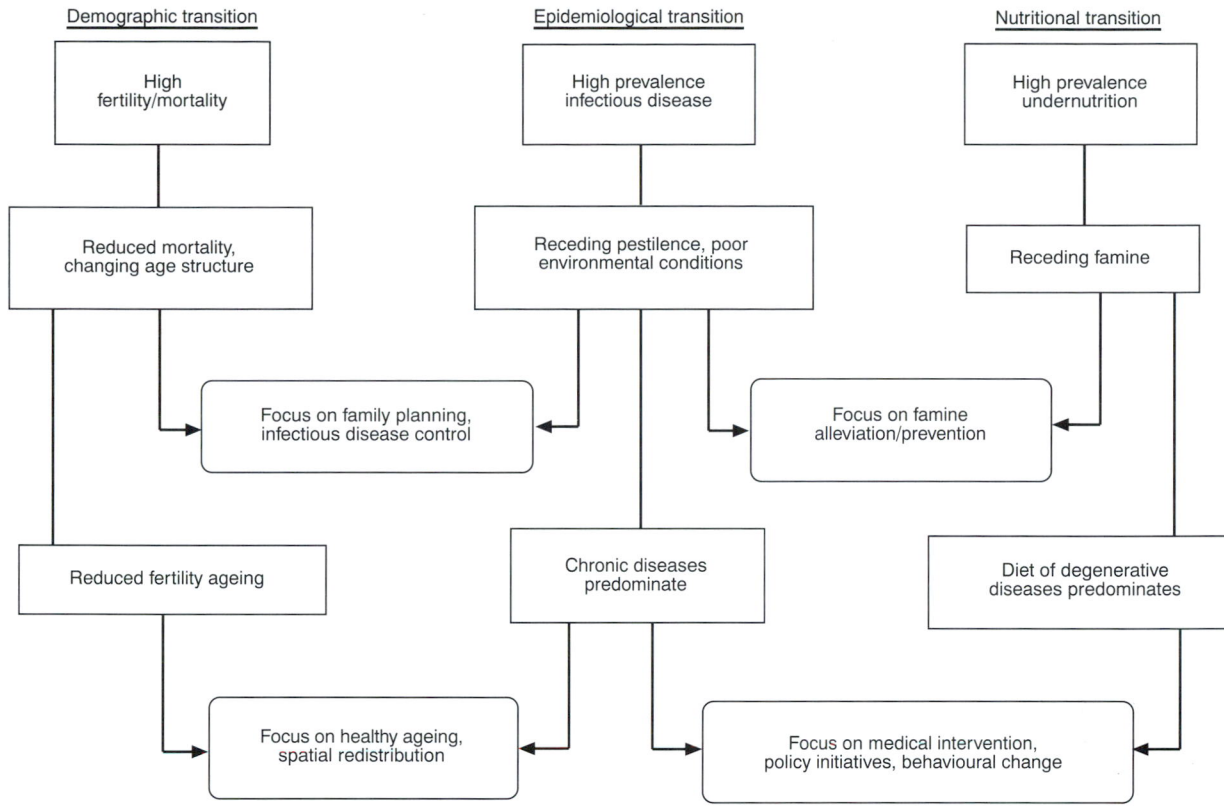

Figure 1 Stages of health, nutritional and demographic change.

People living in urban areas consume diets distinctly different from those of their rural counterparts. City-dwellers have led the movement from the pattern of famine to the patterns of receding famine and of degenerative disease. Compared with rural diets, urban diets show trends toward consumption of the following:

- superior grains (e.g. rice or wheat, rather than corn or millet);
- more milled and polished grains (e.g. rice, wheat);
- food higher in fat;
- more animal products;
- more sugar;
- more food prepared away from the home; and
- more processed foods.

These contrasts between urban and rural eating patterns are more marked in lower-income than in higher-income countries. In higher-income countries, market penetration into rural areas is common, and national integrated food distribution systems exist.

Key dimensions of world urbanization Several major demographic shifts began after World War II; they continue unabated and have even accelerated in some regions. One is the vast increase in the proportion of persons who reside in urban areas. A second is urban agglomeration. A third is the shift of poverty toward the urban areas, particularly toward squatter and slum areas.

Proportion living in cities Urban growth was relatively modest before the Industrial Revolution. Rapid urban development first occurred in the higher-income countries; now, at the end of the twentieth century, lower-income countries are undergoing even more rapid urbanization. In **Table 2** United Nations (UN) population research is used to show that in 1994 the higher-income world comprised predominantly urban residents, while that was not the case for the less developed and poorest, least developed countries. Nevertheless, by the year 2025 urban residency will be the more common form of residence throughout all but the poorest African countries.

The rates of population growth are far greater in urban than rural areas because of the continuation of long-term patterns of in-migration. **Table 3** shows that these patterns will accelerate in the twenty-first century.

Concentrated population growth Urban growth, particularly in lower-income countries, has been skewed toward a few larger cities, often called urban

Table 1 Summary characteristics and broad changes in dietary patterns and their relationship to social and economic factors

Transition profile	Pattern 1: Collecting food	Pattern 2: Famine	Pattern 3: Receding famine	Pattern 4: Degenerative disease	Pattern 5: Behavioural change
Nutritional					
Diet	Plants, wild animals; varied diet	Cereals predominant; diet less varied	Fewer starchy staples; more fruits, vegetables, animal protein; low variety	More fat (especially from animal products), increased carbohydrates, sugar and processed foods; less fibre	Less fat and processing; increased carbohydrates, fruits and vegetables
Nutritional status	Robust, lean, few nutritional deficiencies	Children and women suffer most from low fat intake; nutritional deficiency diseases emerge; stature declines	Continued maternal/child nutrition problems; many deficiencies disappear; weaning diseases emerge; stature grows	Obesity; problems for elderly; many disabling conditions	Reduced body fat levels and obesity; improved bone health
Morbidity	Much infectious disease; no epidemics	Epidemics; endemic disease (plague, smallpox, polio, tuberculosis); deficiency disease begins; starving common	Tuberculosis smallpox, infection, parasitic disease, polio, weaning disease (diarrhoea, retarded growth) expand, later decline	Chronic disease related to diet, pollution (heart disease, cancer); infectious disease declines	Increased health promotion (preventive and therapeutic); decline in coronary heart disease, improvement in age-specific cancer profile
Economy	Hunter-gatherers	Agriculture, animal husbandry, homemaking begin; shift to monocultures	Second agricultural revolution (crop rotation, fertilizer); Industrial Revolution; women join labour force	Fewer jobs with heavy physical activity; service sector and mechanization; leisure exercise grows to offset sedentary jobs	Service sector mechanization, industrial robotization dominate; leisure exercise grows to offset sedentary jobs increases
Household production	Primitive; onset of fire	Labour-intensive, primitive technology begins (clay cooking vessels)	Primitive water systems; clay stoves; cooking technology advances	Household technology mechanizes and becomes more varied	Food preparation technology changes rapidly
Income and assets	Substance; primitive stone tools	Subsistence; few tools	Increasing income disparity; agricultural tools; industrialization rises	Growth in income disparities	Income growth slows; home and leisure technologies increase
Demographic					
Mortality/Fertility	Low fertility, high mortality, low life expectancy	High natural fertility, low life expectancy, high infant and maternal mortality	Mortality declines; fertility static, then declines; cumulative population growth	Life expectancy reaches high levels (60s–70s); fertility low and fluctuating	Life expectancy extends to 70s, 80s; disability-free life expectancy increases
Age structure	Young population	Young; very few elderly	Chiefly young; shift to older population begins	Fertility decline; elderly proportion increases	Increasing proportion of elderly >75 years
Residence patterns	Low density	Rural; a few small, crowded cities	Chiefly rural; move to cities increases; international migration begins; large cities develop	Urban population disperses; rural green space reduced	Lower-density cities rejuvenate; urbanization of rural areas around cities increases
Food processing	Rudimentary	Food storage begins	Storage process (drying, salting); canning and processing technologies; increased food refining and milling	Numerous foods transforming technologies	Technologies create foods and food constituent substitutes (e.g. macronutrient substitutes)

Table 2   Urban population: 1970, 1994 and 2025

Region	Urban population (millions)			Urban share (%)		
	1970	1994	2025	1970	1994	2025
World	1353	2521	5065	36.6	44.8	61.1
Less developed regions	676	1653	4025	25.1	37.0	57.0
Least developed countries	38	122	506	12.6	21.9	43.5
More developed regions	677	868	1040	67.5	74.7	84.0

Source: United Nations, Population Division (1995).

Table 3   Average annual growth rate of urban and rural population, less-developed regions (%)

Region	1965–70	1990–95	2020–25
Less-developed regions			
Urban	3.58	3.51	2.33
Rural	2.18	0.96	−0.28
Africa			
Urban	4.64	4.38	3.34
Rural	1.98	2.03	0.72
Asia			
Urban	3.28	3.68	2.31
Rural	2.34	0.81	−0.57
Latin America			
Urban	3.97	2.60	1.26
Rural	0.81	−0.20	−0.61
Oceania			
Urban	7.26	3.13	3.32
Rural	1.62	1.90	0.22

Source: United Nations, Population Division (1995).

conglomerates. As is seen in **Table 4**, the most explosive growth of these mega-cities is in Asia.

Shift in the proportion of poor to the cities   Concomitant with increased concentration of the population in urban areas is a dramatic shift in the proportion of poor people living in cities. In absolute and relative terms, the majority of the poor of the lower-income world live in cities. At the same time, a disproportionate share of those with middle and

Table 4   Mega-cities[a], 1970–2015

Region	1970	1994	2000	2015
World	11	22	25	33
Less-developed regions	5	16	19	27
Africa	0	2	2	3
Asia	2	10	12	19
Latin America	3	4	5	5
More-developed regions	6	6	6	6

Source: United Nations, Population Division (1995).
[a]Cities with eight or more million residents.

upper incomes in the higher-income countries also live in urban areas.

Proposition 2

Changes in income, patterns of work and leisure activities and related socioeconomic shifts lead to changes in women's roles and shifts in dietary and activity patterns.

A major change in economic structure associated with the nutrition transition is the shift from a preindustrial agrarian economy to industrialization. This transformation then accelerates: the service sector grows rapidly, industrial production is dominated by capital-intensive processes, and time-allocation patterns change dramatically. Associated socioeconomic changes especially important in the nutrition transition are changes in women's roles (especially with respect to patterns of time allocation), in income patterns, in household food-preparation technology, in food production and processing technology, and in family and household composition.

The sectoral distribution of the labour force toward industry and service has accelerated around the world. **Fig. 2** shows earlier data on this pattern. As has been shown often, the most labour-intensive agricultural and industrial work also requires the greatest amount of energy expenditure. One of the most inexorable shifts with modernization and industrialization is the reduced use of human energy to produce goods and services. The result is obviously a marked shift in activity patterns at work, a trend particularly associated with our shift into increasingly capital-intensive production and increasingly sedentary service and commercial work.

Unfortunately, there are few studies of this shift in activity and energy expenditures. One quite simple measure of overall activity has been collected in each survey from 16 000 Chinese as part of the China Health and Nutrition Surveys (CHNS). Activity patterns for Chinese adults shifted remarkably between 1989 and 1993. In particular, urban residents in all

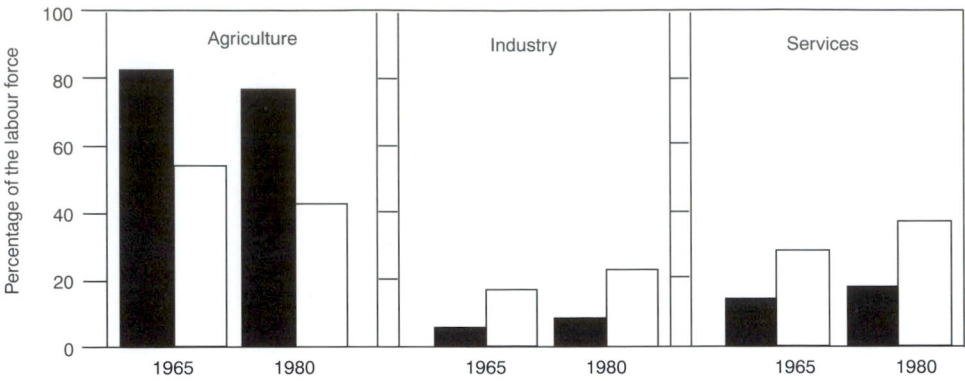

Figure 2 The sectoral distribution of the labour force in low- and middle-income developing countries, 1965 and 1980. Key: ■, low-income countries; □, middle-income countries. Source: World Bank Data.

income groups were more likely in 1993 to have adopted a more sedentary activity pattern (**Table 5**). In contrast, this pattern was not seen in the rural areas. In fact, rural residents, particularly low-income ones, showed a significant change from low and moderate activity patterns toward a high physical activity pattern.

Related to the effect of industrialization and modernization on market production is a similar shift in time allocation and physical effort in home and leisure activities. Possibly an even more astounding shift has come in leisure activities. While there was a time when leisure activities for children meant active play, it may now mean a quite sedentary activity such as viewing television or playing a computer game. Documentation of such patterns across the lower-income world is not available in terms of time spent and the shift in activities. This area cries out for greater focus.

Income patterns Income is an important element in the nutrition transition because it measures control over the flow of goods and services. Income allows one to purchase goods or services that can affect diet, activity and nutritional status. Three key issues relating income to nutrition are: (1) the effect of income changes on dietary structure; (2) the effect of income changes on the amount of energy, protein and fat consumed; and (3) the effect of change in the structure of the economy, particularly the change to commercial agriculture, on the nutritional status and diet of subsistence agriculturalists. The effect of income in purchasing the assets and technologies that in turn affect time use, diet and the activity patterns noted above is equally important but is not discussed here. The classic shift in the structure of diet is shown in **Fig. 3**. These relationships between income and diet have an important culture-specific component.

A second apparent relationship between income

Table 5 Distribution of physical activity of Chinese aged 20–45, by tertile of household income and residence

| | Household income per capita tertiles | | | | | | | | |
| | Low | | | Middle | | | High | | |
Residence and activity (%)	1989	1991	1993	1989	1991	1993	1989	1991	1993
Urban residence									
Lowest level	23.7[b,d]	34.3[b]	42.6	35.5[c]	45.4	42.8	44.5[c]	58.3	55.5[a]
Middle level	49.6[b,c]	30.1	30.2	46.1[c]	39.7[a]	40.6	48.0[c]	34.5	32.0[a]
Highest level	26.7[b]	35.6[b,c]	27.2	18.4	14.9	16.6	7.5	7.2	12.5[a,c]
Rural residence									
Lowest level	15.3[c]	3.9[b]	4.8[b]	16.2[c]	12.3	12.6	23.7[a]	24.8	19.8
Middle level	22.2[b,d]	5.3[b]	7.9[b]	28.9[c]	14.1	13.3	35.2[c]	24.0	26.8[c]
Highest level	62.5[b,d]	90.8[b]	87.3[b]	54.9[c]	73.6	74.1	41.1[c]	51.2	53.4

Data from CHNS (1989, 1991, 1993).
[a]The proportion differs significantly from middle- and high-income groups within same year ($P < 0.05$).
[b]The proportion differs significantly among three income groups within same year ($P < 0.05$).
[c]The proportion differs significantly from corresponding value in other 2 years ($P < 0.05$).
[d]The proportion differs significantly from corresponding value among 3 years ($P < 0.05$).

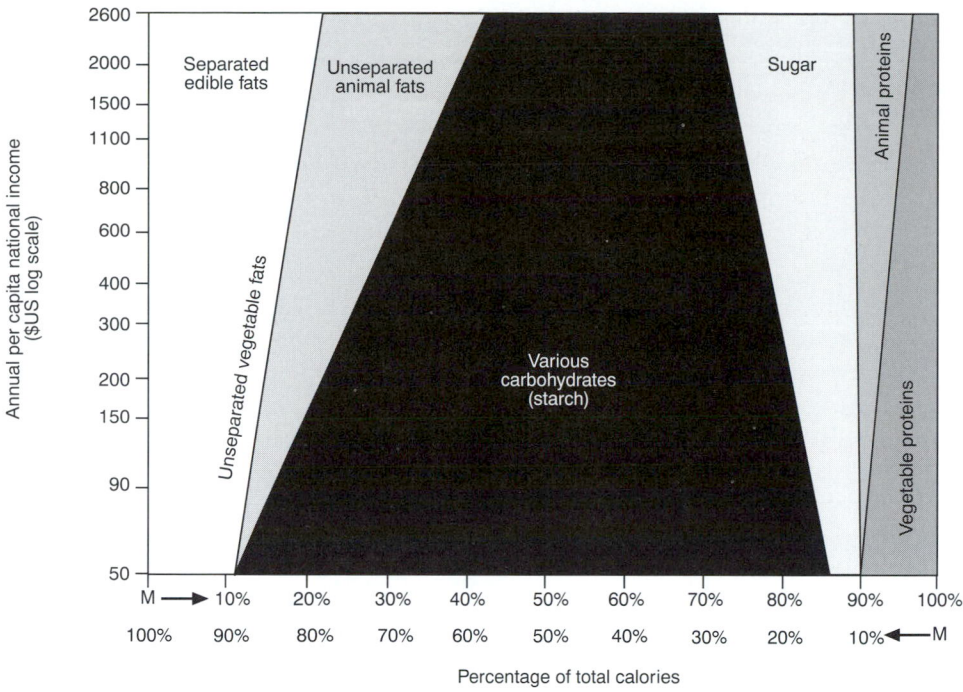

Figure 3 Structure of the diet and income (country-level sources of energy). FAO/UN (1970).

and diet is that as income increases (beyond the point where total food energy needs are met), people spend more per food item, partly to obtain higher quality. As many have shown, food demand is much more price- and income-elastic among the poor than among higher income groups.

Extensive research, including rigorous econometric and ethnographic studies, has focused on the effects of change from a subsistence to a cash economy; the results are varied and difficult to summarize. In most cases, introduction of a cash economy has also substantially increased household incomes, making it difficult to separate the effects of these two economic factors. The most impressive body of knowledge on the dietary effects of commercialization comes from six large case studies conducted by the International Food Policy Research Institute (IFPRI) in the Philippines, Guatemala, the Gambia, Rwanda, Kenya and Malawi. These studies indicate that commercialization substantially helped to alleviate hunger; however, increased income alone did not solve the problems of malnutrition.

For lower-income countries, a crucial dimension of the relationship between socioeconomic status and nutrition is the distribution of chronic disease risk factors by income group. In particular, a 1991 World Bank study on adult health in Brazil indicates that where income constraints among the poor are not too severe, many risk factors for cardiovascular disease will likely be greater among the poor than

among the rich. For example, **Fig. 4** illustrates the negative correlation between income and the risk factors hypertension and obesity in one city in Southern Brazil. In general, this study found that lower socioeconomic situations tended to be associated with higher risk factors for a range of noncommunicable disease risk factors but also found that this was not the case for obesity among men.

Changes in women's role and time-allocation patterns Women perform clear-cut biological, cultural and economic roles in the household: childbearer,

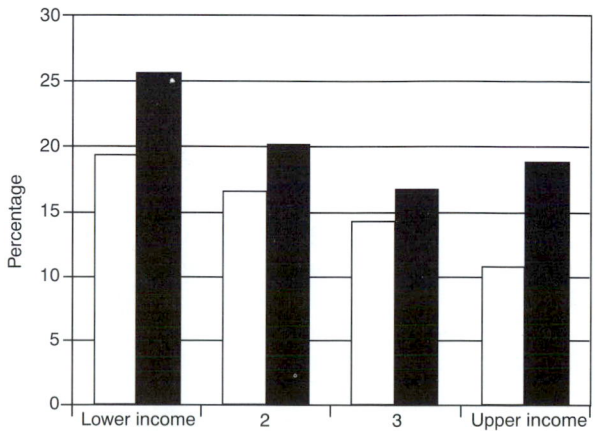

Figure 4 Percentage of population in four income categories at risk for hypertension and obesity in Porto Alegre, Brazil, 1986–87. Key: □, hypertension, ■, obesity.

caretaker of children and the old, gatekeeper responsible for family food preparation, and contributor to the family's economic well-being. Because women are the main decision-makers with respect to family food and nutrition, the ways they allocate their time and the constraints they face have enormous impact on family diet.

Proposition 3

Dietary change is associated with changes in our knowledge base and access to mass media.

Changes might be positive or negative. Gaining an understanding of the profound effects of modern media on the lives of persons in all nations is central to an understanding of development and its impact. The information technology revolution of the twentieth century, combined with increased rates of literacy and education, has fostered rapid communication of information among almost all populations worldwide, including social and private marketing information. The rate of change of diet and body composition in many low-income countries at the end of the twentieth century is far greater than that experienced in the past. The cause is clearly not just more rapid increases in income; there must be some causes lying either in other dimensions of behaviour that affect demand or in the way that food marketers are able to reach populations that is very different from the approaches used in the 1970s or 1980s. Television has certainly played a major role in this shift.

A review prepared in 1989 by *Population Reports* of Johns Hopkins University found from representative surveys of women of child-bearing age in lower-income countries the following:

- Latin America and the Caribbean: there is one television set for every six people;
- the Middle East and North Africa: one television set for every eight people;
- Asia: there is one television set owned for every 13 people;
- sub-Saharan Africa: one television set for every 29 people.

A 1992 estimate from 28 Demographic and Health Surveys places the proportions higher. A majority of married women have radios in their households in all these regions. Television also reaches a large proportion except in sub-Saharan Africa. In 11 countries surveyed, a majority of women have television at home; in Colombia and Egypt at least three-quarters have television. The more urban a nation, the greater the population exposure to all media. Reports or data exist for single countries. For instance, in Pakis-

tan in 1992 close to two-thirds of rural and 90% of urban households viewed television.

Proposition 4

Interaction among epidemiological, socioeconomic and demographic changes determines the nature and pace of the nutrition transition.

Clearly, the patterns of dietary change over time and space that constitute the nutrition transition have occurred concurrently with demographic, socioeconomic and epidemiological changes. The relationships among these factors are complex; the hope is that as we understand more about dietary, nutritional, demographic, epidemiological and socioeconomic patterns, we will come to understand the causal relationships among these factors. In this section, patterns of recent dietary change in several countries in relation to relevant demographic, socioeconomic and epidemiological factors are outlined.

To overcome data constraints, let us focus on the few countries that have systematically studied diet and body composition with larger nationwide surveys, e.g. the USA, China, Russia and Brazil. For China and Russia, data sets collected by this author are used. One must have individual and household data to comprehend fully the shifts in dietary excess and deficit that are occurring.

In the next section, some of the nutrition transitions, particularly in lower-income countries, are presented.

Nutrition Transitions

One of the marked patterns that appears to be emerging around the world is an increase in the consumption of vegetable oils. No matter what stage of development a country is in, there appears to be not only a shift toward this type of oil and away from other types, but also with increased income, oil intake goes up very rapidly. This is shown below for four Asian countries, but one can find this pattern equally in a middle-income country like Brazil or the poorer countries of Africa. The Western model is typified by the USA and Western Europe.

The earlier model of accelerated change: Japan and Korea

For Japan, household food intake data are available to track changes in energy, protein and fat intake for the entire period between 1946 and the present (1997). Since the period of post-World War II food shortages, the Japanese diet has shifted rapidly. Energy intake in Japan increased slowly toward a peak around 1970–75, whereas intake of animal products and fat increased continuously from 1946 to the present. During this period, daily per capita consumption of animal products increased by 257 g, daily per capita total fat consumption increased 341%, and the proportion of energy from fat increased from 8.7% to 24.8%.

South Korea, another Asian country that has achieved remarkably rapid economic growth since the 1960s, experienced a change in dietary structure similar to that of Japan. Trends in the South Korean diet since 1969 include a marked decline in grain and potato consumption and an increase in consumption of fish, meat, eggs and milk (**Fig. 5**). By the late 1980s, total fat intake as a proportion of energy in Korea had reached only 15%; Japan reached this level in 1965 and by 1987 this had increased to 25% of energy from fat. The South Korean diet might be expected to continue changing rapidly in a similar manner, resulting in a transition in disease patterns similar to that experienced by Japan.

The rapidly growing countries of East and Southeast Asia

China and Thailand are the leaders of change among this cluster of countries, whose economies are growing very rapidly, and with this there are marked shifts in diets and activity patterns. The type of diet associated with a pattern of degenerative disease is emerging rapidly. As noted earlier for China, there are equally rapid shifts toward reduced levels of physical activity.

One of the first changes to appear is the increased intake of oils. Food balance data are used here to illustrate, for 1980–90, the proportional change in food available for consumption in four countries with some of the most rapid growth in Asia (**Fig. 6**). In each case, the change in energy intake has been small but there have been large changes in consumption of animal products, sugar and fats. The very large proportion increase in vegetable oil consumption is shown.

Clearly these countries are moving along somewhat different paths toward a diet associated with a degenerative disease pattern. The foods differ among countries and hence one would expect that the resultant long-term health implications will also vary.

The China Health and Nutrition Survey collected 3 days of 24-hour recall dietary data along with anthropometric and detailed socioeconomic status (SES) data from its families. (More detail on the CHNS as well as the actual data sets can be gained by accessing the website for this survey, which can be reached at the following URL: http:www.cpc.unc.edu/projects/china/china_home.html.) The China experience is explored in more detail, not only because of its importance, but also because the trends documented in China appear to be emerging for other Southeast Asian countries which lack the monitoring system China has developed.

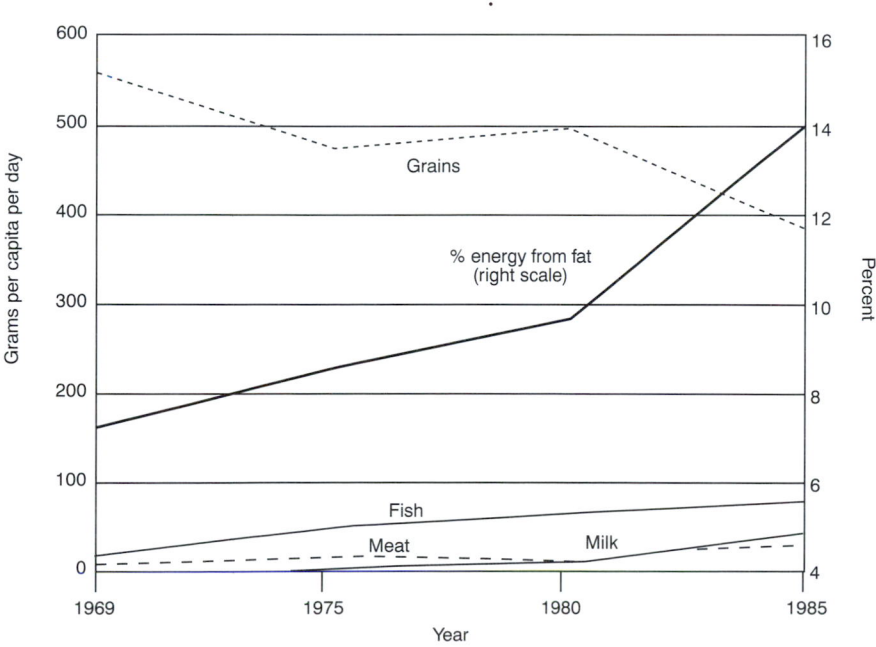

Figure 5 Changes in consumption of selected foods: daily intake and percentage of energy from fats, Korea 1969–85. From Kim, SH (1991) Changing nutritional status affected by rapid economic growth of Korea. *Proceedings of International Symposium on Food Nutrition and Social Economic Development*, pp. 472–478. Beijing: Chinese Academy of Preventive Medicine. Reproduced with permission.

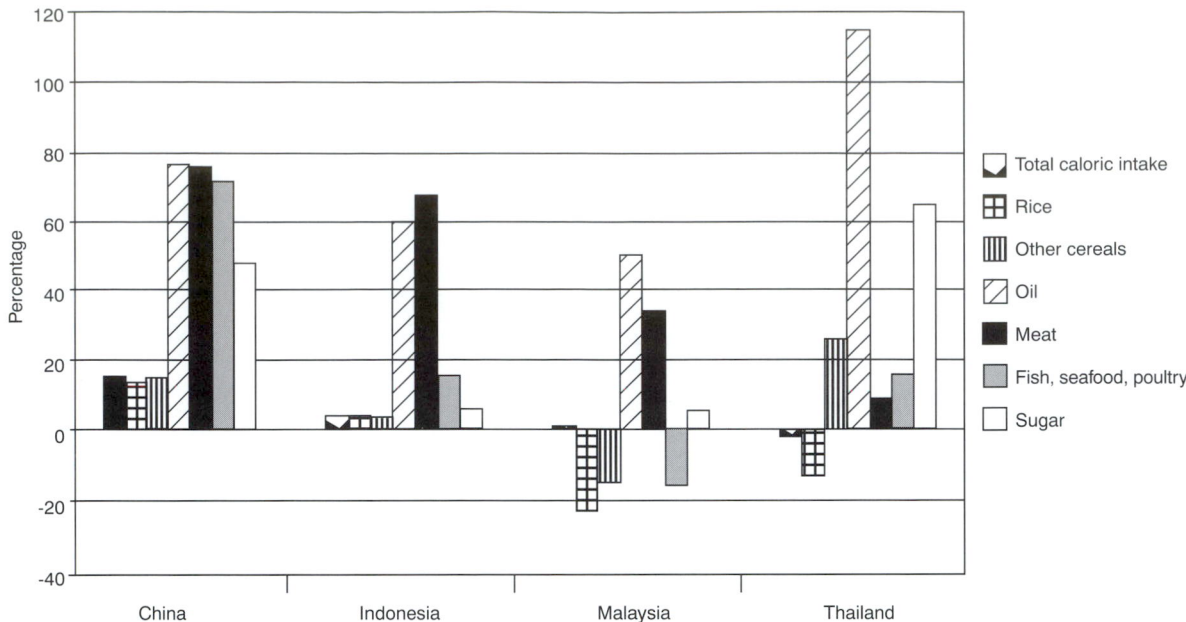

Figure 6 Percentage changes in food available for consumption, 1980–90 (calories per capita per day). Reprinted with permission. All rights reserved. *Nutrition Reviews* **52**:289. ©1994 by the International Life Sciences Institute, Washington, DC. 20036–4810.

While the traditional Chinese diet was felt to be a low-fat one, only a small and rapidly diminishing proportion of the population now follows this traditional low-fat pattern and an ever-increasing proportion is consuming more than 30% of their energy from fat. This high-fat diet was significantly more common in urban and higher-income populations than in rural and lower-income ones (**Table 6**). At the same time, there were decreases in the proportion of adults consuming a low-fat diet among all income groups.

When coupled with the dietary intake changes and the activity changes noted earlier, it is clear that one would expect an increase in obesity in the urban sample and possibly an increase in undernutrition among the low-income rural residents. When these relationships are explored, the weight shifts are indeed significant. The large increase in child obesity is equally concerning.

Thailand Thailand is undergoing an economic transition which began about 5 years after China's and is proceeding at a slower pace. There has been a remarkably rapid increase in obesity in Thailand.

Table 6 Percentages of study population of Chinese aged 20–45 in high and low energy consumed from fat dietary intake categories by tertile of household income

Distribution of sample by % energy from fat	Household income								
	Low			Middle			High		
	1989	1991	1993	1989	1991	1993	1989	1991	1993
% Consuming <10%									
Urban	14.3[a]	10.0[b]	1.5[a,c]	8.6[c]	2.7	0.4	7.1[c]	0.4	0.3
Rural	39.2[b,c]	17.3[b]	14.7[b]	24.7[c]	9.1	9.1	14.8[c]	3.3	3.5
Total	36.5[b,d]	16.4[b]	12.2[b]	18.6[c]	7.1	6.5	11.1[c]	1.8	2.3
% Consuming >30%									
Urban	19.1	25.4[b]	36.4[b,c]	19.1[d]	45.5	51.0	22.8[c]	62.0	66.6
Rural	7.6[b,c]	12.8[b]	12.9[b]	12.0[d]	19.9	24.9	15.3[d]	39.1	44.1
Total	8.8[b,d]	14.3[b]	17.3[b]	14.6[d]	27.7	32.6	18.9[c]	50.7	52.7

Data from CHNS (1989, 1991, 1993).
[a]The proportion differs significantly from middle- and high-income groups within same year ($P < 0.05$).
[b]The proportion differs significantly among three income groups within same year ($P < 0.05$).
[c]The proportion differs significantly from corresponding value in other 2 years ($P < 0.05$).
[d]The proportion differs significantly from corresponding value among the three years ($P < 0.05$).

The increases in obesity in urban areas are found not just in Bangkok, but also in other parts of the country.

Vietnam Large-scale representative surveys of adults seem to indicate that the country has yet to shift out of a pattern of receding famine in rural areas. SES and anthropometric data were collected from 12 800 rural men and women from 10 states. Chronic undernutrition, defined by a BMI below 18.5, was found in over 20% of all age–gender groups. An urban survey would be needed to capture faithfully the effects of the current resurgence of the Vietnamese economy.

One question concerns the inevitability of the transition toward high levels of obesity in Asia. Among large populations in Asia other than China, too little is known yet to understand whether the pattern of body composition found in China and the smaller Thai and Vietnamese surveys will be found elsewhere. The rapid increases in diabetes rates in China and other Asian countries and the dietary and physical activity patterns and obesity information do not present a promising picture for the rapidly growing economies of Southeast Asia.

The slowly emerging Latin American pattern

In Central and South America and the Caribbean, information is available to document the pace and nature of the transition in diet and body composition. In this region, where patterns of dietary change have been much slower, we have begun to face the problem of obesity and other problems of dietary excess among not only the rich, but also the poor. The problem of increased obesity has been carefully documented in Brazil, where equally important increases in undernutrition among the poor are not seen; in fact, there have been significant declines in undernutrition among all income groups. Similar trends and related problems have been documented in Chile and the Caribbean. Overall, it is clear that obesity rates and shifts in diet and activity are probably further along the nutrition transition in Latin America but there is enormous variability in patterns of obesity. One comparative study by International Clinical Epidemiology Network (INCLEN) of four Asian and three Latin American countries found in Asia that the range of adult obesity was 6–38%, while that in Latin America was 32–70%. By the early 1980s obesity levels were high in many Latin American countries. One survey of over 30 000 adults in Cuba in the early 1980s found obesity rates of over 20% in all age–gender groups and over 33% in all adults aged 30 and older. This study found much higher rates in urban areas and among persons with higher levels of education and higher-paid and more sedentary occupations.

Africa and the Near East—the polarized region

There is an extensive literature on undernutrition among children and adults in most North African and sub-Saharan African countries. At the same time, there is an emerging literature that shows extensive adult obesity. The most detailed studies have come from Egypt, Kuwait and Saudi Arabia. Data from the 1994 Egypt Food Consumption Monitoring Survey showed that close to 25% of the rural women and 39% of the urban women consumed more than 30% of their energy from fat and a remarkably small percentage consumed low-fat diets. At the same time, they showed that obesity was very high (above 30% of the women). This risk was higher among urban women. Other careful work has come from South Africa and studies in the Congo and Saudia Arabia.

Emerging Concerns

Several issues have become increasingly important in lower-income countries. These topics seem likely to have significant, adverse effects on the health in lower-income nations or they are important topics about which little is known.

Child obesity

Most of the concern and information regarding the nutrition transition in low-income countries has focused on adults. This focus is misleading and may ultimately have adverse consequences if concern for the factors affecting children is not forthcoming. **Table 7** presents from one study on child obesity and stunting, the child obesity patterns for four countries at different stages of the nutrition transition. These are compared with rates for child obesity in the USA, a country that considers child obesity to be a major public health problem. The values in Table 7 estimate the percentage of persons in each category with BMIs at or above the sex- and age-specific overweight criteria defined by the National Health Examination Survey percentiles. This indicates a serious public health problem among children in several of the world's larger countries.

Early nutritional insults and obesity

A related issue explored in one recent study is the relationship between nutritional insults during pregnancy and infancy. It has been shown that adults with low weight at age 1 or low birthweights have a greater tendency to store fat abdominally. In addition, it has been found that males who

Table 7 Prevalence of children aged 6–8 years[a] with BMI higher than the US reference – NHES 85th and 95th centiles in six countries

NHES centiles	NHANES III (1980–91)[c]	China (1993)	Russia (1994–95)	South Africa (1994) Total	South Africa (1994) Only black and coloured	Brazil (1989)
NHES 95th[b]						
Males	11.7	8.0	11.8	7.4	8.2	4.6
Females	13.7	9.2	8.1	4.1	4.5	3.3
NHES 85th[b]						
Males	21.3	14.1	25.6	25.0	23.0	12.8
Females	24.2	12.2	17.8	20.3	20.9	10.5

[a]Note: 6–8 years is equivalent to 72–108 months.
[b]Source: National Health and Examination Survey BMI standards at the 95th and 85th centiles; personal communications, Richard P Troiano, National Center for Health Statistics, April (1996).
[c]Source of NHANES III data: Troiano RP, Flegal KM, Kuzmarski RT, Campbell SM and Johnson CL (1995) Overweight prevalence and trends for children and adolescents. *Archives of Pediatrics & Adolescent Medicine* **149**:1085–1091.

experienced famine during the first half of gestation were more likely to become obese as young adults. Our research showed that there was a significant likelihood that stunted children would become obese in four large countries. The emergence of the nutrition transition suggests that this relationship might lead to considerable obesity in the first few decades of the twenty-first century, affecting individuals living in environments where current infant-feeding and morbidity patterns during infancy are associated with extensive stunting. Rapid shifts in the structure of diets and activity patterns might lead to a major problem of obesity among these stunted children. This topic needs research attention.

Ageing

A second unique challenge facing Asian and Latin American countries, particularly those such as China, Thailand, Indonesia and several smaller countries (e.g. Sri Lanka), is the ageing of the population, largely driven by rapid reductions in the birth rate. Many of these populations will experience a doubling or a tripling of the proportion of the population aged 65 and older between 1990 and 2025.

Impact of the mass media

Little is understood about the way the penetration of the mass media has affected the shift in diet. It is clear that there has been a rapid rise in television viewing during the 1980s and 1990s. This, coupled with increased liberalization of the air waves, has allowed modern mass advertising and other influences related to exposure to television viewing to reach most persons, particularly the young. Much more attention needs to be paid to the impact of this on the diets and activity patterns of children and other age groups.

See also: **Dietary Surveys**: Surveys of National Food Intake. **Energy**: Energy Requirements. **Epidemiological Studies**: Role and Interpretation. **Exercise**: Diet and Exercise; Beneficial Effects. **Obesity**: Definition, Aetiology and Assessment; Early Obesity and Prognosis.

Further Reading

Al-shoshan AA (1992) The affluent diet and its consequences: Saudi Arabia—a case in point. *World Review of Nutrition and Dietetics* **69**:113–165.

Briscoe J (1990) *Brazil: The New Challenge of Adult Health*. World Bank Country Study. Washington, DC: World Bank.

Galal OM and Harrison GG (1997) Goals for preventive nutrition in developing countries. In: Bendich A and Deckelbaum RJ (eds) *Preventive Nutrition*, pp. 531–541. Totowa, NJ: Humana Press.

McGuire J and Popkin BM (1989) Beating the zero sum game: Women and nutrition in the Third World. *Food and Nutrition Bulletin* **11**:38–63; **12**:3–11.

Milio N (1990) *Nutrition Policy for Food-rich Countries: A Strategic Analysis*. Baltimore: Johns Hopkins University Press.

Omran AR (1971) The epidemiologic transition: A theory of the epidemiology of population change. *Milbank Memorial Fund Quarterly* **49**(4, part 1):509–538.

Popkin BM (1994) The nutrition transition in low-income countries: An emerging crisis. *Nutrition Reviews* **52**:285–298.

Popkin BM and Bisgrove EZ (1988) Urbanization and nutrition in low-income countries. *Food and Nutrition Bulletin* **10**:3–23.

Popkin BM, Siega-Riz AM and Haines PS (1996) A comparison of dietary trends between racial and socioeconomic groups in the United States. *New England Journal of Medicine* **335**:716–720.

Popkin BM, Richards MK and Monteiro C (1996)

Stunting is associated with overweight in children of four nations that are undergoing the nutrition transition. *Journal of Nutrition* **126**:3009–3016.

United Nations Department for Economic and Social Information (1995) *World Urbanization Prospects:* *The 1994 Revision*, ST/ESA/SER.A/150. New York: United Nations.

World Bank (1991) *The World Development Report 1991: The Challenge of Development*. New York: Oxford University Press for the World Bank.

POTASSIUM

Physiology, Dietary Sources and Requirements

M P Navarro, Estación Experimental del Zaidín, CSIC, Granada, Spain

M P Vaquero, Instituto de Nutrición y Bromatología, CSIC-UCM, Madrid, Spain

Potassium is one of the most abundant cations in the body. Almost 98% of the potassium in the body is contained inside the cells making it the major intracellular cation. The remainder is found in the extracellular fluid. The study of potassium physiology and nutrition comprises aspects related to food composition, requirements, intake, absorption, transport, storage and excretion, as well as homeostatic mechanisms that serve to maintain an adequate plasma potassium concentration.

Absorption, Transport and Storage

Absorption

The absorptive capacity of the intestine for potassium is very large and as much as 90% of dietary potassium is absorbed by normal subjects. Faecal potassium excretion changes only slightly as dietary potassium intake is varied over a wide range, thus indicating that absorption rises almost in direct proportion to increasing intake.

In the human small intestine K^+ permeability is high and potassium absorption is thought to take place primarily by passive mechanisms in response to electrochemical gradients and solvent drag. In the proximal small bowel, K^+ is concentrated through the absorption of water, thus providing a driving force for the movement of these cations across the intestinal mucosa and into the blood. The duodenum and jejunum absorb this ion even more rapidly than water. Indeed, shortly after a meal, the potassium concentration ($[K^+]$) in jejunum rapidly reaches plasma levels. In the ileum, the transepithelial electrical potential difference strongly influences the cation movement. Evidence for active transport of K^+ in the small intestine is lacking, but there might be an active process that would most likely be due to an apical membrane H^+/K^+-exchanging ATPase (EC 3.6.1.36). Specific transport mechanisms are explained below.

In the colon, potassium may be either secreted or absorbed: net secretion occurs when the luminal concentration is less than about 20–25 mmol, while net K^+ absorption takes place above 25 mmol. The proximal portion of the colon secretes K^+ whereas the distal colon mainly absorbs K^+. There are two mechanisms for K^+ secretion: a major component is a passive flux, potential-dependent, via transcellular or paracellular mechanisms, and there is also an active serosal to mucosal secretory mechanism of minor quantitative physiological importance. Active K^+ secretion is the result of both an uptake across the basolateral membrane controlled by the enzyme Na^+/K^+-exchanging ATPase (EC 3.6.1.37) and the movement of potassium across the apical membrane through K^+ channels. Active K^+ absorption is also present in the distal colon, in which the K^+ uptake appears to be an exchange for H^+ across the apical membrane.

The availability of potassium in the diet is very high, at 90–95%. Two factors may account for this fact. First, potassium salts are completely soluble because they are wholly ionic, and second, few dietary components have been described that modify its digestive utilization. Among the latter, olive oil is one of the fats that favours potassium uptake, while some fibres and certain ion exchange resins may decrease K^+ absorption.

Transport

Potassium, being an electrolyte, is transported mainly in ionic form in the extracellular liquid.

Plasma concentration reaches 4–5 mmol l^{-1}, of which only 10–20% is bound to proteins. Intracellular potassium concentration lies in the range of about 110–150 mmol per litre of cells. More than 95% of the potassium pool is exchangeable. In erythrocytes, potassium is slowly changeable, whereas in the skeleton, given the small amount present, it is not readily exchanged.

Extra and intracellular sodium and potassium concentrations are maintained by the enzyme Na^+/K^+-exchanging ATPase, which is found in the plasma membrane of virtually all animal cells (**Fig. 1**). This enzyme is a carrier protein that pumps $2K^+$ in and $3Na^+$ out of the cell during each cycle of conformational changes driven by ATP hydrolysis. This process is electrogenic, meaning that one net positive charge is removed from the cell in each pump cycle.

Another system for active K^+ transport is controlled by H^+/K^+-exchanging ATPase which ejects H^+ in exchange for K^+. This pump has an important role

in some gastrointestinal cells and in the renal collecting duct.

Other potassium transport systems are driven by the force of ion gradients rather than by ATP hydrolysis (they are said to be secondary active transports, while those mediated by ATP are said to be primary active transports). The free energy gained during the movement of an inorganic ion down an electrochemical gradient is used as the driving force to pump other solutes against their electrochemical gradient. Thus, the carrier protein acts as a coupled transporter and electroneutrality is maintained. In fact an Na^+-K^+-Cl^--cotransport, carrying $1Na^+$, $1K^+$ and $2Cl^-$ inside the cell, has been found with a K^+-Cl^--cotransport in various renal tubular cells.

Passive transport of K^+ occurs via paracellular and intracellular pathways. The intracellular mechanism involves K^+ channels, which are pores made by a specific protein through the plasma membrane. Channels have 'gates', which open and close in response to specific stimuli. Accordingly, a variety of K^+ channels have been identified as: voltage-gated channels, mechanically gated channels, ligand-gated channels, ion-gated channels, etc. The role of K^+ channels in cell physiology has attracted attention from many research teams. It has been found that the membrane potential depends not only on Na^+/K^+-exchanging ATPase, but also on K^+ leak channels; that voltage-gated channels are responsible for the active potential transmision in a nerve cell; and that some K^+ channels are activated by second messengers such as Ca^{2+}, ATP and G proteins.

Different K transport mechanisms can operate simultaneously in a cell. They are usually interrelated and are also linked with other ion transport systems. Furthermore they can become targets for specific hormones.

Storage

Total body potassium is a function of age, weight, height and sex. A 70 kg adult man contains approximately 135 g of potassium, representing a concentration of 45–55 mmol kg^{-1} of body weight, whereas in women potassium content is 35–40 mmol kg^{-1} of body weight, mainly because of a lower ratio of muscle mass to fat. During childhood and in the elderly these values are lower than those for women. Total potassium is an index of body cell mass. It can be measured with ^{40}K, a natural isotope present as a small fraction of the total potassium, which emits γ rays and can be detected by a sensitive whole body counter. Because potassium is present only in the fat-free compartments of the body, total body ^{40}K can be used as an index of lean body mass.

A decrease in total body potassium has been

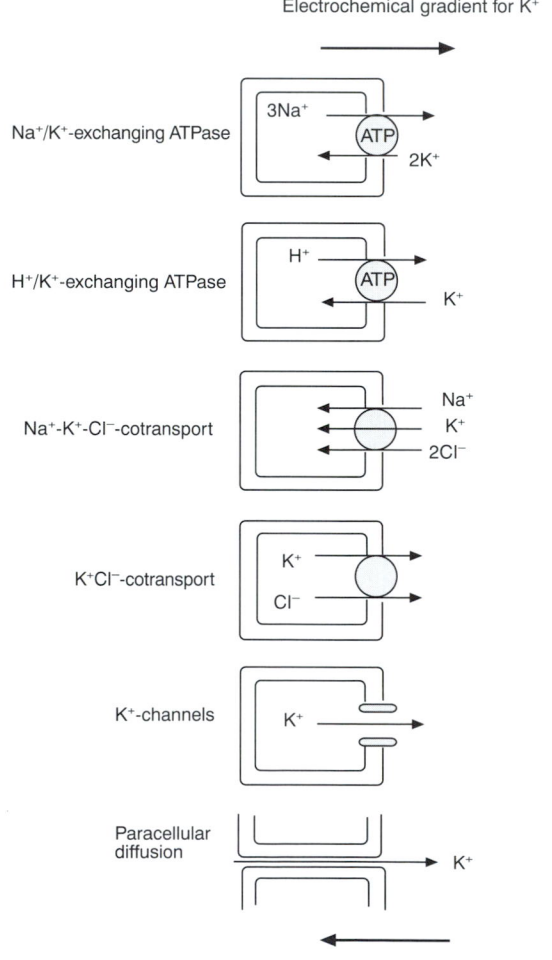

Figure 1 Potassium transport via intracellular and paracellular pathways.

observed in chronic protein–energy malnutrition owing to the reduction in muscle proteins and loss of intracellular potassium. The cellular exchange of sodium and potassium is altered, leading to potassium loss and increased intracellular sodium and water. In contrast, exercise and adequate training increase total lean body mass, thereby causing a rise in the potassium content of the body. Therefore, when the muscular mass has to be increased, in cases of recovery from malnutrition or extreme physical exercise, the storage of this electrolyte also takes place in the muscle. In such cases it is necessary to ingest proteins as well as adequate amounts of potassium and magnesium, the main intracellular electrolytes.

The storage of K in the intracellular environment is a physiological response to an increase of the extracellular potassium. Even a small increase in extracellular potassium may cause a significant rise in plasma potassium concentration, resulting in muscle hypopolarization. However, if such an increase is stored in the cells, then fewer intracellular changes would result, with only a slight difference appearing in potassium concentration across cell membranes. In order to accomplish this 'buffer' function, the major reservoir of potassium is the muscle, followed by the liver and erythrocytes, although each cell possesses the capacity for accumulating potassium.

Metabolism and Excretion

The extracellular potassium concentration must be maintained within narrow limits to prevent dangerous hyperkalaemia, where extracellular $[K^+]$ exceeds 5.5 mmol l^{-1}, or hypokalaemia, where extracellular $[K^+]$ is below 3.5 mmol l^{-1}. This is achieved by two mechanisms: 'internal balance', i.e. distribution of K^+ between intra- and extracellular spaces, carried out by Na^+/K^+-exchanging ATPase; and 'external balance', i.e. intake–output equilibrium, which takes place principally in the kidney but also in the intestine. After a meal, the K^+ is absorbed rapidly and enters the extracellular fluid. The subsequent rise in plasma $[K^+]$ is attenuated by the rapid uptake of K^+ into cells (occurring within minutes). To maintain external K^+ balance, all of the K^+ absorbed and exceeding needs must be excreted slowly by the kidneys.

Excretion

Potassium is mainly excreted in the urine. An average of 65 mmol of K^+ per day is eliminated in this way. Faecal losses of potassium represent approximately 10% of the ingested amount, although this percentage can be somewhat higher in cases of diarrhoea. Vomiting is also a cause of potassium loss.

When dietary potassium is severely restricted, faecal loss of potassium decreases to about 3.5 mmol per day. This presumably represents obligatory faecal potassium loss – that is excretion from intestinal secretions – as K^+ is present in salivary, gastric, biliary and pancreatic secretions. Potassium from desquamated cell and mucus secretion also contributes to total excretion. Potassium concentration in sweat is about 10 mmol l^{-1}. This has little effect on total potassium excretion because sweat losses are negligible provided that temperature and exercise conditions are not extreme.

The kidneys play the main role in maintaining a steady level of potassium in the body. Potassium is freely filterable at the renal corpuscle. Usually, the filtered fraction that is excreted ranges between 5% and 15%, which indicates the existence of tubular potassium reabsorption. The renal tubules are thus capable of reabsorbing and secreting potassium in response to a variety of stimuli.

The proximal tubule is responsible for the reabsorption of approximately 60% of previously filtered potassium. The mechanisms have not yet been fully elucidated, but it seems that the movement of potassium from lumen to the interstitial fluid might be mainly the result of paracellular diffusion through K^+Cl^--cotransport and K^+ channels located in the basolateral membrane, all of these serving to counteract the basolateral Na^+/K^+-exchanging ATPase (**Fig. 2**). In this region the basolateral K^+ channels have higher conductance than the apical ones, which is essential for maintaining a negative intracellular membrane potential and hence promoting reabsorption of sodium and organic substrates, such as glucose and amino acids.

The concentration of potassium increases as the filtrate passes through the loop of Henle, where permeability for K^+ is very high. At the end of the descending limb the amount of K^+ present usually exceeds that of the glomerular filtrate. There is a net secretion of K^+, arising mainly from reabsorption in the collecting tubule and partly from reabsorption in the ascending limb. These pathways of potassium transport establish a 'potassium recycling' process in the renal medulla. In the thick ascending limb potassium is mainly reabsorbed – about 30% of the amount filtered by transcellular and paracellular pathways – but a role for this limb in potassium secretion has also been recognized. The secretion of potassium through apical K^+ channels is important for net Na^+ and Cl^- reabsorption through the Na^+-K^+-Cl^--cotransporter, since the luminal Na^+ and Cl^- concentrations are higher than the luminal K^+

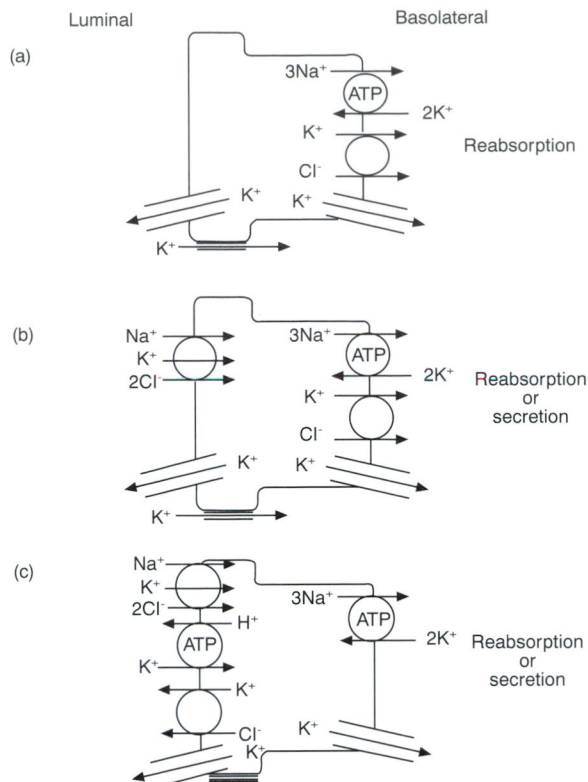

Figure 2 Principal mechanisms of potassium transport in the major tubular segments of the nephron. (a) Proximal tubule, (b) thick ascending limb; (c) distal tubule and collecting duct.

concentration. Aldosterone and antidiuretic hormone (ADH) appear to increase the number of these channels.

In all parts of the nephron preceding the distal tubule, potassium transport is strongly related to the reabsorption of other nutrients. However, the balance control for this element takes place mainly in the most distal portion. Almost all potassium excreted in the urine has been previously secreted by the distal tubule, principally by the cortical collecting duct, although the medullary collecting duct possesses the highest potassium reabsorption capacity. Potassium secretion may be stimulated by Na^+/K^+-exchanging ATPase activity in the basolateral membrane, with subsequent exit of potassium from the cell taking place through the channels located in the apical membrane or through the K^+Cl^--cotransporter. Potassium reabsorption would take place through the Na^+-K^+Cl^--cotransporter, the H^+/K^+-exchanging ATPase pump and through the exit of potassium to the interstitial space by the basolateral K channels. Several regulating systems act at this level. Proton secretion by H^+/K^+-exchanging ATPase, together with that by H^+-ATPase, contribute to acidification of the urine. These enzymes are probably located at the luminal and basolateral sites (not

shown in Fig. 2) and participate in the acid–base balance and potassium status. In potassium repletion, luminal K^+ transported by Na^+/K^+-exchanging ATPase and H^+/K^+-exchanging ATPase recycles back into the lumen, whereas in the case of potassium depletion this 'waste' of potassium through luminal K^+ channels is very low.

Regulation of Potassium Homeostasis

A variety of factors, including the actions of hormones, contribute to potassium homeostasis acting at different levels (**Fig. 3**)

Internal balance

A rise in plasma $[K^+]$ together with the hormones insulin, adrenaline (by activating β_2-receptors) and aldosterone promote the uptake of K^+ into skeletal muscle, liver, bone and red blood cells. In contrast, hypokalaemia and the stimulation of α-adrenergic receptors induce the release of K^+ from the intracellular to the extracellular fluid. Moreover, hyperkalaemia stimulates insulin, aldosterone and adrenaline secretions, while hypokalaemia has the opposite effect.

Other factors also influence K^+ movements across the cell, but these are not normal homeostatic mechanisms. Metabolic acidosis promotes movement of K^+ out of cells, whereas metabolic alkalosis has the opposite effect. An increase in the osmolality of the extracellular fluid enhances K^+ release by cells. Cell lysis causes K^+ release and might produce hyperkalaemia.

External balance

Plasma $[K^+]$ and aldosterone are the major physiological regulators of K^+ excretion. High $[K^+]$ stimulates potassium elimination by the intestine but principally by the kidney, thus promoting secretion in both the distal tubule and collecting duct by different mechanisms: stimulation of the Na^+/K^+-exchanging ATPase pump; increasing permeability to K^+ of the apical membrane; and aldosterone secretion. Hypokalaemia decreases K^+ secretion by antagonist actions.

Aldosterone stimulates Na^+ reabsorption and increases K^+ secretion by the distal tubule and collecting duct in a straightforward manner by increasing the amount of Na^+/K^+-exchanging ATPase in the principal cells. This enzyme is the driving force for K^+ exit and controls the permeability of the apical membrane to K^+. It also increases the amount of K^+ delivered by the small bowel to the colon and stimulates K^+ secretion by colon and rectum.

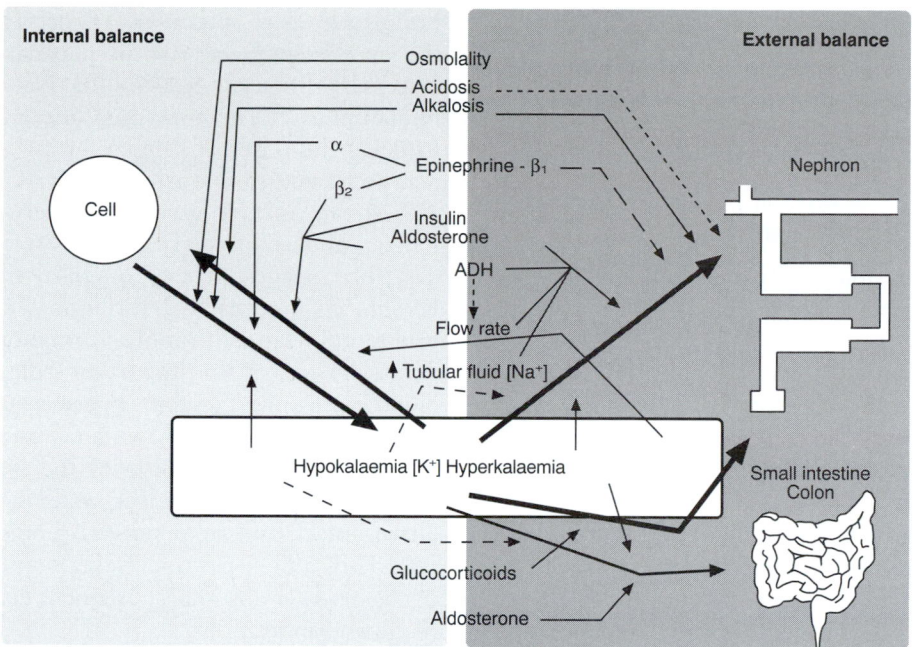

Figure 3 Potassium homeostasis. (——, ——, activation; broken and dotted lines (– – –, · · · ·, —— —— ——), inhibition; ADH, antidiuretic hormone.

There are other phenomena of lesser importance than those mentioned above. Glucocorticoids are kaliuretic, but their effect appear to be controlled by an increase in the glomerular filtration rate, rather than by a direct action on K^+ transport. A rise in the flow of tubular fluid rapidly stimulates K^+ secretion; this means that diuretics enhance urinary K^+ excretion. Accordingly a fall in the flow reduces K^+ secretion. Antidiuretic hormone (ADH) also increases K^+ secretion because, although ADH decreases tubular fluid flow, changes in ADH levels do not substantially alter urinary K^+. Physiological $[Na^+]$ does not alter K^+ secretion but a large $[Na^+]$ in tubular fluid increases K^+ secretion; however a fall in $[Na^+]$ has the opposite effect. Acid–base balance is another factor that regulates K^+ secretion: alkalosis increases secretion, whereas acidosis decreases it.

These processes of regulation allow the human body to maintain a normal plasma $[K^+]$. Moreover, the $[K^+]$ exerts a feedback regulation over most of its own control factors. In spite of these mechanisms, the equilibrium can sometimes be altered, thus causing either hypokalaemia or hyperkalaemia.

Hypokalaemia

Hypokalaemia can be the result of either or both intracellular shift and potassium depletion. Among its clinical sequelae are hyperpolarization of membrane, which affects the activity of nerves and muscles, as well as cardiac, renal and metabolic alterations.

Causes of hypokalaemia

1. Intracellular shift Alkalosis, insulin excess, familial periodic paralysis, catecholamine increase, intoxication (theophyline, barium).

2. Extrarenal causes

- Insufficient potassium intake (starvation, anorexia nervosa);
- Gastrointestinal losses (diarrhoea, vomiting, laxative abuse);
- Skin losses.

3. Excessive renal losses Renal tubular acidosis, hypermineralocorticoidism, syndrome of chloride depletion, diuretic condition.

The mechanisms mentioned in 1 and 2 above can also cause potassium depletion.

Hyperkalaemia

Hyperkalaemia can be the consequence of a potassium shift from cells to extracellular fluid or effect of excessive potassium retention. The first signs are flaccid paralysis, natriuresis and some minor endocrine effects. The most important consequences are ventricular fibrillation and cardiac arrest.

Causes of hyperkalaemia

1. Without potassium excess Caused by potassium shift from cells (acute acidosis, hyperosmolality, insulin deficiency, β-adrenergic blockers, succinylcholine, vigorous exercise).

2. With potassium excess

- Impaired renal excretion (renal failure, aldosterone deficiency, primary tubule dysfunction);
- Inappropriately high oral or parenteral potassium administration.

Metabolic Function and Essentiality

Potassium is physiologically important in many functions of the human body encompassing the muscular, cardiovascular, respiratory, digestive, renal, endocrine and nervous systems. A high intracellular potassium concentration is essential for optimal cellular metabolism: metabolic control; growth and division; DNA, protein and carbohydrate synthesis; and since this element is a cofactor for enzymes of energy transduction, glycogenesis, cellular growth and other pathways. Potassium deficiency causes growth retardation through a decrease in plasma levels of growth hormone and somatomedin C and a concomitant deterioration of protein synthesis; it may also contribute to growth retardation through a relatively organ-specific resistance to some growth factors.

Potassium is also implicated in the metabolism or utilization of several nutrients, particularly in sodium metabolism, so an adequate potassium intake is needed to achieve effective homeostasis of sodium. The enzyme Na^+/K^+-exchanging ATPase provides the driving force for the transport of other solutes, such as amino acids, sugar and phosphate. An increase in dietary potassium reduces urinary calcium and results in a more positive calcium balance.

Many of the functions of potassium are due to its ionic character, whereby it generates gradients of concentration, potential and pressure, and K^+ participates in regulation of the acid–base balance. By virtue of being the predominant osmotically active species within cells, K^+ plays a major role in the distribution of fluids inside and outside the cell and hence in the maintenance of cellular volume.

A difference of potassium concentration across cell membrane is essential for the normal polarization of the cell, and the latter is crucial for maintaining cell excitability and muscle contraction. The transmembrane electrical potential of the cell is determined by the ratio of the intracellular to extracellular potassium and sodium concentrations, mainly potassium. These concentration differences of K^+ and Na^+ across cell membranes are maintained by the specific permeability to each one of these ions and by the operation of Na^+/K^+-exchanging ATPase pump. Thus K^+ is critical for the excitability of nerve and muscle cells.

Potassium released from contracting skeletal muscle cells facilitates ongoing muscle contraction but also leads to muscular fatigue. Training reduces the exercise-induced rise in plasma $[K^+]$ and also increases the total activity of Na^+-K^+ pumps in human muscle. The potassium internal balance helps to delay the onset of fatigue during exercise and to restore homeostasis during recovery.

A strong inverse association between potassium intake and hypertension and stroke has been described, suggesting the possibility that elevation of K^+ inhibits free radical formation, smooth muscle proliferation and thrombus formation. In addition, potassium plays an important role in decreasing blood pressure under hypertensive conditions through some of the following actions: its natriuretic properties; the suppression of the sympathetic nervous and renin–angiotensin systems; a direct vasodilator effect; and an increase in glomerular filtration rate. Thus a high-potassium diet may prevent lesions of the artery walls and subsequent cerebral haemorrhage and infarctions.

Finally, potassium can modify both the mechanical and electrical properties of the heart, because it is critical for the contractility of cardiac cells. In chronic heart failure, potassium can reduce the potentially lethal ventricular tachyarrhythmias. However, as mentioned above, hyperkalaemia can produce a cardiac arrest.

Requirements

Until the 80's, recommended dietary intake for potassium had not been established. Indeed, potassium deficiency arising from inadequate dietary intake is unlikely, given the ubiquity of this element in all kinds of food. Before 1983, only a few countries had set some indications about recommended dietary potassium intake, and they did so only for some population groups So far, no unanimous agreement has been reached and various 'Recommended Intake', 'Estimated Intake' and 'Dietary Reference' values have been accepted.

The Nutrition Working Group of the International Life Sciences Institute of Europe in 1989 proposed a Recommended Daily Intake (RDI) of potassium for a healthy adult male, an amount equivalent to the actual molar sodium intake (100 mmol per day), i.e. 3900 mg of potassium per day. This recommendation was based on epidemiological evidence suggesting that a reduction in sodium intake and an increase in potassium intake were desirable to provide a molar Na/K ratio of 1, defined as beneficial in the prevention of several pathologies.

The subcommittee on the 10th edition of the Recommended Dietary Allowances (RDA) Food and

Nutrition Board of the National Research Council (NRC) in 1989 established that the minimum potassium requirements for healthy persons was 2000 mg per day. In December 1992 the Scientific Committee for Food of Commission of the European Communities (CEC) elaborated a report about nutrient and energy intakes that set the 'Population Reference Intake', a very similar standard to the RDA, as 3100 mg per day for both sexes from 11 years of age.

Calculations of potassium requirements are based on estimates of what is needed for growth and for replacement of obligatory losses: urinary, faecal and other negligible losses, e.g. in sweat. To maintain normal body stores as well as a normal concentration in plasma and interstitial fluid, the minimum requirement is approximately 1600–2000 mg per day. Nevertheless there is considerable evidence of the beneficial effect of dietary potassium in hypertension, therefore NRC suggests raising the daily potassium intake of adults to about 3500 mg (90 mmol). These values are very close to the standards fixed by the Committee of the CEC, which would also cover pregnancy and lactation, given that potassium digestibility might be favoured during these periods.

In infants and children, since this nutrient is a necessary constituent of each body cell, the increase in lean body mass is a major determinant of potassium needs, that is 50–80 mol kg^{-1} of weight gained. Dietary intake of potassium must be higher than the amount required at tissue level to allow obligatory urinary, cutaneous and faecal losses, some of these being higher in children. The requirement for an infant from birth to 15 weeks are estimated on a human milk potassium content basis. Hence lower values are possibly obtained and for this reason the intake should be increased appropriately, always taking into consideration that infants' kidneys are immature and an excess of potassium can be harmful. Some authors have estimated that, in general 186 mg MJ^{-1} (78 mg per 100 kcal) should maintain potassium balance in children of all ages.

In the elderly, potassium depletion is common due to both dietary lack and drug therapy; similarly the hyperkalemia is more frequent as a result of renal insufficiency, also intensified by drug therapy. It appears that the minimum satisfactory potassium intake is around 2000–2300 mg per day.

During exercise potassium needs may be increased owing to higher losses in sweat, especially in hot climates and in unaccustomed individuals. Some athletes may require as much as 3–6 g more potassium per day; this need can be satisfied by eating food rich in potassium and exceptionally by the ingestion of potassium supplements.

Dietary Sources and High Intakes

Potassium is ubiquitous in all kinds of food, but the best dietary sources are vegetables and fruits because they combine a high potassium content with a low sodium concentration (**Table 1**). Among these foods, the legumes stand out because they provide at least 1 g of potassium for 100 g of edible portion (EP). Dried fruits should also be mentioned, since they often exceed 0.5 and even 1 g per 100 g of EP, for example dried apricots, figs and prunes. Nuts such as pistachios and almonds also contain potassium, but the addition of salt during the roasting process upsets the ideal proportion of Na/K that is present in these foods. Banana is known to be one of the fruits richest in potassium, together with coconut, melon, avocado and kiwi fruit. Among the major vegetables sources of potassium are potatoes, spinach and Swiss chard. These foods, combined with

Table 1 Sodium and potassium content of various foods (mg per 100 g edible portion)

Food	Sodium	Potassium
Legumes		
Red kidney beans	18	1370
Soya beans	5	1730
Lentils	12	940
Dried fruit		
Raisins	60	1020
Figs	62	970
Nuts		
Walnuts	7	450
Almonds	14	780
Fruit and vegetables		
Banana	1	400
Melon	5–32	100–210
Potato	11	320
Spinach	140	500
Meat and fish		
Beef, veal, lamb	52–110	230–360
Chicken	81	320
Herring	120	320
Halibut	60	410
Tuna	47	400
Mussels	290	320
Miscellaneous		
Cow's milk	55	140
Chocolate	11	300

Values from Holland B, Welch AA, Unwin ID, Buss DH, Paul AA and Southgate DAT (1994) *McCance and Widdowson's The Composition of Foods*. London: Royal Society of Chemistry. (With the permission of the Controller of Her Majesty's Stationery Office.)

cereals and derived products that have a lower potassium content but are consumed in large quantities, account for almost 75% of potassium ingestion in Western diets. Milk should also be taken into account because of the importance of dairy products in Western nutrition. In particular, milk is the largest dietary source of potassium for infants. Meat and fish also contain a considerable amounts of potassium, but they also provide a much higher sodium content.

Food processing has no significant effect on dietary potassium given that potassium is mainly an intracellular cation. However, the potassium content of food can be depleted as a result of leaching. Indeed processes such as boiling, soaking or canning, particularly if they require the food to be cut into pieces, seem to decrease the potassium content.

Potassium intake varies considerably, depending on food selection; people who eat large amounts of fruit and vegetables have a higher intake of this nutrient. The reported daily intake of potassium by Western populations ranges from 40 to 150 mmol (1560–5850 mg). The Mediterranean diet provides a daily dose of potassium that reaches 3500 mg.

A sudden and significant enteral or parenteral increase in potassium, if not followed by a subsequent elimination, will produce acute intoxication: hyperkalaemia. To avoid hyperkalaemia a suitable potassium intake can be reliably achieved by an appropriate consumption of foods rather than by the use of potassium salts supplement, since the latter measure, if abused, may produce toxicity in individuals with undetected renal insufficiency. Intakes above 450 mmol per day induce symptomatic hyperkalaemia in some normal individuals and can thus be used as threshold for acute toxicity. However, chronic intakes above 5900 mg per day may be dangerous for individuals with impaired renal function. Therefore, since there is no apparent benefit in exceeding 5900 mg of potassium per day, this value is proposed as an upper safe level of intake by the Scientific Committee for Food (CEC).

See also: **Body Composition**: Determination and Physiological Significance. **Cofactors**: Organic Cofactors; Inorganic Cofactors. **Coronary Heart Disease**: Lipid Theory of Coronary Heart Disease; Haemostatic Factors and Coronary Heart Disease; Aetiology; Prevention. **Electrolytes**: Water-Electrolyte Balance; Acid-Base Balance. **Exercise**: Physiology of Skeletal Muscle; Diet and Exercise; Beneficial Effects. **Gastrointestinal Tract**: Structure and Function of the Stomach; Structure and Function of the Small Intestine; Structure and Function of the Colon. **Hypertension**: Physiology; Nutritional Management; Interrelationships Between Hypertension and Diabetes. **Nutrient Requirements**: International Perspectives. **Renal Function and Disorders**: Nutritional Management of Renal Disorders. **Sodium**: Physiology.

Further Reading

Agarwal R, Afzalpurkar R and Fordtran JS (1994) Pathophysiology of potassium absorption and secretion by the human intestine, *Gastroenterology* 107:548–555.

Berne RM and Mattew NL (1992) *Physiology*, 3rd edn, pp 652–716, 719–809. St Louis: Mosby Year Book.

Brenner BM and Rector FC (1991) *The Kidney*, 4th edn, pp 283–317, 805–840. Philadelphia: WB Saunders.

Breyer MD and Ando Y (1994) Hormonal signaling and regulation of salt and water transport in the collecting duct, *Annual Review of Physiology* 56:711–739.

Commission of the European Communities (CEC) (1992) *Nutrient and Energy Intakes for the European Community*, Food Science and Techniques. Reports of the Scientific Committee for Food (31st Series), Directorate-General, Internal Market and Industrial Affairs, EUR.

Eaton SB, Eaton III SB, Konner MJ and Shostak, M (1996) An evolutionary perspective enhances understanding of human nutritional requirements, *Journal of Nutrition* 126:1732–1740.

Jan LY and Jan YN (1992) Structural elements involved in specific K$^+$ channel functions, *Annual Review of Physiology* 54:537–555.

Johnson LR, Alpers DH, Christensen J, Jacobson ED and Walsh JH (1994) *Physiology of the Gastrointestinal Tract*, 3rd edn. New York: Lippincott-Raven.

National Research Council (1989) *Recommended Dietary Allowances*, 10th edn, pp 247–261. Washington DC: National Academy Press.

Navarro MP and Vaquero MP (1993) Potassium physiology. In: Macrae R, Robinson RK and Sadler MJ (eds) *Encyclopaedia of Food Science, Food Technology and Nutrition*, pp 3665–3672. London: Academic Press.

Nutrition Working Group (ILSI) (1990) Recommended daily ammounts of vitamins and minerals in Europe. *Nutrition Abstracts and Reviews*, Series A 60:827–842.

Vander AJ (1995) *Renal Physiology*, 5th edn. New York: McGraw-Hill.

Wang W, Sackin H and Giebisch (1992) Renal potassium channels and their regulation. *Annual Review of Physiology* 54:81–96.

Wingo CS and Smolka AJ (1995) Function and structure of H-K-ATPase in the kidney, *American Journal of Physiology* 269 (*Renal Fluid Electrolyte Physiology* 38):F1–F16.

Poultry *see* **Meat, Poultry and Meat Products**: Nutritional Value.

PREGNANCY

Contents

Energy Requirements and Metabolic Adaptations

G R Goldberg, Dunn Clinical Nutrition Centre, Cambridge, UK

Copyright © 1998 Academic Press

In addition to a woman's usual energy requirements, which depend on her body size and how physically active she is, pregnancy incurs extra energy costs. Some of these are obligatory, others avoidable. The relatively low stress per unit time of human pregnancy enables women to meet the extra costs of pregnancy by using various physiological, metabolic and behavioural strategies. Previous studies, mostly cross-sectional, of energy metabolism during pregnancy, focused on the average weight and fat gains, and birthweights which were associated with the best pregnancy and infant outcomes. More recently the emphasis has been on detailed longitudinal studies in which the various components of the energy cost of pregnancy – changes in basal metabolic rate, body fat and physical activity – have been measured. These studies have shown that there is a very high level of variability both between and within populations. Because of this, the total energy costs, and therefore the energy requirements, of pregnancy are also very variable, and it is impossible to predict the energy requirements of an individual pregnant woman. It should not be assumed that pregnant women will have energy-sparing alterations in metabolism and/or that physical activity naturally decreases. Worldwide, the majority of pregnant women are nutritionally an at-risk group. Future studies will almost certainly focus on specific gestational adjustments in metabolism and long-term consequences for both mother and infant.

Extra Energy Costs of Pregnancy

Tissue deposition

Weight gain during pregnancy is made up of the fetus, placenta and amniotic fluid (the products of conception) and the extra growth of several maternal tissues. The deposition of fat in pregnancy is presumed to help meet the extra energy demands of lactation. The total energy deposited as new tissue, excluding maternal fat averages about 49 MJ (11 700 kcal). If an average maternal fat gain of 2.6 kg is assumed, then estimates of the total energy deposited as new tissue during an average pregnancy is about 174 MJ (41 600 kcal) (**Table 1**).

Maintenance energy costs of pregnancy

Because of the increase in tissue mass the body's oxygen consumption also increases during pregnancy. Estimates suggest that the daily increase in oxygen consumption is equivalent to an extra 187 kJ (45 kcal) at 0–10 weeks, 414 kJ (100 kcal) at 10–20 weeks, 620 kJ (148 kcal) at 20–30 weeks, and 951 kJ (230 kcal) at 30–40 weeks gestation. The total maintenance cost for an average human pregnancy amounts to about 150 MJ (35 800 kcal) (**Table 2**).

Theoretical total metabolic costs of pregnancy

Compared with many other mammals, humans have a relatively small and usually single infant which develops during a long gestation period. The energy stress to the mother is therefore low per unit time. The 49 MJ of energy deposited as the products of conception represent only 4–5 days of food intake for the mother. Humans also differ from most other mammals because their large fat stores can help meet some of these costs. The theoretical total metabolic costs (i.e. due to extra tissue and increased metabolism) of pregnancy amount to about 335 MJ (80 000 kcal), or 1.25 MJ per day (300 kcal per day). This value does not make any allowance for changes

Table 1 Protein and fat deposition during pregnancy for a reference woman (adapted from Prentice *et al.*, 1996)

	Protein		Fat			Total	
Site	kg	MJ (kcal)	kg	MJ (kcal)	Water kg	kg	MJ (kcal)
Fetus	0.44	12.76 (3050)	0.44	20.24 (4840)	2.41	3.29	33.00 (7890)
Placenta	0.10	2.90 (690)	0.04	0.18 (43)	0.54	0.64	3.08 (740)
Amniotic fluid	0.003	0.09 (21)	0.00	0.00	0.79	0.79	0.09 (21)
Uterus	0.17	4.81 (1150)	0.04	0.18 (43)	0.80	0.97	5.00 (1200)
Breasts	0.08	2.35 (560)	0.12	0.55 (130)	0.30	0.40	2.90 (690)
Blood	0.14	3.92 (940)	0.02	0.92 (220)	1.29	1.44	4.84 (1157)
Water	0.00	0.00	0.00	0.00	1.50	1.50	0.00
Subtotal	**0.93**	**26.83 (6400)**	**0.48**	**22.08 (5280)**	**7.63**	**9.04**	**48.9 (11 700)**
Fat stores	0.07	1.94 (460)	2.68	123.10 (29 400)	0.60	3.35	125.04 (29 900)
Total	**0.99**	**28.77 (6900)**	**3.16**	**145.18 (34 700)**	**8.24**	**12.38**	**173.94 (41 600)**

Table 2 Increases in oxygen consumption (ml min^{-1}) during pregnancy (adapted from Hytten, 1991)

	10 weeks	20 weeks	30 weeks	40 weeks
Cardiac output	4.5	6.8	6.8	6.8
Respiration	0.8	1.5	2.3	3.0
Kidneys	7.0	7.0	7.0	7.0
Breasts	0.1	0.6	1.2	1.4
Uterus	0.5	1.2	2.2	3.6
Placenta	0	0.5	2.2	3.7
Fetus	0	1.1	5.5	12.4

(increases or decreases) in energy expended on physical activity. It has been assumed that the majority of the energy costs of human pregnancy are met by behavioural adjustments in energy metabolism rather than increased energy intake (*See:* **Energy**; Energy Requirements). This assumption has formed the basis for energy intake recommendations summarized in **Table 3**. The estimates used by WHO/FAO/UNU may be revised as a consequence of a recent workshop held by the International Dietary Energy Consultative Group (IDECG). Future recommendations may separate the obligatory costs (e.g. by fixed increments) and differences in physical activity (based on PAL values).

Longitudinal Studies of the Energy Costs of Pregnancy

This section summarizes parts of a recent position paper prepared by Prentice *et al.* (1996) for IDECG.

Fat deposition

The increase in maternal fat stores is by far the largest contributor to the energy cost of tissue deposition. It is also the most variable. Although the average increase for a well-nourished woman who has an uncomplicated pregnancy and healthy infant is about 3 kg, a large number of studies have reported ranges of −2 to +8 kg and standard deviations of 2–4 kg. There is also a wide range in fat deposition between different populations, particularly when those from developed and developing countries are compared (**Fig. 1**). Fat is very energy dense and therefore changes in body fat stores have a large impact on the energy costs of pregnancy. A loss of 2 kg saves about 78 MJ (18 600 kcal), while a gain of 8 kg costs about 312 MJ (74 600 kcal). Women most likely to need an energy reserve to help meet the costs of lactation are often those who are least able to deposit spare energy as fat in pregnancy. Conversely, women who store large amounts of fat during pregnancy are least

Table 3 Current recommendations for energy intakes during pregnancy (taken from Prentice *et al.*, 1996)

Recommending body	Trimester(s)	Increment: MJ day^{-1} (kcal day^{-1})	Total for pregnancy: MJ (kcal)	Qualifying comments
FAO/WHO/UNU (1985)	All	1.20 (300)	336 (80 300)	
	All	0.84 (200)	235 (56 150)	For healthy women who reduce activity
UK (1991)	3rd	0.80 (190)	74 (17 000)	Underweight women and those not reducing activity may need more
USA (1989)	2nd and 3rd	1.25 (300)	233 (55 700)	
The Netherlands (1981)	All	0.60 (140)	168 (40 150)	Reduction in physical activity assumed

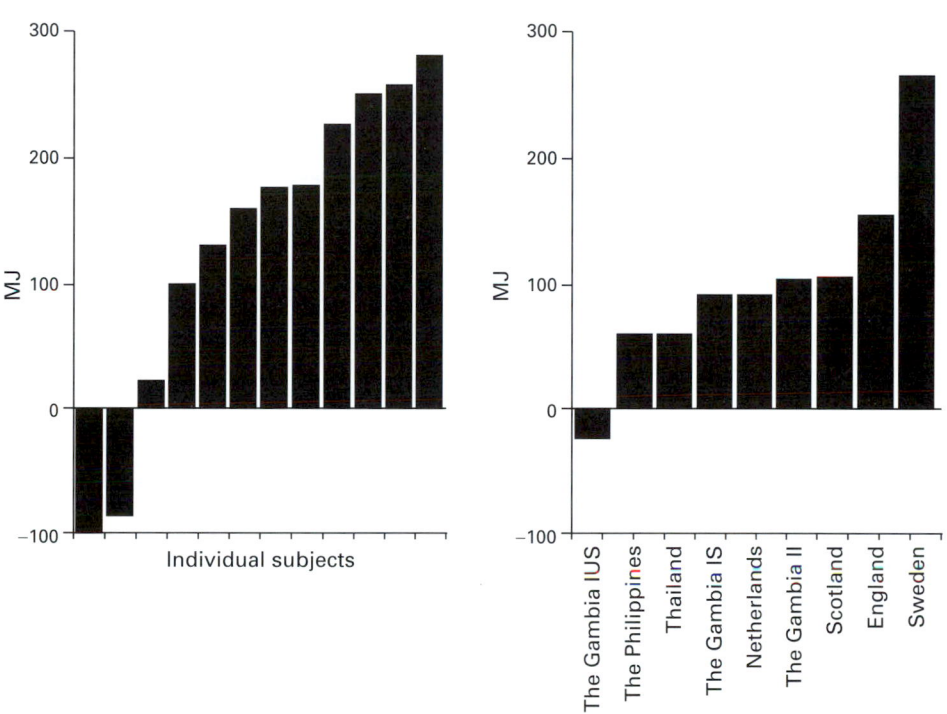

Figure 1 Energy lost or deposited as fat during pregnancy in individual women (left) and in different populations of women (right). U, unsupplemented women; S, supplemented women. (Data from Goldberg *et al.*, 1993 and Poppitt *et al.*, 1994.)

likely to need to use it during lactation. They are often able to increase food intake and/or decrease physical activity instead. Postpartum retention of excess fat has implications for the development of obesity.

Basal metabolic rate

The cumulative increase in basal metabolic rate (BMR) can comprise a large part of the total energy costs of pregnancy. While 150 MJ is a good estimate of the average energy cost of maintenance for a well-nourished woman, there is a very wide range. This has an important influence on the extra daily requirements for individual women. Studies in which BMR

has been measured every 6 weeks from prepregnant to 36 weeks pregnancy have shown very marked differences (**Fig. 2**). In some women there is the expected response to pregnancy – an immediate and progressive increase in BMR. In other women, BMR actually decreases or increases only slightly in the early stages of pregnancy and does not increase substantially until late gestation. In some of these 'energy-sparing' women the early reduction in BMR is sufficient to offset the rise in late gestation. The total net cost of maintenance (calculated by deriving the areas under the curves in Fig. 2) is negative or only very small (**Fig. 3**). Fig. 3 shows data from individual women and illustrates that this between-

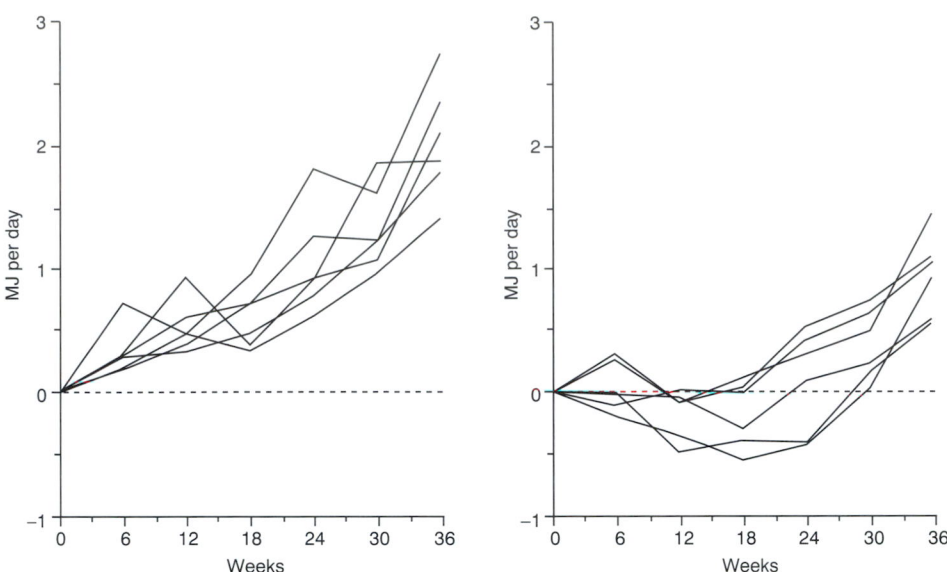

Figure 2 Individual changes in BMR in women measured longitudinally throughout pregnancy. Subjects have been divided according to 'energy-sparing' or 'energy-profligate' responses. (From Goldberg *et al.*, 1993.)

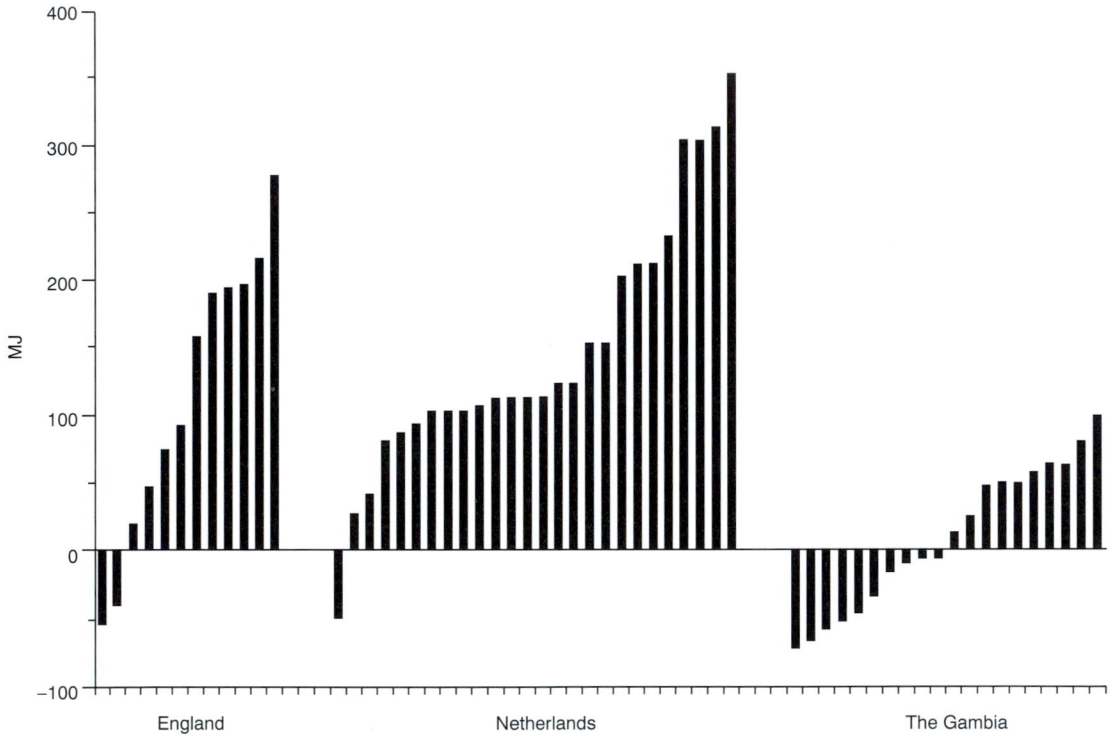

Figure 3 Cumulative costs of BMR in individual women during pregnancy (adapted from Prentice *et al.*, 1996.)

subject variability is found in women from both well-nourished and marginally nourished populations. However, 'energy-sparing' and 'energy-profligate' responses dominate in marginally and well-nourished women, respectively. There is a more than five-fold range between the most 'energy-profligate' and the most 'energy-sparing' woman.

As well as the wide variability in changes in BMR between individual women there are also wide variations between different populations. **Fig. 4** illustrates the *average* changes in BMR using data from over 360 pregnancies in nine studies. The shapes of the curves are similar to those from *individual* subjects in Fig. 2. Well-nourished, affluent women from

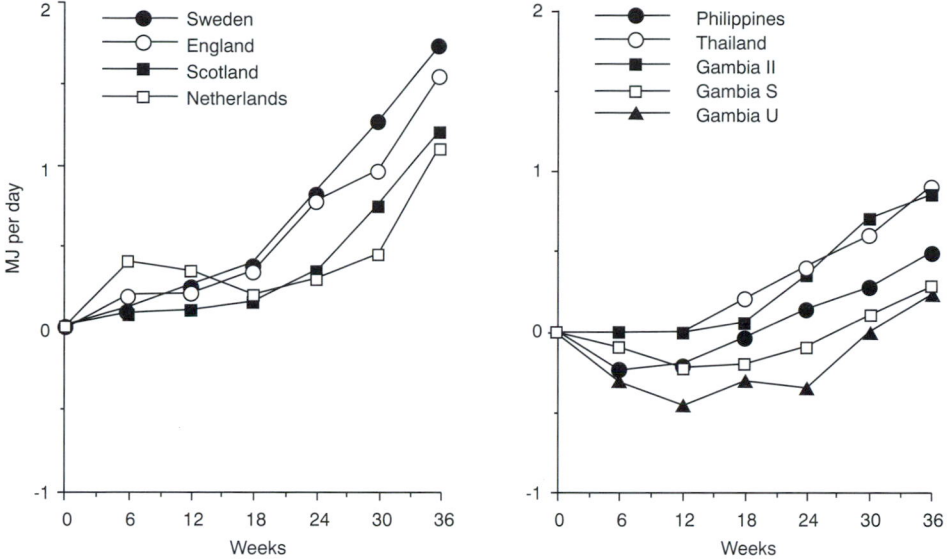

Figure 4   Mean changes in BMR in women from developed and developing countries measured longitudinally throughout pregnancy (adapted from Poppitt *et al.*, 1994.)

developed countries tend to show an energy-profligate increase in BMR. In marginally nourished thinner women from developing countries the increase in BMR is delayed and/or preceded by a fall in early pregnancy. The total maintenance costs of pregnancy in these studies (**Fig. 5**) range from +210 MJ (+50 000 kcal) to −45 MJ (−11 000 kcal)

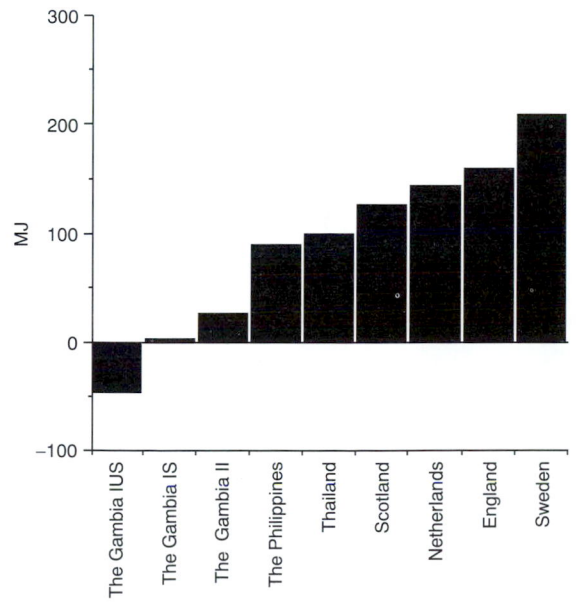

Figure 5   Mean cumulative costs of BMR derived by calculating the areas under the curves in Fig. 4.

Diet-induced thermogenesis

A reduction in diet-induced thermogenesis (DIT) could be a mechanism by which energy is saved during pregnancy. However, when expressed as a proportion of energy intake, DIT remains essentially unaltered and any changes are small and unlikely to be biologically significant.

Energy cost of activities

Results from a number of longitudinal exercise studies have shown that the cost of non-weight-bearing activity changes little until very late pregnancy. From about 35 weeks, the gross costs (which includes changes in BMR) increases by about 11% and net costs by about 6%. The gross and net costs of weight-bearing exercise (treadmill walking and standardized step-testing) remains fairly constant during the first half of pregnancy and then increases progressively by about 15–20% at term.

Behavioural changes in physical activity

It has frequently been assumed that a behavioural reduction in the energy expended on physical activity helps to counteract the increases in expenditure resulting from increased body weight. In some women this leads to saving of energy which largely meets the costs of pregnancy (*See:* **Energy**; Measurement of Energy Intake and Expenditure). However, although only relatively small changes in activity patterns can potentially result in significant energy savings, there is little evidence that this occurs to a large extent. A possible reason for this is that affluent women are habitually so sedentary that there is little scope for further reduction. In contrast, in developing countries habitual levels of physical activity are high and there is therefore more potential for behavioural reductions. However, many women are likely to be unable to reduce their physical activity because of the constraints imposed by a subsistence livelihood.

Between-Country Comparison of the Metabolic Costs of Pregnancy

Fig. 6 illustrates the total metabolic costs of pregnancy (i.e. not including energy expended on physical activity) from the studies illustrated in Figs 1 and 5. The average costs across the different populations range from -30 MJ (-7000 kcal) to 523 MJ (125 000 kcal). These studies have also shown that the amount of prepregnancy body fat is strongly correlated with both the maintenance costs ($r = +0.84$, $P<0.01$) and the total metabolic costs ($r = +0.80$, $P<0.01$) of pregnancy. This flexibility in energy metabolism acts in a protective manner with undernourished women showing significant energy-sparing adaptive strategies which tend to normalize energy balance. Body fat content is one of the measures of

fitness for reproduction; fertility is suppressed in undernourished women. However, future unfavourable conditions cannot be anticipated and pre/early-pregnant fatness may be indicative of overall nutritional status and energy balance during pregnancy. This suggests that the body has some means of detecting energy status and modulating physiological responses. The recent discovery of leptin and its role not only in the regulation of adipose tissue, appetite and metabolic rate, but also in reproductive function, add support to this hypothesis.

Individual Variability in the Total Energy Costs of Pregnancy

Because of the marked differences between individuals in the different components of the energy costs of pregnancy (changes in BMR, body fat, energy expended on physical activity), the total energy costs, and therefore energy requirements, are also very variable. This is illustrated in **Fig. 7** from studies in well-nourished women. The total extra energy costs of pregnancy averaged 418 MJ (100 000 kcal), considerably higher than the estimates in Table 3, and with a huge range from 34 to 1200 MJ (8000 to 287 000 kcal). These values are probably representative of many women in developed countries. They

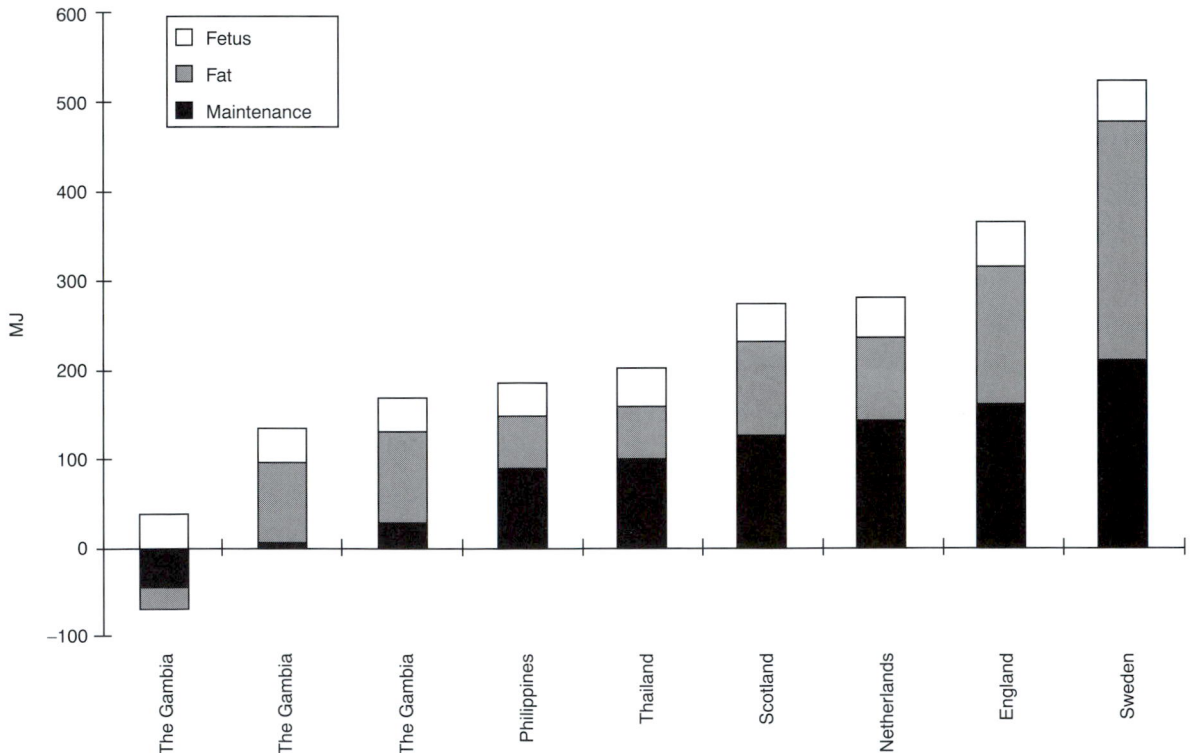

Figure 6 Total metabolic costs of pregnancy in studies illustrated in Figs 1 and 5 and including energy deposited as products of conception (data from Poppitt *et al.*, 1994). Note these costs do not include energy expended on physical activity.

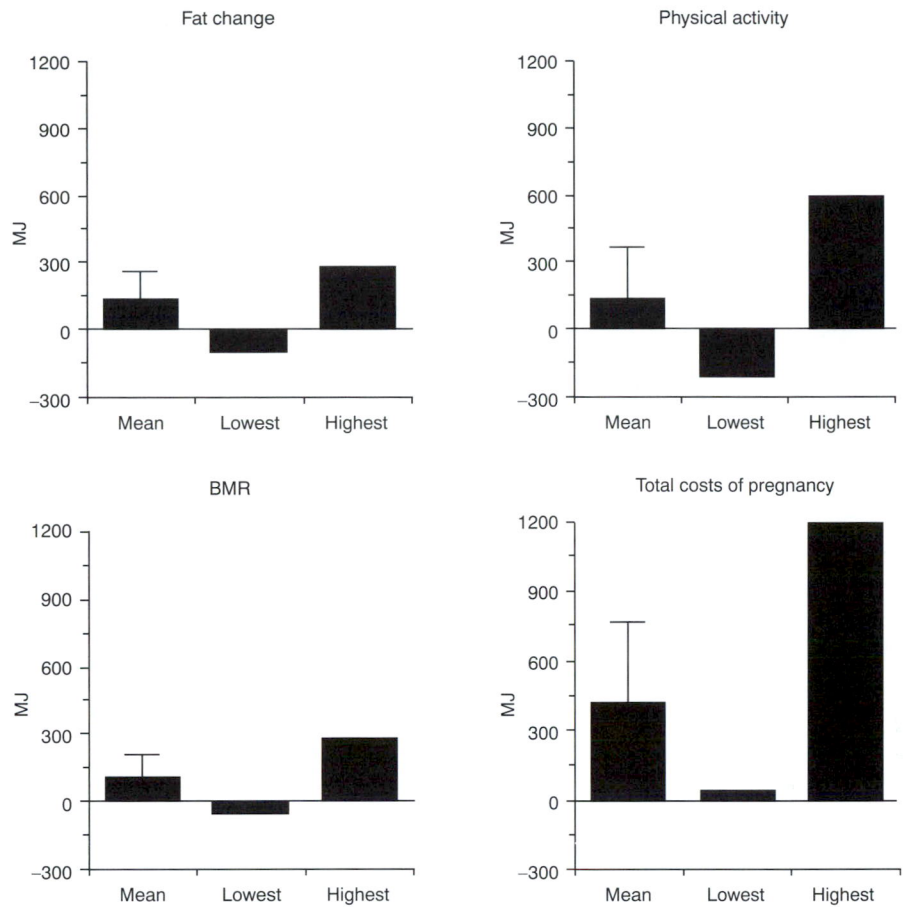

Figure 7 Components of the energy costs of pregnancy and total energy costs of pregnancy (including products of conception) in 12 well-nourished women measured longitudinally throughout pregnancy from a prepregnant baseline. Physical activity was assessed by doubly labelled water measurements of total energy expenditure (TEE-BMR). Means and individual ranges are illustrated. Error bars are SD. (Data from Goldberg *et al.*, 1993.)

show that it is impossible to prescribe energy intakes for individual women since it cannot be predicted how they will respond metabolically (BMR, fat) or behaviourally (physical activity, food intake) to pregnancy. Eating to appetite unless extremes of weight gain occur is the most appropriate advice.

Implications of Energy-Sparing Adaptations for Mother and Infant

Human energy metabolism is particularly adaptable during pregnancy with pre/early-pregnancy body 'fatness' appearing to be a major determinant. The adaptive strategies which maintain energy balance seem to be a mechanism which may work to protect fetal growth under harsh nutritional conditions. However, it must not be assumed that pregnant women will have energy-sparing alterations in metabolism and/or physical activity decreases. Any adaptations that do occur should not be over interpreted as suggesting that pregnant women are not

nutritionally at-risk. The possible long-term detrimental effects must also be considered. The biochemical and physiological processes that are downregulated in the mother to cause the suppression in BMR are unknown and there might be long-term consequences to her health.

The associations between maintenance needs, pregnancy weight gain and prepregnant fatness indicate that a target weight gain of 12.5 kg will be associated with maintenance costs of about 160 MJ (38 000 kcal). Although individual women or populations may have lower maintenance requirements, these may be associated with inadequate weight gain and low-birthweight infants. Birthweight is a much larger percentage of total weight gain in undernourished mothers who struggle to achieve a satisfactory outcome of pregnancy. A major determinant of birthweight is maternal weight gain, and the single most important determinant of infant survival is birthweight. Finally, although birthweight is *relatively* well preserved at different planes of nutrition, weight alone is an inadequate measure of a baby's overall condition at birth. Even subtle nutritional influences on the fetal environment might have long-term consequences.

See also: **Adaptation**: Overview of Adaptive Responses to Malnutrition. **Adipose Tissue**: Structure, Function and Metabolism of Adipose Tissue. **Body Composition**: Determination and Physiological Significance. **Energy**: Energy Requirements; Energy Balance; Measurement of Energy Intake and Expenditure. **Fertility**: Body Fat, Menarche and Fertility. **Fetal Origins of Disease**: Fetal Development and Later Disease. **Nutrient Requirements**: International Perspectives. **Obesity**: Definition, Aetiology and Assessment. **Pregnancy**: Nutrient Requirements; Appropriate Maternal Weight Gain; Safe Diet for Pregnancy. **Seasonality**: Nutritional Implications. **Weight Management**: Weight Maintenance; Weight Cycling.

Further Reading

Barash IA, Cheung CC, Weigle DS, Ren H, Kabigting EB, Kuijper JL, Clifton DK and Steiner RA (1996) Leptin is a metabolic signal to the reproductive system. *Endocrinology* **137**:3144–3147.

Forsum E, Sadurskis A and Wager J (1988) Resting metabolic rate and body composition of healthy Swedish women during pregnancy. *American Journal of Clinical Nutrition* **47**:942–947.

Goldberg GR, Prentice AM, Coward WA, Murgatroyd PR, Davies HL, Wensing C, Black AE, Harding M and Sawyer M (1993) Longitudinal assessment of energy expenditure in pregnancy by the doubly-labelled water method. *American Journal of Clinical Nutrition* **57**:494–505.

Goldberg GR (1997) Reproduction: a global nutritional challenge. *Proceedings of the Nutrition Society* **56**:319–333.

Hytten FE (1991). Nutrition weight gain in pregnancy. In: Hytten F and Chamberlain G (eds) *Clinical Physiology in Obstetrics*, 2nd edn, chaps 6, 7. Oxford: Blackwell Scientific Publications.

IDECG (1996) Energy and protein requirements. Proceedings of an IDECG Workshop, Scrimshaw NS, Waterlow JC and Schurch B (eds). *European Journal of Clinical Nutrition* **50** (supplement 1):S1–S197.

Lawrence M, Lawrence F, Coward WA, Cole TJ and Whitehead RG (1987) Energy requirements of pregnancy in the Gambia. *Lancet* **ii**:1072–1076.

Poppitt SD, Prentice AM, Goldberg GR and Whitehead RG (1994) Energy-sparing strategies to protect human fetal growth. *American Journal of Obstetrics and Gynecology* **171**:118–125.

Poppitt SD, Prentice AM, Jequier E, Schutz Y and Whitehead RG (1993) Evidence of energy-sparing in Gambian women during pregnancy: a longitudinal study using whole-body calorimetry. *American Journal of Clinical Nutrition* **57**:353–364.

Prentice AM, Goldberg GR, Davies HL, Murgatroyd PR and Scott W (1989) Energy-sparing adaptations in human pregnancy assessed by whole-body calorimetry. *British Journal of Nutrition* **62**:5–22.

Prentice AM, Spaaij CJK, Goldberg GR, Poppitt SD, van Raaij JMA, Totton M, Swann D and Black AE (1996) Energy requirements of pregnant and lactating women. *European Journal of Clinical Nutrition* **50** (supplement 1):S82–S111.

Prentice AM and Whitehead RG (1987) The energetics of human reproduction. *Symposia of the Zoological Society of London* **57**:275–304.

Thongprasert K, Tanphaichitre V, Valyasevi A, Kittigool J and Durnin JVGA (1987) Energy requirements of pregnancy in rural Thailand. *Lancet* **ii**:1010–1012.

Tuazon MA, van Raaij JMA, Hautvast JGAV and Barba CVC (1987) Energy requirements of pregnancy in The Philippines. *Lancet* **ii**:1129–1130.

van Raaij JMA, Vermaat-Miedema SH, Schonk CM, Peek MEM and Hautvast JGAJ (1987) Energy requirements of pregnancy in The Netherlands. *Lancet* **ii**:953–955.

Nutrient Requirements

S Greeley, North Dakota State University, Fargo, North Dakota, USA

J C King, Western Human Nutrition Research Center and University of California, Berkeley and Davis, San Francisco, California, USA

Dietary guidance to pregnant women in different parts of the world varies (often widely) in the amounts and the specifics of the recommended nutrients. This 'diversity' of recommendation is more easily understood if one examines the context in which guidelines are proposed. Dietary advice must consider human biological diversity (genetic variation and physiological adaptation) and must account for environmental factors that are present. The chemistry of foods may alter the bioavailability of specific nutrients, reflecting the complex biochemical interaction between plants and humans. Additionally, 'usual dietary intakes' are likely to differ between populations as influenced by the culture (food acceptability, traditions, preferences), food security (accessibility), the economy (food-purchasing power), and so on. There will be inevitable differences in interpretation of available scientific data and clinical findings, based on the education, experience and beliefs of those making the recommendations. Other differences emerge from the specific charge given to the expert consultation group, and that mandate will focus the deliberations and recommendations of the committee.

The intended uses of the nutrient requirements flow logically from the mandate and the deliberative process. Canadian Nutrition Recommendations are intended to 'form the basis for advice to the public ... used by those responsible for planning and providing the national food supply and making appropriate foods available ... without any general need of supplements'.

The European Community Food Committee was charged 'to advise the European establishment of recommended dietary allowances for a number of purposes, including nutrition labeling, community programmes on research and nutrition, and to make recommendations'.

The US Recommended Dietary Allowance (RDA) is applied in a variety of settings. The 1989 RDAs (10th edn) are used to 'plan and procure food supplies, to interpret food consumption records, as guidelines for food assistance and education programs, to evaluate the national food supply, and to develop new foods'. Revisions of the 1989 RDAs are under consideration and 'a plan for the next RDAs will need to have more flexibility to address multiple uses' (*How Should the Recommended Dietary Allowances be Revised?*, 1994).

A 1996 WHO expert Consultation Group (*Trace Elements in Human Nutrition and Health*) stated that 'the final ... aim is to provide scientists and national authorities worldwide with an up-to-date and authoritative review ...'. The WHO/FAO guidelines and standards allow planners to design intervention studies, to compare dietary intakes, to consider relevant physiological and environmental variables, and to inform food manufacturers of community needs.

In summary, published reports can help the reader to understand factors which influence nutrient intake and thus are useful in assorted official and informal settings. Each document will reflect (to a lesser or greater degree) the biological, chemical, economic, social and educational characteristics of the people and the institutions being served.

This article will introduce the reader to six sources that deal with human pregnancy requirements for protein, fatty acids, vitamins, minerals and dietary fibre. Specifically, we will discuss nutrient requirements during pregnancy based on the following reports: Canada (1990), *Recommended Nutrient Intakes (RNI)*; European Community (1993), *Population Reference Intakes (PRI)*; UK (1991), *Reference Nutrient Intakes (RNI)*; USA (1989), *Recommended Dietary Allowances (1989)*; and World Health Organization (1985 and 1996), *Safe Level of Intake for Protein and Vitamins, Normative Requirement for Trace Elements*. The interested

reader is referred to those original documents for more detail.

Protein, Essential Fatty Acids and Dietary Fibre

Approximately 925 g protein are deposited in a woman gaining 12.5 kg during pregnancy and delivering a 3.3 kg infant. However, the rate of deposition is not constant; approximately 0.64, 1.84, 4.76 and 6.10 g protein are gained in the first, second, third and fourth quarters of pregnancy, respectively. These values served as the basis of the recommendations by the WHO, US and Canadian Panels (**Table 1**). The rates of tissue protein deposition have been adjusted for the efficiency with which dietary protein is converted to tissue and for the need to maintain the added lean tissue in pregnancy. The uncertainty about these adjustments contributes to the variance in protein recommendations across the five panels. The UK Panel recommends the lowest total protein intake, 51 g per day; the recommendation for a 60 kg woman by the EC Panel and the WHO Committee is 55 g per day. The US recommends 60 g per day and the Canadians 74 g per day in the third trimester. The Canadian Panel recommended that four times as much protein be added to the diet of a pregnant woman as the UK Panel.

The essential fatty acids are linoleic acid (C18:2 n-6) and α-linolenic acid (C18:3 n-3). Several longer-chain fatty acids that have physiological functions, for example arachidonic acid (C20:4 n-6), are synthesized to a limited extent in the tissues and, therefore, are not strictly essential fatty acids. A deficiency of linoleic acid has been seen in humans when intake is less than 1–2% of the total energy or less than 2–5 g per day of linoleic acid. The UK and EC Panels established dietary standards for linoleic acid of 1.0% and 2% of the total energy intake, respectively (Table 1). The Canadian Panel was the only group to recommend an incremental intake of linoleic acid in pregnancy (0.3 g per day in the first trimester and 0.9 g per day in the second and third). A specific deficiency of α-linolenic acid has not been demonstrated and the recommended intake is about 0.2–0.5% of the energy, or about 1–1.5 g per day. No recommended intakes were established by the US and WHO Panels for essential fatty acids.

Recommended intakes for dietary fibre have not been established.

Fat-soluble Vitamins

Vitamin A is required for cellular differentiation, growth and development of the fetus. A total intake

Table 1 Recommended intakes of protein, unsaturated fatty acids and dietary fibre

Panel	Trimester	Protein (g per day)	Fatty acids (g per day) n-3	n-6	Fibre
Canada, 1990 (RNI)	1	50 + 5	1.2 + 0.05	7 + 0.3	'not possible to determine an RNI'
	2	50 + 15	1.2 + 0.16	7 + 0.9	
	3	50 + 24	1.2 + 0.16	7 + 0.9	
		(0.75 g per kg per day)			
			% of total energy		
EC[a] (PRI)	1	+10	0.5	2	No specific fibre recommendation for pregnancy
	2	+10	0.5	2	
	3	+10	0.5	2	
UK[b] (RNI)	1	45 + 6	0.2	1	No specific fibre recommendation for pregnancy
	2	45 + 6	0.2	1	
	3	45 + 6	0.2	1	
US[c] (RDA)	1	50 + 10	Not established		No specific fibre recommendation for pregnancy
	2	50 + 10	Not established		
	3	50 + 10	Not established		
		(0.75 g per kg per day)			
WHO[d]	1	+1.2			No specific fibre recommendation for pregnancy
	2	+6.1			
	3	+10.7			

[a]European Community (1993) *Population Reference Intake*.
[b](1991) *Reference Nutrient Intake*.
[c](1989) *Recommended Dietary Allowance*.
[d]World Health Organization (1985).

of 700 or 800 retinol equivalents (1 retinol equivalent = 1 μg retinol or 6 μg β-carotene) is recommended for pregnancy by the five panels (**Table 2**). The US and Canadian panels did not recommend an additional increment for pregnancy over the standard for nonpregnant women; the other groups recommended an additional 100 retinol equivalents. Fetal accretion of vitamin A during the third trimester represents a small proportion of maternal liver stores of vitamin A. Accretion of 200 μg per day by the fetus during the last trimester is equivalent to only 9% of the total maternal stores if the maternal liver contains 100 μg vitamin A g^{-1}. The US and Canadian Panels concluded that most women in those countries could provide the additional increment of vitamin A from hepatic reserves. Studies of maternal vitamin A supplementation had little impact on fetal liver vitamin A concentrations.

Retinol is teratogenic. Intakes above 3300 μg per

day have been associated with birth defects. The UK Panel advised pregnant women not to take supplements containing vitamin A unless prescribed by a doctor or health clinic and not to eat liver or products made from it since animal livers can contain on average 13 000–40 000 μg per 100 g, depending on the species.

It has not been determined whether there is an increased need for dietary vitamin D during pregnancy. The Canadian Panel recommended an additional 2.5 μg per day, bringing the total to 5.0 μg per day. The US and UK Panels recommended a total intake of 10 μg per day, or 400 IU. Since vitamin D ensures an adequate absorption of calcium, maternal vitamin D status may improve fetal calcium accretion. In Scotland, infants of women not taking vitamin D supplements had a higher incidence of hypocalcaemia, hyperparathyroidism, and a defect of dental enamel. Dietary intake of vitamin D may be

Table 2 Recommended intakes of fat-soluble vitamins during pregnancy

Panel	Trimester	Vitamin A (RE[a])	Vitamin D (μg)	Vitamin E (mg α-TE[b])	Vitamin K (μg)
Canada	1	800	2.5 + 2.5	7.2 + 2	No RNI
	2	800	2.5 + 2.5	7.2 + 2	No RNI
	3	800	2.5 + 2.5	7.2 + 2	No RNI
EC	1	700	No PRI	No PRI	No PRI
	2	700	No PRI	No PRI	No PRI
	3	700	No PRI	No PRI	No PRI
UK	1	700	10	No RNI	No RNI
	2	700	10	No RNI	No RNI
	3	700	10	No RNI	No RNI
US	1	800	10	10	65
	2	800	10	10	65
	3	800	10	10	65
WHO	1	600			
	2	600			
	3	600			

[a]Retinol equivalents.
[b]Alpha-tocopherol.

more critical in countries like Scotland where exposure to sunlight is more limited.

Vitamin E is an antioxidant that prevents the oxidation of unsaturated fatty acids by trapping peroxyl free radicals. Alpha-tocopherol is the most active form of vitamin E. Three other tocopherols exist in nature – β-, γ- and δ-tocopherol. Only the Canadian and US Panels made a recommendation for vitamin E intake during pregnancy. The Canadian and US Panels recommended an additional 2.0 mg α-tocopherol for a total intake of 9.2 and 10 mg, respectively. The increased rate of metabolism during pregnancy may enhance the production of free radicals and increase vitamin E needs. Maternal circulating tocopherol concentrations rise during pregnancy, in conjunction with rising plasma lipid levels, making more tocopherol available to the fetus.

Data on the dietary requirement for vitamin K are limited. The UK Panel suggested that all adults consume 1 μg per kg per day and made no specific recommendation for pregnancy. The US Panel recommended 65 μg per day, or about 1 μg per kg per day, for nonpregnant, pregnant and lactating women. The usual dietary intake of vitamin K in the US generally exceeds that standard.

Water-soluble Vitamins

All four national panels recommended an additional 10 mg of ascorbic acid (**Table 3**) during pregnancy. If the incremental fetal need for ascorbic acid is equivalent to the requirement per unit of body weight in adults, then the total need of the fetus near term is small, about 3–4 mg per day. Actual requirements are assumed to be higher, however, because fetal turnover rates of ascorbic acid are probably greater than those of adults. To account for those higher rates of turnover and to maintain maternal body pools, 10 mg of additional ascorbic acid are recommended. Since the total recommended daily intake of ascorbic acid for nonpregnant women varied two-fold, from 30 mg by the Canadian Panel to 60 mg by the US Panel, the total daily intake recommended during pregnancy ranged from 40 to 70 mg.

Studies of the urinary excretion of thiamin and erythrocyte transketolase activities show that the requirement for thiamin increases during pregnancy (Table 3). The US Panel recommended an additional 0.4 mg per day to accommodate fetal growth, changes in maternal thiamin utilization and increased energy intakes. The recommendations of the other panels were more modest with either an additional 0.1 mg per day suggested or no change. The EC Panel recommended 100 μg MJ^{-1} (239 kcal equals 1 MJ). The estimated energy requirement for a 65 kg woman with light physical activity is 10.8 MJ, bringing her total daily recommended thiamin intake to approximately 1.0 mg. All of the Panels agreed that thiamin requirements are related to energy metabolism, with need ranging from 95 to 120 μg MJ^{-1} (0.4 to 0.5 mg per 1000 kcal).

The Panels were consistent in their conclusion that the extra need for riboflavin placed on the pregnant mother by the fetus is approximately 0.3 mg per day (Table 3). As pregnancy progresses, urinary riboflavin excretion falls, but the erythrocyte glutathione reductase activity ratio rises, indicating an increased need for riboflavin for that function.

Table 3 Recommended intakes of water-soluble vitamins during pregnancy

Panel	Trimester	Ascorbic acid (mg)	Thiamin (mg)	Riboflavin (mg)	Niacin (NE[a])	Vitamin B_6 (mg per day)	Folate (μg per day)	Vitamin B_{12} (μg per day)
Canada	1	30 + 0	0.8 + 0.1	1.1 + 0.1	15 + 1	15 μg per g protein	180 + 200	1 + 0.2
	2	30 + 10	0.8 + 0.1	1.1 + 0.3	15 + 2	15 μg per g protein	180 + 200	1 + 0.2
	3	30 + 10	0.8 + 0.1	1.1 + 0.3	15 + 2	15 μg per g protein	180 + 200	1 + 0.2
EC	1	45 + 10	100 μg MJ^{-1}	1.3 + 0.3	1.6 μg MJ^{-1}	15 μg per g protein	200 + 200	1.4 + 0.2
	2	45 + 10	100 μg MJ^{-1}	1.3 + 0.3	1.6 μg MJ^{-1}	15 μg per g protein	200 + 200	1.4 + 0.2
	3	45 + 10	100 μg MJ^{-1}	1.3 + 0.3	1.6 μg MJ^{-1}	15 μg per g protein	200 + 200	1.4 + 0.2
UK	1	40 + 10	0.8	1.1 + 0.3	13	1.2	200 + 100	1.5
	2	40 + 10	0.8	1.1 + 0.3	13	1.2	200 + 100	1.5
	3	40 + 10	0.8 + 0.1	1.1 + 0.3	13	1.2	200 + 100	1.5
US	1	60 + 10	1.1 + 0.4	1.3 + 0.3	15 + 2	1.6 + 0.6	180 + 220	2 + 0.2
	2	60 + 10	1.1 + 0.4	1.3 + 0.3	15 + 2	1.6 + 0.6	180 + 220	2 + 0.2
	3	60 + 10	1.1 + 0.4	1.3 + 0.3	15 + 2	1.6 + 0.6	180 + 220	2 + 0.2
WHO	1						370–470	1.4
	2						370–470	1.4
	3						370–470	1.4

[a]NE = niacin equivalent.

Conclusions regarding the dietary need for niacin (Table 3) varied widely among the five Panels reviewed. The UK group and the EC Panel concluded that the additional need for niacin would be met by the increased conversion of tryptophan to niacin during pregnancy, and that an increased intake of niacin was unnecessary. The US Panel agreed that the normal physiological adjustments of pregnancy cause an increase in the ability to form niacin from tryptophan, but recommended an additional 2 niacin equivalents because of the increased energy requirements. (One niacin equivalent equals 1 mg niacin or 60 mg tryptophan.) The EC Panel expressed the recommendation as 1.6 μg MJ^{-1}, which is equivalent to about 17 NE. Recommended total intakes of niacin are either 13 (UK) or 17 NE per day.

All of the Panels concluded that the dietary requirement for vitamin B_6 is related to protein intakes. The Canadian, EC and UK Panels used a conversion factor of 15 μg vitamin B_6 per g protein; the US Panel used a conversion factor of 16 μg per g protein. Based on the recommended increases in dietary protein during pregnancy, the Canadian and EC Panels advise an additional daily intake of 0.36 and 0.15 mg vitamin B_6, respectively (Table 3). The US recommended an additional 0.6 mg per day, whereas the UK concluded that no increase in vitamin B_6 is necessary. Pregnant women tend to have lower levels of vitamin B_6 in the plasma as well as decreased alanine aminotransferase activity compared with nonpregnant women. It is unknown if these changes represent an insufficient supply of dietary vitamin B_6 or if they are simply the normal physiological changes of pregnancy.

Folate requirements increase in late pregnancy to support cell division during this period of rapid growth. Prior to the widespread use of supplemental folate, bone marrow megaloblastosis was prevalent even in otherwise well-nourished populations. An additional 100 or 200 μg of folate are recommended daily for the pregnant woman; the recommended total intakes range from 300 (UK) to 400 μg (Canada, EC and US) (Table 3). The UK Panel concluded that 100 μg per day will maintain plasma and red cell folate levels at or above those of nonpregnant women; the US Panel stated that the equivalent of 200 μg of pteroylglutamic acid (PGA) will prevent folate deficiency in pregnancy among women who start with moderate folate stores. On the basis of a 50% food folate absorption, and additional 200 μg per day was recommended. The WHO group recommends a supplement of 200–300 μg per day. Since 170 μg per day is recommended for the nonpregnant woman, the total intake recommended for pregnancy is 370–470 μg per day.

The incremental need for vitamin B_{12} has been estimated from the vitamin B_{12} content of stillborn infants from normally nourished mothers. This need is approximately 0.1–0.2 μg per day. Normally, maternal body stores are sufficient to provide this additional demand, but all of the Panels except the UK group recommended an additional daily intake of vitamin B_{12} (Table 3). The WHO Panel recommended an additional 0.4 μg per day; the other Panels advised 0.2 μg per day.

Minerals and Electrolytes

The newborn contains about 30 g of calcium, most of which is deposited during the third trimester, leading to a daily deposition of 200–250 mg. Although the rate of calcium absorption increases during pregnancy, the US and Canadian Panels felt that it is prudent to increase the calcium intake during gestation by either 400 or 500 mg per day (**Table 4**). The UK and EC Panels concluded that mobilization of maternal calcium depots will meet the needs for fetal growth. An exception may be the special need for pregnant adolescents where there is an increased calcium demand for both fetal and maternal growth.

The precise requirement for dietary phosphorus is unknown. The EC, UK and US Panels recommended equivalent amounts of dietary calcium and phosphorus and concluded that neither inadequate nor excessive intakes of phosphorus are a problem. The Canadian Panel stated that calcium and phosphorus intakes should be 'in parallel'; they recommended a total of 1300 mg calcium and 1050 mg phosphorus during gestation (Table 4).

A healthy full-term infant contains about 1 g magnesium at birth; most of this is acquired during the last two trimesters at a rate of approximately 6 mg per day. The US Panel estimated an incremental need of 20 mg per day to cover fetal and maternal needs. This value was doubled to 40 mg per day to allow for 50% absorption of dietary magnesium. A total daily intake of 320 mg was recommended. The Canadian and UK Panels also made magnesium recommendations for pregnancy. The UK Panel concluded that the physiological adaptations during pregnancy will meet additional fetal and maternal needs; the Canadians recommended an additional 15 mg per day. The EC Panel recommended that magnesium intakes range from 150 to 300 mg per day.

Recommended iron intakes varied widely among these five groups. The US Panel recommended that iron intake be doubled from 15 to 30 mg per day (Table 4). The UK Panel concluded that 'ideally all women of childbearing age should have sufficient stores to cope with the metabolic demands made by pregnancy . . . However, when iron stores are inappropriately low . . ., supplementation with Fe may be necessary'. A total of 14.5 mg iron per day was recommended for all trimesters. The WHO committee suggested nearly an 8-fold increase in iron between the first and third trimesters in order to provide the total incremental need from diet alone. All Panels agreed that except for well-nourished women who begin pregnancy with adequate iron stores, the increased iron requirement for pregnancy cannot be met by habitual diet and supplemental iron is necessary.

The US and Canadian Panels recommend a total of 15 mg zinc per day throughout pregnancy whereas the EC and UK Panels only recommend 7 mg per day. The WHO Committee suggested that a pregnant woman in the third trimester consume 13.3 mg zinc per day; this is about twice that recommended for a nonpregnant woman (6.5 mg per day). All groups agreed that the need for absorbed zinc rises in parallel with fetal growth rates, but the UK and EC Panels assume that the metabolic adaptations in healthy pregnant women ensures an adequate transfer of zinc to the fetus, obviating any need for a change in dietary zinc. The other groups concluded that an increase in dietary zinc may be necessary since there is no evidence of physiological adaptations in zinc utilization among pregnant women.

An increment of 25 μg iodine per day was recommended by the US and Canadian Panels for a total intake of 175 and 185 μg per day, respectively. The WHO Panel recommended 200 μg per day whereas the EC and UK Panels felt than no increment was necessary for pregnancy (Table 4).

The US Panel recommended an increment of 10 μg selenium per day based on the assumption that a total of 1.25 mg selenium is retained during pregnancy, or about 5 μg per day. A value of 6.5 μg per day was used to allow for variability. If about 80% of the dietary selenium is absorbed, the dietary need is 10 μg per day. The WHO Committee used a similar factorial approach and concluded that an additional 9 μg selenium per day should be consumed. The UK and EC Panels agreed that 'since adaptive changes in the metabolism of Se occur during pregnancy, no advantage is seen in recommending extra Se at this time'. The Canadian Panel felt that there was insufficient evidence to recommend a dietary allowance for selenium.

None of the Panels recommended additional copper for pregnant women. The additional need for copper is estimated to be about 21 mg; it is assumed that this need is met by small increases in copper absorption. Recommended total daily intakes of copper range from 1.1 to 3.0 mg.

See also: **Ascorbic Acid**: Physiology, Dietary Sources and Requirements. **Calcium**: Physiology. **Carotenoids**: Chemistry, Sources and Physiology. **Cholecalciferol and Ergocalciferol**: Rickets and Osteomalacia. **Copper**: Physiology, Dietary Sources and Requirements. **Dietary Fibre (Fiber)**: Physiological Effects and Effects on Absorption. **Fatty Acids**: Metabolism; Health Effects of Saturated Fatty Acids; Health Effects of Monounsaturated Fatty Acids; Health Effects of n-6 Polyunsaturated Fatty

Table 4 Recommended daily intakes of minerals and electrolytes during pregnancy

Panel	Trimester	Calcium (mg)	Phosphorus (mg)	Magnesium (mg)	Sodium (mg)	Potassium (mg)	Iron (mg)	Zinc (mg)	Iodine (µg)	Selenium (µg)	Copper (mg)
Canada	1	800 + 500	850 + 200	200 + 15	NA	NA	13 + 0	9 + 6	160 + 25	NA	NA
	2	800 + 500	850 + 200	200 + 15	NA	NA	13 + 5	9 + 6	160 + 25	NA	NA
	3	800 + 500	850 + 200	200 + 15	NA	NA	13 + 10	9 + 6	160 + 25	NA	NA
EC	1	700	550	150–300	NA	3100	20 + sup	7	130	55	1.1
	2	700	550	150–300	NA	3100	20 + sup	7	130	55	1.1
	3	700	550	150–300	NA	3100	20 + sup	7	130	55	1.1
UK	1	700	550	270	1600	3500	14.5	7	140	60	1.2
	2	700	550	270	1600	3500	14.5	7	140	60	1.2
	3	700	550	270	1600	3500	14.5	7	140	60	1.2
US	1	800 + 400	800 + 400	280 + 40	NA	NA	15 + 15	12 + 3	150 + 25	55 + 10	1.5–3.0
	2	800 + 400	800 + 400	280 + 40	NA	NA	15 + 15	12 + 3	150 + 25	55 + 10	1.5–3.0
	3	800 + 400	800 + 400	280 + 40	NA	NA	15 + 15	12 + 3	150 + 25	55 + 10	1.5–3.0
WHO	1						8[a]	7.3[b]	200	30 + 9	1.15
	2						44	9.3	200	30 + 9	1.15
	3						63	13.3	200	30 + 9	1.15

[a]Based on a 10% bioavailability of dietary iron.
[b]Moderate availability, normative recommendation.

Acids; Health Effects of n-3 Polyunsaturated Fatty Acids; Health Effects of *trans* Fatty Acids. **Folic Acid**: Physiology, Dietary Sources and Requirements. **Iodine**: Physiology, Dietary Sources and Requirements. **Iron**: Physiology, Dietary Sources and Requirements. **Magnesium**: Physiology, Dietary Sources and Requirements. **Niacin**: Physiology, Dietary Sources and Requirements. **Phosphorus**: Physiology, Dietary Sources and Requirements. **Pregnancy**: Energy Requirements and Metabolic Adaptations; Appropriate Maternal Weight Gain; Safe Diet for Pregnancy. **Protein**: Requirements and Role in Diet. **Retinol**: Hypovitaminosis A. **Riboflavin**: Physiology. **Selenium**: Physiology, Dietary Sources and Requirements. **Thiamin**: Physiology. **Tocopherols**: Physiology. **Vitamin B$_6$**: Physiology. **Vitamin K**: Physiology. **Zinc**: Physiology.

Further Reading

Food and Nutrition Board, Institute of Medicine, National Academy of Sciences (1989) *Recommended Dietary Allowances*, 10th edn. Washington, DC: National Academy Press.

Panel on Dietary Reference Values of the Committee on Medical Aspects of Food Policy (1991) *Dietary Reference Values for Food Energy and Nutrients for the United Kingdom*. London: HMSO.

Report of a Joint FAO/WHO Expert Consultation (1988) *Requirements of Vitamin A, Iron, Folate and Vitamin B$_{12}$* FAO Food and Nutrition Series no. 23. Rome: FAO.

Report of a Joint FAO/WHO/UNU Expert Consultation (1985) *Energy and Protein Requirements*, World Health Organization Technical Report Series no. 724. Geneva: World Health Organization.

Report of the Scientific Review Committee, Minister of National Health and Welfare (1990) *Nutrition Recommendations*. Ottawa: Canadian Government Printing Centre.

Reports of the Scientific Committee for Food (1993) *Nutrient and Energy Intakes for the European Community*. Luxembourg: Commission of the European Communities.

World Health Organization (1996) *Trace Elements in Human Nutrition and Health*. Geneva: World Health Organization.

Appropriate Maternal Weight Gain

L Allen, Department of Nutrition, University of California, Davis, California, USA

Since the 1950s there have been dramatic changes in the recommendations for optimal maternal weight gain during pregnancy. In the past it was thought to be necessary to restrict the diet of many pregnant women so as to reduce the perceived risks of higher weight gains. The fetus was thought to be relatively unaffected by this advice. In contrast, the current recommendations in the USA are based on actual weight changes in pregnancy that are compatible with a healthy pregnancy outcome. Because several maternal factors influence the amount of weight gained in pregnancy, these factors have to be taken into consideration when basing recommendations on actual weight gain. The result has been the development of more realistic weight gain guidelines that are based to some extent on the characteristics of the mother. However, there is still much to be learned about the determinants of, and variability in, energy requirements and balance of pregnant women.

Pregnancy Weight Gain Recommendations

In 1970 the National Academy of Sciences (NAS) published guidelines for weight gain during pregnancy in their report 'Maternal Nutrition and the Course of Pregnancy'. The recommended pregnancy gain was 10.9 kg (24 lb), with a range of 9.1–11.4 kg (10–25 lb). The report advised health-care providers and pregnant women not to restrict weight gain – a practice that had been fairly widespread during the previous decade in order to reduce the perceived risks of labour complications, pre-eclampsia and excess weight retention postpartum. In fact many obstetricians had been recommending gains of only 6.8–9.1 kg (15–20 lb).

Even with the more generous recommendations set in 1970, by the 1980s it had become clear that average gains of women in the USA far exceeded these guidelines. An analysis of data from the National Natality Survey in 1980 showed the average pregnancy weight gain to be 13.2 kg (29 lb), and the National Maternal Infant Health Survey in 1988 showed that the average had increased to 14.5 kg (32 lb). The range of gain was very wide, from no gain at all to over 34.1 kg (75 lb).

Based on this realization, in 1990 the weight gain recommendations were revised completely by the Institute of Medicine (IOM) of the National Academy of Sciences. Existing data from a national survey were analysed to determine the weight gain that was compatible with a normal pregnancy outcome. The latter was defined as having a full-term infant of normal birthweight and no pregnancy or delivery complications. It became apparent from these analyses that maternal weight-for-height at conception, expressed as body mass index (BMI: weight in kg

Table 1 Recommendations for pregnancy weight gain by body mass index (BMI) at conception

BMI category	Recommended total gain (kg)
Low (BMI <19.8)	12.8–18.0
Normal (BMI 19.8–26.0)	11.5–16.0
High (BMI >26.0–29.0)	7.0–11.5
Obese (BMI >29.0)	>6.0

Modified from Institute of Medicine (1990).

divided by height in m²), was an important predictor of actual weight gain. Thin women (with a low BMI) gained more weight than fatter women. Different weight gain recommendations were therefore developed for women entering pregnancy with different BMIs (**Table 1**). For thinner women (BMI < 19.8 or <90% of ideal body weight), recommended gains are 12.7–18.2 kg (28–40 lb); for women with a normal BMI (19.8–25.9), gain should be 11.4–15.9 lb (25–35 lb) or 0.45 kg (1 lb) per week; and for overweight women (BMI >29.0 or >135% ideal body weight), gain should be at least 6.8 kg (15 lb) or 0.32 kg (0.7 lb) per week. New weight gain grids were constructed that showed the recommended gains over the course of pregnancy for each BMI group (**Fig. 1**), enabling the adequacy of weight gain to be tracked for individual women. To use the chart, woman's height and weight should be measured as near to the time of conception as possible (because pregnancy causes a temporary reduction in height) and used to obtain her BMI from a table.

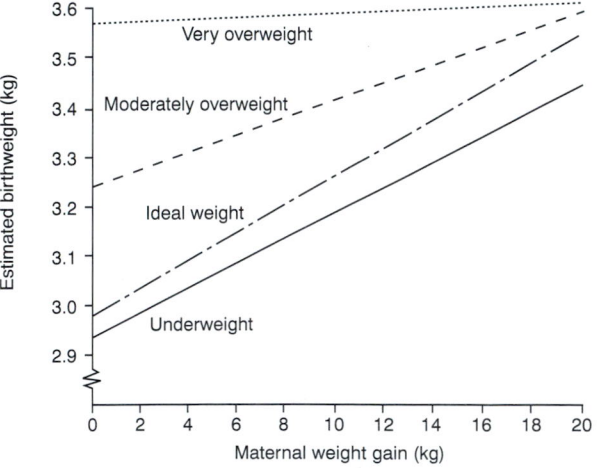

Figure 1 The relationship between maternal pregnancy weight gain and birthweight. From Institute of Medicine (1990).

Pattern of weight gain

Relatively little (1–2.5 kg) of the total weight gain during pregnancy occurs during the first trimester, while gain in the last two trimesters is linear. Nevertheless, it is important to pay attention to the quality of pregnant women's diets during the first trimester, and to ensure that they do not restrict their intake during this time when there is the strongest risk of nutrition-related birth defects and spontaneous abortions. In some studies an association has been noted between low weight gain in the first trimester and increased risk of spontaneous preterm delivery.

Variability in weight gain

The BMI-specific target ranges for gain are relatively narrow, yet a very wide range of gain actually occurs. In a California study for example, only 50% of the mothers who had uncomplicated pregnancy and normal birthweight infants gained the recommended 12.5–18 kg, with the remainder gaining more or less than this.

Maternal Weight Gain and Birthweight

Inadequate weight gain is associated with poor fetal growth even when the contribution of fetal weight and factors such as length of gestation are taken into consideration. Birthweight is an important determinant of child health and survival; low birthweight (<2.5 kg) infants are 40 times more likely to die in the neonatal period. Low weight-for-length at birth may be a risk factor for chronic disease in later life. It has been estimated that in women with normal prepregnancy BMI, each kg of total weight gain has an average effect on birthweight of 20 g. In California, women with pregnancy weight gains below recommendations were associated with a 78% higher risk of the infant being born small, while women who gained in excess of recommendations were twice as likely to give birth to a large infant.

As noted, maternal BMI at conception is strongly inversely related to expected pregnancy weight gain. Nevertheless, heavier women still tend to deliver heavier infants (**Fig. 2**) and thinner women tend to have smaller infants. In thinner women birthweight is more strongly related to pregnancy weight gain. Thus, as is evident from Fig. 2, the greatest risk of low birthweight is for thin women with a low pregnancy weight gain. It is crucial that thin women gain adequate amounts of weight. These associations are not explained by other risk factors associated with thinness, such as smoking.

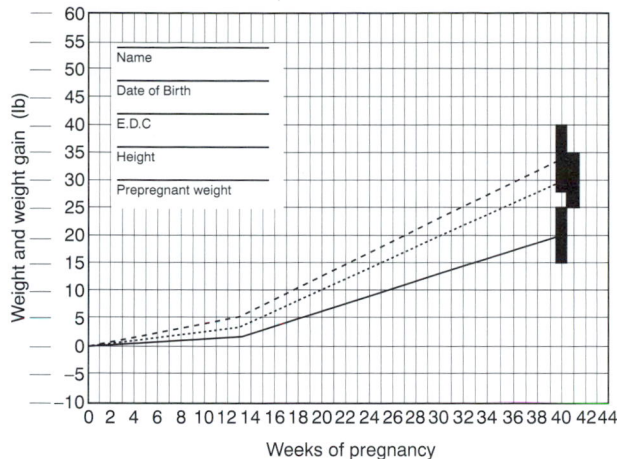

Figure 2 Recommended pregnancy weight gains (in lb) based on BMI at conception. (···), prepregnancy BMI < 19.8; (- - -), prepregnancy BMI 19.8–26.0 (normal); (—), prepregnancy BMI > 26.0. From Institute of Medicine (1992).

Changes in Body Composition and Maternal Energy Status

It used to be assumed that maternal energy intake during pregnancy was the main determinant of the amount of weight gained. While our knowledge of this relationship is still inadequate, newer information indicates that other maternal factors, and especially her body composition, are more important predictors.

The weight gained during pregnancy can be roughly divided into the weight of the fetus, placenta and amniotic fluid (a total of about 5 kg), maternal gain in the uterus, breasts, blood and fluid (about 4 kg), and maternal fat gain. The latter component is the most variable, and explains approximately 70% of the variability in pregnancy weight gain among women. While average fat gain in different studies is about 2–5 kg, values for individual women range from a loss of several kg to a gain of about 12 kg. Even in a group of women with normal BMIs at conception, the range of fat gain was 0.5 to 9.5 kg. Fatter women at conception gained less fat during pregnancy, as would be expected from their lower weight gains. The greater fat gain of thinner women is a potential energy store for the fetus and would afford some protection against maternal malnutrition in late pregnancy – a situation that is not uncommon in some economically disadvantaged countries.

Recent work has demonstrated that maternal BMI at conception influences not only the amount of maternal weight and fat gained during pregnancy, but changes in her basal metabolic rate (BMR). In studies of well-nourished pregnant women BMR has

been reported to increase by about 20–30%. For undernourished women, however, the increment in BMR may be only 20% of that seen in those who are well-nourished. In contrast, in a group of well-nourished Californian women weighing 55 to 116 kg, the BMR of those with higher BMIs was almost twice that of the thinnest women in the group.

Overall, it is clear that fatter women gain less weight and fat during pregnancy and have a higher increase in BMR. It has not yet been determined how these changes translate into energy requirements for women in the different BMI groups used to predict weight gains. Therefore, at present a single value for energy requirements is used for all pregnant women, regardless of their BMI at conception.

Weight Gain for Special Population Groups

Adolescents

Well-nourished adolescents tend to gain at least as much, if not more, weight than adult women. The relationship between BMI, pregnancy weight gain and birthweight is probably no different in this group, but to ensure adequate nutrition for those who are still growing, weight gain in the upper range of BMI-specific recommendations is advised. The effects of this recommendation on weight retention postpartum have not been evaluated adequately.

Short women

Women who are less than 157 cm tall tend to give birth to infants who are large relative to maternal pelvic size, with a subsequently sightly greater risk of a more difficult delivery. These women are therefore advised to gain near the lower end of the weight gain range that is compatible with their BMI.

Ethnic groups

Black women in the USA tend to gain less weight in pregnancy and to produce lower birthweight infants. The reasons for this are not known but it could not be explained by differences in gestational age or other factors that were measured. Adequate weight gain in this group is known to be especially important for the prevention of fetal growth retardation. In one study, 18% of nonobese Black women who gained less than the IOM recommendations gave birth to low-birthweight infants, compared with 10% whose gain was in the ideal range and 4% who gained more than the recommendations. In obese Black women the low-birthweight prevalence was about six times higher than for those who gained less than the recommendations.

Most surveys indicate that Hispanics seem to gain about the same amount of weight as Anglo women. In the National Natality Survey in 1980, Hispanic and non-Hispanic White women gained similar amounts of pregnancy weight, but the risk of low-birthweight infants was twice as high in Hispanics.

Substance abusers

Cigarette smokers tend to gain less weight during pregnancy and to produce smaller infants. This effect is not explained by a lower food intake of smokers. Alcohol and drug use have similar effects. Simply gaining more weight during pregnancy will not compensate for the adverse effects of these practices on fetal outcome or pregnancy complications.

Multiple births

Relatively few data are available from national surveys on which to base weight gain recommendations for women with twins. A weight gain of 15.9–20.5 kg, or 0.7 kg per week, in the second and third trimesters is usually consistent with a healthy pregnancy outcome for these women. No recommendations are available for women carrying more than two fetuses, but it is reasonable to expect that they will increase by at 3.5 kg for each additional infant.

Exercising women

Women who are physically fit at conception appear to be able to continue to exercise during pregnancy without harm to themselves or the fetus, as long as the activity is not too strenuous or prolonged. In several studies it was observed that exercising women gained 2–3 kg less than those who were more sedentary.

Pregnancy Weight Gain and Postpartum Risk of Obesity

On average, well-nourished women retain relatively little weight at about 1 year postpartum – approximately 0.5–1.5 kg. Delivery is followed by a rapid loss of weight in the subsequent 2 weeks owing to fluid loss. This is followed by a slower rate of loss for the next 6 months, so a complete return to pre-conception weight should not be expected in less time than this. In general, weight still retained at 1 year postpartum is unlikely to be lost without lowering intake and/or increasing physical activity. If weight retention is substantial it can add to the risk of obesity in the longer term. Obesity is a major health concern in many countries.

The relatively low average weight retention postpartum obscures the fact that many women do retain excessive amount of weight. Those who retain most are likely to have gained large amounts of weight during pregnancy. At 10–18 months postpartum, weight retention was 2.5 kg for women who gained more than the IOM recommendation, compared with 0.7 kg for White women and 3.2 kg for Black women who gained the advised amount. These large racial differences in weight retention have not been explained and certainly may be a risk factor for the higher prevalence of later obesity in this group.

Most women breast-feed their infants exclusively or partially for a relatively short time. There is little difference in weight loss between women who breast-feed and those who do not, for periods up to 6 months postpartum. This is presumably due to the greater appetite and energy intake of women who are breast-feeding, and perhaps to dieting on the part of non-breast-feeders. One study of women who breast-fed until 12 months postpartum did report a 2 kg greater weight loss in comparison with women who stopped breast-feeding before 3 months. Even more weight was lost by those who breast-fed more often and gave longer feeds.

Women with a high BMI at conception tend to either lose or gain more weight postpartum than those with normal BMI; about one-third end up weighing less than at conception, and one-third weigh substantially more. The reasons for the highly variable weight retention in this group are not understood.

Although inadequate intake of nutrients during lactation can lead to maternal nutrient depletion and lower breast milk content of some nutrients and especially vitamins, breast-feeding women who choose to lose weight can do so by exercising and/or reasonable restriction of energy intake. Exercising through jogging, cycling and aerobics for 45 minutes, four to five times per week, for 12 weeks did not affect the ability of well-nourished mothers to lactate, nor did it influence the composition of their milk. However, it is possible that severe energy deficit in lactation, especially of thinner women, will reduce breast milk volume.

Impact of Supplementation

The benefits of energy and/or protein supplementation for pregnancy weight gain and other outcomes have been explored by numerous investigators. However, relatively few trials have randomly assigned these supplements and used control diets. A statistical analysis was conducted of the 10 such studies that met this criterion in 1995. Most, but not all, of these studies were located in developing countries. Balanced energy and protein supplementation during pregnancy produced no significant effect on weekly gestational weight gain, not even in women who were likely to be undernourished. Likewise, no significant impact of supplementation was seen on birthweight or birth length, head circumference or gestational age. It is not clear why no benefits were seen, but possibilities include a relatively low intake of supplements (which supplied only 556–1792 kJ per day), lack of compliance on the part of the subjects, or inadequate inclusion of micronutrients in the supplements. It is also possible that there were other benefits to maternal or infant function that were not detected. Finally, the dominating influence of maternal prepregnancy BMI may have obscured differences in weight gain between the supplemented and unsupplemented groups.

See also: **Alcohol**: Effects of Alcohol Consumption on Diet and Nutritional Status. **Drugs**: Drug-Nutrient Interactions. **Exercise**: Diet and Exercise. **Lactation**: Dietary Requirements. **Obesity**: Prevention.

Further Reading

Dewey KG and McCrory M (1994) Effects of dieting and physical activity on pregnancy and lactation. *American Journal of Clinical Nutrition* 59 (supplement):439–445.

Hickey C, Cliver S, Goldenberg R, Kohatsu J and Hoffman H (1993) Prenatal weight gain, term birth weight, and fetal growth retardation among high risk multiparous black and white women. *Obstetrics and Gynecology* 81:529–535.

Institute of Medicine, Committee on Nutritional Status During Pregnancy and Lactation (1990) *Nutrition During Pregnancy. Weight Gain. Nutrient Supplements*, Food and Nutrition Board. Washington, DC: National Academy Press.

Institute of Medicine, Committee on Nutritional Status During Pregnancy and Lactation (1992) *Nutrition During Pregnancy and Lactation. An Implementation Guide*, Food and Nutrition Board. Washington, DC: National Academy Press.

Keppel K and Taffel S (1993) Pregnancy-related weight gain and retention: implications of the 1990 Institute of Medicine Guidelines. *American Journal of Public Health* 83:1100–1103.

King JC, Butte NF, Bronstein MN, Kopp LE and Lindquist SA (1994) Energy metabolism during pregnancy: influence of maternal energy status. *American Journal of Clinical Nutrition* 59(supplement):439S–445S.

Kramer M (1993) Effects of energy and protein intakes on pregnancy outcome: an overview of the research evidence from controlled clinical trials. *American Journal of Clinical Nutrition* 58:627–635.

Luke B, Minogue J, Witter F, Keith LG and Johnson TRB (1993) The ideal twin pregnancy: patterns of weight gain, discordancy, and length of gestation. *American Journal of Obstetrics and Gynecology* 169:588–597.

Parker J and Abrams B (1992) Prenatal weight gain advice: an examination of the recent prenatal weight gain recommendation of the Institute of Medicine. *Obstetrics and Gynecology* 79:664–669.

Safe Diet for Pregnancy

L Allen and **J E Casterline**, University of California, Davis, California, USA

During pregnancy there is an increased demand for nutrients for maternal metabolism and growth of fetal and maternal tissues. Nutrition concerns during pregnancy include consumption of a high-quality diet that is dense in micronutrients, and the avoidance of (or a reduction in) intake of substances that are potentially harmful to the fetus or pregnant woman. The majority of additional nutrient requirements can be met by appropriate selection of foods. However, many women consume vitamin and mineral supplements and medications during pregnancy. It is important to understand the risks, as well as the benefits, of these nondietary substances.

Dietary Guidelines for Pregnancy

In general pregnant women should follow the dietary advice provided for the public in general. For example, the dietary guidelines of the US Department of Agriculture are as follows:

- Eat a variety of foods.
- Balance the food you eat with physical activity and maintain or improve your weight.
- Choose a diet low in fat, saturated fat and cholesterol.
- Choose a diet moderate in sugars, salt and sodium.
- If you drink alcoholic beverages, do so in moderation.

Most of the increased requirements for nutrients during pregnancy can be met primarily by an adequate dietary pattern, with a few important changes (**Table 1**). Milk intake should be increased to 1 litre, which will increase energy, protein, calcium and vitamin D intake. For women who are lactose intolerant, dairy products that contain digested lactose should be used. Cheese and yogurt have less lactose than milk and can be substituted. Whole-grain breads and cereals, leafy green and yellow vegetables and fresh fruits should be consumed daily to provide additional vitamins, minerals and fibre. Six to eight glasses of water should be consumed every

Table 1 Daily food pattern for pregnancy

Food	Amount	Protein (g)
Milk, yogurt and cheese	3–4 servings	24–32
Meat, poultry, fish, egg	2 servings (115–170 g, 4–6 oz)	28–42
Vegetables (include dark-green and yellow vegetables)	3–5 servings	6–10
Fruits, fresh or canned	2–4 servings	1–2
Breads and cereals	7 or more servings	>14
Fats and sweets	Moderate intakes	Variable
Total protein		>73
Vegetarian pattern		
Milk, yogurt and cheese	3–4 servings	24–32
Beans, tofu, soya protein	2 servings	14–18
Vegetables (include dark-green and yellow vegetables)	3–5 servings	6–10
Fruits, fresh or canned	2–4 servings	1–2
Breads and cereals	7 or more servings	>14
Fats and sweets	Moderate intakes	Variable
Total protein		>59

day to prevent intestinal stasis, which can occur from reduced activity and the pressure of the enlarging uterus.

Obesity in Pregnancy

Obesity is one of the most common nutritional problems complicating pregnancy in the western world. Complications resulting from obesity include macrosomia in the infant (even when pregnancy weight gain is inadequate), and increased incidence of diabetes mellitus, hypertension, preeclampsia and multiple gestation. Maternal obesity is an important risk factor for failure to diagnose fetal abnormalities, particularly neural tube and cardiac defects, because ultrasonographic visualization of fetal anatomy is impaired. Obese women are also more likely to have delayed labour and repeated caesarean sections.

Dietary recommendations for obese women should include consideration of an optimal maternal weight gain. They do not need to gain as much weight during pregnancy as normal weight or thin women, and in fact their weight gain is usually lower without intentional dietary restriction. In part this is explained by their larger increase in basal metabolic rate during pregnancy, compared with women of normal or low fatness. However, weight gains of 6.8–11.4 kg are recommended to account at least for the weight of the fetus and maternal support tissues. Because obese women may be resistant to the idea of gaining weight, special attention may be required to explain that pregnancy is not a time for weight loss. Some practical guidelines for obese pregnant women are listed in **Table 2**.

Alcohol

There is abundant evidence that associates heavy alcohol consumption with teratogenicity, although the mechanisms by which this occurs are not completely understood. One possibility is that alcohol accumulates to toxic levels in the fetus, which is damaging during blastogenesis and cell differentiation. It has also been hypothesized that dietary deficiencies result from the excess alcohol consumption, specifically of folate, magnesium and zinc. The pattern of abnormalities that occurs is called 'fetal alcohol syndrome', which has the characteristic features of prenatal and postnatal growth retardation, developmental delay, microcephaly, eye changes, facial abnormalities and skeletal joint abnormalities. The impacts of either binge drinking or moderate alcohol consumption have not been satisfactorily evaluated and therefore the recommendation is that women abstain from consuming any alcohol during pregnancy.

Caffeine

Caffeine crosses the placenta to the fetus where it may affect fetal heart rate and breathing. Recent studies of reproductive loss have reported an increase

Table 2 Practical guidelines for overweight or obese mothers

1. Weight loss is not advised during pregnancy
2. For women with a BMI of 26.1–29.0, a weight gain of 6.8–11.4 kg and a normal dietary intake for pregnancy should be recommended
3. Women with a BMI greater than 29.0 should be advised to gain 4.5–6.8 kg during pregnancy
4. Nutritional counselling should focus on lowering intake of energy-dense foods that are low in other nutrients
5. Obese women should be made aware of the increased risk for glucose intolerance. Screening for gestational diabetes should occur at the first prenatal visit, with repeated testing at 28 weeks' gestation if negative
6. Frequent blood pressure monitoring with a cuff of the appropriate size is essential. If the patient has chronic hypertension, appropriate medication and a decreased sodium diet is indicated
7. Weight loss should be encouraged after delivery

Modified from Wolfe and Gross (1994).
BMI, body mass index.

in spontaneous abortions and risk of miscarriages in heavy coffee drinkers. No studies in humans have shown a link between caffeine consumption and birth defects, although massive doses of caffeine given to mice are teratogenic. Reports of an association between prenatal caffeine consumption and motor development in humans have been conflicting. Because it has not been proved without doubt that caffeine does *not* cause birth defects and other problems in humans, the recommendation is that all pregnant and lactating women should consume no more than the equivalent of two 150 ml cups of coffee daily.

Artificial Sweeteners

High doses of saccharin are weakly carcinogenic in rats so it is recommended that this sweetener be consumed in no more than moderate amounts during pregnancy. Safety concerns about the use of aspartame are limited to pregnant women with phenylketonuria; individuals with this condition should not consume aspartame in either the pregnant or nonpregnant state.

Nutrient Supplements

Many pregnant women have special circumstances that prevent them from consuming an adequate diet. These include lactose intolerance, substance abuse, being an adolescent or a strict vegetarian, and having multiple fetuses. For these women a multivitamin and mineral supplement may have positive benefits, including a reduction of the risk of some developmental defects, improvements in immune function, and a reduction in the onset or progression of some cancers. Anaemia is common during pregnancy and justifies treatment with iron supplements. However, some micronutrients commonly taken as supplements are potentially harmful to the developing fetus or, less often, to the pregnant woman.

Vitamin A

Although poor maternal vitamin A status is associated with preterm birth, intrauterine growth retardation and low birthweight in developing countries, vitamin A deficiency is rare in industrialized countries. Moreover, recommended intakes are not increased during pregnancy because maternal stores can easily meet fetal needs. Excessive preformed vitamin A, in an amount more than 10 times the US recommended dietary intake of 8000 μg retinol equivalent, should be avoided shortly before or during pregnancy because of its potential teratogenicity. Fetal vitamin A toxicity and birth defects have also

occurred from ingestion of isotretinoin and etretinate, drugs used for treatment of severe cystic acne. High intakes of carotene (a precursor of vitamin A) do not have the same teratogenic effects.

Vitamin D

Because of its importance in increasing calcium retention during pregnancy, recommended intakes of vitamin D are doubled. Vitamin D deficiency during pregnancy causes disorders of calcium metabolism including neonatal hypocalcaemia and tetany, hypoplasia of infant tooth enamel and maternal osteomalacia. Because the prevalence of vitamin D deficiency during pregnancy is high during the winter months at northern latitudes in regions such as Europe, the USA, Canada and Japan, vitamin D supplements may be necessary for women who live in these regions or who have little exposure to sunlight. High maternal intakes of vitamin D were implicated as the cause of a syndrome that included mental and physical growth retardation and hypercalcaemia in British infants between 1953 and 1957. Excessive amounts of vitamin D taken during gestation have also caused aortic stenosis and abnormal skull development in infants.

Folic acid and vitamin B_{12}

There is a substantial increase in folate requirements during pregnancy because of increased erythropoiesis and fetoplacental growth. Increased folate intakes throughout child-bearing age are recommended to prevent neural tube defects such as spina bifida and anencephaly, the most common birth defects, and to lower the risk of abruptio placentae. To be effective at preventing neural tube defects, increased folate intakes are needed early in pregnancy. The neural tube closes by 28 days of gestation, which is before many women realize that they are pregnant. It is for this reason that increased folate intakes are recommended throughout the child-bearing years. In addition, typical intakes of folate are only about half of the recommended amount. No adverse effects were reported in recent studies in which pregnant women consumed up to 4 mg of folic acid per day during pregnancy.

Vitamin B_{12} supplements are definitely required by pregnant women who are strict vegetarians; the vitamin is found only in animal products and the usefulness of the form of the vitamin found in algae and bacteria is not clear. There is evidence to suggest that an adequate intake of the vitamin during pregnancy is at least as important as the woman's vitamin B_{12} status at conception. Infants born to women with low vitamin B_{12} intakes are at high risk of growth failure and neurobehavioural problems that emerge when the infant is a few months old, and may be permanent. While supplements containing the recommended dietary intake of the vitamin are probably adequate for pregnancy, no adverse effects of consuming higher amounts have been reported.

Vitamin C

Low plasma vitamin C concentrations have been associated with preeclampsia and premature rupture of the membranes. There has been some concern about fetal vitamin C dependency induced by excessive maternal vitamin C intakes, but this is based on only one anecdotal report.

Vitamin K

Usual diets provide adequate amounts of vitamin K for pregnant women. Newborn infants are routinely given a supplement of vitamin K by intramuscular injection because exclusively breast-fed infants are at risk of developing fatal intracranial haemorrhage secondary to vitamin K deficiency. This practice is quite safe.

Iron

Demands for iron are increased by about 700–800 mg during pregnancy and most of this is needed during the last two trimesters. Because the risk of becoming anaemic is greater during pregnancy and there is an increased risk of a compromised pregnancy outcome for anaemic women, the National Academy of Sciences recommends that all pregnant women with a well-balanced diet take a supplement of 30 mg of ferrous iron daily during the second and third trimesters. If iron deficiency anaemia is detected by routine testing, the recommendation is that 60–120 mg of ferrous iron be given in divided doses throughout the day.

Gastrointestinal side effects, mainly heartburn, nausea, upper abdominal discomfort, diarrhoea and constipation, increase with high iron doses and contribute to poor compliance with taking daily iron supplements. Supplements of 15 mg of zinc and 2 mg of copper daily are also recommended for pregnant women taking more than 30 mg iron per day because iron can interfere with the absorption of other minerals. It is therefore important not to exceed recommended intakes of iron during pregnancy. It may be as effective to consume the recommended intakes once a week as it is to take them daily, because daily iron supplements gradually block the absorption of subsequent doses.

Zinc

Typically, zinc intakes are below recommended amounts for pregnancy even in industrialized countries. In populations where zinc deficiency is common the prevalence of malformations and low birthweight is higher, although the causal role of zinc deficiency has not been proved. Zinc supplementation is recommended for pregnant women who ordinarily consume an inadequate diet, smoke, are substance abusers or are carrying multiple fetuses. However, copper absorption may begin to be impaired at zinc intakes of about 18.5 mg per day, and a daily intake of 50 mg zinc impairs both iron and copper absorption.

Sodium

Owing to hormonal changes during pregnancy, sodium metabolism is altered. At one time dietary restriction of sodium was a common treatment for maternal oedema, although it is ineffective. The newborn infants of women who had restricted their sodium intake drastically during pregnancy were observed to have hyponatraemia. In animals, sodium restriction during pregnancy leads to water intoxication along with renal and adrenal tissue degradation of the pregnant animal. Therefore sodium restriction during pregnancy is not advisable.

Iodine

Typically the iodine intakes of pregnant women in the industrialized world easily meet recommended intakes. Maternal iodine deficiency and suboptimal iodine intake have been associated with cretinism, mental development impairments *in utero* and infant mortality. Iodine deficiency before or during early pregnancy has the most severe effects, and in regions of endemic iodine deficiency cretinism should be prevented by eliminating maternal iodine deficiency before or during the first 3 months of pregnancy. Hypothyroidism in the mother and fetus can, however, be corrected by iodine administration in the third trimester. It appears to be safe to administer massive amounts (500 mg iodine) to pregnant women, orally or intramuscularly.

Teratogens

The World Health Organization estimates that 15% of all clinically recognizable pregnancies end in abortion. Of these, 50–60% are due to chromosomal abnormalities. In addition, 3–6% of all offspring are malformed. The causes of these malformations can be divided into three categories: unknown, genetic and environmental. Environmental causes only account for 10% of all congenital malformations and can be further divided into maternal conditions, infectious agents, mechanical problems (deformations) and chemicals (including prescription drugs and high-dose ionizing radiation). Chemical environmental causes include consumption during pregnancy of the teratogenic agents discussed below. These account for less than 1% of all congenital malformations, but are important in that the exposures to these chemicals may be preventable.

Several anticancer drugs cause problems for fetal development. Aminopterin can induce abortion within its therapeutic range, and causes microcephaly, hydrocephaly, cleft palate, meningomyelocele, intrauterine growth retardation, abnormal cranial ossification, and mental retardation. Cyclophosphamide interacts with DNA and can result in cell death. Its use during pregnancy can result in growth retardation, ectrodactyly, syndactyly and cardiovascular anomalies.

Some antibiotics cause abnormal fetal development if taken by the pregnant woman. Streptomycin can cause hearing problems although the risk of this is low. Tetracycline may produce staining of the teeth and bones if taken late in the first trimester or during the last two trimesters.

Anticonvulsants can also cause adverse pregnancy outcomes. Carbamazepine produces minor craniofacial defects, fingernail hypoplasia and developmental delays. Trimethadione (troxidone) causes fetal trimethadione syndrome, characterized by V-shaped eyebrows, low-set ears, a high-arched palate, irregular teeth, central nervous system anomalies and severe developmental delays. Valproic acid causes spina bifida and facial dysmorphology in the fetus of 1% of pregnant users.

Other potentially teratogenic drugs include androgens, which result in masculinization of the embryo and stimulate growth and differentiation of sex steroid receptor-containing tissues. Angiotensin-converting enzyme inhibitors are antihypertensive agents that have detrimental effects during the second and third trimesters. These effects include fetal death, oligohydramnios, pulmonary hypoplasia, neonatal anuria, intrauterine growth retardation and skull hypoplasia. The pregnant woman who uses cocaine risks preterm delivery, fetal loss, intrauterine growth retardation, microcephaly, neurobehavioural abnormalities, vascular disruptive phenomena, cerebral infarctions and certain types of visceral and urinary tract malformations. Coumarin, a vitamin K analogue, is an anticoagulant and in the first trimester can produce malformations including nasal hypoplasia, stippling of secondary epiphyses, intrauterine growth retardation, and anomalies of the eyes, hands, neck and central nervous system. Lithium carbonate, an antidepressant, has teratogenic effects in animals but these have not been confirmed in humans.

Contaminants

Most heavy metals such as lead and mercury are embryotoxic. High maternal serum lead concentrations increase the risk of abortion, and adversely affect the central nervous system of the developing fetus leading to a low IQ and abnormal behaviour of the infant. Polychlorinated biphenyls (PCB) are environmental contaminants that remain in the body up to 4 years after exposure. The fetus of a pregnant woman exposed to PCB is at increased risk of fetal growth retardation, abnormal skull calcifications, deformed nails and pigmentation of gums, nails and the groin. Organic mercury compounds tend to accumulate in fat tissue and cause cell death owing to the inhibition of cellular enzymes. These compounds cause cerebral palsy, microencephaly, mental retardation, blindness and cerebellar hypoplasia in the infant.

Special Conditions

Nausea and vomiting

Morning sickness or nausea is common in the early months of pregnancy. It is rarely a condition to cause alarm, except when there is excessive vomiting. In this situation an acute protein and energy deficit and loss of minerals, vitamins and electrolytes may result. Treatment of this condition is by consuming small, frequent meals and a low-fat, high-carbohydrate diet. Prolonged, persistent vomiting (hyperemesis gravidarum) occurs in about 2% of pregnant women. Hospitalization is usually required, with intravenous fluid and electrolyte replacement to prevent dehydration.

Heartburn

Heartburn is a common complaint during the latter part of pregnancy due to the pressure of the enlarged uterus on the stomach in combination with the relaxed oesophageal sphincter. This can usually be relieved by limiting the amount of food consumed at one sitting and avoiding lying in a reclining position after eating.

Constipation and haemorrhoids

Pregnant women often develop constipation, most frequently during the latter stages of pregnancy. It is caused by reduced gut motility, physical inactivity and the pressure exerted on the bowel by the enlarged uterus. The weight of the fetus and the downward pressure on the veins can lead to haemorrhoid formation. These conditions can be treated with increased consumption of high-fibre foods and dried fruits, and increased fluid intake. Bulk-forming laxatives such as Metamucil can also be used; however, there is a risk of alterations in electrolyte absorption with chronic use of laxatives.

Oedema

Mild oedema (fluid accumulation) is usually present in the hands, feet and legs in the third trimester. It is caused by the pressure of the enlarging uterus on the veins returning fluid from the legs. This fluid is often mobilized in the evening when the woman is lying down. This is a normal condition and does not require any special dietary or other treatment.

Diabetes in pregnancy

For women with diabetes, nutritional counselling should include advice on adequate dietary intake, frequent glucose monitoring, insulin management to meet the growth needs of the fetus, maintaining optimal blood glucose levels, and preventing ketosis and depletion of the mother's nutrient stores. The demands of pregnancy may impose a need for insulin in pregnant women whose condition was controlled through diet alone in the nonpregnant state. Because of hormonal changes during pregnancy, changes to the diet and the insulin dosage may be necessary.

Gestational diabetes occurs only during pregnancy and usually resolves itself after pregnancy. It occurs in 5–10% of pregnancies and most commonly arises after 20 weeks' gestation. Gestational diabetes can be treated largely through nutritional care and moderate exercise to achieve weight control. Nutritional recommendations are to limit protein intake to 15% of total energy, to consume 55% of total energy as carbohydrate, and to limit fat intake to 30% or less of total energy. Cholesterol intake should be 300 mg per day or less, simple carbohydrate intake should be limited, and sodium intake should not exceed 1000 mg per 1000 kcal (4.2 MJ). Insulin is rarely needed, although blood glucose levels should be monitored daily.

Hypertension in pregnancy

Pregnancy-induced hypertension is a syndrome characterized by hypertension, proteinuria and oedema. This condition usually develops in the third trimester and occurs in about 7–8% of pregnant women. It occurs more often in women who are young, pregnant for the first time, or are of low socioeconomic status. The exact cause of this condition is unknown, but most researchers agree that it is associated with a decreased uterine blood flow leading to reduced fetal nourishment. Previous treatments for this condition included sodium restriction and diuretics; however, neither of these has been successful at altering blood pressure, weight gain or proteinuria in this condition.

Multiple births

Women pregnant with twins or multiple fetuses should gain more weight than those with singleton births, about 15–20 kg. Nutrient supplementation should include at least zinc and vitamin B_6 in addition to the iron supplements recommended for all pregnant women.

See also: **Alcohol**: Absorption, Metabolism and Physiological Effects. **Ascorbic Acid**: Physiology, Dietary Sources and Requirements. **Caffeine**: Chemistry and Physiological Effects. **Cobalamins**: Physiology, Dietary Sources and Requirements. **Diabetes Mellitus**: Classification and Chemical Pathology. **Energy**: Energy Requirements. **Fetal Origins of Disease**: Fetal Development and Later Disease. **Folic Acid**: Physiology, Dietary Sources and Requirements. **Hypertension**: Physiology. **Iodine**: Physiology, Dietary Sources and Requirements. **Iron**: Physiology, Dietary Sources and Requirements. **Obesity**: Definition, Aetiology and Assessment. **Protein**: Requirements and Role in Diet. **Retinol**: Physiology. **Riboflavin**: Physiology. **Sodium**: Physiology. **Vitamin K**: Physiology. **Zinc**: Physiology.

Further Reading

Allen LH (1994) Nutritional supplementation for the pregnant woman. *Clinical Obstetrics and Gynecology* 37(3):587–595.

American Diabetes Association (1991) Position statement: gestational diabetes mellitus. *Diabetes Care* 14:5–6.

Institute of Medicine (1987) Committee on Nutrition of the Mother and Preschool Child. *Laboratory Indices of Nutritional Status During Pregnancy*. Washington: National Academy of Sciences.

Institute of Medicine (1989) *Recommended Dietary Allowances*, 10th edn. Washington: National Research Council/National Academy Press.

Institute of Medicine (1990) *Nutrition During Pregnancy*. Washington: National Research Council/National Academy Press.

King JC, Bronstein MN, Fitch WL *et al.* (1987) Nutrient utilization during pregnancy. *World Review of Nutrition and Dietetics* 52:71–142.

Lewis DD and Woods SE (1994) Fetal alcohol syndrome. *American Family Physician* 50:1025–1032.

Neuhouser MLS (1996) Nutrition during pregnancy and lactation. In: Mahan LK and Escott-Stump S (eds)

Krause's Food, Nutrition and Diet, 9th edn. Philadelphia: WB Saunders.

Picciano MF (1996) Pregnancy and lactation. In: Ziegler EE and Filer LJ (eds) *Present Knowledge of Nutrition*, 7th edn. Washington: ILSI Press.

Rosso P (1990) *Nutrition and Metabolism in Pregnancy: Mother and Fetus*. Oxford University Press.

Wolfe HM and Gross TL (1994) Obesity in pregnancy. *Clinical Obstetrics and Gynecology* 37(3):596–604.

Role of Placenta in Nutrient Transfer

Pedro Rosso and **Sofia P Salas**, Department of Pediatrics and Obstetrics and Gynecology, Pontificia Universidad Catolica de Chile, Santiago, Chile

The Fetal 'Supply Line'

The fetus requires a steady supply of oxygen and nutrients. Components of the fetal 'supply line' of these vital elements include the maternal blood and its circulating nutrients; the uterine and maternal placental blood flows; the placental trophoblast; and the fetal placental blood flow.

The placenta is an organ of fetal origin that performs several functions that are considered to be critical to normal fetal growth, including nutrient transport from maternal blood to the fetal circulation. It is composed of two layers of tissue: a multinucleated true syncytium, lacking lateral cell membranes, called the syncytiotrophoblast; and a layer of undifferentiated stem cells underlying this syncytium, called the cellular trophoblast or cytotrophoblast. During gestation, the cells of the cytotrophoblast fuse with each other giving rise to the syncytiotrophoblast, the predominant structure in the placenta near term. The syncytiotrophoblast is the portion of this organ that mediates the maternal–fetal exchange of nutrients, oxygen and waste products (**Fig. 1**).

Some of the components of the fetal supply line are considered to be part of the maternal physiological adjustments of pregnancy. These include a fall in peripheral vascular resistance, blood volume expansion, increased cardiac output and expansion of uterine blood flow. The increased uterine blood flow reflects the progressive expansion of the placental vascular bed and is regulated by short-term and long-term mechanisms. Short-term regulation is based on both locally produced and systemic vasoactive substances, such as prostaglandins, nitric oxide and catecholamines. Long-term regulation involves blood volume expansion and increased cardiac output.

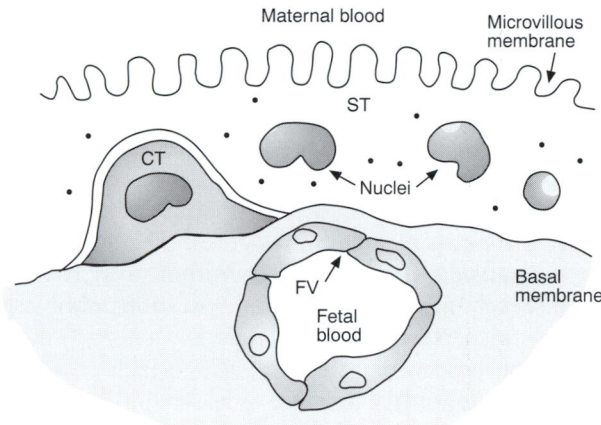

Figure 1 Schematic representation of the human placental villous structure. CT, cytotrophoblast; ST, syncytiotrophoblast; FV, fetal vessel.

The expanded blood volume allows a redistribution of cardiac output to accommodate the greater uterine blood flow without reducing blood supply to other maternal organs and tissues. Near term, approximately 450 ml min^{-1} of blood enters the placenta's intervillous space. This quantity represents approximately 7% of the maternal cardiac output. In the nonpregnant state uterine blood flow is around 10–15 ml min^{-1}.

Nutrients from maternal blood reach the fetal tissues by crossing the placenta and entering the fetal circulation. During gestation fetal–placental blood flow must therefore increase proportionally to maternal blood flow. Transfer of substances from the maternal into the fetal circulation is strongly influenced by the rate of blood flow on either side of the placenta.

Comparative studies have shown that, as well as being affected by blood flow, placental transport is influenced by placental thickness and morphology. During the course of gestation the placental trophoblast becomes thinner and its exchange surface area increases many fold, making it possible to rise the rate of nutrient transfer per gram of placental tissue.

Placental Transport Mechanisms

Substances cross the placenta utilizing either transcellular (transyncytial) or paracellular pathways. Transcellular mechanisms include simple diffusion and transfer by specific transporter systems. Paracellular pathways are wide pores, sparsely distributed, that transverse the syncytiotrophoblast.

Simple diffusion is a passive, non-energy-consuming process, reflecting random thermal motion of molecules across the syncytiotrophoblast and other membranes. The net quantity of molecules transferred depends on the concentration and/or electrochemical gradient between the maternal blood and the fetal blood. Other factors are the diffusibility and physicochemical nature of the molecule, including size, electrical charge and lipid solubility (**Fig. 2**).

Endocytosis is used to transport macromolecules, such as large protein (i.e. antibodies), that cannot pass through cell membrane pores. The substances to be transferred are taken up within invaginations of the cell membrane of the syncytiotrophoblast. Once incorporated into the cytoplasm, these invaginations become microvesicles which cross the syncytiotrophoblast and are released into the fetal circulation.

Transfer by specific transporter systems (mediated transport) involves energy-independent and energy-dependent mechanisms. The energy-independent (facilitated diffusion) and endocytosis mechanisms always proceed in the direction of a concentration gradient, while the energy-dependent ones (active transport) take place against concentration gradients. Many of the energy-dependent systems require maintenance of electrochemical gradients of sodium, potassium, chloride, magnesium and other ions. These gradients provide the driving force for their operation. Other transport systems utilize exchange mechanisms.

The transporters are rather specific membrane-bound proteins located in the microvillous and basal membrane of the syncytiotrophoblast. They recognize the spatial configuration of the molecules, a quality that makes them rather specific to individual substances. For example, D-forms of carbohydrates are transported more rapidly than L-forms. The number of transporters bound to the membrane and their affinity with specific molecules strongly influence the rate of transport. Most of the transport systems can be saturated by a high concentration of their specific molecules. Also, substances with a similar configuration can compete for the same transport system.

Paracellular transport can take place by simple diffusion and by bulk volume flow (ultrafiltration). The driving forces of bulk flow are differences in hydrostatic or osmotic pressure between the maternal and fetal compartments.

Placental Transport of Specific Nutrients

Many aspects of placental transport of nutrients remain unexplored. The available information has considerable gaps and contradictions that future research must elucidate. The information that follows is based only in generally acepted facts concerning nutrient transport in the human placenta (**Table 1**).

Carbohydrates

Glucose, the main metabolic fuel of the fetus, is transported using a facilitated diffusion mechanism. Experimental studies have shown that placental tissue expresses at least two glucose transport isoforms, Glut 1 and Glut 3. Controversy still prevails as to the expression of Glut 4. In pregnant women,

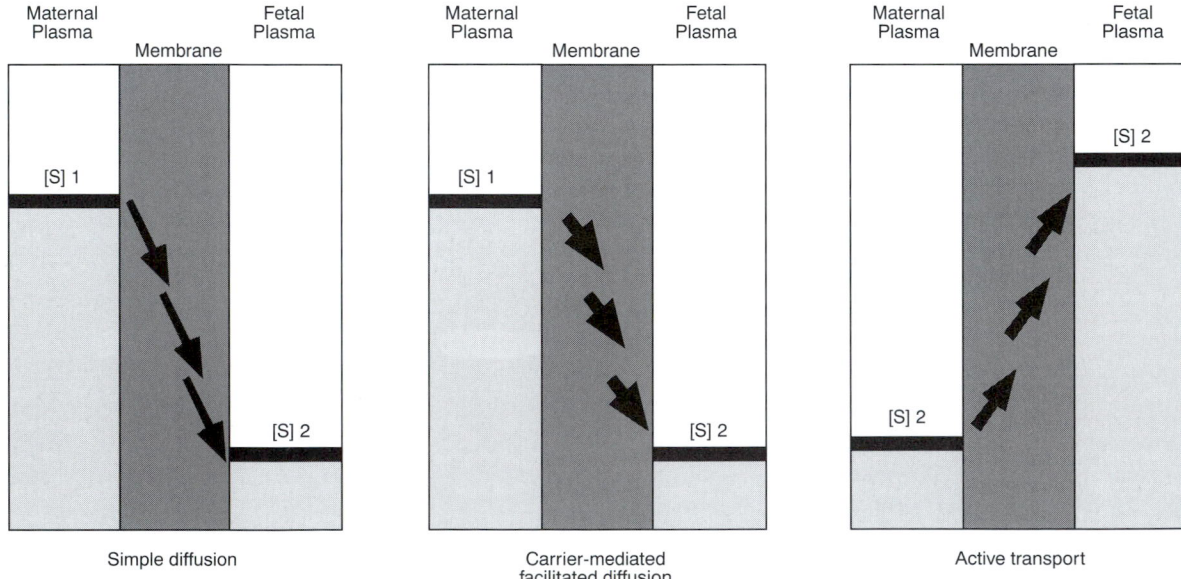

Figure 2 Diagram representing three possible mechanisms of transport between maternal and fetal circulation. Simple diffusion is a passive, concentration-dependent process. Carrier-mediated facilitated diffusion also proceeds in the direction of the concentration gradient, whereas active transport occurs against the concentration gradient.

Table 1 Placental mechanisms for nutrient transfer

Nutrient	Transport mechanism
Carbohydrates	Facilitated diffusion; maternal > fetal gradient
Lipids	Passive diffusion; maternal > fetal gradient
Amino acids	Active transport; fetal > maternal gradient
Water-soluble vitamins	
Ascorbic acid	Active transport; fetal > maternal gradient
Folic acid	Passive? Binding protein
B_6 and biotin	Passive diffusion
Lipid-soluble vitamins	
Retinol	Facilitated diffusion, retinol-binding protein
Vitamin D	Facilitated diffusion, binding protein
Minerals	
Ca^{2+}	Active transport; fetal > maternal gradient
Iron	Receptor-mediated endocytosis

maternal blood levels of glucose are higher than fetal levels. Fetal blood concentration of this metabolite increases linearly if the maternal concentration rises. This concentration curve levels off at $250 \, mg \, dl^{-1}$, when maternal concentration is $450 \, mg \, dl^{-1}$ or higher, indicating saturation of the transport system. Insulin influences the rate of placental transfer of glucose by altering the levels of this metabolite in maternal and fetal blood, but it does not have a direct effect in the glucose transport system.

Lipids

Blood lipid levels are higher in maternal blood than in fetal blood. Therefore, the transplacental passage of lipids takes place in the direction of a concentration gradient. Lipid transport kinetics are also influenced by the capacity of the placenta to metabolize some of these substances. For example, triacylglycerols are hidrolysed and then re-esterified in the syncytiotrophoblast before they are released into the fetal blood. Lipoprotein uptake by human placenta is mediated by high-affinity, low-capacity receptors specific for LDL. Very low-density lipoprotein/apolipoprotein E receptor (VLDLR) is expressed in placenta in a pattern consistent with a role in placental lipid transport.

Amino acids

The primary mechanisms for amino acid transfer across the human placenta are specific transport systems located in the microvillous and basal membranes. The average concentration of most amino acids in fetal blood is several-fold higher than in maternal blood, indicating that they cross the placenta against a concentration gradient. This implies the use of active type of transport mechanism. At least nine of these mechanisms have been described.

Neutral amino acids utilize the sodium-dependent systems A, ASC and N and the sodium-independent I (formerly called L). The A system is found in microvillous membrane and basal membrane, while the ASC system is present only in the basal membrane.

Cationic amino acids mostly utilize the sodium-independent systems y^+ and $b^{0,+}$. The maternal–fetal transfer of these amino acids is a rather complex process and there are still doubts concerning various specific aspects.

Placental concentration of *anionic amino acids* is considerably higher than either the maternal or fetal blood concentrations. Glutamate transport from maternal blood into the syncytiotrophoblast is accomplished by sodium-dependent potassium-coupled transporters located in the microvillous membrane. In this tissue most of the glutamate would be metabolized.

Placental amino acid transfer might be regulated by several mechanisms including substrate availability, protein kinase C activity, and calcium concentration. More recently, the possibility of regulation by insulin and epidermal growth factor has been suggested. A smaller proportion of amino acids also crosses the trophoblast by simple diffusion and, presumably, bulk flow mechanisms.

Water-soluble vitamins

The concentration of water-soluble vitamins is higher in fetal than maternal blood, so that placental transfer of these vitamins would proceed against a concentration gradient. However, water-soluble vitamins are found as either free or bound forms and the proportion of each may differ in maternal and fetal blood. Therefore, while total vitamin concentration could be higher in the fetal blood than in the maternal blood, the opposite may be true for the free form. In the first case transport might seem to proceed against a gradient, while in fact the free vitamin fraction is moving in the direction of the gradient.

Bound and free fractions of *ascorbic acid* have higher concentrations in fetal blood. Placental transfer of this vitamin is carried out by an energy- and sodium-dependent specific transport system. Thiamin, riboflavin and choline also have specific transporters that can be saturated by an excess of these vitamins.

Folic acid (5-methyltetrahydrofolate) is bound to a placental folate receptor, concentrated in the placenta and then passively released into the fetal circulation. JAR human placenta carcinoma cells transport folate using a probenecid-sensitive transporter that is driven by a transmembrane H^+ gradient. In contrast, vitamin B_6 and biotin are transported by passive diffusion.

Lipid-soluble vitamins

Retinol transfer in perfused human placenta suggests a facilitated diffusion mechanism. Apparently this vitamin crosses the placental membrane by a direct transfer of retinol-binding protein (RBP), involving cellular uptake and release of the protein–ligand complex. The steps of this process would include uptake of retinol by a cell surface receptor specific for RBP, transient esterification of retinol, and release of the vitamin into the fetal serum. Binding of RBP to its specific receptor would be obligatory for the subsequent delivery of retinol to the membrane. A similar mechanism is envisioned for vitamin D transfer.

Minerals

Calcium uptake by the human placenta is saturable and concentration-dependent, but sodium-independent. The microvillous membrane does not show any ATP-dependent transport activity while basal plasma membrane uptake is sodium-dependent, energy (ATP)-dependent, and requires the presence of Mg^{2+}.

Magnesium transfer is Na^+-dependent in the rat placenta, but its transport mechanisms in the human placenta have not yet been explored.

Zinc transfer is based on a potassium-dependent transporter. Net flux between maternal and fetal blood is linked to the level of free zinc in the trophoblast.

Iron crosses the placenta using receptor-mediated endocytosis. Placental transferrin receptors, located at the apical side of syncytiotrophoblast, mediate iron uptake.

Placental Transport and Maternal Malnutrition

In underweight mothers, mean birthweight is lower than in women with a normal body mass, thus indicating that the fetus has suffered a moderate degree of growth retardation. The effect of a reduced prepregnancy body weight on fetal growth is still apparent when underweight mothers are able to gain an average amount of weight (12 kg). Thus, the fetal growth retardation of these mothers cannot be directly attributed to a reduced availability of nutrients, but rather to a reduced body mass.

The association between maternal prepregnancy body mass, gestational weight gain and fetal growth has been explained by inadequate haemodynamic adjustments, leading to a smaller than normal maternal plasma volume during the second half of pregnancy and a reduced placental blood flow expansion. Evidence indicates that maternal body mass is strongly correlated with plasma/blood volume. In turn, plasma/blood volume during the second half of gestation influences cardiac output expansion and, indirectly, placenta blood flow, since placental blood flow expansion is proportional to cardiac output.

Throughout pregnancy, underweight women have a smaller plasma volume than normal weight gravidas. Near term, underweight mothers also have a reduced cardiac output and a higher total peripheral vascular resistance (TPVR) than normal weight mothers, although within the normal range. Placental blood flow has not yet been measured in underweight gravidas; however, their higher than normal TPVR values are consistent with the possibility of a reduced placental blood flow. During normal gestation, TPVR falls owing to vasodilation and the low resistance caused by the expanded placental blood flow. In normotensive pregnant women TPVR values near term are inversely correlated with birthweight.

See also: **Amino Acids**: Chemistry and Classification; Metabolism. **Ascorbic Acid**: Physiology, Dietary Sources and Requirements. **Calcium**: Physiology. **Carbohydrates**: Requirements and Dietary Importance. **Folic Acid**: Physiology, Dietary Sources and Requirements. **Iron**: Physiology, Dietary Sources and Requirements. **Lipids**: Chemistry and Classification. **Magnesium**: Physiology, Dietary Sources and Requirements. **Retinol**: Physiology. **Zinc**: Physiology.

Further Reading

Abrams BF and Laros RK (1986) Prepregnancy weight, weight gain and birth weight. *American Journal of Obstetrics and Gynecology* 154:503–510.

Hay WW Jr (1994) Placental transport of nutrients to the fetus. *Hormone Research* 42:215–222.

Kainulainen H, Järvinen T and Heinonen PK (1997) Placental glucose transporters in fetal intrauterine growth retardation and macrosomia. *Gynecology and Obstetric Investigation* 44:89–92.

Kudo Y and Boyd CA (1990) Characterization of amino acid transport systems in human placental basal membrane vesicles. *Biochimica Biophysica Acta* 1021:169–174.

Moe AJ (1995) Placental amino acid transport. *American Journal of Physiology* **268** (*Cell Physiology* 37):C1321–C1331.

Rosso P (1990) *Nutrition and Metabolism in Pregnancy. Mother and Fetus*, pp 133–167. New York: Oxford University Press.

Rosso P and Salas SP (1994) Mechanisms of fetal growth retardation in the underweight mother. *Advanced Experimental Medicine and Biology* 352:1–9.

Rosso P, Donoso E, Braun S, Espinoza R and Salas SP (1992) Hemodynamic changes in underweight pregnant women. *Obstetrics and Gynecology* 79:908–913.

Törmä H and Vahlquist A (1986) Uptake of vitamin A and retinol-binding protein by human placenta in vitro. *Placenta* 7:295–305.

Wilkening RB, Anderson S, Martensson L and Meschia G (1982) Placental transfer as a function of blood flow. *American Journal of Physiology* 242H:429–435.

Preconception Nutrition and Prevention of Neural Tube Defects

P Kirke, The Health Research Board, Dublin, Ireland

Donald G Weir, Department of Clinical Medicine, Trinity College, Dublin, Ireland

John M Scott, Department of Biochemistry, Trinity College, Dublin, Ireland

Neural tube defects (NTDs) are major congenital malformations of the central nervous system resulting in fetal and perinatal death and severe handicap in most survivors. The finding that folic acid can prevent most NTDs ranks as one of the most important medical research discoveries in recent times. In this article the epidemiology of NTDs is reviewed, focusing primarily on the role of folic acid and, to a lesser extent, vitamin B_{12} in the aetiology and prevention of these malformations. The causes of the 30% or so of NTDs that are estimated not to be related to folate are also briefly considered. The mechanisms underlying the link between folate, vitamin B_{12} and NTD aetiology are examined and the growing evidence for a metabolic explanation is reported. The main issues in using folic acid to prevent NTDs are discussed: ways to increase folate/folic acid intakes including the 'high-risk' and 'population' approaches, dose and duration of supplementation, and safety. The role of other nutrients in NTD prevention is considered. Recommendations on using folic acid to prevent NTDs have been issued by various national health authorities and the main points in these recommendations are presented.

Epidemiology

Failure of the embryonal neural tube to close normally between 24 and 28 days after conception gives rise to a group of severe congenital malformations known as neural tube defects (NTDs) which includes spina bifida, anencephalus (approximately 50% and 40% of cases, respectively), encephalocoele and iniencephaly. These anomalies are believed to be caused by an interaction of genetic predisposition and environmental factors and many different factors have been pursued. Evidence of the importance of nutrition has accumulated since the 1960s and the key role of folate/folic acid in the pathogenesis of these malformations was demonstrated conclusively in 1991.

Genetic and environmental factors

Evidence of a genetic component in the aetiology of NTDs includes familial recurrence patterns, ethnic variation and sex variation (commoner in females). More direct evidence of the role of genetic factors is the discovery that the gene encoding for the thermolabile variant of the 5,10-methylenetetrahydrofolate reductase enzyme is more common in individuals with spina bifida than in controls. The most striking environmental, or nongenetic, factors are the marked variations in prevalence over time and between areas. The prevalence rates of NTDs at birth have been falling in most countries, particularly in regions which traditionally had high rates. It is assumed, but not scientifically proven, that better nutrition is a main factor determining this trend. Variations with season, social class (more common in disadvantaged groups), and, to a lesser extent, maternal age and reproductive history, provide further evidence of the role of environmental factors. Several of these factors might be explained in whole or in part on nutritional grounds. (*See:* **Socioeconomic Status**: Relationship with Diet and Nutritional Status).

Folate/folic acid

There is now a vast literature on the role of folate/folic acid in the aetiology and prevention of NTDs. Evidence that folic acid can prevent NTDs comes from two main types of studies: observational studies of dietary folate intake and of supplementation with folic acid preparations, and intervention studies. The strongest evidence on the efficacy of folic acid comes from randomized controlled trials,

Table 1   Intervention studies of periconceptional folic acid supplementation and NTD risk

Study	Design	Daily dose folic acid (mg)	Outcome: number of NTDs	Relative risk	Comments
UK Medical Research Council Trial (1991)	Randomized controlled trial, international	4.0	6/593 suppl.[a] 21/602 not suppl.[a]	0.29	Significant[b]
Laurence et al. (1981)	Randomized controlled trial, Wales	4.0	2/60 suppl. 4/51 not suppl.	0.42	Not significant Small numbers
Kirke et al. (1992)	Randomized controlled trial, Ireland	0.36	0/172 suppl. 1/89 not suppl.	0.00	Not significant Small numbers
Czeizel and Dudas (1992)	Randomized controlled trial, Hungary	0.8	0/2104 suppl. 6/2052 not suppl.	0.00	Significant[b]
Smithells et al. (1983)	Nonrandomized controlled trial, UK	0.36	3/454 suppl. 24/519 not suppl.	0.14	Significant[b]
Vergel et al. (1990)	Nonrandomized controlled trial, Cuba	5.0	0/81 suppl. 4/114 not suppl.	0.00	Not significant Small numbers

[a]Six NTD pregnancies in 593 women supplemented with folic acid and 21 NTD pregnancies in 602 women not supplemented with folic acid.
[b]Statistically significant difference in NTD rate between supplemented and nonsupplemented groups.

notably the Medical Research Council (UK) trial on NTD recurrence and the Hungarian trial on NTD occurrence (i.e. first-time NTDs). These and other intervention studies are summarized in **Table 1**. Following on earlier research, the Medical Research Council trial published in 1991 conclusively established the efficacy of folic acid in preventing NTD recurrence. This trial used a research design to investigate the effects of both folic acid and a combination of other vitamins. The recurrence rate in the groups that received folic acid (1.0%) was significantly lower than that in the groups who did not take folic acid (3.5%), giving a 71% protective effect. Thus, 29% of NTDs were not prevented by folic acid. The multivitamin combination without folic acid had no protective effect. The main observational studies which have examined the effect of periconceptional use of vitamin supplements containing folic acid on NTD pregnancies are illustrated in **Table 2**. All of these studies but one found a marked protective

effect of supplementation against NTD occurrence. In most of the studies of NTD occurrence, the daily dose of folic acid was between 0.4 and 0.8 mg. Studies of dietary folate intake also show a protective effect of high intakes during the periconceptional period. The consistent finding of a protective effect of dietary folate and folic acid supplementation in virtually all of these different types of studies is very striking. Further evidence implicating folate comes from studies linking maternal folate status to pregnancies affected by NTDs. The studies that have been published on serum/plasma folate and red cell folate (RCF) are summarized in **Table 3** and **Table 4**. The differences between affected and unaffected pregnancies are more pronounced in the first trimester of pregnancy.

Vitamin B₁₂

The role of vitamin B_{12} in NTDs is of particular interest because of the close metabolic relationship between this nutrient and folate. The results of studies of maternal levels of serum vitamin B_{12} in NTD pregnancies are shown in **Table 5**. As for folate, lower levels of vitamin B_{12} are seen in affected pregnancies, especially in the first trimester. It is possible that the low levels of vitamin B_{12} just coincide with low levels of folate although the findings of a case–control study in Dublin (described below) suggest that they are independent risk factors. In another smaller study lower levels of vitamin B_{12} in affected pregnancies were not independent of folate levels. On biochemical grounds there is so much interaction between the pathways involving both nutrients that

Table 2   Main observational studies of the effect of periconceptional use of folic acid supplements on NTD risk

Study	Odds ratio
Mulinare et al. (1988)	0.41
Mills et al. (1989)	0.94
Milunsky et al. (1989)	0.29
Werler et al. (1993)	0.60
Shaw et al. (1995)	0.65

Difference between folate-supplemented and unsupplemented groups statistically significant in all studies except Mills et al. (1989).

Table 3 Serum folic acid (SFA) and central nervous system defects

Publication		No. of pregnancies	Mean SFA ($\mu g \, l^{-1}$)	Difference	Statistical significance
Blood taken at antenatal booking					
Hall *et al.* (1977)	Affected	11	6.3	−0.3	No
	Unaffected[a]	>1000	6.6		
Molloy *et al.* (1985)	Affected	32	3.4[b]	0.0	No
	Unaffected	384	3.4[b]		
Kirke *et al.* (1993)	Affected	81	3.5[b]	−1.1	Yes
	Unaffected	247	4.6[b]		
Blood taken in first trimester					
Smithells *et al.* (1976)	Affected	5	4.9	−1.4	No
	Unaffected	953	6.3		
Mills *et al.* (1992)	Affected	89	4.1	−0.2	No
	Unaffected	172	4.3		
Wald *et al.* (1996)	Affected	16	4.3[b]	−1.4	No
	Unaffected	36	5.7[b]		
All women (antenatal booking and first trimester)				−0.6 95% CI (−1.0,−0.2)	Yes (P = 0.005)
Blood taken in second trimester					
Economides *et al.* (1992)	Affected	8	9.8[b]	2.4 95% CI (−0.04,4.84)	Yes (P = 0.054)
	Unaffected	24	7.4[b]		
Blood taken after delivery					
Emery *et al.* (1969)	Affected	19	4.9	0.3	No
	Unaffected	37	4.6		
Yates *et al.* (1987)	Affected	20	2.8	−0.5	No
	Unaffected	20	3.3		
Bower and Stanley (1989)	Affected	61	5.6	−0.1	No
	Unaffected	140	5.7		
Wild *et al.* (1993)	Affected	29	6.2[b]	0.7	No
	Unaffected	29	5.5[b]		
All women (after delivery)				−0.03 95% CI (−0.5,0.4)	No (P = 0.090)

From Wald NJ, Hackshaw AK, Stone R and Sourial NA (1996) Blood folic acid and vitamin B_{12} in relation to neural tube defects. *British Journal of Obstetrics and Gynaecology* **103**: 319–324, Blackwell Scientific.
[a]Unaffected women were those without a neural tube defect pregnancy either before or during the particular study, except for Wald *et al.* (1996) in which women had at least one neural tube defect pregnancy before the study.
[b]Median value.

it is possible that deficiency of either could affect a common event in the closure of the neural tube. The role of vitamin B_{12} in NTDs is discussed further below.

Other nutritional factors

Vitamin C, vitamin A and zinc have also been linked to NTDs. Lower maternal levels of white cell vitamin C were reported in affected compared with unaffected pregnancies in one small study. Large doses of natural or synthetic vitamin A consumed by the mother during pregnancy have been associated with congenital anomalies in her offspring. In a large American study of maternal vitamin A intake before and during early pregnancy a total daily intake greater than 15 000 IU was associated with an increased risk of birth defects, especially of structures arising from the cranial neural crest (craniofacial, central nervous system, thymic and heart defects), but the risk of NTDs was not raised. However these findings have been challenged. Children born to women who take vitamin A supplements at levels found in current multivitamin preparations have not been shown to be at increased risk of birth defects. Although several studies have linked zinc deficiency or abnormalities in zinc metabolism to NTDs, the results have not been consistent. The role of zinc in NTD aetiology requires further clarification.

Table 4 Red cell folic acid (RCFA) and central nervous system defects

Publication		No. of pregnancies	Mean RCFA ($\mu g\ l^{-1}$)	Difference	Statistical significance
Blood taken at antenatal booking					
Kirke et al. (1993)	Affected	81	269[b]	−69	Yes
	Unaffected[a]	247	338[b]		
Blood taken in first trimester					
Smithells et al. (1976)	Affected	6	141	−87	Yes
	Unaffected	959	228		
Wald et al. (1996)	Affected	14	156[b]	−6	No
	Unaffected	26	162[b]		
All women				−77	Yes
(antenatal booking and first trimester)				95% CI (−94,−60)	($P < 0.001$)
Blood taken in second trimester					
Laurence et al. (1981)	Affected	4	238	−43	No
	Unaffected	47	281		
Economides et al. (1992)	Affected	8	435[b]	35	No
	Unaffected	24	400[b]		
All women				5	No
(second trimester)				95% CI (−76,86)	($P = 0.90$)
Blood taken after delivery					
Yates et al. (1987)	Affected	20	178	−90	Yes
	Unaffected	20	268		
Bower & Stanley (1989)	Affected	61	301	−7	No
	Unaffected	140	308		
Wild et al. (1993)	Affected	29	247[b]	24	No
	Unaffected	29	223[b]		
All women				−6	No
(after delivery)				95% CI (−33,21)	($P = 0.66$)

From Wald NJ, Hackshaw AK, Stone R and Sourial NA (1996) Blood folic acid and vitamin B_{12} in relation to neural tube defects. *British Journal of Obstetrics and Gynaecology* **103**: 319–324, Blackwell Scientific.
[a]Unaffected women were those without a neural tube defect pregnancy either before or during the particular study, except for Wald et al. and Laurence et al. in which women had at least one neural tube defect pregnancy before the study.
[b]Median value.

Research in the USA has shown that women who are obese (defined as prepregnancy body weight of more than 80 kg or body mass index of 29 kg m^{-2}) are more likely to have infants with NTDs, and that this association is independent of folate intake. While the underlying mechanism is unclear, these findings suggest that it may involve something other than folate.

Other causes of NTDs

It is estimated from the results of the Medical Research Council trial that about 30% of NTDs are not folate-related. The causes of this group of NTDs are unknown but are likely to include genetic and environmental factors. In this context the recent reports on obesity and NTDs are most interesting. Further research on this subject should result in a better understanding of the complex aetiology of NTDs. Nutritional factors other than folate may be involved, for example vitamins B and C and zinc as noted above, and other nutrients.

Mechanisms

The possible mechanisms underlying the involvement of folate/folic acid in the aetiology and prevention of NTDs are examined in this section.

Functions of folate and vitamin B_{12} and NTD aetiology

Folate acts as the purveyor of methyl groups for two important processes in metabolism, namely the methylation reactions and the synthesis of the nucleic acids, DNA and RNA (**Fig. 1**). The folate cofactor,

Table 5 Maternal serum vitamin B_{12} (SB12) and central nervous system defects

Publication		No. of pregnancies	Median SB12 (ng l^{-1})	Difference	Statistical significance
Blood taken at antenatal booking					
Kirke et al. (1993)	Affected	81	243	−53	Yes
	Unaffected[a]	247	296		
Blood taken in first trimester					
Schorah et al. (1980)	Affected	6	288	−129	Yes
	Unaffected	48	417		
Molloy et al. (1985)	Affected	28	297	20	No
	Unaffected	363	277		
Mills et al. (1992)	Affected	89	483[b]	−37	No
	Unaffected	178	520[b]		
Wald et al. (1996)	Affected	18	230	−10	No
	Unaffected	75	240		
All women				−38	Yes
(first trimester and antenatal booking)				95% CI (−56,−20)	(P < 0.001)
Blood taken in second trimester					
Economides et al. (1992)	Affected	8	205	−25	No
	Unaffected	32	230	95% CI (−58,8)	(P = 0.12)
Blood taken after delivery					
Yates et al. (1987)	Affected	20	300[b]	−20	No
	Unaffected	20	320		
Wild et al. (1993)	Affected	29	449	−40	No
	Unaffected	29	489		
All women				−34	No
(after delivery)				95% CI (−83,15)	(P = 0.17)

From Wald NJ, Hackshaw AK, Stone R and Sourial NA (1996) Blood folic acid and vitamin B_{12} in relation to neural tube defects. *British Journal of Obstetrics and Gynaecology* **103**: 319–324, Blackwell Scientific.
[a]Unaffected women were those without a neural tube defect pregnancy either before or during the particular study, except for Wald et al. (1996) in which women had at least one neural tube defect pregnancy before the study.
[b]Median value.

N^5-methyltetrahydrofolate, acts via the vitamin B_{12}-dependent enzyme, methionine synthase, to remethylate homocysteine to produce methionine which is converted to S-adenosylmethionine (SAM) via S-adenosylmethionine synthase; SAM is the universal methylator which is necessary for the synthesis of essential proteins, lipids such as myelin, and DNA. The folate cofactor also acts via methionine synthase to synthesize tetrahydrofolate which, unlike N^5-methyltetrahydrofolate, can be polyglutamated and thereafter used to produce the nucleic acids, DNA and RNA. Simple deficiency or metabolic impairment in the biochemical functions of either folate or vitamin B_{12} could, by interrupting DNA biosynthesis or methylation reactions, interfere with cell growth and tissue development during a period of very rapid cell proliferation of the fetal neural crest, thereby preventing normal closure of the neural tube.

Folate/folic acid and NTDs: mechanisms

Does folic acid prevent NTDs by correcting simple dietary deficiency, by overcoming a problem in gastrointestinal absorption or by overcoming some type of metabolic block? Recent research has helped to clarify the role of folate/folic acid in the aetiology and prevention of these malformations. Blood samples were collected from women at their first antenatal clinic in the Dublin maternity hospitals and 81 women in this cohort subsequently had babies affected by NTDs. Folate and B_{12} status were compared in these 81 cases and in a control sample of 247 unaffected pregnancies by measuring plasma and red cell folate (RCF) and plasma vitamin B_{12}. While folate levels were significantly lower in the cases than in the controls, more than 91% and 86% of the cases had normal plasma and RCF levels,

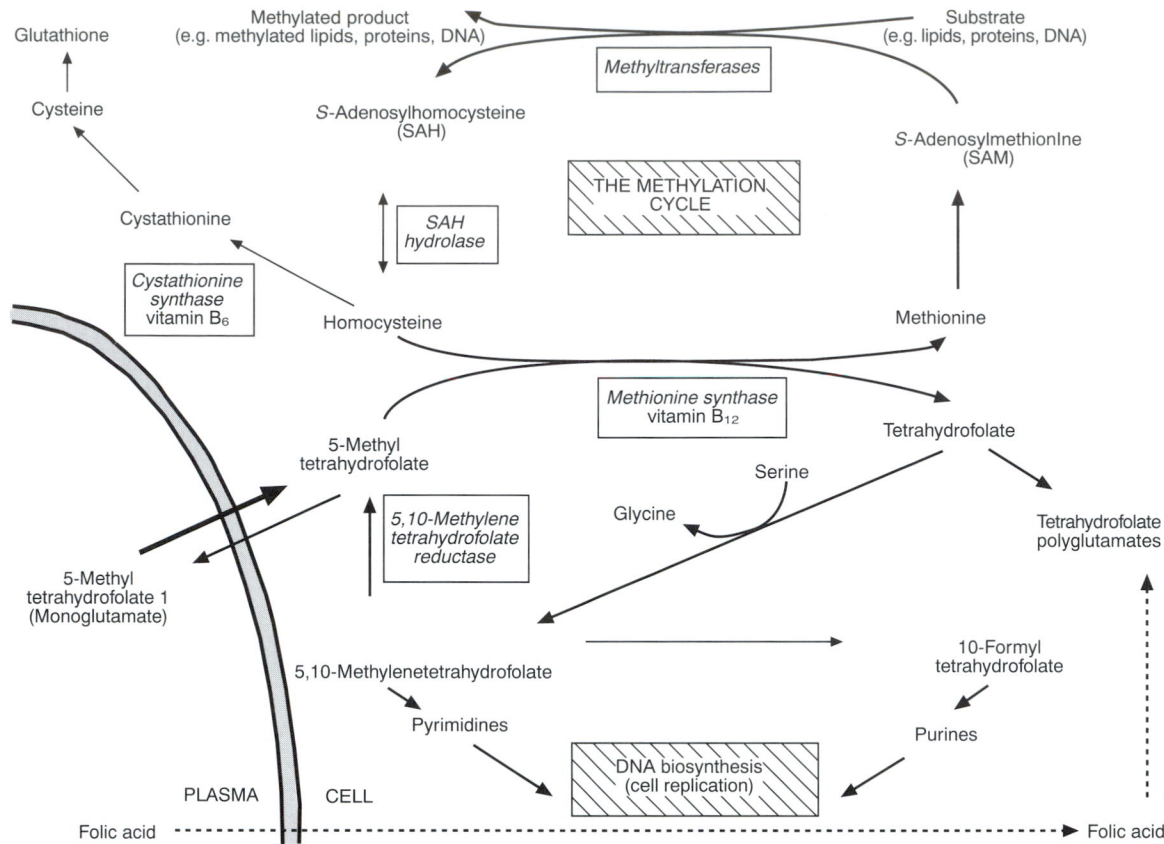

Figure 1 Intracellular pathways of folate and homocysteine metabolism and their relation to vitamin B_{12} function.

respectively. Thus the vast majority of women who had an NTD birth were not folate-deficient, as defined by conventional levels.

It has been suggested that women who have had children with NTDs might have a defect in gastrointestinal absorption of folate or folic acid, but there is no evidence to support this. In a study designed to overcome the methodological problems of earlier investigations, folic acid absorption was similar in a group of nonpregnant women with a history of an NTD pregnancy and in control women with a normal pregnancy history. These findings suggest that the absorption of folic acid routinely consumed in supplements and fortified food products is not impaired in women with a history of an NTD pregnancy.

A woman's risk of having an NTD baby has been shown to be closely related to her early pregnancy levels of plasma folate and RCF, the relationship being stronger for RCF (**Table 6**). There is a strong dose–response effect. Those with RCF levels less than 150 μg l^{-1} have more than eight times the risk of those with levels of over 400 μg l^{-1}. Although the most marked absolute reductions in risk occur by elevating the lower RCF levels, risk continues to fall

as RCF levels increase well beyond what would be considered normal levels, with little further protection apparently being gained at levels beyond 400 μg l^{-1}. Most of the NTDs were born to women whose RCFs would have been considered to be in the normal range (i.e. > 150 μg l^{-1}). Thus, our views on what constitutes desirable levels of RCF need to be reconsidered.

The lack of evidence of a simple dietary deficiency or of malabsorption and the marked dose–response relationship between maternal RCF level and risk of NTD point to a metabolic explanation for the aetiology of these conditions. Since it is estimated that folic acid can prevent up to 71% of NTDs, defects in folate-related enzymes or processes have been candidates for study. There are 16 folate-dependent enzymes in the internal metabolism of mammalian cells. The finding in the Dublin study (mentioned above) of significantly higher plasma homocysteine levels in case mothers than in controls suggested that one or more enzymes involved in homocysteine metabolism might be abnormal. The main folate-related enzymes involved in homocysteine metabolism are illustrated in Fig. 1. Homocysteine levels in the amniotic fluid of women carrying a fetus with

Table 6 Distribution of cases and controls and risk of NTDs by red cell folate level

Red cell folate ($\mu g\ l^{-1}$)	No. (%) of cases	No. (%) of controls	Risk of NTD per 1000 births	95% confidence interval
0–149	11 (13.1)	10 (3.8)	6.6	3.3–11.7
150–199	13 (15.5)	24 (9.0)	3.2	1.7–5.5
200–299	29 (34.5)	75 (28.2)	2.3	1.6–3.3
300–399	20 (23.8)	77 (29.0)	1.6	1.0–2.4
≥400	11 (13.1)	80 (30.0)	0.8	0.4–1.5
Total	84 (100.0)	266 (100.0)	1.9	1.5–2.3

From Daly LE, Kirke PN, Molloy A, Weir DG and Scott JM (1995) Folate levels and neural tube defects – implications for prevention. *Journal of the American Medical Association* **274**: 1698–1702. Copyright © 1995, American Medical Association.

an NTD have been reported as being higher compared with normal pregnancies. Evidence of deranged homocysteine metabolism also comes from metabolic studies conducted in Holland. In a study in which women who had given birth to an NTD baby were given a methionine-loading test, methionine intolerance and very high peak levels of homocysteine were found in a subgroup of the NTD women. Cystathionine synthase levels in skin fibroblasts taken from the methionine-intolerant women were normal.

The findings of the Dublin study already referred to pointed to an abnormality in the methionine synthase enzyme. There was a statistically significant positive correlation between plasma vitamin B_{12} and RCF in the case mothers but not in the controls, so that in the cases, the B_{12} level seemed to influence their ability to make RCF. Plasma folate and vitamin B_{12} were also found to be independent risk factors for NTDs. These findings provide strong evidence for the involvement of methionine synthase, which requires both folate and vitamin B_{12} to function. As already noted in this study, plasma homocysteine levels were found to be higher in the case mothers than in controls, especially when maternal vitamin B_{12} levels were low, offering further support for the involvement of a defective methionine synthase enzyme.

Genetic risk factors

A common variant has recently been identified in one of the folate-related enzymes, 5,10-methylenetetrahydrofolate reductase (MTHFR) (Fig. 1). It is possible to screen for this variant which provides a thermolabile form of the enzyme. In each of three studies in Holland, Ireland and the USA the frequency of homozygosity for this variant was significantly higher in spina bifida cases compared with controls. Based on a pooled analysis of these results and on the assumption that the association between

homozygosity for the variant and the NTDs is causal, it is estimated that 13% of NTDs are attributable to this genetic factor. As it is considered that some 71% of NTDs can be prevented by folic acid, variants in genes coding for other folate-dependent enzymes probably underlie the remainder and await discovery. The MTHFR gene variant is the first specific genetic risk factor to be linked to NTDs. It is the strongest evidence to date for the involvement of a metabolic derangement in the aetiology of these conditions. This breakthrough gives added impetus to the search for other genetically determined risk factors.

An association has been reported between a polymorphism of the T gene and human spina bifida. The human T gene which has recently been cloned and characterized is the human homologue (T) of the mouse T (Brachury) gene. It is believed to be a transcription factor which regulates genes involved in fetal (mesoderm) development. Other genes which are involved in embryonic cranial development, such as the homeobox genes, are being studied in mouse models. Of particular interest is a recent report that the development of NTDs in the mouse embryos can be prevented by prenatal administration of folic acid.

Prevention

In the context of the prevention of NTDs, it is necessary to distinguish between primary and secondary prevention. Primary prevention concerns measures which prevent the development of NTD in the embryo. Secondary prevention refers to screening and termination of affected pregnancies. Primary prevention became a reality following the demonstration of the efficacy of folic acid in preventing NTDs and represented a major public health breakthrough.

A substantial body of research shows that taking extra folate/folic acid before conception and during the early months of pregnancy prevents about 50–75% of NTDs and is effective in preventing both occurrent and recurrent NTDs. All women who are at risk of pregnancy are recommended to take an extra 0.4 mg of folic acid per day for the primary prevention of NTDs. This is in addition to the usual dietary folate intake, which is estimated to be, on average, about 0.2 mg per day in the UK. The most effective ways of using this knowledge to reduce the number of NTD births are discussed below.

'High-risk' and 'population' strategies

The data in the Dublin study already referred to, showing a marked relationship between early pregnancy maternal RCF levels and NTD risk, were used to examine the effectiveness of two different strategies to increase maternal folate levels for the purpose of preventing NTDs: the 'high-risk' and the 'population' strategies. The high-risk strategy involves identifying women at high risk because of low RCF levels and supplementing them with folic acid. In a population strategy the population mean RCF level is increased by fortifying staple foods with folic acid. To take an example under the high-risk strategy, a policy of intervention in women with RCF levels less than 200 μg l^{-1} and a target of increasing levels above this figure would prevent an estimated 17% of folate-responsive NTDs if implementation was complete (i.e. all women with RCF levels less than 200 μg l^{-1} successfully identified and the levels of all women increased above this figure). This figure reduces to 13% if three-quarters of the women achieved the target, and to 9% if the more realistic figure of half of the women reached the target. If the level for RCF intervention was set higher then there would be a larger reduction in NTDs, but at a greater cost in terms of the effort required in screening and in the number of those treated with folic acid. While this high-risk strategy may not be of great benefit to society, the effect for an individual woman of ascertaining her red cell folate status and taking supplements could be dramatic. The authors calculate a woman's risk of an NTD-affected birth for a RCF less than 150 μg l^{-1} to be 6.6 per 1000 and this reduces by some 88% to 0.8 per 1000 births if she increases her RCF status to over 400 μg l^{-1} (Table 6). Alternatively a population strategy could be used. The analysis in this study showed that if, as the result of a general fortification of the diet, all women in a population doubled their red cell folate level, then this would reduce the prevalence of folate-responsive NTDs by some 66%. If this increase was 150%, which could be achievable with sufficient fortification, the level of protection would be 73% of folate-responsive NTDs (equivalent to 53% of all

NTDs). Thus while an individual woman may derive dramatic protection from identifying her folate status and taking folic acid supplements, it seems clear that such a strategy on a population basis would be less effective. Conversely, if the diet was fortified by folic acid being added to one or more staple foods, the increase in folate status that could be achieved would be substantial in almost all women, and could reduce NTD births by more than half.

Experimental evidence that increasing maternal RCF levels is effective in preventing NTDs is available from intervention studies. Clinical trials demonstrating the efficacy of folic acid in NTD prevention have, not surprisingly, reported marked rises in maternal folate levels. In one study where women took 0.36 mg folic acid daily for periods ranging from 11 to 28 weeks, the mean RCF increased from 250 to 478 μg l^{-1}.

The two strategies can be considered as complementary. In view of the marked reduction in NTD risk which may ensue if a woman with a RCF level less than 150 μg l^{-1} were identified and supplemented, consideration should be given to implementing opportunistic screening by the general practitioner. The condition can largely be prevented in high-risk women who, based on this research, can now be easily identified with a blood test (RCF estimation). In terms of reducing the prevalence of NTDs in the population, however, the high-risk strategy, requiring screening for low folate status, is likely to be less effective than the population approach.

Ways of increasing folate/folic acid intake

As already noted, a woman can increase her folate intake in three ways: eating more folate-rich foods, eating foods fortified with folic acid, and taking folic acid as a medicinal or food supplement. While all three methods are known to increase folate status, taking folic acid either as supplements or in fortified foods has been shown to be much more effective in achieving this than eating folate-rich foods. It is very difficult to achieve a total daily intake of 0.6 mg folate/folic acid from folate-rich (unfortified) foods alone. Furthermore, folate in unfortified food is not as bioavailable as folic acid in fortified food or in supplements. The only practical ways of taking an extra 0.4 mg folic acid daily, as recommended, is by consuming fortified foods or folic acid supplements and this should be made clear in the advice given by health professionals to women. However, an improved general diet, especially consuming more vegetables and fruit, should be advocated preconceptionally and during pregnancy because it would result in an increased intake of other vitamins and nutrients which are important for normal fetal development.

Supplementation, which involves an individual regularly taking a tablet containing folic acid, is probably the most efficient method for a high-risk approach but not for a population strategy. In England there have been low levels of compliance with the Department of Health's recommendations to take folic acid supplements periconceptionally. Studies in antenatal clinics reported supplementation rates of between 2% and 18%. Clearly the supplementation approach is only reaching a minority of women. Food fortification is a preferable solution for a population approach. Folic acid is added to one or more staple foods, such as flour, so that consumption increases passively, without any change in dietary habits. The objective of a food fortification policy to prevent NTDs is to increase folate intakes for the target childbearing population as near as possible to the recommended intakes while maintaining safe levels of intake for the entire population.

Dose

The results of the randomized trials and observation studies show that a daily dose of 0.4–0.8 mg of folic acid prevents neural tube defects. The finding that a woman's risk of having a child with an NTD is related to her early pregnancy levels of RCF in a continuous dose–response relationship, suggests that folic acid intake would also be related to risk in a continuous dose–response relationship. It may be that a regular daily intake of lower doses of folic acid might raise the RCF above 400 μg l^{-1} which, as already noted, is associated with a low risk of NTDs. While firm data are not yet available on the effect of different levels of folic acid intake on RCF levels, a study has shown that RCF levels commensurate with a low risk of NTDs can be achieved by daily intakes of 0.2 mg and possibly as low as 0.1 mg. Individuals with folate-related enzyme defects may require higher doses of folic acid.

The 4.0 mg daily supplement recommended by the Departments of Health in the UK and the Department of Health and Human Services in the USA for the prevention of NTD recurrence is based mainly on the unequivocal evidence of the efficacy of this dose in the UK Medical Research Council Trial. In another large nonrandomized intervention study a daily dose of 0.36 mg folic acid seemed to offer similar protection in that the recurrence rate in the treated groups was similar to that in the Medical Research Council trial. So while the recommendation for 4.0 mg to prevent recurrence is quite correctly based on the best scientific evidence, it is likely that a much smaller dose would be equally effective.

Duration of supplementation

Another issue is the minimum duration of supplementation necessary for prevention. While the recommendations of most national health authorities are that women should take the extra folic acid for at least 4 weeks before conception and until the twelfth week of pregnancy, it may be that supplementation for a shorter duration before closure of the neural tube may also be effective. Until more data are available, the official guidelines should be followed. Given the estimate that about half of all pregnancies are unplanned, however, it is important that a woman who has not been taking extra folic acid and who suspects that she may be pregnant should immediately start taking a folic acid supplement. This point requires greater emphasis.

Safety

The main concern about taking folic acid at levels greater than 0.4 mg per day is the possibility that the diagnosis of pernicious anaemia, which is caused by vitamin B_{12} malabsorption and is more common in the elderly, would be missed since folic acid at high levels prevents the development of the anaemia and thus its diagnosis. In this situation nerve damage progresses and becomes irreversible. To ensure that 95% of all women get 0.4 mg of folic acid per day through fortification of staple foods such as bread or cereals would mean that, depending on the diet and differences in eating habits, more than half of the population would get approximately 0.7 mg and 5% would get more than 1.0 mg per day. A compromise is to select a lower target figure for universal fortification which would aim to prevent most folate-responsive NTDs and not put the elderly at risk. This is what the US Food and Drug Administration has done. However, folic acid in the dose range 0.5–1.0 mg may be absorbed in its original unmetabolized form and may be found in this form in the bloodstream. Circulating folic acid would then be taken up by body cells by a vitamin B_{12}-independent mechanism (see Fig. 1) and would have the potential to switch on the megaloblastic bone marrow in a vitamin B_{12}-deficient person thereby preventing the development of the anaemia and masking the B_{12} deficiency. Further research is needed, therefore, to determine the amount of folic acid in fortified food which is safe from this potential hazard.

Adding vitamin B_{12} as well as folic acid to fortified food has been suggested as a solution but this is problematic. The vast majority of cases of vitamin B_{12} deficiency are due to the autoimmune disease, pernicious anaemia. In this condition the absence of intrinsic factor prevents the absorption of physiological amounts of vitamin B_{12}. Thus including vitamin B_{12} at levels of the dietary reference value (DRV) or less cannot benefit such people because it is not absorbed. It has been suggested that if a large enough dose of vitamin B_{12} is added to the diet then a sufficient amount will be absorbed by passive diffusion to prevent vitamin B_{12} deficiency. However, the amounts required to do this would be between 200 and 400 times the DRV for vitamin B_{12} and most experts on the subject would be concerned about adding such a vast excess of an albeit apparently safe nutrient to the food chain.

It is established that anticonvulsant drugs impair folate status and there is concern that folic acid supplements may reduce the efficacy of these drugs, thereby causing a medical management problem for women with epilepsy.

Apart from these two situations, there is no evidence that a daily dose of 0.4 mg of folic acid has any adverse effects.

Other nutrients

As noted above, nutritional factors might be involved in the aetiology of some of the non folate-related NTDs. Although there is growing evidence for the involvement of vitamin B_{12} and lesser evidence for vitamin C and zinc, the available evidence is not strong enough to support dietary supplementation with these or other nutrients.

Because large doses of vitamin A are known to be teratogenic, women at risk of pregnancy and those in the early months of pregnancy should avoid liver products, which can contain high quantities of vitamin A. In order to keep daily vitamin A intake below 10 000 IU, women in these groups should not take a multivitamin tablet that contains a dose of more than 5000 IU.

Recommendations

The Departments of Health in the UK and the Department of Health and Human Services in the USA were the first to issue recommendations on the use of folic acid to prevent neural tube defects (NTDs). The recommendations relate to prevention of occurrent (first-time) and recurrent NTDs and similar recommendations have been adopted by other national health authorities. The main points in these recommendations are given below.

Prevention of NTD recurrence

To prevent NTD recurrence in the offspring of women or men with spina bifida or encephalocoele themselves, or with a history of a previous child with NTD:

- Such women and men should be counselled about the increased risk in subsequent pregnancies and about the protective effect of supplementation with folic acid.
- Women with a previously affected pregnancy should, unless contraindicated, be advised to take 4.0 mg of folic acid daily from at least 4 weeks before conception until the end of the third month of pregnancy. In countries where a 5.0 mg rather than a 4.0 mg preparation is available, the former can be used but the lower 4.0 mg dose should be used as soon as this preparation becomes available.
- The 4.0 mg dose should be taken only under the supervision of a doctor for two main reasons. First, giving high doses of folic acid can complicate the diagnosis of vitamin B_{12} deficiency. Second, epileptic women on anticonvulsant therapy require individual counselling before starting folic acid.
- The folic acid dose should be obtained from pills containing only folic acid and not from multivitamin preparations because of the danger of taking harmful levels of vitamins A and D.

Prevention of NTD occurrence

For the prevention of occurrence of NTDs the US Public Health Service recommends that all women capable of becoming pregnant consume 0.4 mg of folic acid per day and that total folate consumption should not be more than 1.0 mg per day to avoid the possible risks of high intakes. The UK Expert Advisory Group recommends that women should take an extra 0.4 mg of folic acid daily from when they begin trying to conceive until the twelfth week of pregnancy. If a woman who has not been taking this additional amount of folic acid suspects that she may have just started a pregnancy, she should begin taking extra folic acid at once and continue until the twelfth week of pregnancy. The US Public Health Service and the UK Expert Advisory Group outlined the three possible ways of achieving an extra intake of folate/folic acid: eating more folate-rich foods, eating foods fortified with folic acid, and taking folic acid as a medicinal or food supplement. It was recommended that women should use whatever source or combination of sources they preferred to ensure that they obtained the necessary extra folic acid. The effectiveness of these approaches in achieving the recommended increase population intake of folate/folic acid is considered in the section on Prevention.

Food fortification with folic acid

The USA is the first country to introduce mandatory fortification of some food products to prevent NTDs.

In 1996 the Food and Drug Administration issued a rule which requires all food manufacturers to add folic acid to all enriched cereal grain products by January 1998. Specified grain products will be required to be fortified with folic acid at levels ranging from 0.43 mg to 1.0 mg per pound of product (1 pound $\approx$ 454 g). These amounts are chosen to keep daily intakes of folic acid below 1.0 mg because of the concern that intakes above 1.0 mg may mask symptoms of pernicious anaemia. It is estimated that this level of fortification will add an average of 0.1 mg to women's diets in the USA and that a small proportion, perhaps only 2.5% of women of reproductive age, will consume the recommended 0.4 mg as a result of eating the newly fortified foods. The UK Expert Advisory Group was more cautious on the food fortification issue. While they wished to see an increase in the range of breads and breakfast cereals fortified with folic acid, they recommended that there should not be universal fortification of these foodstuffs. The approach to fortification in the UK appears to be nondirective, leaving it to industry to make such additions on a voluntary basis at the prompting of the Departments of Health and Agriculture.

See also: **Bioavailability**: Definition and General Aspects. **Cobalamins**: Physiology, Dietary Sources and Requirements. **Folic Acid**: Physiology, Dietary Sources and Requirements. **Food Fortification**: Importance in the Diet. **Fruits and Vegetables**: Nutritional Value. **Obesity**: Definition, Aetiology and Assessment. **Pregnancy**: Nutrient Requirements. **Vitamin Supplementation**: Role.

Further Reading

Centers for Disease Control (1991) Use of folic acid for prevention of spina bifida and other neural tube defects – 1983–1991. *Morbidity and Mortality Weekly Report* 40:513–516.

Centers for Disease Control (1993) Recommendations for the use of folic acid to reduce the number of cases of spina bifida and other neural tube defects. *Morbidity and Mortality Weekly Report* 41(RR-14):1–7.

Daly LE, Kirke PN, Molloy A, Weir DG and Scott JM (1995) Folate levels and neural tube defects – implications for prevention. *Journal of the American Medical Association* 274:1698–1702.

Elwood JM, Little J and Elwood JH (1992) *Epidemiology and Control of Neural Tube Defects*. Oxford: Oxford University Press.

Expert Advisory Group (1992) *Folic Acid and the Prevention of Neural Tube Defects*. London: Department of Health.

Scott JM, Weir DG, Molloy A, McPartlin J, Daly L and Kirke P (1994) Folic acid metabolism and mechanisms of neural tube defects. In: *Neural Tube Defects*. CIBA Foundation Symposium 181, pp 180–191. Chichester: Wiley.

Scott JM, Kirke PN and Weir DG (1995) Folate and neural tube defects. In: Bailey L (ed.) *Folate in Health and Disease*, chap. 12, pp 329–360. New York: Marcel Dekker.

Wald NJ (1994) Folic acid and neural tube defects: the current evidence and implications for prevention. In: *Neural Tube Defects*. CIBA Foundation Symposium 181, pp 192–211. Chichester: Wiley.

Wald NJ, Hackshaw AK, Stone R and Sourial NA (1996) Blood folic acid and vitamin B_{12} in relation to neural tube defects. *British Journal of Obstetrics and Gynaecology* 103:319–324.

Whitehead AS, Gallagher P, Mills JL, Kirke PN, Burke H, Molloy AM, Weir DG, Shields DC and Scott JM (1995) A genetic defect in 5,10 methylenetetrahydrofolate reductase in neural tube defects. *Quarterly Journal of Medicine* 88:736–766.

Pre-eclampsia and Diet

R Fraser, Department of Obstetrics and Gynaecology, Northern General Hospital, Sheffield, UK

This article provides definitions of pre-eclampsia and the other related hypertensive disorders that complicate pregnancy. The epidemiology of pre-eclampsia is discussed with particular reference to its increased frequency in first pregnancies relative to subsequent pregnancies. The pathophysiology includes the development of abnormal vascular anatomy in the placental bed as the primary pathological feature, a phenomenon which is almost certainly of immunological origin. The secondary features of this disorder are described to explain the progression of the disease and to illustrate the points at which interventions might possibly have beneficial effects. Conventional management of the condition and its complications is outlined. The various nutritional interventions which have been considered as either being aetiological, prophylactic or therapeutic, are then reviewed in detail.

Epidemiology

Definition

The clinical classification given in **Table 1** is typical of the many classification based on reviews of the spectrum of hypertensive disease complicating pregnancy. However, there is some confusion over what obstetricians mean when they use the term 'pre-

Table 1 Clinical classification of hypertensive disorders in pregnancy

Disorder	Definition
Gestational hypertension and/or proteinuria	Hypertension or proteinuria developing in pregnancy, labour or the puerperium in a previously normotensive, nonproteinuric woman
Gestational hypertension	Without proteinuria
Gestational proteinuria	Without hypertension
Gestational proteinuria and hypertension	Pre-eclampsia
Chronic hypertension and chronic renal disease	Hypertension or proteinuria in pregnancy in a woman with chronic hypertension or chronic renal disease diagnosed before, during or after pregnancy
Chronic hypertension	Without proteinuria
Chronic renal disease	Proteinuria with or without hypertension
Chronic hypertension with superimposed pre-eclampsia	Proteinuria developing for the first time in pregnancy in a woman with known chronic hypertension
Unclassified	Hypertension and/or proteinuria found either (1) at first examination after 20 weeks' gestation in a woman without known chronic renal disease or chronic hypertension, or (2) during pregnancy, labour, or the puerperium where information is insufficient to permit classification.
Eclampsia	Generalized convulsions during pregnancy, labour or within 7 days of delivery not caused by epilepsy or other convulsive disorders

After Davey and McGillivray (1988).

eclampsia'. Some talk of pregnancy-induced hypertension (PIH) rather than gestational hypertension and reserve the term pre-eclampsia for pregnancy-induced hypertension in which the woman has also developed proteinuria. The reason for this separation is that the more serious effects both for the mother and fetus are seen almost exclusively in the cases where proteinuria has developed. Obviously nonproteinuric hypertension is a retrospective diagnosis after the pregnancy has been completed. Hypertension complicating pregnancy is recognized when the diastolic blood pressure (DBP) is 90 mmHg or greater, or the systolic blood pressure (SDP) is 140 mmHg or greater, or both. Others have recognized a rise in the DBP of 15 mmHg or in the SBP of 30 mmHg or greater over levels recorded earlier in pregnancy as being diagnostic. Proteinuria is considered to be present if there is more than 300 mg of protein measured in a 24 h urinary collection in subjects who do not have chronic proteinuria. 'Severe pre-eclampsia' is diagnosed when the SBP exceeds a 160 mmHg and DBP exceeds 110 mmHg *and* when proteinuria of greater than 1 g is present in a 24 h collection.

Acute vascular damage (atherosis) is induced by mean arterial pressures above 140 mmHg in a previously normotensive subject. Irrespective of the stage of the pregnancy or the extent of proteinuria, such levels of blood pressure constitute a medical emergency requiring acute therapeutic interventions. The implication of the term 'pre-eclampsia' is that in some cases, if the condition is not treated, it will progress to eclampsia, i.e. the presence of generalized

convulsions. Once eclampsia has developed, if left untreated it is rapidly fatal for both mother and fetus. It is often suggested that the avoidance of eclampsia by skilled diagnosis of pre-eclampsia and appropriate therapeutic interventions is an indicator of high-quality obstetric care being provided to a population.

Pre-eclampsia can be superimposed on pre-existing essential, or renal, hypertension but of course recognizing the development of the secondary disease is in itself a diagnostic achievement. Where prevalence of hypertensive disorders varies between antenatal populations it is usually because of different background rates of chronic renal disease.

Incidence

Hypertensive disorders in total complicate about 8% of pregnancies and 10–15% of first pregnancies. Between 2 and 5% of women develop pre-eclampsia, three-quarters of the cases occurring in first pregnancies. (This is strictly in first pregnancy with the present partner; women who have more than one partner may be exposed to a similar risk of pre-eclampsia with each first pregnancy with each new partner.) The recurrence rate of pre-eclampsia in subsequent pregnancies is approximately 5%.

Pre-eclampsia appears to be additionally more common in pregnancies when there is excessive placental growth such as in poorly controlled maternal diabetes or in multiple pregnancy. It is also said to be more common in women with pre-existing hypertension.

Extensive family studies suggest a genetic

predisposition, pre-eclampsia being more common in the daughters of women who also suffered the condition compared with their daughters-in-law.

Clinical features

In the early stages of pre-eclampsia most women are asymptomatic but examination reveals the presence of hypertension and commonly oedema. Ward testing will confirm the presence of proteinuria. Based on the definitions above, the condition is usually classified as mild or severe.

In severe cases the woman will commonly complain of headache and upper abdominal pain which is thought to be caused by distension of the liver capsule. Visual disturbances in the form of blurring of vision or 'flashing lights' suggest retinal oedema. Peripheral oedema might be manifest by swelling of the fingers leading to difficulty removing rings, etc., and oedema of the face and eyelids. Examination might reveal exaggerated reflexes. Coagulation deficits may be revealed by the presence of spontaneous haemorrhage, typically from the gums or the renal or genital tracts.

Pathophysiology

Hypertensive disorders complicating pregnancy regularly occupy the first or second place in the list of the numerically most important causes of maternal death in the UK. They usually account for about 20% of true maternal deaths (maternal death ascribed solely to complications of pregnancy) and terminal pathological features are renal failure, hepatic or adrenal failure often secondary to interstitial haemorrhage. Pulmonary oedema with or without pulmonary haemorrhage may be terminal events, as may be a picture of cardiomyopathy caused by multiple intramural haemorrhages.

The initiating pathological abnormality can be detected on microscopy of the spiral arteries in the placental bed. In the physiological situation trophoblast cells invade the lining of the arteries and cause the destruction of the smooth muscle layer at between 16 and 20 weeks' gestation. A muscular, narrow lumen high-pressure vessel becomes converted into a low-resistance vessel with slow rate of flow. It is felt that these physiological changes are essential to normal placental perfusion and allow a 10-fold increase in blood supply to the intervillous space of the placenta. In the woman who is going to develop pre-eclampsia the normal extent of arterial invasion by trophoblast is arrested at the decidual layer and does not enter the inner third of the myometrial layer (uterine wall). There is therefore an abnormal narrow arterial segment which later in the

pregnancy is often the site of acute atherosis. Vascular damage leads to interruption of blood flow and placental infarction. Widespread pathological change in the vessels of the placental bed reduces the blood flow which normally perfuses the placenta. The more extensive the anatomical problem, the more likely it is that the disease will manifest early. Reduced placental perfusion triggers a signal from the fetal–placental unit which raises the maternal systemic blood pressure in an attempt to maintain perfusion across the spastic segments of the abnormal spiral arteries.

As the fetus grows the demand for placental perfusion increases, and sooner or later hypertension develops. Because in most cases there is a prolonged preclinical phase, there is widespread feeling that prophylactic and therapeutic intervention in high-risk women might prevent deterioration. However the anatomical abnormality is already present and no known therapeutic intervention is available to restore normal anatomy to the placental bed. The sequences of secondary events and their eventual effects are outlined in **Table 2**.

In summary, the essential pathological feature of pre-eclampsia is widespread spasm of small blood vessels throughout the body. There is reduction in circulating plasma volume leading to an increase in blood viscosity. Increased sensitivity of the arterioles to pressor substances such as angiotensin triggers increased blood pressure. In the early stages of the disease the increased systemic blood pressure compensates for vascular spasm of the placental bed and maintains blood flow, but as the spasm becomes

Table 2 Pathophysiology of pre-eclampsia

Abnormal vascular anatomy	Suppressed aldosterone release
Reduced placental perfusion	Reduced plasma volume
Raised systemic blood pressure	Raised blood viscosity
Abnormal vascular sensitivity to pressor agents (angiotensin)	Placental vascular sludging
Vascular spasm	
Reduced vasodilatory prostaglandins (prostacyclin)	
Increased vasoconstrictor prostaglandins (thromboxane)	
Placental vascular thrombosis	**Tissue thromboplastin release**
Reduced placental perfusion	Disseminated intra-vascular coagulation
	Renal vascular fibrin deposition
	Proteinuria

worse this mechanism eventually fails. Renal biopsies of women with pre-eclampsia have shown a characteristic abnormality with swelling of the endothelial lining of the capillaries. Reduction in the ability of the kidney to filter blood caused by blockage of the capillaries leads to reduced sodium filtration and sodium and water retention. In turn this causes widespread oedema with the swelling of the hands, feet and face which has been described above. The abnormalities of coagulation which occur are initially mild and well compensated and may be diagnosed by a fall in the platelet count accompanied by a slight rise in fibrin degradation products (FDP). In severe cases this may proceed, to disseminated intravascular coagulation (DIC) with local damage, particularly in the brain and the kidneys. This pathological development can be made worse by FDP-induced hypocoagulability. Typically in the complicated cases there is DIC-associated haemorrhage both externally and within tissues such as the kidney, adrenal gland, pituitary gland, liver and brain. Jaundice is a feature of severe cases of pre-eclampsia but is also seen in a variant of pre-eclampsia known as HELLP syndrome which is recognized by the presence of haemolysis, elevated liver enzymes, and a low platelet count.

Before irreversible complications have set in, the process can be reversed and a complete resolution of signs and symptoms obtained by delivering the baby. This is a straightforward option and usually taken up when the baby is mature enough to survive independently. With modern neonatal care, delivery would usually be undertaken in the presence of deteriorating pre-eclampsia from about 32 weeks of gestation onwards. Clinical difficulties arise in the management of the apparently severe case at a gestational age where the fetus might not be expected to survive and a balance between the fetal interest and the maternal interest may be impossible to strike.

In the face of deteriorating pre-eclampsia there is an increase of the perinatal mortality rate (deaths *in utero* + deaths in the first week of life per 1000 births) Some of these babies die before birth as a result of compromised placental blood flow, while others may die of complications of prematurity after medical intervention as described above. Where the disease remains mild, however, there is no increase in perinatal mortality and the pregnancy can usually be prolonged, with or without the use of hypertensive drugs, to a stage at which the baby is capable of survival.

Long-term follow-up has revealed no excess of complications in the newborn over and above those which might be expected as a result of the premature birth, when that has taken place.

Prophylaxis and Treatment

The idea that the complications of pre-eclampsia can be prevented has gained considerable currency since the work of Wallenberg published in 1986 suggested that low-dose aspirin might prevent deterioration of pre-eclampsia in women at risk. The basis of the hypothesis was that aspirin, being a prostaglandin synthetase inhibitor, would prevent the imbalance between prostacyclin and thromboxane in which thromboxane effects predominate, i.e. vasoconstriction and thrombosis (see Table 2). Since this publication extensive international studies have addressed the question as to whether low-dose aspirin can prevent the onset or modify the deterioration and complications of pre-eclampsia. The overall position is genuinely confused. Where the study design has included only primigravid women the balance of evidence favours a reduction in the instance of proteinuric pre-eclampsia. Both of the large studies which have included women in the second and subsequent pregnancies, judged to be at increased risk, demonstrated no clear benefit either in terms of the rate of progression to pre-eclampsia, or indeed in any reduction in perinatal deaths.

In the area of medical treatment a whole series of hypotensive drugs and anticonvulsants have been found to have a place in the management of severe pre-eclampsia or eclampsia itself, but when the condition is severe enough to justify the use of these drugs, then it is likely that delivery is urgent. Chronic use of hypotensive drugs has been considered in three other situations. There seems to be little doubt that in those who have essential or renal hypertension requiring hypotensive treatment their drugs should be continued throughout pregnancy as required. Some modern hypotensive drugs are not safe for use in pregnancy and should be reviewed in the prepregnancy period. The second area for drug treatment which seems to be established is in preventing superimposed pre-eclampsia in women with established mild hypertension in early pregnancy. For instance a pioneering study found that in mild hypertensives treated throughout pregnancy with methyldopa, none of the 117 women on treatment subsequently developed a blood pressure in excess of 180 over 120 mmHg, whereas this occurred in 11 of 122 untreated controls. In terms of treatment of established pre-eclampsia, two studies using β-blocking drugs have shown significant benefits in terms of reduction of blood pressure and in prevention of deterioration of severe pre-eclampsia as well as prevention of the development of proteinuria. General clinical opinion is that a β-blocker or combined α- and β-blocker is appropriate treatment for women with mild pre-eclampsia who are judged to be too early in pregnancy for delivery to be undertaken safely in the fetal interest. No advantage has been shown to the treatment of mild pre-eclampsia in late pregnancy when delivery of the fetus is a safe option.

Nutrition in the aetiology, prophylaxis and treatment of pre-eclampsia

In reviewing the published studies on nutrition and pre-eclampsia it is very important to bear the background of each study in mind. One possibility is that nutritional factors may influence proneness to develop the disease. Some populations or subgroups may be at increased risk because of their habitual diet and so dietary modification might reduce the risk of the disease. Second, dietary modification might reduce the risk of complications in the subject who is going on to develop the disease because the pathological vascular changes described above are already established before diagnosis. This is the situation analogous to the idea of aspirin prophylaxis discussed above. Third, it is possible that in the presence of the established disease with hypertension and/or proteinuria nutritional interventions may beneficially modify the progress of the disease, or indeed alleviate it. Intuitively the second and third areas for research seem more likely to prove fruitful than the first. If there were an environmental factor such as nutrition in pre-eclampsia, then this would certainly have come to light as a result of epidemiological studies, but in fact it is the case that the disease is widespread throughout all human populations with a roughly comparable incidence. Of some interest is the fact that a similar syndrome is not recognized in any animals, with the possible exception of the gorilla.

Interest in nutritional factors in the aetiology of pre-eclampsia stems from three sources. First, reported geographical difference (since reported to be false owing to difficulties in ascertainment, especially in developing countries) in the 1930s suggested that diet may be important. For example, meat-eating Muslims were reported as having higher incidences of pre-eclampsia than Hindus (vegetarian). Second, the lower incidences of pre-eclampsia during wartime (a reduction during World War I and during the Dutch Hunger Winter of 1944–45, followed by an increase after World War II) were assumed to be caused by dietary deficiencies during wartime: other demographic changes were not considered. The fall in pre-eclampsia in 1915 preceded the food shortage, as the rise in 1919 preceded its alleviation; thus dietary restrictions cannot be implicated. The third source of interest came from an apparent association of pre-eclampsia with social class, with the assumption that pre-eclampsia was associated with a poorer diet among lower social classes. This association is now doubtful as again other factors, such as availability of antenatal care, were not considered, but it gave support to proponents of a dietary aetiology.

Advocates of a nutritional basis for pre-eclampsia have had considerable influence in the past, with weight restriction in particular becoming an integral part of antenatal prevention of pre-eclampsia. This view is now not widely held, and has minimal influence on current antenatal practice. Greater influence has been exerted by Thomas Brewer. He maintains that pre-eclampsia is a disease of maternal malnutrition, whose symptoms can be largely eliminated by eating a well-balanced diet with adequate protein, energy, vitamins and minerals. Weight restriction should be avoided. This theory has not been substantiated scientifically, but Brewer's work has been a major influence and source of information, not least through women's self-help groups. It seems certain that in general terms Brewer's advice has been of some benefit in improving the diet of pregnant women and in eliminating widespread weight restriction, or salt or water restriction, but there is no evidence at present that it has led to a reduction in the incidence of pre-eclampsia.

Current scientific knowledge suggests that dietary manipulations have no effect on the prevention of pre-eclampsia, but may be able to prevent or moderate the secondary features of the disease.

Maternal weight

Maternal obesity is associated with an increased risk of essential hypertension and, possibly secondary to this, pre-eclampsia. (Obese women must have blood pressure measurements performed with a large cuff; otherwise artificially high readings will be obtained.)

Underweight women (at least 20% below ideal body weight-for-height) may also be at increased risk, although this has still to be validated.

Maternal weight gain in pregnancy has attracted a lot of attention, with advice to restrict weight gain in the hope of preventing pre-eclampsia being widespread. A higher weight gain in the second half of pregnancy is associated with an increased risk of pre-eclampsia, but the overlap between those remaining normotensive and those with pre-eclampsia is so large that weight gain is not a very useful predictive factor.

The association has led to attempts at prevention of weight gain, with dramatic improvements in pre-eclampsia rates claimed with intensive antenatal care and dietary advice (high-protein, low-carbohydrate, low-weight-gain diet). There is no evidence that it was the dietary advice, rather than intensified antenatal surveillance, which caused the reduction.

Controlled trials have failed to show any effects of dietary restriction. A comparison of two groups of women, one given dietary advice to gain an 'ideal' weight and the other with no dietary advice, resulted in the advice group achieving the ideal weight but with no reduction in pre-eclampsia. Similarly, no benefit in pre-eclampsia rates can be shown with weight reduction in either high weight gainers or obese women, even though a reduction in weight gain can be achieved.

Energy intake

There is no evidence that the overall nutritional intake or energy intake differs between women with and without pre-eclampsia. Interventions aimed at ensuring an optimal diet improved the quality of the maternal diet, but failed to affect the incidence of pre-eclampsia.

Protein

Pre-eclampsia is associated with low protein levels in the maternal plasma, which have an effect on fluid balance in the body. This has led to interest in the effect of protein supplementation in prevention and treatment of disease.

Dietary surveys and biochemical markers of protein intake and development of pre-eclampsia have failed to show an association between protein intake and the development of pre-eclampsia.

Studies on dietary supplementation also provide little evidence. An influential early report concluded that a high-protein diet did not increase the incidence of pre-eclampsia, and this led to support for dietary supplementation to prevent pre-eclampsia. However, despite attempts since then, there have been no scientifically adequate studies establishing or refuting a relationship between protein supplementation and pre-eclampsia.

Salt

Dietary sodium is considered to be an important factor in the development of essential hypertension in nonpregnant subjects. It therefore seems likely that interest will be generated again in the role of salt in the aetiology of pre-eclampsia. At present there is no evidence to suggest a causative role. On the contrary, in theory salt restriction may exacerbate pre-eclampsia by further reducing plasma volume.

Salt restriction was practised widely early in the twentieth century for the treatment of oedema in pregnant and nonpregnant subjects. It was subsequently applied to the prevention of pre-eclampsia, without any scientific basis. Two studies comparing high and low salt intakes failed to show any differences in outcome; one study showed fewer cases of pre-eclampsia in the high-salt group.

Vitamins and minerals

Calcium is considered to be important in the regulation of blood pressure, with the flow of calcium ions into cells being essential for contraction of the muscle cells in blood vessel walls. Blockage of this flow with calcium-blocking drugs may be used for the control of blood pressure in both pregnant and nonpregnant subjects. It would therefore seem theoretically possible that calcium restriction may prevent pre-eclampsia.

Despite this theory there is recent evidence that women with pre-eclampsia may have low calcium intakes, and that calcium supplementation may reduce the levels of hypertension seen in pre-eclampsia. A randomized controlled trial, in which either 1.5 g of elemental calcium per day or placebo was administered to healthy pregnant women in their first or second pregnancy from 26 weeks' gestation, showed a reduction in term SBP and DBP of 4–5 mmHg in the treated group. The incidence of pregnancy-induced hypertension was 11% in the placebo group and 4% in the calcium group, although on the number studied this difference was not statistically significant. The whole question has recently been reviewed in a meta-analysis of 14 published trials of calcium supplementation versus placebo in pregnancy. The pooled estimate in terms of calcium supplementation and reduction of pre-eclampsia was of an odds ratio of 0.38 (95% Cl 0.22–0.65) in those who took a calcium supplement. This would obviously be a worthwhile reduction of considerable clinical importance. A similar reduction was observed in the incidence of hypertension alone, but when other outcomes were considered there was only a small nonstatistically significant reduction in preterm delivery. This might be expected to reflect the major benefit if such treatment were worthwhile. The conclusion was that it might be thought that pregnant women known to be at risk of pre-eclampsia should consider taking a calcium supplement. Since this meta analysis a further randomized study in the USA involved 4589 women in their first pregnancies, given 2 g of elemental calcium or placebo daily from 13–21 weeks of gestation has been reported. Calcium supplementation did not prevent pre-eclampsia, gestational hypertension or adverse perinatal outcomes.

The benefit of calcium supplements in women on calcium deficient diets remains a possibility.

The role of zinc may be important: low plasma zinc concentrations have been found in women with severe pre-eclampsia, and a lower incidence of PIH has been reported among women who had received zinc supplementation, despite the fact that this supplementation did not raise plasma zinc concentrations. A randomized placebo-controlled study in the UK failed to confirm this finding and further studies are needed.

Supplementation with folic acid or vitamin B has been shown to be ineffective, but multivitamins and mineral supplementation may be useful. One study failed to show any beneficial effect of supplementation (cereal plus vitamin A plus vitamin D) but two other studies have suggested a reduction in pre-eclampsia in the group supplemented with multivitamins and minerals. This area requires further scientific investigation.

A large-scale supplementation study was performed by the People's League of Health in the UK in the 1940s. Women taking daily supplements of vitamins and minerals containing iron, calcium, iodine, manganese, copper, vitamin A and D, or no supplement, were compared for their rates of pre-eclampsia, defined as hypertension with albuminuria. There was a significant reduction in the incidence of pre-eclampsia in primiparous women, 4.5% versus 6.4%, but the difference was nonsignificant in the multiparous group, 3.2% versus 4.6%.

Other supplementation studies have shown no significant benefit or have been methodologically unsatisfactory. In retrospect, and in view of the comments above, it is possible that this study also demonstrated a calcium supplementation benefit.

Polyunsaturated fatty acids

Interest has been raised in the relationship between prostaglandins and the development of pre-eclampsia. An alteration in the ratio of these naturally occurring compounds in the body could underlie the spasm of blood vessels seen in pre-eclampsia.

Experimentally, linoleic acid supplements result in a reduction in sensitivity of blood vessels to substances controlling blood pressure. Deprivation of essential fatty acids in pregnant rabbits has been shown to increase this sensitivity; hence there is a theoretical possibility that linoleic acid supplementation may prevent pre-eclampsia.

Fish oil has been thought to interfere with prostaglandin metabolism as a result of its rich n-3 fatty acid content. Dietary supplements result in reduced formation of the less biologically active thromboxane A_3 and increased formation of prostacyclin I_3, whose activity is equal to that of prostacyclin I_2. In PIH the production of thromboxane A_2 is elevated and supplementation with n-3 fatty acids inhibits its production. This suggests a possible role for fish oil in prevention of PIH.

Circumstantial support for a role of prostaglandins comes from the Faroe Islands where the diet is rich in fish oils. The incidence of pre-eclampsia in the Faroes is lower than on the mainland, but again a causative role has yet to be proved. Dietary surveys among pregnant women with and without pre-eclampsia have failed to show any difference in fatty acid intake. A recent publication of a randomized controlled trial of fish oil supplementation in late pregnancy in 533 women, where one group was supplemented with fish oil containing 2.7 g per day of n-3 fatty acids and the controls to olive oil or no oil supplementation in a 1:1 ratio, there were no significant difference in absolute levels of systolic or diastolic blood pressure between the three groups with advancing pregnancy. Mean DBP was 68.3 mmHg in the fish oil group, 68.8 mmHg in the olive oil group, and 68.3 mmHg in the untreated group. Fifteen women developed PIH and five developed pre-eclampsia; eight of the PIH group were in the fish oil group, but none of the pre-eclamptics were. This interesting piece of work suggests that while there is no beneficial effect of fish oil supplementation in terms of reducing blood pressure overall, and indeed it is unlikely that it significantly reduces the incidence of PIH, it may in fact have a significant beneficial effect in prevention of pre-eclampsia. At the time of writing a major multicentre randomized trial is in progress, but has not yet been reported.

Conclusions

It is unlikely that any nutritional aetiology for pre-eclampsia will be identified. The areas currently being explored such as polyunsaturated fatty acid supplementation may very well turn out to be of value in preventing the serious complications of the disease. Indeed, nutritional interventions of this nature may prove more acceptable and easier to implement than the use of pharmaceutical drugs.

See also: **Calcium**: Physiology. **Epidemiological Studies**: Role and Interpretation. **Fatty Acids**: Health Effects of n-3 Polyunsaturated Fatty Acids. **Fish**: Nutritional Value. **Health Foods**: Dietary Supplements - Micronutrients. **Hypertension**: Nutritional Management. **Infants**: Low-birthweight and Preterm Infants. **Pregnancy**: Energy Requirements and Metabolic Adaptations; Nutrient Requirements; Appropriate Maternal Weight Gain; Role of Placenta in Nutrient Transfer. **Prostaglandins and Leukotrienes**: Physiology. **Salt**: Epidemiology. **Zinc**: Physiology.

Further Reading

Boucher HC, Guyatt GH, Cook RJ et al (1996) Effect of calcium supplementation on pregnancy induced hypertension and pre-eclampsia. A meta-analysis of randomised controlled trials. *Journal of the American Medical Association* **275**:1113–1117.

Beroyz G, Casale R, Farrieros A et al (1994) Clasp: a randomised trial of low dose aspirin for the prevention and treatment of pre-eclampsia amongst 9,364 pregnant women. *Lancet* **343**:619–629.

Campbell DM (1983) Dietary restriction in obesity and its effect on neonatal outcome. In: Campbell DM and Gilliner MDG (eds) *Nutrition in Pregnancy*, pp 243–250. London: RCOG Press.

Davey D and MacGillivray I (1988) The classification and definition of the hypertensive disorders of pregnancy. *American Journal of Obstetrics and Gynecology* **158**:892–898.

Green J (1989) Diet and prevention of preeclampsia. In: Chalmers I, Enkin M and Keirse MJNC (eds) *Effective Care in Pregnancy and Childbirth*, vol. 1, pp 281–300. Oxford: Oxford University Press.

Levine RJ, Hauth JC, Curet LB et al (1997) Trial of calcium to prevent pre-eclampsia. *New England Journal of Medicine* **337**:69–76.

MacGillivray I (1983) *PreEclampsia. The Hypertensive Disease of Pregnancy*. London: WB Saunders.

Pickles CJ, Broughton-Pipkin F and Symonds EF (1992) A randomised placebo controlled trial of labetalol in the treatment of mild to moderate pregnancy induced hypertension. *British Journal of Obstetrics and Gynaecology* **99**:964–968.

Salvig JD, Olsen SF and Secher NJ (1996) Effects of fish oil supplementation in late pregnancy on blood pressure: A randomised controlled trial. *British Journal of Obstetrics and Gynaecology* **103**:529–533.

Winick M (1989) *Nutrition, Pregnancy and Early Infancy*, pp 114–119. Baltimore: Williams & Wilkins.

PREMENSTRUAL SYNDROME

Nutritional Aspects and Management

Miriam Coelho de Souza, Departamento de Nutrição, Universidad de Mogi das Cruzes, São Paulo, Brazil

Ann F Walker, Hugh Sinclair Unit of Human Nutrition, The University of Reading, Reading, UK

Premenstrual syndrome (PMS), the common disorder which affects woman of reproductive age, is characterized by changes in mood, behaviour or mental and physical functioning in the luteal phase of the menstrual cycle, and yet has no defined cause for its aetiology. The different hypotheses proposed in the literature indicate several mechanisms and hence a range of possible therapeutic strategies. The involvement of nutritional factors in PMS has allowed a dietary approach for the management and treatment of women experiencing the condition. This article focuses on the definition, classification and prevalence of PMS, emphasizing the hypotheses of aetiology, including dietary factors, in the relief of PMS symptomatology.

Definition, Classification and Prevalence

Premenstrual Syndrome (PMS), or Premenstrual Dysphoric Disorder (PMDD), is an association of distressing physical, psychological, and/or behavioural symptoms which occur in the luteal phase (second half) of the menstrual cycle of sufficient severity to interfere with the normal activities and personal relationships of many women. Although the late luteal phase is the most common time for symptoms of PMS to be experienced, occasionally symptoms may occur as early as ovulation. To be classified as PMS, symptoms must be relieved by the onset of or during menstruation. Indeed, a symptom-free week after menstruation is necessary for differential diagnosis from other gynaecological or psychiatric disorders.

Despite the plethora of research studies on the subject, there exists no commonly agreed definition of PMS among gynaecologists and researchers. The lack of consensus is probably due to the large number of symptoms described. PMS was previously associated only with nervous tension and termed Premenstrual Tension (PMT). However, this term is no longer used as it only describes a limited range of the numerous symptoms experienced by many women. The most commonly mentioned symptoms of PMS are now grouped into psychological and somatic categories (**Table 1**).

Classification

The variable symptoms of PMS have been classified into four main categories by the American clinician and researcher Abraham, in an attempt to facilitate research and elucidate the aetiology of PMS and its links with lifestyle, including diet (**Table 2**). Abraham contended that each PMS category may exist alone or in combination with other categories. For example, PMS-D normally manifests itself in association with PMS-A, which is usually exhibited first.

Although other classification systems for PMS symptoms have been suggested, there is little evidence to suggest any greater merit of them over Abraham's system. In 1992 an attempt was made to systematize criteria and procedures for diagnosing PMS as LLPDD (Late Luteal Phase Dysphoric Disorder) in the *Diagnostic and Statistical Manual of*

Table 1 Summary of the most common premenstrual symptoms

Psychological	Somatic
Aggression	Abdominal bloating
Agitation	Acne/spots
Anorexia	Breast swelling
Anxiety	Breast tenderness
Craving for sweets	Change in bowel habit
Argumentative	Clumsiness
Confusion	Constipation
Crying/easy upset	Cramps
Decreased alertness	Diminished activity
Decreased libido	Diminished efficiency
Depression	Diminished performance
Emotional liability	Dizziness
Forgetfulness	Heart pounding
Hopelessness	Hot/cold flushes
Hunger	Headache
Impulsive behaviour	General pain/aches
Increased appetite	Infections, e.g. cold
Lethargy	Passing water frequently
Insomnia	Migraine
Irritability	Nausea/sickness
Lack of inspiration	Oedema
Loss of attention	Poor concentration
Loss of concentration	Swelling of extremities
Loss of confidence	Weight gain
Loss of self-esteem	
Pessimism	
Loss of self-control	
Nervous tension	
Mood swings	
Sadness	
Violent feelings	
Social isolation	
Suicidal tendency	
Tiredness	

Table 2 Abraham's classification of premenstrual symptoms

PMS category[a]	Symptoms
PMS-A (Anxiety)	Anxiety, irritability, mood swings, nervous tension
PMS-H (Hydration)	Weight gain, abdominal bloating and tenderness, breast tenderness, swelling of the extremities
PMS-C (Craving)	Premenstrual increased appetite, craving for sweets, fatigue, palpitations, headache
PMS-D (Depression)	Depression, withdrawal, lethargy, forgetfulness, confusion, insomnia, difficulty verbalizing

[a]PMS (premenstrual syndrome) is used in place of Abraham's PMT (premenstrual tension).

Menstrual Disorders. Despite this, there remains much confusion surrounding the classification of PMS symptomatology, which has led to difficulties of data interpretation and diagnosis.

In the absence of quantifiable signs of PMS, most studies have relied upon the self-reporting of symptoms. The methods have largely fallen into two categories: the use of a retrospective Menstrual Health Questionnaire (MHQ) or use of a prospective Menstrual Diary (MD). While the MHQ may be helpful in screening prospective volunteers for studies of PMS, the requirements for a useful instrument for assessing PMS must include the use of prospective recording and the quantification of symptoms which identify and exclude psychiatric occurrences.

Prevalence

PMS can first appear at any stage in the reproductive life of a woman. However, the most prevalent age of onset is usually from 28 to 34 years and symptoms may be first noticed following pregnancy or oral contraceptive use. The reported prevalence of PMS differs greatly from 21% to 90% of specific female populations studied. Some of this variability relates to the difficulty of a precise definition of PMS, its classification and the reporting method used. In addition, other factors such as age, parity, race, culture, psychopathology, menstrual characteristics, occupation, social activities, family life, lifestyle and stress may play a part. Indeed, reaction to stress has been advocated by a number of gynaecologists as an underlying cause of PMS.

The Aetiology of PMS

Various hypotheses have been implicated in the aetiology of PMS, including interaction between ovarian steroid hormones, endogenous opioid peptides, central neurotransmitters, eicosanoids, and peripheral autonomic and endocrine secretions. Despite all the investigations relating to these diverse fields, there is no firmly established biological pattern for PMS and its pathophysiology still remains obscure.

Gonadal hormone imbalance

As early as the 1930s, it was suggested that PMS was caused as a result of excessive levels of the female sex hormones in the blood. Later, deficient blood levels of progesterone were blamed, so that by the 1960s PMS treatment was dominated by progesterone administration. Despite this, the findings from several studies showed no clear link between low blood progesterone levels and the severity of the condition.

More recently, attention has been given to the significance of the oestrogen-to-progesterone ratio as a factor triggering PMS. In particular, it has been postulated that women with PMS-A (Anxiety) have increased plasma concentrations of oestrogen relative to progesterone in the luteal phase, compared with normal women. One possible mechanism is that low plasma blood levels of oestrogen and progesterone early in the luteal phase in PMS sufferers lead to an increased secretion of gonadotrophic hormones from the pituitary which, in turn, leads to a rise in oestrogen in the late luteal phase, owing to the stimulation of ovarian follicles. These follicles rapidly regress under the influence of the luteal secretion of progesterone. Excess oestrogen in the luteal phase may be the cause of fluid retention, breast tenderness, changes in carbohydrate metabolism and mood swings associated with PMS. Although the ovarian hormone imbalance hypothesis remains unproven, administration of progesterone in the latter half of the cycle continues to be the first-line treatment for PMS by general practitioners in the UK.

The existence of subgroups of PMS of varying aetiology may account for clinical observations that some women with severe premenstrual depression report, paradoxically, a worsening of symptoms during progesterone treatment. Indeed, such women have been reported to respond to oestrogen treatment. Their condition may be linked to progesterone excess, which has been suggested to occur in some women who experience PMS symptoms at mid-cycle. High luteal progesterone levels may lead to depletion of oestrogen receptors of the hypothalamus, which is consequently less sensitive to oestrogen, requiring a higher mid-cycle oestrogen surge for normal pituitary response. This is followed by an abrupt and pronounced oestrogen drop at mid-cycle which may even result in symptoms of hot flushes.

Angiotensin

It has been demonstrated that symptoms such as irritability, withdrawal, depression, hopelessness, tension, lack of initiative and weight gain are linked to changes in urinary potassium/sodium ratio, which in PMS women is higher 3–4 days before the onset of menses, and lower for the rest of the cycle, compared with that in normal women. The reason for this may lie in the enhanced secretion of angiotensin promoted by higher progesterone levels during the luteal phase of the menstrual cycle.

Angiotensin is a hormone with vasoconstricting properties which acts on the kidneys by constricting efferent arterioles. This reduces blood flow from the kidneys and enhances excretion of the electrolytes sodium and potassium. An electrolyte imbalance occurring in PMS may alter neurotransmitter activity, in particular monoaminergic (noradrenalin and serotonin) and cholinergic neurotransmitters, affecting behaviour and mood regulation. Angiotensin is also known to act directly on the adrenal cortex to promote aldosterone release (see below), and may be involved in stimulating antidiuretic hormone (ADH) secretion by the pituitary. Both of these hormones are directly involved in the maintenance of electrolyte balance.

Aldosterone

Aldosterone, the steroid hormone secreted by the adrenal cortex, promotes retention of sodium and excretion of potassium by the kidneys. An elevated secretion of aldosterone in the luteal phase would tend to lead to sodium retention and, as a result, promote fluid retention. Whether the high aldosterone levels found in PMS are a consequence of direct adrenal cortex stimulation or are promoted by increased adrenocorticotrophic hormone (ACTH) secretion from the pituitary is unknown, although circulating levels of gonadal hormones are known to influence electrolyte homeostasis via the angiotensin–aldosterone system, as stated above.

Prolactin

Fluctuation in prolactin levels has also been suggested as a cause for PMS. Prolactin is a pituitary hormone which regulates mammary gland development in women and is necessary for successful lactation. Latent hyperprolactinaemia is thought to predispose nonlactating women to premenstrual breast pain. Prolactin levels rise acutely due to stress and higher levels promote sodium, potassium and water retention. Noradrenalin has been implicated in promoting prolactin release, while the presence of dopamine reduces it. Both stress and high oestrogen levels promote noradrenalin secretion, while dopamine may be reduced in those consuming a diet low in certain nutrients (see below).

Thyroid stimulating hormone

In one study, a high percentage of women with PMS who were treated with thyrotrophin releasing hormone (TRH) were found to have low thyroid function. As thyroid hormone supplementation has been used in the past as antidepressant therapy, some recent studies have attempted to link thyroid dysfunction to PMS. Indeed, there are suggestions that PMS may be an early symptom of a progressive thyroid disorder and the severity of PMS increases as thyroid dysfunction progresses. Nevertheless, the use of thyroid hormone for the treatment of PMS remains controversial.

Opioids, peptides and endorphins

Opioid and neuropeptides receptors are found in nerve synapses of the brain and the gastrointestinal tract, and their suppression by morphine is known to alter the perception of pain. Endorphins are substances also found in the brain and in the pituitary gland that have opiate-like activity. Indeed, the endogenous opioid of the pituitary, β-endorphin, has been described as the body's own analgesic, absence of which leads to symptoms sometimes described by PMS sufferers: cramping, craving for carbohydrates, insomnia, irritability and nausea. This observation has led to the hypothesis that β-endorphin deficiency may be the cause of PMS. If this is the case, then it is only likely to hold true for a minority subgroup of PMS because although lacrimation, diarrhoea and pupillary dilation are common in β-endorphin deficiency, they are not common in PMS. On the other hand, PMS symptoms such as depression, breast swelling or tenderness, and weight gain are not common features of β-endorphin withdrawal.

Neurotransmitter imbalance

Depression is a commonly reported symptom of PMS. Monoamines, such as noradrenalin and serotonin, are known chemical mediators of mood. Monoamine oxidases (MAOs) and catechol-O-methyl transferase are enzymes that metabolize monoamines and thus decrease the amounts available for neural transmission. Their activity can be affected by the greater fluctuation in progesterone and oestrogen levels found in women with PMS compared with normal women.

Oestrogen suppresses MAO type A activity and increases MAO type B activity. While MAO type A enzymes are involved in the breakdown of adrenalin, noradrenalin, serotonin and dopamine, MAO type B enzymes deactivate only dopamine. Thus suppression of type A and increase in type B enzyme activity results in excess serotonin, adrenaline and noradrenalin and a relative deficiency of dopamine, a situation which may trigger anxiety and depression.

PMS and Dietary Factors

Various reports, many of a preliminary nature, or based on clinical experience, suggest that women suffering from PMS consume more sugar, refined carbohydrate and dairy products and less fibre, B complex vitamins, iron, zinc and magnesium than normal women.

Carbohydrate

Carbohydrate-rich meals have been shown to improve mood in women with premenstrual depression. The reason for this has been indicated in animal studies: the availability of tryptophan to the brain increases following such meals. As tryptophan is a substrate for the synthetic pathway to serotonin, levels of this neurotransmitter rise, while levels of other neurotransmitters are maintained. Hence premenstrual craving has been suggested as a compensatory response to deal with a relative lack of serotonin during this phase of the cycle. Indeed, PMS symptoms of craving, particularly for sweet foods, may be a useful indicator of the cyclical changes that occur in brain neurotransmitters in women.

Increased energy intake due to craving has been shown to range from 380 to 2000 kJ per day (90–500 kcal per day) during the luteal phase compared with the follicular phase in women with PMS. However, there is no obvious pattern of macronutrient intake. Some women consume more carbohydrate, some more fat, and some more protein. As might be expected, the increase in energy intake is accompanied by an increase in certain nutrients, such as magnesium, vitamin D, potassium, phosphorus and riboflavin. Enhanced intake of several of these nutrients has been linked to alleviation of PMS symptoms (see below).

Magnesium

Magnesium deficiency has been proposed as a causative factor in PMS. Magnesium has a sedative effect on neuromuscular excitability and is involved as an enzyme cofactor in many reactions in the body. In the metabolism of essential fatty acids it also acts as a cofactor, working together with vitamin B_6, zinc, niacin and vitamin C. At the cell membrane, magnesium acts as a regulator of both membrane rigidity and ion exchange, helping to maintain electrolyte balance. In addition, it moderates the action of calcium in stimulating cell functions such as hormone secretion.

Modern Western diets high in refined cereals lack magnesium. Many dietary surveys, including those sponsored by governments throughout the Western world, have shown that the mean intake of magnesium for women is below recommended dietary standards, with subgroups having exceptionally low intakes. Decreased intake or absorption or increased renal excretion may lead to a reduced intracellular magnesium. Indeed, perhaps the most consistent physiological abnormality yet found for PMS subjects has been the reduced magnesium level in red blood cells compared with controls.

While severe magnesium deficiency is characterized by a progressive muscle weakness, failure to thrive, neuromuscular dysfunction and tachycardia, symptoms of marginal deficiency are more subtle. Nevertheless, there is accumulating evidence to suggest that magnesium supplementation of the diet can alleviate a variety of conditions in which there is an element of muscular overcontraction, such as hypertension and tension headaches. The stress of modern living plays a part by enhancing magnesium excretion in the urine even in otherwise normal subjects. This sets up a vicious circle, as magnesium deficiency itself increases susceptibility to stress by increasing the secretion of ACTH-mediated adrenal androgen, which is a central nervous system depressant.

Several mechanisms proposed for the development of PMS symptoms have been claimed to be promoted by magnesium deficiency. Low magnesium status may also be responsible not only for exacerbating gonadal hormone imbalance in women, but may promote an increase in the aldosterone-to-oestrogen ratio. Enhanced aldosterone levels promote potassium and magnesium excretion and sodium retention, thus inducing fluid retention as found in PMS-H. In addition, deficient levels of magnesium decrease blood glucose control in two ways: by decreasing the ability of the liver to metabolize glucose and by increasing insulin secretion in response to glucose. Hence, changes in appetite and craving, both common PMS symptoms, may be closely linked to magnesium deficiency through loosening of blood glucose control. A low blood glucose supply to the brain may cause craving as a signal for increased energy intake. Even the decreased brain dopamine levels postulated to be responsible for anxiety and irritability of PMS (see above) may be exacerbated by magnesium deficiency.

In support of some of these hypotheses, several scientific reports have demonstrated a role for magnesium supplementation in relieving symptoms of PMS. In particular, Italian workers have shown that in 32 women, who were given 360 mg magnesium or placebo per day from the 15th day of the menstrual cycle to the onset of menstrual flow, magnesium supplementation was an effective treatment for low mood in PMS.

Vitamin B$_6$

Vitamin B$_6$, in the form of pyridoxal phosphate (PLP), is a cofactor in a large number of important enzymic reactions throughout the body. Therefore it is a cofactor in serotonin and dopamine production in the hypothalamus. High oestrogen levels may lead to a relative deficiency in vitamin B$_6$ by altering tissue distribution and by inducing hepatic enzymes which increase the rate of vitamin B$_6$ breakdown. An oestrogen-induced deficiency in vitamin B$_6$ may reduce the synthesis of both serotonin and dopamine, an action that may alter the delicate balance between the two, normally maintained by adequate synthesis and breakdown. Adequate intakes of vitamin B$_6$ are also thought to be necessary for the maintenance of normal intracellular magnesium levels, as this vitamin plays a fundamental role in the active transport of magnesium through the cell membrane. Thus, a synergetic role for magnesium and vitamin B$_6$ has been suggested, although this remains to be tested.

High doses of vitamin B$_6$ have been found to be effective in treating most of the most common symptoms of PMS in several double-blind, placebo-controlled trials. For this reason administration of dietary supplements is a popular therapy for PMS used by many medical practitioners. However, as large doses have been associated with dependency and sensory neuropathy, doses higher than 50 mg per day should be avoided.

Essential fatty acids

Gamma-linolenic acid (GLA) is thought to be the major active constituent of evening primrose oil (EPO), which is self-administered by many women for the relief of PMS symptoms. GLA is a fatty acid belonging to the n-6 essential fatty acid family. It is formed in the body from linoleic acid (from seed oils such as sunflower). In the body linoleic acid is elongated and further desaturated in a several-step process leading to arachidonic acid. GLA is one of the intermediates in this pathway, which, in response to a stimulus, can act as a substrate for a series of enzyme reactions giving rise to series 1 eicosanoids (biologically active substances, including prostaglandins), which have a broad range of activities in the body.

Under similar circumstances arachidonic acid present in the cell membrane gives rise to series 2 eicosanoids, which tend to be pro-inflammatory unless moderated by the presence of series 1 and 3 eicosanoids (series 3 are from n-3 fatty acids, which are high in fish oils). In people consuming a Western diet, it is common to find that when cell membranes are stimulated (e.g. stressed), production of series 2 eicosanoids is dominant. This is because arachidonic acid can be provided in the preformed state in the diet in meat, and body status of GLA and ω-3 fats can be low. Although low status of the latter may derive from poor diet choice, low GLA status may result because of the slow action of the enzyme δ-6-desaturase, which is involved in the first desaturation step in the metabolism of linoleic acid. Its action is further slowed by viral infection, age, alcohol, stress and lack of magnesium or zinc in the diet.

The suggestion that PMS may be caused by eicosanoid imbalance is based on the assumption that failure of the normal conversion of linoleic acid to GLA results in low levels of prostaglandin E_1 (PGE_1) eicosanoids in relation to the other eicosanoids, and this sensitizes tissues so that they respond abnormally to normal levels of oestrogen and progesterone. In support of this hypothesis, studies from Japan, Finland and the UK have shown that women suffering from PMS have lower blood levels of GLA and DGLA (dihomo-γ-linolenic acid, a compound related to GLA), although linoleic acid levels are higher. Additional support for a therapeutic role of GLA in PMS comes from six double-blind, placebo-controlled studies which have shown a significant improvement in symptoms from a daily supplement of GLA in the form of EPO, although one further study carried out in Australia showed no benefit.

Cyclical mastalgia, or breast pain, in the premenstrual phase may or may not be accompanied by other symptoms of PMS. In any case, similar abnormalities in n-6 fatty acid profile of cell membranes to that described above for PMS have been found in this condition and good response to GLA supplementation has been reported. Indeed, EPO is commonly prescribed by breast surgeons as the first-line treatment for the condition. In one study nearly half of hospital outpatients with this condition showed a benefit of EPO treatment without side effects, although doses of at least 4 g per day are required.

Other nutrients

Apart from those already discussed, a role for deficiency of other nutrients in the aetiology of PMS has been suggested, although few well-designed studies have been reported. Studies in vitamin E-deficient animals suggest that vitamin E supplementation may enhance the production of eicosanoids of series 1 and reduce the release of arachidonic acid from phospholipids. Hence, this combined action would reduce the inflammatory tendency implicated in some forms of PMS. Two double-blind, placebo-controlled studies in the 1980s indicated that supplementation with vitamin E may alleviate PMS symptoms, but at least one other study reported no effect. In one of the positive studies, daily supplements of 300 IU significantly alleviated PMS symptoms of anxiety after 2 months, while 600 IU per day were required for the same duration to reduce PMS symptoms of craving and depression. These levels of vitamin E are far greater than can be obtained through diet.

Zinc deficiency may be involved in the aetiology of PMS. This suggestion stems from observations of low luteal-phase zinc levels in women suffering from PMS. Several mechanisms for involvement of zinc deficiency in PMS have been proposed. Zinc is involved in the regulation of pituitary hormone secretion, influencing, in particular, prolactin and luteinizing hormone activity, which may affect predisposition to PMS. Zinc is a modulator of endogenous opiate-receptor binding in the central nervous system, a system also implicated in the condition. Zinc also takes part in the synthesis of PGE_1 by its involvement in the release of DGLA and hence may influence eicosanoid balance (see above). Nevertheless, no placebo-controlled study has been carried out to show the effects of supplementary zinc as therapy for PMS.

Women with PMS have been reported to have higher intakes of calcium than normal women owing to excessive intake of dairy products. Foods in this group are characterized by having very high calcium-to-magnesium ratios and PMS sufferers have been reported to have diets with higher ratios than normal women. As a high intake of calcium is known to reduce magnesium absorption, a high calcium intake has been proposed to result in a chronic magnesium deficiency and PMS. It has also been postulated that excessive calcium intake may cause the behavioural changes of PMS by calcium interference with glucose breakdown as a source of energy to the brain. However, a controversial placebo-controlled study on 33 women showed that daily supplementation of 1 g of calcium for 3 months significantly reduced PMS symptoms of depression and fluid retention.

Caffeine

Several surveys of unselected women have shown that those who consume large amounts of beverages containing caffeine are more likely to suffer from PMS. Although constant consumption of low doses of caffeine may exacerbate the stress reaction and tendency to PMS, paradoxically, acute, high-dose consumption has been used to treat migraine headaches, although it was not reported whether these headaches were present premenstrually.

Botanicals

There has been renewed increased in recent years in the therapeutic applications of herbal medicine for a wide range of conditions. The active phytochemicals of the majority of commonly used herbs and their physiological effects are well reported. It is only recently, and mostly in Germany, that clinical studies of efficacy in treatment have been undertaken. There is no doubt from the clinical experience of practitioners that phytotherapy has much to offer for treatment of hormone imbalance syndromes in women, including PMS, but more research-based evidence is required.

An important herb used by phytotherapists to treat PMS is the chaste tree (*Vitex agnus-castus* L.). Extracts of the berries have been shown to reduce the abnormally high prolactin secretion of PMS via the ability of certain of its phytochemicals to mimic the action of dopamine by binding to dopamine receptors in the pituitary. Other herbs traditionally used in phytotherapy for PMS contain phyto-oestrogens. These molecules may have oestrogen-like action, either due to the steroidal nature of their active constituents (false unicorn root, *Chamaelirium luteum* A. Gray) or to the spatial similarity of active groups in their constituents, which allow them to bind to oestrogen receptors. Among the latter group are isoflavonoids and lignans, which appear to have 'adaptogenic' properties: they are weakly oestrogenic at low circulating oestrogen concentrations and anti-oestrogenic at high oestrogen concentrations. Isoflavonoids are present in soya bean and its products and in medicinal herbs such as black cohosh (*Cimicifuga racemosa* Nutt.); these show a beneficial effect in reducing symptoms of PMS and the menopause. Lignans are present in high concentration in seed coats, including wheat, and are especially high in linseed (*Linum ussitatissimum* L.). The presence of lignans may explain why women who eat high quantities of wholegrains, fruit and vegetables are less likely to suffer from PMS.

See also: **Appetite**: Psychobiological and Behavioural Aspects. **Behaviour**: Dietary Effects on Mood and Behaviour. **Brain and Nervous System**: Biology, Metabolism and Nutritional Requirements. **Carbohydrates**: Regulation of Carbohydrate Metabolism. **Cofactors**: Organic Cofactors; Inorganic Cofactors. **Health Foods**: Dietary Supplements - Micronutrients. **Hunger**: Overview. **Magnesium**: Physiology, Dietary Sources and Requirements. **Phytochemicals**: Epidemiological Factors. **Vitamin B₆**: Physiology.

Further Reading

Abraham GE (1982) Magnesium deficiency in premenstrual tension. *Magnesium Bulletin* 1:68–73.

Abraham GE and Rumley RE (1987) Role of nutrition in managing the premenstrual tension syndromes. *Journal of Reproductive Medicine* 32:405–422.

Backstrom T and Hammarback S (1986) Endocrinological aspects of the premenstrual syndrome. *Progress of Clinical and Biology Research* 225:421–428.

Brush MG, Watson SJ, Horrobin DF and Manku MS (1984) Abnormal essential fatty acid levels in plasma of women with premenstrual syndrome. *American Journal of Obstetrics and Gynecology* 150:363–366.

Chuong CJ and Dawson EB (1992) Critical evaluation of nutritional factors in the pathophysiology and treatment of premenstrual syndrome. *Clinical Obstetrics and Gynecology* 35:679–692.

Dalton K (ed.) (1984) *Premenstrual Syndrome and Progesterone Therapy*, 2nd edn. London: William Heinemann Medical Books Ltd/Year Book Medical Publishers Inc.

Facchinetti F, Borella P, Sances G, Fioroni l and Nappi RE (1991) Oral magnesium successfully relieves premenstrual mood changes. *Journal of the American College of Obstetrics and Gynecology* 78:177–181.

Gallant SJ, Popiel DA, Hoffman DM, Chakraborty PK and Hamilton JA (1992) Using daily rating to confirm premenstrual syndrome/late phase dysphoric disorder. *Psychosomatic Medicine* 54:149–166.

Janowsky DS, Berens SC and Davis J (1973) Correlation between mood, weight, and electrolytes during the menstrual cycle: a renin–angiotensin–aldosterone hypothesis of premenstrual tension. *Psychosomatic Medicine* 35:143–154.

London RS, Murphy L, Kitlowski KE and Reynolds MA (1987) Efficacy of alpha-tocopherol in the treatment of the premenstrual syndrome. *Journal of Reproductive Medicine* 32:400–404.

Piesse JW (1984) Nutrition factors in the premenstrual syndrome. *International Clinical Nutrition Review* 4:54–81.

Reid RL and Yen SSC (1981) Premenstrual syndrome. *American Journal of Obstetrics and Gynecology* 1:85–104.

Shangold GA (1993) The premenstrual syndrome: theories of etiology with relevance to the therapeutic use of GnRH agonists. *Seminars in Reproduction Endocrinology* 11:172–186.

Wurtman JJ, Brzezinski A, Wurtman RJ and Laferrere B (1989) Effect of nutrient intake on premenstrual depression. *American Journal of Obstetrics and Gynecology* 161:1228–1234.

PROBIOTICS AND PREBIOTICS

Definition and Role

R Fuller, Ryeish Green, Reading, Berkshire, UK

G Gibson, Microbiology Department, Institute of Food Research, Reading, Berkshire, UK

The human gut flora has both beneficial and pathogenic potentials with respect to host health. In recent years there has been much interest in manipulation of the microbiota composition in order to improve the health-promoting aspect. One approach is through dietary supplementation with live microorganisms, often lactic acid bacteria, that are perceived as positive in terms of health promotion. This is the probiotic concept. An alternative is to use selectively fermentable substrates (prebiotics) added to diet that stimulate the growth of the purported beneficial, indigenous bacteria – bifidobacteria or lactobacilli. Both approaches offer the potential for improved human health, either separately or in combination. As probiotics have been used in this respect for some years, it is this concept that will be discussed in greatest detail in this article.

Definition and Development

The sterile newborn infant rapidly becomes colonized by a vast array of microorganisms derived from its mother and the general environment. The gastrointestinal microbiota that results is a complex collection of microorganisms (mainly bacteria, but there may also be fungi and viruses present) which live in symbiotic association with the host. The component microorganisms interact with each other and with the host. The ultimate effects of such interaction can be beneficial: e.g. the gut microflora can aid digestive function, may increase the hosts energy supply through the fermentative production of short-chain fatty acids, as well as improve resistance to colonization by potentially pathogenic bacteria. However, it is possible that changes occur which have a detrimental effect on the host. Some of the postulated factors that can lead to such adverse changes are: emotional and physical stress; transmission of pathogens; compromise of the immune system; and use of medication such as antibiotics.

It is under these conditions that dietary supplementation designed to improve the microbiota composition can have a role to play. Probiotics, prebiotics and synbiotics are all mechanisms by which host health may be improved through fortification of selected bacteria in the gut. The formal definitions of each are given in **Table 1**.

Probiotics

Probiotics are microbial food supplements which are intended to have a beneficial effect on the consumer by changing the composition and/or metabolic activity of the gastrointestinal microflora. Their use embraces traditional yogurt and also more recently developed products such as bioyogurts and 'over the counter' freeze-dried preparations of lactic acid bacteria.

The desired characteristics of a probiotic are as follows:

Table 1 Definition of various mechanisms used to modulate the composition of the human large intestinal microflora

Term	Definition	Reference
Probiotic	A live microbial feed supplement which beneficially affects the host animal by improving its intestinal microbial balance	Fuller (1989, 1992)[a]
Prebiotic	A nondigestible food ingredient that beneficially affects the host by selectively stimulating the growth and/or activity of one or a limited number of bacteria in the colon, and thus improves host health	Gibson and Roberfroid (1995)[b]
Synbiotic	A mixture of pro- and prebiotics which beneficially affects the host by improving the survival and implantation of live microbial dietary supplements in the gastrointestinal tract	Gibson and Roberfroid (1995)[b]

[a]Fuller R (1989) Probiotics in man and animals. *Journal of Applied Bacteriology* **66**: 365–378; Fuller R (ed.) (1992) *Probiotics: The Scientific Basis*. London: Chapman & Hall.
[b]Gibson GR and Roberfroid MB (1995) Dietary modulation of the human colonic microbiota: introducing the concept of prebiotics. *Journal of Nutrition* **125**: 1401–1412.

- exerts a beneficial effect on the consumer, e.g. improved digestion or resistance to disease;
- is nonpathogenic and nontoxic;
- contains a large number of viable 'cells' (the minimum effective dose is not known);
- has the capacity to survive and metabolize in the gut (e.g. resistant to HCl and organic acids); and
- retains its viability during storage and use.

It is also preferable that a consumed strain has been isolated from the same animal species as its intended user. A crucial feature is maintenance of viability, both in terms of shelf life and after administration. This can be arduous to guarantee and it does not help if label specifications cannot always be confirmed. Survival after ingestion is extremely difficult to estimate, especially when the colon is the target organ. The future development of more efficient tagging systems as well as the molecular typing of bacterial genetic material (e.g. 16S ribosomal RNA) should improve the situation.

The history of probiotics is as old as the consumption of fermented milks, records of which exist from over 2000 years ago. However, at the beginning of the twentieth century probiotics were first put onto a scientific basis by the work of Metchnikoff at the Pasteur Institute in Paris. He contended that the normal microflora of the lower gut of humans was having an adverse effect on the host and that consumption of soured milks reversed this effect. Metchnikoff refined the treatment by using pure cultures of what is now called *Lactobacillus delbrueckii* subsp. *bulgaricus*, which in concert with *Streptococcus salivarius* subsp. *thermophilus* is used to ferment milk in the production of yogurt. Subsequently workers in the USA, reasoning that an intestinal isolate would colonize the gut more effectively, used *L. acidophilus*. Over the years many other species of microorganism have been used (**Table 2**). These consist not only of lactic acid bacteria (lactobacilli, streptococci, enterococci, lactococci, bifidobacteria) but also

Bacillus spp. and fungi such as *Saccharomyces* spp. and *Aspergillus* spp. Many of these isolates are of gut origin but some, such as the fungi, are from other sources and cannot grow in the intestine.

Selection of isolates for use in probiotic preparations has, in the past, been made on an *ad hoc* basis. Recently, with the demonstration that adherence to intestinal epithelial cells is an important aid to colonization, strains have been selected on this basis. However, adherence is not essential for successful colonization; fast growth in the gut and/or continuous administration will also allow some establishment. Nevertheless, use of adherent strains is an encouraging sign that producers are employing a more scientific basis for selection.

Probiotic Effects

Research into the potential for beneficial effects of probiotic preparations and products has been focused in the following areas:

- alleviation of the symptoms of lactose malabsorption
- improved natural resistance to infectious diseases of the intestinal tract
- the potential for suppression of cancer
- lowering of plasma cholesterol
- aiding digestion
- production of vitamins
- stimulation of the immune system.

Lactose malabsorption

The most scientifically based claim made for probiotics is alleviation of symptoms caused by lactose malabsorption. These include abdominal distension, excessive flatulence and/or diarrhoea. Over half the world's population is unable to utilize lactose effectively. In those who are lactose intolerant, the ability to digest lactose enzymically is lost after weaning when, under natural conditions, lactose would

Table 2 Lactic acid bacteria used in probiotic products for animals and humans

Lactobacilli	Streptococci (and other Gram-positive cocci)	Bifidobacteria
L. acidophilus	Lactococcus lactis subsp. cremoris	B. bifidum
L. casei	S. salivarius subsp. thermophilus	B. adolescentis
L. delbrueckii subsp. bulgaricus	Enterococcus faecium	B. animalis
L. reuteri	S. diaacetylactis	B. infantis
L. brevis	S. intermedius	B. longum
L. cellobiosus		B. thermophilum
L. curvatus		
L. fermentum		
L. lactis		
L. plantarum		

disappear from the diet. It is now well established that in this so-called 'lactase nonpersistent' group, lactose administered in yogurt can be utilized more efficiently than the same amount given in untreated milk. Results with milk fermented with *L. acidophilus* are more variable and may be strain dependent.

The basis for improved digestibility of lactose in yogurt is unclear, with some research results pointing to lactase activity of the bacteria, whereas other work indicates a stimulation of the host's mucosal lactase activity. A recent study which compared γ-eradicated lactobacilli with strains killed by shear forces concluded that although it was not necessary for the lactobacilli to be alive, it was important for the cells to be intact. The assumption was that the cell wall protected the intracellular β-galactosidase from the inimical effect of the gut. It would seem from this result that the breakdown of lactose by yogurt organisms is of microbial origin.

Intestinal infections

Various claims have been made for beneficial effects of probiotics against infectious diarrhoea conditions caused by bacteria and viruses. In a careful analysis of 14 published studies of the antidiarrhoeal effects of probiotics containing lactobacilli, bifidobacteria or enterococci it was found that only three gave unequivocal positive results. Of the eleven other trials, five were definitely negative but six, although they reported no positive results, were of questionable significance because of a poor experimental design and/or data analysis. Work in the treatment of antibiotic-associated diarrhoea using *Saccharomyces boulardii* is encouraging and may have future potential. Patients treated with antibiotics frequently develop a diarrhoea unrelated to their original disease condition. This is often due to overgrowth with *Clostridium difficile*, which in the untreated gut is suppressed by the normal microflora. Further antibiotic therapy is often unsuccessful and can even exacerbate the condition. In carefully conducted double-blind, placebo-controlled trials the incidence of diarrhoea has been reduced by 50% in those treated with a probiotic containing *S. boulardii*.

The manner in which probiotics may be of some use in the prevention or treatment of intestinal infections may be by:

- production of strong acids
- excretion of antimicrobial compounds
- metabolism of toxins
- occupation of potential colonization sites.

Suppression of cancer

No successful clinical trials using probiotics in cancer therapy have been made. Many of the results published are interesting but the problems of transposing observations from rodents, or *in vitro* cell lines, to humans should be borne in mind.

Bacterial enzymes which convert precarcinogens to active carcinogens are produced in the gut but their involvement in the pathogenesis of cancer is unclear. Nevertheless, these enzymes, which include β-glucuronidase, nitroreductase and azoreductase, do provide an index of the effect that probiotics may have on the metabolic activity of the gut microflora. *L. acidophilus* fed to healthy volunteers was shown to significantly decrease β-glucuronidase, nitroreductase and azoreductase activities. The same strain of *L. acidophilus* fed to rats associated with a human faecal flora significantly decreased β-glucuronidase and β-glucosidase activities.

In rats, several studies have attempted to relate probiotic treatment to chemically induced tumours. At present the results are unconvincing.

Effects on plasma cholesterol

Studies designed to show that probiotic supplementation can reduce plasma cholesterol concentrations and consequently reduce the risk of coronary heart disease have given variable data and no firm conclusions can be drawn. However, this area of research has attracted favour as the results are easily measurable, i.e. any change in plasma total or low-density lipoprotein (LDL) cholesterol levels can be determined in response to dietary intervention. It is critical, however, that such studies are carried out in different population subgroups, with appropriate controls and in a doubly blind manner. Potentially, a probiotic may:

- interfere with cholesterol absorption from the gut (e.g. by deconjugating bile salts)
- directly assimilate cholesterol
- produce metabolites (e.g. propionate) that affect the systemic levels of blood lipids.

Aid to digestion

It is a popular conception that probiotics aid digestion. This activity would be directly related to their viability and ability to colonize effectively. However, it is virtually impossible to demonstrate and therefore quantitate such an effect.

Production of vitamins

In vitro, some probiotic strains (e.g. bifidobacteria) are able to produce vitamins, largely of the B group.

Immune stimulation

One of the most interesting, scientifically, and perhaps most useful aspects of probiotic supplementation is the finding that it can provoke an immune response. It has long been known that γ-globulin levels are higher in conventional compared with germ-free mice, but it has now been shown that specific strains of lactobacilli and bifidobacteria can stimulate immunity in rodents. Some recent preliminary trials in humans have also shown promising results.

In animal models, probiotics have been shown to stimulate the production of antibody (local and systemic), enhance the activity of macrophages, increase γ-interferon levels and increase the concentration of natural killer cells. Obviously, the non-pathogenic nature of the probiotic is a prerequisite.

These findings extend the possible range of activities which could be expected from probiotics. In the past it has been thought that their influence was restricted to the gut, but it may be that probiotics also exert systemic effects.

Mechanisms of Probiotic Activity

The exact manner in which probiotics may achieve their effect(s) is still uncertain, but based on our knowledge of how microorganisms interact in complex populations, it is possible to speculate on the possible mode of action. On this basis we can recognize:

- chemical inhibition or stimulation
- competition for nutrients
- immune clearance
- competition for adhesion receptors.

Biochemical effects

Microorganisms can influence each other by producing chemical substances which have either an inhibitory or stimulatory effect. Many lactic acid bacteria are known to produce antimicrobial compounds. These are often peptides (bacteriocins) and normally have a narrow spectrum of activity, affecting only closely related species. They have not yet been shown to be active in the gut, but could have important ecological consequences by allowing the bacteriocin-producing probiotic organism to grow at the expense of other lactic acid bacteria indigenous to the intestine.

Short-chain fatty acids are common end products of metabolism that may also have a role to play in manifestation of the probiotic activity. It is possible that the intestinal pH may be lowered, in a microniche, to levels below those at which pathogens are able to compete effectively. Butyric acid in particular has been shown to be produced in inhibitory concentrations in the lower gut of rats.

The vitamin supply may also influence the composition of the flora, with some strains producing vitamins which others require.

Competition for nutrients

The gut provides a rich source of nutrients for the growth of microorganisms and it is difficult to imagine a situation where nutrients would become limiting. However, it only requires a lack of one essential nutrient for inhibition to occur. Inhibition of *Cl. difficile* by the indigenous microflora has been shown to depend, at least partly, on competition for glucose, N-acetylglucosamine and sialic acid.

Immune clearance

The immune response has obvious potential as a factor which might control the growth of microorganisms in the gut. Although the role of the immune system in controlling the indigenous flora is not clear, there is evidence that mixtures of *L. casei* and *L. acidophilus* elicit a protective effect against challenge with *Salmonella typhimurium*. This effect seems to be related to higher levels of circulating antibody in lactobacillus-treated mice. Theoretically, immune stimulation by probiotics may occur when culture viability is not in question, i.e. bacteria are antigenic whether they are dead or alive.

Competition for adhesion receptors

Perhaps the most convincing basis for microbial interaction in the gut is provided by work on microbial adhesion to intestinal epithelial cells. It has been established that many intestinal pathogens must adhere to the gut wall if they are to colonize and produce adverse effects. This enables them to counter the flushing effect of peristalsis which would otherwise remove them from the gut before they could have any effect. There is evidence to support the suggestion that probiotic organisms can pre-empt adhesion sites on the gut wall and thus prevent certain pathogens from adhering and subsequently colonizing.

In vitro studies, with human enterocyte-like Caco-2 cells, have shown that although different species of bifidobacteria had different adhesion abilities, a strain of *Bifidobacterium longum* which adhered well was also a good colonizer of the human gut, as measured by its appearance in large numbers in the faeces after administration.

Future Developments

The future development of probiotics is dependent on obtaining more evidence for and more information about how probiotics produce beneficial effects. When the biochemical basis of the probiotic effect is known, it may be possible to reproduce the effects using nonviable chemical preparations. This would be of great help to producers who have the task, unique to pharmaceutical preparations, of having to manufacture a product with a sustainable viable count of microorganisms.

There is already a move in that direction with the development of prebiotics. These are supplements administered specifically to stimulate probiotic microorganisms already resident in the lower gut. The definition of a prebiotic is given in Table 1 and the concept shown schematically in **Fig. 1**. An early example of a prebiotic was lactulose, which was used to stimulate bifidobacteria in the gut of formula-fed infants. Later, it was used to encourage growth of lactobacilli which lowered the pH and in turn reduced ammonia absorption, thus eliminating symptoms of hepatic encephalopathy.

More recently, the emphasis has been on oligosaccharides. The four types currently being exploited are:

- *trans*-galactosylated oligosaccharides (TOS)
- fructo-oligosaccharides (FOS)
- soya bean oligosaccharide extract (SOE)
- galacto-oligosaccharides (GOS).

Animal trials have also been undertaken with a manno-oligosaccharide. Inclusion in the diet improved the efficiency of food utilization and growth rate of turkeys. It has also been suggested that this oligosaccharide can block colonization sites often occupied by pathogens, stimulate a nonspecific immune response and adsorb mycotoxin. However, its efficacy in humans has not been tested.

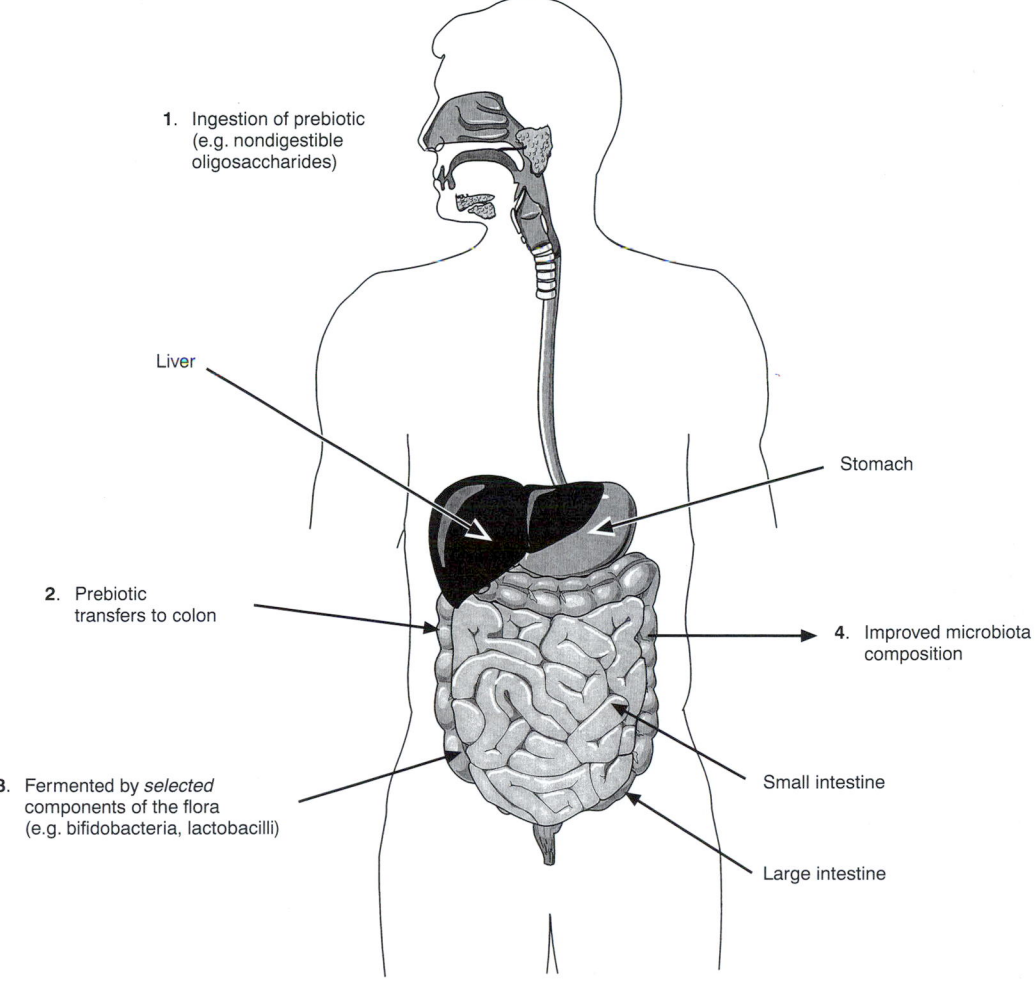

1. Ingestion of prebiotic (e.g. nondigestible oligosaccharides)

Liver

Stomach

2. Prebiotic transfers to colon

4. Improved microbiota composition

3. Fermented by *selected* components of the flora (e.g. bifidobacteria, lactobacilli)

Small intestine

Large intestine

Figure 1 Schematic representation of the prebiotic concept. (1) The prebiotic is ingested as a dietary supplement. (2) It transfers to the colon in an intact form. (3) A selective fermentation occurs which is directed towards 'health-promoting' microorganisms. (4) The microbiota composition is altered such that a potentially healthier community exists.

Similar oligosaccharides occur naturally in certain vegetables such as artichoke, chicory, garlic, leek and onion, but the low concentrations (never more than 20%) mean that the oligosaccharides are unlikely to be ingested in sufficient quantities to achieve dietary modulation of the gut flora. An alternative is the supplementation of common foodstuffs with purified preparations. Fructo-oligosaccharide addition (15 g per day) to the diet targets bifidobacteria in the colon. *In vitro* and *in vivo* human studies show that although other microorganisms (e.g. lactobacilli) are increased to a small degree, by far the most statistically significant effect is in the numbers of bifidobacteria, such that these bacteria become numerically predominant in faeces. This is because bifidobacteria possess enzymes that allow a preferred metabolism of the fructo-oligosaccharides.

Bifidobacteria have been shown to have a number of characteristics which have the potential to affect the health and wellbeing of the host. Bifidobacteria:

- produce organic acids (e.g. acetate) as metabolic end products which lower pH. This can be antibacterial, but may also protonate the potentially toxic NH_3 to form NH_4, which is less well absorbed from the gut;
- excrete antimicrobial agent(s) directed towards the activities of a variety of gut pathogens;
- produce B vitamins and digestive enzymes such as human casein phosphatase and lysozyme;
- stimulate the immune system, possibly to control harmful bacteria and malignant cells;
- restore indigenous flora after antibiotic treatment;
- lower blood lipid levels (shown in experiments with rats).

An enhanced bifidobacterial count in the lower gut may therefore have desirable effects on the host.

A further development is the use of synbiotics, where probiotics and prebiotics are combined. Thus, the live microbial additions would be used in conjunction with a specific substrate for growth. As such, improved survival and growth of the probiotic would occur. This approach offers increased efficacy to the probiotic concept, where strain survival is required and can be in doubt. The functionality of the prebiotic component would be directed both towards the live food addition as well as selected components of the indigenous flora.

Conclusions

The use of dietary supplementation to improve human health is an attractive concept. The targeting of beneficial microorganisms is a noninvasive approach that might be useful for the treatment and prophylactic management of some human diseases.

Extrapolations from animal or laboratory studies are only useful to define possible probiotic mechanisms and generate tools (e.g. genotypic bacterial probes) for use in volunteer trials. It is therefore important that carefully controlled human trials, involving modern methods of detection, are carried out in terms of probiotic/prebiotic survival and effect. In this way the potential for health promotion through microbiological means will be realized.

See Colour Plate 7.

See also: **Cancer**: Diet in Cancer Treatment. **Cholesterol**: Sources, Absorption, Function and Metabolism; Factors Determining Blood Cholesterol Levels. **Coronary Heart Disease**: Prevention. **Dairy Products**: Nutritional Value. **Diarrhoeal (Diarrheal) Diseases**: Nutritional Factors. **Food Intolerance**: Types and Incidence. **Immunity**: Physiological Aspects.

Further Reading

Fuller R (1989) Probiotics in man and animals. *Journal of Applied Bacteriology* **66**:365–378.

Fuller R (ed.) (1992) *Probiotics: The Scientific Basis*. London: Chapman & Hall.

Conway PL (1989) Lactobacilli: fact and fiction. In: Grubb R, Midvedt T and Norin E (eds) *The Regulatory and Protective Role of the Normal Microflora*, pp 263–281. Basingstoke: MacMillan Press.

Gibson GR and Roberfroid MB (1995) Dietary modulation of the human colonic microbiota: introducing the concept of prebiotics. *Journal of Nutrition* **125**:1401–1412.

Gilliland SE (1990) Health and nutritional benefits from lactic acid bacteria. *FEMS Microbiology Reviews* **87**:175–188.

Hamilton-Miller JMT, Shah S and Smith CT (1996) 'Probiotic' remedies are not what they seem. *British Medical Journal* **312**:55–56.

Hughes DB and Hoover DG (1991) *Bifidobacteria*: their potential for use in American dairy products. *Food Technology* **45**:74–83.

Huis in't Veld JHJ and Havenaar R (1991) Probiotics and health in man and animals. *Journal of Chemistry, Technology and Biotechnology* **51**:562–577.

Lee YK and Salminen S (1995) The coming age of probiotics. *Trends in Food Science and Technology* **6**:241–245.

Metchnikoff E (1907) *The Prolongation of Life*. New York: Putnam & Sons.

Sanders ME (1993) Effect of consumption of lactic cultures on human health. *Advances in Food and Nutrition Research* **37**:67–130.

Sanders ME (1993) Summary of conclusions from a consensus panel of experts on healthy attributes of lactic cultures: significance of fluid milk products containing cultures. *Journal of Dairy Science* **76**:1819–1828.

Savage DC and Fletcher M (1985) *Bacterial Adhesion:*

Mechanisms and Physiological Significance. New York: Plenum Press.

Simon G and Gorbach SL (1984) Intestinal flora in health and disease. *Gastroenterology* 86:174–193.

Tannock GW (1995) The role of probiotics. In: Gibson GR and Macfarlane GT (eds) *Human Colonic Bacteria: Role in Nutrition, Physiology, and Pathology*, pp 257–271. Boca Raton: CRC Press.

Processed foods *see* **Food Processing**: Nutritional Influences.

PROSTAGLANDINS AND LEUKOTRIENES

Physiology

S Katayama, Saitama Medical School, Saitama, Japan

James B Lee, State University of New York, Buffalo, New York, USA

Prostaglandins (PGs) were discovered in the 1930s and were first chemically isolated and identified in sheep seminal vesicles and renal medulla in the 1960s. Although, together with thromboxanes (TXs) and leukotrienes (LTs), the PGs possess the most potent and most divergent biological activities of any naturally occurring compounds, their true physiological role in many instances remains unknown. From a pathophysiological viewpoint, an absolute or relative deficiency of PGs relative to TXs has been implicated in the aetiology of hypertension, thrombosis and atherogenesis for many years. Since PGs and TXs are derived from essential fatty acids, the role of dietary intake of these fatty acids in PG and TX production, particularly in relation to the cardiovascular system, will be examined. The possible role of dietary essential fatty acids on LT and PG production in relation to inflammation, the immune system and gastric function will also be discussed.

Chemistry

In the 1930s it was reported that fresh human semen caused rhythmic contractions of human endometrium. These observations were confirmed in sheep seminal vesicles and the active substance was called 'prostaglandin'. In the 1960s, PG was determined to be a mixture of biologically active compounds which were isolated from sheep seminal vesicles and identified as PGE_{1-3} and PGF_{1-2}. These compounds were independently isolated from extracts of rabbit kidney medulla and identified as PGA_2, PGE_2 and PGF_{2a}. Later, in 1975, the compound TXA_2, which is a potent vasoconstrictor and platelet aggregant, was isolated, while in 1976 prostacyclin (PGI_2) was discovered. Prostacyclin is synthesized mainly by endothelial cells, prevents platelet aggregation and is vasodilatory. Studies of the slow-reacting substance of anaphylaxis (SRS-A) showed that it was composed of certain LTs which are products of leucocyte membrane arachidonate.

The PGs are composed of a basic 20-carbon fatty acid chain containing a cyclopentane ring, the so-called hypothetical prostanoic acid. The carbons are numbered 1 to 20 from the carboxyl to the terminal methyl group. The designations of PGE_1, PGE_2 and PGE_3 refer only to the number of double bonds in the aliphatic side chains. The PG_2s are the most abundant naturally occurring class. For PG_1s the precursor is 8,11,14-eicosatrienoic acid (dihomo-γ-linolenic acid), and for PG_2s the precursor is 5,8,11,14-eicosatetraenoic acid (arachidonic acid). The PG_3s can be formed from 5,8,11,14,17-eicosapentaenoic acid (EPA).

The LTs were named because they were discovered in leucocytes and because the common structural feature is a conjugated triene. Various members of the group have been designated alphabetically and the subscript denotes the number of double bonds.

Analysis of Prostaglandins and Leukotrienes

Prostaglandins and leukotricenes are present in many different biological samples including plasma. However, eicosanoid quantification in the peripheral circulation does not accurately reflect *in vitro* biosynthesis and disposition because of rapid turnover, low concentration, metabolism by lung and liver, and sample processing problems. For example, plasma concentrations of PGE_2 and TXB_2 determined by gas chromatography have been reported to be 12 and several pg ml^{-1}, respectively. Urinary samples can be utilized to evaluate *in vivo* PGs or LTs for the kidneys, while pleural fluids or bronchial lavages can be used to evaluate for pulmonary production. The most accurate reflection of local synthesis is obtained by incubations of slices or homogenates of specific cells and/or tissues with measurement of PG, TX or LT production *in vitro*.

The most precise method to determine PGs and LTs is undoubtedly gas chromatography linked to mass spectrometry. However, this type of analysis is not widely available. Radioimmunoassay using a specific antibody against various PGs or LTs and [3]H- or ^{125}I-labelled tracer are available, highly specific, sensitive and relatively inexpensive and have been widely utilized for eicosanoid analysis.

Prior to radioimmunoassay, extraction of arachidonic acid metabolites from plasma, urine or tissue homogenates may be required. The most common method is to extract acidified aqueous solution with an organic solvent such as diethylether or ethyl acetate, followed by purification by column chromatography with a octadecylsilyl (ODS) silica (SEP-PAK C_{18})® cartridge, silicic acid or sometimes by high-performance liquid chromatography (HPLC).

Biosynthesis of Prostaglandins and Leukotrienes

Arachidonic acid and its metabolite by-products (the arachidonic acid cascade) are important mediators of a number of physiological phenomena. As shown in **Fig. 1**, the rate-limiting step in the formation of the metabolites of arachidonic acid seems to be the initial step, i.e. the release of free arachidonic acid from the cell membrane phospholipid pool mediated through activation of phospholipase A_2. Phospholipase C may play another role in arachidonic acid release through liberating a diglyceride, which is then hydrolysed by another lipase to yield arachidonic acid. Following the release of arachidonic acid, enzymes are involved in its subsequent metabolism. Prostaglandin synthetase (PGS), i.e. cyclooxygenase, is a key enzyme in controlling the extent of prostanoid biosynthesis. It possesses two enzymatic activities: cyclooxygenase activity, the conversion of arachidonic acid (AA) to PGG_2; and peroxidase activity, the conversion of PGG_2 to PGH_2 catalysing a two-electron reduction of PGG_2 to PGH_2. PGH_2 is the common precursor for a number of biologically important prostanoids, i.e. PGI_2, TXA_2, PGE_2, PGD_2 and $PGF_{2\alpha}$, formation of which occurs through the action of the respective synthetases called PGI synthetase, TXA synthetase, PGE synthetase, PGD synthetase and PGF synthetase. Cyclooxygenase is distributed in most mammalian tissues. Two isoforms of cyclooxygenase have been identified and cloned. Cyclooxygenase 1, originally cloned from ram seminal vesicles and subsequently from mouse tissues and human endothelial cells and platelets, is considered to be constitutive, while cyclooxygenase-2, cloned from chicken embryonic fibroblasts and mouse 3T3 fibroblast, is highly inducible. Cyclooxygenase-1 activity is inactivated by aspirin through acetylation of the serine residue and inhibited by other non-steroidal anti-inflammatory agents, whereas cyclooxygenase-2 is inhibited by glucocorticoids. Various biological activities are due to binding of prostanoids to the receptors on the cell surface. With the advent of molecular biology techniques, eight prostanoid receptors have been cloned so far: TP, IP, FP, DP and four classes of EPs (EP_1, EP_2, EP_3 and EP_4). Prostanoid receptors have seven transmembrane domains and are members of the superfamily of the rhodopsin receptor. These receptors are classified into three groups: IP, DP, EP_2 and EP_4 are the stimulatory receptors which generate cAMP, resulting in vasodilation; TP, FP and EP_1 are the G protein-linked receptors which increase intracellular Ca^{2+} concentration, resulting in vasoconstriction; and EP_3 is an inhibitory receptor which inhibits the elevation of cAMP, resulting in vasodilation.

In the second pathway of arachidonic acid metabolism, 5-lipoxygenase forms a series of products named LTs, as illustrated in **Fig. 2**. 5-Hydroperoxyeicosatetraenoic acid (5-HPETE) may be enzymatically dehydrated to LTA_4 ((5S)-*trans*-oxido-7,9-*trans*-11,14-*cis*-eicosatetraenoic acid). Subsequent enzymatic hydrolysis of LTA_4 results in LTB_4 ((5S, 12R)-dihydroxy-6-*cis*-8, 10-*trans*-14-*cis*-eicosatetraenoic acid). LTA_4 also reacts with sulfhydryl compounds by addition of gluthathione (Glu–Cys–Gly) by glutathione-(S)-transferase, yielding LTC_4 ((5S)-hydroxy-(6S)-glutathionyl-7,9-*trans*-11, 14-*cis*-eicosatetraenoic acid). LTD_4 can be then produced from LTC_4 through elimination of glutamyl residue by a γ-glutamyl transpeptidase. The remaining peptide bond in LTD_4 is hydrolysed to give LTE_4 by a dipeptidase.

Physiological Action of Prostaglandins and Leukotrienes

The relative amounts of compounds formed depend

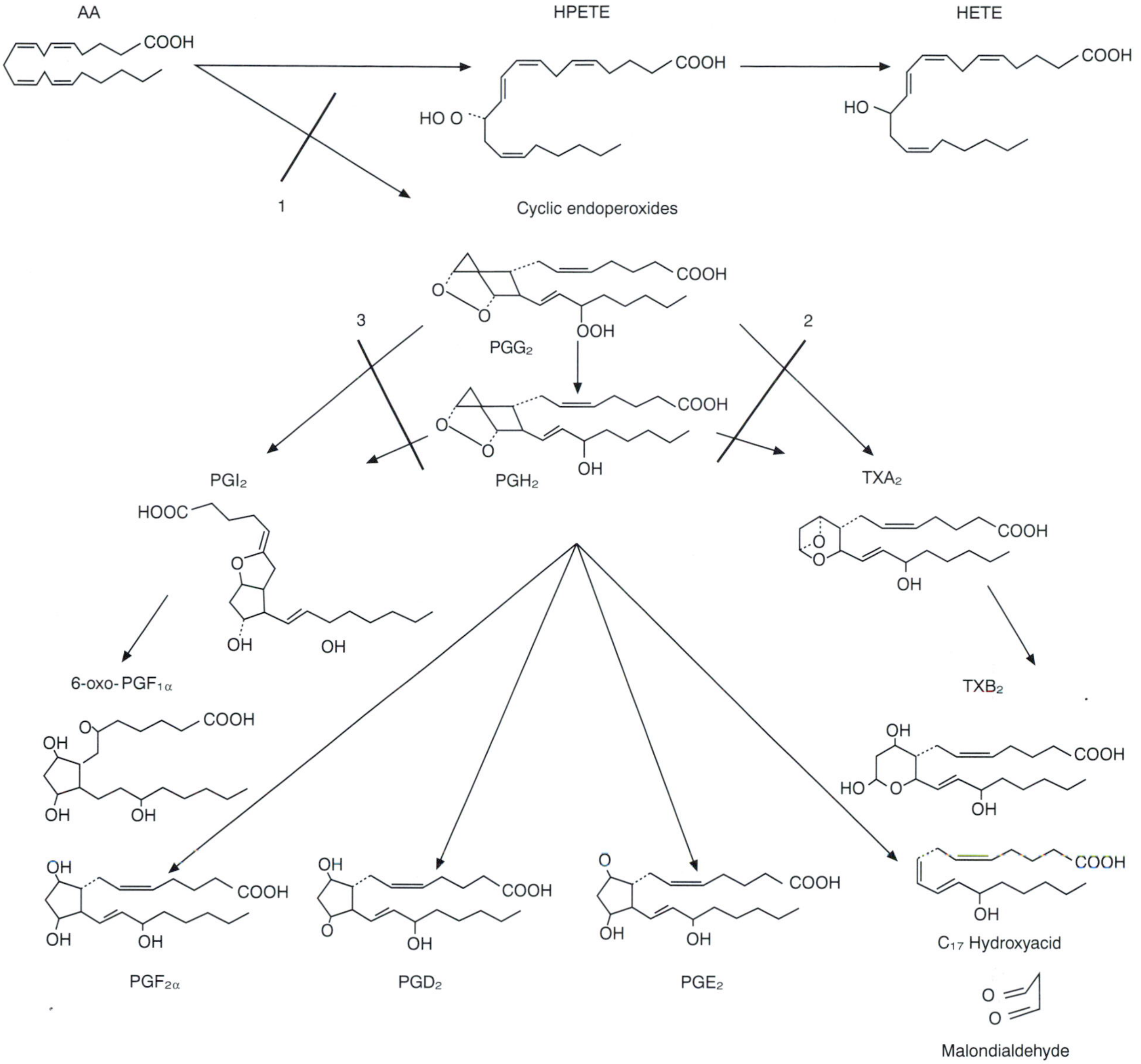

Figure 1 Metabolic pathways of prostaglandin (PG) biosynthesis from arachidonic acid. Sites where cyclooxygenase inhibitors (aspirin-like drugs), thromboxane synthetase inhibitors (imidazole and 1-methyl imidazole) and prostacyclin synthetase inhibitors (15-hydroperoxyarachidonic acid and 13-hydroperoxylinoleic acid) act are indicated by the numeral 1, 2 and 3, respectively. AA, arachidonic acid; HETE, 12-hydroxyarachidonic acid; HPETE, 12-hydroxyperoxyarachidonic acid; PGI_2, prostacyclin: TXA_2, thromboxane A_2; TXB_2, thromboxane B_2. From Moncada S and Vane JR (1978) Unstable metabolites of arachidonic acid and their role in haemostasis and thrombosis. *British Medical Bulletin* **34**:129–135. Reproduced with permission from Churchill Livingstone.

on the tissue or cell being studied. When platelets are activated by collagen or thrombin, unstable TXA_2 is predominant, resulting in a rapid and irreversible aggregation of platelets and contraction of vascular smooth muscle cells. However, vascular endothelial cells form unstable PGI_2 which has a potent vasodilating and antiaggregatory action similar to stable PGE_2. Neutrophils as well as monocytes or macrophages produce PGE_2, while PGD_2 is formed in mast cells and basophils. In the kidney, renal interstitial cells and collecting duct cells synthesize PGE_2, the renovasculature endothelia synthesize PGI_2, while

glomerular mesangial endothelia form $PGF_{2\alpha}$. In addition to PGE_2, other PGs are also produced in the gastrointestinal tract. PGE_1, PGE_2 and their analogues, administered exogenously, suppress gastric acid secretion and possess the property of protecting the gastric mucosa against necrotizing agents such as absolute ethanol or hydrochloric acid (cytoprotection).

Prostaglandins play many physiological roles in human reproduction, e.g. menstrual regulation, pregnancy and induction of labour. PGE_1, PGE_2 or their analogues are now widely used clinically for

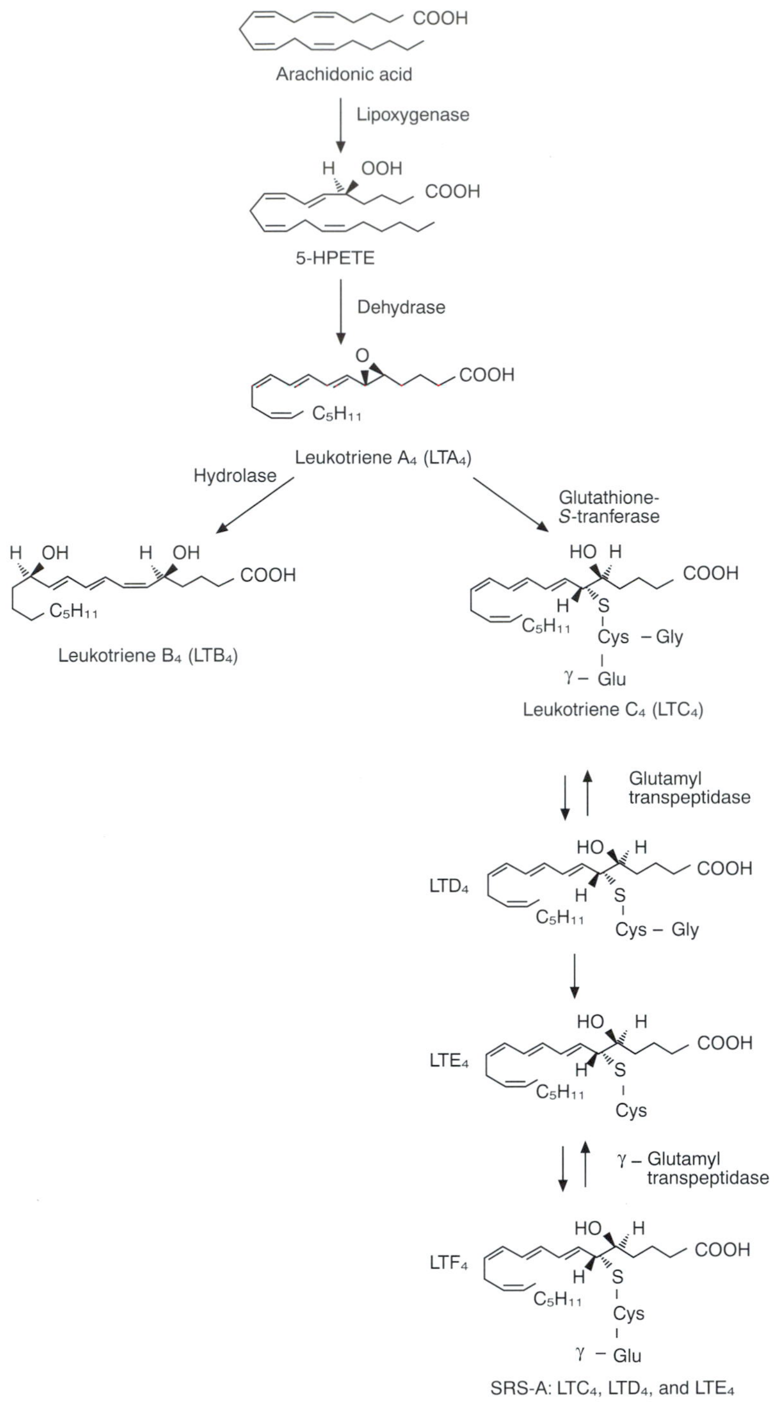

Figure 2 Formation of leukotrienes from arachidonic acid by way of 5-lipoxygenase pathway. From Samuelsson B (1983) Leukotrienes: mediators of immediate hypersensitivity reaction and inflammation. *Science* **220**:568–575. Copyright by the Noble Foundation, 1983. Reproduced with permission from The American Association for the Advancement of Science.

induction of labour or abortion. PGE_2 and PGI_2 produce or augment vasodilation and enhance bradykinin or serotonin-induced pain, resulting in redness, heat, swelling and pain in the inflammatory processes. PGs as such as PGE_2 and PGI_2 have also been shown to increase during pyrogen-induced fever. In fact, PGE_2 administered into the hypothalamus

increases body temperature while PGD_2 deceases body temperature, indicating a possible role of PGs in human thermoregulation. PGs and TXs, and some monohydroxy derivatives of arachidonic acid (hydroxyeicosatetraenoic acids) also have chemotactic effects on polymophonuclear leukocytes. LTB_4 is not only chemotactic for neutrophils and eosinophils but also for monocytic macrophages. These phenomena are considered to be the initial events of the inflammatory response. Polymorphonuclear leucocytes only survive for hours in the inflammatory area, while monocytes may stay for weeks and finally may be transformed to fibroblasts, initiating the repair process of the wounds. Furthermore, monocytes can present antigens to cells capable of producing antibodies and can synthesize all the members of the arachidonic acid cascade. Monocytes are also capable of forming interleukin, interferon, complement and protease, all of which participate in tissue disruption. The lipoxygenase system is more important in subacute and chronic inflammation, whereas the cyclooxygenase system produces or modulates acute inflammation. The anti-inflammatory action of aspirin, indomethacin and other non-steroidal anti-inflammatory agents is produced almost entirely by PG synthesis inhibition, as shown by studies revealing inhibition of PG cyclooxygenase with aspirin.

LTC$_4$, LTD$_4$, LTE$_4$ and their *trans* isomers do not have any effects on chemotaxis, enzyme release or leucocyte aggregation. However, they possess potent biological activities, which were formerly attributed to SRS-A release from sensitized lungs treated with a specific antigen. These compounds may be important mediators in asthma and other acute hypersensitivity reactions. Contraction of guinea pig ileum and other smooth muscle by LTs exhibits a slow onset and relaxation, which is the basis of the original designation as SRS-A. This distinguishes these substances from histamine, bradykinin and PGF$_{2\alpha}$. LTC$_4$ and LTD$_4$ are respectively about 200-fold and 20 000-fold more potent than histamine in promoting small airway contraction. In addition, these LTs cause rapid arteriolar contraction and promote plasma leakage in postcapillary venules. They also slow the rate of mucus clearance from the airways of patients with asthma after the inhalation of antigen, and increase the amount of mucous glycoprotein synthesis in the airways.

With the advent of cloning of various prostanoid synthetases and their receptors, vast numbers of prostanoid analogues synthesized so far will be retested. Diverse physiological actions of various prostanoids will be shortly reevaluated and reclassified based on their specific receptors using a specific agonist and antagonist. For example, inhibition of vasopressin-induced water reabsorption in kidney or histamine-induced gastric acid secretion can be explained by EP$_3$-mediated inhibition of adenylate cyclase. Furthermore, genetic engineering such as prostanoid receptor knockout mice may be able to clarify a specific physiological role of PGs and LTs.

Effects of Diet on Prostaglandin Formation

Polyunsaturated fatty acids

It was first shown in 1974 that dietary deficiency of essential fatty acids in animals results in hypertension that depends on a high sodium intake, thus being very similar to renoprival hypertension or experimental 'salt-sensitive' hypertension. This was later confirmed in 1983 and the blood pressure response was attributed to a dietary deficiency of linoleic acid. However, it would appear unlikely that this is a cause of human hypertension since selective deficiency of essential fatty acid in the human diet is rare.

A low prevalence of atherosclerosis and a low mortality from myocardial infarction among greenland Eskimos, despite a diet high in fat and cholesterol, suggested that dietary fish may have some properties that could prevent coronary artery disease. The Eskimos consume 5–10 g daily of the long-chain n-3 polyunsaturated fatty acids EPA (C_{20}; 5n-3) (**Fig. 3**) and docosahexaenoic acid (C_{22}; 6n-3) which are present in fish oils. When n-3 fatty acids are included in the diet, EPA inhibits conversion of linoleic acid and competes with arachidonic acid for the 2-acyl position in membrane phospholipids, reducing plasma and cellular levels of arachidonic acid. In addition, EPA competes with arachidonic acid as the substrate for cyclooxygenase. The platelets produce biologically inactive TXA$_3$ instead of TXA$_2$. However, PGI$_2$ synthesis in endothelial cells is not markedly inhibited and any newly synthesized PGI$_3$ has the same potency as PGI$_2$. Thus diet abundant in EPA may inhibit platelet aggregation and cause vascular dilatation, resulting in blood pressure reduction. In fact, a meta-analysis including 1356 subjects from 31 placebo-controlled trials confirmed the blood pressure lowering effects of dietary fish oils. The hypotensive effect was dose-dependent; there was little change in blood pressure at doses lower than 3 g per day (corresponding to 250 g salmon) but, above this, a 0.66 mmHg fall in systolic blood pressure was demonstrated per 1.0 g increase in n-3 polyunsaturated fatty acid. The hypotensive effect appeared greater in patients with hypertension,

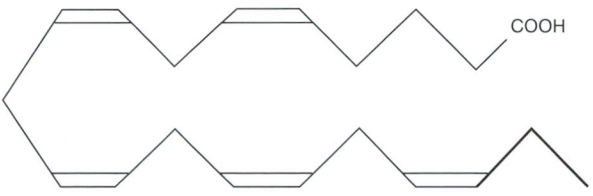

Figure 3 Eicosapentaenoic acid (EPA).

hypercholesterolaemia or coronary heart disease. Mechanisms by which n-3 polyunsaturated fatty acids may act might be attributed to attenuated constrictor responses to vasoactive agents, such as noradrenaline and angiotensin II, an attenuated sympathoadrenal stimulation, and/or modulated production or release of nitric oxide from vascular endothelial cells. However, the safety and long-term benefits of this treatment have been questioned because PGE_2 synthesis is inhibited and replaced by PGE_3 from EPA in the fish oils. Since renal blood flow is dependent on PGE_2 in renal disease and during volume contraction, any decrease in PGE_2 might result in more severely compromised renal function.

The other merit of dietary fish or fish oil supplements may be its lowering effect on plasma lipid. The principal effect has been found to be a reduced production of triacylglycerols and very low-density lipoprotein (VLDL) in the liver. Because VLDL is a precursor of low-density lipoprotein (LDL), a secondary reduction in LDL-cholesterol is also seen. Such conditions are considered to reduce the atherogenicity of lipoprotein particles. Furthermore, n-3 fatty acids have been reported to improve insulin sensitivity in skeletal muscle, possibly through a decrease in triacylglycerol accumulation. However, fish oil supplementation to diabetic patients resulted in no change in glycaemic control in one study and an actual deterioration in glycaemic control in another study.

Increased intake of polyunsaturated fatty acids has also been reported to result in reduced gastric acid secretion and an increase in gastric mucosal protection. Diets enriched in fish oil or dihomo-γ-linolenic acid also reduce LTB_1 formation in leucocytes or monocytes, suggesting a possible role for fish oil diets in suppressing inflammation in such disorders as rheumatoid arthritis or systemic lupus erythematosus.

Proteins

Protein intake has profound effect on renal haemodynamics and excretory function. High protein intake has been shown to have deleterious effects on the kidneys, especially in pre-existing renal disease, indicating a rationale for dietary protein restriction to lessen renal parenchymal damage. However, not all proteins are equipotent in relation to their renal effects. Lower glomerular filtration rate and renal plasma flow, as well as reduced excretion of albumin and some proteins, have been reported in vegan and lactovegetarian individuals compared with omnivorous subjects. In fact, acute (more than 80 g) or chronic loading (more than 1 g per kg of body weight per day) with animal proteins resulted in an increase

in renal plasma flow and glomerular filtration associated with a higher clearance of albumin than that found in individuals on vegetable protein diets. Vasodilatory PGs such as PGI_2, which may be partly dependent on a rise in glucagon secretion from the pancreas, have been proposed as possible mediators of such renal effects of animal proteins since the administration of indomethacin was found to abolish the renal response to a meat meal.

Minerals

The isolation and identification of renal PGE_2 and PGA_2 between 1965 and 1967 provided biochemical support for the renal anitihypertensive–endocrine function. Numerous studies in humans and animals thereafter showed that PGE_2 has a potent vasodilatory and natriuretic action and hence a pivotal role in sodium homeostasis. In fact, PGE_2 administration augments renal blood flow and urinary sodium excretion. In addition, PGE_2 stimulates renal renin secretion and inhibits vasopressin-mediated water reabsorption. During a low sodium intake the renin–angiotensin axis is activated by volume depletion resulting in antinatiuresis and vasoconstriction. Renal PGE_2 synthesis is stimulated by elevated circulating angiotensin II, which then counteracts the action of angiotensin II, leading to normalization of renal blood flow, blood pressure and sodium excretion (**Fig. 4**). This is the rationale for the beneficial effects of a low-sodium diet on these cardiovascular parameters. The same can be said for diuretic therapy, since the renomedullary synthesis of PGE_2 from arachidonic acid is directly stimulated by furosemide. The natriurietic and antihypertensive effects of furosemide are mediated by this newly synthesized PGE_2, since both effects are inhibited by indomethacin.

Dietary potassium deficiency leads to hypokalaemia and impairment of maximal urinary concentrating ability. Since PGE_2 antagonizes vasopressin-induced water reabsorption, an increase in renomedullary PGE_2 production was postulated to underlie this concentrating defect. However, during chronic dietary potassium depletion secondary to dietary potassium deprivation in animals, PGE_2 synthesis by the renal medulla is markedly reduced, and thus current evidence does not support a role for PGs in hypokalaemic polyuria.

Oral calcium supplementation has been reported to decrease blood pressure in some patients with essential hypertension and hypertensive rats. However, in other studies calcium supplementation produced no effect on blood pressure in normotensive or hypertensive subjects. Although calcium supplementation has been shown to increase urinary PGE_2

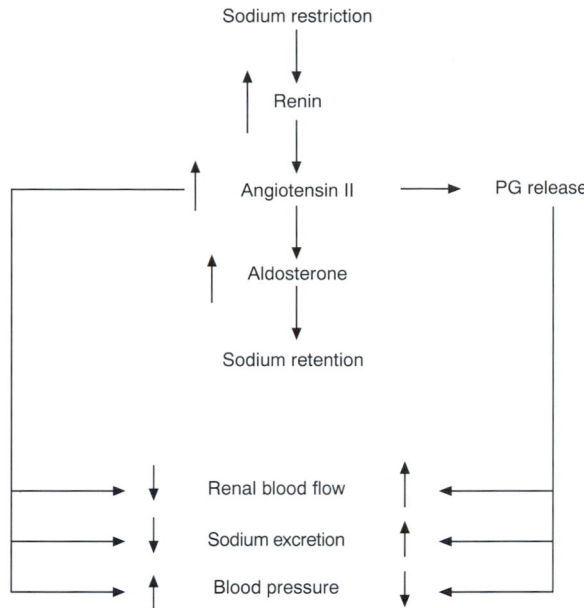

Figure 4 Scheme whereby volume depletion secondary to dietary sodium restriction leads to an increase in PG release from the renal medulla and resultant physiological antagonism of the antinatriuretic and hypertensive actions of angiotensin II. From Lee JB (1980) Prostaglandins and the renin–angiotensin axis. *Clinical Nephrology* **14**:159–163. Reproduced with permission of the publisher.

excretion in normotensive women, there was no associated fall in blood pressure.

Spices

Spices have been consumed by many cultures for thousands of years. In fact, in classical Indian (Ayurvedism), Chinese or Graeco-Arabic systems of medicine some spice-containing plant materials were used to prevent or treat some diseases. Some spices have been shown to inhibit platelet aggregation. These include onion, garlic, ginger, cloves, omum, cumin and turmeric. Extracts from these spices were found to inhibit platelet cyclooxygenase, allowing less TXA_2 to be produced. As cyclooxygenase is inhibited, more substrate (arachidonic acid) becomes available to the lipoxygenase pathway, as shown by the observation that 12-HPETE increases in platelets treated with extracts from ginger, cloves, cumin and turmeric. On the other hand, onion extracts have been demonstrated to inhibit the 5- or 12-lipoxygenase in platelets. This might at least partially explain the observation that crude ethanolic extracts of onion prevented allergen-induced bronchoconstriction in animals and humans. Ginger, which is demonstrated to have antihistaminic and antioxidant action, also inhibits both the cyclooxygenase and 5-lipoxygenase pathway. Garlic extracts have been also demonstrated to inhibit cyclooxygenase activity and LTC_4 formation.

See Colour Plate 11.

See also: **Calcium**: Physiology. **Fatty Acids**: Metabolism; Health Effects of Saturated Fatty Acids; Health Effects of Monounsaturated Fatty Acids; Health Effects of n-6 Polyunsaturated Fatty Acids; Health Effects of n-3 Polyunsaturated Fatty Acids; Health Effects of *trans* Fatty Acids. **Fish**: Nutritional Value. **Hypertension**: Physiology; Nutritional Management. **Potassium**: Physiology, Dietary Sources and Requirements. **Renal Function and Disorders**: Nutritional Management of Renal Disorders. **Sodium**: Physiology.

Further Reading

Bergstrom S, Ryhage R, Samuelsson B and Sjovall J (1962) The structure of prostaglandin E_1, F_1, and F_2. *Acta Chemica Scandinavica* **16**:501–507.

Chin J and Dart AM (1995) How do fish oils affect vascular function? *Clinical and Experimental Pharmacology and Physiology* **22**:71–81.

Coleman RA, Smith WL and Narumiya S (1994) VIII International Union of Pharmacology. Classification of prostanoid receptors: Properties, distribution, and structure of the receptors and their subtypes. *Pharmacological Review* **46**:205–229.

Dusing R, Scherhag R, Glanzer K, Budde U and Kramer HJ (1983) Effect of changes in dietary prostaglandin precursor fatty acids on arterial blood pressure and vascular prostacyclin synthesis. In: Samuelsson B, Paoletti R and Ramwell P (eds) *Advances in Prostaglandin. Thromboxane and Leukotriene Research*, Vol. 12. New York: Raven Press.

Fioretto P, Trevisan R, Valeriho A, Avogaro A, Borsato M, Doria A, Semplici A, Sacerdoti D, Jones S, Bongneti E, Viberti GC and Nosadini R (1990) Impaired renal response to a meat meal in insulin-dependent diabetes: role of glucagon and prostaglandins. *American Journal of Physiology* **258**:F675–F683.

Funk CD (1993) Molecular biology in the eicosanoid field. *Progress in Nucleic Acid Research and Molecular Biology* **45**:67–98.

Hamburg M, Svensson J and Samuelsson B (1976) Novel transformations of prostaglandin endoperoxides: formation of thromboxanes. In: Samuelsson B and Paoletti R (eds) *Advances in Prostaglandin and Thromboxane Research*. New York: Raven Press.

Katayama S, Maruno Y, Inaba M, Itabashi A, Inaba M, Akabane S, Tanaka K, Tanaka K, Shibuya M, Kawazu S, Ishii J, Kusuhara R, Wakabayashi T and Kagawa Y (1991) Effect of dietary calcium on renal prostaglandins. *Postaglandins, Leukotrienes and Essential Fatty Acids* **42**:197–200.

Knapp HR and Fitzgerald GA (1989) The antihypertensive effects of fish oil. *New England Journal of Medicine* **320**:1037–1043.

Kontessis P, Jones S, Dodds R, Trevisan R, Nosadini R, Fioretto P, Borsato M, Sacerdoti D and Viberti G

(1990) Metabolic and hormonal responses to ingestion of animal and vegetable proteins. *Kidney International* **38**:136–144.

Kurzrok P and Lieb CC (1930) Depressor substance in seminal fluid. *Chemistry and Industry* **28**:268–272.

Lee JB, Covino B, Takman BH and Smith ER (1965) Reno-medullary depressor substance, medullin: isolation, chemical characterization and physiological properties. *Circulation Research* **7**:57–77.

Lee JB and Katayama S (1985) Prostaglandins, thromboxanes and leukotrienes. In: Wilson JD and Foster DW (eds) *Williams Textbook of Endocrinology*. Philadelphia: WB Saunders.

Moncada S, Gryglewski R, Bunting S and Vane JR (1976) An enzyme isolated from arteries transforms prostaglandin into an unstable substance that inhibits platelet aggregation. *Nature* **263**:633–665.

Morris MC, Sacks F and Rosner B (1993) Does fish oil lower bood pressure? A meta-analysis. *Circulation* **88**:523–533.

Oates JA, Fitzgerald GA Branoh RA, Jackson EK, Knapp HR and Roberts LJ (1988) Clinical implications of prostaglandin and thromboxane A_2 formation. *New England Journal of Medicine* **319**:689–698; 761–767.

Samuelsson B (1983) Leukotrienes: mediators of immediate hypersensitivity reaction and inflammation. *Science* **220**:568–575.

Smith WL and Willis AL (1971) Aspirin selectively inhibits prostaglandin production in human platelets. *Nature New Biology* **231**:235–237.

Vane JR (1971) Inhibition of prostaglandin synthesis as a mechanism of action for aspirin-like drugs. *Nature New Biology* **231**:232–235.

PROTEIN

Contents
Digestion and Bioavailability
Quality and Sources
Requirements and Role in Diet
Synthesis and Turnover
Deficiency

Digestion and Bioavailability

Zulfiqar A Bhutta, The Aga Khan University, Karachi, Pakistan

Proteins are the principal nitrogenous constituents of the protoplasm of all animal and plant tissue and it is estimated that almost half of the dry weight of animal cells is composed of proteins. Proteins are crucial for the synthesis of body tissues and regulatory proteins, and it is also recognized that almost 90% of all cellular proteins are present as enzymes.

The basic structural units of proteins are the amino acids, which are characterized by the presence of an amino (NH_3) component and an acid or carboxyl group. Nitrogen thus comprises roughly 16% of all proteins by weight. Most naturally occurring amino acids are of the L-configuration. These amino acids are in turn linked together by peptide bonds. Units of two or three amino acids are called dipeptides or tripeptides, respectively, whereas by convention any protein structure of less than 100 amino acid residues is called a polypeptide. The primary structure of a protein refers to the chains of amino acids constituting it, whereas the secondary structure is formed by the linkages between close amino acids by hydroxyl or sulfide bonds. More complex proteins have a tertiary structure owing to the amino acids being held together by strong interatomic forces. The quarternary structure of a protein refers to the manner of association or binding between different units.

Dietary proteins are the major sources of protein intake and constitute on average about 10–20% of daily energy intake. In addition, they are the main source for the essential amino acids (*See:* **Amino Acids**), which cannot be synthesized by humans. Despite wide variations in dietary composition, the average daily protein intakes in different populations of the world range from 50 to 70 g, although it must be recognized that the intake may be much lower in deprived populations, in both qualitative and quantitative terms. Almost half of the total protein entering the gsatrointestinal tract daily is derived from endogenous sources, mainly intestinal secretions and cellular desquamation. Salivary, gastric, biliary, pancreatic and intestinal secretions contribute approximately 20–30 g per day, while desquamated villus epithelial cells contribute a further 30 g, and a relatively smaller amount (2 g) is derived from plasma proteins leaking into the lumen.

An intricate and coordinated system of digestion ensures that under normal conditions, almost 95% of ingested protein is digested and absorbed.

Digestion

The purpose of digestion is to hydrolyse proteins to small peptides and amino acids so that these can be absorbed. The daily protein load requiring digestion within the gastrointestinal tract includes both the exogenous protein derived from the food consumed, as well as that from endogenous intestinal enzymes and cellular debris. The latter could constitute almost 40% of the total gastrointestinal protein load, approximately 160–170 g daily. The digestion of proteins in the gastrointestinal tract involves a coordinated series of events at different levels, with sequential digestion by proteolytic enzymes to a form that can be absorbed into the bloodstream. **Fig. 1** is a sequential representation of the various sites of protein digestion and absorption in the gastrointestinal tract. The main gastric and pancreatic proteolytic enzymes and their physiological functions are summarized in **Table 1**.

Stomach peptic activity

The digestion of proteins begins in the stomach by the actions of pepsins, which are secreted as the pre-cursor form pepsinogen by the gastric mucosa chief cells. The release of pepsinogen is stimulated by gastrin, histamine and cholinergic stimulation and is closely linked to acid secretion. In acid pH the pepsinogens are converted to the active form, pepsin, by the loss of a small basic peptide. Pepsins remain active in the acid pH of the stomach and have a broad proteolytic specificity, splitting peptide bonds mostly involving phenylalanine, tyrosine and leucine. The level of peptic activity and acid production is lower in premature infants and increases in relation to gestational age; pepsin activity increases almost two-fold between infancy and adulthood (**Fig. 2**). Immunohistochemistry indicates two distinct forms of pepsinogen: pepsinogen I is only found in acid-secreting regions of the stomach, whereas pepsinogen II is also found in the mucous cells of the oxyntic and pyloric regions of the stomach, as well as in the duodenal Brunner's glands. Although these two forms of pepsinogen have slightly different pH optima, their substrate specificity is very similar and both are rapidly inactivated by the alkaline pH beyond the pylorus.

A gelatinase liquefying gelatin is also found in the stomach. There is controversy regarding the presence of rennin (a peptidyl peptide hydrolase) in the stomach of young infants, however the milk-clotting activity in human infants is fairly rapid.

The completeness of gastric protein digestion is dependent on several factors including the rate of gastric emptying, the pH of intragastric contents and the type of protein ingested. Given the significant buffering capacity of food, it is unlikely that gastric proteolysis plays a major role in protein digestion. This is also verified by the fact that neither patients

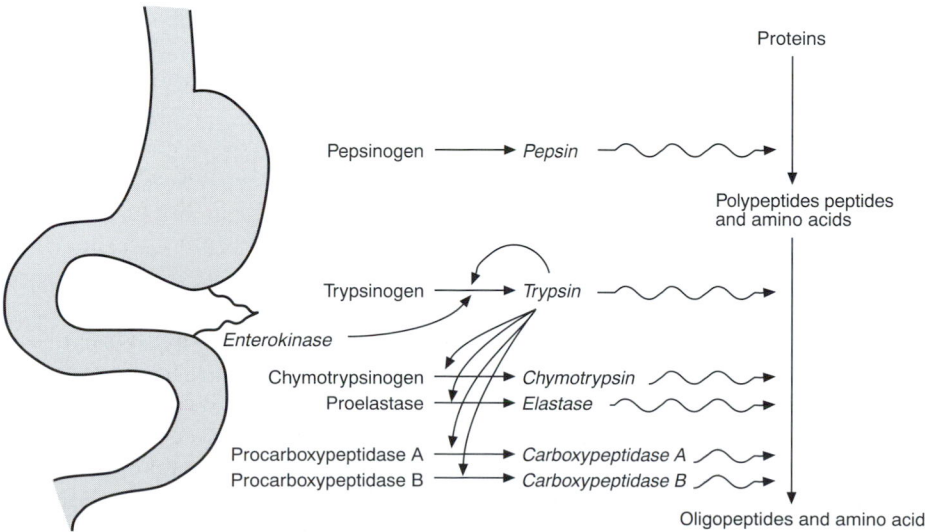

Figure 1 Cascade of protein hydrolysis in the gastrointestinal tract.

Table 1 Proteolytic enzyme activity in the gastrointestinal tract

Enzyme	Precursor	Products	Catalyst	Substrate	Action
Stomach					
Pepsins	Pepsinogens	Polypeptides of diverse sizes and some amino acids	Acid pH	Protein	Hydrolyse bonds between aromatic amino acids, e.g. phenylalanine or tyrosine and another amino acid
Pancreatic proteases					
Trypsin	Trypsinogen	Oligopeptides	Enterokinase	Proteins	Cleaves internal bonds at lysine or arginine amino acids; cleaves other pancreatic proenzymes
			Trypsin	Polypeptides	
Chymotrypsin	Chymotrypsinogen	Oligopeptides	Trypsin	Protein	Cleaves bonds of aromatic or neutral amino acids
				Polypeptides	
Elastase	Proelastase	Oligopeptides	Trypsin	Elastin	Cleaves bonds of aliphatic amino acids, e.g. alanine, glycine and serine
				Other proteins	
Carboxypeptidase A	Procarboxypeptidase A	Aromatic amino acids and peptides	Trypsin	Polypeptides at the free C terminal end of the chain	Cleaves aromatic amino acids from C terminal end of protein and peptides
Carboxypeptidase B	Procarboxypeptidase B	Arginine, lysine and peptides	Trypsin	Polypeptides at the free C terminal end of the chain	Cleaves arginine or lysine from carboxyl terminal end of protein and peptides

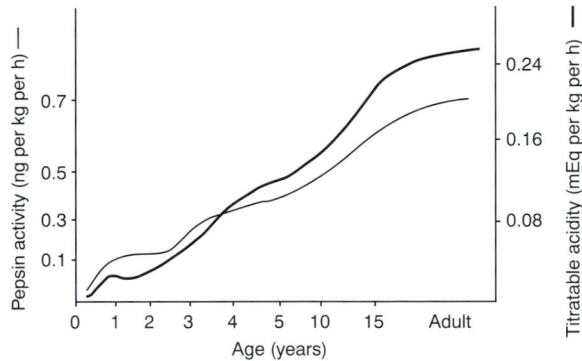

Figure 2 Postnatal development of gastric pepsin secretion and titratable acidity. Modified from Koldovsky (1987) Digestion and absorption of carbohydrates, proteins and fat in infant, and children. In: Walker WA and Watkins JB (eds) *Nutrition in Pediatrics*. Boston: Little, Brown. Reproduced with permission from Little, Brown & Company.

with achlorhydria nor those recovering from major gastric surgery appear to have a major problem with protein digestion.

Pancreatic proteases

The pancreatic proteases are secreted as proenzymes and are activated in the lumen. The enteropeptidase (also called enterokinase) released from the brush border membrane removes a hexapeptide from the N terminal end of trypsinogen, converting it to the active form trypsin. Trypsin in turn activates the other protease proenzymes and also autocatalytically promotes further activation of trypsinogen. The pancreatic proteases include the endopeptidases trypsin, chymotrypsin and elastase, primarily splitting peptide bonds located within the protein molecules resulting in the production of short-chain polypeptides. These are further hydrolysed by the exopeptidases carboxypeptidase A and B, acting on aromatic/aliphatic C terminals or basic C terminals, respectively, to remove single amino acids. The end product of this coordinated intarluminal digestion by these endopeptidases and exopeptidases is a mixture of neutral and basic amino acids (30%) with peptides chains varying in length from two to six amino acids (70%). The presence of excess amino acids in the lumen can further limit peptide hydrolysis (product inhibition).

The activity of enterokinase is noticeable after 26 weeks gestation and its activity at term is approximately 10% of that of adults. However, although pancreatic trypsin levels are substantial in both preterm and term infants, the secretory response to secretin and pancreozymin stimulation is somewhat blunted at birth compared with that at 2 years of age. However, such comparatively lower levels of protease activity in newborn infants do not appear to limit protein digestion significantly.

Brush border membrane and cytoplasmic peptidases

An important step in the final hydrolysis of peptides is their proteolysis to amino acids, either at the level of the intestinal brush border or within the cytoplasm of the intestinal mucosa. An important physiological observation is that protein absorption can occur both as amino acids as well as peptides, indeed absorption as peptides is considered a more efficient way of amino acid absorption compared with single amino acids (**Fig. 3**). Even when a di- or tripeptide is subject to rapid hydrolysis by brush border peptidases, almost 30–50% of it is directly absorbed unconverted. This recognition that peptides are the main physiological route of entry of amino acids into the enterocytes is a point of fundamental importance in the formulation of special protein hydrolysates and enteral feeds.

A range of peptidases are present at the level of the brush border membrane or cytoplasm with the capability of hydrolysing oligopeptides of up to eight amino acid residues (**Table 2**). These oligopeptidases are synthesized in the rough endoplasmic reticulum of enterocytes and, after transfer through the Golgi apparatus, are transported to the brush border and extruded by exocytosis. There is little posttranslational processing of these peptidases and they are attached to the brush border membrane by short anchoring pieces. The brush border peptidases differ in several ways from the cytoplasmic peptidases; the bulk of the hydrolysis of tetrapeptides and longer peptides occurs at the brush border, whereas the converse is true for dipeptidase activity, which is primarily within the cytoplasm. Most oligopeptidases are aminopeptidases, acting at the N terminal amino acid. The brush border proteolysis rate is most rapid for tripeptides and least for dipeptides, whereas the rates of hydrolysis of tetrapeptides and pentapeptides is somewhat intermediate. The brush border peptidases are capable of hydrolysing all peptide bonds except those with proline at the C terminal.

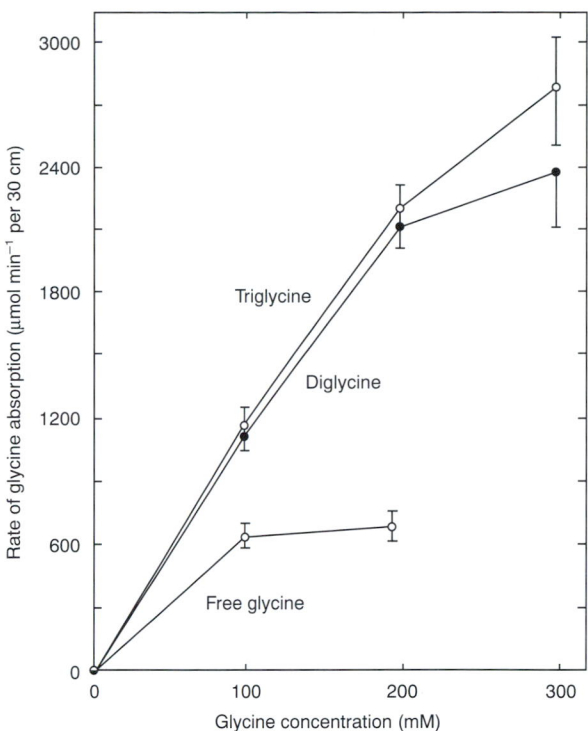

Figure 3 Rates of glycine absorption (mean ± SEM) from perfusion solutions containing equivalent amounts of glycine in free or peptide form. From Adibi SA, Morse EL, Masilamani SS and Amiu P (1975) Evidence from two different modes of tripeptide appearance in human intestine: uptake by peptide carrier systems and hydrolysis by peptide hydrolases. *Journal of Clinical Investigation* **56**:1355–1363. Reproduced with permission from the American Society for Clinical Investigation.

In general, the cytoplasmic peptidases are more heat-labile than brush border peptidases. Of the cytoplasmic peptidases, the most abundant is a dipeptidase which cleaves neutral dipeptides, whereas the aminotripeptidase has a high specificity towards tripeptides with N terminal amino acids or those containing proline terminally.

Very little is known about the developmental aspects of brush border and cytoplasmic proteases. However, the activity of many of these proteases is discernible by 10–16 weeks gestation and progressively increases during development. In contrast, γ-glutamyl transpeptidase activity decreases with increasing gestational age, but the significance of this transition is unknown.

Colonic digestion

Although colonic digestion and fermentation is an important mechanism for energy production in plant-eating animals, its role in human nutrition is of minor importance. Colonic fermentation may lead to the production of short-chain fatty acids from undigested starch, nonstarch polysaccharides or

Table 2 Peptidases present at the brush border membrane and cytoplasm of villous epithelial cells

Peptidase	Action	Products
Brush border membrane peptidases		
Aminooligopeptidases (at least two types)	Cleaves amino acids from C terminal of 3–8 amino acid peptides	Amino acids and dipeptides
Aminopeptidase A	Cleaves dipeptides with acidic amino acids at N terminal	Amino acids
Aminopeptidase I	Cleaves dipeptides containing methionine	Amino acids
Aminopeptidase III	Cleaves glycine-containing dipeptides	Amino acids
Dipeptidyl aminopeptidase IV	Cleaves proline containing peptides with free C terminal	Peptides and amino acids
Carboxypeptidase P	Cleaves proline containing peptides with free C terminal	Peptides and amino acids
Angiotensin I converting enzyme (ACE)		
γ-Glutamyl transpeptidase	Cleaves γ-glutamyl bonds and transfers glutamine to amino acid or peptide	γ-Glutamyl amino acid or peptide
Endopeptidases (two, including PABA peptidase)		
Folate conjugase	Cleaves pteroyl polyglutamates	Monoglutamate
Cytoplasmic peptidases		
Endopeptidases (several including gly–leu dipeptidase)	Cleaves most dipeptides	Amino acids
Aminotripeptidase	Cleaves tripeptides	Amino acids
Proline depeptidase	Cleaves X-Pro bonds in proline-containing depeptides	Proline and amino acids

PABA, para aminobenzoic acid.

proteins reaching the colon, providing approximately 5–10% of daily energy requirements from this source. The contributory role of colonic protein digestion may become important for people with reduced small intestinal function such as short bowel syndrome.

Absorption

As already indicated, although the final end product of protein digestion is amino acids, small peptides are the dominant form of entry of amino acids into enterocytes, where they are further hydrolysed into amino acids and absorbed into the bloodstream (**Fig. 4**). Thus the vast majority of products of protein digestion that reach the bloodstream are single amino acids. Amino acid transport systems develop *in utero* by the end of the first trimester, whereas peptide transport systems can be demonstrated by the beginning of the second trimester.

It is recognized that the intestinal permeability of the preterm and newborn infant may be high, allowing the entry of small amounts of undigested proteins. The maternal antibodies from colostrum can enter the newborn's bloodstream relatively unaltered by a process of endocytosis and subsequent exocytosis. Although the intestinal permeability decreases with age, adults can still absorb larger proteins under abnormal circumstances. However, the predominant form of absorption and presentation of larger foreign proteins is through the specialized microfold or M cells overlying the lymphoid Peyer's patches. This mode of absorption of intact proteins or polypeptides is, however, nutritionally insignificant.

Peptide absorption

Di- and tripeptides can cross the brush border membrane as such by a main peptide transport system with broad specificity. This carrier protein can transport dibasic as well as diacid peptides and peptides consisting of up to three amino acid residues. However, there is some stereospecificity for this transporter, as the longer the length of the amino acid side chain on the peptides, the easier the absorption. The transporter system also has greater affinity for

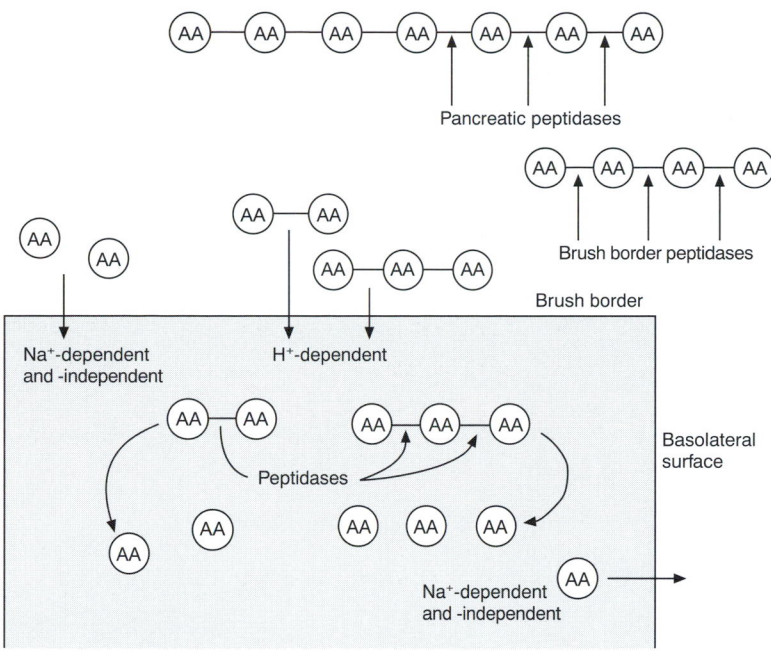

Figure 4 Small intestinal protein digestion and absorption. After Shulman RJ (1996) Intraluminal digestion and absorption in the small intestine. In: Gluckman PD and Heyman MA (eds). *Pediatrics and Perinatology: The Scientific Basis*, 2nd edn. London: Arnold. Reproduced with permission from Arnold (UK).

dipeptides than tripeptides, and the acidic and basic amino acid residues in dipeptides lower the affinity for the transport system compared with neutral amino acids. In general, the absorption of L-isomers of amino acids in dipeptides is preferred over the D forms. The peptide transport system is coupled to the proton pump system rather than the sodium gradient. The oligopeptide transporter (Pept-1) in the brush border membrane is the major mechanism for protein absorption in the human intestine and is primarily responsible for the transport of di- and tripeptides. Several factors may determine the levels of Pept-1 such as insulin, which may stimulate membrane insertion of the oligopeptide transporter from a preformed cytoplasmic pool, and cholera toxin, which decreases the activity of Pept-1 through an increase in the intracellular concentration of cyclic AMP.

Once in the absorbing cell, the di- and tripeptides are further hydrolysed to the constituent amino acids by the cytoplasmic peptidases before absorption. The only small peptides that are known to enter the portal blood directly are those from gelatin that contain proline and hydroxyproline, and those from certain meats containing carnosine and anserine. However, their relative proportion in comparison to amino acids is inconsequential.

Amino acid absorption

Although some diffusion of amino acids does occur, they are mostly absorbed by active transport. Unlike peptides, which are absorbed equally well in both proximal and distal small intestine, amino acids are absorbed more rapidly in the duodenum and jejunum. Also in contrast to the parsimonious peptide transport system, there are multiple transport mechanisms for various amino acids at both the luminal end and the basolateral membrane of the enterocyte (**Table 3**). At the luminal end, the transporters are mostly located at the villous enterocytes. The villous enterocytes utilize some 10% of the absorbed amino acids for their own protein production, whereas the crypt cells derive their amino acid supply from the portal circulation. Of various amino acids, glutamine appears to have a major role in the nutrition and regeneration of enterocytes, and it is now recognized that in the human intestine the predominant mechanism for assimilation of glutamine dipeptides is absorption as intact dipeptide rather than hydrolysis.

There are at least five different sodium-dependent transport systems for amino acid uptake. The sodium-dependent transport is facilitated by energy derived from Na^+/K^+-exchanging ATPase at the basolateral membrane. Most energy-dependent

Table 3 Major amino acid transport systems in the intestinal epithelial cells

Transport system	Substrates	Sodium gradient-dependent
Brush border membrane		
B	Dipolar α-amino acids	+
$B^{0,+}$	Dipolar α-amino acids Basic amino acids Cystine	+
$b^{0,+}$	Dipolar α-amino acids Basic amino acids Cystine	–
y^+	Basic amino acids, e.g. lysine Cysteine	–
IMINO	Imino acids, e.g. proline β-Alanine	+
X^-_{GA}	Acidic amino acids, e.g. glutamate, aspartate	+
β	β-Amino acids, e.g. alanine	+
Basolateral membrane		
L	Broad selectivity	–
A	Broad selectivity	–
ASC	Neutral amino acids, e.g. alanine, serine Cysteine	+
N	Glutamine, histidine, asparagine	+

Modified from Shulman RJ (1996) Intraluminal digestion and absorption in the small intestine. In: Gluckman PD and Heyman MA (eds) *Pediatrics and Perinatology: The Scientific Basis*, 2nd edn. London: Arnold.

transporters are coupled either to cotransport of Na^+ or Cl^- or to the countertransport of K^+. An additional system of sodium-independent facilitated diffusion also exists, and is predominantly geared towards basic and dipolar α-amino acids. These passive transporters are either facilitated transporters or channels.

Digestibility

The digestibility of a protein is a measure of the amount of protein available from it for absorption after digestion; this is usually obtained from estimates of dietary nitrogen, faecal and urinary nitrogen. Digestibility is different from the other measures of protein quality such as the amino acid or chemical scores and biological value, which respectively represent the essential and nonessential amino acid composition of the protein and the proportion of available nitrogen retained for growth or maintenance. Thus a protein-based diet of high amino acid or chemical score may be poorly digested and thus of limited nutritional value. The digestibility of a protein is also dependent on the physical shape of the protein and the relative ease with which peptide bonds can be hydrolysed. Fibrous proteins with long polypeptide chains such as collagen, keratin and elastin are relatively insoluble. In contrast globular proteins, which are coiled and tightly packed, are comparatively soluble and thereby more digestible. Such proteins are insulin, enzymes, haemoglobin and albumin.

The apparent protein digestibility is a measure of the amount of protein intake (%) available for absorption and is usually calculated by estimation of fecal nitrogen and corresponding dietary intake:

Apparent digestibility =

$$\frac{(\text{dietary nitrogen} - \text{faecal nitrogen})}{\text{dietary nitrogen}} \times 100$$

However, since not all faecal nitrogen is of dietary origin and some is derived from obligatory endogenous intestinal losses, a more appropriate measure is that of 'true protein digestibility'. This is derived as:

True protein digestibility =

$$\frac{[\text{dietary nitrogen} - (\text{faecal nitrogen} - \text{obligatory faecal nitrogen})]}{\text{dietary nitrogen})} \times 100$$

The obligatory faecal intestinal protein losses have been variably estimated to range from 20 mg per kg per day in young infants and preschool children to approximately 12 mg per kg per day in adults.

Table 4 gives the true digestibility values for several common foods and diets. In general milk and eggs have the highest true digestibility values of about 97%, followed closely by meats, fish and poultry. Plants and legumes have comparatively lower protein digestibility values ranging from 75 to 85%. Thus in mixed diets, increasing the relative amounts of animal proteins compared with plant-based proteins increases the protein digestibility of the diet. However, some fibrous animal proteins such as keratin and collagen are relatively indigestible. A useful approximation is to assume a protein digestibility of 75–80% for diets based upon whole-grain cereals and vegetables, 95% for diets based on refined cereals and animal proteins, and roughly 85–90% for mixed diets. In general the lower the true digestibility of a protein, the greater is the amount required to achieve nitrogen equilibrium.

In addition to the differences in the nature of proteins highlighted above, several other factors affect protein digestibility of a diet. These include the presence of additional dietary factors such as fibre, polyphenols and natural inhibitors such as trypsin inhibitors. The latter may be present in certain foods such as navy beans and soya beans, and can be largely inactivated by heating, thus improving protein digestibility. Although moderate heating can promote digestibility by promoting breakdown of peptide crosslinkages and inactivation of protease inhibitors in natural foods, strong heating, especially in the presence of a carbohydrate or oxidized lipids, may make the protein resistant to enzymatic hydrolysis. The Maillard or 'browning reaction' occurs after high, usually prolonged heating of a protein in the presence of a reducing sugar such as lactose or glucose, resulting in crosslinkages of the sugar with the free side chain of the lysine residues. This may make up to 30% of the lysine biologically unavailable. These changes are of particular importance in situations of marginally sufficient protein intake, where cooking procedures may further aggravate protein malnutrition. The effect of heat treatment on the protein digestibility of a formulation was highlighted by a study using an elegant suckling rat model to investigate the digestibility of different infant milk formulations. The data indicate that proteins from ultraheat-treated milk formulae were most rapidly digested (84%), resulting in an amino acid profile closest to breast-milk-fed pups, whereas the digestibility from powdered formulations (77–82%) and soya milk-based formulae was slower. The slowest digestion of protein was found in sterilized milk formulae (72–74%), where the canned formulation was exposed to high temperatures for extended time periods.

Despite several limitations, the digestion and absorption of ingested proteins is remarkably complete, with only a small fraction (3–5%) of ingested protein nitrogen escaping hydrolysis and excreted in the stools. In the context of infant nutrition, while breast milk is well digested, some proteins such as secretory IgA, lactoferrin and α_1-antitrypsin escape digestion.

See also: **Amino Acids**: Chemistry and Classification; Metabolism. **Protein**: Quality and Sources; Requirements and Role in Diet; Synthesis and Turnover; Deficiency.

Further Reading

Adibi SA, Morse EL, Masilamani SS and Amin PM (1975) Evidence from two different modes of tripeptide appearance in human intestine: uptake by peptide carrier systems and hydrolysis by peptide hydrolases. *Journal of Clinical Investigation* 56:1355–1363.

Castanga M, Shayakul C, Trotti D, Sacchi VF, Harvey WP and Hediger MA (1997) Molecular characteristics of mammalian and insect amino acid transporters: implications for amino acid homeostasis. *Journal of Experimental Biology* 200:269–286.

Gaudichon C, Mahe C, Luengo C, Laurent C, Meaugeais P, Krempf M and Tome D (1996) A ^{15}N-leucine-dilution method to measure endogenous contribution to luminal nitrogen in the human upper jejunum. *European Journal of Clinical Nutrition* 50:261–268.

Table 4 Illustrative values of protein digestibility in humans

Protein source	True digestibility (%)	Digestibility relative to reference protein (%)
Eggs	97	100
Milk and cheese	95	100
Meat and fish	94	100
Maize	85	89
Oatmeal	86	90
Whole wheat	86	91
Refined wheat	96	101
Polished rice	88	93
Soya flour	86	91
Soya bean isolate	94	99
Millet	79	83
Peanut butter	95	100
Beans	78	82
Chinese mixed diet	94	99
Brazilian mixed diet	78	82
Guatemalan mixed diet	79	83
Indian rice and milk diet	87	92
Mixed American diet	96	101

Modified from Torun B (1985). Reproduced with permission from Raven Press.

Hopfer U (1987) Membrane transport mechanisms for hexoses and amino acids in the small intestine. In: Johnson LR (ed.) *Physiology of the Gastrointestinal Tract*, 2nd edn. New York: Raven Press, p 1499.

Koldovsky O (1987) Digestion and absorption of carbohydrates, protein and fat in infants and children. In: Walker WA and Watkins JB (eds) *Nutrition in Pediatrics*. Boston: Little Brown, pp 257–277.

Lonnerdal Bo (1994) Digestibility and absorption of protein in infants. In: Raiha NCR (ed.), *Protein Metabolism During Infancy*. New York: Raven Press, pp 53–65.

National Research Council (1989) *Recommended Dietary Allowances*, 10th edn. Washington, DC: National Academy Press.

Nordgarrd I and Mortensen PB (1995) Digestive processes in the human colon. *Nutrition* **11**:37–45.

Proteins and amino acids. In: Robinson CH, Lawler MR, Chenoweth WL and Garwick AE (eds), *Normal and Therapeutic Nutrition*, 17th edn. New York: Macmillan, pp 44–63.

Shulman RJ (1996) Intraluminal digestion and absorption in the small intestine. In: Gluckman PD and Heyman MA (eds) *Pediatrics and Perinatology: The Scientific Basis*, 2nd edn. London: Arnold, pp 634–637.

Torun B (1985) Proteins: chemistry, metabolism, and nutritional requirements. In: Brunser O, Carraza F, Gracey M, Nichols B and Senterre J (eds). *Clinical Nutrition of the Young Child*. New York: Raven Press, pp 99–119.

Turnberg LA and Riley SA Digestion and absorption of nutrients and vitamins. In: Sleisenger MH and Fordtran JS (eds) *Gastrointestinal Disease: Pathophysiology/ Diagnosis/Management*, 5th edn. Philadelphia: WB Saunders, pp 993–997.

Quality and Sources

Benjamin Torun, Institute of Nutrition of Central America and Panama, Guatemala City, Guatemala

Food proteins differ in their capacity to provide nitrogen and essential amino acids for utilization in the human body, depending on their amino acid composition and on the efficiency with which they are digested and their constituent amino acids are absorbed. This capacity, known as *protein quality*, influences dietary requirements: the lower the quality, the higher the required dietary protein intake. The nutritive value of a protein source is also influenced by its *protein concentration* and the *bioavailability* of its amino acids. The latter can be affected by some forms of food storage and processing.

This article examines the ways of assessing the protein quality of foods and diets and the character-istics used to classify protein sources. The following terms will be used frequently.

- Protein (or nitrogen) digestibility – the proportion of dietary nitrogen that is absorbed. 'True' protein digestibility takes into account endogenous or obligatory faecal nitrogen losses in the calculations (**Table 1**).
- Essential amino acids (EAA) (also called 'indispensable amino acids') – amino acids that humans cannot synthesize from components present in the diet, at a rate commensurate with normal bodily needs.
- Amino acid scoring pattern – amino acid composition of a hypothetical 'ideal' protein that contains all EEAs in the amounts necessary to satisfy requirements.
- Limiting amino acids – essential amino acids that have a value lower than 100, when their content in 1 g of a food protein is calculated as a percentage of the same amino acid in the amino acid scoring pattern (or lower than 1.00, when using fractional values) (Table 1).
- Amino acid score (also called 'chemical score' or 'protein score') – value of the limiting amino acid with the lowest score in a protein ('most limiting amino acid'). A protein is assigned a percentage score of 100 (or a fractional score of 1.00) when none of its EAAs is limiting.

Assessment of Protein Quality

The most accurate assessment of protein quality of foods for humans is through clinical (metabolic) studies that measure growth and/or nitrogen balance and other metabolic functions. Because of their cost and time requirements, clinical studies are done mainly to evaluate new, nonconventional protein sources and novel food processes that might affect protein quality. Other methods that can predict protein quality for humans rapidly and at low cost are used to evaluate diets and conventional foods routinely.

For many years, biological assays in laboratory animals were used, based either on the ability of a protein to support growth in young rats (e.g. protein efficiency ratio, PER) or on nitrogen retention (e.g. net protein utilization, NPU). It is now known that those assays underestimate the value of some vegetable and animal proteins for humans. For example, the proteins of pulses and milk casein have a lower quality for rats than for humans, owing to the higher requirement of the rat for sulfur-containing amino acids. Thus, application of rat assay results to human nutrition can result in large quantitative errors. The discrepancy generally has economic rather than

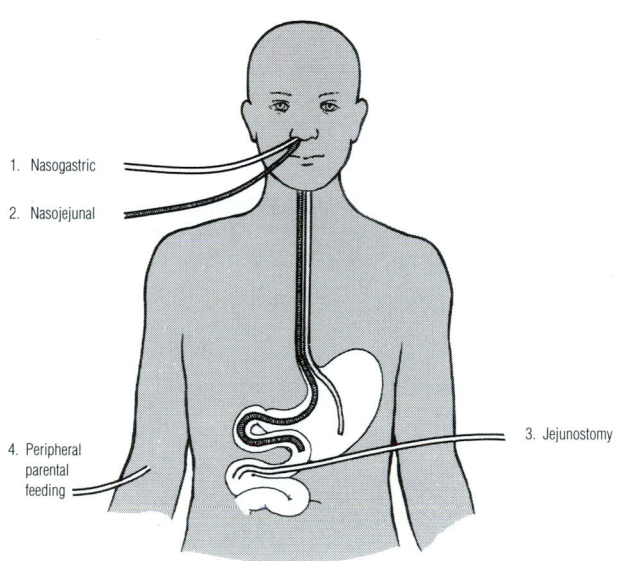

Plate 1 Nutrition labelling. Example of a full label (EC Nutrition Labelling Directive) on a can of baked beans. The information can be of use to different people. People following medical advice to eat a low-salt diet may watch the sodium content of foods, slimmers may count calories. Nutrition labels can help everyone to choose a healthy diet. (With permission from MAFF).

Nutrition Information		
	Typical values	
	per 100 g	per serving 210 g
Energy	312 kJ 75 kcal	655 kJ 158 kcal
Protein	4.7 g	9.9 g
Carbohydrate	13.6 g	28.6 g
of which Sugars	6.0 g	12.6 g
Fat	0.2 g	0.4 g
of which Saturates	0.1 g	0.2 g
Fibre	3.7 g	7.8 g
Sodium	0.5 g	1.1 g

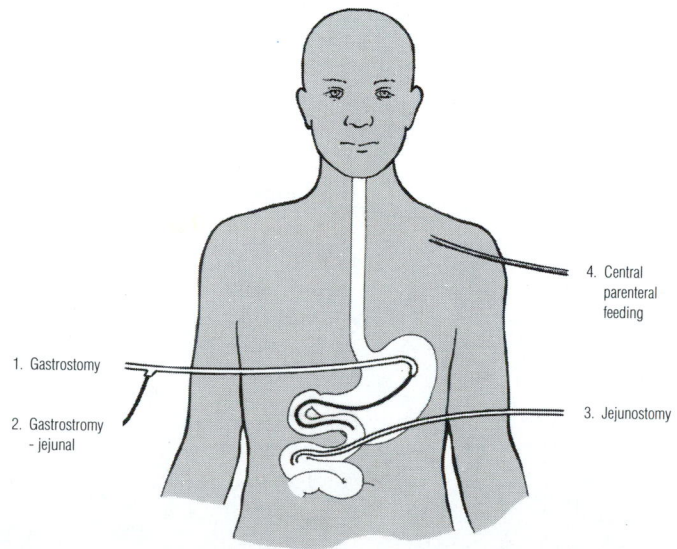

1. Nasogastric
2. Nasojejunal
3. Jejunostomy
4. Peripheral parental feeding

Plate 3 Routes of short-term (< 4 weeks) nutritional support. (With permission from Fresenius Ltd).

1. Gastrostomy
2. Gastrostromy - jejunal
3. Jejunostomy
4. Central parenteral feeding

Plate 4 Routes of long-term (> 4 weeks) nutritional support. (With permission from Fresenius Ltd).

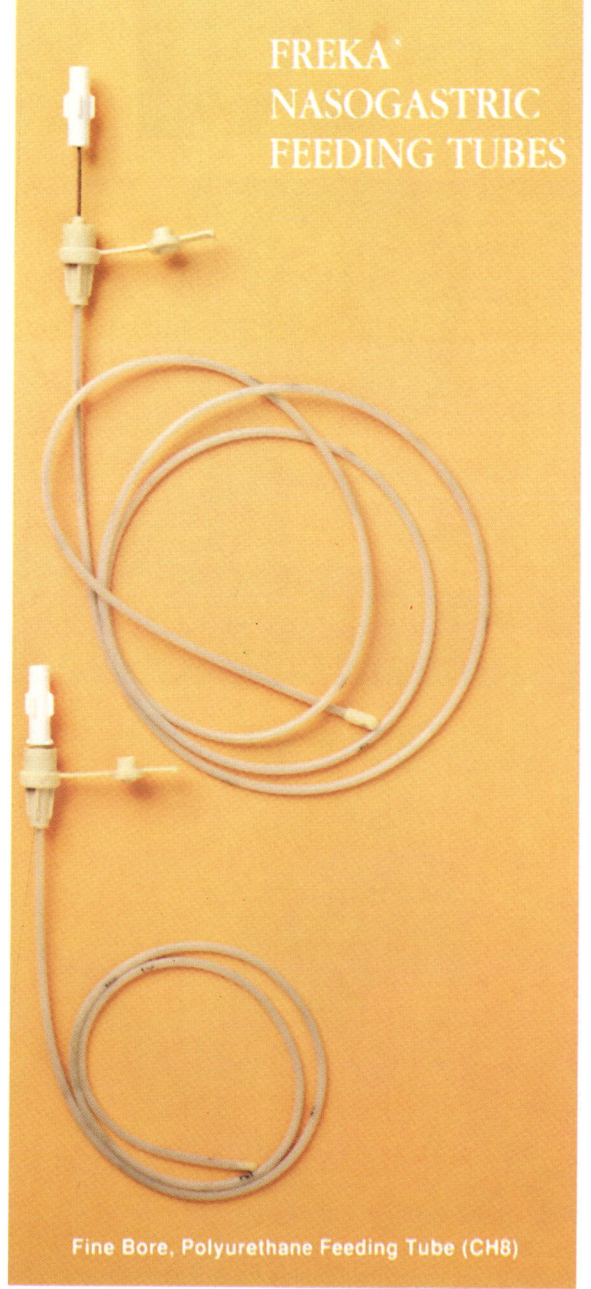

FREKA* NASOGASTRIC FEEDING TUBES

Fine Bore, Polyurethane Feeding Tube (CH8)

Plate 2 Nutritional support. Polyurethane nasogastric feeding tube (CH8). (With permission from Fresenius Ltd).

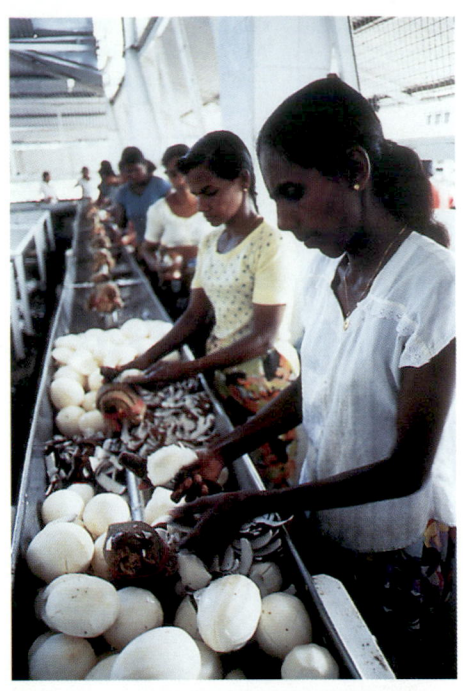

Plate 5 Workers in a coconut factory. The large, hard-shelled seed of the coconut palm, *Cocas nucifera*, is enclosed in a thick husk. It contains an edible white meat and a milky liquid known as coconut milk. (With permission from CTC/Zeneca).

Plate 6 *(below)* **Obesity.** A pair of callipers is used to measure the skinfold thickness of the waist *(left)* and upper arm *(right)* of an obese man to assess body fat content. About a third of the UK adult population is considered overweight, but only 5% is obese. The cause of obesity is not always clear: some people simply eat too much while others are thought to become obese due to genetic factors, low metabolic rates or physical inactivity. The condition raises the risk of stroke, heart disease, diabetes and some cancers, and aggravates osteoarthritis. (With permission from Dr P. Marazzi/Science Photo Library).

Plate 7 *(bottom right)* **Probiotics.** Tablets containing probiotic bacteria which are claimed to have beneficial health effects. The grainy tablets contain *Lactobacillus acidophilus* bacteria and the plain ones, *salivarious*. Probiotic products are claimed to colonize the gastro-intestinal tract with probiotic bacteria that may help to counter pathogenic bacteria, may improve the recovery of intestinal disorders, and stimulate the immune system. Healthy people have many bacteria in their intestines, but the numbers of benificial bacteria may become depleted due to a poor diet or the use of antibiotics and other drugs. (With permission from Cordelia Molly/Science Photo Library).

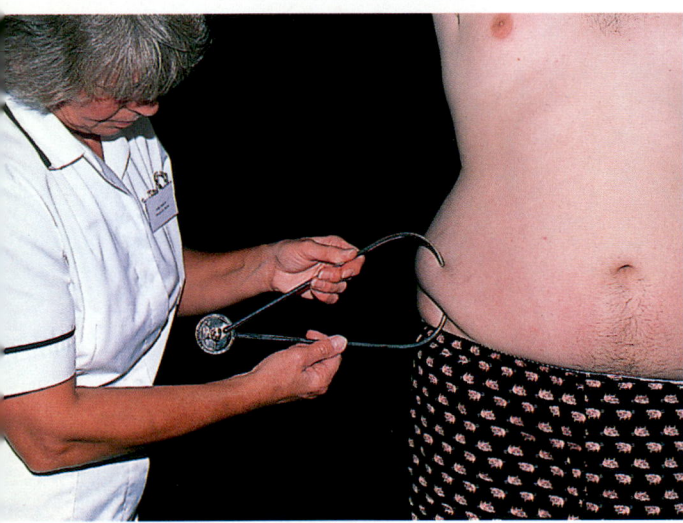

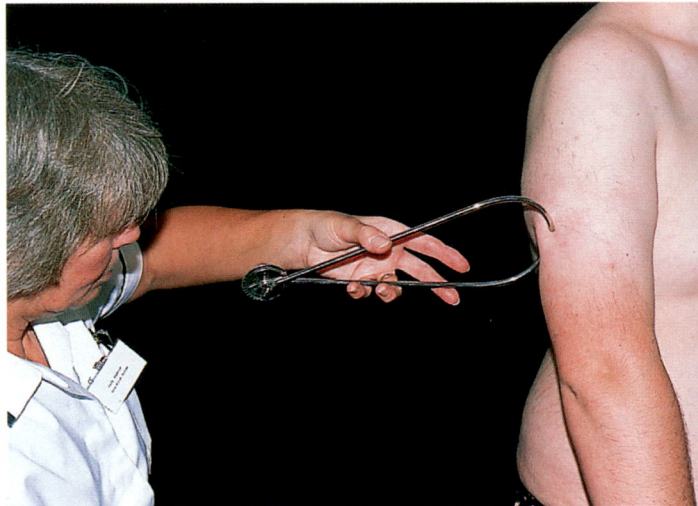

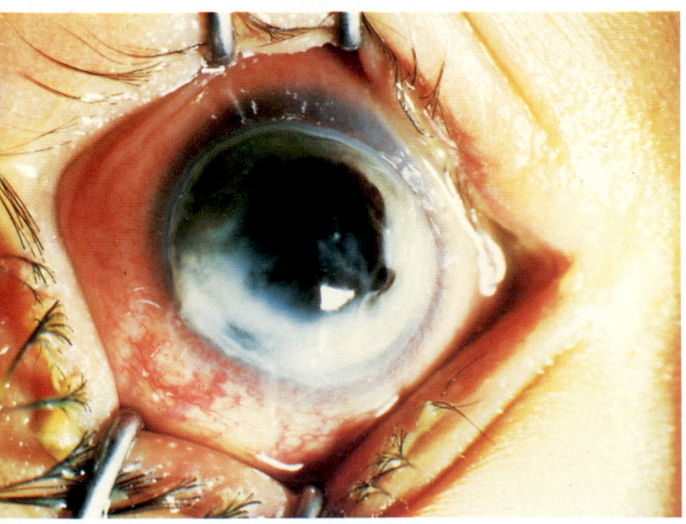

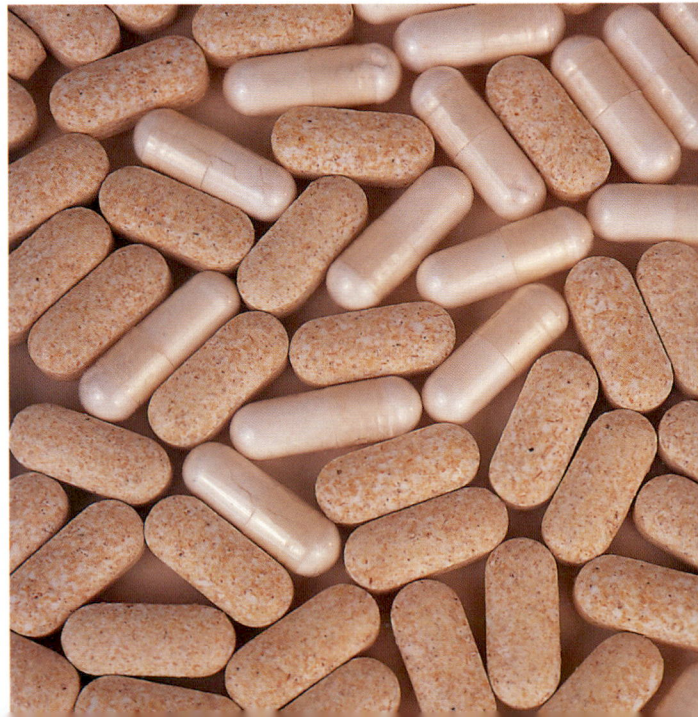

Plate 8 *(above)* **Hypovitaminosis A.** Keratomalacia in a 3 year old Indonesian child. The cornea is dissolved. The brown iris is bulging through opaque, whitish material. (Kindly provided by Professor A. Sommer).

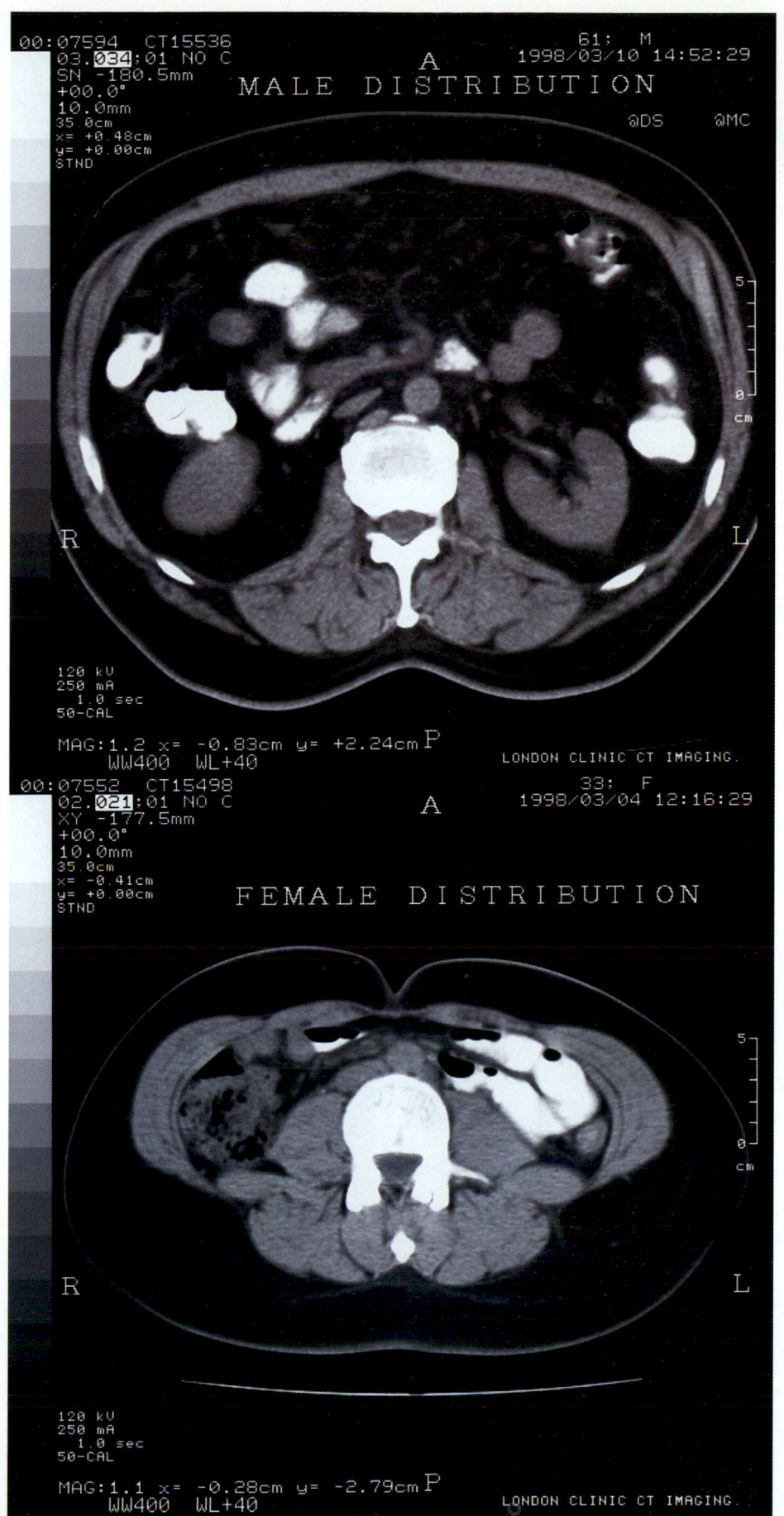

Plate 9 Fat distribution in humans. Male fat distribution *(top)* and female fat distribution *(bottom)*. (With permission from The London Clinic).

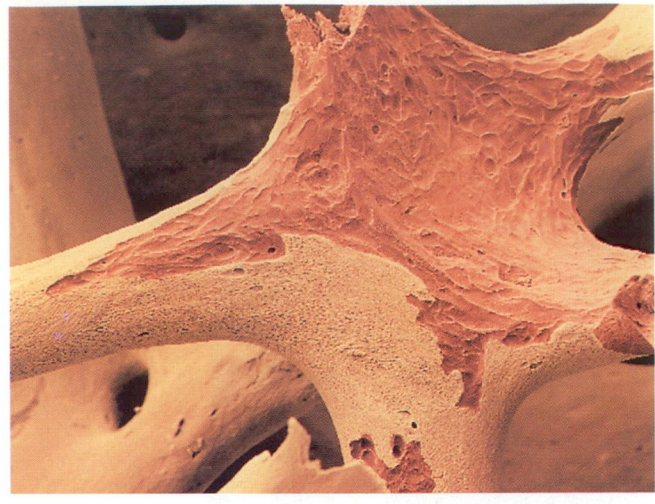

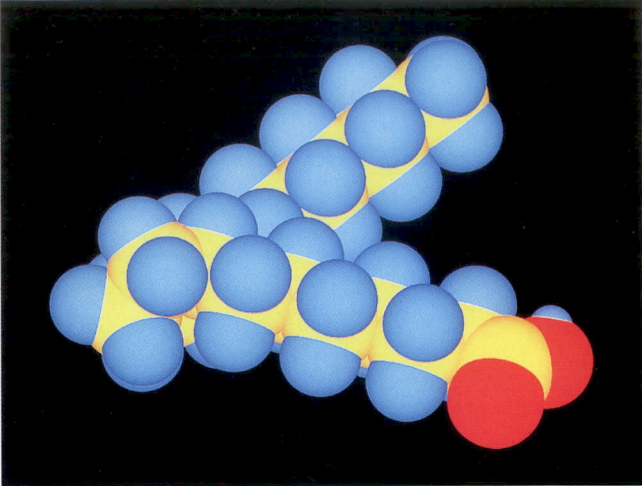

Plate 10 Osteoporosis. Coloured Scanning Electron Micrograph (SEM) of the brittle and spongy fractured thighbone (femur) from a patient with *osteoporosis*. The lighter areas of this bone have a grainy, spongy appearance with dark areas being where the bone mineral has been reabsorbed by the body. Osteoporosis, also known as brittle bone disease, is the loss of the protein matrix from bone causing it to become brittle and easily fractured. The condition is seen most commonly in the thigh and backbones of post-menopausal women, where it is associated with a reduction in oestrogen-hormone production. (With permission from Dr Tony Brain/Science Photo Library).

Plate 11 Prostaglandin. Computer graphic of a molecule of prostaglandin, a hormone-like chemical. It is an unsaturated fatty acid or lipid that has a broad range of physiological activity. The molecule's atoms are colour coded: carbon is yellow, hydrogen is blue and oxygen is red. There are many types of prostaglandins, each with 20 carbon atoms, that are continually produced in mammal tissues. Their effects include lowering blood pressure, causing contractions of smooth muscle, regulating cell function and fertility, promoting inflammation, and affecting the platelet cells that form blood clots. (With permission from Alfred Pasieka/Science Photo Library).

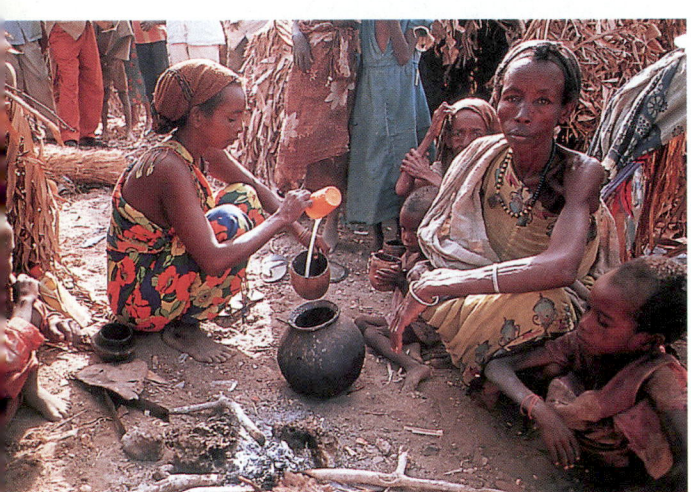

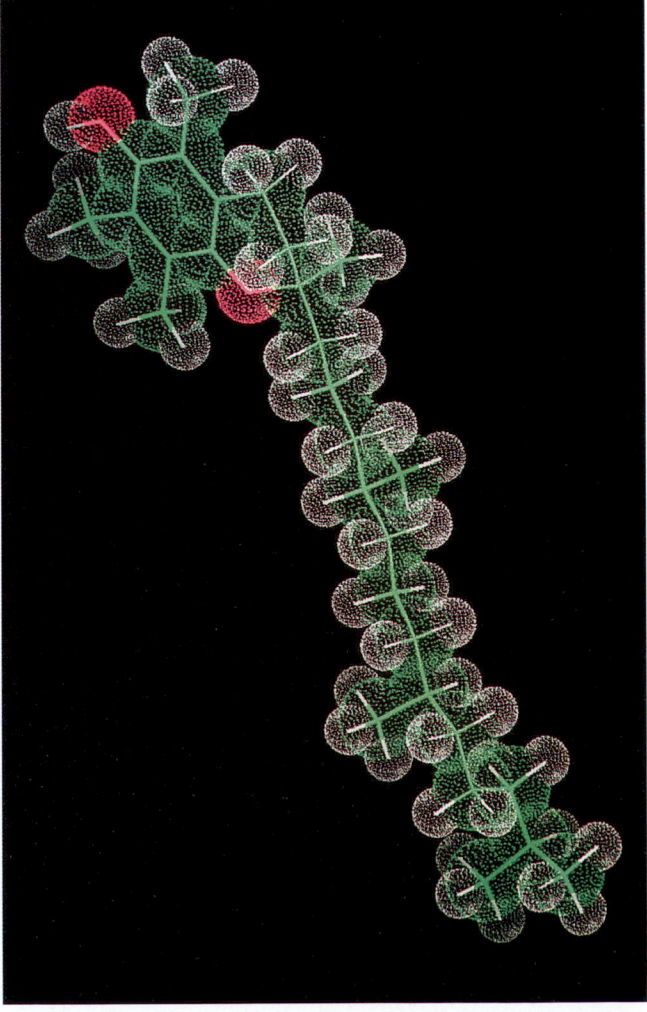

Plate 12 Lunch in a refugee camp. A woman distributes a drink to her family in a refugee camp. The drink is made by boiling available grains. Some camps may also provide small rations of dietary supplements. (With permission from Peter Menzel/Science Photo Library).

Plate 13 Molecular graphic of vitamin E. Green spheres represent carbon atoms, white spheres represent hydrogen and red spheres represent oxygen. Solid lines represent bonds. Vitamin E is found in vegetable lipids and animal fats. It protects unsaturated fat from oxidation and is thus thought to stabilise cell membranes. It is essential for fertility and reproduction in animals. (With permission from Alfred Pasieka/Science Photo Library).

Table 1 Calculations of working definitions; these can be multiplied by 100 and expressed as percentages

Definition	Calculation
Apparent digestibility	$\dfrac{I_N - F_N}{I_N}$
True digestibility	$\dfrac{I_N - (F_N - F_E)}{I_N}$
Amino acid score	$\dfrac{\text{mg of EAA in 1 g of food protein}}{\text{mg of EAA in 1 g of reference protein (}or\text{ EAA scoring pattern)}}$
Limiting amino acid	EAA with a score <1.00 (or $<100\%$)

EAA, essential amino acid; F_E, endogenous faecal nitrogen; F_N, total faecal nitrogen; I_N, nitrogen intake.

public health implications because rat assays usually err by underestimating protein quality for humans, although they can overestimate the value of certain animal proteins because of higher efficiency of utilization by the rat.

Since protein quality is largely dependent on its provision of essential amino acids, the concept of assessing it on the basis of a protein's constituent amino acids was introduced in the Late 1940s. It was later suggested that the calculations be corrected by the protein's digestibility. The validity of this approach and its correlation with results of clinical studies were initially limited by lack of accurate procedures to measure tryptophan and sulfur amino acids, insufficient information on digestibility of proteins from various sources, and uncertainty about human amino acid requirements to prepare an adequate scoring pattern. Significant scientific and technological advancements now allow the use of an amino acid scoring procedure adjusted for digestibility as a good and practical predictor of protein quality for humans.

Amino Acid Score Adjusted for Digestibility

This method is recommended by expert committees of the World Health Organization (WHO), United Nations Food and Agriculture Organization (FAO), United Nations University (UNU) and the Codex Committee on Vegetable Proteins (CCVP), as well as by regulatory agencies of several countries, for routine evaluation of protein quality for humans. The elements required for its application are: knowledge about the amino acid composition and digestibility of the food protein(s) under evaluation and a scoring pattern based on human amino acid requirements.

Amino acid analysis of food proteins

Modern methods that involve acid or alkaline hydrolysis of the protein followed by separation and quantification of the released amino acids by ion exchange, gas–liquid or high-performance liquid chromatography, and other chemical and microbiological methods for specific amino acids, such as lysine, methionine, cystine and tryptophan, provide data with a repeatability within laboratory of about 5% and a reproducibility between laboratories of about 10%. Several national and international food composition tables have published amino acid contents of foods, the largest being that compiled by FAO in 1970. Nevertheless, owing to technical shortcomings and the considerable variability between the reported values, especially for tryptophan, cystine and methionine, it is recommended that analytical results from a reliable laboratory be used unless there is trustworthy data for specific proteins or foods.

Amino acid data should be calculated as mg amino acid per g protein. If they are reported as mg amino acid per g nitrogen, they can be converted to the protein equivalents multiplying by a factor of 6.25. To calculate the amino acid content of a combination of food proteins, as in a processed food based on several protein sources or in a mixed diet, a weighted mean of the published or analytical results of each component should be used, as illustrated in **Table 2**.

Amino acid scoring pattern

All international groups associated with the United Nations and related to food, health and nutrition (WHO, FAO, UNU, CCVP) have agreed that for infants younger than 1 year the scoring pattern should be based on the amino acid composition of breast milk. Some EAAs in human milk probably exceed requirements for infants of this age. For example, infants consuming cow's milk proteins, which have less sulfur-containing amino acids than human milk, show adequate growth and nitrogen balance. However, although the use of a scoring pattern based on human milk composition may somewhat underestimate the protein quality of some

Table 2 Calculating the lysine (lys) content of a rice, lentil and chicken mixture

1. Protein sources in 100 g of the cooked mixture:

   10 g dry polished rice
   10 g dry lentil
   20 g raw white chicken meat

2. Chemical composition:

	Rice	Lentil	Chicken
Protein (g per 100 g food)	7.0	23.7	19.2
Lysine (mg per 100 g food)	255	1739	1590

3. Lysine content of the mixture (mg per g protein):

Food	mg lys per g protein		g component per100 g mixture
Rice	(255/7.0)	×	10
Lentil	(1739/23.7)	×	10
Chicken	(1590/19.2)	×	20

Weighted mean = (364 + 734 + 1656)/(10 + 10 + 20) =
69 mg lys per g protein.

foods for infants, there is a consensus to err on the side of safety for this highly vulnerable age group.

The international groups also agree that the scoring pattern proposed in the 1980s for preschool children, which is based on studies of amino acid requirements at the Institute of Nutrition of Central America and Panama and on recommendations of protein intake by FAO, WHO and UNU, is robust and represents the best available estimates of EAA requirements for this age group. Proteins with an EAA content and pattern that meet the needs of young children will also be adequate for older children and adults, whereas the converse may not be true. Thus, in the absence of reliable experimental data for older children and on all EAAs for adults, it was agreed that, at present, the preschool child scoring pattern should be used for all ages over 1 year. Recent studies in adults on the oxidation and turnover of some EAAs suggest that the use of that pattern is satisfactory and will not lead to important underestimations of protein quality for the older age groups.

Table 3 shows the internationally accepted patterns for amino acid scoring; the composition of high-quality animal foods is shown for comparison. The content of each EAA in a food protein is compared with the scoring patterns, as described in Table 1. All EAAs that exceed requirements, thereby obtaining a score greater than 100% in relation to the pattern, are assigned a value of 100. The EAA with the lowest percentage value determines the protein's amino acid score.

The only EAAs that are likely to limit the protein quality of mixed diets for humans are lysine, the sulfur-containing amino acids (methionine and cystine), threonine and tryptophan. Consequently, when there are technical or financial constraints to obtain information on the content of all EAAs in a diet, protein quality can be estimated on the basis of its score for those four amino acids.

Correction for protein digestibility

A protein may have an amino acid composition similar to the scoring pattern, but if it is not fully digested or if its constituent amino acids are not absorbed, its capacity to provide nitrogen and EAAs for utilization in the body will diminish. Not all food proteins are digested, absorbed and utilized to the same extent because of inherent differences in their source (e.g. inside vegetable cells with indigestible membranes), their physicochemical nature (e.g. protein configuration, amino acid bonding), the presence of food constituents which modify digestion (e.g. dietary

Table 3 Amino acid scoring patterns for infants under 1 year and for older children and adults (mg amino acid per g protein). Composition of animal proteins shown for comparison

Amino acid	Infant <1 year	Older children and adults	Egg, cow's milk and beef protein
Histidine	26	(19)[a]	22–34
Isoleucine	46	28	47–54
Leucine	93	66	81–95
Lysine	66	58	70–89
Methionine + cystine	42	25	33[b]–57
Phenylalanine + tyrosine	72	63	80–102
Threonine	43	34	44–47
Tryptophan	17	11	12[b]–17
Valine	55	35	50–66

[a]Essentiality of histidine not clearly determined after 1 year of age.
[b]Cow's milk proteins have less sulfur-containing amino acids and tryptophan than human milk.

Table 4 True protein digestibility of selected foods and diets

	True protein digestibility (%)
Egg white	97
Whole egg, milk, beef, poultry, fish	95
Wheat, refined flour	95
Soya protein isolate	94
Polished rice	88
Soya flour	86
Wheat, whole	86
Maize products	85
Rice, whole	84
Beans	69
Mixed diets	
USA	96
China	94
Colombia, high-income	93
Philippines, urban	88
Chile, middle class	82
Mexico, rural	80
Guatemala, rural	79
Brazil, rural	78
India, vegetarian	78

fibre, tannins and other polyphenols), the presence of antiphysiological factors that interfere with protein breakdown (e.g. trypsin inhibitors, lectins) and processing conditions that alter the nature or release of amino acids (e.g. Maillard reaction, formation of polyamino acids and methylmercaptan). Consequently, amino acid scores as predictors of protein quality must be adjusted for protein digestibility and amino acid availability.

The standard for obtaining digestibility data is through clinical (metabolic) studies in humans, in which the nitrogen excreted in the faeces is subtracted from the amount ingested with the diet and expressed as a percentage of intake. This apparent digestibility value must be corrected for the amount of faecal nitrogen excreted when a person is consuming a protein-free diet to calculate 'true' digestibility (Table 1). Ethical constraints and practical complexities do not permit determining obligatory faecal nitrogen losses on a protein-free diet in all age and

physiological groups. It is then recommended that existing published values for daily obligatory faecal losses in preschool children (around 20 mg N kg^{-1}) and adults (around 14 mg N kg^{-1}) be used to correct apparent protein digestibility values.

Established digestibility values of well-defined foods and diets may be taken from published reliable data. **Table 4** shows some examples. When such data are not available for a mixed diet, a weighted average can be calculated from the true digestibilities of its constituent protein sources, as illustrated in **Table 5**. For new or novel products or processes, digestibility must be determined, preferably in humans. When cost and practicality do not permit performing metabolic studies in humans, a standardized faecal balance method in rats has been recommended. This method has given true protein digestibility values of 93–100% for animal foods or food products (casein, beef salami, skim milk, tuna, chicken sausage) and soya protein isolate; 86–92% for beef stew, chick peas, rolled oats, and whole-wheat cereal; and 70–85% for lentils and different types of beans. These value ranges are similar to data from human studies. Nevertheless, rat data must be used with caution for foods and diets which are known or suspected of being handled differently by the human and rat intestines. *In vitro* procedures have also been developed, using combinations of trypsin, chymotrypsin, peptidase and bacterial protease. Some look promising but further research is needed to validate their use as predictors of protein digestibility in humans.

Calculations and examples

Protein quality of individual foods can be calculated from laboratory analysis and clinical studies or from reliable published data of their protein content, amino acid profile and true digestibility. The percentage or fractional value of the most limiting EAA (non-corrected amino acid score) is multiplied by the percentage of fractional value of the true protein digestibility to obtain the corrected score. Proteins that have no limiting amino acids are assigned a non-corrected amino acid score of 100% (or 1.00), even when all the EAAs have a value greater than 100%

Table 5 Calculation of true digestibility of a mixed diet of rice, beans, wheat and egg

Diet	True protein digestibility (%)	Proportion of total protein (g per 100 g protein in whole diet)
Polished rice	88	40
Black beans	69	35
Whole wheat	86	15
Whole egg	95	10
Estimated digestibility of whole diet:	$(0.88 \times 40) + (0.69 \times 35) + (0.86 \times 15) + (0.95 \times 10) =$ **82%**	

in comparison with the amino acid scoring pattern. Similarly, if the clinical or experimental assessment of 'true' protein digestibility gives a value greater than 100% due to experimental variability, a digestibility correction factor of 100% (or 1.00) is used. The corrected amino acid score is equivalent to protein quality. This is sometimes expressed in relation to a 'standard' protein, usually casein or an animal food (milk, egg, beef). **Table 6** shows examples of calculations for a single protein source. The same procedure can be used for food mixtures. When there are no laboratory or published data for a food mixture, the corrected amino acid score can be calculated by a weighted average procedure based on the protein content, amino acid composition and digestibility of the individual components. **Table 7** is an example of those calculations; for simplicity, only the four EAAs that usually can be limiting are shown.

Improvement of Protein Quality

Amino acid profile

The amino acid profile of a food or diet can be improved by increasing the amount of constituent amino acids in its proteins, adding synthetic amino acids or combining foods in proportions that result in a better amino acid pattern.

Genetic handling   This has resulted in cereals with higher contents of the amino acids that limit its protein quality. For example, varieties of Opaque-2 corn have around 50% more lysine and 35% more tryptophan, both of which are limiting amino acids in native corn.

Fortification and enrichment   The addition of synthetic amino acids, as in lysine-enriched wheat flour, eliminates or reduces the effect of limiting amino acids.

Complementation   The combination of a food that has one or more limiting EAAs with other food(s) that have a surplus of those amino acids results in

an improved combined amino acid profile. A double complementation effect has been achieved in the formulation of vegetable mixtures based on protein sources with different limiting amino acids, as illustrated in **Fig. 1**.

Digestibility and bioavailability

Various food processing procedures can improve protein digestibility by removing food constituents that reduce digestibility (such as dietary fibre), breaking down poorly digestible vegetable cell membranes, destroying or neutralizing antiphysiological factors and increasing the food surface area that can come in contact with gastrointestinal enzymes. For example, soya protein isolate, polished rice, and refined wheat flour have higher protein digestibilities than soya flour, whole rice and whole wheat, respectively (Table 4).

Food storage and processing under adverse circumstances can reduce protein quality by making some of its EAAs unavailable for use in the human body. These conditions should be avoided to preserve protein quality. Some examples are the storage of dried milk under mild–moderate heat and humidity, which renders lysine side chains unavailable after reacting with the reducing sugar, lactose (Maillard or 'browning' reaction); the severe treatment of protein with alkali, which causes lysine and cysteine residues to react and form lysinoalanine; and the treatment of proteins with oxidizing agents, which can result in a loss of methionine. Severe heating conditions in the presence of reducing sugars or oxidized lipids can make some food proteins resistant to digestion, thereby reducing the availability of all its amino acids.

Protein concentration

The amount of protein per unit of food also contributes to the overall protein quality and nutritive value of a protein source. This can be especially important for young infants and elderly persons whose small gastric capacity or poor appetite limit the amount of food they eat.

Table 6 Calculation of amino acid scores of single protein sources corrected for digestibility and in relation to the protein quality of cow's milk

Food	Most limiting amino acid	Noncorrected amino acid score	True protein digestibility	Corrected amino acid score	Protein quality relative to milk
Cow's milk	None	>100 → 100%	× 95%	= **95%**	–
Polished rice	Lysine 36 mg per g protein	(36/58) × 100 = 62%	× 88%	= **55%**	(55/95) × 100 = **58%**
Egg white	None	>100 → 100%	× 97%	= **97%**	(97/95) × 100 = **102%**

Table 7 Calculation of protein quality of a mixed diet based on whole wheat, polished rice and chicken breast

| Raw ingredients | Data from analysis or literature | | | | | | | Quantities calculated for the mixed diet | | | | |
	Weight (g) A	Protein (g per 100 g) B	Lys[a] (mg per g protein) C	SAA[a] D	Th[a] E	Trp[a] F	True digestibility (%) G	Total protein (g) $H = A \times B/100$	Lys (mg) $I = H \times C$	SAA (mg) $J = H \times D$	Thr (mg) $K = H \times E$	Trp (mg) $L = H \times F$
Whole wheat	300	11	28	37	29	11	86	33	924	1221	957	363
Polished rice	200	7	36	38	33	13	88	14	504	532	462	182
Chicken breast	150	19	83	38	40	12	95	28.5	2366	1083	1140	342
Totals								75.5	3794	2836	2559	887

M Weighted mean digestibility of the mixed diet (sum of $(G \times H)$ for each   **0.90**
   food component divided by total protein, H)

N mg amino acid per g protein (totals for I, J, K or L divided by total H)   50   38   34   12

P Amino acid scoring pattern, mg amino acid per g protein   58   25   34   11

Q Score for each amino acid in the mixed diet (N/P)   0.86   1.52   1.00   1.09

R Amino acid score adjusted for digestibility (Q of the limiting amino acid $0.86 \times 0.90 = $ **0.77** (or **77%**)
   multiplied by M)

Lys, lysine; SAA, sulfur-containing amino acids; Thr, threonine; Trp, tryptophan.
[a]Values given as mg per g protein.

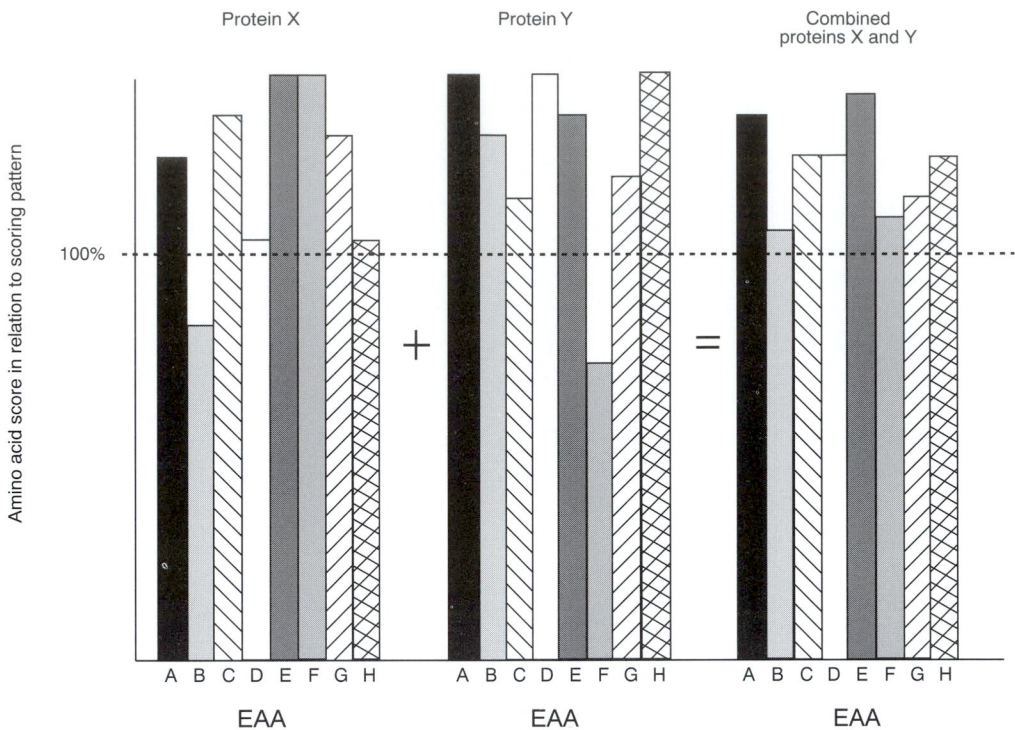

Protein X   Protein Y   Combined proteins X and Y

Figure 1 Amino acid complementation: when the two proteins are combined, protein X compensates the deficiency of amino acid F in protein Y, and protein Y compensates the deficiency of amino acid B in protein X (EAA = Essential Amino Acids). From Torun B, Menchu MT and Elias LG (1994) *Recomendaciones Dietéticas Diarias del INCAP*. INCAP publication ME/057. Guatemala: Institute of Nutrition of Central America and Panama.

Protein concentration can increase by genetic selection of protein sources, as in improved varieties of rice that have about 30% more protein than native rice, by the use of nitrogen-containing fertilizers that can raise the protein contents of several cereals, or by industrial and home processing that reduce the water content of food preparations. Addition of concentrated protein sources, such as casein, soya protein isolates, soya flour, milk powder or dehydrated egg, will also increase the protein concentration of foods and diets, as well as their amino acid score in some instances.

Evaluation of a food on the basis of its protein concentration must be done in ready-to-eat preparations. Protein concentration of raw foods can be misleading, since food processing and dilution can result in significant changes, as illustrated in **Table 8**. Meats, poultry and fish usually have a higher concentration of protein after cooking or frying, whereas vegetable food preparations contain less protein than the raw products.

Dietary Sources

Foods of animal origin, such as milk and milk products, eggs, meats, poultry and fish, have an excellent amino acid profile with a score of 100% and true

Table 8 Protein concentration in selected raw and ready-to-eat foods (g protein per 100 g food)

Food	Ready-to-eat		Raw
Beef, lean	36.8	(cooked)	21.4
Fish	31.8	(fried)	20.0
Wheat flour	12.0	(white bread)	11.0
Egg, hen	11.3	(hard-boiled)	11.3
Lentils	7.1	(cooked)	23.7
Common beans	6.2	(cooked)	22.0
Maize	4.2	(tortilla)	9.4
Milk powder, cow	3.2	(12% in water)	26.1
Rice	2.5	(boiled)	7.2
Potato, no skin	1.1	(cooked)	1.8

protein digestibility of 95–98%. In addition, their protein concentrations often increase after cooking. Consequently, they are used as the reference for comparison of protein quality, provided that they are processed in ways that will not decrease amino acid bioavailability.

Almost all vegetable foods have one or more limiting amino acids. Soya beans and soya products are notable exceptions. In general, proteins in natural vegetable foods have digestibilities of 70–85%. Vegetable protein isolates, flours and extruded products have higher digestibilities.

Among vegetables, pulses have the highest protein

concentrations, ranging from 20–25% in most raw beans and peas, to about 36% in soya beans. Pulses usually have limiting sulfur-containing amino acids.

Cereals and cereal products are the largest source of proteins in most parts of the world because of their large production and consumption. Cereal grains and flours contain around 7–12% protein. Protein quality is limited by their lysine content and, in many instances, also by threonine and/or tryptophan. Although deficient in lysine and threonine, rice has one of the best amino acid profiles among cereals, while sorghum and native maize (i.e. not genetically improved) are among the lowest.

Most nuts and edible seeds contain 8–18% protein. Many oil seeds have 12–20% protein and the cake that remains after oil extrusion can have as much as 30–40% protein.

See also: **Amino Acids**: Chemistry and Classification; Metabolism. **Protein**: Digestion and Bioavailability; Requirements and Role in Diet; Synthesis and Turnover; Deficiency.

Further Reading

Bach-Knudsen KE, Wisker E, Daniel M, Feldheim W and Eggum BO (1994) Digestibility of energy, protein, fat and non-starch polysaccharides in mixed diets: comparative studies between man and the rat. *British Journal of Nutrition* 71:471–487.

Bodwell CE, Carpenter KJ and McDonough FE (eds) (1989) A collaborative study of methods of protein evaluation: introductory paper. *Plant Foods in Human Nutrition* 39:3–11.

FAO (1970) *Amino Acid Content of Foods and Biological Data on Proteins*. FAO Nutrition Studies no. 24. Rome: Food and Agriculture Organization of the United Nations.

FAO/WHO (1991) *Protein Quality Evaluation*. FAO Food and Nutrition Paper no. 51. Rome: Food and Agriculture Organization of the United Nations.

FAO/WHO/UNU (1985) *Energy and Protein Requirements*. WHO Technical Report Series no. 724, pp 64–70, 117–127. Geneva: World Health Organization.

McDonough FE, Sarwar G, Steinke FH, Slump P, Garcia S and Boisen S (1990) In vitro assay for protein digestibility: interlaboratory study. *Journal of the Association of Official Analytical Chemists* 73:622–625.

McDonough FE, Steinke FH, Sarwar G, Eggum BO, Bressani R, Huth PJ, Barbeau WE, Mitchell GV and Phillips JG (1990) In vivo rat assay for true protein digestibility: collaborative study. *Journal of the Association of Official Analytical Chemists* 73:801–805.

Pineda O, Torun B, Viteri FE and Arroyave G (1981) Protein quality in relation to estimates of essential amino acid requirements. In: Bodwell CE, Adkins JS and Hopkins DT (eds) *Protein Quality in Humans: Assessment*

and In Vitro Estimation, pp 29–42. Westport: AVI Publishing Co.

Sarwar G and McDonough FE (eds) (1990) Evaluation of protein digestibility-corrected amino acid score method for assessing protein quality of foods. *Journal of the Association of Official Analytical Chemists* 73:347–356.

Torun B (1990) Current concepts on requirements of essential amino acids. In: *New Era! Global Harmony Through Nutrition*. 14th International Congress of Nutrition: Symposium Lectures, pp 87–91. Seoul: Ewha Womans University.

Torun B, Menchu MT and Elias LG (1994) *Recomendaciones Dietéticas Diarias del INCAP* ('INCAP's Recommended Daily Dietary Allowances'), pp 16–32. INCAP Publication ME/057. Guatemala: Institute of Nutrition of Central America and Panama.

Torun B, Pineda O, Viteri FE and Arroyave G (1981) Use of amino acid composition data to predict protein nutritive value for children with specific reference to new estimates of their essential amino acid requirements. In: Bodwell CE, Adkins JS and Hopkins DT (eds) *Protein Quality in Humans: Assessment and In Vitro Estimation*, pp 374–393. Westport: AVI Publishing Co.

Young VR, Bier DM and Pellett PM (1989) A theoretical basis for increasing current estimates of the amino acid requirements in adult man, with experimental support. *American Journal of Clinical Nutrition* 50:80–92.

Requirements and Role in Diet

D J Millward, University of Surrey, Guildford, UK

Estimation of Protein Requirements

Terminology

Protein requirements are best discussed in terms of metabolic demand, dietary requirement and dietary allowances. *Metabolic demand* is determined by the nature and extent of those metabolic pathways (e.g. net protein synthesis) that consume amino acids, and which vary with the phenotype and the developmental and physiological state of the individual. The *dietary requirement* is the amount of protein or its constituent amino acids that must be supplied in the diet in order to satisfy the metabolic demand. The requirement will usually be greater than the metabolic demand because of factors influencing the efficiency of protein utilization: these are factors associated with digestion and absorption, which affect the digestibility and consequently the amount of dietary nitrogen lost in the faeces, and the cellular bioavailability of the absorbed amino acid pattern in relation to cellular needs, which affects the biological value. *Dietary allowances* are a range of intakes derived from estimates of individual requirements which are designed to meet the dietary requirements of the population and which take into account the variability between individuals in that dietary requirement. In the UK these allowances are described in terms of *dietary reference values* (DRVs).

Metabolic role

The metabolic demand for dietary protein is to provide amino acid precursors for the synthesis of tissue proteins and a range of nonprotein products.

Tissue proteins are diverse; they include structural or fibrous insoluble proteins and soluble globular proteins, with characteristic properties and functions determined by their amino acid sequence. All proteins are in a dynamic state of constant turnover, i.e. breakdown to constituent amino acids and resynthesis, although for the structural proteins this is slow or minimal.

Nonprotein products include nucleic acids and a diverse range of smaller molecules such as creatine, taurine, glutathione, hormones (e.g. catecholamines and thyroxine), neurotransmitters (serotonin, dopamine) and nitric oxide, a key regulator of blood flow and other physiological processes.

With continuous and extensive amino acid interconversion, dietary amino acids need not match the composition of tissue proteins exactly because some amino acids are dispensable and can be replaced by other amino acids or nitrogen sources. However, amino acids that are not interconverted or which are formed only slowly from other amino acids need to be provided in the diet and are classified as indispensable. Traditionally, dietary proteins have been classified in terms of their nutritional value (quality) measured in terms of their ability to provide for tissue growth in rapidly growing rats. With these criteria marked differences are observed between most animal proteins and plant protein sources, with the relative nutritional values reflecting mainly the relative amounts of indispensable amino acids. The similarity between overall tissue protein amino acid composition and that of most animal dietary protein sources and the contrast with plant protein sources resulted in clear distinctions between their quality. In particular, cereal proteins tend to have low levels of lysine and tryptophan, while legumes have low levels of sulfur-containing amino acids. When plant proteins are combined, however, it has been recognized that they can provide the appropriate balance of essential amino acids.

However, in human nutrition with growth occur-

ring very slowly after the first few months of life the nutritional demand for indispensable amino acids for tissue growth is much less and may be minimal. While considerable protein synthesis continues as part of the turnover of body protein, this generates little metabolic demand for amino acids because of amino acid recycling. Some net protein synthesis occurs associated with continuing growth of skin and hair, and the synthesis of gastric secretions (e.g. threonine-rich mucus glycoproteins) which pass into the colon to be utilized for bacterial metabolism. At nitrogen equilibrium the metabolic demand is for the maintenance of normal function and composition. In this case nutritional needs are more complex and reflect the rates at which amino acids are needed for the various metabolic pathways other than protein synthesis. Thus the qualitative nature of the metabolic demands for amino acids for growth, mainly the amino acid pattern of tissue protein, is quite different from that required for maintenance. Contrary to general opinion, the distinction between dietary protein sources in terms of the nutritional superiority of animal protein over plant protein is much more difficult to demonstrate and less relevant in human nutrition. This was recognized by The World Health Organization in a joint report with the Food and Agriculture Organization in 1991, and there are currently, no universally agreed values for the requirements for indispensable amino acids in the human diet; and different views exist about the relative importance of dietary protein quality in human nutrition. National bodies reviewing the issue have stressed that in most mixed, nutritionally balanced diets sufficient indispensable amino acids will be provided regardless of the relative amounts of plant and animal protein sources.

The diverse biological demands for amino acids for maintenance represent an essential but probably small intrinsic metabolic demand for protein as indicated by the magnitude of the obligatory nitrogen loss. In subjects fed a protein-free but otherwise nutritionally adequate diet nitrogen losses fall, reaching a stable and reproducible low level after 7–14 days with the subject losing body protein at a constant daily rate. These losses, the obligatory nitrogen losses (ONL), are assumed to represent nitrogen end products of amino acids derived from body protein and utilized for the obligatory metabolic demand. In normal adult men the obligatory urinary, faecal and surface losses of nitrogen are about 37 mg kg^{-1}, 9 mg kg^{-1} and 8 mg kg^{-1} respectively, i.e. 54 mg per kg per day, in total equivalent to a protein loss of 0.34 g per kg per day. The ONL is a function of body weight and, when normalized to 'metabolic body size' ($W^{0.75}$, where W is the body weight in kg), varies little with age. It is likely that the true metabolic demand for protein for maintenance is even less than 0.34 g per kg per day. This amount of tissue protein lost each day will include both amino acids required to provide the maintenance metabolic demand and other amino acids not actually needed but which cannot be returned on their own to the tissue protein pool. Thus, when individual amino acids such as threonine, tryptophan and the sulfur-containing amino acids are fed as part of the protein-free diet, the net loss of tissue protein falls considerably.

The ONL at a rate of protein loss of 0.34 g per kg per day is only 50% of current estimates of the daily protein requirement (0.6 g kg^{-1}) and the nature of this additional need (the difference between 0.34 and 0.6 g protein) has been the cause of considerable confusion. Traditionally, maintenance protein requirements were defined in terms of metabolic demands represented by the ONL and an inefficiency of utilization which accounted for additional need, although why proteins such as those in milk, egg or meat were not utilized more efficiently was always puzzling. It is now known that the additional need represents an actual metabolic demand generated in response to the presence of protein in the diet at levels in excess of minimal metabolic needs.

Since amino acids can only be stored as protein, for which the body's storage capacity is limited, excess dietary amino acids are oxidized and converted to glucose or fat. Many amino acids, especially the branched-chain, aromatic and sulfur-containing amino acids, represent a potentially toxic challenge to the organism and are maintained at very low levels in the tissue free amino acid pools. After a meal, these amino acids, if not deposited in protein, are rapidly removed by oxidative catabolism, mediated by high-capacity, sensitively regulated pathways. Furthermore, the capacity and activity of these pathways adapt to match the protein levels in the diet to ensure rapid postprandial disposal. Most importantly, because this adaptation of oxidative catabolism to a change of protein intake is relatively slow, the extent of postprandial oxidative catabolism reflects mainly the habitual rather than actual protein intake in meals. In effect, the habitual level of protein in the diet creates a level of oxidative amino acid catabolism sufficient to avoid accumulation of toxic concentrations of certain free amino acids, and this becomes part of the metabolic demand. Furthermore, this habitual protein intake-dependent, regulatory oxidative catabolism occurs in both the postprandial and postabsorptive state (e.g. at night) with a postabsorptive loss of tissue protein, and this generates a metabolic demand for postprandial tissue protein

repletion. It would appear that during slow growth or at weight maintenance, in order to be able to dispose rapidly of dietary protein in excess of minimal needs, pathways of oxidative amino acid catabolism are in effect primed to operate at the appropriate rate set by habitual protein intakes, and this rate continues regardless of the actual acute intake, utilizing tissue protein if the dietary level falls or during the postabsorptive state, for as long as it takes to adapt to the lower level of intake. As a result there is a diurnal cycle of postabsorptive losses and postprandial gains with an amplitude which increases with the increasing habitual level of protein intake.

The overall metabolic scheme is shown in **Fig. 1**. The dietary protein contributes amino acids to the tissue free amino acid pool which is in a state of dynamic exchange with the protein pool through protein turnover. The metabolic demand includes both net protein synthesis (i.e. the repletion of postabsorptive losses and any growth), and irreversible amino acid metabolism and oxidative metabolism. The latter component is shown divided into three parts: (1) the metabolic demands for nonprotein products which eventually give rise to an obligatory nitrogen loss; (2) adaptive oxidative amino acid catabolism which is also part of the metabolic demand; and (3) any additional oxidative amino acid catabolism due to an inefficiency of protein utilization. Within this metabolic framework the determination of protein requirements is a problem of assessing both intrinsic, fixed metabolic demands and the adaptive oxidative catabolism, which together define the metabolic demand; assessment of the latter component accounts for the major practical and conceptual difficulties in applying nitrogen balance techniques to the study of protein requirements.

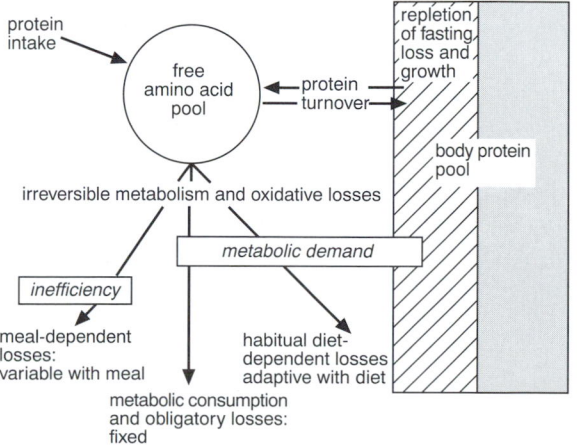

Figure 1 Metabolic fate of dietary protein in terms of the metabolic demand for net protein synthesis, and irreversible amino acid metabolism and oxidative catabolism.

The diurnal cycle of postabsorptive losses and postprandial gains of increasing amplitude with increasing habitual protein intakes is shown in **Fig. 2**. This also includes the concept that the body protein mass is regulated at a fixed upper limit – a mechanism that has been described as a 'protein-stat'.

Nitrogen Balance

Nitrogen balance studies were initiated in the mid nineteenth century by Carl Voit and such studies have been central to the definition of protein requirements ever since. The aim of nitrogen balance studies is simple, i.e. to define the relationship between intake and all losses (urinary, faecal and surface: mainly sweat, skin, hair, breath ammonia and nail clippings), so that the intake which allows equilibrium and provides for all losses can be identified. Thus, when the intake equals the requirement,

$$balance = intake - losses = 0$$

As indicated above, the lowest level of nitrogen losses observed, the ONL, is about 54 mg per kg per day, equivalent to a daily loss of protein of 0.34 g per kg per day. When such subjects are refed with protein, losses of body protein fall as the dietary protein provides for some of the metabolic demand. However, nitrogen losses increase with intake, so that the requirement intake for balance is more than the ONL. The main objective of nitrogen balance studies has been to define how much extra protein above the ONL must be fed to achieve equilibrium. Despite the numerous reports on human nitrogen balance studies, this objective has not been satisfactorily resolved.

Some of the difficulties reflect the practical problems that arise in performing nitrogen balance studies. Measurements of nitrogen balance (i.e. N intake minus all N losses) are relatively imprecise, with balance a small value compared with the much larger

values of nitrogen intake and excretion, resulting in considerable error in the prediction of balance. Typical errors are in the range of ± 11 mg per kg per day, more than the entire miscellaneous nitrogen losses (8 mg kg^{-1}).

Other difficulties stem from the nonlinearity of the balance curve. Since body protein content is regulated at a characteristic maximum size, in feeding trials starting at low intakes, losses rise to match intakes when body protein reaches the maximum level. The intake–balance curve must be curvilinear, with balance increasing asymptotically towards zero with intake as losses increase to eventually match intake. In fact there is a further complication with the common finding that at high intakes balance is usually overestimated, with unrealistic positive balances for reasons not explained. This means that there is no simple term to define the overall shape of the balance curve allowing prediction of the requirement (as the zero balance intake). Feeding trials are time-consuming and laborious, and in practice, few different intakes can be fed, and the design of feeding trials with intakes close to the requirement avoiding complex curve fitting has proved most difficult. Prediction of a zero balance–intake intercept from a few balance points by linear regression will result in requirement values that will vary according to where the intake values lie on the balance curve. Thus, studies conducted at low intakes will underestimate requirements, while studies conducted with intakes exceeding maintenance levels will overestimate requirements (**Fig. 3**). Reliable balance studies are therefore those conducted with intakes very close to the actual requirement, and studies with intakes based on preconceived requirement values will tend to confirm such preconceptions. With the coefficient of variation within nitrogen balance studies being high, e.g. 36% within a study with similar subjects

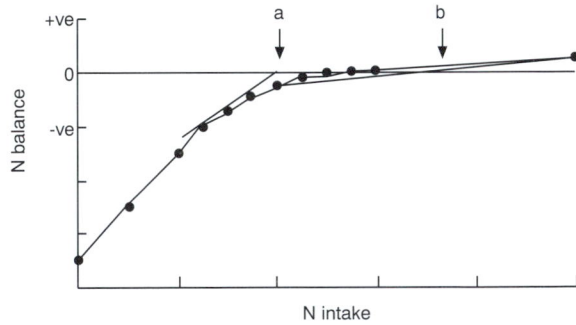

Figure 3 Nitrogen balance curve showing curvilinear relationship between intake and balance. Prediction of a zero balance-intake intercept from a few balance points at low intakes by linear regression (a) will underestimate requirements, while studies conducted with intakes in excess of maintenance requirements (b) will overestimate requirements.

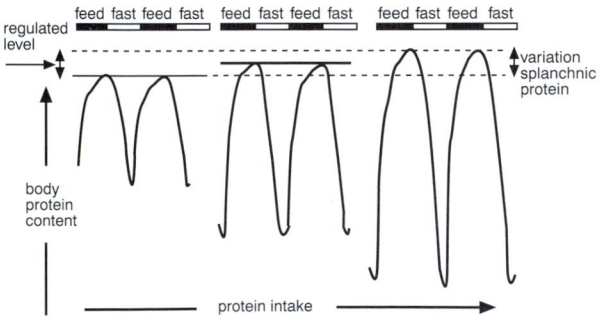

Figure 2 Balance regulation throughout the diurnal cycle in relation to increasing habitual protein intakes.

fed the same diets, in part because of day-to-day variation in the balance achieved, it is clear that the nitrogen balance method is a very blunt tool for establishing protein requirements. The main difficulty with the nitrogen balance method is reconciling an apparently simple objective with the complex adaptive behaviour of amino acid and nitrogen homeostasis to variation in intake.

Adaptation

With the metabolic demand for amino acids including both fixed and variable demands, the relationship between intakes and balance will be a function of time and the rate of adaptation. This is undoubtedly why the determination of human protein requirement by nitrogen balance has proved to be so difficult.

As indicated above, subjects normally consuming high protein intakes and exhibiting high rates of amino acid oxidation and nitrogen excretion will continue to do this for a considerable time after switching to lower intakes, resulting in loss of body protein and negative nitrogen balance (**Fig. 4**). Balance at the lower intake will only be restored when oxidative catabolism has fully adapted to the new lower level. This can take several weeks, with slower changes occurring over periods of months. Indeed, some have argued that with time adaptation to intakes equal to the ONL was eventually possible (although this view is not widely accepted). Since balance trials necessarily involve relatively short-term periods of adaptation, complete adaptation to new intakes is unlikely within the trial. Thus it is

likely that much of the variation in balance observed between individuals on similar intakes reflects differences in the extent of their adaptation to the feeding levels. With habitual protein intakes from the mixed diets consumed in developed countries 2–3 times higher than average requirements, balance trials attempting to define minimum requirements for such populations will require considerable adaptive reductions in amino acid oxidative catabolism to occur and this may require more time than can be practically allowed for in feeding trials.

Energy–protein Interactions

Energy intake has long been known to influence the amount of protein needed for balance. If dietary energy is below the requirement, dietary protein will be utilized for energy, will not meet the amino acid metabolic demand and such diets will require more protein to allow balance if it occurs at all. When excess energy is fed and there is weight gain with some protein deposition, balance can be achieved at lower intakes. Thus the choice of energy level at which balance trials are conducted – adequate but not excessive energy intakes – becomes an important consideration.

The quantitative relationship between energy intake and nitrogen balance has been investigated in several studies. Multiple regression of daily nitrogen balance (NB) in mg kg^{-1} on daily energy intake (EI) in kcal kg^{-1} and nitrogen intake (NI) in grams of protein per kilogram indicates that

$$NB = 0.171NI + 1.006EI - 69.13$$

This means that the protein requirement (i.e. the intake for zero nitrogen balance) varies with the energy intake (**Table 1**).

Since NB varies as a function of energy intake it might be argued that protein requirements can only be defined in terms of a specified energy intake level. The problem then becomes one of defining the appropriate energy intake. Energy equilibrium is not easily measured and weight maintenance alone is inadequate since the energy intake for weight

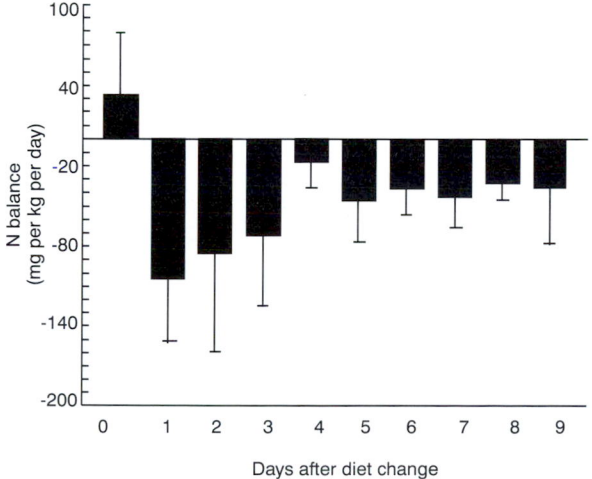

Figure 4 Nitrogen balance in subjects consuming a high protein intake (2 g per kg per day) and after switching to a lower daily intake of 0.75 g kg^{-1}. Balance at the lower intake requires oxidative amino acid catabolism to adapt fully to the lower level, which can take several weeks.

Table 1 Variation of protein requirement with energy intake

Energy intake		Protein requirement	
(kcal kg^{-1})	*(kJ kg^{-1})*	*Nitrogen (mg kg^{-1})*	*Protein (g kg^{-1})*
30	125	227.8	1.42
45	188	139.5	0.87
60	250	51.3	0.32

maintenance varies with the protein intake. In fact the question raises several major issues. Should protein requirement recommendations be increased for populations in the developing world with marginal energy intakes and lowered in the developed world because of the higher energy intakes? Protein intakes of developing populations are already lower than in the industrialized countries through generally lower intakes of animal foods. These are difficult questions with no simple answers.

Functional significance of intake level for zero balance

With appropriate resources and with sufficient time for adaptation a minimum protein requirement to which humans can ultimately adapt can be identified, and this will be between the intake from normal diets (i.e. 0.8–1.5 g per day) and the 0.34 g protein per day equivalent of the ONL. Values ranging from 0.45 g to 0.7 g have been reported. Such studies are identifying in effect a *minimal* requirement. However, since natural diets providing sufficient energy and other nutrients always provide more protein than this, the magnitude of this minimal requirement becomes to some extent an issue of scientific curiosity only. It has been suggested that the requirement for balance is less important than the functional consequences of particular levels of protein in the diet. In other words, the key issue is that of an *optimal* requirement which not only allows balance but also supports optimal body function (e.g. optimal immune function, and minimal long-term deterioration of renal function).

While the issue of an *optimal* protein requirement is generally recognized as important, there is little qualitative or quantitative information. In growing animals dietary protein intakes in excess of those associated with maximum efficiency of protein utilization have been shown to increase rates of bone growth through hormonal mechanisms involving insulin and insulin-like growth factor I. This has resulted in the concept of an 'anabolic drive' of dietary protein exerted by protein intakes in excess of minimal needs. The extent to which this is important in human growth has yet to be explored.

The importance of dietary protein for the maintenance of the immune system has also been suggested, with dietary protein influencing the response to infection through several mechanisms. One mechanism is the maintenance of gut barrier function, through provision of threonine, cysteine and other amino acids involved in synthesis of mucus glycoproteins. Another is maintenance of general immunocompetence through provision of specific amino acids for synthesis of cellular proteins of the immune system

and to support the hepatic acute-phase protein response. In particular glutathione, a key free radical scavenger synthesized from glutamate (glutamine), glycine and cysteine, is depleted in hepatic and intestinal mucosa in protein-restricted animals, in the erythrocytes of infants suffering from kwashiorkor, and in low-birthweight infants who have low circulating levels. The reduced level in rats is restored by providing cysteine in the diet. The influence of protein intake on glutamine levels is also a possible factor. Glutamine is strongly concentrated in skeletal muscle, appears to play a specific role in maintaining function of rapidly proliferating cells such as lymphocytes and mucosal enterocytes, and also regulates muscle protein turnover. Under conditions of infection and trauma, muscle concentrations of glutamine fall and this may limit the provision of glutamine for the immune system or to the splanchnic bed where it appears to play a specific role in maintaining glutathione synthesis during trauma. Taurine, a β-aminosulfonic acid derived from cysteine, appears to be an effective scavenger of peroxidation products (particularly those containing the oxychloride groups) and acts as a neuromodulatory agent. Taurine is specifically concentrated in skeletal musculature and in the central nervous system. Creatine, a compound that is crucial for energy flow within skeletal muscle, is synthesized from glycine, arginine and a suitable source of methyl groups, and is concentrated in skeletal muscle and brain; it is lost from muscle during infection and trauma, with a deterioration of muscle contractile function. Because glutamine, creatine and taurine are maintained at substantial concentrations in the free amino acid fraction of milk, it is thought that provision of all three compounds is important in supporting postnatal development. Finally, provision of arginine is important in relation to the immune system. This may relate to its role as precursor for nitric oxide synthesis, a key regulator of a variety of physiological processes which include the regulation of hepatic protein metabolism, macrophage killer function and interactions between macrophages, and lymphocyte adhesion and activation. It is currently argued that:

1. The metabolic end products of specific amino acids are crucial intermediates in maintaining a variety of physiological functions.
2. These functions bear only an indirect relationship to protein metabolism.
3. Precursors for synthesis of these compounds are often nonessential (e.g. glutamate, glutamine) or conditionally essential amino acids (e.g. glycine, arginine and cysteine).

Notwithstanding the growth in research in this

area, details of nonessential and conditionally essential amino acid synthesis and metabolism *in vivo* remain fragmentary, and most importantly it is as yet not possible to define an optimal protein requirement in terms of the amounts of dietary protein needed to provide for these additional needs.

Recommendations for Protein Intakes

Current dietary reference values for protein in the UK (**Table 2**) derive from 1985 recommendations by the Food and Agriculture Organization, World Heath Organization and United Nations University (FAO/WHO/UNU). The *estimated average requirement* (EAR) defines the notional mean requirement for the population group. The *recommended nutrient intake* (RNI) is defined according to the range of interindividual variability and is 2 standard devi-

Table 2 Dietary reference values for protein published by the UK Department of Health

Age	Weight (kg)	EAR[b] (g per day)	RNI (g per day)
0–3 months	5.9	–[c]	12.5
4–6 months	7.7	10.6	12.7
7–9 months	8.8	11.0	13.7
10–12 months	9.7	11.2	14.9
1–3 years	12.5	11.7	14.5
4–6 years	17.8	14.8	19.7
7–10 years	28.3	22.8	28.3
Males			
11–14 years	43.0	33.8	42.1
15–18 years	64.5	46.1	55.2
19–50 years	74.0	44.4	55.5
50+ years	71.0	42.6	53.3
Females			
11–14 years	43.8	33.1	41.2
15–18 years	55.5	37.1	45.4
19–50 years	60.0	36.0	45.0
50+ years	62.0	37.2	46.5
Pregnancy[a]			+6
Lactation:			
0–6 months			+11
6+ months			+8

From UK Department of Health (1991).
EAR, estimated average requirement; RNI, reference nutrient intake.
[a]To be added to adult requirement through all stages of pregnancy and lactation.
[b]Milk or egg protein. These figures assume complete digestibility. For diets based on high intakes of vegetable proteins, a correction may need to be applied to take account of reduced digestibility.
[c]No figures were given by WHO for infants aged 0–3 months, therefore no EAR has been derived. The RNI is calculated from previous UK Department of Health recommendations.

ations (SD) above the EAR. The RNI (or recommended dietary allowance) is thus an intake which will meet the requirement of most of the population assuming normal distribution of requirements, and is therefore a 'safe' allowance. The *lower nutrient reference intake* (LNRI), which is 2 SD below the EAR, defines the lowest intake that will meet the requirement of some of the population. The values derive from balance studies and have not taken into account functional consequences of the level of protein intake, because of lack of information. These aspects have only been considered in relation to the definition of a safe upper limit.

Maintenance requirements derive from short-term and long-term nitrogen balances in adults, which indicated a rounded value for protein of 0.6 g per kg per day (96 mg per kg per day of nitrogen) for the EAR. For infants and children, a much more limited range of short-term balance studies indicated a maintenance value for nitrogen of 120 mg kg^{-1} which was assumed for children up to 12 months of age, with values for intermediate ages (1–20 years) interpolated between this and the adult value (96 mg kg^{-1}). Growth requirements were calculated from accretion rates of protein in the bodies of infants and children, adjusted to take account of the efficiency of utilization (70%) and daily variation in growth rates (an addition of 50%), indicating a requirement calculated as $(1/0.7) \times 1.5 = 2.14$ times the metabolic demand. Interindividual variability was assumed as 1 SD = 12.5% (for all except children less than 18 months old for whom values up to 17.5% were used on the basis of a higher coefficient of variation for growth). Thus the RNI was 25% greater than the EAR (35% for infants).

The protein requirements for pregnancy allow for protein retention in the products of conception and in the maternal tissues associated with the birth of an infant weighing 3.3 kg, assuming protein gain in the maternal tissues in the early part of pregnancy and in the fetus mainly in the latter stages, so that the metabolic demand is uniform throughout pregnancy. Thus a single daily additional amount throughout pregnancy is recommended.

The protein requirements for lactation are based on estimates of the protein content of breast milk of healthy mothers (milk nitrogen × 6.25), assuming that daily breast milk protein content is constant for the first 6 months and falls thereafter. The requirement values are shown in Table 2.

In the case of the elderly, the RNI has been assumed to be the same as for younger adults. However, because of the smaller amount of lean body mass per kilogram of body weight in the elderly, this will result in a higher RNI per unit of lean body mass than in younger adults.

In the UK and USA the issue of a safe upper limit has been considered, because of growing concern that excessive intakes of protein may be associated with health risks. Potential problems associated with deterioration of renal function and demineralization of bone have been identified, as well as the fact that populations consuming vegetarian diets and consequently lower protein intakes exhibit lower blood pressure. From these admittedly scant data it has been concluded that it is prudent for adults to avoid protein intakes of more than twice the current safe allowance (i.e. 1.5 g kg^{-1} of protein).

Definitions of protein requirements have historically been problematic and controversial; the current values are no exception and are under review. Most concern exists in relation to the protein requirement of infants and children, with some authors arguing that the currently recommended protein requirements for infants must be overestimates. This argument is based on a comparison of the requirement values with the protein intake of the breast-fed infant. Thus, using the methodology discussed above, a calculation of the EAR for the 3-month old infant indicates a value which is the same as the average protein intakes of the breast-fed infant. If the National Center for Health Statistics standards are taken as representing desirable rates of growth, then it is the case that infants of healthy, well-nourished mothers, consuming habitual amounts of breast milk, can satisfy this target during the early months of life. This indicates that the average breast milk protein intake is, in effect, the safe level, i.e. similar to the RNI and higher than the EAR. New estimates have been suggested (but not yet endorsed) based on lower maintenance and growth values, which result in EAR and RNI values at 3 months of age for protein of 1.06 g kg^{-1} and 1.37 g kg^{-1} respectively. Thus the RNI value would be similar to the mean protein intake of the breast-fed infant (1.44 g kg^{-1}). However, at this age of most rapid growth the nitrogen in breast milk is utilized with unusual efficiency – an indication of the special properties and qualities of breast milk which are poorly understood. Because of this it might be proposed that formula-fed infants require more protein because of less efficient protein utilization. Indeed, some have questioned whether the breast-fed infant is the ideal model for protein requirements, with breast milk protein levels a compromise between feeding the baby and minimizing losses of maternal protein stores.

See also: **Amino Acids**: Metabolism. **Energy**: Energy Requirements; Energy Balance. **Lactation**: Dietary Requirements. **Older People**: Nutritional Requirements. **Pregnancy**: Nutrient Requirements.

Further Reading

FAO/WHO/UNU (1985) *Energy and Protein Requirements*. Report of a joint expert consultation. WHO Technical Report Series 724. Geneva: WHO.

FAO/WHO (1991) *Protein Quality Evaluation*. Report of a joint FAO/WHO expert consultation. FAO Food and Nutrition Paper 51. Geneva: FAO.

Hegsted DM (1976) Balance studies. *Journal of Nutrition* **106**: 307–311.

Millward DJ (1995) A protein-stat mechanism for the regulation of growth and maintenance of the lean-body mass. *Nutrition Research Reviews* **8**: 93–120.

Millward DJ and Rivers JPW (1988) The nutritional role of indispensable amino acids and the metabolic basis for their requirements. *European Journal of Clinical Nutrition* **42**:367–393.

Millward DJ, Jackson AA, Price G and Rivers JPW (1989) Human amino acid and protein requirements: current dilemmas and uncertainties. *Nutrition Research Reviews* **2**: 109–132.

National Research Council (1989) *Recommended Dietary Allowances*. Washington: National Academy Press.

Pellet P and Young VR (1992) Protein energy interactions. In: Scrimshaw NS and Schurch B (eds) *Protein–Energy Interactions*, pp 63–81. I/D/E/C/G. Lausanne: Nestlé Foundation.

Price GM, Halliday D, Pacy PJ, Quevedo MR and Millward DJ (1994) Nitrogen homeostasis in man: 1. Influence of protein intake on the amplitude of diurnal cycling of body nitrogen. *Clinical Science* **86**: 91–102.

Quevedo MR, Price GM, Halliday D, Pacy PJ and Millward DJ (1994) Nitrogen homeostasis in man: 3. Diurnal changes in nitrogen excretion, leucine oxidation and whole body leucine kinetics during a reduction from a high to a moderate protein intake. *Clinical Science* **86**:185–193.

Reeds PJ and Becket PR (1996) Protein and amino acids. In: Ziegler EE and Filer LJ (eds) *Present Knowledge in Nutrition*, 7th ed, chap. 8, pp 67–86. Washington: ILSI Press.

UK Department of Health (1991) *Dietary Reference Values*. London: HMSO.

Synthesis and Turnover

D J Millward, University of Surrey, Guildford, UK

Whole-body Protein Homeostasis

The regulation of the protein mass of the body requires mechanisms that control the protein content within cells, organs and tissues, and which coordinate this control during growth and body weight maintenance. With all intracellular proteins exhibiting turnover, regulation of the cellular protein content involves control of both protein synthesis and proteolysis. For some proteins such control is understood in considerable detail. Less is known about the coordinated control of intracellular protein turnover to maintain an appropriate cellular composition and even less about whole-body coordination. There are two aspects of this coordination: acute control during feeding and fasting, and chronic control during growth and long-term maintenance.

The diurnal cycle of feeding and fasting characteristic of human nutrition results in gains and losses of body protein in subjects in overall nitrogen balance. Furthermore, such diurnal cycling occurs with an amplitude that increases with increasing dietary protein intakes. These oscillations in body protein content involve changes in whole-body and tissue protein synthesis, proteolysis and amino acid oxidation, and much effort has been invested in identifying the control mechanisms.

Long-term homeostasis is a less well-understood phenomenon. For the slow-growing, long-lived human, most of the life span involves a constant body weight, and the remarkable phenomenon of this long-term constancy of body protein at a characteristic mass is a particularly challenging problem. We know that regulatory mechanisms exist which allow restoration of body weight and especially protein content to its target size after an insult that induces wasting (i.e. catch-up growth), and which prevent the continuation of growth after that target size has been reached, but such mechanisms are poorly understood.

One approach to the problem has involved the concept of a 'protein-stat' mechanism, the central feature of which is an interaction between linear growth of bone, protein deposition in skeletal muscle and dietary protein intake, with the growth of most other organs secondary to this interaction. Thus, whole-body protein content is controlled through an aminostatic appetite mechanism, acting primarily to maintain skeletal muscle mass at a level set by the linear dimensions of the organism (**Fig. 1**). Bone lengthening occurs at rates determined by genetic programming and an appropriate hormonal anabolic drive, exerted by dietary protein. Bone lengthening controls (by passive stretching) net protein deposition in skeletal muscle, mainly through the regulation of new connective tissue synthesis which controls muscle volume. Some level of muscle activity is also required for maximal muscle size. Provision of amino acids to allow muscle to accumulate myofibrillar protein and increase to its phenotypic size is regulated through appetite stimulation which in some way monitors net amino acid flow into muscle. This is most obvious in catch-up growth. After muscle wasting with loss of myofibre protein there is potential for expansion within the preexisting connective tissue framework. Muscle growth ceases in the absence of passive stretch when bone length growth ceases. The growth of most other organs is secondary to this main interaction, determined primarily by the level of protein intake and the consequent metabolic work and functional demand for the organ, and is not specifically limited in size.

Protein turnover

Protein turnover occurs because of the presence within cells of proteolytic systems which degrade

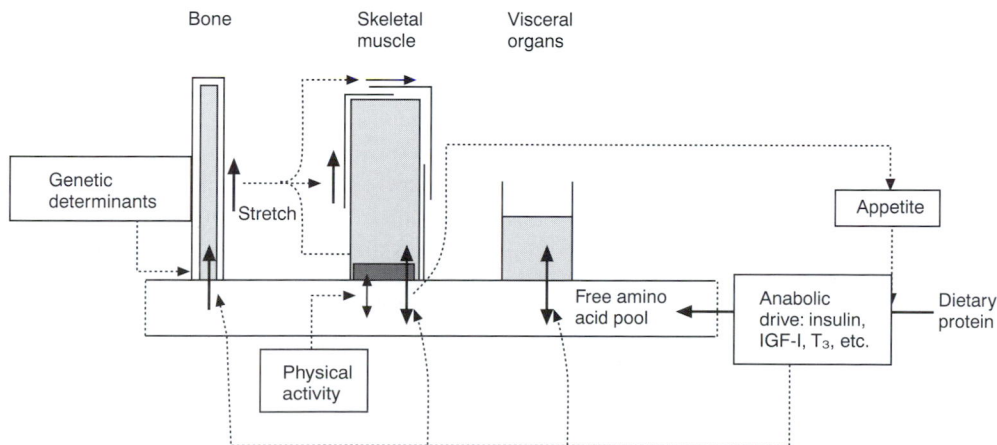

Figure 1 Protein-stat mechanism for coordinated control of body protein growth and maintenance. The protein content of skeletal muscle is controlled by long-bone growth and dietary protein intake, with the growth of most other organs secondary to this interaction. IGF-I, insulin-like growth factor I; T3, triiodothyronine. Adapted from Millward (1995a).

proteins for a variety of reasons, ranging from the removal of proteins with an incorrect primary amino acid sequence ('error' proteins) to the provision of free amino acids during nutrient deprivation. However, the half-lives of individual proteins vary over at least 3 orders of magnitude within the same cells, identifying the process as specific. The nature and control of proteolysis is poorly understood. The physicochemical structure, especially hydrophobicity and ionic charge, influences susceptibility to proteolysis. Also an amino acid sequence (PEST – proline, glutamate, serine and threonine) influences susceptibility to proteolysis and occurs in several rapidly degraded proteins. The molecular basis for this remains largely unknown. The heterogeneous turnover of proteins within structures such as mitochondria, myofilaments and multienzyme complexes while functional integrity, is maintained requires complex coregulation, with evidence for the involvement of at least three different systems in the case of skeletal muscle.

The lysosomal-autophagic system is present in all cells and involves acid proteinases (cathepsins) within a distinct vacuolar structure capable of engulfing and degrading complete organelles and ribosomes, as well as individual intracellular proteins and proteins entering cells via endocytosis. Lysosomal proteolysis is complete and most is known about hepatic macroautophagy.

The ubiquitin-proteosome system is widely distributed among tissues, with a relatively broad protein specificity, catalysing the complete hydrolysis of protein to free amino acids and exhibiting an ATP dependency. It involves two components. One is a recognition system involving the protein ubiquitin, which is responsible for targeting the protein substrates toward degradation via an ATP-dependent formation of a covalent link between the protein and ubiquitin, catalysed by four proteins which may confer substrate specificity. The other is a large molecular weight, multifunctional protease, the proteosome, comprising two closely related particles which, together with three other protein factors, mediate proteolysis. The relative importance of the two main systems capable of complete proteolysis – the lysosome and the proteosome – in various tissues remains uncertain.

The calpain-calpastatin system is a calcium-activated proteolytic pathway which can initiate (but not complete) proteolysis. Two main calpain isoforms occur, active at low and high calcium concentrations respectively, and subject to inhibition by the protein calpastatin. Their role in turnover is not yet established.

Models and Tracer Methods for the Study of Protein Turnover

Study of protein turnover has utilized isotope tracer techniques, radioactive tracers (^{14}C, ^{35}S) in animals and stable isotopes (^{13}C, ^{15}N and ^{2}H) in human studies. Most studies use simplified models, the simplest and most widely used (**Fig. 2**) based on the measurement of the amino acid flux through the plasma amino acid pool. An example is the primed continuous intravenous infusion of [^{13}C1] leucine. During the infusion, the tracer isotopic enrichment is diluted by unlabelled amino acid from proteolysis (D) and the diet (I). At isotopic equilibrium constant labelling of the tracee is achieved, the magnitude of which, as tracer dilution or tracer/tracee ratio, in relation to the infusion rate (i), indicates the flux (Q), the total entry or exit rate of leucine through the pool. With the free leucine pool relatively small and turning over rapidly, isotopic equilibrium can be reached in 2–4 h if a priming dose is given.

At isotopic and metabolic equilibrium, rates of entry and exit from the free leucine pool are equal for both labelled and unlabelled leucine so that Q is the rate of appearance or irreversible loss. Appearance is partitioned into dietary intake which is known (I) and entry from proteolysis of body protein (D) – i.e. no *de novo* synthesis of leucine occurs. Loss is partitioned into protein synthesis (S), and oxidative catabolism (O), to carbon dioxide and urinary nitrogen. The rate of leucine oxidation (O), is calculated from measurement of the production of labelled ^{13}CO$_2$ in the breath and the labelling of the leucine or its keto acid in the plasma. This allows the components of protein turnover (D and S) to be calculated. From knowledge of the leucine content of tissue proteins rates of leucine appearance and loss can be converted into rates of whole-body protein synthesis and proteolysis.

The tracer [^{13}C1]leucine is especially useful since (1) leucine is essential, enabling D to be calculated; (2) it has a small pool, enabling equilibrium to be achieved in a short period; (3) decarboxylation is the first irreversible step in its catabolism releasing ^{13}CO$_2$ quantitatively; and (4) its transamination product α-ketoisocaproate (KIC) appears in the plasma and can serve as a measure of the labelling of the intracellular pool.

This last advantage of leucine is especially important since the problem of definition of isotopic enrichment of the precursor amino acid pool for protein synthesis is the most serious area of uncertainty in these studies. Thus in the body amino acid pools are compartmentalized, and the isotopic enrichment of tRNA-bound amino acids is lower than the

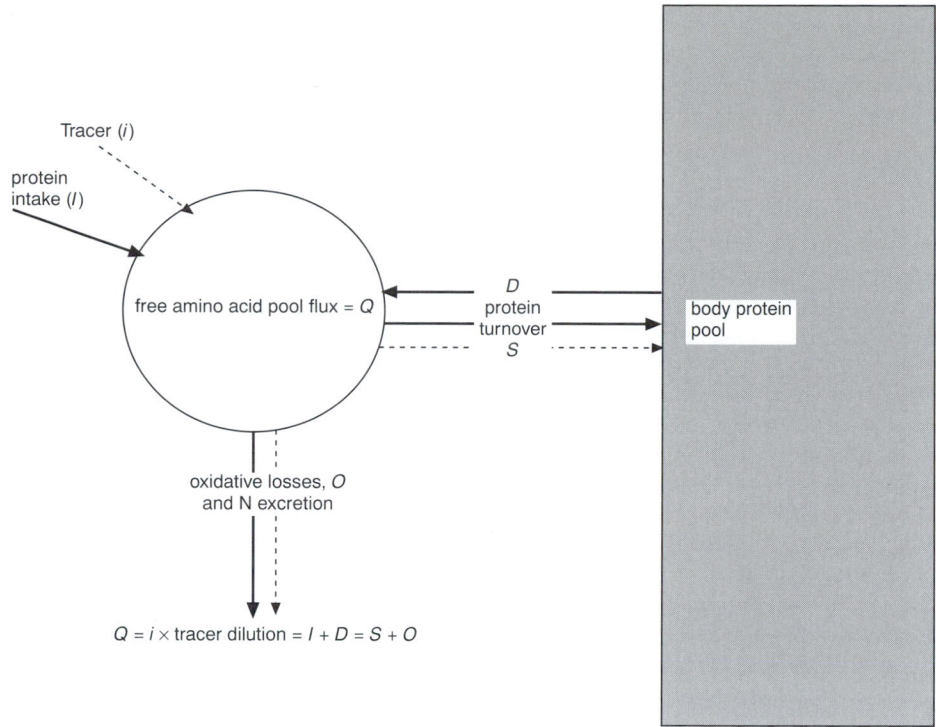

Figure 2 Single pool model for study of amino acid flux and protein turnover by trace-labelled amino acid infusion.

measurable extracellular amino acid pool. Because it is extremely difficult to measure labelling of amino acyl tRNA, a variety of indirect approaches have been used in an attempt to circumvent the problem. In addition to the measurement of plasma KIC, equilibrium labelling of apolipoprotein B-100 has also been used to measure isotopic enrichment of hepatic amino acids. Because apo B-100 turns over with a half-life of less than 1 h, during an infusion of several hours the protein labelling will reach a plateau level representative of the hepatic precursor pool, and this has indicated a complex relationship between plasma and precursor enrichments for phenylalanine and leucine.

Flux rate measurements define whole-body rates of protein synthesis and proteolysis, and each measurement is subject to error associated with the precursor assumption. Alternative methods have attempted to measure protein synthesis and proteolysis separately. In animal studies a 'flooding large dose' measurement of protein synthesis has been developed, which enables all free pools to become equally labelled. Protein synthesis rates are calculated from measurement of isotope uptake into protein and free amino acid labelling during short periods after the dose. The method has been adapted for human use with a stable isotope but there is evidence that the large quantities of the single amino acid stimulates protein synthesis.

Quantification of rates of proteolysis is especially problematical. In animal studies it can be estimated from values for the rates of synthesis and growth of tissue protein and with careful design proteolysis rates can be measured over relatively short periods (e.g. 6 h following the administration of an endotoxin). Urinary excretion rates of 3-methylhistidine, a posttranslationally modified amino acid not metabolized in the organism and excreted quantitatively in the urine, were proposed as a measure of myofibrillar protein degradation. However, the substantial contribution of small, rapidly turning over pools in microfilaments invalidates this approach. Nevertheless, its release from incubated or perfused muscle can be used to determine myofibrillar protein degradation.

Simultaneous determination of protein synthesis and degradation can be made, in principle at least, from organ tracer balance studies – i.e. measurements of concentrations and isotopic enrichments of tracer amino acids across tissues such as the leg or forearm, combined with measurements of 3-methylhistidine release. Such studies have identified a selective inhibitory effect of insulin on nonmyofibrillar protein degradation.

All these methods allow study of turnover of individual amino acids in protein and their nonprotein metabolic fate (e.g. oxidation). A somewhat different approach is to use [^{15}N]glycine to study overall amino nitrogen turnover. Because of transamination, this label acts as a tracer for total free amino nitrogen, rather than for any individual amino acid. The whole-body nitrogen flux is estimated from the relative proportion of administered tracer excreted in the end product. This is then resolved into protein synthesis and proteolysis from measurements of nitrogen intake and excretion. The application of the method can be made simple by giving the ^{15}N label orally as a single dose. While simple in concept, this approach is metabolically complicated, with two end products of nitrogen metabolism in the urine – urea and ammonia – each deriving from different pathways and each giving different flux values.

The choice of method must depend on the questions asked and circumstances of the subjects under study. Labelling with ^{13}C is more suited to short-term (4–24 h) clinical measurements where frequent blood and breath sampling is possible. Thus the efficiency and mechanisms of postprandial protein utilization during meal feeding can be measured by means of [^{13}C]leucine balance and turnover measurements. Methods using ^{15}N are more suitable for free-living subjects and patients, when urine sampling is possible but regular blood and breath sampling are inconvenient, and such a method has been used in an unassisted Antarctic crossing. Both methods involve many assumptions, but in practice the two approaches have been shown to give similar results.

Applications

Extent and physiological implications of protein turnover

In the human adult about 300 g of protein turnover occurs each day (4 g per kg per day), i.e. 3–4 times the daily dietary intake. Rates vary between tissues with rapid turnover in visceral tissues and slow turnover in muscle. Liver and intestine account for about 8% of the lean body mass and up to 50% of whole-body protein turnover, with skeletal muscle, at 55% of the lean body mass, accounting for only about 25% of total protein turnover. Thus whole-body protein turnover varies with body composition, and this largely explains developmental changes. In the infant turnover rates are much higher, in the range 10–20 g protein per kilogram per day, consistent with the higher proportion of metabolically active tissue and lower muscle mass. However, animal studies indicate a developmental fall in protein turnover in skeletal muscle which may be an additional component of the marked fall in protein turnover with age. In the elderly there is little evidence of any change other than that associated with the fall in lean body mass.

Protein turnover constitutes an appreciable fraction of the maintenance energy expenditure. On the basis of 5 mol ATP/GTP per mole of protein turnover (4 mole per peptide bond with an extra mole for amino acid transport, RNA turnover and proteolysis), an energy cost of 22 kcal (92 kJ) per mole of ATP, and a molecular weight of 110 per mole of peptide bond, this is equivalent to about 1 kcal g^{-1} (4.2 kJ g^{-1}) protein turnover. Thus, in the normal adult, protein turnover at 300 g per day accounts for about 20% of the basal metabolic rate. Because of this, changes in the protein turnover and metabolic rate would be expected to occur in parallel to some extent, and this is observed. Thus the fall with age in both protein turnover and metabolic rate from birth to adulthood involves a factor of 3–4 in each case.

As to protein turnover and protein requirements, there is no *a priori* reason for any interrelationship and little evidence of any. Thus turnover does not consume amino acids and amino acid catabolism is not linked to turnover. Maintenance protein requirements fall relatively little with age (< 20%) compared with the 3 to 4-fold fall in turnover.

Regulatory mechanisms of protein turnover control

The physiological importance of protein turnover is undoubtedly the regulatory flexibility it allows. With opportunities for control of both synthesis and proteolysis, the number of potential control sites is increased. In addition, because of the continuing turnover in the steady state, changes in amounts of protein can be achieved with low energy costs through inhibition of proteolysis to allow growth or inhibition of synthesis to allow mobilization.

At the molecular level regulation of protein synthesis is necessarily complex at both transcriptional and translational levels. Advances in molecular biology have revealed many examples of transcriptional control. Notable examples include control of hepatic export protein synthesis. Thus the downregulation of albumin synthesis in response to protein deficiency involves reductions in the albumin mRNA. Also, the acute-phase response whereby cytokines such as interleukin 6 (IL-6) induce hepatic acute-phase protein synthesis and inhibit synthesis of albumin and other normal hepatic export protein synthesis, is mediated largely at the level of transcriptional control of mRNA levels.

The concentration of ribosomes in tissues

determines the capacity for protein synthesis and in this way controls overall tissue protein turnover rate and the changes associated with postnatal development. Cellular ribosome concentrations can change both acutely, e.g. during the diurnal cycle of feeding and fasting, and chronically in response to protein and energy intakes, increased functional demand, and hormones such as insulin, thyroid, growth hormone and the glucocorticoids. Furthermore, these influences are tissue specific, with glucocorticoids for example increasing hepatic ribosome concentrations (as part of the hepatic acute-phase response), and decreasing ribosome concentrations in muscle. In contrast, thyroid hormones increase the concentration of ribosomes (and proteolytic enzymes) in both muscle and liver, in association with a generalized increase in protein turnover.

Acute regulation of translation is exerted mainly through initiation, with reversible phosphorylations known to regulate at least four separate steps of the initiation cycle enabling very rapid changes in protein synthesis. Peptide hormones (insulin and insulin-like growth factor I), glucocorticoids and amino acids have all been implicated in such regulation, although the specific targets of such control remain uncertain. Furthermore, major differences exist between the mechanisms observed in the young, rapidly growing animal compared with the adult. Thus in skeletal muscle in the young rat, an insulin-mediated stimulation occurs. In adult human muscle insulin is relatively ineffective, with amino acid levels the main stimulatory influence. Indeed, with insulin inhibiting proteolysis and lowering amino acid levels, insulin alone appears to inhibit protein synthesis in human muscle.

As to the regulation of proteolysis, most is known about lysosomal proteolysis especially hepatic autophagy, with both amino acids and insulin having inhibitory roles. Leucine, alanine and insulin interact in regulating this pathway with a leucine-sensitive, receptor-mediated inhibitory pathway identified in liver. In the case of the ubiquitin-proteosome system its activation in skeletal muscle during fasting and following glucocorticoid treatment does support a role in the physiological regulation of protein turnover. On the other hand, both lysosomal and calcium-activated proteolysis are activated under the same conditions. Similarly, in response to protein deficiency when protein turnover rates generally fall in tissues, in part through the decrease in thyroid hormone levels, the activities of all three systems fall. A control mechanism has been discovered that involves changes in cell volume: swelling acts like a proliferative anabolic signal, inhibiting proteolysis, while cell shrinkage is catabolic, stimulating proteo-

lysis. These effects have been shown in liver and with some evidence for such a mechanism in skeletal muscle.

Postprandial protein utilization

With overall nitrogen homeostasis maintained within the diurnal cycle of postprandial protein gain and postabsorptive loss of increasing amplitude with increasing habitual protein intake, the key questions are how both acute and chronic protein intakes mediate such responses. The mechanisms for nutritional regulation of protein turnover and amino acid oxidation involve both hormonal responses to food intakes and direct substrate influences. While interactions between insulin, thyroid hormones and insulin-like growth factor I (IGF-I) mediate the anabolic drive of dietary protein on muscle and bone growth in the growing animal, the control mechanisms involved in the transient gains and losses of protein during diurnal cycling differ, since neither thyroid hormones nor IGF-I levels vary from meal to meal or in relation to habitual protein intakes. On the basis of several studies with either insulin or amino acids alone or variation in meal protein levels, it appears that insulin and amino acid substrate supplies act as main acute regulators.

The mechanisms involved are best understood in the context of the interrelationships between the free and protein-bound amino acid pools. Many indispensable amino acids are potentially toxic and are maintained at very low concentrations in tissues. After a protein meal two pathways for disposal exist. The first comprises the various high-capacity, finely regulated catabolic pathways activated by a protein meal. In most cases rates of catabolism are influenced by their tissue concentrations (generally similar to the K_m of the rate-limiting enzymes), together with substrate activation and covalent enzyme modification. Examples are phenylalanine hydroxylase and branched-chain keto acid dehydrogenase (BCKADH), both regulated by substrate binding and reversible phosphorylation and dephosphorylation. The second pathway is protein deposition which removes amino acids after a meal. This can be achieved by stimulation of protein synthesis or inhibition of proteolysis, so that a regulatory link between postprandial hyperaminoacidaemia and both responses might be expected and does indeed exist.

For protein synthesis, amino acids cannot exert simple kinetic concentration-related influences, since the low K_m of amino acyl tRNA synthesis means they are usually fully charged. Nevertheless there is ample evidence for a regulatory stimulation by amino acids, which remains poorly understood but which most probably involves regulation of the initiation process. However, stimulation of protein synthesis through increased amino acid levels may also stimulate amino acid catabolic pathways as discussed above, and while this allows effective removal of amino acids, in the context of an efficient protein utilization this would not be a preferred mechanism.

For proteolysis, amino acids exert an inhibitory influence as described above, and this inhibition will reduce endogenous amino acid supply. This prevents undue increases in amino acid levels and therefore minimizes amino acid oxidation and maximizes dietary protein utilization. Furthermore, since inhibition of proteolysis and lowering of intracellular amino acid levels can be achieved by receptor-mediated mechanisms involving insulin as well as specific amino acids (e.g. leucine), this allows the postprandial increases in plasma amino acid concentrations to mediate substantial amino acid transport into cells, allowing protein deposition without any increase in intracellular amino acid levels and with minimal increases in amino acid oxidation. Thus as a strategy for mediating postprandial protein utilization, inhibition of proteolysis would be predicted to be more efficient.

Studies using [^{13}C]leucine have provided clear experimental support for such a mechanism. In a study of the meal protein-dependent responses of protein synthesis, proteolysis and leucine oxidation in adult subjects fed isoenergetic meals with a protein daily intake increasing from $0.36\,\text{g kg}^{-1}$ to $2.07\,\text{g kg}^{-1}$ (**Fig. 3**), an inhibition of proteolysis occurred at all levels of protein intake, but to an increasing extent with intake. However, the direction and magnitude of the response of protein synthesis reflected

the level of dietary protein intake, with slight inhibition or no change at low intakes and stimulation at high intakes. Such studies clearly establish the importance of proteolysis as a regulator of tissue protein balance in the postabsorptive and postprandial state. Further evidence for this inhibition of proteolysis mechanism of postprandial protein utilization is shown in **Fig. 4**. The separate influences of energy (low protein, LP) and protein meals (HP) is shown during a single three-phase (postabsorptive, low protein, high protein) 9 h [^{13}C1]leucine infusion. With isoenergetic, constant-carbohydrate meals throughout, insulin levels were constant but amino acid levels varied from low to high so that the protocol in effect examines the response to insulin alone (LP meals) and amino acids with insulin (HP meal). The negative postabsorptive leucine balance becomes less negative during LP meals and positive with the HP meals owing to an inhibition of proteolysis by both insulin and amino acids. The fall in protein synthesis and oxidation with the LP meals and the increase with HP meals are consistent with free amino acid levels mediating the changes.

Thus these two nutritional studies, together with other studies with insulin or amino acids alone, indicate a combined influence of insulin and tissue amino acid levels on proteolysis, protein synthesis and amino acid oxidation. They suggest a mechanism in which the major target of insulin is inhibition of proteolysis with amino acids acting both to enhance the inhibition of proteolysis and to stimulate synthesis and oxidation (**Fig. 5**). With tissue amino acid levels controlled by both diet and endogenous supply from proteolysis, inhibition of proteolysis will minimize any increase in amino acid levels, minimize oxidation and maximize protein utilization. Since protein synthesis and amino acid oxidation appear to be

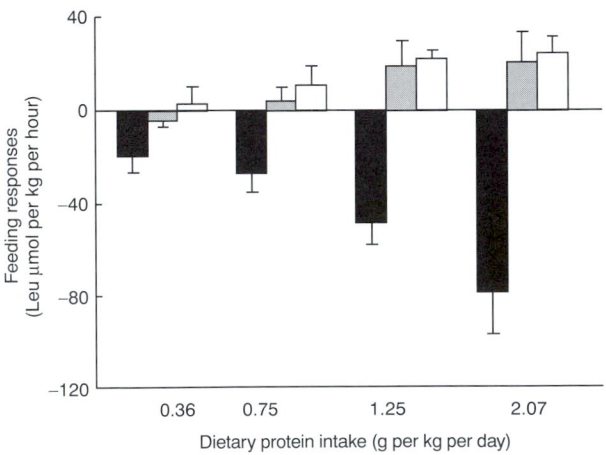

Figure 3 Feeding-induced responses of leucine kinetics shown as protein synthesis (shaded bars), proteolysis (solid bars) and leucine oxidation (open bars). Meals were isoenergetic, frequent, small meals of increasing protein intake equivalent to daily intakes as shown. Adapted from Pacy *et al.* (1994).

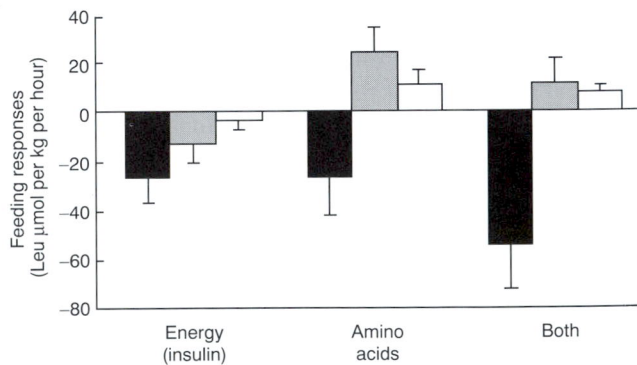

Figure 4 Separate influences of insulin, induced by energy (as low-protein meals), amino acids plus insulin (as high-protein meals), and the combined responses to the high-protein meals. Open bars, oxidation; shaded bars, synthesis, solid bars, proteolysis. Adapted from Gibson *et al.* (1996).

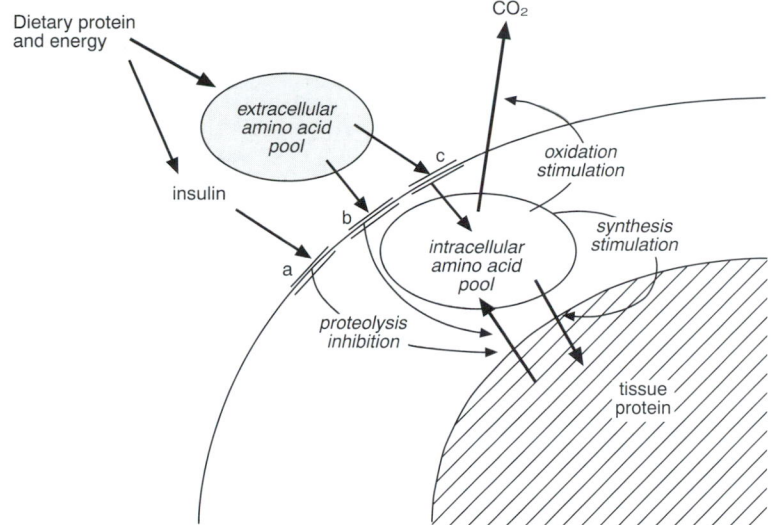

Figure 5 Scheme for the action of insulin and amino acid supply on postprandial protein utilization. Insulin and extracellular amino acids exert inhibitory influences on proteolysis through receptor-mediated mechanisms (a, b), while amino acid uptake (c) and proteolysis regulate intracellular amino acid levels, amino acid oxidation and protein synthesis in parallel. Maximal inhibition of proteolysis and maintenance of low intracellular amino acid levels is the optimal response. Modified from Millward *et al.* (1996).

stimulated in parallel, the optimum strategy for maximum efficiency of postprandial protein utilization would appear to involve maximal inhibition of proteolysis and minimal postprandial increases in tissue amino acid levels.

In summary, postprandial protein utilization appears to be mediated by an insulin-mediated, protein-conserving influence of dietary energy which inhibits proteolysis, lowers amino acid levels and reduces oxidation, with dietary amino acids augmenting the inhibition of proteolysis. The response of protein synthesis will be primarily determined by the resultant intracellular amino acid levels which reflect the balance between the falling endogenous supply following insulin-mediated inhibition of proteolysis and the increasing exogenous supply as dietary protein intake increases, stimulating protein synthesis and increasing oxidation when amino acid dietary supply exceeds the capacity for its net deposition.

See also: **Amino Acids**: Metabolism. **Bone**: Composition, Metabolism and Bone Growth. **Protein**: Requirements and Role in Diet.

Further Reading

Gibson NR, Fereday A, Cox M, Halliday D, Pacy PJ and Millward DJ (1996) Influences of dietary energy and protein on leucine kinetics during feeding in healthy adults. *American Journal of Physiology* 33:282–291.

Haussinger D and Lang F (1992) Cell volume and hormone action. *Trends in Pharmacological Science* 13:371–373.

Millward DJ (1995a) Insulin and the regulation of amino acid catabolism and protein turnover. In: Cynober (ed.) *Amino Acid Metabolism in Health and Disease*, pp 127–136. Boca Raton: CRC Press.

Millward DJ (1995b) A protein-stat mechanism for regulation of growth and maintenance of the lean-body mass. *Nutrition Research Reviews* 8:93–120.

Millward DJ and Rivers JPW (1989) The need for indispensable amino acids: the concept of the anabolic drive. *Diabetes Metabolism Reviews* 5:191–212.

Millward DJ, Fereday A, Gibson NR and Pacy PJ (1996) Postprandial protein metabolism. *Baillière's Clinical Endocrinology and Metabolism* 10:533–549.

Pacy PJ, Price GM, Halliday D, Quevedo MR and Millward DJ (1994) Nitrogen homeostasis in man: 2. The diurnal responses of protein synthesis, degradation and amino acid oxidation to diets with increasing protein intakes. *Clinical Science* 86:103–118.

Waterlow JC, Garlick PJ and Millward DJ (1978) *Protein Turnover in Mammalian Tissues and in the Whole Body*. Amsterdam: Elsevier/North-Holland.

Deficiency

Claus Leitzmann, Justus-Liebig University, Giessen, Germany

Protein deficiency indicates a lack of body protein or a relative deficiency of one or several essential amino acids. Thus protein deficiency is synonymous with a negative nitrogen balance. The deficiency can result from a protein-deficient diet or other events, such as diseases, and it must be distinguished from the multi-factorial syndrome of kwashiorkor. However, the clinical features and physiological effects are generally similar to those of kwashiorkor.

Causes and Groups At Risk

Causes

Although the main cause of protein deficiency is a protein-deficient diet, frequently seen in children in developing countries, it can also occur in patients suffering from various diseases. In this sense, protein deficiency (as well as other nutritional deficiencies) is a secondary consequence of the particular disease.

Secondary protein deficiencies can be ascribed to six causes:

1. Irregular food habits, e.g. in the case of chronic alcoholics. The diet of alcoholics can be severely deficient in protein.
2. Inability to digest and absorb the protein that is consumed; this occurs in patients with chronic gastrointestinal disorders, such as coeliac disease or enteritis.
3. A disturbed protein metabolism, which may exist in patients with cirrhosis of the liver, but also in patients with hormonal disorders or in some cases of diabetes.
4. A continuous loss of protein; this predominates in patients with diseases such as chronic renal disease, bleeding or exudative gastroenteropathy. High losses of albumin into the urine are indicators of the nephrotic syndrome.
5. An increased protein turnover, which is characteristic in cases of infection, fever or gastroenteritis.
6. Enhanced catabolism of protein, with increased nitrogen losses, seen in patients with severe injuries, especially burns, or in postoperative stress.

Protein losses after operations depend on the kind of surgery (**Table 1**). If patients are unable to eat nor-mally, then insufficient food intake worsens the protein deficiency.

Groups at risk

The groups at risk can be classified according to the causes of protein deficiency (see above) or better according to socioeconomic parameters. According to socioeconomic parameters, by far the largest group is the poor population in developing countries, primarily children in the second year of life. This group is at risk from primary protein deficiency because of a protein-deficient diet, caused by economic, ecological and political factors. In developed societies, groups at risk are those who adhere to extreme diets or suffer from anorexia nervosa or bulimia nervosa.

Clinical Features

Fatty liver

Protein deficiency contributes to fatty infiltration of the liver and results in hepatomegaly. This can be seen in healthy subjects receiving a low-protein diet as well as in protein-deficient animals fed adequate quantities of other nutrients. Because of a decreased synthesis of β-lipoproteins needed for the transport of triacylglycerols, the fat accumulates in small droplets within the cells, first in the periphery of the lobules and then spreads to the centre of the lobules. In spite of this, the liver functions are well maintained.

Muscle wasting

Because of increased protein catabolism, skeletal muscle is often wasted, and subjects limit their physical activity. In many cases the parallel prevailing oedema conceals the wasting.

Oedema

Oedema is a frequent sign in protein deficiency. It generally causes swelling of the tissues, but usually appears in the feet and lower legs. The aetiology of oedema has not been completely clarified. Protein deficiency or, rather, hypoalbuminaemia, is only one of the factors.

Other common features of protein deficiency are changes in the hair; it becomes easily plucked and there are changes in texture and colour. Also common are skin changes, with areas of desquamation, hypo- and hyperpigmentation. Protein deficiency also leads to mental changes, lethargy, fatigue, anorexia and some degree of anaemia and is frequently associated with infections. In children, severe protein deficiency leads to growth retardation.

Table 1 Postoperative protein losses

Operation	Loss (g per day)
Stomach removal	110–112
Strumectomy	72
Cholecystectomy	71
Herniotomy	11
Amputation of the breast	9–18
Fractures of long bones	86–312
Skull injuries	67
Hip joint dislocation	17

From Welsch A (1986) Krankenernährung, 5th edn, p 410. Stuttgart: Georg Thieme Verlag.

Physiological Effects

Organs and systems can be changed in protein deficiency, and this may alter their physiological functions.

Cardiovascular system

Muscle wasting in the heart leads to reduced cardiac output and poor circulation. As a result, the pulse rate of many patients is low and even impalpable, and the extremities are cold and pale.

Renal function

Structural abnormalities of the kidney have not been observed, but the glomerular filtration rate may be diminished. The concentrating power can also be impaired, which may be attributable to a low blood urea concentration or an accompanying potassium deficiency.

Pancreas

Atrophic changes and fibrosis of the pancreas have been observed both in children dying of protein malnutrition, and in animals fed low-protein diets. The atrophy affects the acinar cells, responsible for exocrine secretion, but not the islets, responsible for hormone (glucagon and insulin) production. A reduced number of secretory granules has also been observed. These changes result in impaired pancreatic function with a diminished secretion of pancreatic enzymes into the intestine. Glucagon and insulin secretion are also lowered in severe cases of protein deficiency.

In another abnormality of the pancreas in protein-deficient animals the protein content and phospholipid levels are reduced, and triacylglycerols and cholesteryl ester levels are increased. This altered pancreatic lipid composition in protein-deficient animals may lead to changes in the integrity of pancreatic membranes and can predispose to injury.

Gastrointestinal tract

The mucosal epithelial cells of the small intestine make up the tissue with the highest turnover rate and are therefore very vulnerable to protein deficiency. The intestine wall becomes thin, the mucous membrane is smooth and atrophic, and the villi are frequently flattened. The enzyme-secreting cells and the pancreatic acinar cells may be affected in a similar way. As a result, the production of digestive enzymes, primarily the disaccharidases, is reduced and the absorptive and digestive capacity of nutrients is impaired.

A feature seen in biopsis after protein deficiency is the intense cellular infiltration in the mucosa and submucosa, especially with lymphocytes and plasma cells. The colon can be less affected, but the muscle coats may also be atrophic and the surface epithelium may show infiltration of plasma cells.

Endocrine system

The pituitary gland responds effectively to the stimulus of protein deficiency; thus the secretion of human growth hormone is normal or possibly supranormal and the thyroid-stimulating hormone is elevated.

The thyroid may be atrophic with reduced colloid tissue, and the vascular cells are flattened and inactive. The thyroid function appears to be normal, but there are data suggesting a reduced function of the thyroid gland. The concentrations of thyroxine-binding proteins and of thyroxine are reduced.

The adrenal gland appears atrophic but, nevertheless, plasma cortisol levels are elevated and may lead to metabolic disturbances. A reduced insulin secretion, as seen after glucose tolerance tests, can also be predominant in protein deficiency.

Immunological system

In protein deficiency the lymphoid tissue – primarily the thymus gland, but also lymph nodes and spleen – is atrophic. First, the production of thymus-dependent lymphocytes (T cells) is reduced and is responsible for the diminished cell-mediated immunity to infectious agents, as demonstrated in specific tuberculin skin tests. In addition, the phagocytic activity of neutrophils and antibody formation are reduced. The body, therefore, becomes more susceptible to infections which can be fatal.

Treatment

The dietary treatment of protein deficiency depends on the cause of the deficiency. In patients with nephrotic syndrome, characterized by massive losses of albumin into urine, the intake of protein should be increased to 90–120 g per day for adults when hepatic synthesis of albumin can compensate in part the urinary losses.

In cases of acute renal failure, the protein intake should be only 20 g per day. This reduces protein metabolism and the production of urea. In patients with liver cirrhosis the protein intake should also be reduced because a high-protein diet can precipitate hepatic encephalopathy.

Special feeding methods

Protein deficiency can be treated by tube feeding, intravenous feeding or supplementary feeding. Tube feeding is indicated in patients with severe malnutrition who are unable to eat. Parenteral nutrition is essential when the small intestine is unable to digest and absorb nutrients, or after severe injuries such as burns.

In mild protein deficiencies an increased oral intake of protein is sufficient to meet dietary needs. Several special preparations containing high levels of protein are available on the market.

Complications

Since protein deficiency is frequently accompanied by infections, dehydration and deprivation of vitamins and electrolytes, these conditions need special attention. In most cases of severe protein deficiency, therefore, treatment has to start with fluid replacement and, if indicated, with antibiotic therapy.

Adaptation to Low-protein Intakes

Waterlow (1986) described two possibilities of nutritional adaptation, which he called the first and second line of defence. The first line of defence is the ability to achieve nitrogen balance at various levels of protein intake. The second line of defence is necessary after the capacity to economize nitrogen is exhausted, resulting in a reduced lean body mass or reduced growth rate in children. In this section, only the first line of defence is discussed.

Nitrogen balance

Nitrogen equilibrium is a state in which, for a given intake of nitrogen, an equivalent amount of nitrogen is lost from the body via urine, faeces, skin, sweat, etc. When protein intake is low, dietary protein is used more efficiently; this is exemplified by the excretion of nitrogen, particularly in the form of urea, which is reduced and so contributes to the restoration of nitrogen balance. In this situation the pathways of amino acid synthesis predominate.

The liver plays an important role in the adaptive process since it is the only organ which can transform the nitrogen from amino acids into urea. The alterations in the nitrogen pathway are mainly brought about by changes in the activity of liver enzymes. Experiments with animals have shown that in protein deficiency urea cycle enzymes, such as argininosuccinase, are low and the amino-acid-activating enzymes are high. **Table 2** shows this finding in children with severe protein malnutrition, soon after admission to hospital and after recovery.

The metabolic activity of the gastrointestinal tract is important in the adaptive process. Normally, one third of the urea produced is passed into the bowel and can be hydrolysed by the gut microflora. Thus

Table 2 Enzymatic activity of the livers of children with malnutrition

	Amino-acid-activating enzymes	Arginino-succinase
Soon after admission	1.44	1.06
1–2 months later	0.91	1.46

The figures for the amino-acid-activating enzymes are the mean of 18 measurements and are expressed in μmol phosphorus exchanged per mg protein; for argininosuccinase the figures are the mean of 11 measurements and expressed in μmol urea per mg protein. The changes on recovery are statistically significant. From Passmore R and Eastwood MA (1986), p 52. (With permission from Churchill Livingstone).

urea nitrogen becomes available for metabolic interaction, e.g. for the synthesis of nonessential and essential amino acids. However, the necessary carbon skeletons can be the limiting factor in adaptation. In protein deficiency a greater proportion of urea is retained by the body.

Recent investigations have shown that the colon is permeable to urea and amino acids, thus supporting the view that hydrolysis of urea plays an important nutritional role.

Plasma albumin

Plasma albumin reacts very sensitively to a reduced protein intake. Although the albumin turnover is reduced by about 36% in studies with adults, the plasma albumin concentration is reduced by only about 7%. This maintenance of intravascular circulating albumin mass is attributable to a reduced breakdown and a shift of albumin from the extravascular to the intravascular compartment.

Factors affecting adaptation

Among the factors that can affect the adaptation to low protein intake are infections, diarrhoeal diseases, and injuries. In infections, protein from muscle and skin is needed for the immune response, and this leads to a negative nitrogen balance. In diarrhoeal diseases the malabsorption has a negative influence on the adaptive process; in patients with injury the severe losses of nitrogen have the same effect.

Energy balance is also essential for nitrogen balance because of its nitrogen-sparing effect. Thus if protein deficiency is accompanied by energy deficiency, the adaptation to a low protein intake cannot be achieved completely.

Table 3 Relative losses of protein in different organs and tissues from rats over 7 days

Organ or tissue	Loss (percentage of primary content)
Liver	40
Prostate gland	29
Seminal vesicle	29
Gastrointestinal tract	28
Kidney	20
Blood plasma	20
Heart	18
Muscle, skin, skeleton	8
Brain	5
Eyes	0
Testicle	0
Adrenal gland	0

From Kraut H (1981), p 148.

Protein Reserves

The body of a human adult (65 kg) contains 12 kg of protein, about 50% of which is found in muscles. The amount of body protein depends on, among other things, the dietary protein and carbohydrate intake; if carbohydrate is lacking, the amino acids are utilized for gluconeogenesis.

Protein reserves are not comparable to special fat depots, and not all body proteins can serve as protein reserve. Reserves are primarily organs which contain labile body protein such as liver, plasma (with proteins such as albumin and enzymes) and the gastrointestinal tract which has an assessed protein content of about 700–800 g. Although the protein turnover rate in muscle is very slow, this tissue is a very important protein reserve owing to its large mass.

In protein deficiency the labile body proteins are metabolized first; when deficiency is long-term, all organs are affected to various extents (**Table 3**). The well-fed human adult can lose about 3 kg of protein without disturbances to his or her health.

See also: **Burns Patients**: Nutritional Management.

Coeliac Disease: Aetiology and Nutritional Management. **Glucose**: Chemistry, Dietary Sources and Glycaemic Index; Metabolism and Maintenance of Blood Glucose Level; Glucose Tolerance. **Immunity**: Physiological Aspects; Role of Iron and Zinc. **Malnutrition**: Definition, Classification and Epidemiology; Primary Malnutrition; Secondary Malnutrition. **Microflora of the Intestine**: Role and Effects. **Protein**: Deficiency. **Renal Function and Disorders**: Nutritional Management of Renal Disorders. **Surgery**: Perioperative Feeding; Long-term Nutritional Management of Patients.

Further Reading

Elmadfa I and Leitzmann C (1990) *Ernährung des Menschen*, 2nd edn. pp 139–162. Stuttgart: Verlag Ulmer.

Jackson AA (1990) The aetiology of kwashiorkor. In: Harrison GA and Waterlow JC (eds) *Diet and Disease in Traditional and Developing Societies*, pp 76–113. Cambridge: Cambridge University Press.

Kraut H (ed.) (1981) *Der Nahrungsbedarf des Menschen: I – Stoffwechsel. Ernährung and Nahrungsbedarf, Energiebedarf, Proteinbedarf*, pp 140–153. Darmstadt: Steinkopff Verlag.

Latham MC (1990) Protein–energy malnutrition. In: Brown ML (ed.) *Present Knowledge in Nutrition*, 6th edn, pp 39–46. Washington. DC: International Life Sciences Institute – Nutrition Foundation.

Passmore R and Eastwood MA (1986) *Human Nutrition and Dietetics*, 8th edn, pp 40–53, 279–291, 403–407, 452, 482–501. Edinburgh: Churchill Livingstone.

Siegenthaler W, Kaufmann W, Hornbostel H and Waller HD (eds) (1984) *Lehrbuch der Inneren Medizin*, pp 14.17–14.19. Stuttgart: Georg Thieme Verlag.

Trowell HC, Davies JNP and Dean RFA (1982) *A Nutrition Foundation's Reprint of Kwashiorkor*, pp 122–160. New York: Academic Press.

Waterlow JC (1986) Metabolic adaptation to low intakes of energy and protein. *Annual Reviews of Nutrition* 6:495–526.

Waterlow JC (1992) *Protein-energy Malnutrition*. London: Edward Arnold.

Pulses *see* **Legumes**: Types and Nutritional Value.

QUASI-VITAMINS

Definition and Examples

A E Bender, Leatherhead, Surrey, UK

Thirteen vitamins have been established as being essential in the diet of human beings; strictly speaking, two of these – vitamin D, which can be synthesized through the action of sunlight on the skin, and niacin, which can be synthesized in the body from tryptophan – are not dietary essentials. However, it was not until 1954 and 1962 respectively that vitamin B_6 and vitamin E were shown to be essential for humans, and other substances, discussed below, have been shown to be essential for other organisms but not for human beings. The early definition of the term 'vitamin' would have included these latter compounds. In addition, certain organic compounds present in foods are regarded by some as being borderline substances, and it has been claimed that some non-nutrient organic compounds found in food have beneficial effects on health. Food components with biological activity or suggested activity can be classed as follows:

1. The thirteen established vitamins: during the investigation of dietary factors various authors coined names for substances that were subsequently shown to be identical, so that some vitamins have had a variety of names (**Table 1**). A number of technical and historical errors are listed in **Table 2**.
2. Substances essential for certain organisms but not for human beings.
3. Substances that are conditionally essential, i.e. may become essential under special circumstances.
4. Several 'pseudovitamins', exploited as so-called 'health supplements'.
5. Chemicals found particularly in plant foods, sometimes called 'phytochemicals'.

Classification

Established vitamins

The established vitamins were shown to be essential through two lines of investigation: firstly, from evidence that experimental animals could not develop normally when fed a purified diet without the addition of other foods or extracts subsequently proved to be dietary essentials for humans, and secondly, the cure of diseases that were shown to be due to a dietary deficiency (e.g. beriberi, rickets). It is often difficult to demonstrate essentiality since in some instances, e.g. vitamins A and B_{12}, it can take a long time before a dietary deficiency becomes evident. Also, the fact that blood levels of a substance fall when it is excluded from the diet may not be evidence, since 'normal' blood levels may be higher than required for normal function.

As discussed below, flavonoids have been termed 'partly essential' and in the *Geigy Scientific Tables* flavonoids, choline, inositol, lipoic acid and essential fatty acids are classed as 'vitamin-like substances' or 'vitaminoids'.

Table 1 Multiple nomenclature of vitamins

Accepted name	Historic names
Folic acid (folacin)	Citrovorum factor (CF), leucovorin, rhizopterin, *Streptococcus lactis* factor, Wills factor, vitamin M, vitamin B_c, factors U, R and S
Niacin	Nicotinic acid, nicotinamide, vitamin PP (pellagra-preventing), vitamin B_2, lactoflavin
Vitamin B_6	Pyridoxine (the hydro compound previously called pyridoxol), pyridoxal (the aldehyde) and pyridoxamine (the amine); yeast eluate factor, factor I, factor Y, adermin

Table 2 Compounds at one time assigned vitamin nomenclature

B_3	Assigned to a compound which was probably pantothenic acid; incorrectly used for niacin
B_4	Assigned to what was later identified as a mixture of arginine, glycine and cysteine
B_5	Assigned to what was later assumed to be either vitamin B_6 or nicotinic acid, also used for pantothenic acid
B_7	Never assigned
B_8	Never assigned
B_9	Never assigned
B_{10}	Assigned to what was later identified as a mixture of folic acid and vitamin B_1
B_{11}	Assigned to what was later identified as a mixture of folic acid and vitamin B_1
B_{13}	Orotic acid – not a vitamin, but an intermediate in pyrimidine synthesis
B_{14}	Assigned to a substance in urine which increases proliferation of bone marrow in culture
B_{15}	Pangamic acid, no established vitamin function
B_{16}	Never assigned
B_{17}	Amygdalin or Laetrile, a cyanogenic glycoside with no established vitamin function
B_c	Obsolete name for folic acid
B_p	Assigned to the 'antiperosis' factor for chickens, can be replaced by choline and manganese
B_T	Carnitine, a growth factor for the mealworm, but not a vitamin
B_W	Assigned to a factor which was probably biotin
B_x	Obsolete name for p-aminobenzoic acid, required for folic acid synthesis in microorganisms, not a vitamin. Also used at one time for pantothenic acid
F	Essential fatty acids – not classified as vitamins
G	Obsolete name for riboflavin
H_3	Gerovital – procaine hydrochloride, promoted without evidence as alleviating the symptoms of diseases associated with ageing. Not recognized as a vitamin
L	Factor in yeast claimed to promote lactation, not established as a vitamin
M	Obsolete name for folic acid
P	Bioflavonoids, pharmacologically active but not vitamins
PP	Obsolete name for niacin (pellagra-preventing vitamin)
Q	Ubiquinone
T	Assigned to a mixture of folic acid, vitamin B_{12} and nucleotides
U	Methylsulfonium salts of methionine. May have pharmacological actions, but not a vitamin

Pseudovitamins

Some substances are called 'vitamins' as a marketing ploy and there are usually public figures willing to provide testimonials and so promote sales.

Vitamin B_{17} 'Vitamin B_{17}' is the most notorious of the pseudovitamins, having no possible justification for use of the title. It was widely sold at one time, particularly in the USA, as a cure for cancer. It is a combination of glucose with cyanide originally isolated from fruit stones and named 'amygdalin', with 'prunasin' as a variant. A number of such glycosides of cyanide are found in the stones of apricots, almonds, peaches, cherries and plums, and to a lesser extent in cassava, butter beans, linseed and bamboo shoots.

The compound Laetrile is an extract of apricot kernels, although the name was originally given to a derivative of amygdalin, a cyanogenic glucoside containing benzaldehyde. It was widely promoted in the USA as a cure for cancer, with the suggestion that the cyanide present kills the cancer cells without affecting the rest of the body. In fact there were several cases of illness and even some deaths from cyanide poisoning. As a sales ploy it was suggested that

cancer is due to a vitamin deficiency and Laetrile was given the name vitamin B_{17}.

Laetrile was banned from interstate commerce in the USA in 1971, but its popularity forced 27 states to allow its sale to continue. The death of a baby who swallowed between one and five tablets was reported in the *New England Journal of Medicine* in February 1979, yet Laetrile took such a hold on the US public that the compound was smuggled in from Mexico.

Laetrile was sold in health-food shops in the UK with the claim that it is virtually absent from 'civilized' diets and contributes towards the mythical longevity of the people of the Hunza Valley, a region of India reputed to have extraordinarily long-lived inhabitants. Sales in the UK were restricted in 1984 through the Medicines (Cyanogenetic Substances) Order and over-the-counter sales were banned. The freedom of medical practitioners to follow their beliefs, however, limited the effectiveness of this ban.

Vitamin B_{15} A substance found to be involved in oxidation processes *in vitro* was named 'vitamin B_{15}', but it is not a human dietary essential so the term is incorrect. The substance is question is pangamic acid, the N-diisopropyl derivative of glucuronic acid. It was discovered in 1951 in apricot kernels and rice bran and is also present in brewers' yeast and many cereals. The name 'pangamic acid' was coined because the product is so widespread (Greek *pan*, universal) and is found in so many seeds ('gamic').

Vitamin B$_{13}$ Orotic acid (uracil-4-carboxylic acid) is an intermediate in the synthesis of pyrimidines which is readily formed from aspartic acid and has no known effect in humans. It has been shown to be an essential growth factor for certain bacteria. It has been sold as a 'vitamin-mineral bridge' in the form of iron, magnesium and other metallic salts, but without evidence of any effect.

Growth factors

Some 'vitamins' were first identified as growth factors for one or more organisms, but the term was dropped when they were subsequently found not to be dietary essentials in humans.

Choline Choline or N-trimethylethanolamine is present in cell membranes as phosphatidylcholine (lecithin) and in the central nervous system as sphingomyelin; acetylcholine is a transmitter at neuromuscular junctions. Lecithin is normally synthesized in the body in adequate amounts. It is naturally present in many foods and is added to some processed foods as an emulsifying agent, so it is most unlikely that any dietary deficiency occurs in humans. The crude lecithin preparations marketed as dietary supplements are of no physiological value.

In the 1930s choline was shown to be essential for experimental animals, in that a deficiency resulted in fatty infiltration of the liver owing to defective synthesis of specific plasma proteins with failure to transport triacylglycerols from the liver.

Although choline is not a dietary essential for humans there is some evidence that conditions can arise where the synthesis of acetylcholine is limited. Supplements of phosphatidylcholine may increase the rate of acetylcholine turnover and result in some improvement in cognitive function in patients suffering from senile dementia and tardive dyskinesia. Long-term total parenteral nutrition can result in a fall in plasma concentration of choline with subsequent impaired liver function.

Inositol Inositol is a hexahydric sugar alcohol (hexahydroxycyclohexane) with nine possible isomers, of which only *myo*-inositol (*meso*-inositol) has biological activity. It functions mainly as a constituent of phospholipids and is widespread in fruits, meat, milk, nuts and vegetables; it also occurs in relatively large amounts in cereals as the hexaphosphate, phytic acid.

Inositol is a growth factor for newly born mice where deficiency symptoms include 'spectacled eye' and alopecia, and for chicks. It has a lipotropic action similar to that of choline. It is also essential for human cells in tissue culture, and supplementary doses in preterm infants with respiratory distress syndrome during the first weeks of life have been associated with increased survival.

There is no evidence that inositol is a dietary essential for healthy humans. On the contrary, there is evidence that high intracellular concentrations of inositol may impair nerve conduction. Abnormalities in the metabolism of *myo*-inositol have been implicated in diabetes mellitus, renal disorders and some forms of cancer. Although supplementation has been shown to be helpful in diabetes, this is not the case for renal disease, and inositol may even be toxic in these circumstances.

***Para*-aminobenzoic acid** *Para*-aminobenzoic acid (PABA) is a growth factor for certain microorganisms and an antagonist to the bacteriostatic action of sulfonamide drugs. It forms part of the folic acid molecule and this may be why it is a dietary essential for organisms that do not require preformed folic acid. It has been used to treat certain rickettsial diseases, possibly because it inhibits *p*-oxybenzoic acid which is essential for these microorganisms.

Vitamin Q Vitamin Q, also known as ubiquinone or coenzyme Q$_{10}$ is one of the electron carriers in mitochondria and therefore has an essential function in all energy-yielding metabolism. It may also have a general antioxidant role in membranes. It is readily synthesized in the body and there is no evidence that it is a dietary essential nor that supplements serve any useful purpose.

Lipoic acid Lipoic acid is also called thioctic acid, protogen and acetate replacement factor. It is an essential growth factor for the protozoon *Tetrahymena geleii* and for *Streptococcus faecalis*. Its chemical name is 6,8-dithiooctanoic acid. It is associated with thiamin in the initial decarboxylation of α-keto acids but has not been shown to be a dietary essential for humans or experimental animals.

Carnitine Carnitine or β-hydroxy-γ-butyrobetaine was isolated from Liebig's extract of meat in 1905 but only examined for biochemical function half a century later. It was identified as a substance found to be essential for the development of the mealworm

Tenebrio molitor and certain microorganisms, and was called vitamin B_T. Carnitine is synthesized in the body from lysine and methionine with the aid of vitamins C, B_6 and niacin, and is involved in the transfer of fatty acids into the mitochondria where they are oxidized.

Carnitine depletion is seen only where there is general protein–energy malnutrition (and hence deficiency of methionine and lysine). Depletion can also follow the administration of some anticonvulsant drugs which increase the excretion of carnitine. This can give rise to liver dysfunction which is improved with carnitine supplementation. Carnitine may be required by premature infants where the synthetic capacity is low, and low blood levels have been reported in adults maintained for long periods on total parenteral nutrition (TPN). Apart from these special circumstances it does not appear to be a dietary requirement; strict vegetarians who ingest only about one-tenth of the average intake of 100–300 mg per day have carnitine levels within the average range.

Carnitine was marketed under the name of Bicarnesine (a double molecule) in Belgium in the early 1950s with the claim that it stimulated appetite and promoted growth in children and experimental animals, but this claim was never confirmed. Carnitine is also the subject of a US patent claim as a treatment of obesity 'when taken with an energy-restricted diet', but without presenting evidence. Unverified claims have been made for an effect of carnitine on increasing work capacity because of the ability of muscle to oxidize fatty acids.

It has been suggested that the depletion of muscle carnitine in scurvy as a result of impaired ascorbic acid-dependent hydroxylase activity may account for the lassitude and fatigue that precede clinical signs of ascorbic acid deficiency.

Taurine   Taurine or 2-aminoethane sulfonic acid is a nonprotein amino acid. For many years its only known function was the conjugation of bile acids to form taurocholic acid. Later it was found to be a dietary essential for kittens, in whom low intakes of taurine give rise to retinal degeneration which is cured by administering taurine.

Taurine has not been established as a dietary essential for humans since it is normally synthesized in adequate amounts from cysteine and is excreted in the free form in urine, and as taurine conjugates and taurocholic acid. However, children maintained on TPN for long periods without added taurine suffer changes in the electrical conductivity of the retina. Adult patients on long-term TPN without added taurine or cysteine (which is unstable in solution)

show changes in the electroretinogram when plasma taurine levels fall below about 30 μmol l^{-1} compared with the reference range of 55–70 μmol l^{-1}.

There are very few plant sources of taurine yet the low intake of strict vegetarians gives rise to plasma concentrations that are only slightly lower than those of carnivores (40–50 μmol l^{-1} compared with 55–70 μmol l^{-1}).

The relatively high concentration of taurine in the central nervous system and the rapid fall between birth and weaning suggest that it may have a role in the development of the central nervous system and postnatal development of synaptic connections. Since breast milk contains a high concentration of taurine it has been suggested that preterm infants may require preformed taurine. There is a large body of literature showing functional benefits of added taurine for formula-fed infant. Taurine has been classed as conditionally essential and is added to some infant formulae.

Conditionally essential amino acids

Amino acids are classed as essential and nonessential; however, some nonessential ones may become essential in the absence of their precursors. For example, arginine and citrulline play an essential role in the urea cycle and may not be synthesized in adequate amounts when there is a high intake of amino acids. Tyrosine and cystine are classed as nonessential because they can be synthesized from phenylalanine and methionine respectively, but with an inadequate supply of the latter two essential amino acids a dietary supply of tyrosine and cystine becomes necessary. Similarly, the nonessential amino acid glycine is excreted in conjugated form in the urine and may not be synthesized in adequate amounts when there is a high intake of substances that require conjugation.

Certain metabolic disorders can limit the synthesis of nonessential amino acids thereby making them essential, but these conditions are extremely rare.

Phytochemicals

Vitamin P   The existence of vitamin P was postulated in 1936 by Szent-Györgyi and coworkers who concluded that extracts of red peppers and lemon juice were more effective in the treatment of vascular fragility than ascorbic acid itself. The active factor was named 'vitamin P' (for 'permeability'), but curative claims could not be confirmed.

Flavonoids   Flavonoids were classed by Kuhnau as semiessential food components. The substances in question are present in fruits and green leaves conjugated with sugars and organic acids, and are now termed 'bioflavonoids'; some 2000 have been identified. Epidemiological evidence has shown that diets rich in fruits and vegetables have a protective action against some forms of cancer and coronary heart disease, and this has been attributed to a range of substances that function as antioxidants and scavengers of free radicals. It is suggested that these plant substances should be considered as a new class of nutrients: flavonoids. They include flavonones, flavones, flavonols, flavylium compounds (anthocyanins and anthocyanidins), flavan diols and catechins (flavan-3-ols).

Flavonoids contain the 2-phenylbenzo-γ-pyrane (flavane) nucleus which cannot be synthesized by animals. It is difficult to ascertain whether they are dietary essentials since they are so widespread in foods – the average intake is around 1–3 g per day. The bioavailability is not known and flavonoids are both altered by the intestinal bacteria and, if absorbed, rapidly metabolized in the body. They may be essential for some living organisms, for example butterflies, but even here they may simply accumulate from the diet of caterpillars.

Rutin, partly replaceable by hesperidin, appears to be essential for the cricket, *Acheta domestica*, and other flavonoids have a special function in silkworm larvae and some species of beetles. In addition there is some growth-promoting activity in young rats after a diet poor in flavonoids and in human cells in tissue culture. Flavonoids can reverse chemically induced carcinogenesis in animal models. In addition there are some hundred glucosinolates in plants of the *Brassica* genus, alliins in the *Allium* genus, and phytooestrogens including isoflavones, lignans, coumestans and resorcyclic acid lactones – the last offering protection against hormone-dependent cancers, such as breast cancer.

Polyamines (putrescine, spermine, spermidine) are found in all living organisms and so are ingested in the diet, as well as being formed by intestinal flora and synthesized in the body from ornithine and methionine. They are believed to be essential for cell growth and differentiation in humans.

Flavonoids such as quercetin, kaemferol, myricetin, apigenin and luteolin occur in tea, red wines and onions and there are indications that they offer some protection against certain forms of cancer; resveratrol in red and white wines reduces the oxidation of low-density lipoprotein and platelet aggregation *in vitro* and it has been suggested that it may be responsible in part at least, for the lower incidence of coronary heart disease in Mediterranean countries.

It has been claimed that allicin, found in onions and garlic, catechins in green tea and indoles in green vegetables reduce levels of blood cholesterol, enhance immunity and enhance production of glutathione S-transferase, but more evidence is needed to substantiate these claims.

Apart from epidemiological observations, most of the evidence for the effects of this range of substances comes from experiments *in vitro* and animal models. Many of the benefits are difficult to interpret. For example, while glucosinolates have some beneficial effects, they can cause sterility in livestock. Saponins (in beans) are claimed to offer protection against some cancers but have an adverse effect in retarding growth of animals and altering the permeability of the intestinal mucosa. Some of the naturally occurring antioxidants can be prooxidants at different concentrations, and individual flavonoids at high concentrations can be potential mutagens *in vitro*.

This is a relatively new field of enormous complexity and any claims must be regarded with caution.

See also: **Antioxidants**: Diet and Antioxidant Defence; Observational Epidemiology; Intervention Studies. **Cancer**: Epidemiology and Associations Between Diet and Cancer. **Carotenoids**: Epidemiology. **Cofactors**: Organic Cofactors; Inorganic Cofactors. **Epidemiological Studies**: Role and Interpretation. **Food Folklore**: Overview. **Fruits and Vegetables**: Nutritional Value. **Functional Foods**: Definition and Potential for Nutritional Role. **Health Foods**: Dietary Supplements - Micronutrients.

Further Reading

Bender AE (1985) *Health or Hoax?* Goring-on-Thames, England: Elvendon Press.

Hertog MGL (1996) Epidemiological evidence on potential health properties of flavonoids. *Proceedings of the Nutrition Society* 55:385–397.

Johnson IT, Williamson G and Musk RR (1994) Anticarcinogenic factors in plant foods; a new class of nutrients? *Nutrition Research Reviews* 7:175–204.

Kuhnau J (1976) The flavonoids; a class of semi-essential food components; their role in human nutrition. In: Bourne GH (ed.) *World Review of Nutrition and Dietetics*, 24, pp 117–191. Basel: Karger.

Okuba T *et al.* (1992) In vivo effects of tea polyphenol intake on human intestinal microflora and metabolism. *Bioscience, Biotechnology, Biochemistry* 56:588–591.

Pierpoint WS (1990) Flavonoids in human food and animal feedstuffs. In: Das NP (Ed.) *Flavonoids in Biology and Medicine*, vol. 3, pp 497–514. Current Issues in Flavonoid Research. National University of Singapore.

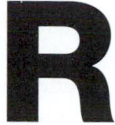

REFUGEES

Nutritional Management

C J K Henry, School of Biological and Molecular Sciences, Oxford Brookes University, Oxford, UK

Refugees Today

The refugee phenomenon is not new. It has existed since antiquity. Adam and Eve may be described as the first refugees when they were expelled from paradise. Today refugees are of a different kind. They have committed no crime. Their only 'crime' is to come from societies and countries that have repressive governments.

Statistics on refugees and other uprooted people are often inexact and controversial. One country's refugee is another country's illegal alien. Today's internally displaced person may be tomorrow's refugee. In 1970 there were 2.5 million refugees in the world. In 1980 the number was 11 million. By 1995 the number had risen to approximately 16 million. While government statistics cannot always be trusted to give full and unbiased accounts of refugee movements, the statistics presented in **Table 1** is a compilation from the US. Committee for Refugees.

Further examples of major movement of refugees and internally displaced persons during 1996 are listed below:

Table 1 Number of refugees and asylum-seekers worldwide

Year	No. of refugees and asylum-seekers
1987	13 300 000
1988	14 400 000
1989	15 100 000
1990	16 700 000
1991	16 600 000
1992	17 600 000
1993	16 300 000
1994	16 300 000
1995	15 300 000
1996	14 500 000

- Rwanda – 1.3 million Rwandans repatriated
- Liberia – 300 000 Liberians newly uprooted
- Zaire – At least 400 000 uprooted in civil war
- Bosnia and Herzegovina – 200 000 displaced Bosnians relocated
- Burundi – At least 150 000 Burundians flee to Tanzania
- Iraq – 75 000 Iraqis flee temporarily to Iran

The scale and complexity of today's refugee crises are a reflection of the instability of the period in which we live. The collapse of the old order has given rise to a more hostile world in which new refugee movements are likely to continue to occur. There are estimated to be about 24 million internally displaced people in the world today. Some of them are trapped by conflict and have no possibility of seeking asylum across an international border, but many of them are potential refugees. Significantly, about 80% of these uprooted people are women and children.

Definition of a refugee

The term refugee has been defined by the UN Convention Relating to the Status of Refugees as a person who:

> owing to a well-founded fear of being persecuted for reasons of race, religion, nationality, membership of a particular social group or political opinion is outside the country of his nationality and is unable or, owing to such fear, is unwilling to avail himself of the protection of that country; or who, not having a nationality and being outside of his former habitual residence as a result of such events, is unable or, owing to such fear, is unwilling to return to it.

The definition has been extended in Africa, through a Convention approved by the Organization of African Unity (OAU), to cover any person who 'owing to external aggression, occupation, foreign domination or events seriously disturbing public order in either part of or the whole country, is compelled to seek refuge outside his country of origin'.

Because refugee status inherently implies movements across international borders, a joint responsibility between international organizations and national governments has existed for many years and has been codified in international law. Primary responsibility for refugee protection and assistance lies with the UN High Commissioner for Refugees (UNHCR).

Distributing relief assistance to refugees

In addition to UNHCR, the World Food Programme (WFP), the UN Children's Fund (UNICEF), the UN Development Programme (UNDP), the World Health Organization (WHO) and the International Labour Organization (ILO) are also called upon to provide expertise in matters related to their areas of interest. In addition, nongovernmental organizations (NGOs), e.g. Oxfam, Médecins sans Frontières (MSF) and Save the Children Fund (SCF), have traditionally played an important role as partners in implementing programmes for refugees.

Collaboration between WFP and UNHCR

Close collaboration between the two organizations has existed for many years. More recently, the WFP and UNHCR signed a Memorandum of Understanding. This memorandum included provision for: (a) better assessment of the numbers and needs of refugees, (b) a clearer role for WFP in final distribution of food, (c) the need to monitor the food pipeline closely, (d) sharing timely information and taking early joint action on shortfalls in deliveries.

The salient points of the memorandum are:

1. WFP and UNHCR will seek to ensure the restoration and maintenance of a sound nutritional status through a food basket that meets the assessed requirements, is nutritionally balanced and is culturally acceptable.
2. Promotion of self-reliance through programmes to develop food production or self-employment.

The two organizations have also divided their tasks and responsibilities. UNHCR is largely responsible for assessing the nutritional status of refugees and for the implementation of selective feeding programmes. Moreover, UNHCR is responsible for mobilizing local fresh foods, spices, tea and 'dried and therapeutic milk'. WFP is responsible for mobilizing other commodities, whether for general or selective feeding: cereals, oils, pulses, blended foods, salt, sugar and biscuits. WFP is also responsible for the provision of blended foods 'or other fortified commodities' to prevent or correct micronutrient malnutrition.

Refugee rations are normally composed of *basic foods* and *complementary foods*. Their broad definitions are listed below.

Basic foods Commodities which constitute the bulk of general rations, provide the greatest part of the requirements of the beneficiaries in terms of energy, protein and fat. The commodities include cereals, protein-rich food (usually pulses but occasionally some quantities of canned fish or meat), edible oil or fat, salt, sugar and fortified cereal blends (also known as blended foods).

Complementary foods Food items which are required in addition to and in smaller quantities than basic foods, in order to provide additional nutrients, increase palatability, and for cultural reasons. These include fresh or dried vegetables, fish or meat, fruit, eggs, spices and condiments (other than salt), coffee and tea, DSM/DWM (dried skim milk/dried whole milk) and high-protein biscuits.

Nutritional Deficiencies Amongst Refugees

A typical refugee ration per day is usually composed of 400–500 g cereals (wheat, rice, corn), 30 g legumes or lentils, 20 g oil, and a small quantity of sugar (5 g). Dried skimmed milk powder is now rarely given routinely as part of the refugee ration. Where refugees are unable to supplement their rations by obtaining work or by cultivation, they must live on these rations alone.

Table 2 shows the average vitamin and iron content of a typical refugee ration, and compares it with that of an average pet food. The refugee ration is not only devoid of vitamins C and A, but it is also low in riboflavin, niacin and iron. The only vitamin in any physiologically acceptable level is thiamin, and even that may be inadequate if the cereals are milled inappropriately. By contrast, pet food is not only balanced, but also has an excellent micronutrient composition.

Classical vitamin depletion studies, conducted in humans, may be used as a guide to assess the potential time needed for the appearance of vitamin deficiencies within populations living on refugee rations. These are 6–8 weeks for the appearance of niacin deficiency, 12–19 weeks for riboflavin deficiency, 3–5 weeks for thiamin deficiency, and 10–13 weeks for vitamin C deficiency. Deficiency of vitamin A took 18 months to develop during experimental deprivation studies of healthy British adults, but many populations in developing countries have dangerously low vitamin A stores in the 'normal' state. The extra stress of infections such as measles and diarrhoea that plague refugee camps can precipitate malnutrition-induced blindness within a few weeks. These depletion times indicate that aid agencies and nongovernmental organizations

Table 2 Comparison of vitamin and iron content in refugee rations and pet food

Food item	Quantity (g)	Thiamin (mg)	Riboflavin (mg)	Niacin (mg)	Folic acid (μg)	Vitamin C (mg)	Iron (mg)
Refugee ration							
Wheat flour	400	1.28	0.08	8	40	0	6.8
Kidney beans	30	0.16	0.05	1.6	39	0	2
Vegetable oil	20	0	0	0	0	0	0
Sugar	5	0	0	0	0	0	0
Total	**455**	**1.44**	**0.13**	**9.6**	**79**	**0**	**8.8**
Pet food	455	1.07	1.62	22.5	52	0	44
RNI		1.01	1.3	17	200	40	14.8

Source: Modified from Tomkins A and Henry CJK (1992) Comparison of refugee rations with pet food. *Lancet* **340**:368.

working with refugees need to be vigilant for potential outbreaks of micronutrient deficiencies among those who have been on standard refugee diets for 2–3 months.

A review of data collected from 1985 to 1987 by relief programmes in five refugee camps in Somalia and one in Sudan had shown scurvy (vitamin C deficiency) as a serious public health problem for refugees dependent on standard relief food. The outbreaks of clinical scurvy occurred among refugees in all the camps between 3 to 4 months after their arrival. The risk was higher among the females of child-bearing age and among an elderly population. A range of nutritional deficiencies which could be caused in people dependent on refugee rations for prolonged periods of time is shown in **Table 3**. These deficiency diseases, without treatment, can lead to permanent disability and eventually to death.

Refugees are also prone to anaemia because the food rations are often low in vitamin C and are high in polyphenols and fibre; both factors reduce iron absorption. Moreover, the diets rarely contain the bioavailable form of haem iron found in meat, poultry and fish. Refugees also have diseases such as hookworm and malaria that increase iron loss.

Niacin deficiency (pellagra)

Outbreaks of pellagra have been reported in 1988–1989 in refugee camps in Ethiopia, Malawi, Zimbabwe and other African countries. Pellagra occurs where maize, which is low in both niacin and tryptophan, has been the primary relief grain and where little complementary food rich in protein has been given. The lead time for developing this disease in about 2–3 months.

Table 3 Summary of selected reports of nutritional deficiency diseases in refugee camps

Disease and location	Date	Prevalence (%)	Main groups affected	Remarks
Scurvy				
Somalia	1984–1987	5.6–45.2	Total population	Camps installed in a very
		1–28.8	Children	poor environment
Sudan	1985	22	Women 45 years	
Eastern Ethiopia	1988	1–2	–	
Xerophthalmia				
Sudan	1985	6.70	Children	
Anaemia				
Somalia	1987	17.6–21.3	Children, women	
Pellagra				
Zimbabwe	1988	1.54	Adults	
Malawi	1989	1.17		
Beriberi				
Thailand	1980	8	Adults	

Source: as summarized in Berry Koch (1990). Alleviation of nutritional deficiency diseases in refugees. *Food and Nutrition Bulletin* **32**(2):107. With permission.

Thiamin deficiency (beriberi)

Thiamin deficiency can occur where the diet consists mainly of white (milled) cereals, including polished rice and starchy staple foods such as cassava and tubers. A diet deficient in thiamin produces lethargy, moodiness, mental fatigue, insomnia and anorexia. Beriberi can develop within 12 weeks of deficient intake. Outbreaks of all these types of beriberi have been reported in camps in southeast Asia, although no formal surveys have been conducted except in Thailand.

Methods to Combat Nutrient Deficiencies in Refugees

Until now, the control of deficiency diseases in refugee populations has largely depended on the following methods:

1. distribution of supplementary tablets
2. distribution of additional foods (e.g. fruits, dried fish, meat) containing the required nutrients to the rations.

As a strategy, the distribution of tablets has been unsatisfactory because of the large populations involved and the difficulty of securing adequate compliance. Moreover, it is unsatisfactory for any population to depend upon medicines for its long-term survival. In specific cases, deficiency diseases have been controlled, at least intermittently, by procuring appropriate foodstuffs. In Malawi, for example, pellagra was controlled by the distribution of groundnuts, which are a rich source of niacin and other micronutrients. These, however, are in short supply and expensive. The possibility that nutrient deficiencies in refugee diets might be prevented by adding the nutrient to a food item has often been suggested. Some processed food supplied to refugees, for example corn-soya-milk, are fortified with some nutrients. However, these foods are used almost entirely as supplementary rations for malnourished children: they are rarely available in the quantities required for general distribution. As an alternative, the possibility of using nutrient fortification of bulk food aid commodities to improve the quality of refugee rations has been successfully exploited in Malawi and other African countries.

Food fortification may be broadly defined as the process whereby one or more nutrients are added to food to maintain, improve or enhance the quality of a diet consumed by a group, community or population. The term fortification is sometimes used loosely to include the terms 'enrichment' or nutrification. In all these operations the primary objective is to enhance the nutritional quality of the food by direct addition of various nutrients. The major attraction of food fortification as a nutritional intervention is that it does not entail major changes in the existing diet or lifestyle. In contrast to other interventions, it can be technically implemented over a relatively short timescale. This may be an important consideration in certain groups such as referees.

In the refugee context, the potential vehicles to which micronutrients might be added are cereals, oil, pulses, salt and occasionally sugar. However, in many locations only cereals are consistently supplied, other commodities being supplied more or less intermittently. Cereals may, therefore, prove to be the only feasible vehicle for food fortification. However, in specific locations where distribution and consumption may be closely monitored, it is possible to consider oils and pulses as potential vehicles for micronutrient additions as these foods will be consumed by the whole population reasonably consistently. Special foods such as corn-soya-milk might be used as a vehicle aimed at selected groups, particularly children under 5 years of age.

The following generalizations may be made about refugee foods:

- cereals are potential vehicles for the addition of most B vitamins, iron, calcium and zinc;
- oil can be used for the addition of vitamin A;
- sugar can be used for the addition of iron, vitamin A.

A newly released report commissioned by the Canadian International Development Agency (CIDA) on the fortification of foods for refugee feeding has raised concerns about the micronutrient inadequacy of refugee rations. The report recommends the fortification of refugee rations, especially grain-based commodities, as a method to improve the micronutrient intake of refugees.

Guidelines for Calculating Food Rations for Refugees

Guidelines (WFP memorandum: WFP/PO/227, 1991) and sample food rations for refugee populations have been agreed upon by the WFP and the UNHCR. The food items required may be provided from a variety of sources: by the refugees themselves, host governments, nongovernmental organizations and by the international community. The following is a summary of these guidelines.

1. In order to meet the nutritional requirements of refugees, food rations should complement any food which the refugees are able to obtain

themselves through agricultural or income-generating activities. If such activities are restricted or impossible, the food ration should, as far as possible, meet all essential nutritional requirements, including micronutrients.

2. When refugees depend to a greater extent on the provision of food from external sources, the food basket provided should consist of a variety of basic food items and, to ensure nutritional adequacy and palatability, complementary foods should be included.

3. Where dependency on externally provided food exists, the total food available to refugees from all sources should include both basic and complementary foods. They should provide an intake of no less than 8000 kJ (1900 kcal) of energy per person per day. At least 8% should be in the form of protein and 10% in the form of fat. **Table 4** provides examples of variations of the 8000 kJ ration. This food requirement can either be increased or decreased, depending on the circumstances of the population and according to a variety of physiological and/or climatic conditions.

The nutritive value of food commonly used in refugee feeding

Local food   Organizations in charge of food distribution should be familiar with what is usually eaten in different countries and regions in order to choose appropriate commodities for distribution amongst refugees. Local foods should be chosen as far as possible, rather than unusual (or even unfamiliar) foods.

Cereals, pulses and legumes   Cereals (rice, wheat, sorghum, maize, millet) can serve as staple foods and as the main source of carbohydrates (food energy) and protein. Cereals contain a range of protein (7–

15%) which are of relatively good quality. Limiting amino acids (i.e. those present in the lowest concentration relative to needs) are lysine, leucine and tryptophan. These can be corrected by combining cereals with other foods such as legumes or pulses. Since major vitamins and minerals of the cereal grain are mainly located in the outer layers and the germ, when the grains are polished and milled into flour, these vitamins and minerals are largely lost. Pulses (beans, peas, lentils, chickpeas, soya beans, peanuts) have a very high protein content (20–30% on average; soya up to 40%). Their protein is of relatively good quality and combines ideally with cereal protein so that some mixtures reach the protein quality of milk protein. Pulses also contain large amounts of iron and B vitamins; quite high amounts of carotenes (provitamin A) are found in beans, peas and lentils. Oilseeds (sesame, sunflower seeds) also have a remarkably high protein and a very high fat/oil content.

Oils and fats   Oils and fats are concentrated sources of food energy and increase the energy content of any meal considerably. Milk fat (but not vegetable fat) contains vitamin A and small amounts of vitamin D. An exception is red palm-oil with its very high content of carotene. It is an important source of provitamin A in some West African countries.

New products   The term 'new products' refers to various foodstuffs developed more or less directly for use against nutritional deficiencies (mostly protein, but also vitamins and minerals). It is possible to classify them roughly into food blends, enriched foods and concentrates. Food blends contain slightly processed foodstuffs (ground or dried) using pulses (20–30%) and cereals (60–70%), with an additional 5–10% dry skim milk, vitamins and minerals. These products are usually designed as baby, weaning and infant food and are produced in many developing countries. They can also be in biscuit form, such as the 'Oxfam Energy Biscuit'.

Factors which may increase average nutritional requirements in refugees

Age and gender   If the target population has a significantly greater than normal proportion of males, the per capita rations should be increased in energy content by approximately 10%.

Health/nutrition and physiological status   If the population has been subjected to nutritional stress (such as severe food shortages), or if there is widespread illness and/or general undernutrition, the ration should provide a higher food intake for an

Table 4   Examples of 8000 kJ rations

Items		Rations (quantity in g)		
		1	2	3
Wheat flour/maize meal/rice		400	400	400
Pulses		60	20	40
Oils/fats		25	25	25
Fortified cereal blend[a]		–	25	–
Canned fish/meat		–	–	20
Sugar		15	20	20
Salt		5	5	5
Approximate food value:	Energy (kJ)	8000	8000	8000
	Protein (g)	45	45	45
	Fat (g)	45	45	30

[a]Such as corn soy blend, wheat soy milk, likuni phala, faffa, etc.

initial period of 6 months. Supplementary and therapeutic feeding programmes should also be implemented for malnourished children, pregnant and lactating women, and for other individuals specifically identified as being nutritionally at risk. **Table 5** provides examples of the enhanced rations.

Physical activity level For refugees engaged in heavy physical activity (such as clearing land for agricultural crops or infrastructure works), an increase in dietary energy for those involved is recommended. Increasing the cereal component of the ration to 500 g is a first option. The vitamin and mineral content of diet may also need to be increased.

Climate For populations exposed to cold climatic conditions, energy provisions need to be increased by 5% (i.e. approximately 420 kJ, or 100 kcal) for every 5°C below 20°C (thermoneutral temperature).

Factors which may decrease food aid requirements

Access to additional foods Some of the target population may be able to produce a proportion of their own food from farming, gardening, livestock/poultry raising, hunting and fishing. In such cases, the corresponding food items may be withdrawn from the ration.

Income-generating opportunities Certain groups of refugees at times have possibilities of earning some cash income. Refugees in camps who engage in some economic activity and have access to markets may therefore have smaller basic rations.

Table 5 Examples of enhanced rations

		Rations (quantity in g)	
Items		400	450
Wheat flour/maize meal/rice		40	50
Pulses		25	25
Oils/fats		30	50
Fortified cereal blend[a]		60/40	30
Canned C fish/dried fish		20	20
Sugar		15	15
Salt		5	–
Vegetables/fruit		150	–
Condiments/spices		As available	
Approximate food value:	Energy (kJ)	9450	9770
	Protein (g)	65	80
	Fat (g)	55	45

[a]Such as corn soy blend, wheat soy milk, likuni phala, faffa, etc.

Other considerations

When designing and distributing food to refugees the following considerations must be borne in mind.

Food habits The staple food should be one that the target population is familiar with; they must be able to process and prepare it. The source of protein also needs to be acceptable; legumes and pulses, for example, are not well known to all populations.

Nonfood needs The availability of adequate supplies of essential nonfood items such as water and cooking fuel must be assured. Whenever whole grains (wheat, maize, sorghum) are supplied, grinding facilities and utensils should be available. Appropriate cooking facilities may also be required.

Food processing considerations Losses may be expected as a result of household-level processing or due to milling costs of whole grain cereal. These should be taken into consideration in determining the quantity to be included in the ration.

Food safety A system of quality control for all commodities must be implemented to ensure that foods distributed to refugees are of good quality and safe for human consumption.

WFP Provisional Guidelines for Selective Feeding Programmes

In an emergency, there are three types of feeding programmes: (a) General Food Distribution (GFD), and two types of selective feeding programmes, (b) Supplementary Feeding Programmes (SFP) and (c) Therapeutic Feeding Programmes (TFP). An SFP provides extra food in addition to the basic ration, as dry take-home rations or wet on-the-spot feeding, in order to meet the additional needs of nutritionally and physiologically vulnerable people. SFPs can be further distinguished into two main categories:

1. A Generalized Supplementary Feeding Programme (GSFP) which provides a food supplement for all children of a certain age in order to prevent an increase in the number of malnourished children.
2. A Targeted Supplementary Feeding Programme (TSFP) which aims at the rehabilitation of malnourished children/adults.

The objectives of these selective feeding programmes, as detailed in guidelines issued by Médecins sans Frontières, are listed in **Table 6**.

An adequate general ration is considered a

Table 6 Objectives of selective feeding programmes from MSF guidelines

Programme	Objectives	Target group
Targeted SFP	Reduction of % of severe acute malnutrition in under 5s	W/H 70–80% or −3 to <−2 Z scores (moderately malnourished children under 5 years)
	Reduction of under 5 mortality rates	Malnourished individuals above 5 years
		Children discharged from TFP
Generalized SFP	Prevention of further deterioration in nutritional situation	Children under 5 in general
	Reduction of under 5 mortality rates	Pregnant and lactating women
		Socially and/or medically needy individual cases
		Elderly persons

W/H, weight-for-height.

precondition for the set up of such programmes. If the general ration is inadequate, supplementary feeding of vulnerable groups will be of limited value. The need for SFPs has been frequently debated. As a policy, supplementary programmes should be temporary, targeted and the criteria for termination of the programmes should be defined from the beginning. The current tendency is to favour targeted feeding programmes to restore nutritional status of those individuals who are malnourished. Supplementary feeding programmes should under no circumstances replace the provision of adequate basic rations to the whole family.

Current guidelines for supplementary feeding programmes

Generalized supplementary feeding programme A GSFP for prevention purposes maybe implemented in the absence of a full ration, under one or a combination of the following circumstances:

- Problems in the delivery/distribution of the general ration.
- Prevalence of acute malnutrition among children under 5 years (weight-for-height above 15–20%. Z score <−2 or <80% of reference median).
- Prevalence of acute malnutrition among children under 5 years above 10–15%. (weight-for-height Z score <−2 or 80% of reference median) plus aggravating factors.
- Malnutrition problems linked to seasonality.

Targeted supplementary feeding programme The implementation of SFPs for selected individuals in vulnerable groups is required under the following circumstances:

- Prevalence of acute malnutrition among children under 5 years above 10% (weight-for-height Z score <−2 or <80% of the reference median).
- Prevalence of acute malnutrition among children under 5 years above 5–9% (weight-for-height Z

score <−2 or <80% of the reference median), plus aggravating factors.
- Existence of TFP established to respond to a high percentage of severely malnourished children.

Aggravating factors to be considered are the following: crude mortality above 1 per 10 000 per day, epidemic of measles and high prevalence of respiratory or diarrhoeal disease, poor sanitation environment and unreliable food distribution system. **Fig. 1** illustrates the entry and exit to and from supplementary feeding programmes as outlined by Médecins sans Frontières.

Foods used in supplementary feeding programmes (from CONCERN Worldwide guidelines)

The diets are based predominantly on porridges, local foods and family diet. Most foods should provide energy intakes of 400–800 kJ (100–200 kcal) per 100 ml. The percentage of energy from protein should be approximately 12–16% to allow for catch-up growth to occur.

Supplementary porridges Supplementary porridges, made up to 650–850 kJ (150–200 kcal) per 100 ml, can be made up in the feeding centres using blended cereals or milled staples with legumes or rice. Most blended cereals provide approximately 1500–1700 kJ (350–400 kcal) per 100 g of dry product.

If available, mineral and vitamin mixes for supplementary feeding should be added to porridges which are not prefortified.

Milks High-energy milk (HEM) (420 kJ, 100 kcal) and 2.9 g protein per 100 ml) can be given in wet SFPs (see **Table 7**). Minerals and vitamins should be added to milks. To make up 1 litre use 900 ml of water. Dry milk powders should not be distributed as a dry ration on their own; milk powder can be added to a premix for distribution. The composition of a dry ration premix in described below.

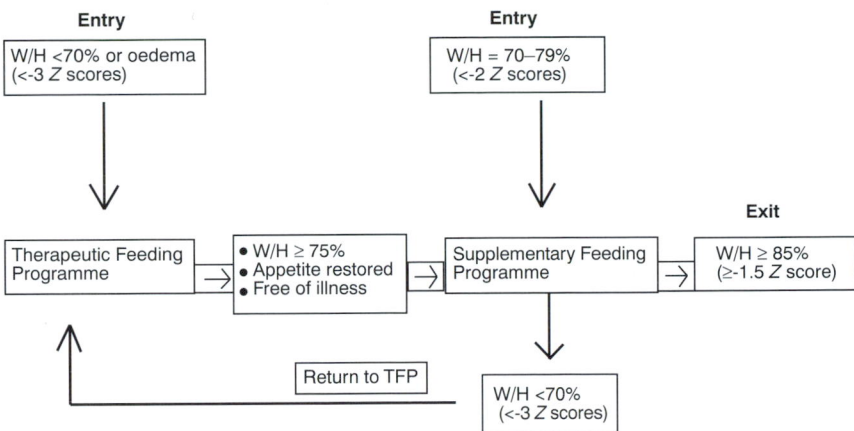

Figure 1 Criteria for entry and exit to and from SFPs according to MSF guidelines. W/H, weight-for-height.

Table 7 Nutrient composition of feeds

	Phase 1 milk	HEM (phases 2 and 3)
DSM (g l⁻¹)	a	80
Oil (g l⁻¹)	a	60
Sugar (g l⁻¹)	a	50
Protein per litre of milk (g)	10–12	28.8
Energy per litre of milk (kJ)	3150	4200+

ᵃNo information available for recipe, use commercial product. HEM, high-energy milk.

Therapeutic feeding programmes

Therapeutic Feeding Programmes (TFP) are strictly for life-saving and rehabilitation purposes and are directed to the most seriously malnourished children who need specific and intensive nutritional/medical attention. The severely malnourished child has to be admitted to a special feeding centre, hospital or clinic where the child is given several feeds throughout the day and, when needed, medical treatment.

Energy protein requirement The size of the daily supplement will depend on the general situation and on the method used. On-site feeding or wet ration distribution involves distribution of cooked food at feeding centres. Rations for on-site feeding should provide 1200–2100 kJ (300–500 kcal) of energy per person per day, including at least 10–15 g of protein. Take-home or dry ration distribution involves the distribution of a ration to be prepared at home. Take-home rations should provide 4200–6300 kJ (1000–1500 kcal) and at least 25 g of protein. Food must be culturally appropriate, palatable, energy dense and low in bulk. Usually a blended food such as CSB, Unimix or one blended locally will be used

(addition of 10 g sugar and 10 g oil per 100 g of CSB may be required). Emergency food such as high-energy biscuits and/or BP5 biscuits can also be used in combination. Energy density is an important feature of a suitable food for targeted feeding programmes. To be considered energy dense more than 20% of the energy has to come from fat. This means that dry foods such as porridge mixes, blended food or biscuits should contain at least 10 g fat per 100 g. Unimix, Faffa and CSB have very high fat contents and all the mixes should have oil/fat added during preparation.

Treatment of malnutrition in refugee camps Low-protein diets are recommended for treating severe childhood malnutrition. In the recovery phase, the diet may be higher in protein and energy, to produce rapid weight gain. A formula of 80 g dried skimmed milk, 50 g sugar, 60 g oil, minerals and vitamins per litre of feed (energy density 4.2 kJ ml⁻¹ (1 kcal ml⁻¹) is sufficient for catch-up growth when fed to appetite. The same formula may also be given orally or by a nasogastric tube, in the early stages of treatment, if diluted 3:1 with water. About 100 ml per kg per day of the formula (total 133 ml with water) should be given in the first few days, when the children are anorexic, and then very much more of the undiluted feed (about 200 ml per kg per day) once appetite has returned.

The diet must also contain adequate potassium, magnesium, zinc, copper, selenium, iodine and each of the vitamins. In the case of diets not specifically preformulated for treatment of malnutrition, addition of minerals and vitamins is feasible only from ready-made sachets (or stock solutions). For stability, the minerals and vitamins have to be packaged separately.

More recently (1994) a commercial company

Nutriset (France) has developed three specifically formulated milk-based product for the treatment of severe malnutrition. F75 (phase 1 milk) is designed for use in the initial phase of the recovery process from severe malnutrition when metabolism is abnormal. F75 formula is enriched with a high concentration of minerals and vitamins to correct associated deficiencies. In the Nutriset range of products F75 formula is designated a phase 1 therapeutic milk.

F100 (phase 2 milk) is a high-energy milk with added minerals and vitamins. It is intended for the treatment of severely malnourished children once their condition has been stabilized (in phase 2 therapeutic feeding) and is designed to maximize weight gain and reduce mortality rates. This formula allows the child to grow at 10–15 g per kg per day, which is 10–20 times faster than well-nourished children of the same age. Nutriset claims that the F100 formula corresponds to therapeutic milk.

SP450 is a porridge fortified with vitamins and minerals. It can be used in phase 2 of therapeutic feeding and in supplementary feeding programmes. It is suitable for all ages.

Local foods and family diets Emphasis should be placed on providing a supplementary diet based on local foods. If possible vegetables purchased or grown locally should be included.

A variety of recipes should be prepared with the community for wet-feeding purposes. These recipes can be adapted to ensure they have adequate energy and protein content. Ease of use, accessibility and supply are important factors in selecting products for use in such recipes.

Dry premix should be prepared using blended cereals that are available locally.

High-energy and high-protein biscuits High-energy and high-protein biscuits are suitable for use in SFPs. These biscuits increase the energy content of the supplementary diet significantly and are particularly useful in the beginning of the emergency operation.

Biscuits are a valuable commodity on the market and efforts should be made to prevent them being sold; they should be crushed or broken before being added to the dry ration premix.

Long-term dependence on high-energy and high-protein biscuits should be avoided; biscuits are expensive and should not be given priority over locally available products. If is unlikely that families can afford these biscuits once food aid is no longer

being provided. Every attempt should be made to use locally available foods.

Fruit If available, fruit is a suitable supplement in a wet SFP and is a good source of vitamins. Children in therapeutic feeding programmes should have priority access to bananas.

Conclusion

Thousands of refugees are still dying of macro- and micronutrient deficiencies. All methods to alleviate their suffering must be vigorously pursued. Supplementary and therapeutic feeding along with food fortification are effective ways to bring nutritional relief and benefits to millions of refugees the world over.

See Colour plate 12.

See also: **Ascorbic Acid**: Scurvy. **Famine**: Population Responses. **Food Aid**: Overview. **Food Aid Organizations**: History and Role. **Food Fortification**: Importance in the Diet. **Malabsorption Syndromes**: Nutritional Management. **Malnutrition**: Definition, Classification and Epidemiology; Primary Malnutrition. **Niacin**: Pellagra. **Thiamin**: Beriberi. **United Nations Children's Fund**: History and Role. **World Health Organization**: Role.

Further Reading

Boerhart M, Davis A and Lelin B (1995) *Nutrition Guidelines*, 1st edn. Paris: Médecins sans Frontières.

Briend A and Golden M (1993) Treatment of severe malnutrition in refugee camps. *European Journal of Clinical Nutrition* 47:750–754.

Golden M (1995) Severe malnutrition. In: *Oxford Textbook of Medicine*, pp 1278–1295. Oxford: Oxford University Press.

Henry CJK (1995) Improving food rations for refugees: a case for food fortification. *Postgraduate Doctor Middle East* 3:84–89.

Refugee Studies Programme (1991) *Responding to the Nutrition Crisis among Refugees: The Need for New Approaches*. Report of an international symposium, 17–20 March 1991, Oxford. Oxford: Refugee Studies Programme.

Toole M and Waldman R (1990) Prevention of excess mortality in refugee and displaced populations in developing countries. *Journal of the American Medical Association* 263:3269–3302.

UNHCR (1982) *United Nations High Commissioner for Refugees Handbook for Emergencies*. Geneva: UNHCR.

RELIGIOUS CUSTOMS

Influence on Diet

P Fieldhouse, Faculty of Nursing, The University of Manitoba, Winnipeg, Manitoba, Canada

This article discusses the nature, function and origins of food practices associated with religious beliefs. A review of historical and contemporary dietary practices in major world religions includes Christianity, Islam, Judaism, Hinduism and Buddhism, and is followed by a brief account of dietary tenets of Jainism, Sikhism and the Baha'i faith.

The Function and Nature of Religious Food Practices

What people need to eat to survive as biological organisms and what they choose to eat as human beings are two different matters. While practically any food combination which supplies the requisite nutrients to meet physiological needs is adequate for biological purposes, this is clearly not the case for cultural purposes. People make choices from the foodstuffs available to them which reflect a constellation of social, economic, political and cultural influences, as well as personal preferences. Religion is one such influence, and religious adherents around the world are more or less circumscribed in their food choices by the teachings of their chosen faith.

Religious dietary laws serve a number of different functions. They can provide a way for people to demonstrate their faith – to show that they accept religious authority. As a mark of group identity they strengthen feelings of belonging, and in this way act as a material reflection of the spiritual bonds which link co-religionists.

Conversely, dietary rules may serve to demonstrate separateness by clearly demarcating cultural boundaries between religions. Foregoing food during religious fasts is a form of self-denial, showing that one is more interested in spiritual than in worldly values. Through sacrifices or sacrificial meals, food is used as a means of communicating with God or other supernatural forces. Offerings may be made to placate the God and so forestall disaster, or to seek favours and good fortune. Finally, religious practices may serve, incidentally or purposefully, to encourage ecological sustainability through conservation and judicious use of scarce resources.

Cultural food practices are rich in examples of foods which are not allowed for consumption though they be freely available, and religious codes often exclude whole categories of foods from consumption. What must not be eaten may be determined by characteristics of individuals such as age, gender, social or physiological status, or by external constraints such as time of day or time of year (**Table 1**). Prescriptive rules of what must be eaten, when and how, are the counterpart of prohibitions. Religious food practices often require the use of specific foods in specific situations, especially during special celebrations such as feasts or fasts, where particular foods often have important symbolic values.

Religious food customs originate in three main ways. Some are required by God and are described in scriptures; others are decreed by religious or political leaders; still others arise through adaptation or co-option of pre-existing food practices. Pagan festivals were frequently assimilated and given new meanings as modern religions assumed dominance over older forms of worship. Indeed, religious food practices are far from static; they are subject to continuous adaptation and re-interpretation. Changes may occur as result of religious reform or revisionism, acculturation, individual, family or community adaptations.

Immigration provides a good example of how changing circumstances may result in changing attitudes to food. Through the process of acculturation dietary practices are modified in the light of availability of foodstuffs and as an adaptation to new cultural rules, customs and expectations.

Continued compliance with traditional rules may depend on social contexts. Adherents who are strict when with members of their own religious group may be willing to be more lax when alone or with a different social group. Even without such external forces, adherence to religious dietary laws or guidelines varies on a national, regional, community, family or individual level. In many cases religions have developed several branches, sects or schools of thought which make different demands on members. Such variability in practice should be kept in mind when reading the following descriptions of normative customs. **Table 2** summarizes the size and distribution of contemporary religious followings.

Table 1 Comparative examples of religious dietary strictures

Religion	Dietary stricture
Food restrictions	
Judaism	Eat only animals with cloven hooves and which chew the cud, i.e. cattle, sheep, goats, deer
	Eat only forequarters of animal
	Eat only fish with scales and fins
	No blood
Islam	No blood
	No pork
	No intoxicating liquor
Sikhism	No beef
Hinduism	Must not kill or eat any animal
Days of the year	
Christianity	No meat on Fridays during Lent (Catholics)
	Fast on Wednesday and Friday (Greek Orthodox)
Judaism	No food preparation on Sabbath
Time of day	
Islam	Foods may not be eaten between sunrise and sunset during Ramadan
Buddhism	Monks do not eat after midday
Preparation of food	
Judaism	Ritual slaughtering of animals
	Separate utensils for meat and dairy products
Islam	Ritual animal slaughter
Hinduism	Ritual bathing and donning of clean clothes by Brahmins before eating
Fasts	
Christian	40-day Great Lent fast before Easter and a 40-day Advent fast (Greek Orthodox)
Islam	Month of Ramadan
	13th, 14th and 15th of each month

Reproduced with permission from Fieldhouse P (1995) *Food and Nutrition: Customs and Culture*, 2nd edn, p 124. London: Chapman & Hall.

Dietary Practices in Selected World Religions

Christianity

Early Christians observed Mosaic dietary laws. However, the concept of uncleanliness described in Leviticus was rejected by St Paul and, as Christianity spread across cultural and geographical boundaries, dietary laws largely disappeared (except in the Eastern Orthodox Church). Food, rather than being a way of marking separateness, became a symbol of the communality of religious experience. The celebration of the Eucharist, or Communion, with ritual sharing of bread and wine, though it varies in form from the austere to the elaborate, has retained an underlying significance as a meal shared by the followers of Jesus. The saying of a short prayer before and after eating, establishing a direct connection between God and good food, is also common amongst Christian groups.

Notwithstanding the general de-emphasis of dietary laws, certain strictures persisted. Until 1966, Roman Catholics were required to abstain from eating meat on Fridays (since applied only to Fridays during Lent) in symbolic remembrance of the death of Christ. The historic consequence of meat avoidance on Fridays was the regular consumption of fish; fish on Fridays became identified with Roman Catholicism and sometimes fish was deliberately avoided by some other Christian sects who did not wish to be mistaken for Catholics.

In modern times, some Christian sects have established new dietary rules. Seventh Day Adventists are a Protestant sect who emphasize healthful living through eating the right foods and taking exercise and rest. Most Adventists are lacto-ovo-vegetarians.

Table 2 Worldwide adherents of all religions by six continental areas, mid 1995

	Africa	Asia	Europe	Latin America	Northern America	Oceania	World	%	Number of countries
Christians	348 176 000	306 762 000	551 892 000	448 006 000	249 277 000	23 840 000	1 927 953 000	33.7	260
Roman Catholics	122 108 000	90 041 000	270 677 000	402 691 000	74 243 000	8 265 000	968 025 000	16.9	249
Protestants	109 726 000	42 836 000	80 000 000	31 684 000	123 257 000	8 364 000	395 867 000	6.9	236
Orthodox	29 645 000	14 881 000	165 795 000	481 000	6 480 000	666 000	217 948 000	3.8	105
Anglicans	25 362 000	707 000	30 625 000	1 153 000	6 819 000	5 864 000	70 530 000	1.2	158
Other Christians	61 335 000	158 297 000	4 795 000	11 997 000	38 478 000	681 000	275 583 000	4.8	118
Atheists	427 000	174 174 000	40 085 000	2 977 000	1 670 000	592 000	219 925 000	3.8	139
Baha'is	1 851 000	3 010 000	93 000	719 000	356 000	75 000	6 104 000	0.1	210
Buddhists	36 000	320 691 000	1 478 000	569 000	920 000	200 000	323 894 000	5.7	92
Chinese folk religionists	12 000	224 828 000	116 000	66 000	98 000	17 000	225 137 000	3.9	60
Confucians	1 000	5 220 000	4 000	2 000	26 000	1 000	5 254 000	0.1	12
Ethnic religionists	72 777 000	36 579 000	1 200 000	1 061 000	47 000	113 000	111 777 000	2.0	104
Hindus	1 535 000	775 252 000	1 522 000	748 000	1 185 000	305 000	780 547 000	13.7	94
Jains	58 000	4 804 000	15 000	4 000	4 000	1 000	4 886 000	0.1	11
Jews	163 000	4 294 000	2 529 000	1 098 000	5 942 000	91 000	14 117 000	0.2	134
Mandeans	0	44 000	0	0	0	0	44 000	0.0	2
Muslims	300 317 000	760 181 000	31 975 000	1 329 000	5 450 000	382 000	1 099 634 000	19.2	184
New-Religionists	19 000	118 591 000	808 000	913 000	956 000	10 000	121 297 000	2.1	27
Nonreligious	2 573 000	701 175 000	94 330 000	15 551 000	25 050 000	2 870 000	841 549 000	14.7	226
Parsees	1 000	184 000	1 000	1 000	1 000	1 000	189 000	0.0	3
Sikhs	36 000	18 130 000	490 000	8 000	490 000	7 000	19 161 000	0.3	21
Shintoists	0	2 840 000	1 000	1 000	1 000	1 000	2 844 000	0.0	4
Spiritists	4 000	1 100 000	17 000	8 768 000	300 000	1 000	10 190 000	0.2	30
Other religionists	88 000	98 000	443 000	184 000	1 068 000	42 000	1 923 000	0.0	182
Total population	728 074 000	3 457 957 000	726 999 000	482 005 000	292 841 000	28 549 000	5 716 425 000	100.0	262

Tea, coffee, alcohol and tobacco are also avoided. Eating between meals is discouraged on the grounds that the body needs sufficient time to assimilate what is eaten at mealtimes. The religiously inspired food practices, which emphasize cereals, fruits, vegetables and pulses, has conferred nutritional benefits on the Seventh Day Adventists, who, as a group, have a lower prevelence of chronic diet-related diseases such as heart disease than the general population.

Like the Seventh Day Adventists, members of the Church of the Latter Day Saints (Mormons) assert the importance of eating a well-balanced diet in order to nourish the body as the temple in which the soul resides. Vegetables and herbs are emphasized while meat should be used sparingly. Tobacco, alcohol and caffeine are avoided. A 24 h fast for those in sound health occurs once a month, and money or food saved is contributed to the welfare of the poor. The fast is a religious discipline and is not a dietary requirement.

In contrast to Western Christianity, Eastern Orthodoxy imposes substantial dietary strictures on its adherents. Dietary laws revolve around fasting. There are two 40-day fasts at Lent and Advent, two shorter summer fasts, and regular fasts on every Wednesday and Friday in the year, excepting the two preceding Ascension Day. Fasts do not require total abstinence but rather prohibit the consumption of all animal products and fish except shellfish. The avoidance of olive oil (historically stored in casks lined with calf stomach) during fast periods is a symbol of true sacrifice and devoutness.

The Great Lent fast commemorates Christ's 40-day fast in the desert, and is replete with symbolism. In preparation for the resurrection feast following the fast, hard-boiled eggs are dyed red to symbolize Christ's blood. These eggs are considered to be tokens of good luck and are broken open on Easter morning, representing the opening of Christ's tomb. On Good Friday, lentil soup is eaten to symbolize the tears of the Virgin Mary; often it is flavoured with vinegar as a reminder of Christ's ordeal on the cross. The Great Lent fast is broken after a midnight service on Easter Saturday with a lamb-based soup, olives, bread and fruit.

Islam

It is probable that the prophet Mohammed, the founder of Islam, adopted existing Jewish practices, for example the prohibition of pork, as a way of encouraging Jewish converts to Islam and to distinguish Muslims from their Christian rivals. The Qur'an, a Holy Book given to Mohammed by Allah, contains dietary regulations which echo those of Judaism. Flesh of animals that are cloven hooved and those that chew the cud is lawful. Pigs, blood, carrion and foods offered to other idols are forbidden, though one who eats these foods under constraint does not sin. Carnivorous animals and birds which seize their prey with talons are forbidden, as is the flesh of the domestic ass.

Alcohol is prohibited. Fish must be alive when taken from the sea or river, and only fish which have fins and scales are allowed, thus excluding shellfish and eels. To be acceptable to a Muslim an animal must be bled to death while the words 'Bismi 'llahi. Allah Akbar' (I begin with God's name. God is great) are spoken. Such meat is 'Halal', or lawful, and is stamped with a Halal seal.

Fasting is one of the Five Pillars of Islam and is an important duty of Muslims. It is a way of expressing piety, self-restraint and freedom from worldly desire, and is a means of reaping spiritual rewards. Except for a few holy festival days Muslims may voluntarily fast whenever they wish. Strict adherents fast on Monday and Thursday of every week and on the 13th, 14th and 15th of each month.

Ramadan, falling in the ninth lunar month, is the major fast of the Muslim year, and is one of the most strictly observed of Islamic practices. The word is derived from 'ramz', meaning 'to burn', and may derive either from the fact that the fast was first observed in the hot season, or because it was believed that fasting would burn away sins. The Ramadan fast involves abstinence from food and water between sunrise and sunset for the whole month, and is prescribed for all who have reached the 'Age of Responsibility' (12 years for girls; 15 years for boys). The day's fast should be broken as soon after sunset as possible and this often takes place at a mosque or at house parties, for it is highly commendable to provide food to others, especially the poor. A morning meal should be eaten as late as is possible prior to sunrise. The end of Ramadan is signalled by the sighting of the new moon, and is celebrated with prayers and with feasting.

Certain groups are exempted partially or totally from the Ramadan fast. Anyone who is sick, on a journey, or engaged in hard labour may break the fast, but must make up the days later. Women who are menstruating or are in childbirth are similarly exempted, while pregnant or nursing women and elderly persons in poor health may defer fasting until later in the year or may 'substitute fast' by feeding the poor. Younger children are expected to undertake short fasts in preparation for when they reach the Age of Responsibility.

Judaism

The first five books of the Old Testament, known collectively as the Torah, contain what are probably the most detailed dietary directions of any major religion. These biblical injunctions have been interpreted, elaborated and added to by rabbis over the past 2000 years. The term 'kashruth', meaning 'acceptable', is used to describe anything permitted by Jewish dietary laws. While pig-avoidance has become the hallmark symbol of Judaism, it is but one of many restrictions. Only animals having cloven hooves and that chew the cud are permitted. Thus cows, sheep, oxen and goats may be eaten, whereas pigs, hares and camels may not be. Permitted fish must have fins and scales, which excludes shellfish. Other forbidden foods include teeming winged insects, except locusts, certain birds of prey and bats.

To avoid confusion and to obviate the need to make difficult discriminations between animals, the prohibition was later extended by the rabbis to include all insects and birds of prey. Neither blood nor internal organ fat of otherwise permitted animals may be eaten. The sciatic nerve may not be eaten and, as its removal is difficult, often only the forequarters of an animal is used. The rest of the meat may be sold to non-Jews. Rabbinic additions to the Biblical laws decreed that milk from non-kosher animals is forbidden as it has the same qualities as the animal from which it comes.

Animals dying of natural causes or of disease are not permitted for consumption. Meat must be obtained from animals which have been ritually slaughtered under the supervision of a rabbi. A trained butcher, or shochet, slashes the animals throat with a single cut so as to allow the blood to drain completely from the body. The animal is examined for internal irregularities which might render it unfit for consumption and, if acceptable, is given a seal of approval. Following slaughter, soaking, draining and salting of the meat ensures that all traces of blood are removed. Historically, Jewish migration was dependent on the availability of kosher meat and thus of access to the services of a shochet.

A prohibition against mixing meat and dairy products is based on the biblical injunction 'You shall not boil a kid in its mother's milk.' (Exodus 23: 19). After eating milk, hand washing and mouth rinsing is all that is necessary before eating meat; however, depending on local custom, from 1 to 6 hours must elapse after eating meat and before eating milk. Margarine and milk and cream substitutes have made this particular law easier to follow: nevertheless many observant Jews view the use of such substitutes as being spiritually wrong. In Israel, there has been a continuing historical struggle over the banning of pig-rearing and pork-eating. However, these practices continue today, pork being eaten by Christians and non-observant Jews.

There are many fasts in the Jewish calendar, some of scriptural or rabbinical origin and others which mark private events such as family deaths. Fasting is a way of showing repentance, of teaching self-discipline, or of preparing to seek divine guidance. Generally fasts are observed by boys over the age of 13 years and 1 day, and by girls over the age of 12 years and 1 day.

The Sabbath being a day of rest, all food preparation is carried out on Friday. Challah is a traditional Sabbath bread and, in a modern adaptation of an historical practice, two loaves are used to symbolize the double portion of manna provided by God to the Israelites on Fridays during their 40 years in the wilderness. Other festivals, including Rosh Hashannah, the Day of Judgement, and Yom Kippur, the Day of Atonement, are rich in food symbolism, but it is the major festival of Passover that perhaps sees the most elaborate food practices. All leavened products must be removed from the house, reflecting the fact that Jews did not have time to let bread dough rise when they were driven from their homes into exile. Pieces of bread may be deliberately hidden around the house, to be 'discovered' and removed. Unleavened bread called matzah is prepared or bought commercially.

On the eve of Passover it is customary for the first-born to fast in symbolic remembrance of the historic sparing of the first-born. On the first and second night a special family meal, the seder, is eaten, which is itself a testimony to the symbolic power of food. Seder means order, and the meal indeed has a very definite structure which gives it its ritual character. Partaking in this food event is an important way of transmitting culturally valued knowledge from generation to generation.

Hinduism

While vegetarianism and the specific prohibition on eating cows are two of the dietary hallmarks of modern Hinduism, early Hindu writings reveal that beef was eaten freely. Beef prohibition may have arisen as a response to the challenge of Buddhism, which was critical of Brahminism and its cattle-sacrificing practices, and so Brahmins championed the sacred cow concept in order to maintain their own position. It was perhaps subsequently strengthened by the need for Hindus to distinguish themselves from their new Muslim neighbours. Certainly by the time of the

Rigveda, around 1000 CE, the prohibition was firmly ensconced.

For modern Hindus, the cow is a revered animal, a symbol of motherhood and fertility. The duty to protect cows is enshrined in the Constitution of India; slaughter of cows is prohibited by religious custom and in some provinces by legal bans. In villages and towns cows wander freely, foraging where they may; there are even special government-run homes for old and infirm cows.

Observance of dietary prohibitions is strictest in the upper Brahmin caste while beef (and pork) eating is tolerated amongst lower castes, for whom it may be an important source of supplementary protein. For these castes, giving up meat eating is one way to attempt to improve their social status. The caste system is an excellent example of the way in which social structure influences food practices. Concepts of purity and pollution determine who may eat what with whom and who may accept what food from whom. Eating with, or accepting food from, members of a lower class is polluting. In the hot–cold classification system used in traditional healing raw foods are considered to be 'hot' and are therefore purer than cooked foods, which are 'cold'. Brahmins who accept food cooked by a lower caste person lose ritual purity and thus caste status; however, they may accept ghee (clarified butter) and milk – for these are products of the sacred cow and cannot be polluted by touch.

Devout Hindus are vegetarian; meat, fish and often eggs are avoided, the latter especially by women. An exception is made for the Ksatriya warrior caste, who may consume meat without loss of status, a concession probably related to notions of meat, strength and military prowess. Most castes will eat fish, though its actual consumption varies dramatically from region to region. Where fish is eaten, white fish is preferred for it is least like meat. Abstention from eating food is a much praised virtue. Some Hindus may fast 2 or 3 days a week, during which time they may eat only pure foods such as milk, fruit, nuts, starchy roots and vegetables. Fasts are associated with calendric, caste, family and personal events as well as with religious celebrations.

There are literally thousands of festival days celebrated by Hindus in different parts of India. Some are national, some regional and some purely local. On festival days there may be great processions, when people visit shrines to pray and make offerings. Only food which is pacca (contains ghee) may be offered; it thereby becomes blessed, and is then distributed to the waiting crowd. Ghee, as a product of the cow, is sacred and is an important component of many rituals. For example, during marriage ceremonies a ritual flame is kept burning with ghee.

The modern Indian festivals of Dussatra and Divali illustrate the agricultural origins of many contemporary celebrations. Dussatra marks the end of the rainy season when agricultural labour must begin again, as well as commemorating the legendary hero, Rama. It includes a ritual quest for alms by people carrying small fresh stalks of barley plants. Divali, known as the festival of lights, is a new year festival celebrating the sowing of winter crops. Lamps are lit and gifts are exchanged.

Buddhism

Founded in the sixth century BCE by Siddartha Gautama, Buddhism became the state religion of India in 250 BCE, though it is now a minority religion there. Buddhism has been the most influential of religious forces in spreading the practice of vegetarianism, and has developed in different ways in many parts of the world, especially Southeast Asia, Tibet, China, Japan and Korea.

Buddhism championed the concept of Ahimsa – noninjury to all living creatures – and had a profound influence on the subsequent development of Hinduism through its stand against cruelty toward animals and animal sacrifice. Buddhists refrain from eating meat or from harming any living creatures, though the prohibition is observed strictly only by monks and the devout laity. Lay Buddhists may eat meat, or may raise meat for sale to non-Buddhists. Animals found dead may be eaten, as may fish (which are not 'killed' but merely removed from the water).

In contrast to other religions, Buddhism places emphasis on wrongful killing rather than wrongful eating. Thus flesh may be eaten if it was not procured for eating purposes or supposed to have been so. Monks personify the ideal. Food is obtained through begging, and it is meritorious for the laity to voluntarily provide food to the monks, thereby assisting in their own spiritual progress.

Other religions

Jainism is an ascetic Asian religion whose adherents advocate ahimsa, or noninjury, both as an ethical and philosophical goal, and whose example has had a strong admonitory influence on non-Jains. The Jaina monastic community has a number of characteristic practices which evince an extreme regard for life. Monks carry a small brush with which they carefully sweep the floor before sitting or lying so as to avoid crushing any insects. They may wear masks to prevent inadvertent inhalation of small creatures, and strain their drinking water. Wild honey is avoided, as bees may be killed during its collection.

Ascetics have few or no possessions, and must beg for food. Some choose in old age to die through ritual fasting. Most Jainas are not ascetics, although some strive to imitate monastic ideals by pursuing a progressive path of renunciation, leading to rebirth as an ascetic. The nonmonastic Jaina community practices vegetarianism and opposes the killing of animals. Because of this, agricultural and military occupations are not suitable to Jainas, who historically have chosen instead to enter the professions or to take up business interests.

Sikh means disciple, a follower of the ten gurus. Sikhism was founded in the fifteenth century CE by the guru Nanak who proclaimed: 'There is no Hindu; there is no Muslim'. Nanak rejected the social distinctions of the Hindu caste system, and required his followers to eat together as a symbol of unity. Sikhs retain the Hindu reverence for cows, and thus do not eat beef. Other meat may be eaten, although some Sikhs are vegetarians. Permitted animals must be killed with a single blow, 'jhatka', literally a sudden shake or jerk. Generally, Sikhs are not rigid about adherence to dietary laws, and readily adapt to the food customs of other cultures.

Food plays a part in the *Baha'i* religion through fasts and feasts and through dietary injunctions which favour vegetarianism and abstention from alcohol. Vegetarianism is held to be a compassionate practice and one which is in line with God's will, though meat is not actually prohibited. Fasting is viewed as a spiritual undertaking and is symbolic of abstinence from selfish and carnal desires. It is deemed to have both physical and spiritual benefits. A nineteen-day fasting period occurs in March, during which there must be complete abstention from food and drink between sunrise and sunset. Exemptions are granted for travellers, the sick, pregnant and nursing women, while those engaged in heavy work may also be excused. Children under the age of 15 years and elderly persons over 70 years of age are not required to fast, but may choose to do so. Obeying the fast is a matter for individual conscience and is not enforced; if food is eaten 'unconsciously' during the fast it is deemed to be an accident rather than a breaking of the fast. Unlike in Islam, there is no making up of fast days missed as the fast can only be kept during the designated time.

Nineteen Day Feasts (so called because they are held on the first day of each of the 19-day-long Baha'i months), bring Baha'is together to consult and discuss and to offer suggestions to their Local Spiritual Assembly. At a feast, which is entered into with right thinking, the 'heavenly food' of knowledge, understanding, love and kindness is present, providing members with a sense of spiritual restoration. The significance of providing food at these gatherings appears to be related to the Baha'i injunction to serve one's fellows – rather than to the social solidarity of sharing food. The absence of guidelines or restrictions on what may be served indicates that it is the act of serving which is symbolic, not the food itself.

See also: **Cancer**: Epidemiology and Associations Between Diet and Cancer. **Coronary Heart Disease**: Aetiology. **Food Choice**: Factors Influencing Food Choice. **Socioeconomic Status**: Relationship with Diet and Nutritional Status. **Vegetarian Diets**: Practice.

Further Reading

Douglas M (1970) *Purity and Danger: An Analysis of the Concepts of Pollution and Taboo.* Harmonsworth: Penguin.

Fieldhouse P (1995) *Food and Nutrition: Customs and Culture,* 2nd edn. London: Chapman & Hall.

Grivetti LE (1991) Nutrition past – nutrition today: prescientific origins of nutrition and dietetics. *Nutrition Today,* Jan/Feb 13–24; July/Aug 18–29; Nov/Dec 6–17.

Khare RS and Rao MSA (eds) (1986) *Food, Society and Culture: Aspects in South Asian Food Systems.* Durham: Carolina Academic Press.

Sherman S (1991) The Passover seder: ritual dynamics, foodways, and family folklore. In: Humphrey TC and Humphrey LT (eds) *We Gather Together: Foods and Festival in American Life.* Ann Arbor: UMI Research Press.

Simoons FJ (1994) *Eat Not This Flesh,* 2nd edn. Madison: University of Wisconsin Press.

RENAL FUNCTION AND DISORDERS

Nutritional Management of Renal Disorders

F Pender, Queen Margaret College, Edinburgh, Scotland, UK

According to biochemical criteria, subclinical deficiency states may be widespread amongst populations of patients with advanced renal disease. It is generally accepted that impaired nutritional status is associated with increased morbidity and may contribute to poor rehabilitation and quality of life. The principal aims of therapeutic intervention include achieving acceptable biochemical control and adequate reversal of metabolic disturbances. This is achieved through appropriate medical and dietary intervention resulting in a well, ambulatory patient. A knowledge of the basic pathology, intervention strategies, treatment outcomes and patient compliance assist the understanding of the management of patients with advanced renal disease. This article takes the reader through these complex issues.

Definition and Aetiology

Renal failure occurs when the kidney cells are progressively and irreversibly damaged. This is usually a chronic disease process and the renal disorders which most commonly result in chronic renal failure (CRF) are glomerulonephritis, pyelonephritis, nephrosclerosis and polycystic disease of the kidneys. CRF may also occur as a complication of hypertension, diabetes mellitus and as a consequence of infection or autoimmune disease, nephrotoxic drugs and chronic obstruction of the urinary tract. In most patients the disease runs a slow, insidious course.

Renal failure can be described as the stage of renal function in which the kidney is no longer able to maintain homeostasis. End-stage renal failure (ESRF) is defined as irreversible kidney disease causing abnormalities in patients who require renal replacement therapy (RRT) by dialysis or kidney transplant for survival. The combination of signs, symptoms, biochemical and metabolic changes that occur in renal failure is referred to as uraemia or the uraemic syndrome.

The factors directly responsible for the uraemic syndrome remain obscure, but it is generally accepted that the causative agents are dietary protein and the end products of endogenous nitrogen metabolism (low molecular weight toxins), parathyroid hormone and so-called 'middle molecules' (high molecular weight toxins), the chemical nature of which has yet to be fully explained. A number of mechanisms may be implicated and include the accumulation of nitrogenous metabolites, alteration in metabolic pathways producing abnormal constituents in the blood, biochemical disturbance of acid–base equilibrium, inhibition of enzyme activity due to the presence of urea or other metabolites, and tissue hyperosmolarity.

The insidious development of chronic uraemia tends to produce an ill but ambulatory patient in whom long-term metabolic disturbances predominate over acute biochemical changes; disordered carbohydrate, fat, protein and calcium metabolism are common findings. Clinical assessment of renal function is usually made using sequential measurement of glomerular filtration rate (GFR). In practice, GFR is assessed by the clearance of endogenous creatinine.

Prevalence

Chronic renal disease occurs at any age but is much more common in middle-age. In a recent study (UK), there were 96 new patients per million population over the age of 65 years and 38 new patients per million population under the age of 55 years. Specific conditions affect different age groups: nephrotic syndrome is the commonest nephrological problem in children (2–3 years of age) at about 18 new cases per million of the population.

Clinical Pathophysiology

A constellation of signs and symptoms are present in the patient with CRF due largely to the disordered physiology and complex biochemical abnormalities. A number of distinctive and well-documented clinical phenomena arise including: metabolic acidosis, hyperkalaemia, disorders of electrolyte and fluid balance, disturbances in amino acid and protein metabolism, disturbances in carbohydrate, calcium and phosphate metabolism, hyperlipidaemia and atherosclerosis and anaemia. The essential pathology and clinical significance of these are considered.

Metabolic acidosis occurs due to the inability of

the remnant tubular mass to restore body buffers by regenerating bicarbonate and consequent failure to eliminate an excess of hydrogen ions formed in the metabolism of the sulfur-containing amino acids and of certain phosphate esters. Metabolic acidosis leads to an increased rate of muscle protein breakdown and enhanced urea generation. Acidosis may contribute to the metabolic bone disease of uraemia by dissolving buffer salts from the skeleton.

Hyperkalaemia arises partly because of the metabolic acidosis and in part through enhanced cell catabolism. As GFR decreases and urinary output falls, potassium is retained. Plasma potassium concentration may rise sharply and cause cardiac dysrhythmias and cardiac arrest owing to ventricular fibrillation.

As glomerular filtration of water and electrolytes falls, homeostasis is sharply compromised. Sodium may initially be depleted through polyuria and excessive intake of fluid, causing twitching, tetany and convulsions. However at ESRF sodium retention occurs causing peripheral oedema and congestive cardiac failure which aggravate hypertension.

Primary or secondary hypertension contributes to loss of function in kidneys with established disease. Hypertension damages the kidney by increasing arteriolar wall thickness, which leads to ischaemia and subsequent glomerulosclerosis. Control of hypertension is considered a management priority as it reduces the rate of progression of renal disease and preserves GFR. The treatment of choice is usually angiotensin-converting enzyme (ACE) inhibitors. This group of drugs may be superior to other antihypertensive drugs because, as well as controlling systemic hypertension, reducing proteinuria and slowing the progression of renal failure, they appear to reduce intraglomerular pressure.

Patients with advanced renal disease commonly demonstrate negative nitrogen balance. Impaired protein synthesis together with accelerated protein catabolism contribute to a poor protein status which results in a reduction in lean body mass. Uraemic toxicity results in anorexia and poor exogenous protein intake, which exacerbates the poor plane of protein nutrition. Proteinuria occurs in most patients and some evidence suggests that the proteinuria may accelerate glomerular injury.

Carbohydrate intolerance is clinically demonstrated in most patients who present with increased fasting blood glucose levels and normal or increased fasting insulin concentrations. The aetiology of this phenomenon is largely unknown but evidence suggests tissue insensitivity to the action of insulin. The unusual metabolism of carbohydrate may in part be responsible for increased incidence of atherosclerotic complications in individuals with renal failure.

Hyperphosphataemia and hypocalcaemia are significant findings in patients with advanced renal failure. These are found in concert with raised concentrations of parathyroid hormone (PTH). As GFR falls, phosphorous retention occurs. This in turn mediates the development of secondary hyperparathyroidism through calcium depletion. PTH inhibits the reabsorption of phosphorus and stimulates release of bone calcium. Hyperparathyroidism also inhibits the hydroxylation of 25-hydroxyvitamin D. Thus, failure to synthesize 1,25-dihydroxyvitamin D results in inefficient intestinal absorption of calcium and thus status of this nutrient is also hampered. These factors contribute to development of a group of bone diseases prevalent in patients with advanced renal disease.

Glomerulosclerosis has many pathological similarities to atherosclerosis and thus increasing attention is paid to reversal of these pseudoathersclerotic lesions. Dietary cholesterol encourages the development of glomerulosclerosis. The hyperlipidaemia associated with some renal diseases strongly favours the development of cardiovascular disease – a low concentration of high-density lipoproteins, an increase in plasma cholesterol (total) concentration and an increase in low-density lipoprotein concentration. Hypertriacylglycerolaemia is also a common finding. Abnormalities in apolipoprotein composition of plasma lipoproteins have also been identified in patients with advanced renal disease. Factors known to be implicated in this increased atherosclerotic risk are decreased removal of trigacylglycerols because of reduced activity of tissue and plasma lipoprotein lipase.

Anaemia is almost universally found in all patients with advanced renal disease. Uraemic toxins are thought to inhibit erythropoiesis and cause premature ageing of the red blood cells, but the most significantly reported factor resulting in anaemia is probably a decreased production of erythropoietin. Blood loss via the gastrointestinal tract contributes to the presence of anaemia. Aluminium overload, resulting from long-term use of aluminium-containing phosphate binders (prescribed to inhibit uptake of intestinal phosphorus), and folate deficiency also contribute to the situation.

In summary, the patient with advanced renal failure has severely disordered pathology. Fortunately, many of the systems affected respond to medical and pharmacological and dietary intervention. The essential medical intervention strategy for patients with renal disease includes control of hypertension, prevention of extrarenal complications, treatment of the underlying disorders, and control of fluid and electrolyte balance.

Clinical Features

These arise as a result of the disordered pathophysiology related to development of uraemia. Essentially, a number of systems are affected.

Gastrointestinal system

Anorexia, nausea, vomiting and diarrhoea are frequently reported. The presence of urea in the mouth favours poor condition of gums, infection and bleeding; stools are blood-spattered (melaena) and patients may cough, spit or sneeze blood. Gastrointestinal bleeding is commonplace; bleeding from old gastric ulcers is typical.

Cardiovascular system

Oedema, salt and water overload may be features of late renal failure. Hypertension leads to many of the complications in renal failure such as angina and pulmonary oedema. There is an increased incidence of cerebrovascular accident.

Neuromuscular system

Hypertension and salt and water overload can cause convulsions and fitting behaviour. There may be paraesthesia or burning in the extremities. Hyponatraemia may cause muscular cramp and tetany. Some patients become anxious and confused. Hallucinations and coma are not infrequent complications.

Anaemia

As previously mentioned, anaemia is always a feature of progressive renal disease. Patients are typically pale and have a lemon-grey pallor. Anaemia results from defective production of red blood cells as urea is toxic to bone marrow. Haemolysis is prevalent and clotting factors are antagonized and the resulting bleeding tendency aggravates anaemia.

Bones, joints and connective tissue

Bone disease is common, particularly if the uraemia is long-standing. The calcium-to-phosphate ratio is disturbed and resistance to vitamin D occurs. Failure to produce 1,25-dihydroxyvitamin D seriously hampers calcium status and 'renal rickets' may be a feature resulting in osteoporosis and osteomalacia. Patients may complain of generalized bone pain, though for the most part it remains asymptomatic.

Endocrine system

Amenhorrea is common and even mild uraemia leads to lowered fertility and increased rate of spontaneous abortion in women. In children, there is growth inhibition due to impairment of growth hormone secretion. Impaired glucose tolerance results from insulin resistance.

Nutritional Management

The nutritional management of renal disease has long been recognized as an effective part of the care of the patient with kidney disease. Nutritional therapy minimizes the work of excretion and thus spares the function of the diseased organs.

Nutritional goals

The principal aim in the management of renal disease is the reduction of blood urea nitrogen. In addition a number of nutritional goals are essential: maintenance of optimal nutritional status, preservation of lean body mass, maintenance of near-normal concentrations of significant clinical chemistry, reduction of risk of nutrition-related diseases such as cardiovascular disorders, and retarding the progression of the renal failure.

Initially, treatment is by conservative measures (diet and drugs) but as the patient approaches ESRF more aggressive measures are necessary (RRT).

Specific therapeutic strategy

It is important to recognize that requirements for nutrients differ from patient to patient and vary according to the nature of the disease, stage of the disease and degree of residual renal function. Thus dietary regimens must be flexible to take account of individual patient requirements. Dietary prescriptions or guidelines for adults (UK) are indicated in **Table 1** and are based on requirements per kg ideal body weight per day.

Energy

Requirements for energy are increased for the patient with advanced renal disease, principally owing to the catabolic nature of the disease. Additional energy is usually given in the form of carbohydrate and fat. Inadequate supply of this non-nitrogen energy may cause the patient to lose lean body mass and further aggravate the uraemia. Simple carbohydrates are usually the prime source of energy, though care is required in patients with distorted glucose tolerance. Fat intake should primarily come from mono- and polyunsaturated sources (e.g. sunflower, corn or olive oils; oily fish such as herring, mackerel and

Table 1   Renal disorders: dietary guidelines. Nutrient prescriptions are based on requirements per kg ideal body weight per day

	Protein (g)	Energy (kcal)	Phosphorus (mg)	Potassium (mmol)	Sodium (mmol per day)	Notes
Pre-dialysis	0.6	35–40	5–10	*	NAS	Saturated fat not encouraged. Protein intake should favour intake of high biological value sources (70%) – see text.
Nephrotic syndrome	0.8–1.0	30–35	*	*	NAS	Saturated fat not encouraged. Intake of complex carbohydrates encouraged (18–20 g per day).
Haemodialysis	1.0–1.25	30–35	<12	1	NAS	<35% of dietary energy to come from fat with emphasis on PUFA/MUFA. 50% of dietary protein to come from high biological value sources.
CAPD	1.2–1.5	25–35	<12	*	NAS	High intake of complex carbohydrates recommended (18–20 g per day). 30–40% of dietary energy to come from fat with emphasis on PUFA/MUFA. 50% of dietary protein to come from high biological value sources. Calcium intake recommended is between 800 and 1000 mg per day.
Transplant:						
<1st month	1.3–1.5	30–35	*	*	NAS	50% of dietary energy to come from carbohydrate. 30% of dietary energy to come from fat with emphasis on PUFA/MUFA.
>1st month	1.0	for optimal weight maintenance				

*, intake relates to individual patient clinical chemistry.
NAS, No Added Salt Diet (Table 2).
PUFA, polyunsaturated fatty acids.
MUFA, monounsaturated fatty acids.
CAPD, continuous ambulatory peritoneal dialysis.

trout; avocado pears). A good supply of energy also favours good use of exogenous protein and thus spares protein. Energy-dense diets are strongly indicated when serum creatinine begins to rise. This indicates catabolism which is, at least in part, corrected by good intake of energy.

Protein

Increased concentrations of plasma urea or serum creatinine are hallmarks of impaired renal function and excessive intake of protein, therefore, has the potential to exacerbate this position. Thus, the prudent intervention plan is to restrict protein intake to minimize production of end products of nitrogen metabolism, yet supply an appropriate amount to ensure a good plane of nitrogen nutrition to favour positive nitrogen balance. The conceptual basis for lowering the protein intake is that small amounts of high biological value proteins with sufficient energy allow excess blood urea to be utilized for the synthesis of nonessential amino acids. Thus, blood urea nitrogen will be reduced, encouraging utilization of essential amino acids from the permitted high biological value foods.

The optimal level of protein intake is a source of debate. The general agreement is that intake of dietary protein should be individualized in an attempt to maintain nitrogen balance and prevent wasting due to catabolism. Both quality and quantity of dietary protein are important. It is suggested by most authors that 50–75% of the total protein intake should come from high biological sources (small quantities of dairy products, eggs, fish and meat). In practice, protein consumption is self-restricted as the patient may be anorexic. Recent work suggests that circulating peptides may cause a feeling of early satiety but the principal effects of anorexia are mediated as a direct consequence of uraemia and as an indirect effect of anaemia. The intake of protein is frequently monitored; a stable creatinine concentration accompanied by a sustained elevation in plasma urea concentration indicates excessive protein intake and steps should be taken to reduce it. Lower protein intakes also induce hypofiltration and may therefore spare kidney function.

Sodium and fluid

The optimal intake of sodium depends on the nature and stage of the condition but is essentially dictated by serial serum measurement. The sodium intake of all patients must be restricted to prevent sodium retention with consequent oedema. Also, a modest sodium restriction prevents undue thirst and its consequent effect on fluid intake. It seems prudent that all patients receive at least mild sodium restriction (**Table 2**). Sodium restriction may also contribute to the control of hypertension. Fluids are usually restricted and the prescription relates to urine output.

Potassium

It is necessary to individualize dietary potassium intake. Commonly, as urinary output falls, there is a danger of hyperkalaemia and foods high in potassium must be restricted (**Table 3**). Hyperkalaemia is most often a consequence of metabolic acidosis and thus treatment for the latter should alleviate the need for intensive potassium restriction. Most dietary potassium come from fruit and vegetables and therefore curtailing intake of these foods is useful. As a general rule of thumb, the more water the item contains, the less potassium is present. Thus, bananas and dried fruit are high sources and apples are low sources. Aggressive restriction of dietary potassium commences with a serum potassium concentration of greater than 5 mmol l^{-1}. Control of hyperkalaemia reduces the risk of development of cardiac arrhythmia, which is potentially fatal.

Phosphorus and calcium

Under normal circumstances, an equilibrium exists between these two minerals and vitamin D. The bowel is notoriously poor at absorbing calcium with advancing age and in advanced renal disease. Dietary

Table 2 Basic sodium-restricted diet

The daily intake of sodium is usually restricted to 2–3 g (80–100 mmol) per day.
Three *basic modifications* to the diet are necessary:

1. NO salt should be added to meals at the table.
2. Foods high in sodium (salt) should be avoided.
3. Salt should be used sparingly in cooking.

Foods to be avoided

Salt	
Meats	Bacon, ham, salted beef, canned meats, tongue, corned beef, meat pastes, meats wrapped in pastry
Fish	Smoked, salted or canned fish, e.g. kippers, bloaters, sardines, fish pastes, shellfish
Fats	Salted butter, margarine, single cream
Cheese	All kinds, including cheese spreads
Soup	All canned and packet soup, including bouillon
Vegetables	All canned vegetables, spinach, beetroot, celery
Fruit	Dried fruit, e.g. figs, raisins, sultanas, prunes, olives
Beverages	Savoury drinks (meat/vegetable extracts), malted drinks, cocoa, drinking chocolate, soda water, tomato juice, sports drinks
Confectionery	Toffee, chocolate, fudge, liquorice, fruit gums, fruit pastilles
Miscellaneous	Canned and packet foods, gravy powders, pickles, bottled sauces, chutney, syrup, lemon curd, mincemeat, tomato puree, peanut butter, nuts, crisps and packet snacks

Foods in moderation

Milk and dairy products
Eggs
Unsalted butter

intake of calcium may be poor as the prescribed diet is low in dairy products (to effect reduction of dietary phosphorus intake). In addition, the kidney fails to convert (hydroxylate) the parent vitamin D (25-hydroxyvitamin D) to the active metabolite (further hydroxylation to 1,25-dihydroxyvitamin D) and a vitamin D deficiency state arises. The combination of defective intestinal absorption and low intake of dietary calcium usually causes negative calcium balance. Low GFR allows phosphorus to be retained therefore a disequilibrium occurs between the major minerals. Management of calcium and phosphorus imbalance involves four treatment approaches. Patients are given activated forms of vitamin D (calcitriol). Phosphate binders are used to chelate dietary phosphate and prevent absorption or uptake by the gastrointestinal tract. Phosphate binders have traditionally been high in aluminium and exert a

Table 3 Basic potassium-restricted diet

Fruit and vegetables contain large amounts of potassium. About four small servings of most fruit and vegetables per day is usual. Certain cooking methods, especially boiling, reduce availability of potassium and should be used where possible. Intake of raw and salad vegetables and fruit require to be restricted. Canned items are fine (sodium permitting) but potassium leaches into the juice. Discard juice.

Foods in moderation

Milk   <300 ml per day
Yogurt   <2 pots per week

Foods to be avoided

Blackcurrant drinks	Muesli
Bran, bran cereals	Nuts, peanut butter
Brown sugar	Pure fruit juices
Chocolate	Salt substitues
Chutney	Savoury drinks
Curry powder	(meat/vegetable extracts)
Dried fruit	Soya flour
Evaporated milk	Tomato juice
Instant coffee	Tomato sauce/brown sauce
Low-sodium products	Treacle
	Wheatgerm products

toxic effect but less toxic preparations are now in use clinically (calcium carbonate, magnesium carbonate). While they do not have the same potency they are now considered more ethical if less therapeutic in activity. Dietary phosphorus restriction (reducing intake of dairy products and meat) is also implemented (**Table 4**), usually when plasma phosphate concentration exceeds 2 mmol l^{-1}. Calcium supplements are given or a calcium-enhanced intake is encouraged (> 1000 mg per day).

Table 4 Basic phosphorus-restricted diet

Foods to be avoided

Baked beans	Malted bread, drinks
Broad beans	Mushrooms
Brussel sprouts	Nuts
Cauliflower	Oats
Cheese	Oranges
Chocolate, chocolate drinks	Pulses
Chocolate sweets	Raspberries
Cocoa	Sardines
Cod/herring roe	Savoury drinks
Crispbreads	(meat/vegetable extracts)
Dried fruit	Shellfish
Eggs	Whitebait
High fibre breakfast cereals	Wholemeal bread
Kidney	Wholemeal flour
Liver	Yogurt

Saturated fat and cholesterol

Since high intakes of saturated fat and cholesterol are known to cause atherosclerotic lesions in normal individuals and high serum lipid profiles are thought to assist in the progression of renal disease, it seems appropriate to take a sensible approach to intake of fats. A diet similar to that advocated for the general public is a useful therapeutic recommendation: emphasis should be placed on fats of vegetable origin (polyunsaturated and monounsaturated) and intake of total fat limited to between 30 and 35% of the total energy intake.

Vitamins and minerals

Status of water-soluble vitamins is reported to be low in renal disease. This is, in part, due to increased requirements. In addition, water-soluble vitamins are lost during the dialytic process (haemodialysis) and overly restricted diets may compromise intake of essential vitamins and minerals. Thus, individuals with advanced renal failure are routinely prescribed vitamin and mineral supplements. There is general agreement that supplements of water-soluble vitamins (B and C) are useful and an increase in requirements noted particularly for thiamin, riboflavin, pyridoxine and ascorbic acid.

Anaemia is more marked in the patient underdialysing (noncompliant with the dialysis instruction and receiving much less dialysis than prescribed) or in the anephritic patient. Nutritional therapy may include oral iron and folate therapy though the use of recombinant human erythropoietin has revolutionized the treatment of anaemia. This drug is very successful in the correction of anaemia but, because it is very expensive, it is usually reserved for the patient with severe anaemia (Hb < 6–8 g dl^{-1}).

Monitoring

The dynamic nature and progression of renal disease requires the patient to be monitored frequently and both the clinical condition and plane of nutrition examined routinely by anthropometric and biochemical measurement. Compliance with dietary and medical instruction requires regular encouragement and a self-motivated patient is the key to successful rehabilitation.

In summary, the basis of nutritional management of the patient with advanced renal disease is an individually tailored protein and energy intake according to requirements. All other restrictions or dietary modifications tend to be modest in the first instance and tighter clinical control may be appropriate subsequently, each nutrient being modified as necessary.

Progression of Renal Disease

By the late 1920s, experimental work suggested that diets rich in protein caused kidney damage in normal rats. Increasing the protein intake in rats with renal disease caused greater interstitial histological damage with worsening hypertension and higher mortality. This 'theory of hyperfiltration', that is, that a high-protein diet may be nephrotoxic, strongly suggests that earlier dietary intervention in humans may be beneficial. It is well established that a protein restriction is effective in ameliorating uraemic symptoms, but there is accumulating evidence that a dietary protein and phosphorus restriction, implemented early in the course of the disease, can slow the rate of loss of renal function and therefore extend the period of freedom from dialysis or other renal replacement therapy (RRT). Thus a protein- and phosphorus-restricted diet has been accepted by most authors to begin with a tentative GFR of 70 ml min^{-1} or less. Increasingly, attention to the diet of the patient is instituted on diagnosis. This may result in a compliance issue as this group of patients is relatively asymptomatic and patients may not see the immediate clinical benefit of dietary restriction in the absence of overt symptomatology.

Renal replacement therapy

Where renal function deteriorates to a point where conservative measures (diet and drugs) are no longer able to manage the patient within clinically defined parameters and metabolic chaos begins to return (severe hypertension, acute rise in serum potassium, patient in coma or where clinical chemistry is grossly disturbed), then more aggressive medical intervention is required. RRT is indicated; either dialysis or renal transplant. Similar principles of nutritional management are applied, but the nutritional prescription will vary with the treatment modality (Table 1).

Prognosis

Restoration of good nutritional status will not only prolong life but will also improve the quality of life by controlling the effects of the biochemical abnormalities and thus alleviate the effects of some of the symptoms. Improvements in both drug regimens and dialysis technology have afforded the patient with advanced renal disease greater clinical control without increasing the level of restriction. Advances in monitoring strategy have allowed the patient greater self-monitoring with increased dietary freedom and thus allows increasing responsibility for part of the management. Thus, the prognosis in recent years has improved, resulting in a well-nourished, clinically stable patient who enjoys increased feeling of wellbeing.

See also: **Aluminium**: Occurence and Toxicity. **Anaemia (Anemia)**: Iron-Deficiency Anaemia. **Bone**: Composition, Metabolism and Bone Growth. **Calcium**: Physiology. **Cholecalciferol and Ergocalciferol**: Physiology, Dietary Sources and Requirements; Rickets and Osteomalacia. **Hypertension**: Physiology. **Phosphorus**: Physiology, Dietary Sources and Requirements. **Protein**: Synthesis and Turnover. **Sodium**: Physiology. **Thirst**: Physiology. **Vitamin Supplementation**: Role.

Further Reading

Alvestrand A and Bergstrom J (1988) Renal diseases. In: Kinney JM, Jeejeebhoy KN, Hill GL and Owen OE (eds), *Nutrition and Metabolism in Patient Care*, pp 531–557. Philadelphia: WB Saunders.

Brenner BM and Rector FC (1986) *The Kidney*, 3rd edn. vol 2. Philadelphia: WB Saunders.

Cramp DG, Moorhead JF and Wills MR (1975) Disorders of blood lipids in renal disease. *Lancet* i:672–673.

Hatano M (1991) *Nephrology*. Proceedings of the XIth International Congress of Nephrology, vols I and II. Tokyo: Springer-Verlag.

Jacobson HR (1991) Chronic renal failure: pathophysiology. *Lancet* 338:419–423.

Klahr S (1991) Chronic renal failure: management. *Lancet* 338:423–427.

Kopple JD (1984) Causes or catabolism and wasting in acute of chronic renal failure. In: Robinson RR (ed.) *Nephrology*. Proceedings of the IXth International Congress of Nephrology, vol. II. Basel: Springer-Verlag.

Lutz CA and Przytulski KR (1994) *Nutrition and Diet Therapy*. Philadelphia: FA Davis Company.

Mitch WE and Klahr S (1993) *Nutrition and the Kidney*. Boston: Little, Brown and Co.

Respiratory diseases *see* **Cancer**: Epidemiology of Lung Cancer. **Therapeutic Dietetics**: Lung Diseases.

RETINOL

Contents
Physiology
Hypovitaminosis A

Physiology

H C Furr, University of Connecticut, Storrs,
Connecticut, USA

Absorption, Bioavailability, Transport and Distribution

'Vitamin A' is the collective term for compounds that show the biological properties of retinol, including maintenance of epithelial tissue and visual function. This classification includes retinol, retinyl esters and retinal (vitamin A aldehyde); retinoic acid is included even through it does not sustain visual function. These are isoprenoid compounds, having in common an 11-carbon polyene chain attached to a trimethyl-substituted cyclohexenyl ring (**Fig. 1**). The term 'retinoids' refers to all compounds, natural or synthetic, that show some biological activity typical of vitamin A, such as promoting differentiation of cells in culture; not all retinoids can support all the functions of vitamin A, e.g. some are unable to contribute to vision. Vitamin A compounds are not found as such in plant tissues, but rather are characteristic of the animal kingdom; the notable exception is 13-*cis*-retinal, which serves as a chromophore in the purple membrane of certain halobacteria.

Dietary vitamin A comes from two sources: preformed vitamin A, and provitamin A carotenoids. Preformed vitamin A (mostly as esters of retinol with long-chain fatty acids) comes from animal products or from dietary supplements; retinyl esters, e.g. retinyl acetate and retinyl palmitate, are more stable chemically than is free retinol. Provitamin A carotenoids arise mostly from plant products: β-carotene is the most active and is widely distributed in plants, but other carotenoids (such as α-carotene and β-cryptoxanthin and β-apocarotenals) can be important sources of vitamin A from particular foods. The relative importance of these sources of vitamin A is very dependent on diet. Other carotenoids, such as lycopene and xanthophylls, are major carotenoids in some foods and may have other important physiological functions, but they have no provitamin A activity.

Typical estimates of dietary vitamin A absorption efficiency are 70–85%. Estimates of carotenoid absorption are usually much lower, but are confounded by slow intestinal absorption and rapid metabolism; there is considerable species variability in absorption efficiency and in metabolism of carotenoids. Animal feeding studies show that the biological matrix of food carotenoids has profound effects on their bioavailability.

Since both vitamin A and carotenoids are lipids, intestinal micelle formation with bile acids is essential for their absorption. Human subjects with impaired bile acid formation or flow (e.g. with biliary atresia) may require intramuscular supplementation with vitamin A and the other fat-soluble vitamins. Within the intestinal lumen, vitamin A esters (retinyl esters) are hydrolysed to free retinol and are absorbed as such; this free retinol is promptly re-esterified within the intestinal cells (**Fig. 2**). Provitamin A carotenoids, such as β-carotene, are often cleaved within intestinal cells; whether this metabolism is by central cleavage (mediated by the enzyme carotene 15,15′ dioxygenase) or by asymmetric cleavage followed by chain shortening is uncertain. Retinal (vitamin A aldehyde), the final product of carotenoid cleavage, is enzymatically reduced to retinol and is then esterified. The physiological ligand for this esterification process seems to be retinol bound to an intracellular retinol-binding protein (CRBP II, M_r approximately 14 600 Da, one of several small cellular retinoid-binding proteins); the primary retinyl ester-synthesizing activity transfers fatty acid from phosphatidyl choline (lecithin-retinol acyltransferase; LRAT), although an acyl-coenzyme-A-dependent esterifying activity (acyl-CoA-retinol acyltransferase; ARAT) is also present.

Regardless of their dietary source, the retinyl esters are incorporated in the core of chylomicra and transported in the lymph. After removal of triacylglycerols by lipoprotein lipase as the lipoprotein particle circulates through peripheral tissues, the chylomicron remnants are rapidly taken up by the liver, and the vitamin A esters are hydrolysed by retinyl ester hydrolase there. The resulting retinol is then either re-esterified (primarily by LRAT, although ARAT

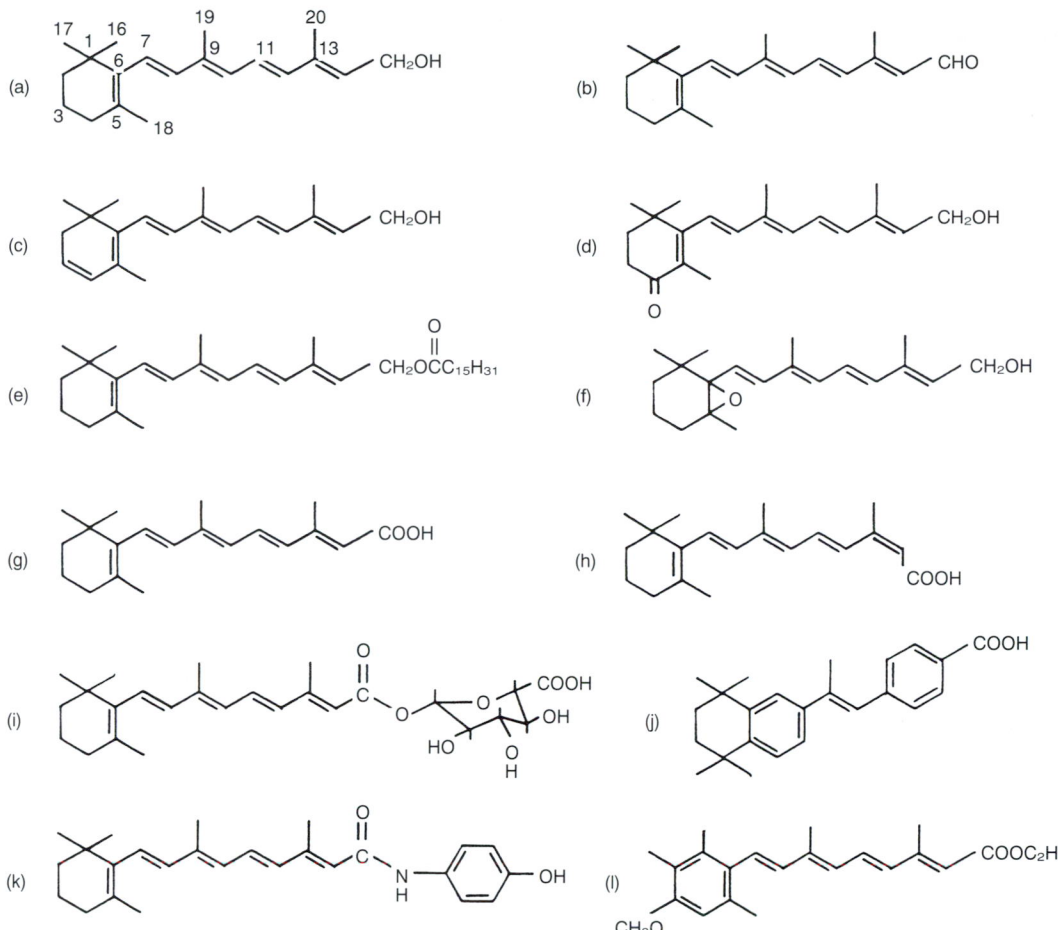

Figure 1 Some naturally occurring retinoids: (a) all-*trans*-retinol (vitamin A alcohol), showing the conventional numbering system for the carbon atoms; (b) all-*trans*-retinal (vitamin A aldehyde); (c) all-*trans*-3,4-didehydroretinol (vitamin A$_2$ alcohol); (d) all-*trans*-4-oxoretinol (also called 4-keto-retinol), a metabolite of vitamin A; (e) all *trans*-retinyl palmitate (vitamin A palmitate), a major storage form of vitamin A; (f) all-*trans*-5,6-epoxy retinol, a metabolite of vitamin A; (g) all-*trans*-retinoic acid (vitamin A acid, tretinoin); (h) 13-*cis*-retinoic acid (also called isotretinoin, Accutane, Ro 4-3780); (i) all-*trans*-retinoyl β-glucuronide, a naturally occurring metabolite. Some synthetic retinoids tested for dermatological or anticancer uses: (j) tetrahydrotetramethylnaphthalenylpropenylbenzoic acid, abbreviated TTNPB and trivially termed an 'arotinoid'; (k) 4-hydroxyphenylretinamide (4-HPR, *N*-retinoyl-4-aminophenol); (l) 'Acetretin', a trimethylmethoxyphenyl analogue of ethyl retinoate (also called Etretinate, Tigason, Ro 10-9359).

activity may be important at high retinol concentrations) and stored in the liver, or released into the plasma as a complex with plasma retinol-binding protein.

Because most forms of vitamin A are hydrophobic, the transport, metabolism and function of vitamin A are dependent on a series of binding proteins, each specific for its ligand and tissue. The M_r of plasma retinol-binding protein (RBP) is typically approximately 21 000 Da in mammalian species; the complete amino acid composition has been determined for several species, and the gene from some species has been cloned. Retinol-binding protein binds retinol with 1 : 1 stoichiometry. The hydrophobic retinol molecule fits into a 'barrel' within the protein, shielded from interactions with the aqueous environment. In turn, holo-RBP binds transthyretin (TTR;

formerly called prealbumin) in plasma; it seems that a TTR tetramer can bind up to four molecules of RBP. Usual concentrations of human plasma RBP are 1.9–2.4 μmol l^{-1} (40–50 μg ml^{-1}); typically, total circulating RBP is 80–90% saturated with retinol ligand. Although retinol, retinal and retinoic acid bind to RBP with similar affinity, retinol is present in highest concentrations and is the predominant ligand. Retinyl esters have much less affinity for RBP and are transported by serum lipoproteins instead.

The release of holo-RBP from liver is carefully controlled to maintain levels of circulating retinol within narrow limits, but the mechanism of this control is not yet clear. In the absence of adequate vitamin A, apo RBP accumulates in the liver, ready to be released as soon as vitamin A is available (this is the basis of the relative dose–response assay for

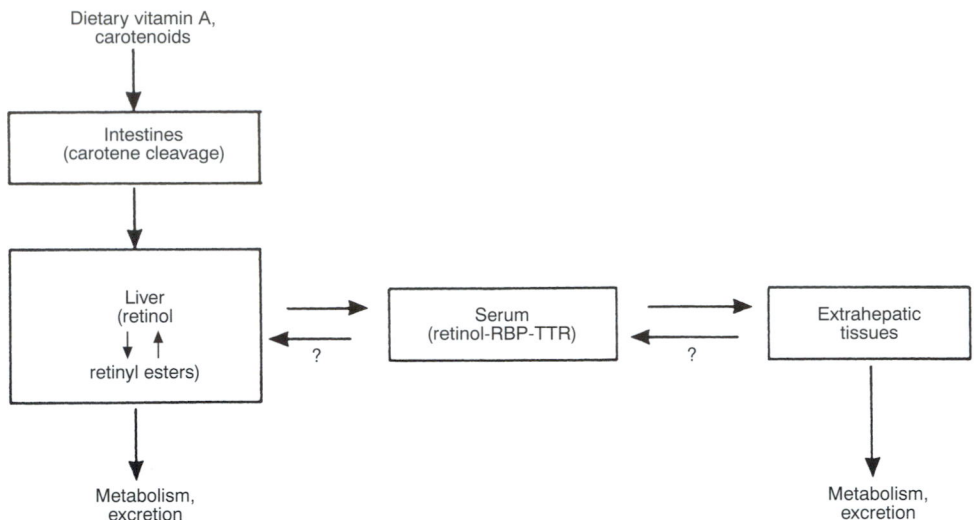

Figure 2 Outline of vitamin A metabolism. RBP, retinol-binding protein; TTR, transthyretin, formerly called prealbumin.

vitamin A deficiency, as discussed below). Clearly, this mechanism has developed because of the dichotomy of vitamin A action: vitamin A is essential, in small amounts, for proper differentiation and maintenance of epithelial cells, but excesses of vitamin A are toxic and must be controlled by the organism.

Metabolism, Storage and Excretion

Vitamin A in excess of immediate requirements is stored in the liver as esters of long-chain fatty acids (Fig. 2); the ratio of liver retinol to retinyl esters decreases as total liver vitamin A increases, but 95% of total liver vitamin A is typically present as the esters. Retinyl palmitate is the primary ester in liver of the human, rat, cow, sheep, rabbit, cat, frog, trout and polar bear, although significant amounts of other esters are found (especially oleate and stearate), and liver retinyl ester composition can be affected by dietary fatty acid composition. (Remarkably, the predominant vitamin A ester in rat adrenal cortex is retinyl stearate.) Liver frequently contains as much as 90% of total body vitamin A, although other organs, such as kidney, testes and adrenal glands, also contain detectable retinyl esters. The efficiency of liver storage of vitamin A is particularly noteworthy in the polar bear, where concentrations as great as 36 µmol g^{-1} of liver tissue (10 380 µg g^{-1}) have been reported. Typical values for human liver vitamin A (autopsy specimens) are 0.44–0.74 µmol g^{-1} (126–211 µg g^{-1}) in the USA.

The two cell types involved in liver vitamin A metabolism are the hepatocytes (parenchymal cells) and the lipocytes (also called stellate cells, Ito cells, or fat-storing cells). The hepatocytes are the major site of RBP synthesis and retinol-RBP release; some

retinyl esters are also found here. The lipocytes store retinyl esters in cytoplasmic lipid droplets which also contain triacylglycerols and some cholesteryl esters within a phospholipid coat. It has been suggested that RBP transfers vitamin A, as retinol, between lipocytes and hepatocytes.

Kinetic studies carried out in rats have shown that there is extensive cycling of liver vitamin A stores, and extensive recycling of vitamin A between liver and other tissues. It is certain that retinol-RBP is the major form of transport from liver to peripheral tissues; it is not yet clear whether the transport of vitamin A from other tissues back to the liver is via retinyl esters transported by lipoproteins (normally present at about 5–10% of the serum concentration of retinol-RBP) or via retinol on RBP synthesized in the outlying tissues (messenger ribonucleic acid, or mRNA, for plasma RBP has been detected in a number of other tissues in addition to liver). In vitamin A-deficient rats the recycling is even more extensive, and catabolism of vitamin A is markedly diminished.

Catabolism of vitamin A in the rat is by oxidation of the cyclohexenyl ring (particularly at the 4-position), epoxide formation at the 5,6-positions, hydroxylation of the ring methyl groups, and chain shortening (some examples of metabolites are shown in Fig. 1). The resulting metabolites are generally inactive, although some may have a little biological activity. These more polar retinoids are excreted in the urine and in the bile.

Retinol can be reversibly oxidized to retinal (vitamin A aldehyde); retinal can be oxidized to retinoic acid but retinoic acid cannot be converted back to the other forms. Thus retinol, retinyl esters, and retinal have equal biological activity because they are freely interconverted; retinoic acid fills some (but not all) of the functions of retinol, but it and its derivatives are not stored. Typical human serum concentrations of retinoic acid are 5–10 nmol l^{-1} (1.5–3 ng ml^{-1}), compared with typical retinol concentrations of 1–2 μmol l^{-1}. Retinoyl β-glucuronide and retinyl β-glucuronide (formed in the liver from retinoic acid and retinol, respectively) are secreted into the bile but can be hydrolysed and reabsorbed in the intestine (enterohepatic circulation); both these compounds have vitamin A activity in a variety of tests; they are found in human blood, and may have regulatory roles in vitamin A function.

Roles in the Body

The major roles of vitamin A are in vision, differentiation of epithelial tissues, and in the immune system. Metabolism of vitamin A in the retina of the eye is unique, in keeping with the unusual role of vitamin A in that tissue. Vitamin A is stored in the retinal pigment epithelium as retinyl esters. All-*trans*-retinyl esters are simultaneously hydrolysed and isomerized to 11-*cis*-retinol, a compound unique to the eye. 11-*cis*-Retinol is then oxidized to 11-*cis*-retinal. 11-*cis*-Retinal is transferred from the pigment epithelium to the rod cells by interstitial retinoid binding protein (IRBP), a distinct binding protein (140 000 Da). In the rod cells, 11-*cis*-retinal binds (as a Schiff base with the ϵ-amino group of a specific lysine residue) to the protein opsin to form the visual pigment, rhodopsin. When a photon of light is absorbed by a rhodopsin complex, the 11-*cis*-retinal is isomerized to all-*trans*-retinal and released from the protein complex; the resulting conformation change of the protein initiates a cascade of reactions, resulting in a neural signal to the brain. The protein opsin is then available to bind another molecule of 11-*cis*-retinal for another round of the visual cycle. The all-*trans*-retinal which was released from the protein complex is transferred back to the pigment epithelium via IRBP, enzymatically reduced to all-*trans*-retinol, and esterified again. In contrast to the high turnover rates of vitamin A in other tissues, vitamin A in the eye is highly conserved, with little leakage back to the liver. Prolonged vitamin A deficiency, however, leads to reduced sensitivity to light, usually first noted as impaired vision at night (night blindness). These effects of vitamin A deficiency are generally reversible by subsequent vitamin A supplementation.

In a very different role, the cornea of the eye depends on vitamin A for proper cell differentiation and for secretion of protective glycoproteins. In vitamin A deficiency, these tissues are susceptible to attack by opportunistic bacteria; such attack may not be reversible and, especially on the corneal surface of the eye, may result in permanent scarring and permanent vision loss. These effects of vitamin A deficiency, unlike those in the retina, may not be reversible by subsequent vitamin A supplementation. Such vitamin A-dependent corneal degeneration (given the general name 'xerophthalmia') accounts for an estimated 500 000 new cases of blindness in preschool children in the world each year.

The action of retinoids in differentiation is manifest in various systems, including maintenance of epithelial tissue (e.g. the lung, intestines and skin, and the cornea of the eye). In the absence of adequate vitamin A, cells of these tissues do not differentiate normally, but change structure (becoming stratified and cornified) and lose the ability to secrete glycoproteins. The common mechanism underlying these roles of retinoids in diverse tissues seem to involve the binding of retinoic acid (and perhaps retinol) to specific proteins associated with nuclear deoxyribonucleic acid (DNA). These nuclear retinoic acid receptor proteins (RARs), which are distinct from the cytoplasmic 'cellular retinoic acid binding proteins' (CRABPs), can then bind to specific regions of DNA, either promoting or inhibiting transcription of specific genes. A number of RARs have now been identified, perhaps explaining in part the variety of effects shown by retinoids on different cell types. The RARs identified to date all belong to a superfamily of nuclear proteins that includes steroid-binding receptors and thyroxine-binding receptors; all act by a common mechanism, but differ in specific DNA binding.

It has been argued, without conclusive proof as yet, that retinoic acid is the active form of vitamin A required for cellular differentiation. Retinoic acid is an endogenous metabolite of vitamin A. Animals maintained on retinoic acid as sole source of vitamin A seem to grow normally and maintain good health, but become blind (because retinoic acid cannot be converted to retinal); some but not all species also show loss of testicular function. Retinoic acid (all-*trans*- and 13-*cis*-isomers) and other acidic retinoid analogues have been found to ameliorate various skin disorders, including acne. Synthetic retinoids (Fig. 1) have been developed to reduce detrimental side effects, which include irritation of the skin, increased serum cholesterol concentrations, and teratogenic consequences.

Retinoids have been shown to inhibit cancer development in a variety of tissues. Again, this seems to be through the role of vitamin A in promoting differentiation of epithelial tissues, in as much as cancer may be thought of as the proliferation of undifferentiated cells.

Although animal studies have long shown a necessity for vitamin A in immune function, the molecular action of retinoids is still unknown. It also seems that some carotenoids function as such in immune function, and perhaps additionally as precursors of vitamin A.

Requirements and Recommended Intakes

Because of confusion among the various units for presenting vitamin A values, the concept of the Retinol Equivalent (RE) has been proposed: 1 RE is equal to 1 µg of all-*trans*-retinol, either free or as the retinyl component of a retinyl ester; 1 RE is also equal to 3.33 IU (international units) of vitamin A, or 3.5 nmol retinol or retinyl ester. Although the exact vitamin A value of carotenoids depends on several factors, the RE has been defined as 6 µg of all-*trans*-β-carotene or 12 µg of other provitamin A carotenoids (10 IU of provitamin A carotenoid).

Liver concentrations provide the best appraisal of vitamin A status. Human liver specimens are difficult to obtain, but analysis of autopsy specimens can be useful in evaluating the vitamin A status of a population. As indicated above, serum retinol levels are maintained nearly constant and are not generally useful in assessing vitamin A status, except when liver vitamin A reserves fall well below $0.07\,\mu mol$ g^{-1} of liver ($20\,\mu g\ g^{-1}$). Serum (or plasma) retinol levels are normally $1\text{--}2\,\mu mol\ l^{-1}$ ($290\text{--}570\ ng\ ml^{-1}$) across a wide range of mammalian species.

Because liver concentrations of vitamin A are not readily measured and serum retinol values are not an adequate indicator of an individual's vitamin A status, several indirect methods have been developed.

Conjunctival impression cytology (CIC) evaluates the development of squamous metaplasia (enlarged epithelial cells) and loss of goblet cells from the conjunctiva of the eye by histological examination of cells transferred from the cornea to filter paper.

The relative dose–response (RDR) depends on the release of retinol-RBP from liver into serum after a large oral dose of vitamin A (typically, 450 µg of retinyl acetate in human studies); as described above, apo RBP accumulates in liver in vitamin A depletion. The RDR is calculated as follows:

$$RDR = (A_5 - A_0/A_5) \times 100\%$$

A_5 represents serum retinol concentration at 5 h after the oral dose, and A_0 represents fasting serum retinol at the time of the dose. Studies in both humans and rats indicate that an RDR value greater than 20% indicates liver vitamin A reserves less than $0.07\,\mu mol$

g^{-1} of liver ($<20\,\mu g\ g^{-1}$), i.e. inadequate vitamin A status. The RDR assay requires, of course, that the oral dose be normally absorbed (an intramuscular injection has been used in human subjects with biliary atresia), and that protein metabolism is normal: protein deficiency or zinc deficiency or liver cirrhosis impairs the dose response.

An alternative approach, the modified relative dose–response (MRDR), uses the vitamin A analogue 3,4-didehydroretinol (vitamin A_2, a form found in some freshwater fish and also found in very low levels in human skin). The ratio of vitamin A_2 to vitamin A_1 in serum retinol at 5 h after an oral dose is used as a measure of vitamin A status, with high values (ratio >0.03 after an oral dose of 100 µg per kg of body weight) indicating poor vitamin A status. Chlorinated vitamin A analogues have been used in a similar fashion.

The RDR and MRDR, as well as CIC, have been used successfully in human population studies. Isotope dilution of tracer-labelled vitamin A (radioactive or stable isotope labelling) has been used to estimate human vitamin A status, but technical difficulties have so far prevented general use of the technique.

Nutritional requirements for vitamin A have not been well defined because of the diversity of vitamin A functions. In animal studies, daily intakes of 3–8 RE (10–28 nmol) per kg of body weight cure deficiency symptoms, and daily intakes of 30–60 RE (100–210 nmol) per kg of body weight produce optimal growth. Kinetic studies of vitamin A metabolism in rats show that irreversible loss of vitamin A is decreased on low vitamin A intakes. Studies on vitamin A requirements have not yet addressed functional criteria such as immune function and possible anticancer effects.

To provide an adequate and safe human intake, current WHO/FAO (World Health Organization, Food and Agriculture Organization) dietary recommendations (1988) and suggested Recommended Dietary Intakes (RDIs) for adults are based on intakes of 9.3 RE (33 nmol of vitamin A) per kg of body weight per day. In contrast, the Recommended Dietary Allowances (RDAs) of the US National Research Council (1989) attempt to set an optimal intake level, and so recommend a higher human male intake of 1000 RE per day, 800 RE for women (because of lower body weight).

Toxicity

Over 600 individual cases of human vitamin A toxicity have been reported, attributable either to acute (single or a few large doses ingested over a brief period of time) or chronic intake (moderately high doses taken frequently for periods of months or years). Acute toxicity in human adults is reported from doses of 300 000 to 10 000 000 RE; chronic doses of 15 000–300 000 RE have produced hypervitaminosis A. Symptoms include headache, vomiting, diplopia, alopecia, dryness of mucous membranes, desquamation, bone abnormalities, and liver damage. On the other hand, single oral doses of 60 000 RE in oil have been successfully used in vitamin A intervention programmes for preschool children, with transient toxic symptoms observed in no more than 3% of subjects. Massive doses of β-carotene are not toxic, but may be less efficiently absorbed and used than vitamin A itself. Rodent animals have been extremely valuable in elucidating vitamin A requirements and metabolism, but the rat seems to be much less susceptible to hypervitaminosis A than is the human.

The toxic effects of high vitamin A intakes are mediated by serum retinyl esters; retinol-RBP concentrations are maintained at normal levels in hypervitaminosis A, but serum retinyl esters are markedly elevated, bypassing the normal homeostatic controls on vitamin A transport. Some carnivores, including the dog, are unusual in having high fasting levels of serum retinyl esters, presumably reflecting differences in lipoprotein metabolism in these species; the implications of this for vitamin A metabolism and for resistance to hypervitaminosis A are not clear.

The most tragic consequences of excessive vitamin A intake are teratogenicity (malformations of the cranium, face, heart, thymus, and central nervous system) and embryotoxicity. Acidic retinoids, such as those that have been used in dermatology, are particularly potent, as they can attain high serum levels and readily pass the placental barrier. Although large intakes of vitamin A itself (>7500 RE, or 26 μmol, per day early in human pregnancy) can cause birth defects (possibly as a result of metabolism of retinol to retinoic acid), serum concentrations of retinol and retinyl esters are normally maintained at moderate levels during pregnancy. It is assumed that these teratogenic effects are related to the important role of retinoids in differentiation of cells and that these effects are mediated via the nuclear receptor proteins. (Interestingly, the retinoid β-glucuronides are less teratogenic than retinoic acid.) In view of these teratogenic effects occurring at less than 10 times the recommended daily intakes, the consensus of several professional organizations is that women should avoid vitamin A supplements during the first trimester of pregnancy, and that subsequent supplements, if taken at all, should be limited to 1500–3000 RE (5.5–11 μmol) per day.

Continuing challenges in vitamin A research include the following: (1) the development and confirmation of indirect indices of vitamin A status; (2) elucidation of the mechanism of control of serum retinol-RBP concentrations; (3) more exact determination of vitamin A requirements for specific functions (not only growth and prevention of blindness, but also immune function and cell differentiation in individual tissues); (4) definition of the role of vitamin A in differentiation in specific tissues, perhaps leading to chemical design of distinctive retinoids to prevent specific cancers and dermatological diseases.

See also: **Antioxidants**: Diet and Antioxidant Defence. **Cancer**: Diet in Cancer Treatment. **Carotenoids**: Chemistry, Sources and Physiology; Epidemiology. **Immunity**: Physiological Aspects; Role of Iron and Zinc. **Retinol**: Hypovitaminosis A.

Further Reading

Blomhoff R, Green MH, Berg T and Norum KR (1990) Transport and storage of vitamin A. *Science* 250:399–404.

Ganguly J (1989) *Biochemistry of Vitamin A*. Boca Raton, Florida: CRC Press.

Olson JA (1991) Vitamin A. In Machlin LJ (ed.) *Handbook of Vitamins*, 2nd edn, pp 1–57. New York: Marcel Dekker.

Sporn MB, Roberts AB and Goodman DS (eds) (1994) *The Retinoids*. New York: Raven Press.

Hypovitaminosis A

K West Jr, Johns Hopkins University, Baltimore, Maryland, USA

Hypovitaminosis A is an extensive nutritional problem, the leading cause of paediatric blindness and a key determinant of child mortality in many developing countries. Globally, vitamin A (VA) deficiency afflicts 125–250 million children in 90 listed countries throughout the Third World (**Fig. 1**). The largest numbers of VA-deficient children live in South and Southeast Asia, where each year an estimated 5 million children develop xerophthalmia, a half million of whom progress to potentially blinding corneal disease. Worldwide, the annual number of cases of xerophthalmia is likely to be 8–10 million. VA deficiency also impairs host defences, predisposing individuals to increased severity of infection and consequent risk of mortality. Approximately 1–2.5 million child deaths occur annually, presumably

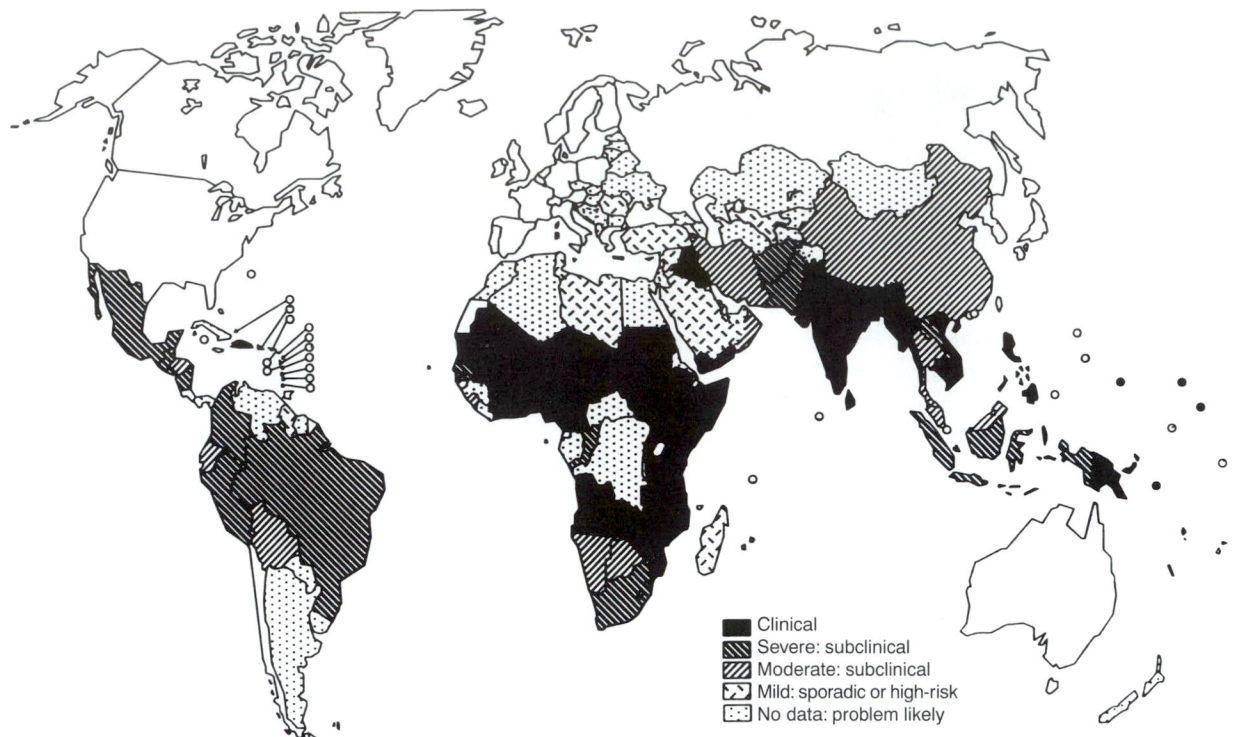

Figure 1 Global geographic distribution of hypovitaminosis A as a public health problem. Source: World Health Organization.

from infection, that can be attributed to underlying hypovitaminosis A. It also appears to explain a substantial proportion of maternal mortality in high-risk regions of the world. Understanding its patterns of occurrence, causes, risk factors and health consequences is fundamental to effective treatment and control of hypovitaminosis A as a public health problem.

Epidemiology

The epidemiology of VA deficiency is understood mostly in relation to xerophthalmia (**Table 1**),

especially the noncorneal stages of night blindness and conjunctival xerosis with Bitot's spots. These mild and readily diagnosed ocular manifestations are common, highly specific to VA deficiency, and are likely to exhibit patterns of risk that parallel those of more widespread, subclinical stages of hypovitaminosis A.

Prevalence

Severe hypovitaminosis A in childhood, manifested by potentially blinding corneal xerophthalmia (**Fig. 2**), rarely affects more than 0.1% of children. It is most likely to strike children late in the second to

Table 1 WHO classification and minimum prevalence criteria for xerophthalmia and vitamin A deficiency as a public health programme

Definition (code)	Minimum prevalence	Highest-risk groups
Night blindness (XN)	1.0%	Children 2–6 years; Pregnant/lactating women
Conjunctival xerosis (XIA)	–	
Bitot's spots (X1B)	0.5%	
Cornea xerosis (X2)		
Corneal ulceration (X3A)/keratomalacia (X3B)	0.01%	Children 1–3 years
Xerophthalmic corneal scar (XS)	0.05%	Cumulative >1 year
Serum retinol <0.35 μmol l^{-1}	5.0%	

Adapted from the joint World Health Organization (WHO)/International Vitamin A Consultative Group (IVACG)/UNICEF (1997) *Guidelines for the Detection and Treatment of Vitamin A Deficiency*.

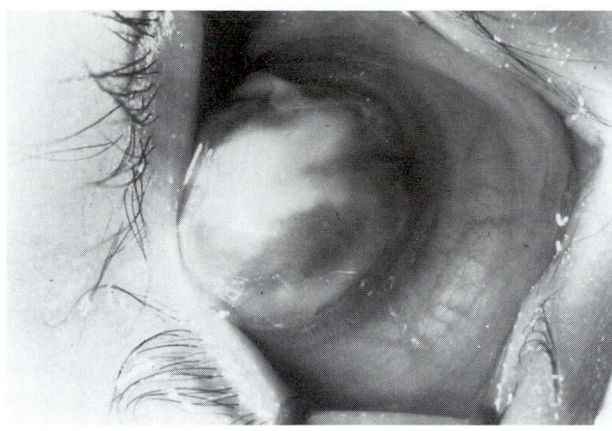

Figure 2 Keratomalacia. From Sommer (1995).

fourth years of life following an acute infection, such as measles, which exacerbates a chronically wasted and vitamin A-deficient state. In contrast, milder xerophthalmia can affect 1–5% of young children. The prevalence of both night blindness and Bitot's spots usually rises from about 1 year of age throughout the preschool and, in some cultures, into the school-aged years. During this period children in traditional societies wean from VA-containing breast milk to a household diet chronically lacking vitamin A.

Hypovitaminosis A, however, persists through adolescence and into adulthood. This is evident in frequent reports of low serum retinol level ($<0.70 \, \mu\text{mol l}^{-1}$) in approximately 25% and night blindness in 5–20% of pregnant or lactating women in endemically deficient areas. Deficiency presumably results from increased nutritional demand during periods of late gestation and postpartum lactation superimposed on a chronically poor intake and vitamin A status of women. While rarely blinding, maternal night blindness is associated with hyporetinemia, anaemia, wasting malnutrition and increased risks of morbidity and mortality.

Location

Vitamin A deficiency tends to cluster by geographical area, often paralleling indices of underdevelopment and low availability of food sources of vitamin A. Risk tends to follow a socioeconomic continuum: cases of xerophthalmia arise more from households of low socioeconomic status. Also, villages where cases are detected tend to be poorer than xerophthalmia-free communities (**Table 2**). In Africa and Asia preschool children incur an approximate two-fold higher risk of having or developing xerophthalmia in villages where at least one other child has been diagnosed with the condition compared with villages where xerophthalmia has not been previously seen (**Table 3**). More striking is a 7- to 13-fold higher risk of xerophthalmia in siblings of children with eye signs compared with children in previously xerophthalmia-free households. An epidemiological link between maternal night blindness and childhood xerophthalmia likely exists but remains to be established. Spatial patterns of risk seem to arise mostly from shared dietary practices in homes and villages rather than other exposures that lead to common infections.

Periodicity

Occurrence of xerophthalmia can follow predictable, though not parallel, seasonal patterns in different parts of the world. Typically, a seasonal peak in VA deficiency emerges from a convergence of causal risk factors. In South Asia, for example, a distinct peak in the incidence of mild xerophthalmia occurs during the late dry and early monsoon seasons (April–July). This peak follows a postharvest growth spurt in the cool dry season. It also coincides with a general scarcity of provitamin A-rich vegetables and fruits and a seasonal rise in the incidence of diarrhoea, respiratory infection and measles. Such periodicity, where it exists, can help identify causes and target prevention to specific times of the year. A decade-long decline in corneal xerophthalmia has been noted

Table 2 Household characteristics of xerophthalmia cases, controls and the remaining Aceh study population

Household characteristic	Cases (%) (N = 466)	Village-matched controls (%) (N = 466)	Aceh study households (%) (N = 15 915)
Unprotected water source	47.5	43.8	41.1[a]
No private latrine	86.7	83.6	71.3[a]
Bamboo house walls	47.1	33.5	31.6[a]
Household head farms	57.3	55.5	53.4
Mother has <6 years of education	94.3	86.6	80.3[a]
History of child death	12.1	9.7	7.5[a]

Adapted from Mele *et al.* (1991). [a]Significant linear trend in proportions, $P < 0.001$.

Table 3   Age-adjusted village and household odds ratios for risk of xerophthalmia among preschool children[a]

	Malawi		Zambia		Indonesia		Nepal	
	N	OR[b]	N	OR	N	OR	N	OR
Village	50	1.2 (1.0–1.5)[c]	110	1.7 (0.9–3.2)	460	1.8 (1.4–2.2)	40	2.3 (1.6–3.4)
Household	2899	7.3 (3.2–16.7)	2449	7.9 (3.5–17.8)	16 337	10.5 (7.0–15.7)	2909	13.2 (6.0–29.0)

Adapted from Katz *et al.* (1993).
[a]Numbers of children <6 years of age in each country: Malawi (*N*=5441); Zambia (*N* = 4316); Indonesia (*N*=28,586); and Nepal (*N*=4764).
[b]Pairwise odds ratio (OR) based on alternating logistic regression.
[c]95% confidence intervals in parentheses.

recently, possibly resulting from effective interventions coupled with dietary and other public health measures in some countries. The trend has been less apparent for milder stages of hypovitaminosis A.

Breast-feeding and diet

Dietary risk in children refers to inadequate breast-feeding and consumption of VA-rich foods from the household diet. A low dietary fat intake (e.g. ≤ 5% of calories) may also restrict absorption of provitamin A carotenoids from food and thus play a role in predisposing individuals to deficiency. Studies in Asia and Africa show that breast-fed children are 10–35% as likely to have or develop xerophthalmia than non-breast-fed peers of the same age. Xerophthalmic children have been shown to begin weaning earlier (by about 1 month) and to have been weaned from the breast approximately 6 months earlier than non-xerophthalmic children, reflecting the potential benefit to be achieved by effective breast-feeding promotion. Even among breast-fed children, the more frequent the daily feeds, the greater the reduction in risk of xerophthalmia.

Complementary feeding affects childhood risk of VA deficiency. Indonesian preschoolers were at a 2- to 6-fold higher risk of xerophthalmia if food sources of vitamin A such as dark green leaves, mango or papaya, egg, meat or fish with liver, and milk and other dairy products were not routinely given during their first year of weaning (**Fig. 3**). However, infrequent dietary intake of foods with preformed vitamin A or precursor carotenoids persists for children through their preschool years in high-risk households (**Fig. 4**). In Nepal, an inadequate dietary intake was one of many manifestations of poor care in the home of xerophthalmics. Siblings of cases shared a similar pattern of low dietary vitamin A intake and child neglect compared with children in families with no history of xerophthalmia. These pat-

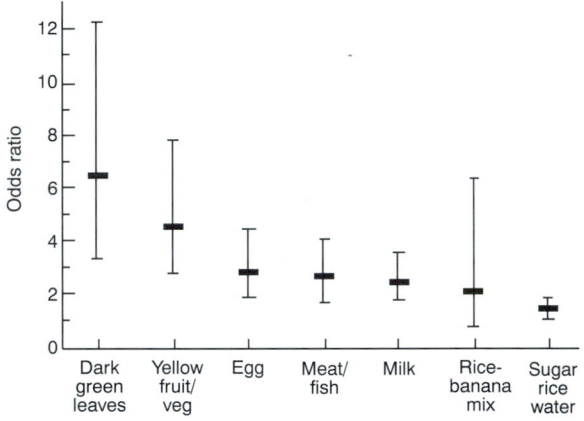

Figure 3   Odds of xerophthalmia in preschool years when foods were not regularly included in the weaning diets of Indonesian children relative to children given such foods. Vertical lines denote 95% confidence intervals. Reproduced with permission.

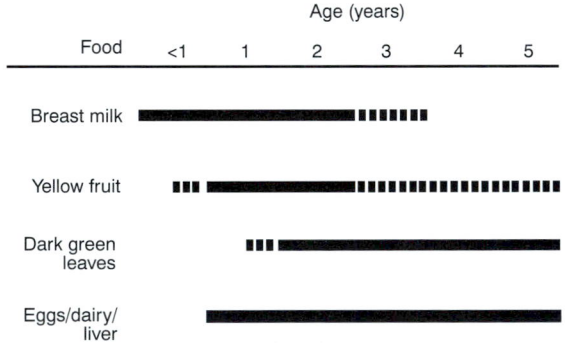

Figure 4   Foods that protect against hypovitaminosis A (xerophthalmia), based on numerous studies. Dark line, strong evidence; dashed line, suggestive evidence. Reproduced with permission.

terns signal the need to improve both child care and dietary practices in high-risk homes in order to sustain adequate VA status.

Infectious morbidity

A bidirectional relationship exists between hypovitaminosis A and infection, each exacerbating the other, representing a classic 'vicious cycle'. Cross-sectionally, xerophthalmia or severe hyporetinaemia has been consistently associated with elevated risks of diarrhoea, fever or other infections, though directionality is difficult to parse from such evidence. Prospective studies show that severe infections, including measles, chickenpox, diarrhoea and acute respiratory illness, induce hypovitaminosis A. In Indonesia, young children with diarrhoea and acute respiratory infections were twice as likely to subsequently develop mild xerophthalmia (XN or X1B) than apparently disease-free children. Reasons for this may include decreased absorption of vitamin A, increased metabolic requirements, impaired retinol transport and greatly increased renal excretion during the acute phase response, and slow normalization of these mechanisms coupled with a chronically decreased dietary VA intake during extended recovery or repeated illness.

On the other hand, hypovitaminosis A raises the risk of infection. In Asia, preschoolers with mild xerophthalmia (XN, X1B and both conditions) have been found to be twice as likely to develop acute respiratory infection and, in Indonesia, three times more likely to develop diarrhea over subsequent 3- to 6-month periods. It follows that such children also exhibit an excessive risk of dying. This was so among Indonesian preschool children whose risk of mortality rose with increased severity of mild eye signs (**Fig. 5**). In Nepal, siblings of cases were more likely to develop xerophthalmia (Table 3) but were also at a two-fold higher risk of dying than children living in xerophthalmia-free households. Data from children and animals support the plausibility of these findings. VA-deficient children show increased bacterial adherence to respiratory epithelium, low lymphocyte counts and T helper to cytotoxic/suppressor cell ratios, and a weaker delayed-type hypersensitivity response compared with non-xerophthalmic children. In animals, VA deficiency produces keratinizing metaplasia of epithelial linings that may affect 'barrier' defences. It also compromises acquired immunity, indicated by lymphoid atrophy, reduced numbers of circulating lymphocytes, impaired blast transformation responses to antigen, T cell-dependent antibody responses and natural killer cell activity, and a greatly increased risk of infection and death.

Manifestations

Vitamin A is essential in maintaining normal retinal function and differentiation of rapidly dividing, bipotential cells. These regulatory roles give rise to specific manifestations of hypovitaminosis A, such as: poor photoreceptor function leading to night blindness; metaplasia and keratinization of mucosal epithelial surfaces leading to conjunctival and, in severe deficiency, corneal xerosis; and failure in the development or functioning of the immune system that can weaken host defenses against infection.

Biochemical depletion

Tissue depletion of vitamin A precedes the functional consequences of deficiency. In uncomplicated hypovitaminosis A, plasma retinol tends to be homoeostatically controlled until body (i.e. liver) stores are low, after which plasma concentration declines. Plasma retinol may also decline during the acute-phase response to clinically significant infection reflecting, in part, urinary loss, increased tissue delivery and reduced mobilization of vitamin A from the liver via restricted release of retinol-binding protein. Plasma retinol gradually normalizes during recovery if there are adequate hepatic stores of the vitamin. Despite these nondietary influences, plasma or serum retinol measurement remains the most common biochemical index of vitamin A status. Hypovitaminosis A is diagnosed at serum retinol levels below a cutoff of 0.70 μmol l^{-1} (20 g dl^{-1}), below which 20% to >50% of concentrations lie in a VA-deficient population compared with <3% of well-nourished populations. A serum retinol <0.35 μmol l^{-1} is indicative of severe deficiency. Decrements in serum retinol concentration below these cutoffs are associated with marked increases in risk of xerophthalmia and infection which can exacerbate the vitamin A-deficient

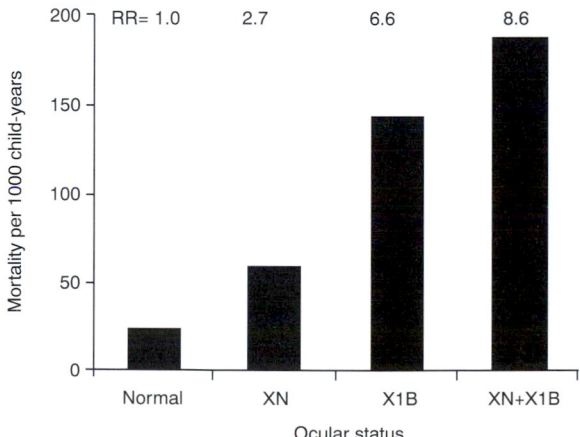

Figure 5 Risk of mortality among approximately 3500 Indonesian preschool children by ocular status at the outset of each 3-month interval. RR, relative risk of mortality. Adapted from Sommer et al. (1983).

state. Other indices of tissue retinol depletion include the relative dose–response, which indirectly reflects hepatic retinol adequacy, breast milk retinol concentration for assessing maternal status and intake adequacy of breast-fed infants, and stable isotopic methods to assess the total body vitamin A pool.

Xerophthalmia

When conjunctival and corneal epithelium is deprived of vitamin A, these surfaces undergo keratinizing metaplasia. Columnar epithelial cells become squamous and mucus-producing goblet cells disappear, providing the histopathologic mechanisms for deficiency-induced xerosis (drying) and destruction of ocular surfaces. Vitamin A is also required for rod vision in dim light. VA deficiency-induced night blindness often occurs with changes on the ocular surface. Thus, night blindness and clinical eye signs are classified as xerophthalmia (Table 1).

Night blindness Vitamin A is an essential cofactor in the generation of rhodopsin. This is a photosensitive pigment in rod photoreceptors of the retina that responds to light (it is 'bleached') by releasing vitamin A, and initiating neural impulses to the brain that permits vision under conditions of low illumination. The utilization and recycling of vitamin A in this process is known as the 'visual cycle'. Hypovitaminosis A restricts rhodopsin production which, in turn, raises the scotopic (low light) visual threshold. Gradually, a perceptive threshold is reached that leads to the recognition of night blindness (XN), the earliest symptom of xerophthalmia. It is marked by an inability to move about in the dark. Young children and pregnant and lactating women appear to be at greatest risk of XN. Where endemic, there is often a local term for XN that translates into 'evening' or 'twilight' blindness or 'chicken eyes' (chickens lack rod cells in their eyes and also cannot see, or move about, at night), making the condition readily detectable by history.

Conjunctival xerosis and Bitot's spots Early xerosis of the conjunctiva can be detected subclinically by filter paper impression cytology, showing distorted, enlarged and noncontiguous sheaths of epithelial cells and disappearance of goblet cells. In advanced vitamin A deficiency, xerosis appears clinically as a dry, unwettable surface of the bulbar conjunctiva (X1A). The affected areas are usually overlaid with superficial white, cheesy or foamy patches of triangular or oval shape that consist of desquamated keratin and bacteria (often the Xerosis bacillus). These are known as Bitot's spots (X1B). They are nearly always bilateral, found temporal (and, in more

advanced cases, also nasal) to the corneal limbus and are more reliably diagnosed than X1A. Bitot's spots are not blinding but are reflective of chronic moderate to severe systemic depletion of vitamin A.

Corneal xerophthalmia Corneal xerophthalmia is manifested as stages of increasingly severe, potentially blinding, ocular disease due to hypovitaminosis A. The earliest corneal epithelial defects appear as superficial punctate defects, evident with a slit lamp, which with advanced deficiency become more numerous and concentrated. The cornea is considered xerotic (X2) when punctate keratopathy covers large areas of the surface, rendering a hazy, unwettable, lustreless and irregular appearance on handlight examination. Stromal oedema may be present. In more severe cases, thick, elevated xerotic plaques may form. Usually both eyes are affected. Corneal ulcers (X3A) can be sharply demarcated, round or oval defects that are usually shallow but may also perforate the cornea. Healed ulcers form a leukoma (scar) or adherent leukoma if the iris has plugged the perforated ulcer. Most ulcers occur peripheral to the visual axis and, thus, may not threaten central vision if treated in time. Keratomalacia (X3B) refers to a full-thickness softening and necrosis of the corneal stroma, which can cause protruding, opaque, yellow-to-grey lesions to form (Fig. 2). These tend to collapse or slough off, leaving a descemetocele following VA treatment. Keratomalacia usually causes blindness in the involved eye, although the degree of visual loss depends on the location, thickness and extent of corneal necrosis. Owing to the generally malnourished and ill state of children with corneal xerophthalmia, fatality of hospitalized cases ranges from 4 to 25%.

Impact of Interventions

Hypovitaminosis A may be prevented through direct supplementation, fortification of commonly eaten food items or through other food-based interventions that include home gardening and various forms of nutrition education. Most evaluation efforts have assessed the impact of direct supplementation, and occasionally fortification, on vitamin A status, xerophthalmia, survival and other health outcomes. Data on the efficacy of dietary regimens are limited to change in vitamin A status.

Vitamin A status The impact of vitamin A prophylaxis on status varies by indicator, dosage and mode of delivery of the supplement, level of initial deficiency and other risk factors. A single, high-potency supplement (210 μmol, 60 mg retinol equivalents or 200 000 IU) has been shown to elevate serum retinol in deficiency-prone populations for periods of 1–6 months. Continuous intake of a half to full recommended allowance of vitamin A through fortified foods gradually improves and sustains an adequate distribution of serum and breast milk retinol levels. Regular consumption of provitamin A food sources (dark green leaves, yellow vegetables and fruits) has variable effects on vitamin A status. Dietary carotenoid intake appears most efficacious in raising serum retinol from deficient concentrations to minimally adequate levels in children and women, but often fails to optimize vitamin A status. Food matrix, methods of storage and preparation, the presence of preformed vitamin A and fat in the diet, and host factors such as initial vitamin A status and gut integrity appear to affect dietary efficacy.

Xerophthalmia

Delivery of high-potency vitamin A to preschool children every 4–6 months is about 90% efficacious in preventing both corneal and noncorneal xerophthalmia. Prophylactic failure (~10%) may reflect inadequacy of dosage for children at very high risk, study-related factors, or other reasons. Xerophthalmia virtually disappears in populations consuming adequate amounts of vitamin A-fortified foods. Supervised dietary treatment alone has been reported to cure or improve noncorneal xerophthalmia, although field trials to show the impact of diet change in preventing xerophthalmia have not been carried out.

Mortality

The impact of vitamin A supplementation on preschool child mortality has been firmly established through the conduct of eight controlled community trials, involving approximately 160 000 children on three subcontinents, in a period of a decade (**Table 4**). In six trials, children 6 months to 6 years of age were supplemented every 4–6 months with an oral dose of vitamin A containing 60 mg retinol equivalents (RE) (or 200 000 IU). Half this dosage was provided to children <12 months of age. One study, in India, provided a small weekly dose to children, while the other, in Indonesia, supplied half of a recommended allowance of vitamin A to children in treatment villages through a routinely marketed fortified monosodium glutamate product (a flavour-enhancer). Rates of mortality in supplemented groups were compared with rates among children in concurrent control groups. Six of the eight trials showed reductions of 19% to 54% in preschool child mortality beyond either 6 or 12 months of age. Meta-analyses of data from these trials have estimated the reduction in mortality to range from 23% to 34%, with the latter value likely applicable to South Asia. The estimates are remarkably consistent, given differences in study designs and analytical approaches. Cumulative mortality curves from trials with positive results show a characteristic departure in mortality experience from control groups shortly after initiation of vitamin A supplementation (**Fig. 6**). Notably, the largest mortality impacts have occurred

Table 4 Vitamin A child mortality prevention trials

Location	VA dosage[a]	No. children	% change[b]
Aceh, Indonesia[c]	60 mg RE/6 months	29 236	↓ 34%*
West Java, Indonesia[d]	0.81 mg RE/day	11 220	↓ 46%*
Tamil Nadu, India[e]	2.5 mg RE/week	15 419	↓ 54%*
Hyderabad, India[f]	60 mg RE/6 months	15 775	↓ 6%
Sarlahi, Nepal[g]	60 mg RE/4 months	28 640	↓ 30%*
Jumla, Nepal[h]	60 mg RE/5 months	7 197	↓ 29%*
Khartoum, Sudan[i]	60 mg RE/6 months	29 615	↑ 6%
Northern Ghana[j]	60 mg RE/4 months	21 906	↓ 19%*

From Sommer and West (1996).
[a]RE = retinol equivalents; trials providing 60 mg RE gave a half dose to infants < 12 months.
[b]Per cent change in mortality rate among vitamin A recipients comparred to controls for children ≥ 6 months or ≥ 12 months of age, depending on study.
[c]Sommer A et al. (1986) Lancet **1**:1169–1173.
[d]Muhilal PD et al. (1988) American Journal of Clinical Nutrition **48**:1271–1276.
[e]Rahmathullah L et al. (1990) New England Journal of Medicine **323**:929–935.
[f]Vijayaraghavan R et al. (1992) Lancet **340**:1358–1359.
[g]West KP, Jr et al. (1991) Lancet **338**:67–71.
[h]Daulaire NMP et al. (1992) British Medical Journal **304**:207–210.
[i]Fawzi WW et al. (1993) Journal of the American Medical Association **269**:898–903.
[j]Ghana VAST Study Team (1993) Lancet **342**:7–12.
*Indicates statistically significant differences (P < 0.05).

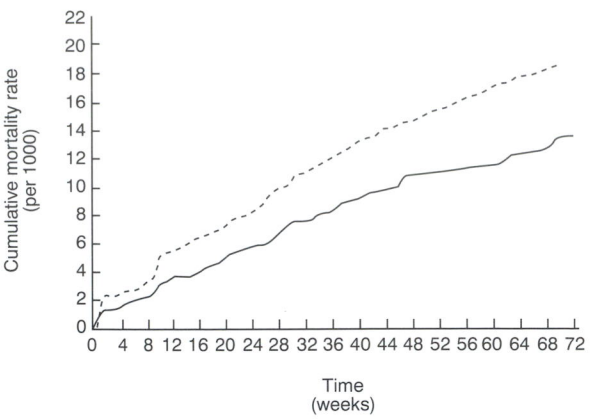

Figure 6 Cumulative mortality of children randomized to 4-monthly placebo control (dashed line) versus 200 000 IU of vitamin A (solid line) during a large community trial in Sarlahi District, rural Nepal. From Sommer and West (1996).

in the two trials that mimicked a normal dietary intake of vitamin A compared with its periodic delivery as a bolus. Investigations into illnesses and events prior to death suggest that vitamin A reduced mortality associated with measles, diarrhoea and acute wasting malnutrition. A lack of apparent impact on mortality attributable to acute respiratory infection has been a perplexing, although consistent, finding across these trials. In contrast, vitamin A administration prior to acquiring measles, or on hospital admission for severe measles infection, has been shown to lower case fatality by about 50%.

Little, if any, impact of vitamin A can be expected on the risk of mortality for children less than 5 months of age. This age difference may relate to a shift in the cause of death from acute respiratory infection in early infancy to diarrhoea, wasting malnutrition, measles and other causes responsive to vitamin A in later infancy and early childhood.

Morbidity

Unlike the impact on mortality, effects of VA on 'morbidity' have been more difficult to establish. This may be due to variation in disease sensitivity to vitamin A and inherent problems in measuring incidence, duration and severity of morbidity. Vitamin A interventions exert only a modest, if any, impact on the prevalence of common childhood morbidities as typically obtained by history. In contrast, VA appears to reduce the severity of potentially fatal infections such as measles, persistent diarrhoea, dysentery and (falciparum) malaria, especially in the presence of wasting malnutrition. The protective effect becomes stronger with episode severity. Thus, febrile illnesses appear to be more responsive to vitamin A than nonfebrile events. Illnesses for which care is sought show a response to vitamin A. In

Ghana, vitamin A supplementation was associated with decreased clinic attendance for illness (relative risk (RR) = 0.88), hospitalization rates for severe disease (RR = 0.62) and severity of illness among children admitted for diarrhoea compared with placebo recipients. In Brazil, prior vitamin A receipt had no effect on children's diarrhoeal episodes of 1–2 days' duration (RR = 0.97) but was increasingly protective against episodes of ≥ 3 days with ≤4 stools per day (RR = 0.91) and episodes of ≥3 days with ≥5 stools per day (RR = 0.80). Vitamin A treatment of measles has led to fewer and less severe complications, and enhanced immunological and clinical recovery. However, as with ALRI-associated mortality, multiple treatment trials report little effect of vitamin A on recovery from childhood pneumonia. This remains a paradox, given decades of experimental animal evidence linking vitamin A deficiency to extensive metaplasia and keratinization and, presumably, greater susceptibility to pathogen invasion and infection of the respiratory epithelium.

Management

Treatment

Children with xerophthalmia and measles should be treated immediately with oral, high-potency vitamin A (200 000 IU) according to WHO guidelines (**Table 5**) and provided with other supportive nutritional and medical therapy, as indicated. Corneal lesions should be topically treated with a suitable antibiotic (e.g. tetracycline or chloramphenicol) to prevent bacterial infection. Corneal xerophthalmia shows improvement with VA treatment within a week and complete resolution within 4 weeks, depending on the size, thickness and location of the lesion, and nutritional and health status of the patient. Night blindness typically is cured within 24 h of VA treatment. Most Bitot's spots begin to respond within 2–5 days and disappear within 2 weeks, though some may persist, particularly in older children. High-potency vitamin A is indicated for women of reproductive age with corneal disease. For milder lesions, smaller daily (5000–10 000 IU) or weekly (≤25 000 IU) doses are recommended for at least a month. Children presenting with severe diarrhoea, dysentery, respiratory infection and exanthematous infections, especially if also moderately to severely protein–energy malnourished, should also be given a single, large oral dose (200 000 IU) of vitamin A.

Prevention

Hypovitaminosis A is prevented by increasing intakes of preformed vitamin A or provitamin A

Table 5 Vitamin A treatment and prevention schedules

| Age | Treatment at diagnosis[a] | Prevention[b] | |
		Dosage	Frequency
< 6 months	50 000 IU	50 000 IU	every 4–6 months
6–12 months	100 000 IU	100 000 IU	every 4–6 months
≥ 1 year	200 000 IU	200 000 IU	every 4–6 months
Women	200 000 IU[c]	200 000 IU	≤ 8 weeks after delivery

Based on WHO/UNICEF/IVACG (1997).
[a]Treat all cases of xerophthalmia and measles with the same age-specific dosage the *next day* and *at least 2 weeks later*.
[b]Exclude children known to have received a high dose of vitamin A within the past 30 days, either prophylactically or as treatment for measles, diarrhoea, respiratory disease, chickenpox, other severe infections, or severe protein–energy malnutrition.
[c]For women of reproductive age, give 200 000 IU only for corneal xerophthalmia, for milder eye signs (night blindness or Bitot's spots) give women 5000–10 000 IU per day or ≤ 25 000 IU per week for ≥ 4 weeks.

carotenoids to levels that maintain adequate status. This can be done through direct supplementation of targeted risk groups, food fortification or dietary approaches that protect breast-feeding and improve the quality of the home diet.

Administration of high-potency, oral vitamin A, adjusted according to age (Table 5), on a 4 to 6-monthly basis, is a common preventive approach in many developing countries. A half-dose is dispensed to infants aged 6–11 months and a quarter dose given to younger infants to minimize risk of toxicity in high-risk areas. The intervention rests on the principle that a large dose of vitamin A is stored primarily in the liver from where it is mobilized as needed. Beyond treatment, supplements can be provided during routine health care (e.g. for growth monitoring, immunization, other extension services) or more extensively and systematically in targeted populations on a regular basis.

Providing mothers a single 200 000 IU dose of vitamin A as soon after birth as possible (but always within 8 weeks to avoid excessive periconceptional exposure) is a safe and effective way to improve vitamin A status of mothers and their breast-fed infants. Otherwise, supplements of ≤10 000 IU per day or ≤ 25 000 IU per week offer safe prophylaxis to women against hypovitaminosis A during their reproductive years.

Increasingly, developing countries are fortifying staple food items with a quarter to a full day's recommended allowance of vitamin A to prevent deficiency in high-risk populations. Potential food vehicles should be technically fortifiable at required concentrations, and consumed within a range that could be both effective in target groups yet safe in the entire population. Fortification has been effectively carried out with nonfat milk powder in food assistance programmes; sugar in Central America and, increasingly, in other developing regions; monosod-

ium glutamate in Indonesia and the Philippines; and with a variety of other products such as nonrefrigerated margarine and wheat flour in the Philippines. This trend will likely continue with increased use of processed foods and as the food industry becomes involved in helping to solve problems of vitamin A and other micronutrient deficiencies.

Dietary diversification is widely held to be the most culturally appropriate and potentially sustainable approach to preventing hypovitaminosis A, although data on effectiveness are generally lacking. Dietary intakes can be improved through home and school gardening initiatives, nutrition education and social marketing of locally available food sources of vitamin A. However, effective dietary change requires a thorough understanding of local cultural, food system and behavioural factors that give risk to hypovitaminosis A.

See Colour Plate 8.

See also: **Children**: Nutritional Requirements of School Children. **Food Fortification**: Importance in the Diet. **Lactation**: Dietary Requirements. **Malnutrition**: Definition, Classification and Epidemiology; Primary Malnutrition; Secondary Malnutrition. **Retinol**: Physiology.

Further Reading

Beaton GH, Martorell R, Aronson KJ, Edmonston B, McCabe G, Ross AC and Harvey B (1993) *Effectiveness of vitamin A supplementation in the control of young child morbidity and mortality in developing countries*. ACC/SCN State of the Art Series Nutrition Policy Discussion Paper, no. 13. Geneva: WHO.

Christian P, West KP, Jr, Khatry SK, Katz J, Shrestha SR Pradhan EK, LeClerq SC and Pokhrel RP (in press) Night blindness of pregnancy in rural Nepal – nutritional and health risks. *International Journal of Epidemiology*.

Ghana VAST Study Team (1993) Vitamin A supplementation in northern Ghana: effects on clinic attendances, hospital admissions, and child mortality. *Lancet* **342**:7–12.

Gillespie S and Mason J (1994) *Controlling Vitamin A Deficiency*. A report based on the ACC/SCN Consultative Group Meeting on Strategies for the Control of Vitamin A Deficiency, United Nations Administrative Committee on Coordination, Subcommittee on Nutrition, Ottawa, Canada, 1993. Geneva: WHO.

Gittelsohn J, Shankar AV, West KP Jr, Ram R, Dhungel C and Dahal B (1997) Infant feeding practices reflect antecedent risk of xerophthalmia in Nepali children. *European Journal of Clinical Nutrition* **51**:484–490.

Katz J, Zeger SL, West KP, Jr, Tielsch JM and Sommer A (1993) Clustering of xerophthalmia within households and villages. *International Journal of Epidemiology* **22**:709–715.

Mele L, West KP Jr, Kusdiono, Pandji A, Nendrawati H, Tilden RL and Tarwotjo I (1991) The Aceh Study Group. Nutritional and household risk factors for xerophthalmia: a case–control study. *American Journal of Clinical Nutrition* **53**:1460–1465.

Sommer A (1995) *Vitamin A Deficiency and Its Consequences: A Field Guide to Detection and Control*, edn. Geneva: WHO.

Sommer A and West KP Jr (1996) *Vitamin A Deficiency: Health, Survival and Vision*. New York: Oxford University Press.

Sommer A, Tarwotjo I, Hussaini G and Susanto D (1983) Increased mortality in children with mild vitamin A deficiency. *Lancet* **2**:585–588.

West KP, Jr and Sommer A (1987) *Delivery of oral doses of vitamin A to prevent vitamin A deficiency and nutritional blindness. A state-of-the-art review.* Nutrition Policy Discussion Paper no. 2. June, 1987. Rome: United Nations Administrative Committee on Coordination, Subcommittee on Nutrition.

WHO (1996) *Indicators for Assessing Vitamin A Deficiency and Their Application in Monitoring and Evaluating Intervention Programmes*. Micronutrient Series, WHO/NUT/96.10. Geneva: WHO.

WHO (1997) *Vitamin A Supplements: A Guide to Their Use in the Treatment and Prevention of Vitamin A Deficiency and Xerophthalmia*, 2nd edn. Prepared by a WHO/UNICEF/IVACG Task Force. Geneva: WHO.

RIBOFLAVIN

Physiology

C J Bates, MRC Dunn Nutrition Unit, Cambridge, UK

Absorption, Transport and Storage

Riboflavin is not synthesized by higher animals. It is therefore an absolute dietary requirement for the synthesis of certain essential coenzymes that are needed for intermediary metabolism in nearly all living cells. Riboflavin must be transported from the food sources within the gastrointestinal tract, across the gut wall into the circulatory system, and thence into the cells of each organ. This transport process frequently needs to occur against a concentration gradient in order to ensure the efficient retrieval of the very small amounts which occur in many foods, and thence from the low concentrations in blood plasma to a milieu of higher concentrations inside living cells. There must therefore be a mechanism, acting to achieve this cellular trapping or assisted transfer. By the fundamental laws of thermodynamics, this must be an energy-dependent process.

The mechanisms and characteristics of the transport systems that occur in the gastrointestinal tract have been studied by means of three alternative models. These models have made use of controlled perturbations, and probes of radioactively labelled vitamin to determine the biological characteristics and requirements of the transport process. One model used a partly isolated segment of the small intestine within a living, anaesthetized animal; a second has used an isolated excised segment, usually everted (i.e. inside-out) and placed in a physiological bathing solution, to study transfer of the labelled vitamin. The third model has used minute sacs or 'vesicles', prepared in a special way from the 'brush border' or absorptive surface of the gut, in order to retain the essential characteristics of the intact organ.

Studies with these model systems have shown that the transport of riboflavin at low (e.g. micromolar) concentrations is temperature- and energy-dependent (it is inhibited by inhibitors of ATP production from energy substrates); it becomes saturated as the concentration of riboflavin increases, and it is sodium ion-dependent. These characteristics are shared with many other types of small molecules that are actively transported across the gut wall. More specifically for riboflavin, the active transport mechanism involves phosphorylation (to riboflavin phosphate, also known as flavin mononucleotide, or FMN) followed by dephosphorylation, both occurring within the intestinal cells (**Fig. 1**). This latter process is not shared by several other B vitamins, but it is one of a number of common strategies which the gut may use to entrap essential nutrients, and then relocate them, in a controlled manner and direction. A similar strategy is employed at other sites in the body to ensure entrapment of circulating riboflavin by cells whose nascent flavin-dependent enzymes need a supply of the vitamin from beyond their borders.

Although the active transport of riboflavin across the gut wall and across other cell membrane barriers within the animal is a saturable process, if large pharmacological amounts are present then the slower and less efficient, but nonsaturable, process of passive absorption predominates and contributes significantly to the total mass-transfer.

Although some of the available riboflavin in natural foods may be present as the free vitamin, ready for intestinal transport, a larger fraction is present in the form of phosphorylated coenzymes – FMN and flavin adenine dinucleotide (FAD) – and there may also be very small amounts of a glucoside of the vitamin. These forms are all efficiently converted to free vitamin by enzymes secreted into the gut lumen, and they are therefore highly available for absorption. There are also small amounts of covalently bound forms of riboflavin present in enzymes, such as succinate dehydrogenase (succinate: ubiquinone oxidoreductase EC 1.3.5.1), which cannot be released by the hydrolytic enzymes in the gut and are therefore

unavailable for absorption. Also unavailable (or very poorly available) in humans is the riboflavin synthesized by the gut flora of the large bowel. Certain animal species, such as rodents, can utilize this riboflavin source by coprophagy.

A wide variety of unnatural analogues of riboflavin have been prepared in order to explore the structural versus functional essentials of the molecule. Some of these analogues have riboflavin-like activity; others are inactive, while others again are antagonists and can cause functional deficiency. These structural changes affect absorption in some instances; in others they affect the conversion of riboflavin to its coenzyme forms within the body. Certain drugs which are used for purposes unrelated to riboflavin function, such as the phenothiazines used as antipsychotic drugs, may also have sufficient structural similarity to riboflavin to act as antagonists in some situations.

Absorption by human subjects

Studies of riboflavin absorption by human subjects require a combination of a test dose, usually taken by mouth, and a sampling procedure to estimate the amount absorbed, and possibly also its subsequent fate. The sampling compartment is generally the urine, since plasma has proved generally unsatisfactory. Faecal sampling is also useless because of the synthesis of riboflavin by bacteria in the large bowel. Although the use of riboflavin labelled with radioactive or stable isotopes is theoretically possible, this has not yet been applied to human studies. The majority of reported studies have relied on relatively large 'bolus' oral doses of riboflavin, comprising at least several milligrams, with urinary monitoring over the subsequent few hours. Riboflavin can be

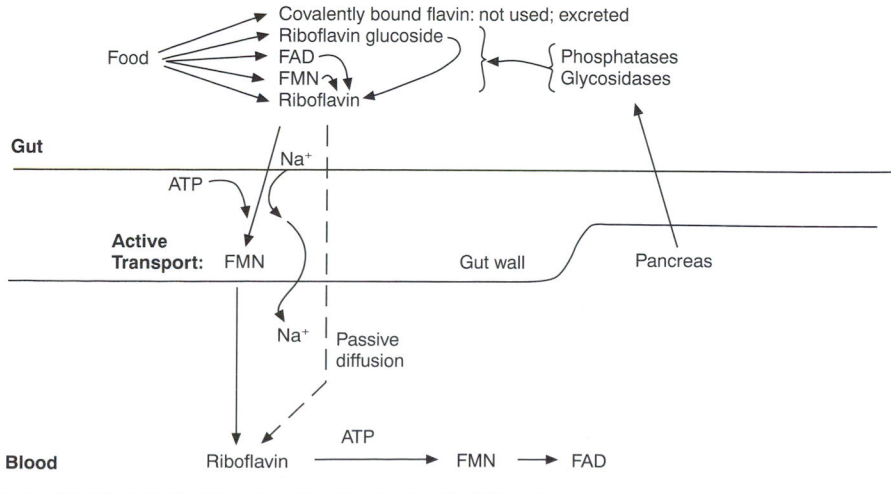

Figure 1 Characteristics of the absorption process for riboflavin and its coenzymes.

quantitated in urine by its very characteristic fluorescence, or by microbiological assay, and high-performance liquid chromatography-based assays have been developed for very accurate work.

For the maximum absorption of a test dose of riboflavin, the duration of exposure within the upper ileum is critical, since this is the region of greatest absorptive efficiency. There is little evidence to suggest that slow-release forms of the vitamin can enhance its absorption, but there does appear to be some absorptive advantage for certain synthetic lipophilic esters, such as the tetrabutyrate ester, which is hydrolysed to the free vitamin during or after absorption. These have been shown to possess beneficial (e.g. antioxidant) properties in some model systems, but their usefulness in human medicine is still at a very early stage of assessment. The concomitant presence of food can enhance absorption, possibly by increasing the transit time. There is little evidence that the efficiency of absorption varies markedly with age or sex in humans.

Although the urinary response to a test dose has been the most commonly used approach to studies of intestinal absorption in humans, it suffers from the potential disadvantage that physiological intakes, and especially low intakes of riboflavin from 'poor' food sources, cannot be measured by this technique. However, such studies of small doses are needed in order to determine the factors which modulate riboflavin absorption in developing countries, where dietary sources of riboflavin are minimal and clinical signs of riboflavin deficiency are common. A much more sensitive biochemical marker of riboflavin status at low intakes is the index known as 'erythrocyte glutathione reductase activation coefficient' (EGRAC), which will be discussed in greater detail later in this article. It is possible to achieve a graded response to graded intakes of riboflavin, and studies of absorption efficiency using this alternative marker as the outcome measure may become feasible (and useful) in the future.

Riboflavin transport at other sites and storage of riboflavin

As mentioned earlier, nearly all tissues require riboflavin. The free vitamin is trapped as one of its phosphorylated coenzyme forms, which then become specifically associated (and in a few cases covalently linked) to the protein chains of catalytic flavoenzymes. If not already covalently linked, the flavin coenzyme can often be liberated by extremes of pH or by other nonphysiological manoeuvres in the test tube. In a few biological locations, such as the mature red cell, a flavoenzyme such as glutathione reductase (NADH: oxidized glutathione oxidoreductase EC 1.6.4.2) may exist – partly in the apoenzyme form (i.e. without its flavin coenzyme and therefore without its normal enzyme activity) – if the animal becomes riboflavin-deficient. A fresh supply of riboflavin will then permit the missing coenzyme (in this case FAD) to be synthesized, and glutathione reductase enzyme activity is restored by combination with the intact apoenzyme protein.

Different enzymes and different tissue sites differ in the tenacity with which they can retain flavin coenzymes in times of riboflavin deficiency, so there is a characteristic 'pecking order' for flavoenzyme protection which appears to reflect the metabolic importance of the different metabolic pathways affected. Apart from this 'pecking order', however, there cannot be said to be any significant repository of unused or nonfunctional riboflavin which could act as a 'store' in times of dietary deficiency. Although some organs (such as liver) have relatively high concentrations of flavin enzymes, all of the flavin in them seems to be present as coenzyme moieties of flavin holoenzymes, which are fully functional. Each tissue has a characteristic 'ceiling' level of riboflavin at saturation, and a 'floor' level characteristic of severe depletion; these are determined, respectively, by the total amount of apoflavoprotein, and the amount of 'resistant' holoenzyme which cannot be depleted of its cofactor during riboflavin deficiency.

Riboflavin is secreted into milk, the concentration being species-specific and to a moderate extent dependent on maternal status and intake. Riboflavin is also required by the developing fetus, which implies a need for active transport from the maternal to the fetal circulation during pregnancy, the flavin concentration being greater on the fetal side. Studies from India have identified a specific riboflavin carrier protein (RCP) present in bird (e.g. chicken) eggs, which is considered to be specific for riboflavin, and is essential for normal embryological development. If this protein is rendered ineffective (e.g. by immuno-neutralization) by treatment of the bird with a specific antibody, then embryonic development ceases and the embryo dies. A genetic mutant lacking RCP is likewise infertile. A homologous protein, which can be rendered ineffective by the antibody to pure chicken riboflavin carrier protein, has been shown to occur in several mammalian species, including two species of monkeys, and also in humans. Termination of pregnancy has also been demonstrated by immuno-neutralization of RCP in monkeys. There remains some controversy over the interpretation of these data and other, less specific, riboflavin binders in blood may also play an important role. These studies have provided an intriguing example of the role of specific vitamin-transporting mechanisms, designed to ensure that the vitamin needs of the developing embryo will be efficiently met. Further evidence of the special needs of developing embryos has been provided by the demonstration that riboflavin analogues can cause teratogenic changes, even in the absence of any detectable damage to maternal tissues.

Metabolism and Excretion

The interconversions of riboflavin with its coenzyme derivatives are depicted in **Fig. 2**. Clearly the 'high-energy nucleotide', ATP, is cosubstrate and driving force (in energy terms), for both stages of the conversion to FAD. Some flavoenzymes specifically require FAD; others specifically require FMN, and it is difficult to account for this dichotomy. **Table 1** lists the broad categories of flavoenzymes found in living tissues: the range of reaction types is considerable, but all of them clearly centre around redox processes involving hydrogen transfer. This fact reflects the central biochemical reaction of the flavin coenzymes,

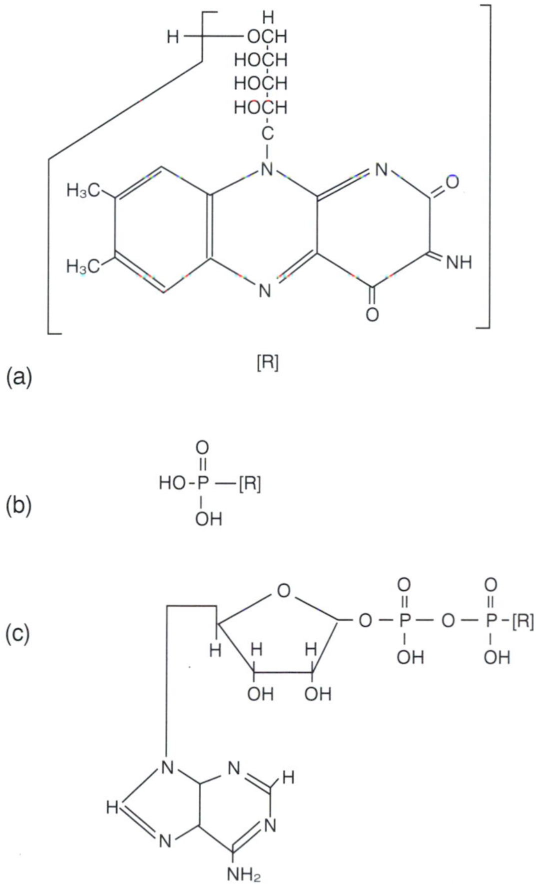

Figure 2   Structure of riboflavin and its coenzyme derivatives. (a) Riboflavin; (b) riboflavin phosphate (flavin mononucleotide, FMN); (c) flavin adenine nucleotide (FAD).

Table 1   Categories of flavoenzymes[a]

Category (subcategory)	Example
1-electron transferases	Mitochondrial electron-transfer flavoprotein
Dehydrogenases	
Pyridine nucleotide dehydrogenases or reductases	Mitochondrial NADH dehydrogenase
Non-pyridine nucleotide dehydrogenases	Mitochondrial succinate dehydrogenase
Pyridine nucleotide-disulfide oxido-reductases	Glutathione reductase
Dehydrogenase-oxygen reductases	
Flavoprotein oxidases $[O_2 \rightarrow H_2O_2]$	Monoamine oxidase
Flavoprotein mono-oxygenases $(1/2\ O_2 \rightarrow H_2O)$	
Internal (α-hydroxy fatty acid $\rightarrow$ fatty acid $(n-1) + CO_2$)	Bacterial lactate mono-oxygenase
External (RH $\rightarrow$ ROH)	Microsomal FAD-containing mono-oxygenase

[a]Source: Merrill AH *et al.* (1981) Formation and mode of action of flavoproteins. *Annual Review of Nutrition* **1**: 281–317.

which is the interconversion of the reduced, dihydro form of the flavin ring and the more stable oxidized form. One of the most important sites of action of flavoenzymes within higher animals is that of the electron transport chain in the mitochondria. The flavins which form part of succinic dehydrogenase and of NADH dehydrogenase form an essential redox link between the oxidizable energy-rich substrates of aerobic metabolism, and the cytochrome chain leading to molecular oxygen, which can generate around 38 moles of energy-rich ATP per mole of glucose oxidized.

Hormone status can affect riboflavin economy in a number of important ways, and there is also some evidence that riboflavin status can affect hormone production. One important control valve for riboflavin economy is thyroid hormone status: hypothyroidism leads to reduced tissue levels of flavin coenzymes, and hence to inactivation of certain flavoenzymes, thus resembling the effects of dietary riboflavin deficiency. Both flavokinase (ATP: riboflavin 5′-phosphotransferase EC 2.7.1.26) and FAD pyrophosphorylase (ATP: FMN adenyltransferase EC 2.7.7.2) are sensitive to thyroid hormone status. In the kidney, synthesis of flavokinase, and hence of flavin coenzymes, is controlled by aldosterone in a similar manner.

The amount of absorbed riboflavin which can remain within the body and the circulation (in blood plasma) is strictly regulated by glomerular and tubular filtration and tubular reabsorption in the kidneys. The latter is an active, saturable, sodium-dependent transport process, with characteristics similar to those of active transport in the gastrointestinal tract. It is responsible for the very sharp and characteristic transition between minimal urinary excretion of riboflavin at low intakes and a much higher level of excretion, proportional to intake, at higher intakes. This transition point has been extensively used to define and to measure riboflavin status and requirements (see below), and to permit studies of intestinal absorption *in vivo* (see above). Excretion of riboflavin is affected by some chemicals (such as boric acid, which complexes with it) and by certain diseases and hormone imbalances.

In addition to the excretion of unchanged riboflavin, there are also small amounts of hydroxylated breakdown products of the vitamin which arise through normal turnover, either within the tissues of the body or in the gastrointestinal tract from bacterial action before absorption. The rate of destruction of riboflavin by this turnover pathway is very low in all species examined to date, and riboflavin within the mammalian body seems to be remarkably efficiently conserved, apparently throughout many cycles of cell turnover.

Metabolic Function and Essentiality

This section will deal in detail with the question: 'what goes wrong when deficiency of riboflavin is encountered, and how does riboflavin interact with other nutrients, or with biochemical and physiological processes, thus producing characteristic functional effects?'

Fatty acid oxidation

The first example of serious metabolic disturbance, seen in moderate riboflavin deficiency, is the disturbance of fatty acid oxidation. The normal first stage in the spiral process of β-oxidation of fatty acids within the mitochondria is the removal of two hydrogen atoms from the two carbons located α and β to the activated carboxyl end of the chain. The fatty acyl coenzyme A substrate is acted upon by one of several fatty acyl-CoA dehydrogenase flavoprotein enzymes (e.g. long-chain acyl-CoA: (acceptor) 2,3-oxidoreductase EC 1.3.99.13), each of which is specific for a small range of acyl chains. The second stage in this process involves transfer of the electrons

via another flavoenzyme, known as 'electron transferring flavoprotein dehydrogenase' (electron-transferring-flavoprotein: ubiquinone oxidoreductase EC 1.5.5.1), and thence to the cytochrome chain and to oxygen. These flavoenzymes, unlike the flavoenzymes that are linked to carbohydrate oxidation, are highly sensitive to dietary riboflavin depletion. Characteristic disturbances of lipid metabolism can therefore be detected in riboflavin-deficient tissues and organisms.

Disturbances in fatty acid oxidation by isolated mitochondria, e.g. from livers of deficient animals, have been demonstrated, and one of the most characteristic metabolic changes, observed even in a mild deficiency state in experimental animals, is the appearance of abnormal dicarboxylic acids, and their derivatives, in the urine. These products seem to arise because fatty acyl intermediates become diverted away from the usual pathway of mitochondrial β-oxidation towards abnormal partial oxidation in the peroxisomes (which are less severely affected by the riboflavin deficiency state).

Genetically normal human subjects have not yet been shown to accumulate these abnormal urinary products, but in contrast, humans who bear an abnormal gene resulting in dicarboxylic aciduria do quite frequently respond to riboflavin supplements, showing a reduction in their excretion of abnormal fatty acid products. It seems that additional dietary riboflavin can help to overcome the inherent genetic abnormality, presumably by providing more of the coenzyme, and thereby making sure that all of the residual fatty acid oxidation machinery is working at its optimum capacity. Interestingly, the accumulation of dicarboxylic acids in urine is characteristic of riboflavin-deficient mammals but not of birds; chick embryos deprived of riboflavin via the genetic lesion of riboflavin carrier protein seem to die in hypoglycaemic shock, but do not exhibit dicarboxylicaciduria.

Iron economy

An important interaction of riboflavin with iron economy has been suspected for many years, partly because iron-deficient animals failed to respond readily to iron supplements if they were also riboflavin-deficient, and also because the redox system involving riboflavin and its coenzymes has been shown to interact very readily with the redox system between ferric and ferrous iron.

Some studies in experimental animals have shown that not only is there evidence for some impairment of absorption of iron in riboflavin-deficient animals, and of its distribution between discrete compartments within the body, but also – more surprisingly and strikingly – a major increase in rates of iron loss from the intestinal mucosa, resulting in impaired retention of the body iron stores. This enhanced rate of iron loss is accompanied by hyperproliferation of crypt cells and increased cellular transit along the villi, leading to an excessive proportion of immature villi, and probably also to a reduction in absorptive area. These studies begin to explain how a combination of iron deficiency and riboflavin deficiency, which is frequently encountered in human populations in many developing countries, may lead to a gradual deterioration of iron status, which is often accompanied by other intestinal lesions and by impaired gut function.

Malaria

Low dietary riboflavin intakes are frequently encountered in malarious areas of the world, and in a small number of studies there has arisen the apparently paradoxical observation that biochemical riboflavin deficiency is associated with a lower level of blood cell parasitaemia, than is encountered in riboflavin-replete subjects. Although neither animal nor human studies have indicated that riboflavin deficiency protects from the life-threatening sequelae of malaria, there does appear to be some interaction between the parasite and flavins within the blood cells, which is not yet fully understood. Interestingly, too, some of the prophylactic drugs used to prevent malaria infection have riboflavin-like structures.

Cataract

Several micronutrients, especially those which can have antioxidant functions in living tissues, have recently been investigated in relation to possible protection against degenerative eye diseases such as cataract. Studies in animal models have suggested, albeit indirectly, that riboflavin status may be important here, and several epidemiological studies, including an intervention study in one region of China, have supported the suggestion that good riboflavin status, or riboflavin supplements, may be protective. Although the evidence must be considered as tentative and incomplete at the present time, this possibility clearly deserves further study.

Vitamin B_6

There are several metabolic interrelationships between riboflavin and vitamin B_6, and some investigators have argued that riboflavin deficiency lesions may arise as the direct result of a disturbance of vitamin B_6 metabolic pathways. The conversion of pyridoxine or pyridoxamine phosphates to pyridoxal phosphate is catalysed by a flavoenzyme (pyridoxaminephosphate oxidase EC 1.4.3.5), so that a deficiency of riboflavin may, at certain key sites, result in a secondary deficiency in B_6-dependent pathways. More evidence is needed to clarify the extent and importance of these interactions.

Physical activity and neuromuscular function

Several studies have documented an apparent increase in riboflavin requirements accompanying an increase in physical exercise in human subjects. This may reflect the fact that anabolic influences and the accretion of new lean body mass creates a demand for the vitamin, for mitochondrial accretion. Intriguingly, there is now also some preliminary evidence that indices of neuromuscular function, as illustrated by 'hand-steadiness', may be influenced by riboflavin status, in communities where riboflavin deficiency is endemic. If confirmed, this might raise the possibility that peripheral neurological function could be affected by riboflavin status in mammals, including humans, just as it has been clearly shown to be in birds.

Assessment of Riboflavin Status

Assessment of status for specific nutrients such as riboflavin is closely bound up with the estimation of requirements in human individuals and groups of subjects, and with the monitoring of human populations for evidence of the adequacy of their intakes. It is usually cheaper, easier and more accurate to collect a sample of blood or urine from an individual and carry out biochemical analyses which determine *status*, than to carry out reliable measurements of *intake* over a period of time, since the latter requires considerable cooperation from the subject, and is also affected by the inevitable uncertainties of food table nutrient values in relation to specific foods and diets.

Biochemical status estimates are generally based upon urinary excretion, or measurements of erythrocyte glutathione reductase (NADPH: oxidized glutathione oxidoreductase EC 1.6.4.2) and its reactivation with flavin adenine dinucleotide (FAD) in red cell lysates. Other biochemical indices, such as total red cell riboflavin concentrations, have been considered but are not widely used, and functional indices, reflecting the competence of flavin-dependent biochemical pathways, are likewise not in common use, except for the investigation of errors of metabolism or rare diseases. The two principal status tests are considered below.

Urinary excretion

As noted earlier, the amount of riboflavin excreted in the urine is negligible at low intakes of the vitamin; as the dietary level rises there is slow increase to a transition point, above which the slope of the excretion rate increases very sharply, and then remains linearly proportional to intake until absorption is saturated. For use in population studies, it has been found convenient to use the creatinine excretion rate as the denominator. The suggested interpretation of urinary riboflavin excretion rates is thus <27 μg riboflavin per g creatinine, deficient; 27–79 μg riboflavin per g creatinine, low; >80 μg riboflavin per g creatinine, acceptable. Detailed studies of the relation between intake and excretion rate have shown that this index is sufficiently sensitive to distinguish riboflavin requirements between people on low-fat, high-carbohydrate diets and the slightly higher requirement associated with high-fat, low-carbohydrate diets. Metabolic states associated with general tissue catabolism can sometimes result in liberation of riboflavin during cell turnover; this increases its urinary excretion even though dietary intake may be low.

The glutathione reductase test

One rather serious drawback of the urinary excretion index for the assessment of riboflavin status is that it is relatively insensitive at low-to-moderate intakes, because the rate of excretion changes slowly and not very predictably with increasing intake in this region of dietary intake. Another important practical drawback is that 24 h urine samples are not easy to collect and excretion rates may fluctuate over short time periods. A more stable index was therefore sought and was identified in the degree of unsaturation of the red blood cell enzyme, glutathione reductase (NADPH: oxidized-glutathione oxidoreductase EC 1.6.4.2), with respect to its flavin cofactor, flavin adenine dinucleotide (FAD) (**Fig. 3**).

As noted earlier, an inadequate supply of dietary riboflavin results in low circulating levels, and hence a gradual progressive loss of cofactor from this red cell flavoenzyme, over a period of several weeks. Since the enzyme protein (apoenzyme) remains intact and reactivable by FAD, it is possible to remove a small sample of blood; collect, wash and haemolyse the red cells; and then measure glutathione reductase activity in the test tube, with and without the FAD cofactor. If the individual is riboflavin-replete, then the added FAD has almost no effect and the 'activation coefficient', or ratio of FAD stimulated to unstimulated activity (EGRAC), is between 1.0 and 1.3–1.4. If the individual is deficient, then added FAD produces a larger stimulation and the 'activation coefficient' is higher. For people living in communities with very low intakes of riboflavin and a significant prevalence of clinically recognizable deficiency, activation coefficients as high as 2.0–3.0 are quite common. In Western countries, however, few values as high as 2.0 are usually encountered.

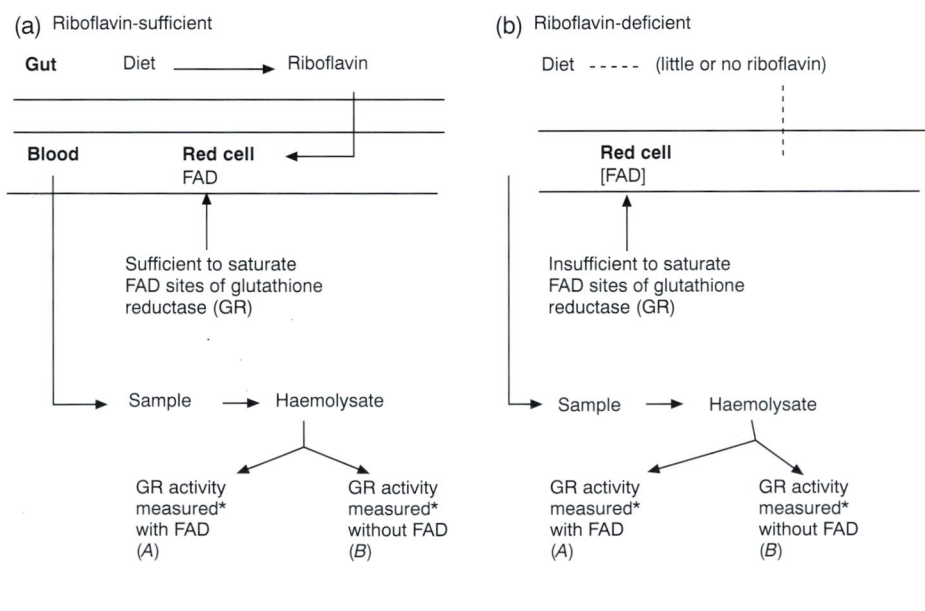

Figure 3 Basis of the glutathione reductase test for riboflavin status. *Reaction of oxidized glutathione with reduced nicotinamide adenine dinucleotide phosphate.

This test has the advantage in that it is highly sensitive to, and predictive of, the extent of tissue depletion in the range of severe-to-moderate deficiency; it is robust and requires only a small sample of blood, and it can be automated by modern enzyme rate reaction analysers. Riboflavin supplements, given to deficient subjects, result in rapid and reproducible restoration of the saturated condition of the enzyme, and graded supplements can be given to estimate human requirements.

There are minor operational differences between different published versions of the analytical procedure for EGRAC which result in small between-laboratory differences in the interpretation of the normal range and there are also some instances of specific factors which cause ambiguity of interpretation. The best known of these is the human genetic variant resulting in glucose-6-phosphate dehydrogenase (D-glucose-6-phosphate: NADP$^+$ 1-oxidoreductase EC 1.1.1.49) deficiency. Both homo- and heterozygotes are affected, and in them erythrocyte glutathione reductase becomes almost saturated with FAD, even in riboflavin-deficient individuals. Other tests of status are required for such individuals.

Some groups of people have increased requirements for riboflavin, related to special metabolic states. There is, for instance, a progressive increase in requirement during pregnancy, followed by a decrease during lactation. Babies exposed to phototherapy for neonatal jaundice also have increased requirements. In certain circumstances the use of oral contraceptives may increase requirements, but the evidence is conflicting. The largest and most dramatic increases in requirements have been seen (as noted earlier) in a subgroup of people with inborn metabolic errors leading to dicarboxylicaciduria and associated clinical abnormalities. Although certain drugs are known to affect riboflavin status indices, there is no clear consensus on the question of the need for supplements by people who are prescribed such drugs – clearly this needs further study.

Requirements

As with most micronutrients, the evidence on which requirement estimates are based, can be subdivided into the following broad classes of criteria:

1. prevention of clinical (pathological) deficiency;
2. attainment of specified blood levels, or tissue stores of riboflavin;
3. titration to the urinary excretion threshold;
4. tests based on cofactor saturation of one or more accessible, diet-sensitive, flavin-dependent enzymes, such as erythrocyte glutathione reductase;

5. physiological function.

Of these five classes of criteria, the first has been useful in defining 'minimum' requirements, but it has several practical drawbacks. First, clinical signs of deficiency in human communities tend to be non-specific and multifactorial. Second, studies involving clinical deficiency in controlled trials would be ethically unacceptable. Use of physiological functional indices in relation to riboflavin deficiency (analogous to dark adaptation for vitamin A, clotting factors for vitamin K, etc.) has not proved possible because the analogous riboflavin-sensitive physiological processes are insufficiently specific, controllable or easily measurable for use in population studies. Of the other three possible indices, urinary excretion and the flavin-dependent enzyme, erythrocyte glutathione reductase, are generally considered to be the front-runners in the race for acceptance in human studies. These have been described in the previous section.

For avoidance of clinical deficiency signs in normal healthy adults, the basic requirement for riboflavin is 0.55–0.8 mg per day. The UK reference nutrient intake for riboflavin is 1.3 mg per day for men and 1.1 mg per day for women, rising to 1.6 mg per day during pregnancy and lactation. For formula-fed infants, the reference intake is 0.4 mg per day.

Dietary Sources and High Intakes

Table 2 lists the riboflavin content of some commonly consumed foods in Western countries. As is the case with most other B vitamins, the richest food sources comprise items such as offal and yeast extract, with meat and dairy products also providing quite generous amounts; fruit and vegetables provide somewhat less, with the smallest amounts, in relation to their energy content, being present in ungerminated grains and seeds, such as nuts. There is an enormous difference in intakes and in status observed between that found in most Western countries, where the basic dietary intake tends to be quite generous, and that in many developing countries, where populations have to depend largely on monotonous and riboflavin-poor staple diets such as polished rice. In developing countries, riboflavin deficiency tends to be widespread. Although even a severe riboflavin deficiency is less obviously life-threatening than some other types of malnutrition that are commonly encountered in the Third World, it can nevertheless be a major source of debility, through skin lesions and metabolic dysfunctions, and riboflavin nutrition thus deserves an important place in future public health programmes.

As with most other B vitamins, riboflavin and its cofactors are remarkably nontoxic even at high

Table 2 Riboflavin content of selected (cooked) foods

	mg per 100 g wet weight	mg per 1000 kcal[a]
Meat, offal and fish		
Stewed mince beef	0.33	1.4
Grilled pork chop	0.2	0.6
Calf liver, fried	4.2	16.5
Lamb's kidney, fried	2.3	14.8
Cod, grilled	0.06	0.6
Dairy products		
Cow's milk, full cream	0.17	2.6
Cheese, cheddar	0.4	1.0
Yogurt (whole milk, plain)	0.27	3.4
Boiled chicken's egg	0.35	2.4
Human milk	0.03	0.4
Fruits		
Apples, eating flesh and skin	0.02	0.4
Oranges, flesh	0.04	1.1
Pears, flesh and skin	0.03	0.7
Strawberries, raw	0.03	1.1
Dried mixed fruit	0.05	0.2
Vegetables		
Potatoes, boiled, new	0.02	0.3
Carrots, boiled, young	0.01	0.3
Brussel sprouts, boiled	0.09	2.6
Cauliflower, boiled	0.04	1.4
Onion, fried	0.01	0.1
Grains, grain products, nuts, beans		
White bread	0.06	0.3
Wholemeal bread	0.09	0.4
Rice, boiled, white	Trace	Trace
Cornflakes (Kellogg)	1.3	3.6
Baked beans in tomato sauce	0.06	0.7
Peanuts, plain	0.10	0.2
Other		
Marmite (yeast hydrolysate)	11.0	64
Bovril (beef hydrolysate)	7.4	44

Compiled from Holland B, Welch AA, Unwin ID, Buss DH, Paul AA, and Southgate DAT (1991) *McCance and Widdowson's The Composition of Foods*, 5th edn. London: Royal Society of Chemistry and MAFF. (With the permission of the Controller of Her Majesty's Stationery Office).
[a]Or mg per 4130 kJ.

intakes. The reasons for this are probably associated with limitations on absorption, once the active transport process has become saturated in the gut, coupled with very effective urinary excretion of any absorbed vitamin which is in excess of cellular requirements.

See also: **Fatty Acids**: Metabolism. **Iron**: Physiology, Dietary Sources and Requirements. **Vitamin B$_6$**: Physiology.

Further Reading

Bates CJ (1987) Human riboflavin requirements, and metabolic consequences of deficiency in man and animals. *World Review of Nutrition and Dietetics* 50:215–265.

Bro-Rasmussen F (1958) The riboflavin requirement of animals and man and associated metabolic relations. 1. Technique of estimating requirement, and modifying circumstances. 2. Relation of requirement to the metabolism of protein and energy. *Nutrition Abstracts and Reviews* 28:1–23;369–386.

Friedrich W (1988) Vitamin B$_2$: riboflavin and its bioactive variants. In: *Vitamins*, chap. 7, pp 403–471. Berlin: Walter de Gruyter and Co.

Merrill AH, Lambeth JD, Edmondson DE and McCormick DB (1981) Formation and mode of action of flavoproteins. *Annual Review of Nutrition* 1:281–317.

McCormick DB (1989) Two inter-connected B vitamins: riboflavin and pyridoxine. *Physiological Reviews* 69:1170–1198.

Powers HJ (1995) Riboflavin-iron interactions with particular emphasis on the gastrointestinal tract. *Proceedings of the Nutrition Society* 54:509–517.

Ross NS and Hansen TPB (1992) Riboflavin deficiency is associated with selective preservation of critical flavo-enzyme-dependent metabolic pathways. *Biofactors* 3:185–190.

White HB and Merrill AH (1988) Riboflavin-binding proteins. *Annual Review of Nutrition* 8: 279–299.

Rickets *see* **Cholecalciferol and Ergocalciferol**: Rickets and Osteomalacia.

Roughage *see* **Dietary Fibre** : Physiological Effects and Effects on Absorption; Potential Role in the Aetiology of Disease; Role in Nutritional Management of Disease.

S

SALT

Epidemiology

C P Sánchez-Castillo, National Institute of Nutrition, Mexico

W P T James, Rowett Research Institute, Aberdeen, Scotland, UK

Occurrence in Nature

The terms salt, sea salt or table salt relate primarily to the compound sodium chloride. Sodium is the sixth most abundant element in the Earth's crust, of which it constitutes 2.8%. Sodium is a reactive element and is always found in compound form. There is a huge variety of salts containing sodium and many of these are found in food. Sodium chloride is very soluble in water and in seawater comprises about 80% of the dissolved matter. Salt in food is used mainly for its preservative, functional and seasoning properties.

A History of Salt Intake

The fundamental importance of salt has been recognized from the earliest times when humans evolved in a hot African environment with scarce sources of salt. In common with other terrestrial animals, humans have special taste and salt appetite systems and have evolved an effective intestinal, urinary and skin conservation system to minimize losses so that fundamental requirements for salt can be met.

Evidence has been found of salt use during the Neolithic Age and the Egyptian, Babylonian and Chinese civilizations all had special culinary uses for salt that are well documented. Evidence for the exploitation of saline slicks in the Austrian Tyrol dates from the Bronze Age. For the Indians in Central America, salt was so precious that to please their gods they abstained from eating salt, and Mexican civilizations offered sacrifices to the Goddess of Salt, Vixtocioatl. In the USA, the Cherokee people placed a cup or glass of salt on the chest during burial. Arab cultures still offer salt to visitors as a sign that their guest is safe; even a Bedouin robber will not violate the laws of hospitality once he has tasted his host's salt.

In pre-Roman times, the principal road started at the salt works near the mouth of the Tiber River and cut through the Italian peninsula towards the Adriatic. In North Africa the caravan route linked the salt oases, while salt roads were a feature of several South American countries. From remote parts of South America, such as the Amazon and Argentina, trails of more than 1000 miles were linked to form the famous 'Cerro de Sal'. In the sixteenth century, sea salt crystals were traded from the sea through the Andes, gradually becoming more expensive further from the sea so that at distances of over 300 km it was used only by tribal chiefs. The common people made do with salt processed from palms and human urine. Salt from springs near Bogota was traded over a distance of 200 km to the north and south. When the first Spaniards arrived in South America in 1537, they found Indians exploiting local salt reserves on a large scale. In Mexico, during the Classic Period there had been a salt trade between the Peten and Yucatan, and by Post-Classical times the island of Cozumel served as an important stopping point in the salt trade between Yucatan, Belize and Honduras.

The financial structure of Venice was also substantially affected by the salt trade, which contributed to the emergence of Venetian capitalism and the vast fortunes of some Venetian merchants. In France salt became a political issue in the fourteenth century; the tax on salt was the most hated of all taxes and a major issue prior to the French Revolution. At that time England, Germany and Italy also taxed salt.

During the earliest period of British rule in India the supply of salt was contentious, often a monopoly, and then taxed. Gandhi emphasized the essential nature of common salt for human and animal wellbeing, especially in a tropical country like India. Cereals and green foods were known to be particularly low in salt, so the vegetarians and rice eaters of

Indian labourers required 'the consumption of salt per head for maintaining a decent standard of health and hygiene'. Gandhi's 'salt march' to the sea broke the monopoly on salt use and led to his arrest and jailing. The following revolt, with 100 000 arrests, brought a change in the law to allow people to produce salt for their own use. Indian salt consumption ranged between 11 and 14 g per head per day, whereas English adults enjoyed 30 g per day. The cost of family salt was equal to about one-sixth of an Indian's annual earnings, whereas a Bengali or Madras soldier on foreign service received up to 55 g per day of salt with salt fish provided in addition. Adulteration of salt with earth became a common practice in India and some salts contained only 3% sodium chloride and were mostly (80%) sodium sulfate.

The Production of Salt

The production of salt was a major industry in China for centuries. The Chinese had sophisticated methods for obtaining salt: coastal saltworks boiled seawater, but solar evaporation was also used. Shallow salt fields were filled with seawater which was shifted from field to field until salt crystallization began. In low areas canals led to the sea. Inland wells were dug and sea or underground salt water was lifted into the fields by windmill or by two men using a wooden bucket. In Egypt salt was extracted in the Nile Delta from seawater and also from lakes near Memphis. Egyptians paid both a salt tax and a sales tax.

Salt in Food Technology

Salt modifies flavour, controls microbial growth, and alters nutrient availability and the texture/consistency of food. It also aids extraction methods, food formulation and aids the malting and fermenting of foods. In the production of some foods, e.g. pickles, cheese and fermented sausages, salt acts to withdraw water and various nutrients from the pickled tissue and provides an appropriate environment for growing the specific salt-resistant bacteria required for the fermentation or pickling process.

The early discovery of salt's inhibition of microbiological spoilage was a significant development in the earliest recorded food technology. Sodium is also important in forming the texture of cheese, limiting bacterial growth and dehydrating cheese, thereby helping to form the rind. Most processed meats, e.g. ham and bacon, have added salt to season and cure the meat. Salt also inhibits bacterial growth and helps to emulsify the fat in sausages.

Sodium nitrate is used as a curing agent to prevent botulism as well as to provide the cured taste and red colour of such meat products. Sodium polyphosphate is added to poultry and fish fingers to increase their water-holding capacity and to bind the product. Salt is also effective in binding meat together by altering protein structure and dissolving some proteins. Salting fish has both a flavouring and a preservative role and fish is treated in brine before being smoked.

In baking, salt enhances other flavours in the product; it also controls the rate of fermentation of yeast-leavened products and prevents the development of undesirable 'wild' types of yeast which would lead to uncontrolled fermentation rates and variable products. Salt strengthens the gluten in bread doughs, thus helping to ensure good dough-handling and reducing the rate of water absorption. Sodium acid pyrophosphates are used in many industrial baking powders for speciality products. Salting of canned vegetables is primarily for flavour, but it can be used to separate mature, starchy green beans or peas, which will sink, from the younger, fresher beans, which float.

Some fruits and vegetables can be peeled using a sodium hydroxide or lye solution, but subsequent washing reduces the residual sodium levels. Some processed 'snacks' are also heavily salted, as are processed cereals. Sodium-containing ingredients are added to many processed foods (**Table 1**), with sodium chloride accounting for about 90% of the sodium used by the food industry.

Table 1 Sodium-containing additives used in food processing

Additive	Use
Sodium citrate	Flavouring, preservative
Sodium chloride	Flavouring, texture, preservative
Sodium nitrate	Preservative, colour fixative
Sodium nitrite	Preservative, colour fixative
Sodium tripoliphosphate	Binder
Sodium benzoate	Preservative
Sodium eritrobate	Antioxidant
Sodium propionate	Preservative
Monosodiumglutamate	Flavour enhancer
Sodium aluminosilicate	Anticaking agent
Sodium aluminium phosphate acidic	Acidity regulatory, emulsifier
Sodium cyclamate	Artificial sweetener
Sodium alginate	Thickener and vegetable gum
Sodium caseinate	Emulsifier
Sodium bicarbonate	Yeast substitute

Other uses of salt

Salt is not used for food processing alone. It is also a good antiseptic, which is why the Roman word for the salt crystals (sal) originates from Salus, the Goddess of Health.

The universal use of common salt has allowed it to be used as a vehicle for combating widespread iodine deficiency by fortifying the salt with iodine, and fluoride has also been added as a preventive measure against dental caries. Chloroquine or pyrimethamine salt mixtures have been used to suppress the sporozoites responsible for vivax malaria.

The impact of refrigeration

Salt intake varies widely across the world. Some agricultural communities, e.g. the Yanomano Indians from Brazil and the Chimbus of New Guinea, do not consume salt other than that found in natural food sources. The Kamtschadales and the Tungouses nomadic tribes from the north of Russia and Siberia are also averse to added salt, whereas the Japanese have traditionally consumed large quantities of salt in pickled salted fish and vegetables.

Without food preservation it would be impossible to supply urban populations with food in any systematic way. A fall in salt consumption has occurred in most countries (**Table 2**) as refrigeration has taken over from salting as a method of preserving food. In Japan, intakes as extreme as the 60 g intake of a farmer in 1955 and the usual 27–30 g per person per day have fallen dramatically to 8–15 g per person per day in 1988. Refrigerators were introduced on a mass scale from the 1960s onwards. In the USA, however, salt intake probably started to decline in the 1920s as ice-boxes and refrigerators became widely available.

Changes in Mineral Composition of Food Induced by Industrialization and Urbanization

Historically salt was not only used as a preservative,

Table 2 Salt intake as NaCl (g per day)

Before 1982[a]	Year	Intake	From 1988[b]	Year	Intake
Communities not using added salt					
Brazil (Yanomamo Indian)	1975	0.06			
New Guinea (Chimbus)	1967	0.40			
Solomon Island (Kwaio)		1.20			
Botswana (Kung Bushmen)		1.80			
Polynesia (Pukapuka)		3.60			
Alaska (Eskimos)	1961	<4.00			
Marshall Islands in Pacific		7.00			
Salt-using communities					
Kenya (Sambura nomads)		5–8	Mexico (Tarahumsa Indian)		3–10
Mexico (Tarahumsa Indian)	1978	5–8	Mexico Rural (Nalinalco)	1992	5.7
			Mexico Urban (Tlalpan)	1991	7.18
Denmark		9.8	Denmark	1988	8.00
Canada (New Foundland)		9.9	Canada		8–10
New Zealand		10.1			
Sweden (Gotenburg)		10.2			
USA (EvansCountry, Georgia)		10.6	USA (Chicago)		7.7
Iran		10.9			
Belgium	1966	11.4	Belgium	1988	8.4
UK (Scotland)		11.5			
Australia		12.0			
India (North)		12–15	India		9–11.4
Federal Republic of Germany		13.1			
Finland (East)		14.3	Finland		10.6
Bahamas		15–30			
Kenya (Samburus, Army)	1969	18.6			
Korea		19.9			
Japan					
Japan (farmer)	1955	60.3	Japan	1988	8–15
Japan (Akita)		27–30			
Japan	1964	20.9			

[a]Source: Intersalt.
[b]Source: Pietinen.

Table 3 Salting of foods in Western societies

	Na	K	Ca	Mg
Maize-based products				
Corn	4	284	55	41
Tortilla, rural	11	192	177	65
Breakfast cereals	866	101	3	11
Processed snacks	838	197	102	56
Wheat-based products				
Natural cereals	39	1166	94	343
Tortillas, wheat	622	73	11	17
Breakfast cereals	855	869	81	236
Processed bread (urban)	573	126	47	31
Salted bread, made locally (rural)	410	92	10	74
Sweet bread, made locally (rural)	97	93	87	18
Processed bread (rural)	344	79	213	18
Processed biscuits	582	80	16	17
Pulses				
Unprocessed, cooked	53	373	50	41
Processed, canned	354	371	27	79

but also for flavouring, to add variety to bland or monotonous diets, and to encourage the consumption of food, such as a sausage from meat by-products, that might otherwise be wasted. Once established, such foods (**Table 3**), became embedded in the culture. Thus, in Mexico City, the process of industrialization and urbanization has affected the nutritional value of many of the more traditional foods (**Table 4**). Although corn and maize tortillas, together with beans, formed the staple traditional diet, tortillas are now being produced differently, both industrially and by individuals at small market stalls.

The concentrations of the major nutrients sodium, potassium, calcium, magnesium and phosphorus in unprocessed foods vary within narrow limits, but in

Table 4 Effects of industrialization in the composition of Mexican foods

Food	Salt content (mmol (g per 100 g fresh weight))		
	Na	K	Ca
Maize foods			
Corn	4	284	55
Tortilla	11	192	177
Breakfast cereals	866	101	3
Snacks	838	197	102
Beans			
Beans, cooked	14	470	67
Beans, processed	354	371	26

Source: Sanchez-Castillo *et al*. (1994, 1995).

processed or cooked foods, where salt (NaCl) or additions of other sodium-containing ingredients are common, the concentration range of sodium is higher. A large proportion of processed food has salt added; as more processed foods are eaten, the saltier the diet becomes. **Table 3** shows that the maize in its original form contains a very small concentration of sodium but is rich in potassium. Once the grain is milled, fractionated and processed to produce tortillas, then the nutrient composition alters. Potassium is lost during the initial washing procedure. Limestone is added to release the niacin from its bound form; this also induces a 3-fold increase in calcium content. Salt is not commonly added during tortilla preparation in the country, but a remarkable 70 to 200-fold increase is found in breakfast cereals and processed maize snacks with substantial potassium losses. Almost no calcium is found in breakfast cereals whereas traditionally prepared tortillas have almost 60 times more calcium.

Salt and Disease

A long-term excess intake of salt is regarded as an inducer of hypertension and thus a risk for stroke and coronary heart disease. An excess of dietary salt may also affect three other conditions/diseases: gastric cancer, osteoporosis and bronchial hyperreactivity.

Salt intake and blood pressure

The importance of salt in inducing high blood pressure is based on animal experiments in investigations at the cellular level, clinical studies and dietary intervention trials as well as population analyses of blood pressure in relation to salt intake. Some evidence suggests that chloride may play a pivotal role in the regulation of renin release and hypertension when sodium chloride is fed, but in practical terms the discrimination between sodium and chloride intakes in man is unnecessary since sodium and chloride intakes are closely matched. Attempts have been made to look at the differential intake of salt in those with and without overt clinical hypertension. **Table 5** shows that studies have sometimes found a modest increase in the salt intake of hypertensives.

Part of the difficulty in demonstrating a link between salt intake and hypertension is the wide range of individual salt sensitivity, the complications arising from the age-related increases in blood pressure and the interactions of other factors. These include altered maternal nutrition with a programming of subsequent tissue sensitivity to high salt intakes, the effects of weight gain, the impact of excess alcohol intakes, and the modulating effects of

Table 5 Sodium expressed as salt excretion in g per day as an index of salt intake in adults with and without hypertension

Author	Men		Women		Combined sexes	
	Hypertensive	Normotensive	Hypertensive	Normotensive	Hypertensive	Normotensive
Ljungman (1981)	10.2 ± 3.2	10.0 ± 3.7				
Simpson (1978)	10.3	10.0	8.0	8.1		
Miall (1959)			7.1 ± 2.3	7.9 ± 2.8		
Phear (1958)	9.1 ± 3.2	8.9 ± 2.7				
Tuomilehto (1980)	11.4 ± 4.3	11.4 ± 4.4	10.0 ± 3.1	10.4 ± 3.2		
Beevers[b] (1980)	10.6 ± 4.0	11.4 ± 3.6	8.4 ± 3.4	10.0 ± 3.1		
Berglund (1976)	10.2 ± 3.2	11.5 ± 2.5				
Dahl (1958)	11.6 ± 3.1	10.5 ± 3.5				
Doyle[a] (1976)						
Bing (1979)					8.2 ± 3.2	6.8 ± 3.2
Morgan[a] (1975)					9.0 ± 0.6	8.8 ± 3.9

Amplified from Watt and Foy (1982).
[a]Studies with higher excretion in hypertensive patients.
[b]Studies with higher excretion in normotensive patients.

high potassium intakes and other modest ionic effects, e.g. of high calcium intakes.

Rural–urban differences in salt intake and blood pressure In most countries rural–urban differences in diet and blood pressure exist, with higher prevalences of hypertension in urban than in rural communities. This is shown in a classic migrant study undertaken in Uganda, where adults migrating to urban societies begin to manifest a rise in their blood pressure within weeks and later an increasing prevalence of hypertension. **Table 6** shows some of the differences between those individuals living in their original environment and those who have migrated to more complex societies.

More recent studies, e.g. in Mexico (**Table 7**), also show the impact of dietary change so these original African studies are not isolated observations.

Interaction of sodium, potassium and calcium

Both epidemiological and clinical evidence suggest that dietary deficiencies of potassium or calcium potentiate sodium chloride induction of high blood pressure. Thus the ratio of urinary sodium to potassium (Na : K) is a stronger correlate of blood pressure than either sodium or potassium alone. Results of clinical trials suggest that an increased potassium intake decreases blood pressure in patients with hypertension and the antihypertensive effect of potassium is more pronounced in persons consuming a high sodium chloride intake.

Primitive societies living on a low-salt diet often ingest large quantities of potassium and have blood pressures which are not only low in early adult life but are maintained at this level throughout life. With acculturation, primitive societies tend to both increase the sodium intake and reduce the potassium content of their diet. The combination of a high potassium with a high-salt diet is, therefore, somewhat unusual but has been found in the Aomori prefecture of Japan where there is a lower blood pressure and a reduced mortality from strokes despite high salt intakes. Potassium loading also prevents or ameliorates the development of sodium chloride-induced hypertension in several animal models.

There is also an inverse association within and

Table 6 Migration studies which assess rural–urban differences in Africa

	Villager	Migrant
Mean systolic blood pressure (mmHg)[a]	112	124
Systolic blood pressure/age slope[b]	0.15	0.64
Urinary Na (mmol l⁻¹)[b]	82.4	108.6
Urinary K (mmol l⁻¹)[b]	67.4	38.4
Skinfold thickness[a]	11.0	13.5

[a]Shaper et al. (1969) (Samburu's from Kenya).
[b]Mugambi (1986) (African Luo's).

Table 7 The urinary 24-hour output of electrolytes and the associated blood pressure (BP) differences in rural and urban Mexico

	Men		Women	
	Rural n = 24	Urban n = 19	Rural n = 54	Urban n = 58
Na (mmol per day)	103.3	133.1	93.3	114.7
K (mmol per day)	41.6	56.7	36.9	50.4
Na/K	2.64	2.51	2.67	2.44
NaCl (g per day)	5.99	7.72	5.41	6.65
Systolic BP (mmHg)	110.4	114.3	104.4	113.8
Diastolic BP (mmHg)	73.3	75.6	67.0	72.8

among populations between dietary calcium and blood pressure. A low calcium intake may amplify the effect of a high sodium chloride intake on blood pressure, and calcium supplementation blunts the effect of a high sodium chloride intake on blood pressure. High dietary calcium also preferentially lowers blood pressure or attenuates the development of hypertension in sodium chloride-sensitive experimental models.

Some evidence in rodents also suggests that sucrose potentiates the sodium chloride sensitivity of blood pressure, but the interaction between sucrose and sodium chloride has not been evaluated in humans.

Salt sensitivity

Rats have different blood pressure responses to salt so it is possible to breed salt-sensitive and salt-resistant colonies. Salt infusion and deprivation studies in humans also suggest marked differences in sensitivity. Young adults from families with hypertension have a greater rate of sodium excretion after a salt load than adults from normotensive families. Twin studies also provide convincing evidence for a hereditary component to salt sensitivity and Blacks are considered to be more salt-sensitive than Whites living in the USA. Molecular genetics is therefore now being used to identify the range of genes responsible for salt sensitivity. Nevertheless, environmental factors are crucial, as shown by the remarkable increase in blood pressure between rural and urban Blacks in the Cameroons, with higher rates in their distant relatives in St Lucia, Jamaica and Barbados. The highest levels of blood pressure are then found in American Blacks.

Genetic influences

Children with a family history of hypertension are 30% more likely to remain in the upper quartile of systolic blood pressure than their peers. However, the effect of family history decreases with age as other environmental factors, e.g. weight gain, modifies the risk (**Table 8**).

Age-related changes in blood pressure

The rise of blood pressure with age occurs exclusively and invariably in salt-eating societies. This age-related rise is absent with sodium intakes of <40 mmol per day and is rare at mean sodium excretion rates of < 100 mmol per day.

Intersalt studies

A major transnational study of over 10 000 men and women described the association between urinary excretion of sodium chloride (as a measure of salt intake) and blood pressure. After adjustments for body weight, alcohol intake, sex and age, a higher sodium intake of 100 mmol per day was linked with a systolic blood pressure rise of 3–6 mmHg in adults aged 40 years but one of 10 mmHg 30 years later. Updated results suggest that the association between sodium excretion and blood pressure is stronger when not adjusted for body weight, but the relationship is present whether or not the adjustment is made.

Animal data suggest that excess salt may be particularly deleterious if given in early life. The age-dependent increase in blood pressure may occur because stretching of an artery induces the synthesis of elastin, which is the dominant fibrous form of

Table 8 Genetic and environmental contributions to disease: the enhanced risk if a relative or parent has genetic vascular disease or dies from a variety of conditions

Relative with disease	Increased risk for:		
	Males under 55	Females under 65	Children of adoptive parents
Ischaemic heart disease			
Male under 55	5.2	2.8	–
Female under 65	6.4	6.9	–
Death of parent under 55	Males and females under 58		
All causes	1.71		1.0
Natural causes	1.98		1.0
Infections	5.81		1.0
Cardiovascular and cerebrovascular disease	4.52		3.02
Cancer	1.19		5.16

From Barclay et al. (1991).

connective tissue in the inner arterial wall. As the elastin mass enlarges the artery is less able to stretch. Blood pressure percentile charts specified in relation to age or height are available with height being the more reliable reference. Defining the cut-off of normality may be taken as 135/85 for the systolic and diastolic blood pressures, i.e. the 95th centiles, or two standard deviations above the mean, but the traditional health cut-off point is 140/90 for specifying hypertension.

Table 9 shows the estimated changes with age in blood pressures as the salt intake is increased by 100 mmol sodium per day. Epidemiologists concerned with the subtle but substantial population effects are mostly of the opinion that salt is an important causal factor in determining the steady increase in average blood pressure and in the prevalence of hypertension in Western societies.

Adults with episodic high blood pressure, e.g. as a response to mental stress, have a greater tendency to develop persisting hypertension. The higher the blood pressure level becomes, the greater the further increase in blood pressure. Thus, the age-dependent increase in blood pressure may be a particularly important factor to measure in both individuals and the community.

Salt reduction in pre-existing hypertension

Salt deprivation became the major means of treating hypertension in the early part of the twentieth century. The low-salt diets were notoriously unpalatable to patients, who became semistarved, and the consequent weight loss helped to reduce blood pressure. A large number of trials of salt restriction have been

conducted since then on both hypertensive and normal subjects and the overall analyses show that the greater the blood pressure, the more marked the fall in blood pressure, particularly if the sodium intake reduction is marked and persists. These data have been interpreted to suggest that the effect of a universal moderate reduction in dietary salt would substantially reduce mortality from stroke and ischaemic heart disease. This impact could be far greater than that achieved by drug treatment of those with high blood pressure. Thus the World Health Organization (WHO) and most national dietary guidelines now call for a lowering of salt intake to 6 g per day on average or less.

Gastric cancer and stroke

There is a strong geographical correlation between stomach cancer and stroke mortality, both of which correlate with salt intake. There are four recognized major aetiological factors for gastric adenocarcinoma: infection with *Helicobacter pylori*, excessive salt intake, low intake of ascorbic acid and low intakes of carotenoids or more generically of vegetables and fruits. Sodium chloride induces atrophic gastritis and enhances the mutagenic effect of nitrosated foods. Salt may also play a role in the later steps involving the transformation of mucosal dysplasia to carcinoma. The salted pickles and salted fish of Japanese cultures appear to be strongly linked to the development of stomach cancers.

Osteoporosis

It has been known for many years that sodium intake is one of the major determinants of urinary calcium excretion. Experimentally sodium intake increases calcium excretion but also induces markers of bone resorption. It is hypothesized that trabecular demineralization may occur, leading to postmenopausal changes and an increased risk of vertebral fractures and cortical erosions.

Bronchial hyper-reactivity

There have been no large-scale epidemiological studies, but a positive relationship between asthma mortality and regional purchases of table salt per person have been shown. In a randomized double-blind crossover trial in subjects with moderately severe asthma, the airway response to histamine was related to urinary excretion of sodium in a dose–response way, but only in men. A low-salt diet is regarded as having a potentially favourable effect in patients with asthma and may help to reduce the need for antiasthma drugs.

Table 9 Predicted change in systolic and diastolic blood pressure (mmHg) for each 100 mmol per 24 h change in sodium intake for various centiles of blood pressure distribution

Age (years)	Centile				
	5th	20th	50th	80th	95th
Systolic					
15–19	3	4	5	6	7
20–29	2	4	5	6	8
30–39	2	4	6	7	9
40–49	2	4	7	9	11
50–59	4	6	9	12	15
60–69	6	8	10	13	15
Diastolic					
15–19	1	1	2	2	3
20–29	1	2	3	3	4
30–39	1	2	3	4	5
40–49	2	3	4	4	5
50–59	2	3	5	6	7
60–69	2	3	4	6	7

Sources of Salt Intake

Various approaches to measuring the daily salt intake in individuals have been tried. Salt comes from: (1) salt in natural products; (2) salt added during industrial processing; (3) salt from catering; (4) other sodium-containing sources: (5) discretionary salt – cooking and table salt; and (6) sodium in drinking water. **Table 10** shows some assessments of Finnish statistics on sodium intakes, based on various traditional approaches. Traditional methods of estimating salt intake, e.g. with economic data, lead to marked errors and usually substantial overestimates. These are now set aside in favour of more modern methods.

The problem with the older methods for measuring personal salt use came when defining the amount of salt derived from sources over which the person had little or no control, i.e. 'nondiscretionary' sources. Most old studies also failed to consider the losses of salt from manufactured foods during cooking. Thus, for example, salted processed vegetables have a high sodium content, but this can be expected to fall once the vegetables are cooked in water. It is therefore important to take account of salt losses and potential salt gains during cooking.

Estimating salt intakes

The principal method for estimating sodium intake is to measure sodium excretion rates in individuals who are asked to collect one or more complete 24-hour urinary outputs. Until recently, however, there was no way of establishing how much of the 24-hour sodium intake was derived from different sources, without the use of traditional weighing and analytical methods. A new technique, involving the use of lithium, has allowed a new approach. The lithium method is novel and involves the fusing of Li_2Co_4 with the NaCl to be used as a tracer. One preliminary 24-hour collection and three full 24-hour urinary collections are required.

The lithium technique provides completely new opportunities for studying the sources of salt intake. Lithium and sodium are not treated equivalently by the sweat gland, as shown by the fact that lithium output in sweat does not mirror increases in sodium output. This means that lithium is probably a very reliable food marker of tagged salt or food intake, whatever the climate or activity status of the subject. In regions where sweat losses may be considerable, lithium remains a valid marker of the specified intake derived from the tagged salt source of interest. The

Table 10 Sources of salt in the Finnish diet

Calculated salt source	Source of information	Amount (g per person per day)	
Crude statistical estimates			
Average salt intake per head per day[a]	Food commodities (1980)	6.9	
	Salt marketing firms (1980)	4.8	
	Sitra (Anon, 1979)	1.0	
Total salt intake		12.7	
Refined statistical estimates			
Naturally occurring sodium (g NaCl per day)	Finnish mineral food tables (Varo, 1981)	1.5	
Salt sold per household	Salt marketing firms	4.8	
Salt in foodstuffs manufactured in Finland	Survey of the Finnish food industry federation (Anon, 1981)	3.5	
Salt from bakery products	Salovaara (1981)	1.8	
Catering	Sitra (Anon, 1979)	1.0	
Total salt intake		12.6	
Dietary survey		Men	Women
NaCl intake (g per head per day)		12.1	8.6
		13.7[a]	9.7[a]
From urine measurements		10.7	8.0
		12.6[a]	10.1[a]

[a]From Seppanen et al. Calculations are those of Pietinen.

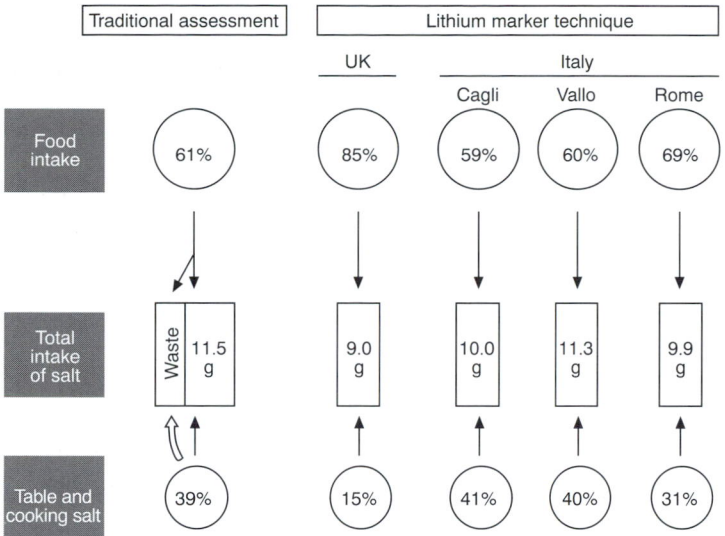

Figure 1 Assessing the sources of dietary salt.

total sodium intakes may, however, be underestimated. Thus, whereas skin sodium losses normally amount to < 10 mmol per day, intense exercise in cool climates may induce salt losses of 60–70 mmol per day. Unacclimatized subjects sweating with heavy physical activity in a tropical environment can lose nearly 60 mmol Na^+ per day; however, within a week of acclimatization this loss will fall very substantially.

Since lithium does not track salt losses in sweat, the ratio of lithium to sodium in urine reflects both the diluting effects of additional sodium ingested from nontagged sources and the effects of the selective loss of sodium from the skin during sweating. Lithium-tagged salt can be used in the prepared food or other source of interest. The amount of cooking salt eaten can then be measured because the tracer lithium tracks the sodium through the cooking and eating processes. After first measuring the back-

ground urinary recovery of ingested lithium, the proportions of lithium in the tagged cooking salt and the lithium and sodium urinary outputs allow the calculation of the actual amount of cooking salt eaten.

Gains and losses of salt during cooking Only a small proportion of the salt added to water for cooking foods is, in practice, eaten. A value of 24% was obtained by the lithium method for the average intake per head of the 'purchased' cooking salt used in cooking. The only other data using traditional methods comes from Hungary where 41% of the salt purchased by households was actually ingested.

The assessment of total discretionary salt use **Figure 1** compares the traditional and lithium marker techniques for assessing both total salt intake and the distribution of its sources. When table and cooking

Table 11 Sources of dietary salt in different countries assessed by traditional methods (g per head per day)

Country	Total	Nondiscretionary sources			Discretionary table and/or cooking
		Natural	Processing	Catering	
England	9.5		7.9		1.6
Britain	9.7	0.9	5.7	–	3.1
Britain	11.7	8.1[a]	–	1.6[a]	2.0
Sweden	11.1	1.0	5.3	–	4.8
USA	14.5	–	8.0	–	6.5
Finland	12.6	1.5	5.3	1.0	4.8
Finland	10.7	1.4	4.7	–	4.6
Finland	11.7	–	7.4	–	4.3
Mexico (State)					7.0

[a]Some cooking salt is included in this value for food consumed at home. For catering and table salt use, a value has been added.

Table 12 Estimates of the use of table salt

Subjects	Number of subjects	Salt intake (g per head per day)		
		Total	Table salt	Table salt as % total
Men				
White and black[a]	24	9.8–16.5	1.5 (0.3)	9–15
White[b]	3	11.0	0.44	4
Black[b]	3	8.9	0.27	3
White[d]	33	10.6	1.6 (1.0)[c]	11
Women				
White and black[a]	13	4.4–4.9	0.9 (0.3)	18–20
White[b]	3	6.4	0.64	10
Black[b]	4	6.5	0.13	2
White[d]	50	7.4	0.73 (0.74)[c]	10
White adolescents	8	7.4	0.95	13
Family studies[e]	15	11.7	1.35[c]	11.6

From James *et al*. (1987). With permission.
[a]Total intake of the subjects was varied systematically in a metabolic ward.
[b]Salt intake assessed with the use of a dietary history and food model.
[c]Value based on the use of normal, not lithium-tagged salt. Where necessary values are recalculated to give the mean (SD).
[d]Study conducted in England; all other studies conducted in the USA.
[e]A complex and less satisfactory approach was used.

salt are combined to form a single value, then the percentage contribution of the discretionary pool to the total intake measured by the lithium marker technique is significantly lower in the UK compared with that assessed by traditional methods which do not consider salt losses during cooking and at the table. This intake in the UK seemed unusually low, but when discretionary sources (table and cooking salt) were assessed in various regions of Italy using the lithium marker technique, salt intake from this source varied between 31% and 41% of the total intake. In Japan, salt is ingested in large amounts as pickled and salted fish and vegetables. These distinctive items may be considered discretionary sources of salt, as may specific foods, e.g. salted meat and vegetable extracts, that are used for flavouring in Western societies. This raises a host of new issues about how best to allow consumers to monitor their salt intake.

Pore size in salt cellars Traditional data on table salt use are given in **Table 11** and new estimates in **Table 12**. The pore size and hole number is important in determining the amount of salt actually shaken onto food. Smaller shaker hole areas lead to a marked fall in salt consumption, for example to about a quarter of the maximum value.

Conclusions

Evidence suggests that sodium intake is an important determinant of blood pressure in the population as a whole, and there is evidence that it influences the rise in blood pressure with age. Accurate amounts of the total salt intake or that coming from a particular source are needed, both for physicians who need to consider the salt intake of their patients and for public health workers who are charged with the implementation of public health programmes.

The predominant source of salt will vary from country to country. In the UK, for example, while some reduction of salt intake can be made by reducing salt in cooking or added at the table, at least as great a potential effect would be possible from reducing the salt content of manufactured food. A different public health approach would apply to Italy, whose discretionary intake of salt is two to three times greater than that of the UK.

See also: **Calcium**: Physiology. **Cancer**: Epidemiology and Associations Between Diet and Cancer. **Food Processing**: Nutritional Influences. **Hypertension**: Physiology; Nutritional Management. **Osteoporosis**: Aetiology; Treatment and Prevention. **Potassium**: Physiology, Dietary Sources and Requirements. **Sodium**: Physiology.

Further Reading

Dietary Sodium and Health (1997) *American Journal of Clinical Nutrition* 65(supplement):2(s).

Denton D (1982) *The Hunger for Salt.* New York: Springer-Verlag

Elliot P, Stamler J, Nichols R, Dyer AR, Stamler R, Kesteloot H and Marmot M (1996) Intersalt revisited: further analyses of 24 hour sodium excretion and blood pressure within and across populations. *British Medical Journal* 312:1249–1253.

Frost CD, Law MR and Wald NJ (1991) By how much does dietary salt reduction lower blood pressure? II. Analysis of observational data within populations. *British Medical Journal* 302:815–818.

Hanneman RL (1996) Intersalt: hypertension rise with age revisited. *British Medical Journal* 312:1283–1284.

James WPT, Ralph A and Sanchez-Castillo CP (1987) The dominance of salt in manufactured food in the sodium intake of affluent societies. *Lancet* 1:426–429.

Law MR, Frost CD and Wald NJ (1991) By how much does dietary salt reduction lower blood pressure? I. Analysis of observational data among populations. *British Medical Journal* 302:811–815.

Law MR, Frost CD and Wald NJ (1991) By how much does dietary salt reduction lower blood pressure? III. Analysis of data from trials of salt reduction. *British Medical Journal* 302:819–824.

Multhauf RP (1978) *Neptune's Gift.* Baltimore and London: The John Hopkins University Press.

Sanchez-Castillo CP, Branch WJ and James WPT (1987) A test for the validity of the lithium-marker technique for monitoring dietary sources of salt in man. *Clinical Science* 72:87–94.

Sanchez-Castillo CP, Solano ML, Flores J, Franklin MF, Limon N, Martinez del Cerro V, Velazquez C, Villa A and James WPT (1996) Salt intake and blood pressure in rural and metropolitan Mexico. *Archives of Medical Research* 27:559–556.

Sanchez-Castillo CP, Warrender S, Whitehead T and James WPT (1987) An assessment of the sources of dietary salt in a British population. *Clinical Science* 72:95–102.

Satiety *see* **Appetite**: Physiological and Neurobiological Aspects.

Saturated fat *see* **Fatty Acids**: Health Effects of Saturated Fatty Acids.

SEASONALITY

Nutritional Implications

A Ferro-Luzzi, Human Nutrition Unit, Rome, Italy

P S Shetty, London School of Hygiene and Tropical Medicine, London, UK

Seasonal variations of climatic conditions are present worldwide, although they differ widely in timing, intensity and other characteristics which depend mostly on the latitude of the area, the altitude and various other complex local environmental features. Climatic conditions have an enormous influence on the agricultural potential of a site; they regulate the vegetative cycle, the biomass production, the labour input required and the outcome in terms of food or cash crops. Biomass has been defined as any 'structured organic matter, living or dormant, and sometimes even dead, comprised within the plant kingdom, the animal kingdom and microbiological organisms, its production is primarily through photosynthesis and represents a good measure of renewable resource potential. It appears obvious, therefore, that climatic seasonality will be an important factor ruling many aspects of the life of rural populations whose survival is closely dependent upon food security.

Besides the food security aspect, climatic seasonality impinges – especially in Third World communities living in rural areas – on the life and health of the human population by periodical exposure to increased pathogens (viruses, microbes, protozoa, worms, etc.) and their vectors. It often happens that exposure to peaks of seasonal demand for agricultural labour overlap with the period when exposure to infectious diseases is heightened and occurs at a time when the food stores are at their lowest just before the new harvest. The ensuing concurrence of strains is called 'the hungry season'; in French, it is referred to as *la soudure*, which aptly describes the time between the exhaustion of previous year's food stores and their replenishment with the products of the new harvest. The hungry season generates a situation of nutritional stress which is experienced by most Third World rural populations, especially small-scale farmers and pastoralists.

This cycle of seasonal stress recurring regularly over the centuries has taught human societies to live with them, adjust and survive by developing appropriate avoidance and coping mechanisms. By these mechanisms, nutritional vulnerability may remain latent and the threshold of biological damage not overstepped. It is when events become unpredictable in intensity, duration or causes, or when there are additional adverse conditions, as in famines, that the coping mechanisms are exceeded and damage of an economic and/or biological nature, often irreversible, is suffered. This in turn leads towards increasing destitution and dependency upon external support. The impact of seasonal cycling of food security on various aspects of human society (production, economy, behaviour, health), displayed as flow diagram in **Fig. 1**, has been an object of interest and research since early 1970. The ecological setting where seasonality is most pronounced is encountered in the tropical regions of the world, for reasons that are explained below.

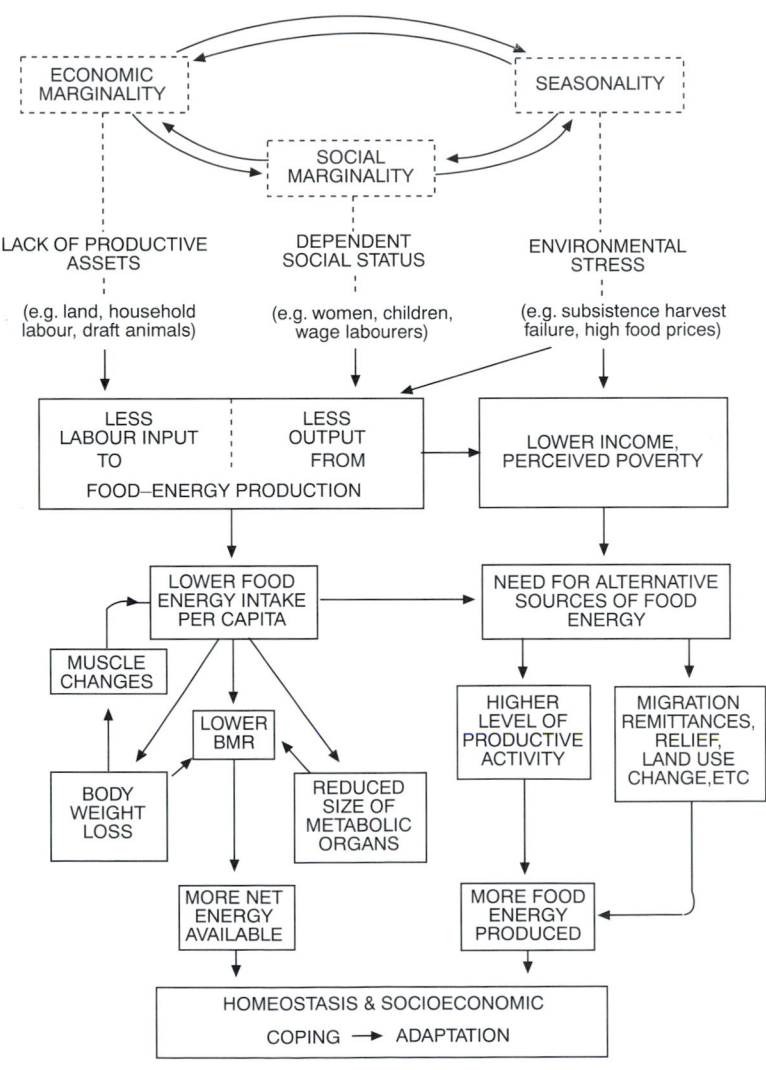

Figure 1 Interaction between the physiological and socioeconomic processes of adaptation to seasonality. From Bayliss-Smith TP (1990) The integrated analysis of seasonal energy deficits: problems and prospects. *European Journal of Clinical Nutrition* **44** (supplement 1): 113–121.

Agro-climatic Seasonality

To appreciate the extent to which climatic seasonality impacts on the life of rural populations, a full understanding of the climatic context is required. Rural communities rely heavily on the annual production of biomass – for direct consumption, as fodder for their livestock or as cash crops. Biomass production, especially in the rural tropical environment, is markedly influenced by environmental and climatic seasonality. The three climatic variables that most strongly influence biomass production are rainfall, evaporation and solar radiation. Evapotranspiration is defined as the amount of water that is lost by green crops. It, therefore, represents a measure of the amount of water needed by any given crop to grow to ripeness. The most extreme climatic conditions are encountered in the tropics. Tropical climates can be broadly characterized as having a strong unimodal distribution of rainfall, with an extended dry season when water is insufficient to sustain the growth of the vegetation and a short wet season with a single summer rainfall peak. In the equatorial or near-equatorial region the rainfall peaks twice in coincidence with the equinoxes. Several attempts to define and classify the climatic context have been made by agronomists and several indices have been developed, mostly based on rainfall regimens (Jackson method, Walsh method). Some of these include a reliability factor (the more marked the seasonality of the rainfall, the less reliable the rainfall during the rainy season), the calculation of potential evapotranspiration (Thornthwaite system) or the estimated temperature limits of different types of plants (Koeppen system). However, to understand fully the food security implications of climatic seasonality, it is necessary to include in the seasonality index a measure of its impact on biomass production. A new index has therefore been developed to take into account the overall influence of climate variables (potential evapotranspiration, rainfall, moisture-retention capacity of the soil and number of days over the year capable of supporting the vegetative cycle). This new index, called the Index of Agro-Climatic Seasonality (IACS), ranges between 0, when there is no seasonality and plants can grow the whole year around, and 1, which is when no growth is possible and there are 365 dry days in the year. On this basis, four levels of seasonality have been proposed: low seasonality, allowing a vegetative season of >200 days per year (IACS 0.00 to 0.44); moderate seasonality, allowing a vegetative period of 200 to 120 days per year (IACS 0.45 to 0.65); severe seasonality, whose vegetative period is restricted to <120 days per year (IACS 0.66 to 0.80); and the desertic environment, with practically no vegetative growth and incapable of supporting rain-fed agriculture (IACS> 0.80). The relevant regions of the world have been classified according the IACS index and are shown in **Fig. 2**.

The IACS classification has been found to correlate well with seasonal weight loss of the resident rural population, body weight loss being taken as a measure of the strain (negative energy balance) imposed by access to food insufficient to meet the energy requirement (**Fig. 3**). Even better results might be obtained, explaining up to 85% of the variance in the amount of weight lost seasonally, if the meterological variables, such as the mean and range of local temperatures, the wind and total radiation, are entered separately in a multiple regression equation. The regression shows that there is practically no seasonal cycling of body weight in areas where the index is 0.2 or lower, but it starts to increase steadily with increase in IACS index, reaching a maximum in those areas where the IACS exceeds 0.6.

Human Adaptive Responses to Agro-climatic Stress

The concept of stress, coping and adaptation

The seasonality of the agricultural cycle translates into a fluctuation of the amount and quality of food available, creating a seasonal alternation of restricted and unrestricted access to food energy. The restriction may be absolute, such as when there is simply not enough food, or relative, such as when the demand for physical labour input rises to its annual peak in coincidence with the work of harvest. The historical exposure of rural societies living in the tropics to seasonal cycling of their food supply has been a regular phenomenon throughout history. They have learned how to face and survive food shortage by developing appropriate strategies. These strategies have been studied in considerable detail by sociologists, economists and nutritionists. It is possible to define broad patterns consisting of a set sequence of actions and behaviours that range from avoidance of the stress generated by the seasonal insufficiency of the supply of food, to coping with it and adapting to it, and finally, to tolerating a certain degree of unavoidable damage. The avoidance and coping strategies become incapable of eliminating or limiting the stress when this exceeds the 'regular' seasonal threshold or persists over a period of time well beyond the limit of tolerance. Famine is then the inevitable outcome, with a breakdown of the system and total dependence for survival on external intervention. A model has been proposed that describes how human societies respond to the progression of

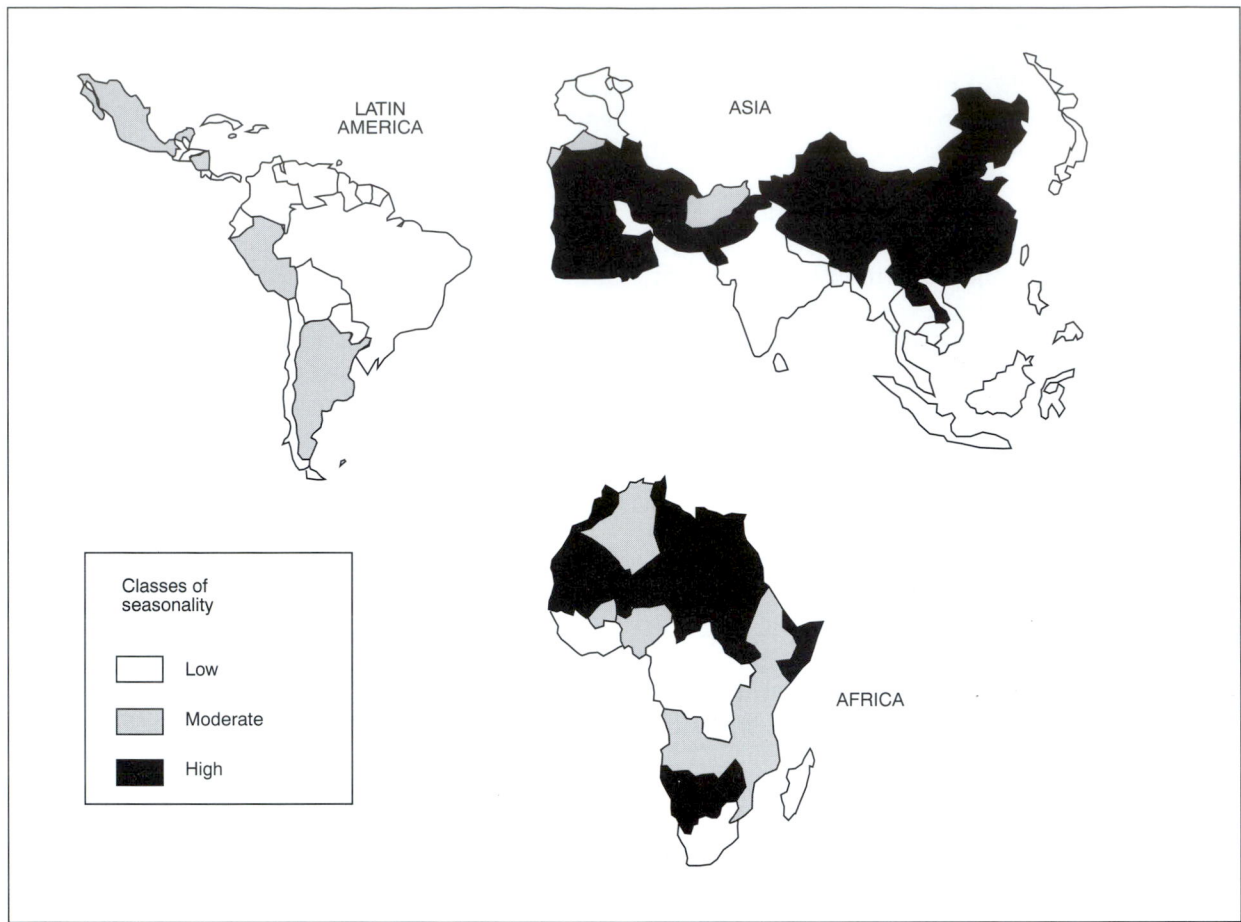

Figure 2 The distribution of agro-climatic seasonality in Asia, Africa and Latin America. The classes of seasonality are based on IACS intervals. Low seasonality, IACS <0.45; moderate seasonality, 0.45≤IACS ≤0.65; high seasonality, IACS >0.65.
From Ferro-Luzzi A, Branca F and Pastore G (1994) Body mass index defines risk of seasonal energy stress in the Third World. *European Journal of Clinical Nutrition* **48** (supplement 3): S165–S178.

a stressing challenge. The initial exposure to the challenge (shortage of food) will trigger activities directed to avoid the stress; should avoidance be unsuccessful, stress will be experienced, and responses of a biological and behavioural nature will escalate. With persistence of the challenge, first strain and later damage being inflicted on the individual or the social system, the response strategy will begin to collapse and some resistive mechanism at first, and then pure passive tolerance, will be the only possible responses. This approach merges the socioeconomic and behavioural responses with the biological ones which – although closely intertwined – are better considered separately.

Biological adaptation to energy stress

Biological responses come into play only after the challenge has reached the stage of stress, more precisely of energy stress, the latter being defined as a sustained negative energy balance following a pro-

longed shortage of food. A negative energy balance cannot be tolerated for any appreciable length of time by the body. When this happens, therefore, there is an immediate response. There are only three biologically possible options (**Fig. 4**): the mobilization of the energy stored in the body; the abatement of the physical activity; and, finally, an increase in the efficiency with which the cells of the body handle the limited energy supply.

The mobilization of the energy reserves of the body is the earliest response, in the absence of which the other two will not be activated. The body stores excess energy as fat in the adipose tissue, to be used when the need arises. The storage as fat rather than as protein or carbohydrates is very convenient since, for the same weight, fat yields more than twice the energy of either protein or carbohydrates. Given that the deposition and removal of fat from the body are fully physiological processes, no detrimental effect should be expected in principle from these responses.

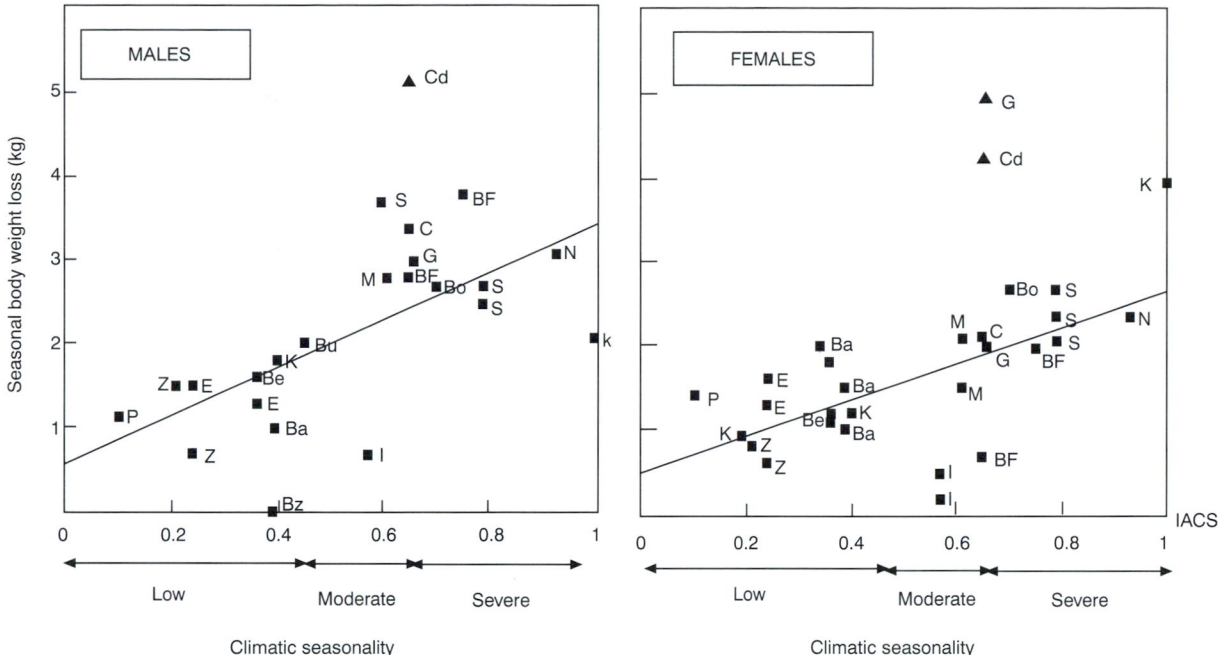

Figure 3 Linear regressions between IACS and seasonal body weight loss of adults in rural communities of developing countries. The triangles represent three outliers not included in the regression. Regression equations:
Men: Δ body weight (kg) = 0.56 + 2.89 IACS, r=0.67, P<0.001;
Women: Δ body weight (kg) = 0.48 + 2.22 IACS, r=0.65, P<0.001.
Key to countries: Ba, Bangladesh; Be, Benin; BF, Burkina-Faso; Bo, Botswana; Bu, Burma; C, Cameroon; Cd, Cameroon during drought; E, Ethiopia; G, The Gambia; K, Kenya; I, India; M, Mali; N, Niger; P, Papua; S, Senegal; Z, Zaire.
From Ferro-Luzzi A, Branca F and Pastore G (1994) Body mass index defines risk of seasonal energy stress in the Third World. *European Journal of Clinical Nutrition* **48** (supplement 3): S165–S178.

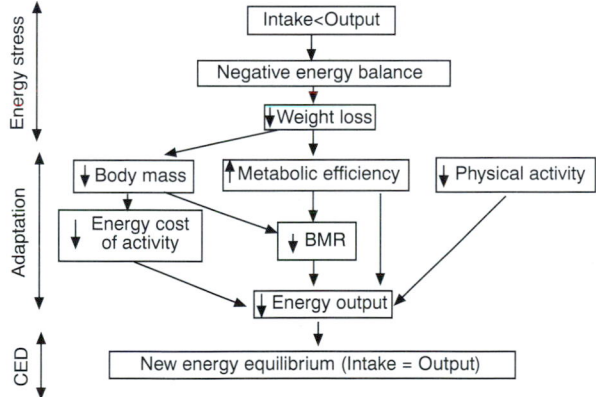

Figure 4 Biological strategies adopted in response to energy stress to restore energy equilibrium. CED, chronic energy deficiency. Modified from: Ferro-Luzzi A (1986) Range of variation in energy expenditure and scope for regulation. In: Taylor TG and Jenkins NK (eds) *Proc. XIII International Congress of Nutrition*. London: J Libbey Press, pp 393–399.

However, two aspects need to be considered, the first being that any loss of fat from the body is accompanied by a simultaneous loss of body proteins as well, and that the proportion of proteins lost depends on the amount of fat present in the body. Therefore, if the person undergoing the weight loss is obese or of normal fatness, the proportion of protein lost is significantly lower than if the weight loss is experienced by a thin person. The protein that is lost derives from the small labile pool of the body but, in the presence of a sustained loss, protein is lost from visceral organs of great metabolic importance such as liver, gut and muscles. Thus any such loss should be avoided or limited as much as possible. The second consideration relates to the fact that the rural population living in the tropics are usually very thin to begin with, which means that any loss of body weight will involve an undesirable wastage of important protein-rich tissues. This will inevitably have repercussions on metabolic performance and functional integrity. The implications are far-reaching and invest areas of concern such as the intergenerational perpetuation of stunting and impaired resistance to infectious diseases.

Limited energy resources may be conserved by reducing physical activity. This is an apparently straightforward and efficient strategy given that the amount of total energy that is spent in bodily movements might be – especially in rural populations – quite large. The level of mechanization of agricultural labour input is very low in the Third World and physical energy is required for work such as tilling the soil, weeding, sowing, harvesting, fertilizing, etc. For example, it has been calculated that energy corresponding to 154 person-days' work will be necessary for cultivating the amount of land (1.156 ha) required for producing the 1170 kg rice necessary to meet the energy needs of one household for 1 year. The implication of this reasoning is that recourse to cutting down physical activity as a means for sparing energy may not be implemented by Third World farmers as it entails a loss of productive potential, is unsustainable, is the least reversible strategy and is likely to lead to extensive and irreparable damage.

This leaves the third type of response to exposure to long-term energy stress. This consists of an improved efficiency of the usage of energy within the body. It has been described under experimental laboratory conditions in previously well-fed young adults in response to acute and pronounced starvation. There is some uncertainty whether this response is observed under real-life conditions of chronic energy deficiency. However, this response affords only a modest saving of about 15% of basal metabolic rate (BMR) – which might represent no more than 5% of total energy requirement – and is a signal of severe biological distress rather than a mechanism for saving energy. It is therefore, of academic interest and should not be relied on as an acceptable means for sparing energy.

Sociobehavioural responses to food insecurity

A combination of conditions recurs yearly in the pre-harvest period. For the farmers in the tropics, this seasonal contingency consists in the peaking of the demand for agricultural labour, the early depletion of household food stores owing to the unimodal climatic pattern, and the exposure to the transmission of infections favoured by climatic conditions (rain and temperature) that accelerate the proliferation of pathogenic organisms and the breeding of vectors. The people's ability to withstand, with minimum strain, this combination of stresses varies widely, and will depend largely on the severity of the challenge and on the prolongation or recurrence over several successive years. Poverty, however, is probably the single factor that most affects the likelihood of emerging unscathed or with limited damage from the hungry season.

The adverse conditions created by poverty, which compound the seasonal stress, are several and interacting, often forcing poor farmers down through successive spirals into total destitution. The high energy demand for agricultural work comes at the worst time of the year when food is scarce, its price highest and food consumption at its lowest, thus exacerbat-

ing the energy requirements. The extra heavy agricultural workload of women will cause a reallocation of their time, leading to meals being prepared quickly and in bulk with attendant losses of nutrients, less time available for gathering of wild foods, fuel and water, a deterioration in domestic hygiene and less time dedicated to child care. Mothers may stop breast-feeding at such times. Malnutrition, in turn, influences susceptibility to infections, resulting in reduced resistance to disease. Coming at this time of the year, when exposure to infections is most pronounced, this lowered resistance leads to higher morbidity. The economic cost of incapacitating diseases is not easily estimated in terms of the foregone agricultural production. However, it can be reasonably inferred from the fact that small farmers rely wholly on their own labour. Missing a critical period in the farming calendar, especially in the tropics where the windows of opportunity may be very short, may mean a smaller harvest or even no harvest at all. Thus illness of the breadwinner during the busy agricultural season will have a disproportionate impact on household economic survival and is likely to create permanent impoverishment. The ratchet effect of illness of the breadwinner at critical times of the year in the downward spiral of poverty has been reported in urban slums in Bangladesh, where there was almost three times as much child malnutrition in the families where the male breadwinner had been incapacitated for work because of disease than in families where diseases were less frequent. In the Southern Highlands of Peru, illnesses were found to affect farming production through a reduction in the number of fields planted as well as through reduced yields and increased work time per field; the majority of the illness episodes occurred during the planting and post-planting season and least illness occurred during harvest and post-harvest. The impoverished farmers in the tropics may therefore be forced down cyclically in their poverty, often past an irreversible threshold. The relative significance of health ratchets in processes of impoverishment can be expected to vary according to the levels of other contingencies, the degree of poverty, the incidence and seriousness of the disease, the availability and efficacy of curative facilities, and the direct and indirect cost of treatment.

A set of socioeconomic and behavioural strategies enacted in response to seasonal contingency has been described progressing from avoidance actions to reapportioning and beyond. The earliest and most practised measures usually consist in a diversification of the cropping patterns in relation to the urgency and priority of food crops over other crops, directed to maximize profit while minimizing risk. Because of narrow backstop margins, the tropical farmer is usually unwilling to jeopardize food security by substituting high-yield crops with greater dependence from rainfall for low-yield low-variance crops. Farmers will rather diversify their cropping patterns, rely more on secondary crops such as household gardening, or contingency non-staple root crops such as cassava, and gather more wild food such as a variety of leaves, nuts and berries known as 'famine foods', for buffering against famine. There will be an attempt to diversify household income sources such as brewing and selling sorghum beer, waged work, petty manufacturing, temporary migrant labour, reduction of meal size and number and disposal of small livestock. With the prolongation of the food shortage or in anticipation of it, other distress measures will be implemented in succession, progressively moving towards the threshold of irreversibility with the disposal of household property, mortgaging or sale of farmland, bartering or sale of oxen for ploughing and of breeding livestock. There is no clear-cut demarcation of the progress from seasonal contingency to famine emergency, but a number of events highlight the condition of severe famine distress such as large-scale migration, prostitution, theft, sale of children, and finally the breakdown of the entire societal and household system and total dependency on outside aid.

Biological Outcomes of Energy Stress

The nutritional outcomes of exposure to seasonal cycling of food supply differs according to intrinsic biological features such as age, sex and specific physiological functions and roles (such as pregnancy and lactation).

Children

The poor environmental hygiene, the restricted access to health services that characterize rural poverty, and the low priority ranking of children's needs under the pressure of conflicting demands of agricultural activities, all concur to make seasonal cycling in food availability a particularly threatening period in the life of the child. Children are particularly vulnerable and they suffer disproportionally when exposed to stress situations. In part this is because of the child's relatively greater energy and nutrient needs which, although small in absolute amounts, are greater than those of an adult when expressed per unit of body weight. Growth, development and even survival are, therefore, particularly dependent upon the provision of nutritionally adequate food. The child's nutritional vulnerability differs from that of the adult also because, besides the immediate and measurable outcomes of malnutrition, long-term irreversible consequences are likely to occur, causing not only permanent stunting and smaller body size, but also impairing brain development and cognitive capacities as measured by development indicators. For the same given level and duration of nutritional deprivation, the younger the child, the more severe and more permanent the damage; however some reversibility has been described, provided appropriate curative action is undertaken as promptly as possible. There appear to be critical periods of life when the deficits that arise are not made up. WHO has identified eight developmental stages: peri-conceptual, prenatal, delivery, neonatal (0–27 days), postnatal (1–11 months), toddler (1–3 years), pre-school (4–5 years) and school age (6–9 years). Each stage has different nutritional needs.

The child's nutritional vulnerability is compounded by the liability to communicable diseases and parasitism, given the well-known synergistic relationship between malnutrition and ill-health. The nutrition–infection link has been discussed elsewhere. The 'ratcheting effect' of seasonal deterioration of health and nutritional status of children has been suggested to be at the basis of an intergenerational vicious cycle of a malnourished female child growing to become a handicapped adult woman, who is, in turn, more likely to have low-birthweight children.

Seasonal deceleration in physical growth of infants and children has been reported in many affluent societies. This phenomenon should not be confounded with the seasonal growth-faltering recorded in most tropical and subtropical regions where malnutrition is endemic. The mechanism of seasonal growth deceleration and the accompanying 'staircase effect' of compensatory acceleration of Western countries has not been fully elucidated and the cause has been variously attributed to the effects of day length and temperature on growth and metabolism. On the other hand, stunting of the Third World child is considered to be an indication of the failure to attain full genetic potential for physical growth and has been associated, in infants and toddlers, with higher morbidity and mortality rates, reduced mental development and reduced work capacity and endurance. A three-way causation is considered responsible for the seasonal slowing or arrest of the child's development, represented by the pre-harvest limitation of food supply, in coincidence with higher disease prevalence and a reallocation of the mother's time away from child care. Therefore, in rural Bangladesh, the growth of children younger than 5 years undergoes cyclical accelerations and decelerations that appear to follow closely the fluctuations of the

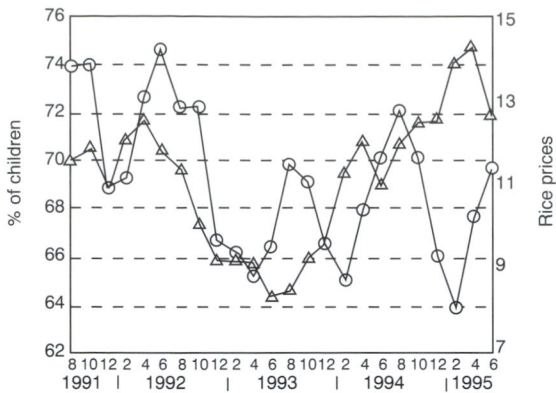

Figure 5 Seasonal fluctuations in the prevalence (%) of underweight children (aged below 5 years) (○) and in the average rice price (△) in rural areas of Bangladesh. From Keller H (1996) International Bangladesh Report of Round 40–Rural–of the Nutrition Surveillance Project (NSP), October 1996.

market price of rice, the staple food of those communities which provides more than 70% of calorie intake at the household level (**Fig. 5**).

It is very difficult to separate the contributions made by the various environmental conditions that may affect the child's nutritional wellbeing: the situation is made more complex by the variable combinations that are possible in any given setting. Therefore, for example, the increase in the prevalence of wasting during the lean pre-harvest among Ethiopian children living in a moderately seasonal, food-deficit area, was directly related to the socioeconomic level of their household, with the children belonging to poorer households suffering a greater and earlier weight loss than the adults of the same family, and recovering to a lesser degree (**Fig. 6**).

In Thailand, the seasonal increase in wasting and prevalence of underweight children seemed to reflect the higher rate of morbidity during the rainy season and reduced caring time by the mothers at the

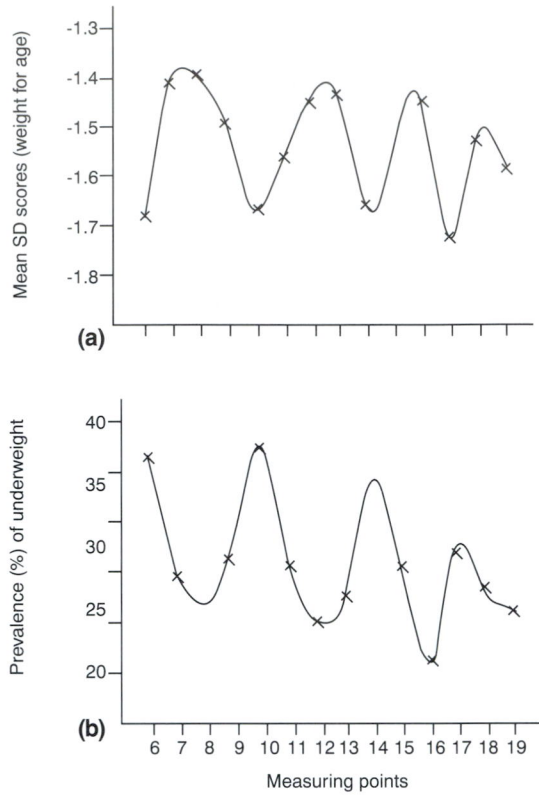

Figure 7 Seasonal variation of the nutritional status (a) of preschool children of rural villages in North Thailand observed longitudinally every 3 months from June 1982 to September 1985. (a) Mean weight for age; (b) prevalence of underweight (weight for age > -2.00 standard deviations). Measuring points: 6, June 1982; 7, September 1982; 8, December 1982; 9, March 1983; 10, June 1983; 11, September 1983; 12, December 1893; 13, March 1984; 14, June 1984; 15, September 1984; 16, December 1984; 17, March 1985; 18, June 1985; 19, September 1985. Modified from Schelp FP, Sornmani S, Pongpaew P, Vudhivai N, Egormaiphol S and Bohning D (1990) Seasonal variation of wasting and stunting in preschool children during a three-year community-based nutritional intervention study in northeast Thailand. *Tropical Medicine and Parasitology* **41**: 279–285. Stuttgart: Georg Thieme Verlag. (With permission).

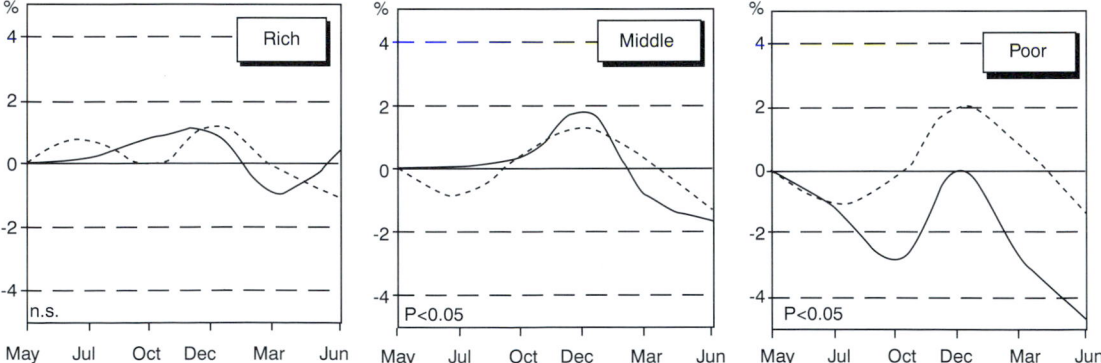

Figure 6 Seasonal fluctuations of household cumulative weight of children (—) and adults (---) by socioeconomic level in rural Ethiopia. From Pastore G, Branca F, Demissie T and Ferro-Luzzi A (1993) Seasonal energy stress in an Ethiopian rural community: an analysis of the impact at the household level. *European Journal of Clinical Nutrition* **47**:851–862.

peaking of the agricultural season rather than the availability of food in the house, which remains unchanged throughout the year (**Fig. 7**).

Child labour might represent an additional stress, contributing to seasonal growth retardation. Children may be obliged by circumstances to continue carrying out critical, energy-costing activities such as looking after younger siblings, pasturing cattle, collecting firewood and fetching water, even when food becomes short in supply. Child labour is widely practised in Third World rural areas, and children contribute in a tangible way to household maintenance and production. In the Peruvian Andes, children as young as 6–7 years have been found to spend up to 50% of their time in productive activities. This implies that the older, school-age child, may be at an even greater seasonal stress than the younger child and other members of the household.

Adults

Seasonal weight cycling is also seen in the adults living in rural areas of the tropics. An overview of the seasonal weight loss as recorded worldwide over a period of decades is presented in **Fig. 8** in terms of changes of body mass index BMI, kg/(height in m)². The weight loss is usually moderate, the maximum between the two yearly extremes being about 4 kg, but mostly in the region of 4–5% of body weight.

This has been calculated to correspond to a change of BMI in the range of <1 to close to 2 units. Pastoralists tend to have larger weight losses and there is a modest but appreciable gender difference, with women having smaller losses. As adults are less prone than children to infectious diseases and have a better command over food resources, their weight losses may be a good indicator of pure energy shortage, uncomplicated by the interference of aspecific stressors and confounding variables.

The appreciation of the significance of such a relatively modest weight loss needs to take into consideration the rate of weight loss as well as the size of the body energy stores; the faster the loss and the smaller the stores, the greater the likelihood of a deterioration of the functional and metabolic integrity of the individual. Smaller seasonal fluctuations of weight have been consistently recorded in groups with smaller BMI than in people with higher BMI. **Fig. 9** illustrates the seasonal cycling of body weight of Beninese women, according to their BMI. There is no satisfactory interpretation of this phenomenon as yet, but it may be interpreted as reflecting the earlier recourse by those whose body fat stores are lower to strategies other than mobilizing body fat, in the attempt to safeguard their already marginal functional integrity.

As discussed above, although a modest saving can

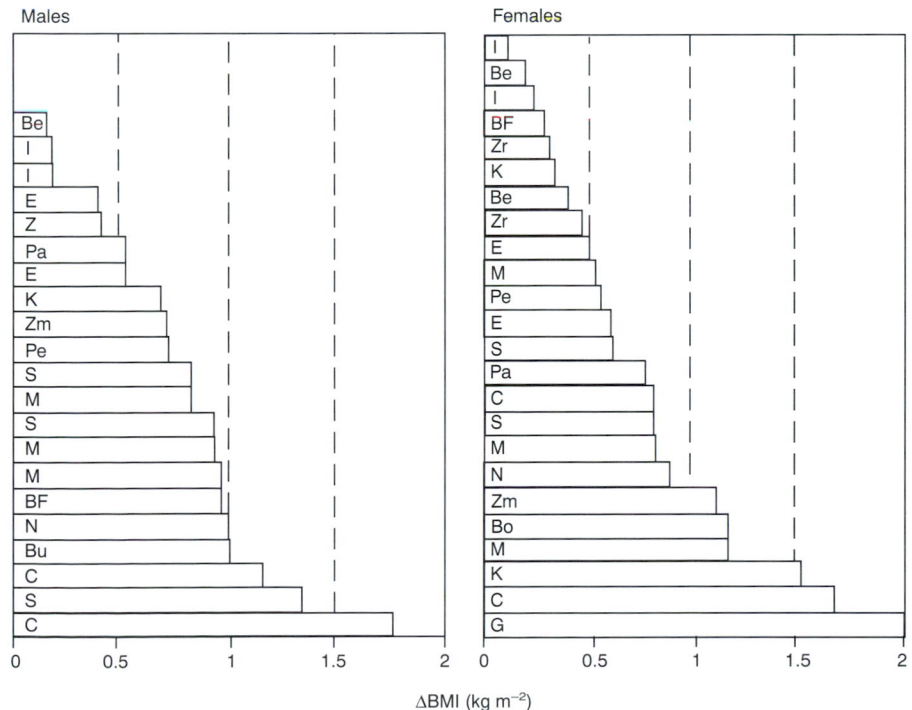

Figure 8 Magnitude of seasonal BMI changes observed in communities of developing countries. Key: Be, Benin; BF, Burkina-Faso; Bo, Botswana; Bu, Burma; C, Cameroon; E, Ethiopia; G, The Gambia; K, Kenya; I, India; M, Mali; N, Niger; Pa, Papua; Pe, Peru; S, Senegal; Za, Zambia; Zr, Zaire. From Ferro-Luzzi A, Branca F and Pastore G (1994) Body mass index defines risk of seasonal energy stress in the Third World. *European Journal of Clinical Nutrition* **48** (supplement 3): S165–S178.

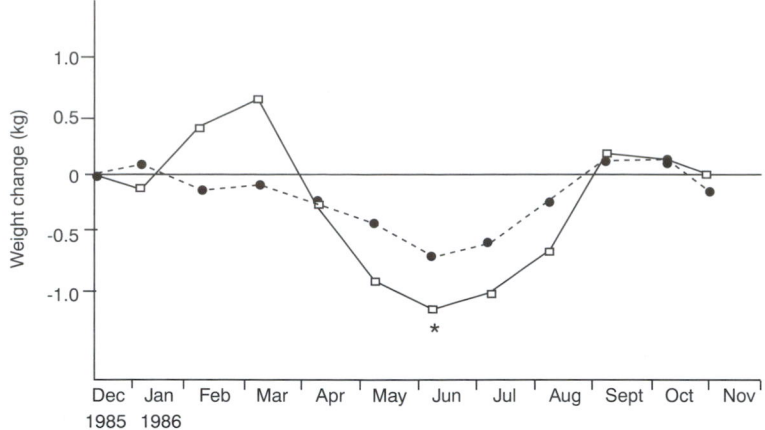

Figure 9 Body weight changes throughout the year of women with initial BMI less than 18 (●) or greater than 18 (□). An asterisk indicates a statistically significant difference from the December value ($P<0.01$). From Schultink WJ, Klaver W, Van Wijk H, Van Raaij JMA and Hautvast JGAJ (1990) Body weight changes and basal metabolic rates of rural Beninese women during seasons with different energy intakes. *European Journal of Clinical Nutrition* **44**: 31–40.

be made through an increase in the metabolic efficiency of energy use at the cellular level, significant conservation of energy resources can only be achieved through a decrease in voluntary physical activity. The implications of this form of energy sparing, however, are likely to be detrimental to long-term survival, given that a decline in physical activity would interfere with the productivity of the individual and lead, by a ratcheting effect, downward into an 'energy trap'. This progressive stepwise descent aptly describes how seasonal stress operates to keep the poor people poor (**Fig. 10**).

Despite the enormous importance that such a strategy is likely to have, there is surprisingly little evidence to substantiate the claim that the distress response of low BMI people consists, in effect, of a reduction in physical activity and energy expenditure, and no firm conclusions can be drawn on this issue. Some earlier observations recorded a synchronous countertendency of weight loss and

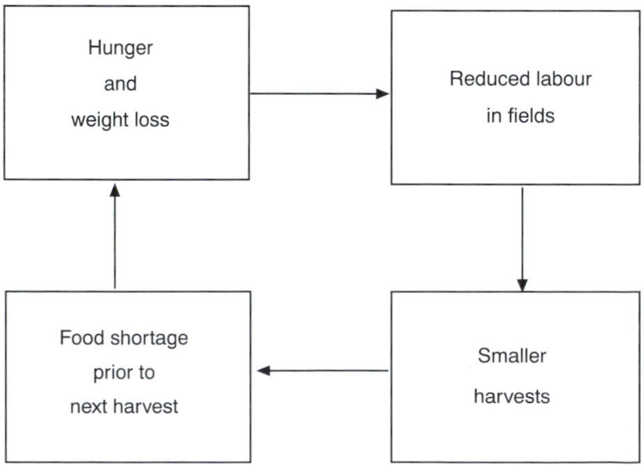

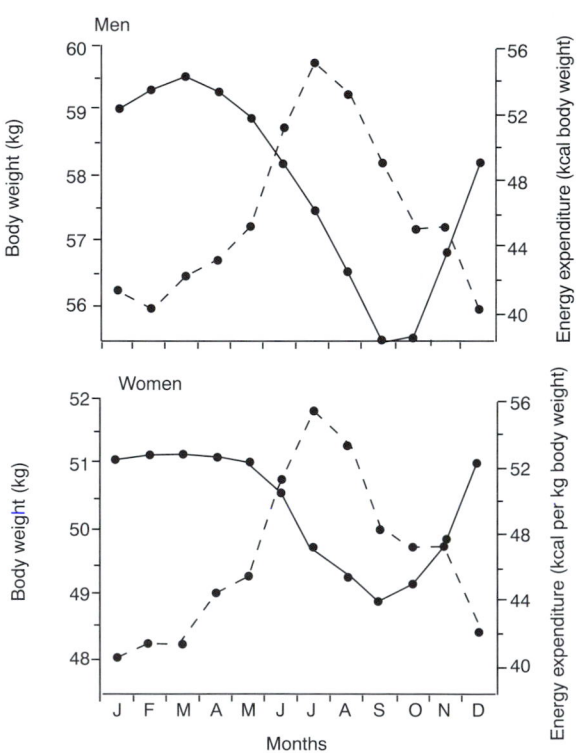

Figure 11 Seasonal fluctuation of mean daily energy expenditure (---) and body weight (—) of adult men and women in Burkina-Faso (former Upper Volte). 1 kcal ~ 4.18 kJ. From Ferro-Luzzi A, Branca F and Pastore G (1994) Body mass index defines risk of seasonal energy stress in the Third World. *European Journal of Clinical Nutrition* **48** (supplement 3): S165–S178.

Figure 10 Vicious cycle through which nutritional constraints on agricultural labour are hypothesized to perpetuate seasonal hunger. From Jenike MR (1996) Activity reduction as an adaptive response to seasonal hunger. *American Journal of Human Biology* **8**:517–534.

Table 1 Distribution of Third World adult population in three classes of seasonality

	Seasonality class		
	Low IACS <0.45 (millions)	Moderate IACS 0.45–0.65 (millions)	Severe IACS >0.65 (millions)
Africa	53	120	58
Asia	337	1121	92
South and Central America	150	72	0
Total	540	1313	150
Only rural	301	840	84

From Ferro-Luzzi A, Branca F and Pastore G (1994) Body mass index defines risk of seasonal energy stress in the Third World. *European Journal of Clinical Nutrition* **48** (supplement 3): S165–S178.

increase in energy expenditure in Burkina-Faso (**Fig. 11**) and in The Gambia, while in Zaire and in Ethiopian farmers, a reduction of activity was recorded only after weight loss. In some cultures, existing constraints appear to prevent any significant curtailment of physical activity, as observed in Nepalese and in Beninese women. Some evidence suggests that the activities that are curtailed first might be those that are the least crucial for short-term survival.

The World Dimension of Seasonal Food Insecurity

Concern and attention has been increasingly directed to the issue of seasonality; this reflects the growing awareness that the climatic fluctuations of the world have recently exceeded its capacity to adjust and that progressively larger regions of the world appear to be at risk of, or actually experience, drought and suffer from the ensuing famines. In early 1980s climatic seasonality was very roughly estimated to affect about 200 million people in Africa south of Sahara, and another 600 million in the Indian subcontinent.

More recently, another more refined estimate of the world dimensions of seasonality has been performed combining – in a stepwise approach – the assessment of agro-climatic exposure with a realistic calculation of the biological risk associated with any given loss of body weight. Using the IACS, which reflects the potential for biomass production and therefore the food security of marginal farmers, and United Nation statistics, 75% of the one and a quarter billion adults living in rural areas of the Third World in the 1980s, inhabited areas affected by moderate (IACS 0.45–0.65) or severe (IACS>0.65) seasonality (**Table 1**).

As IACS has proved to be a reliable predictor of seasonal weight loss of the resident rural populations in developing countries, it is possible to predict the average seasonal weight loss likely to occur in these populations. Only a proportion of these populations will be, on the basis of the criteria of the likely size of the loss of weight combined with the additional constraints of their starting BMI, at risk of functional impairment involving substantial erosion of their health and functional competence. On the basis of

Table 2 The adult population of the rural Third World and the number of individuals at risk of seasonal energy stress

		Individuals at risk of seasonal energy stress	
	Rural population (millions)	Moderate risk (millions)	Severe risk (millions)
Africa	104	28	33
Asia	785	158	371
South and Central America	27	3	4
Total[a]	917	189	408

[a]The enumeration is related only to countries for which the mean BMI of the population can be estimated (917 million out of 1223 million).
From Ferro-Luzzi A, Branca F and Pastore G (1994) Body mass index defines risk of seasonal energy stress in the Third World. *European Journal of Clinical Nutrition* **48** (supplement 3): S165–S178.

this approach, a total of about 600 million people are at some risk of functional impairment from seasonal cycling of their food security; of these 189 million are at moderate risk and 408 million at severe risk (**Table 2**). Most of these people are to be found in Asia owing to the unique combination of a very large rural population and their low BMI.

See also: **Children**: Nutritional Requirements of School Children. **Energy**: Energy Requirements; Energy Balance. **Famine**: Population Responses. **Immunity**: Role of Iron and Zinc. **Infants**: Nutritional Requirements. **Infection**: Nutritional Interactions. **Lactation**: Dietary Requirements. **Pregnancy**: Energy Requirements and Metabolic Adaptations; Nutrient Requirements.

Further Reading

Chambers R, Longhurst R and Pacey A (1981) *Seasonal Dimensions to Rural Poverty*. London: Frances Pinter Ltd.

Ferro-Luzzi A (ed.) (1990) Biology of adaptation to seasonal cycling of energy intake. *European Journal of Clinical Nutrition* 44 (supplement 1):S1–S125.

Ferro-Luzzi A, Brance F and Pestore G (1994) Body mass index defines risk of seasonal energy stress in the Third World. *European Journal of Clinical Nutrition* 48 (Supplement 3):S165–S178.

Ferro-Luzzi A and Branca F (1998) Coping with poverty: the biological impact of nutritional insecurity. In: Livi Beca M and De Sontis G (eds) *Population and Poverty in the Developing Countries*. Oxford: Clarendon Press.

Gillespie S and McNeill G (1992) *Food, Health and Survival in India and Developing Countries*. Delhi: Oxford University Press.

James WPT and Ralph A (1994) *The Functional Significance of Low Body Mass Index (BMI)*, IDECG edn. Lausanne: United Nations University/Nestlé Foundation.

Norgan NG and Ferro-Luzzi A (1995) Human adaptation to energy undernutrition. In: Fregly M and Blatteis CM (eds) *Handbook of Physiology*, pp 1391–1409. Oxford: Oxford University Press.

Payne P and Lipton M (1994) *How Third World Rural Households Adapt to Dietary Energy Stress. The Evidence and the Issues*, Food Policy Review edn. Washington DC: International Food Policy Research Institute.

Sahn DE, (1989) *Seasonal Variability in Third World Agriculture*, IFPRI edn. Baltimore and London: Johns Hopkins University Press.

Schurch B and Scrimshaw N (eds) (1987) *Chronic Energy Deficiency: Consequences and Related Issues*. Lausanne: United Nations University/Nestlé Foundation.

Shetty PS and James WPT (1994) *Body Mass Index: A Measure of Chronic Energy Deficiency in Adults*, FAO Food and Nutrition Paper 56. Rome: FAO.

Seeds *see* **Nuts and Seeds**: Nutritional Value.

SELENIUM

Physiology, Dietary Sources and Requirements

C Reilly, Enstone, Chipping Norton, UK

Occurrence, Chemistry and Uses

Selenium (Se) was discovered by the Swedish chemist Jöns Jacob Berzelius in 1817. Though one of the rarest of the elements, it is widely distributed in small amounts in the Earth's crust. However, there are some areas in which it occurs in high concentrations in soil. Low levels of Se are found in most animal and plant tissues.

Se is classified chemically as a metalloid, sharing properties of both metals and nonmetals. Its atomic number is 34 and atomic weight 78.96. It occurs in group VIA of the periodic table, between the elements sulfur (S) and tellurium (Te). Its chemical properties are very similar to those of S. It combines with other elements to form inorganic selenides, selenites and selenates. It forms oxides and oxyacids, such as the dioxide (SeO_2) and selenic acid (H_2SeO_4), as well as organic compounds corresponding to the S-amino acids and proteins.

Its physical properties account for its increasing

industrial use in electronic equipment, chemicals, pigments, alloys, in agriculture as feed supplements and fertilizers, and in pharmaceuticals. As a result Se has become a potential health and environmental hazard of significance.

This article will concentrate on recent findings about Se in human nutrition, with particular reference to selenocysteine and the functional selenoproteins. Its role in the prevention of certain diseases will be discussed, as well as recommended intakes and dietary sources, including supplements. Se status and methods for its assessment will also be considered.

Absorption, Transport and Storage

Absorption of dietary Se in humans takes place mainly in the small intestine. Uptake of the element and its subsequent fate are summarized in **Fig. 1**. Both organic and inorganic forms of Se are readily absorbed, but organic forms are absorbed more efficiently than inorganic compounds. For example, more than 90% of selenomethionine is taken up compared with about 60% of selenite. Uptake is affected by several factors, such as the presence of vitamins A, E and C. It is higher if the element is supplied in the form of food rather than as a supplement.

Inorganic Se is transported across the intestinal brush border in a passive process in competition with inorganic S. In contrast, absorption of seleno-

methionine is active, using the same enzyme transport system as methionine. It is probable that selenocysteine is absorbed in a similar manner, using the cysteine transport system.

Se is transported in blood, mainly bound to protein. A small amount is attached to albumin, with most of the remainder bound to the very low-density β-lipoprotein fraction. Distribution between the different proteins appears to depend on the composition of the diet.

Se is deposited in several organs and tissues where its concentration is related to the total amount and chemical form ingested. An order of priority exists between different organs for Se accumulation. This is highest in liver and kidney when dietary intake is high; at lower intakes levels in liver may be markedly reduced, while remaining high in the kidney. Because of its total bulk, muscle tissue accounts for the highest proportion of Se related to total body content and may be a major storage compartment for the element. The total amount of Se in the body of an adult ranges from approximately 15 mg in the USA to about 3 mg in New Zealand.

Whole-blood Se levels can vary significantly between different populations, depending on dietary intakes (**Table 1**). Levels in plasma and serum can be affected by a variety of diseases (**Table 2**).

Metabolism and Excretion

The two main forms of Se found in food are selenomethionine, principally in plants, and selenocysteine in animal foodstuffs. Inorganic Se occurs normally only in dietary supplements. The different forms of the element are incorporated into the body in a variety of ways. Some of the ingested Se is methylated, after an initial reduction to selenide, mainly to di- and trimethyl selenide. Methylation is important for detoxification of the element.

Most dietary Se is incorporated into proteins, either nonspecific *Se-binding proteins*, in which

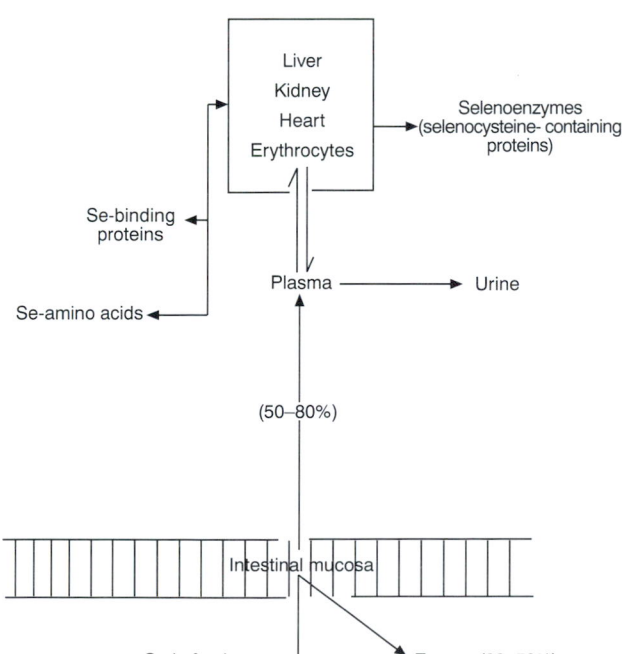

Figure 1 Se transport and absorption in the gastrointestinal tract.

Table 1 Whole-blood selenium levels in relation to dietary intakes of people living in different countries

Country	Intake (μg per day)	Blood Se (μg ml⁻¹)
China (Se-deficient area)	9–11	0.01–0.02
New Zealand (South Island)	28–32	0.05–0.10
Australia	58–87	0.11–0.21
UK	60	0.08–0.32
USA	62–216	0.15–0.40
China (seleniferous area)	3000–6690	0.44–3.20

After Reilly C (1996) *Selenium in Food and Health*. London: Blackie Academic and Professional.

Table 2 Plasma and serum selenium levels in different disease states

Disease	Se levels in plasma or serum ($\mu g \, ml^{-1}$) (control)
Alcoholic liver cirrhosis	0.058 ± 0.011 (0.080 ± 0.011)
Cancer (gastrointestinal)	0.0486 ± 0.015 (0.0543 ± 0.016)
Diabetes (childhood)	0.074 ± 0.008 (0.065 ± 0.008)
Myocardial infarction	0.055 ± 0.015 (0.078 ± 0.011)
Renal disease	0.078 ± 0.016 (0.103 ± 0.018)

After Reilly C (1996) *Selenium in Food and Health*. London: Blackie Academic and Professional.

selenomethionine and selenocysteine substitute for their *S*-analogues, or selenocysteine-containing *selenoproteins*, which are specific for Se and are encoded by a UGA codon in mRNA.

The identification of the selenoproteins and elucidation of their synthetic pathways represent an outstanding achievement of molecular biology. It began with the finding that the gene for the selenoenzyme glutathione peroxidase (EC 1.11.1.9) in the mouse contains an in-frame UGA codon which directs the cotranslational insertion of selenocysteine into protein. Previously the only amino acids known to be incorporated into protein during translation were the 20 'standard' *S*-amino acids. Selenocysteine could thus be considered to be the 21st amino acid, in terms of ribosome-mediated protein synthesis.

Synthesis requires the presence of a specific transfer ribonucleic acid (tRNA^{Sec}) which possesses an anticodon complementary to UGA and is capable of joining to the amino acid serine to form seryl-tRNA^{Sec}. This, after conversion to aminoacrylyl-tRNA^{Sec}, is combined with an activated form of Se, formed by the reduction and phosphorylation of selenide, to give selenocysteyl-tRNA^{Sec}. In the final stage of the synthesis, the selenocysteyl-tRNA^{Sec} is incorporated into a growing polypeptide chain to produce selenoprotein. This occurs at the ribosome complex where the selenocysteyl-tRNA^{Sec} is brought into contact with the UGA codon.

Se is excreted by three different routes: (1) in urine, via the kidneys, largely in the form of the trimethyl-selenonium ion; (2) in faeces, as unabsorbed dietary selenium and in biliary, pancreatic and intestinal secretions; (3) in expelled air, as volatile dimethyl-selenide. A small amount of selenium is lost in hair and nails. It also passes from the mother to her infant in breast milk.

Metabolic Function

Several different types of selenoprotein are synthesized. Nine of these have been characterized in animals by cDNA cloning and full or partial purification (**Table 3**).

Glutathione peroxidase

Glutathione peroxidase (cGSHPx) was the first selenoenzyme to be identified; in 1973 it was shown to contain Se as a functional component. It occurred in erythrocytes, where its role was apparently to protect haemoglobin against oxidative damage by hydrogen peroxide (H_2O_2). It was later shown that GSHPx is not a single enzyme, but has several forms with different, though related functions.

Cytosolic intracellular glutathione peroxidase

Cytosolic intracellular glutathione peroxidase (cGSHPx) was the first of the different forms of GSHPx to be clearly classified. It consists of four identical 22 kDa subunits, each of which contains one selenocysteine residue. It can metabolize a wide range of hydroxides, though not if they are esterified to phospholipids. It is the major selenoprotein in mammalian cells, accounting for about 60% of total Se in Se-adequate animals. In Se-deficient rats, however, hepatic cGSHPx can fall to less than 1% of levels in controls, without any ill effects. Consequently, it is believed that the major role of cGSHPx may be as a buffer to provide Se for other selenoproteins which are more important for maintaining health, rather than as a cellular antioxidant.

Table 3 Selenocysteine-containing functional proteins

Glutathione peroxidases:
   cytosolic (cGSHPx)
   extracellular (eGSHPx)
   gastrointestinal (giGSHPx)
   phospholipid hydroperoxide (phGSHPx)

Iodothyronine deiodinases:
   type 1 (IDI)
   type 2 (IDII)
   type 3 (IDIII)

Selenoprotein P (SeP)

Selenoprotein W (SeW)

Sperm capsule selenoprotein (SCSe)

Thioredoxin reductase (TR)

Gastrointestinal glutathione peroxidase

Gastrointestinal glutathione peroxidase is similar in structure, but not identical with cGSHPx. It is believed to have an antioxidant function specific to intestinal tissue in which it mainly occurs.

Phospholipid hydroperoxide glutathione peroxidase

Phospholipid hydroperoxide glutathione peroxidase (PGSHPx) is a monomer of 20–23 kDa, similar to the subunits of other GSHPx enzymes, but unlike them it can metabolize fatty acid hydroperoxides esterified to phospholipids. It is associated with cell membranes and is involved, along with vitamin E, in the protection of membranes against oxidative damage. It may also have a more general role in cellular metabolism, possibly through involvement in eicosanoid metabolism.

Extracellular glutathione peroxidase

Extracellular glutathione peroxidase (eGSHPx), also a tetramer of four identical 22 kDa subunits, each containing a selenocysteine residue, is a glycoprotein. It is synthesized mainly in the kidneys and is thought to protect extracelluar spaces from oxidative damage.

Selenoprotein P

Selenoprotein P (Se-P) is a single polypeptide chain containing 10 selenocysteine residues. Between 70 and 80% of plasma Se may be in this form. Its function has not yet been elucidated but it may have an antioxidant role in plasma and extracellular spaces.

Selenoprotein W

Selenoprotein W (Se-W) is a low molecular weight protein with a single selenocysteine residue per molecule. It is found in animal muscles and its loss is associated with myopathy in Se deficiency. It may also have antioxidant functions.

Sperm capsule selenoprotein

Sperm capsule selenoprotein contains three selenoprotein residues per molecule. It appears to be required for sperm development and may play a structural role in the sperm tail. Se deficiency can cause abnormal sperm formation and infertility in male rats.

Iodothyronine deiodinases

The iodothyronine deiodinases are a class of 'nonantioxidant' selenoproteins which are involved in thyroid metabolism. Type 1, type 2 and type 3 iodo-thyronine deiodinases (ID-I, ID-II and ID-III) are responsible for the regulation of the interconversion of active and inactive forms of iodothyronines. All three enzymes have selenocysteine at their active sites, but show considerable differences in their sensitivities to the effects of various inhibitors. They also are affected to different extents by Se deficiency.

Thioredoxin reductase

Thioredoxin reductase has recently been identified as a selenoprotein. It is involved in redox regulation of a range of enzymes and transcription factors and is required for the expression of several different proteins.

Essentiality

An early indication of the essentiality of Se was the discovery by Schwarz in 1957 that the element could prevent liver necrosis in vitamin E-deficient rats. Subsequently Se was found to be important in the prevention of several other diseases in animals. The use of Se in rations and fertilizers has had a major impact in reducing levels of incidence of Se-dependent conditions such as white muscle disease (WMD). It was not until 1973 that a satisfactory explanation for the role of Se was proposed following the discovery by Rotruck and his colleagues that the element is an integral part of the antioxidant enzyme GSHPx.

Evidence that Se deficiency was also responsible for specific diseases in humans began to appear in the late 1970s when Chinese scientists reported an association between low Se intake and Keshan disease (KD). This is a cardiomyopathy which affects children and women of child-bearing age. It occurred in epidemic proportions in areas of China where the soil is deficient in Se. Large-scale intervention trials, involving more than 1.5 million children, demonstrated the value of Se in preventing the disease.

While Se deficiency is probably not the only factor involved in KD, it seems clear that it disposes people to its development. A similar situation occurs with Kashin-Bek disease (KBD), a chronic osteoarthropathy which most commonly affects growing children. It occurs in parts of Siberian Russia and in China, where it overlaps with KD. Oral supplementation with Se is effective in preventing KBD, though it is likely that other factors besides Se deficiency are involved.

In addition to KD and KBD, several nonendemic Se-responsive conditions occur in humans. These include cardiomyopathies and muscular problems in patients receiving total parenteral nutrition (TPN) where there is inadequate Se in the infusion fluid.

Symptoms, which are similar to those of KD, usually respond to Se supplementation.

Normal function of the thyroid gland is dependent on an adequate supply of dietary selenium. It has been shown that the myxoedematous cretinism which occurs in regions of endemic goitre in tropical Africa is related to a combined deficiency of both Se and iodine (I). It is believed that Se deficiency increases some indicators of hypothyroid stress associated with inadequate dietary I. The connection between the two elements is complex and is not yet fully understood.

Associations between Se status and various chronic degenerative diseases, including cancer and cardiovascular disease, have been reported. There is some epidemiological evidence linking low intake of Se with some cancers. Animal experiments show that Se, at least at high levels of intake, may protect against certain chemically or virally induced tumours.

It is postulated that damage to the arterial endothelium caused by free radicals produced by peroxidation of lipids can initiate formation of atheromatous plaques leading to coronary vascular disease (CVD). There is some evidence that antioxidant nutrients, including Se, can reduce peroxidation, and thus have a protective effect against CVD.

Se plays a part in the body's response to infection and contributes to the integrity of the immune system. In children with Down syndrome, for instance, who are particularly prone to bacterial infection, Se supplementation has been shown to increase levels of serum IgG_2. Se supplementation may also help to prevent age-related immunosuppression. Decreased immunocompetence in patients suffering from kwashiorkor may be related to low serum Se.

As many as 40 other health conditions have been postulated as having a link with Se. These include age-related macular degeneration of the retina, cataract, cystic fibrosis, multiple sclerosis and sudden infant death syndrome. For some of these, evidence for an involvement of Se is not convincing; for others it is reasonably strong.

The recent inclusion of Se among trace nutrients for which official intake recommendations have been established in many countries, indicates the growing recognition of the nutritional importance of this element by health authorities. Se supplements are available without prescription in most countries and are consumed in considerable quantities. Finland has gone so far as to legislate for the addition of Se to all multielement fertilizers used in agriculture, with the express intent of increasing dietary intake in the belief that this will result in improved health in the community.

Assessment of Selenium Status

There is no one method for assessment of Se status that is entirely satisfactory. Four different approaches that are frequently reported are: (1) measurement of dietary intake of Se; (2) determination of Se concentrations in blood, or its fractions; (3) measurement of GSHPx in blood or its fractions; and (4) measurement of Se levels in other body fluids and tissues. Simple measures of dietary intake, while indicative of the general status of a population, are not sufficient for determining Se status in individuals. This is because of variations in levels of the element between foodstuffs and uncertainty about the availability for absorption of the different forms of the element.

Whole-blood Se measurements are useful in large-scale epidemiological studies because little pretreatment of samples is required. There are certain advantages in using blood fractions. Plasma and serum levels, which respond rapidly to Se supplementation, are indices of short-term status. However, plasma Se may not reflect other body fractions, especially in muscle. Erythrocyte Se is an index of longer-term status and is not subject to sudden changes in dietary intake.

Good correlation exists between blood GSHPx activity and blood Se levels up to about 1.0 mg Se per litre. At higher levels, activity of the enzyme levels off. Nevertheless, at least in populations with a relatively low Se intake, GSHPx activity is a useful index of Se status. The measurements are made relatively easily, usually using a modification of the coupled enzyme assay procedure of Paglia and Valentine. Problems may be caused by the presence of haemoglobin and glutathione-S-transferase. This can be avoided by using platelets rather than whole blood. Though preparation is time-consuming, platelet GSHPx activity has been found to provide a precise measure of short-term Se status.

Urinary secretion of Se was formerly employed, especially by toxicologists, as a measure of exposure to the element, but is now mainly of historical interest. Determination of Se in hair, and in finger- and toenails, to assess Se status, is also used. These tissues have the advantage, especially for field studies, of ease of collection and storage. Evidence of strong correlations between whole-blood Se and both hair and toenail Se has been presented by a number of investigators. However, sample collection and preparation methods have not been well standardized, and external contamination of samples may occur. This is particularly true of hair since the use of Se in shampoos is common.

Requirements

The first recommendation regarding intake of Se was made by the Food and Nutrition Board (FNB) of the US National Research Council in 1980 as an Estimated Safe and Adequate Dietary Intake (ESADI) of 50–200 μg per day for adults. This was largely based on extrapolation from data derived from animal studies.

From the end of the 1980s sufficient data had been accumulated from studies on humans to allow a number of countries to publish recommended daily intakes (RDIs) or allowances (RDAs). These data included results of dietary intakes and balance studies which indicated levels necessary to maintain equilibrium under a variety of conditions. However, since humans can apparently adjust their Se requirements over a wide range of intakes, balance studies alone are insufficient for this purpose. Of more use have been measurement of intakes in areas with and without Se deficiency. Studies in KD endemic regions of China found that when supplements were given to people whose Se status was naturally depleted and their repletion monitored over several months, GSHPx activity plateaued at similar levels for men receiving approximately 40 μg Se per day, which was taken to be their physiological requirement. Using this figure as a basis for calculation, with extrapolation for differences in weight and incorporating a safety factor of 1.3, the FNB estimated the RDA for North American adults.

The US recommendations are compared with those of the UK, with which they closely correspond, in **Table 4**. Unlike the US figures, the British recommendations do not make extra allowance for pregnant women. This is on the grounds that adaptive changes in Se metabolism occur after conception which ensure that the Se needs of both mother and fetus are met by the normal adequate intake of women. During lactation additional Se is, however, required.

Dietary Sources and High Intakes

Se levels in plant-based food reflect concentrations of the element in the soil on which the crops were grown. Since this is subject to considerable regional variations, Se levels in individual foodstuffs can show a wide range even within a single country, such as Australia, as shown in **Table 5**. Variations in levels of Se in foods produced in different countries and regions are reflected in the range of dietary intakes reported worldwide (**Table 6**).

The relationship between Se in soil and in foods, and how dietary intakes can be affected by changes in agricultural practices are indicated in **Table 7**. The data compare Se levels in staple foodstuffs produced in Finland before and after Se enrichment of fertilizers was made mandatory in 1984.

Bioavailability

It should be noted that values quoted here, as in most published studies on Se levels in foods, are in terms of total content of the element. Because of analytical difficulties, few data have been published on levels in foods of the different chemical forms of Se. Since bioavailability is related to the chemical species of

Table 4 Dietary reference values/recommended allowances for Se (μg per day)

Age	UK	USA
0–3 months	10	10
4–6 months	13	10
7–9 months	10	15
10–12 months	10	15
1–3 years	15	20
4–6 years	20	20
7–10 years	30	30
Males		
11–14 years	45	40
15–18 years	70	50
19–50 years	75	70
50+ years	75	70
Females		
11–14 years	45	45
15–18 years	60	50
19–50 years	60	55
50+ years	60	55
Pregnancy	–	65
Lactation	+15	75

After Department of Health (1991) *Dietary Reference Values for Energy and Nutrients for the UK*. London: HMSO; National Research Council (1989) *Recommended Dietary Allowances*, 10th edn. Washington, DC: National Academy of Sciences.

Table 5 Range of selenium levels in different food groups

Food group	Se content (mg per kg wet wt)
Cereals, cereal products	0.01–0.31
Eggs	0.06–0.40
Fish	0.05–0.54
Meat (muscle)	0.06–0.42
(organ)	0.05–1.33
Milk, dairy products	<0.001–0.13
Vegetables, fruit	<0.001–0.022

After Reilly C (1996) *Selenium in Food and Health*. London: Blackie Academic and Professional.

Table 6 Dietary selenium intakes worldwide

Country (region)	Se intake (μg per day)
Australia	57–87
Canada	98–224
China (Keshan county)	3–22
China (Enshi county)	3200–6690
Greece	110–220
Mexico	10–223
New Zealand (Dunedin)	6–70
Portugal	10–100
Russia	60–80
UK	30–60
USA	62–216

After Reilly C (1996) *Selenium in Food and Health*. London: Blackie Academic and Professional.

Table 7 Changes in selenium levels in foods following introduction of Se-enriched fertilizers in Finland

	Se levels (mg per kg dry wt)	
Food	Pre-1984	Post-1984
Beef	0.04	0.46
Broccoli	<0.01–0.01	0.27–1.70
Milk	0.02	0.19
Pork	0.20	0.70
Wheat	<0.004–0.016	0.150–0.485

Data from Eurola M, Ekholm P, Ylinen M (1989) Effects of selenium fertilization on the selenium content of selected Finnish fruits and vegetables. *Acta Agriculturae Scandinavica* **39**: 345–350.

the element as consumed, this shortage of data is not without significance. While all forms of Se are relatively easily absorbed, there is evidence that not all species are used in the same way by the body. Blood Se levels, for instance, are higher when selenomethionine rather than selenite or selenate is consumed. Similarly selenomethionine intake increases nonspecific incorporation of Se into tissue protein more than does inorganic Se. In contrast, erythrocyte GSHPx activity is raised to the same level by both organic and inorganic Se.

High Intakes and Toxicity

Se toxicity, or selenosis, caused by excessive intake, has been well documented in farm animals, but less is known about it in humans. It has occurred on a large scale in seleniferous regions of China where Se-contaminated foods are consumed. There have also been reports of selenosis in individuals who consumed excessive amounts of Se supplements. The most common symptoms are loss of hair and deform-

ity and loss of nails. Skin lesions, peripheral neuropathy, diarrhoea, fatigue, irritability and a garlic-like odour on the breath and in body secretions have also been reported. Blood Se levels may be significantly higher than normal. However, as yet there is no sensitive and specific biochemical test for selenosis.

There is also uncertainty about levels of intake that will cause Se toxicity. Findings in China suggest that about 3–5 mg per day are sufficient to do so. Residents of seleniferous regions in South Dakota in the USA who consumed approximately 700 μg per day showed no symptoms of poisoning. The US Environmental Protection Agency has proposed an oral reference dose (RfD) of 5 μg per kg body weight per day, or 350 μg per day for a 70 kg adult male.

See also: **Antioxidants**: Diet and Antioxidant Defence; Observational Epidemiology; Intervention Studies. **Iodine**: Physiology, Dietary Sources and Requirements; Iodine Deficiency Disorders. **Tocopherols**: Physiology.

Further Reading

Arthur J (1997) Non-glutathione peroxidase functions of selenium. In: Lyons TP and Jacques KA (eds) *Biotechnology in the Feed Industry*, pp 143–154. Loughborough, UK: Nottingham University Press.

Diplock AT (1993) Indexes of selenium status in human populations. *American Journal of Clinical Nutrition* 57:256S–258S.

Eurola M, Ekholm P, Ylinen M, Koivistoinen P and Pertti V (1989) Effects of selenium fertilization on the selenium content of selected Finnish fruits and vegetables. *Acta Agriculturae Scandinavica* 39:345–350.

Ge K and Yang G (1993) The epidemiology of selenium deficiency in the etiological study of endemic diseases in China. *American Journal of Clinical Nutrition* 57:259S–263S.

Paglia DE and Valentine W (1967) Studies on the quantitative and qualitative characterisation of erythrocyte glutathione peroxidase. *Journal of Laboratory and Clinical Medicine* 70:159–169.

Reilly C (1996) *Selenium in Food and Health*. London: Blackie Academic and Professional.

Rotruck JT, Pope A, Ganther HE, Swanson AB, Hafeman D and Hoekstra WG (1973) Selenium: biological role as a component of glutathione peroxidase. *Science* 179:588–590.

Schwartz K and Foltz CM (1957) Selenium as an integral part of factor 3 against dietary necrotic liver degeneration. *Journal of the American Chemical Society* 79:3292–3293.

Thomson CD and Robinson MF (1980) Selenium in human health and disease with emphasis on those aspects peculiar to New Zealand. *American Journal of Clinical Nutrition* 33:303–323.

Senescence *see* **Ageing**: Biological Aspects.

Short bowel syndrome *see* **Therapeutic Dietetics**: Short Bowel Syndrome.

Skinfold thickness *see* **Nutritional Status**: Anthropometric Assessment.

SMOKING

Effects on Diet and Nutritional Status

R L Thompson and **B Margetts**, Institute of Human Nutrition, University of Southampton, Southampton, UK

A A Jackson, Institute of Human Nutrition, University of Southampton, Southampton, UK

Smoking is one of the largest preventable causes of mortality. In economically developed countries, about 3 million people die each year from the effects of smoking, half of them before the age of 70 years. Younger people are more likely to smoke than older people. Despite an overall downward trend in rates of smoking in Northern Europe, the rate continues to increase in younger women. The prevalence of smoking in Eastern Europe and economically developing countries is increasing at an alarming rate. The disease risk of smoking is likely to be more important in the future. The Global Burden of Disease Survey revealed that by 2020 tobacco is expected to cause more premature death and disability than any single disease, accounting for about 12% of the world disease burden.

Precise definitions of smoking status vary between studies. Smokers include those currently smoking cigarettes, but may also include pipe and cigar smokers. Nonsmokers are those people not currently smoking and include people who have never smoked and past smokers. In some studies they may also include pipe, cigar or infrequent smokers. Some studies present data separately for smokers, those who have never smoked and ex-smokers. This article concentrates on cigarette smoking and does not discuss pipe or cigar smoking as a separate classification; here the term 'smokers' is used to describe cigarette smokers.

People who smoke cigarettes differ in many respects from those who do not smoke. Alcoholism is about 10 times higher among smokers than non-smokers; smokers are also more likely to have accidents and less likely to take part in health-related activities than nonsmokers. The factors responsible for the increased disease risk associated with smoking cigarettes are not fully understood. Smokers may be at higher risk of disease because of:

1. a direct effect of smoking on metabolic processes;
2. their dietary habits and lifestyle put them at higher risk; or
3. their psychological and socio-demographic characteristics increase their risk.

It is likely that the disease risk in smokers is elevated because of complex interactions among some or all of the above factors. This article covers the association between diet and smoking and includes the effects of cigarette smoking in humans on dietary intakes, body weight and nutritional requirements, and also the effects of cigarette smoking on physiology and disease risk. It is outside the scope of the article to look in detail at the mechanisms for differences in dietary intake and body weight by smoking status.

Dietary Intakes of Smokers

Meal patterns and food and nutrient intakes differ between smokers and nonsmokers. Few studies have assessed the diets of smokers before they started to smoke. It is, therefore, difficult to establish whether people who eat a certain way are more likely to become smokers, or whether taking up smoking alters dietary patterns. Smoking may either affect food choice directly, or indirectly by, for example, altering physiological processes related to smell, taste or appetite. It is possible that other factors (such as age, gender, socioeconomic group) that are related independently to diet and smoking influence the relationships reported. Smokers' diets are less likely to comply with current dietary guidelines for a healthy diet than those of nonsmokers. Smokers have higher saturated fat and sugar intakes, and lower polyunsaturated fat, fibre and antioxidant intakes than nonsmokers. For a short time immediately upon giving up smoking quitters eat more, thus increasing energy intake transiently. However, after 1 year or more the diets of quitters start to become like those of people who have never smoked.

The available evidence comes from a variety of study designs. First there are cross-sectional studies which compare the dietary habits of current smokers and nonsmokers, where nonsmokers may include those who have stopped smoking for a number of years and those who have never smoked. There are also prospective studies which look at the dietary changes that occur when smokers stop smoking. These studies can be divided into those which look at changes that occur within 1 year of smoking cessation and those which examine changes that occur in the long term.

The food frequency questionnaire and diet record are the most popular methods for assessing diet in cross-sectional studies, while the diet record (weighed or unweighed) is widely used for prospective studies. Most studies adjust for the confounding effects of age, gender and socioeconomic group, and some also adjust for alcohol in their analysis.

The data for food patterns and nutrient intakes have been reviewed separately. The differences in food patterns and nutrient intakes are summarized in **Table 1** and **Table 2**.

Food patterns

Food patterns differ between smokers and nonsmokers. Studies are consistent worldwide from Northern Europe, the USA and Mediterranean countries to

Table 1 Summary of differences in food patterns between smokers and nonsmokers

Smokers consume more:	Smokers consume less:
Whole milk	Skimmed milk
Fried foods	Fruit
Cured meats and sausages	Vegetables
Sugar	Salad
	Wholegrain cereals

Table 2 Summary of differences in nutrient intakes between smokers and nonsmokers

Smokers consume more:	Smokers consume less:
Saturated fat	Protein
Sugar	Fibre
Alcohol	Polyunsaturated fats
	Antioxidant vitamins
	(e.g. vitamin C)

Japan. In comparison with nonsmokers, smokers more frequently consume fried food, processed meats, whole milk and sugar, while smokers less frequently consume fruit, fruit juice, vegetables, salads, skimmed milk and wholegrain cereals (such as wholemeal bread in preference to white bread). Meal patterns also differ by smoking status, with smokers eating breakfast less frequently than nonsmokers.

There is limited information on changes in food patterns upon quitting smoking, except that there may be an increase in snacking between meals. If this is true, it may lead to an overall increase in macronutrient intake after giving up smoking. The Multiple Risk Factor Intervention Trial (MRFIT) showed increased fruit and vegetable consumption for those smokers who gave up smoking compared with nonsmokers or continuing smokers at the 6 year follow-up.

Nutrient intakes

Male smokers consume similar or slightly higher energy intakes than male nonsmokers. The situation in women is less clear, with some studies showing higher, and others lower, energy intakes for smokers compared with nonsmokers. This may be because some women use cigarette smoking to control their body weight and energy intakes. Protein intakes tend to be lower in smokers compared with nonsmokers. In general there are only small differences in carbohydrate and total fat intakes by smoking status.

Larger nutrient differences are observed for type of fat consumed, with smokers consuming less polyunsaturated fat and having a lower polyunsaturated-to-saturated fat ratio compared with nonsmokers. Some, but not all, studies have shown higher saturated fat intakes in smokers compared with nonsmokers. Both men and women smokers consume more alcohol than nonsmokers. Dietary fibre intakes are reported to be lower in smokers than in nonsmokers. The main differences in macronutrient intakes between smokers and nonsmokers are observed for alcohol, polyunsaturated fats, saturated fat and dietary fibre.

Larger differences in nutrient intakes by smoking status have been observed for micronutrients.

Smokers consume lower intakes of β-carotene, ascorbic acid, vitamin E, thiamin and folate than nonsmokers. Some studies have investigated the effect of the number of cigarettes smoked on dietary intake. Consumption of antioxidant vitamins appears to be inversely related to the number of cigarettes smoked. Therefore, light smokers consume higher intakes of micronutrients than heavy smokers.

MRFIT, a longer-term prospective study, also showed that quitters compared with either smokers or nonsmokers decreased energy, total fat and saturated fat intakes and increased fibre, β-carotene and vitamin E intakes.

The studies that report nutrient intake changes after stopping smoking have been grouped by length of follow-up. Studies that focus on immediate changes (within 1 month) after giving up smoking, are consistent in showing statistically significant increases in daily energy intake (range 840–1670 kJ; 200–400 kcal). This consistency is surprising considering the range of subjects and methods of dietary assessment. The medium-term studies of more than 1 month follow-up are not so consistent and tend to show smaller differences in energy intake attributable to smoking cessation. Short- and medium-term prospective studies of macronutrient and micronutrient intakes have shown mixed results, with some showing transient increases and other showing no changes.

Effects of Smoking on Body Weight

Smokers tend to be less overweight than nonsmokers. Immediately upon giving up smoking quitters start to gain weight and continue to do so for at least 1 year. However, several years later some of this excess weight is lost, possibly through dieting.

Energy intakes of smokers do not appear to differ appreciably from those of nonsmokers. Therefore, based upon energy intake alone, differences in body weight between smokers and nonsmokers would not be expected.

In contrast to the expectations from the dietary data about body weight, cross-sectional studies tend to show that smokers weigh less than those who have never smoked. Ex-smokers have been shown to have similar weights or weigh more than those who have never smoked. In general, cross-sectional studies show that nonsmokers weigh, on average, 3.5 kg more than smokers.

Long-term prospective studies report similar weight differences between smokers and ex-smokers to cross-sectional studies. The quitters in MRFIT were divided into those who were early quitters (quit after 1 to 2 years) and late quitters (quit during years

3 to 6). The quitters who had stopped smoking for longer showed a smaller weight gain (2.5 kg) than those who had quit more recently (3.3 kg).

Several studies have looked directly at the effect of giving up smoking on body weight. Most, but not all, people gain weight after giving up smoking. The length of time since quitting seems to influence weight gain (**Fig. 1**); the longer the time of quitting (up to 1 year), the greater the weight gain. There is also a gender difference, with women gaining more weight than men. The increase in body weight after smoking cessation is often regarded as a barrier to giving up smoking. It may also cause people who have recently stopped smoking to start again. The inclusion of a physical activity component or dietary counselling as part of a smoking cessation programme may help limit weight gain and thus improve success in stopping smoking.

Larger differences in weight have been observed in short-term prospective studies (up to 8 kg) than cross-sectional studies or longer-term prospective studies (3.5 kg) where subjects have quit smoking for many years. MRFIT shows that weight gain is less in those quitters who have stopped smoking for longer. Initial weight gain seems to be followed by weight loss. Dietary changes do not seem to account for the increase in weight or differences between smokers and nonsmokers. It is possible that other mechanisms are responsible for the differences in body weight between smokers and nonsmokers.

Possible mechanisms

Several mechanisms have been put forward to explain why smokers eat as much as or more than nonsmokers, despite having a lower body weight. If a person is in energy balance (neither gaining nor losing body weight), then energy intake is equal to energy expended. Therefore, a lower body weight may be due to either an increase in energy expended (such as higher activity levels) or a decrease in energy

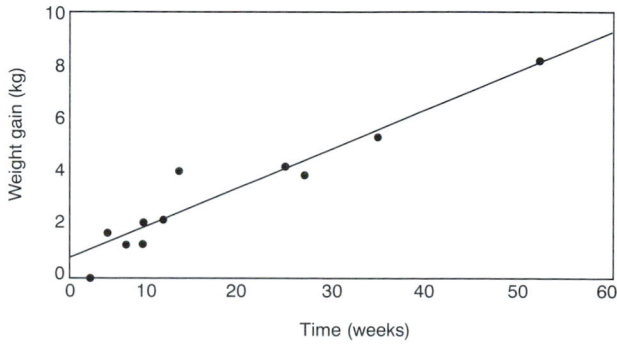

Figure 1 Weight gain after giving up smoking by time since quitting.

intake (eating less), or both. Smoking may increase energy expenditure by increasing metabolic rate. The slightly higher energy intakes shown in some studies are unlikely to account for a large difference in body weight. There is no evidence to suggest that smokers are more physically active than nonsmokers; in fact smokers may exercise less. The short-term increases in energy intake observed immediately after smoking cessation may be a result of people coping with the withdrawal symptoms of nicotine by substituting cigarettes with food.

Effects of Smoking on Nutritional Needs

At the same level of dietary intake, smokers appear to have lower circulating levels of antioxidants. This suggests that smoking affects the metabolic demands for these nutrients. The most likely explanation is through increased free radical load; cigarette smoke contains high levels of free radicals. The body produces free radicals as a result of normal physiological reactions and the body has developed its own defence system to protect against tissue damage. A part of this defence system is antioxidant vitamin intake. If the free radical load exceeds the ability of host defences to deal with this demand, tissue damage will occur. Smokers may therefore be liable to tissue damage owing to an imbalance between free radical production and the antioxidant defence system. The effect of smoking on blood levels of micronutrients independently of dietary intake is reviewed, and the points for and against supplementation are given.

Ascorbic acid

Smoking reduces ascorbic acid levels in plasma and leucocytes. It has been shown that if smokers and nonsmokers consume a similar intake of ascorbic acid, the serum level of ascorbic acid is lower in smokers than nonsmokers. To reach a given serum concentration of ascorbic acid, an increased dietary intake is needed for smokers compared with nonsmokers. In addition, smokers have a decreased intake and absorption of ascorbic acid which contributes to lowered ascorbic acid status. Even passive smoking may increase the requirement for ascorbic acid. Evidence suggests that within 4 weeks of giving up smoking plasma ascorbic acid concentration rises. There may be a beneficial physiological response for ascorbic acid supplementation. This includes improved lung and heart function, as well as decreased oxidation of plasma lipoproteins, these actions having relevance to the antioxidant potential of ascorbic acid. Dietary recommendations set in the UK in 1991 included a recommendation of 120 mg

of ascorbic acid for smokers, an increase of 80 mg over the level recommended for nonsmokers. This level was thought to be sufficient to maintain smokers' body pool and circulating levels of ascorbic acid near those of nonsmokers. In the US, 1989 RDAs (Recommended Dietary Allowances) recommended that regular cigarette smokers should ingest at least 100 mg of ascorbic acid daily. Other studies have suggested levels of 200 mg per day are required.

Dietary supplementation with ascorbic acid is not without its critics. It has been suggested that addition of large amounts of ascorbate drive nicotine out into the urine, thereby prompting smokers to smoke more. Others feel that the scientific evidence does not support a specific protective effect of ascorbic acid against chronic disease, and in certain cases, ascorbic acid stimulates neoplastic growth. Increasing ascorbic acid intake may further increase smokers' already enhanced risk of heart disease by enhancing both iron absorption and mobilization of iron reserves. Others believe that a modest increase may not be sufficient.

Other nutrients and antioxidant vitamins

There has been debate over the potential advantages of recommending higher intakes of other antioxidants and nutrients for smokers. Those arguing for supplementation state that physiological levels of vitamin E and β-carotene are inadequate (owing to lower intake and increased turnover) to deal with smoking-related oxygen stress and that adequate protection is achieved only when these agents are present in supra-physiological amounts. Supplementation with β-carotene in smokers has been shown to have beneficial effects on antioxidant status, regulating activity of phagocyte-derived oxidants, increased respiratory function and reduced risk of oral cancer. Opponents stress that conclusions of experimental and epidemiological studies on effects of reduced nutrient levels are tenuous and do not justify increasing current recommendations.

Exposure to cigarette smoke appears to cause a reduction of folate levels in serum and in erythrocytes. This reduction could render the bronchial epithelia susceptible to neoplastic transformation by carcinogens in cigarette smoke. Supplementation with folate and vitamin B_{12} has been shown to reduce bronchial squamous metaplasia.

Three randomized controlled trials have been carried out looking at the effect of vitamin A supplementation. One trial was conducted on a population of smokers, another on smokers, former smokers and asbestos workers, and a third where only 11% were current smokers. All trials supplemented with β-carotene and one with β-carotene and retinol. The subjects were followed up for between 4 and 14 years. The trial with only 11% of smokers showed no reduction in number of deaths from all causes, lung cancer and cardiovascular diseases. The two other studies showed increased relative risks for death from any cause, death from lung cancer and cardiovascular disease in the treatment group compared with the control group. These trials raise the possibility that these supplements may have harmful as well as beneficial effects, at least at the doses given.

Recommending that smokers consume higher intakes of polyunsaturated fats may not be advantageous. Evidence suggests that people with high intakes of polyunsaturated fats are more susceptible to free radical damage such as oxidation of plasma low-density lipoprotein (LDL). Smokers consuming a diet higher in polyunsaturated fat may increase the imbalance between free radical production and antioxidant defence, unless recommendations also include an increase in antioxidant intake.

Effects of Smoking on Physiology

Smoking cigarettes results in altered lipid metabolism, blood coagulation and an increased inflammatory response. This section reviews the evidence for the physiological effects on substances other than the micronutrients discussed in the previous section.

The high free radical load and relatively low antioxidant status in smokers may result in an imbalance between free radicals and antioxidants that may render lipoproteins more atherogenic. There is some evidence to suggest that cigarette smoke is able to modify LDL and increase its atherogenicity. Blood lipids and lipoprotein concentrations have been measured in both smokers and nonsmokers. In general smokers have higher concentrations of cholesterol (3%), triacylglycerols (9%), LDL cholesterol (2%) and significantly lower serum levels of high-density lipoprotein (HDL) cholesterol (6%) and apolipoprotein A-I (4%) compared with nonsmokers.

Raised fibrinogen is a recognized independent risk for coronary heart disease. Cross-sectional data have shown that smokers on average have higher plasma fibrinogen levels than nonsmokers. A decreased serum albumin has been associated with an increased mortality from cardiovascular disease and cancer. Serum albumin levels are reduced in smokers compared with never and ex-smokers. The low albumin levels may be a marker of an inflammatory response. This is also consistent with a higher white cell count in smokers compared with nonsmokers. Smokers have a slightly lower blood pressure, both systolic and diastolic, than nonsmokers.

Although smokers are less likely to be obese than nonsmokers, they have a higher waist-to-hip ratio. A higher waist-to-hip ratio is a risk factor for coronary heart disease.

Studies have shown that after giving up smoking HDL cholesterol, LDL cholesterol and apolipoprotein A-I concentrations return to the levels found in nonsmokers. Prospective data from smokers who become ex-smokers indicate that although fibrinogen levels appeared to fall quite soon after quitting, it may take 5 years or more to reach levels of people who have never smoked. Another clotting agent, factor VIIc, increases after smoking cessation; however, this may be a result of weight gain or an increased fat intake. Blood pressure tends to increase after smoking cessation. The increase in body weight may be at least partially responsible for this.

Possible mechanisms

Nicotine may stimulate the release of adrenaline leading to an increase of free fatty acids observed in smokers. Free fatty acids stimulate hepatic secretion of very low-density lipoprotein and hence triacylglycerol. High-density lipoprotein concentrations vary inversely with very low-density lipoprotein concentration in serum. It is possible that cigarette smoking initiates an inflammatory response that may lead to both decreased albumin levels and increased acute-phase proteins such as plasma fibrinogen.

The lower body weight of smokers may at least partially explain the unexpected lower blood pressure in smokers compared with nonsmokers. This would also explain the increase in blood pressure after smoking cessation, when body weight increases. The differences in body fat distribution may be a result of changes in hormone levels associated with smoking.

Effects of Smoking on Disease Risk

Cigarette smoking is a major risk factor for many diseases including heart disease and cancer, the major causes of death in the developed world. Giving up smoking reduces this excess risk, but it takes many years for the disease risk to return to the level of those who have never smoked. There are several possible mechanisms by which the physiological effects reported above lead to an increased risk of certain diseases.

Disease risk

Smoking is recognized as a causative factor in cancers of eight sites: lung, upper respiratory tract, bladder, pancreas, oesophagus, stomach, kidney and blood (leukaemia). Smokers are also judged to be at increased risk of six other potentially fatal diseases: respiratory heart disease, chronic obstructive lung disease, stroke, pneumonia, aortic aneurysm and ischaemic heart disease. Smokers compared with those who have never smoked are two to three times more likely to die from these diseases. Nonfatal disease, such as peripheral vascular disease, cataracts, diabetes, hip fracture and periodontal disease, which cause appreciable disability, cost and inconvenience, are also associated with smoking. In pregnancy, smoking increases the risk of limb reduction defects, spontaneous abortion, ectopic pregnancy and low birthweight. About 20% of all deaths in developed countries are attributed to smoking.

Possible mechanisms

There are some possible explanations for the increased risk of coronary heart disease in cigarette smokers. These include altered blood coagulation, damage to the arterial wall and changes in blood lipid and lipoprotein concentrations. The increased risk for cancer may be a result of products of lipid peroxidation causing damage to DNA. Inflammatory reactions in the lung may result in pulmonary diseases. Risk of stroke may be related to cigarette smoking by development of carotid artery atherosclerosis or by increasing arterial wall stiffness, altered pattern of arterial blood flow and decreased pulsatility index.

Effect of giving up smoking and reduction in disease risk

Giving up smoking appears to increase life expectancy by approximately 3 years in both men and women. The increase in life expectancy is observed at all ages but depends on the number of years smoked. The reduction in risk of coronary heart disease starts immediately after stopping smoking and continues for many years. One-third of the excess risk for coronary heart disease disappears within 2 years of cessation. However, it takes 10 to 14 years following smoking cessation before coronary risk returns to the level of those who have never smoked.

Conclusions

The dietary habits of smokers are less in line with current dietary guidelines for a healthy diet than those of nonsmokers. In particular, smokers consume less fruit, vegetables and salads, less fibre but more saturated fat and alcohol than nonsmokers. The decreased antioxidant intake, increased saturated fat intake and the physiological effects of ciga-

rette smoking lead to an increased risk of several diseases including cancer and coronary heart disease.

See also: **Alcohol**: Absorption, Metabolism and Physiological Effects; Disease Risk and Beneficial Effects; Effects of Alcohol Consumption on Diet and Nutritional Status. **Antioxidants**: Diet and Antioxidant Defence. **Ascorbic Acid**: Physiology, Dietary Sources and Requirements. **Cancer**: Epidemiology and Associations Between Diet and Cancer; Epidemiology of Breast Cancer; Epidemiology of Colorectal Cancer; Epidemiology of Lung Cancer; Epidemiology of Gastrointestinal Cancers Other Than Colorectal Cancers; Diet in Cancer Treatment. **Coronary Heart Disease**: Aetiology; Prevention. **Folic Acid**: Physiology, Dietary Sources and Requirements. **Pregnancy**: Energy Requirements and Metabolic Adaptations. **Vitamin Supplementation**: Role.

Further Reading

Bendich A and Langseth L (1995) The health effects of vitamin C supplementation: A review. *Journal of the American College of Nutrition* **14**:124–136.

Bornstein NM (1994) Lifestyle changes: smoking, alcohol, diet and exercise. *Cerebrovascular Disease* **4**:59–65

Diana JN and Pryor WA (eds) (1993) Tobacco smoking and nutrition: influence of nutrition on tobacco-associated health risks. *Annals of the New York Academy of Sciences* **686**:1–360.

Ernst E (1995) Haemorheological consequences of chronic cigarette smoking. *Journal of Cardiovascular Risk* **2**:435–439.

Grimble RF (1990) Nutrition and cytokine action. *Nutrition Research Reviews* **3**:193–210.

Mayne ST (1996) Beta-carotene, carotenoids, and disease prevention in humans. *FASEB Journal* **10**:690–701.

Omvik P (1996) How smoking affects blood pressure. *Blood Pressure* **5**:71–77.

Perkins KA (1992) Effects of tobacco smoking on caloric intake. *British Journal of Addiction* **87**:193–205.

Porkka KVK and Ehnholm C (1996) Smoking, alcohol and lipoprotein metabolism. *Current Opinion in Lipidology* **7**:162–166.

Preston AM (1991) Cigarette smoking – nutritional implications. *Progress in Food and Nutrition Science* **15**:183–217.

Stamler J, Rains-Clearman D, Lenz-Litzow K, Tillotson JL and Grandits GA (1997) Chapter 14. Relation of smoking at baseline and during trial years 1–6 to food and nutrient intakes and weight in the special intervention and usual care groups of the Multiple Risk Factor Intervention Trial. *American Journal of Clinical Nutrition* **65** (supplement): 374S–402S.

Thompson RL, Margetts BM, Wood DA and Jackson AA (1992) Cigarette smoking and food and nutrient intakes in relation to coronary heart disease. *Nutrition Research Reviews* **5**:131–152.

Wald NJ and Hackshaw AK (1996) Cigarette smoking: an epidemiological overview. *British Medical Bulletin* **52**:3–11.

Social class *see* **Socioeconomic Status**: Relationship with Diet and Nutritional Status.

SOCIOECONOMIC STATUS

Relationship with Diet and Nutritional Status

E Dowler and **J Pryer**, London School of Hygiene and Tropical Medicine, London, UK

In most societies there is an inverse relationship between socioeconomic status and nutritional status, whether the former is measured as income, assets or social class, and the latter as food consumption or body dimensions. Socioeconomic status is difficult to define consistently. The problems include how to define and measure basic subsistence; whether to look at the status of individuals or households; how to define and interpret social class differences; and how to understand differences in status between societies, and in one society over time. People's circumstances often change, and sometimes the process of change may affect nutritional outcomes as well as the conditions themselves.

Basic subsistence usually means a level of living that enables people to survive and reproduce. Reproduction here means both physiological (women of child-bearing age are menstruating and can conceive and carry children to term) and economic (a household has the means to feed, clothe and house its members and take part in minimum social and economic exchange). Quantifying this basic level can be difficult: people disagree over the cutoff levels to define minimum energy or nutrient intakes for survival or reproduction, over the rates of child growth that are healthy, and how much money or its equivalent is needed for a household to survive. Resolving these controversies depends partly on technical decisions, and partly on agreed social value judgments.

Disentangling what happens within the household – who owns or has access to what assets and resources – is difficult. Even someone living alone may be entitled to resources or a share of production from another household. However, most surveys use household data on consumption or asset ownership, and then divide these by the number of household members to estimate individual shares. This approach ignores differences within a household over the control and management of resources, and assumes everything is shared equally. (What would 'equally' mean for nutrients? Everyone eating the same, or everyone eating what they need?)

Social class and status are affected by social and cultural conditions as well as economic conditions; most classifications try to incorporate all three factors. Some of the work described here uses proxy measures of socioeconomic status, as an alternative to income. These proxies can be single indicators, such as mother's educational level or head of household's occupation. Alternatively, they can be composite indices, often drawing on census data, which combine single indicators, such as crowding, occupation, car access, housing tenure or employment status, into one index (an example would be the Carstairs index in the UK). All these indicators describe the socioeconomic status of households rather than individuals.

Current social and economic changes which are associated with increasing socioeconomic differentials, in developed countries include the growth in unemployment or insecure employment, unstable family structures, homelessness, migrancy and reductions in welfare provision. Similar factors are in force in developing countries, with the addition of economic structural adjustment and globalization of production and trade. There is debate over the relationship between socioeconomic status, nutrition (food and growth) and work productivity. Some argue undernutrition contributes to poverty at the household level and potentially at national level, because an inadequate diet can reduce an individual's work capacity – either through a direct effect of food, or indirectly over time because a person is small and/or thin. Reduced work capacity results in lower productivity and economic return, which in turn contribute to increasing poverty and malnutrition: a 'vicious circle'. These effects may be seen both in an individual and in their immediate household, or as part of the reduction in human capital in malnourished populations, across generations.

Socioeconomic Status and Disease Risk and Mortality

In the 1970s, the World Fertility Survey documented very large socioeconomic differentials in child mortality in most of the 41 developing countries participating. **Table 1** shows socioeconomic differentials in mortality rates during the first 5 years of life in nine of the countries participating in the World Fertility Survey. Over the subsequent two decades overall child mortality rates fell by around 50%, but socioeconomic differentials in child survival have remained, and in some cases have widened.

Reduction in infant and child mortality rates and concomitant decline in fertility in many developing countries have led to changes in population age structure, overall health status and mortality patterns. A shift towards an older population means a parallel shift to diseases of adults rather than children. In many developing countries populations seem also to be moving from a predominantly environmental exposure to infectious diseases (from poor water, sanitation and insecure food supply) to one for noncommunicable diseases (motor vehicles, unsafe workplaces, air pollution, smoking, alcohol, increased fat and sugar intakes and decreased social support). Current hypotheses on the fetal origins of some chronic diseases highlight the role of the early nutritional environment for the risk of adult hypertension and cardiovascular disease. Those in low socioeconomic groups in developing countries, where low birthweight and inadequate infant nutrition are common experiences, may face the double risk of infectious disease or death in childhood, and, where children survive, of noncommunicable diseases in adulthood.

These shifts in demographic, disease and risk profiles, often referred to as the epidemiological transition, are occurring at different rates in most developing countries, although reliable cause-specific mortality data are rare. **Table 2** shows estimated and projected mortality rates by major cause, sex and region from 1970 to 2000. Poorer adults certainly die younger than richer adults, but why this should be so is less clear. For example, in Porto Alegre, Brazil, the poorest men had higher death rates from cancer and cardiovascular disease than wealthier men. Conversely, large population-based surveys in India suggested the prevalence of coronary heart disease was nearly four times greater in those from higher socioeconomic groups than in those from lower groups. Do poorer people suffer more from infectious and parasitic disease, and the wealthier more from noncommunicable diseases, or do the poor face greater risk of both?

There is also a growing literature on the inverse relationship between socioeconomic status and differential morbidity or premature mortality in developed countries. These differentials are seen in the main causes of mortality – coronary heart disease and cancers – and they have particularly widened in countries where income inequality has increased. The differences seem to be cumulative: those born into low socioeconomic groups, and who remain in them throughout childhood and adulthood, have higher mortality risk than those who move up a class during their lifetime.

Studies have used various socioeconomic indicators: occupational class, employment status, housing tenure, car access. The mortality differentials are large and can be located in terms of people and places: in **Table 3**, for instance, the matching between mortality and spatial indicators of economic and social advantage or disadvantage is very strong. However, the increasing polarization of wealth and poverty between households in the UK (a growth in two-earner and no-earner households) and places, means that lower death rates occur where richer people are concentrated, and higher death rates occur where disadvantaged people are concentrated. It is not just a matter of 'unhealthy places'.

Finally, there is evidence of a gradient of health and mortality, rather than a threshold below which everyone does badly and above which most are reasonably healthy. The UK Whitehall longitudinal studies of civil servants showed those in the second highest grade (not a low socioeconomic group) had worse health and mortality risk than those in the highest grade. However, those in the lowest grade had the worst health and mortality risks, and studies in several countries have shown the long-term unemployed to have high mortality risks.

Current thinking about why these differentials occur is that artefactual distortions or social selection cannot account for them, but that social conditions or material factors, perhaps partially mediated by life circumstances, beliefs and behaviour, offer the best explanations. Money is clearly important: having enough to meet basic needs, but also for a sense of security. Psychosocial factors and the control people have over their working or social environment also play an important part. Indeed, increasing income inequality and insecurity, as much as absolute poverty, may be important predictors of mortality differentials.

Socioeconomic Differences in Food Consumption

The socioeconomic status of a household can affect

Table 1   Mortality rates during the first 5 years of life (per thousand births) for nine countries participating in the World Fertility Survey

	Mortality rate per 1000 births											
Country	Mother's education (years)				Husband's occupation				Husband's education (years)			
	0	1–3	4–6	7+	Agriculture	Skilled/unskilled	Sales/service	Professional	0	1–3	4–6	7+
Lesotho	(224)[a]	215	185	169	(157)	193	(214)	(116)	185	212	196	169
Kenya	181	164	128	111	183	172	148	101	185	208	159	127
Sudan	146	109	109	109	158	138	127	95	155	152	104	84
Peru	237	171	98	55	218	157	123	59	241	217	150	75
Mexico	153	118	87	50	143	103	98	61	155	121	96	53
Panama	134	90	52	43	84	61	53	40	100	91	60	45
Bangladesh	222	198	186	(122)	216	236	208	152	230	221	191	176
Philippines	130	118	94	53	106	82	64	46	118	122	96	62
Malaysia	67	64	56	18	72	59	48	40	88	59	60	40

Data from Hobscraft et al. (1984).
[a]Rates based on fewer than 500 births are shown in parentheses.

Table 2 Estimated and projected mortality rates (per 100 000), by major cause, sex and region, 1970–2000

	1970 Estimated mortality rate (per 100 000)		2000 Projected mortality rate	
Region and cause	Male	Female	Male	Female
Latin America and Caribbean				
All causes	1097	903	677	557
Infections	366	301	100	86
Neoplasms	79	76	94	86
Circulatory	238	214	242	215
Pregnancy	0	12	0	4
Perinatal	61	42	40	28
Sub-Saharan Africa				
All causes	2163	1882	1196	1024
Infections	1070	937	498	430
Neoplasms	52	57	54	55
Circulatory	243	226	182	169
Pregnancy	0	27	0	17
Perinatal	200	157	119	90
Asia				
All causes	1280	1342	784	736
Infections	506	577	149	176
Neoplasms	70	70	101	87
Circulatory	230	227	268	235
Pregnancy	0	17	0	10
Perinatal	98	91	42	32

Data from Bulatao RA (1993) Mortality by cause 1970–2015. In: Gribble and Preston (1993).

Table 3 Age-standardized death rates per 100 000, by area, UK 1990–2 (ranked by male rates, ages 0–74 years)

Areas[a]	Males Rate per 100 000	Females Rate per 100 000
Prosperous wards	443	306
Established owner-occupied	470	316
Rural areas	483	327
Rural areas/mixed economies	530	358
Suburbia	549	365
Metropolitan professionals	624	380
Industrial and manufacturing towns	712	468
Deprived city areas	731	450
Deprived industrial areas	829	538
Purpose-built, inner city estates	868	528

Adapted from Charlton J (1996) Which areas are healthiest? *Population Trends* 83:17–24.
[a]Provisional names assigned by the Office of Population Censuses and Surveys (now Office of National Statistics) to groupings of electoral wards which are similar in terms of socioeconomic characteristics of their population.

the diet of its members in a number of ways. In general, those with higher incomes tend to spend a smaller proportion of that income purchasing food, although they may spend a larger absolute amount than those with lower incomes. Secondly, the kinds of foods richer people buy will be different in quality (less contamination, better processed or packaged) and in nutrient density. Richer people are generally 'less efficient' purchasers of energy than poor people: richer people can afford to buy foods that provide sufficient energy in total but in foodstuffs that are more pleasant to eat, or which are less energy-dense. Poor people have to maximize the energy and nutrients they can obtain for as little cost as possible. However, many studies have shown that even the poorest do not eat a theoretical 'least-cost diet': everyone tries to satisfy cultural demands for taste or tradition in food type or preparation methods. When low-income groups obtain more money, they are often observed to spend it on more expensive foods than hitherto, which are sometimes less energy-dense than commodities bought previously, but which carry higher status (such as meat), or are more tasty (such as fruit). Thirdly, those who are poor tend to obtain most of their energy from basic staple foods, particularly roots and tubers, or coarse grains (millets and sorghums); these starchy foods cost less in land or labour to produce than other foodstuffs. Poorer people also eat monotonous diets based on few food types. As people move up the income scale, they substitute higher-value grains (maize, rice or wheat) and more processed or desirable versions of those grains (bread made from highly milled flour). They also obtain more energy from nonstaple foods, and eat a more varied diet, including foods of animal origin, which in wealthier groups provide between 33% and 40% of total energy. People can also afford to express more health consciousness in food choice, buying leaner meat, more fresh produce and (somewhat perversely) expensive, less refined foods.

Variations in individual nutrient intake by income are usually less than variations between income groups in quantities and patterns of food purchased may suggest. Those who are poorest, whether by income or assets (such as landless labourers), tend to be very sensitive to food prices and will purchase substitute commodities as prices vary. However, people may also exhibit relative price inelasticity for a highly prized staple (for instance, they will buy rice, however expensive).

In developing countries, particularly those undergoing national economic changes through structural adjustment programmes, there is evidence of deteriorating household food security among those whose incomes are declining, and for whom reductions in welfare and food price subsidies have most significance. Those whose social and economic entitlement base is the least secure are most vulnerable to reduced food intakes following economic change. In general, energy and protein intakes, as well as micronutrient intakes, tend to vary inversely with income group, land-holding or asset measures of socioeconomic status, although the degree depends on local social and economic circumstances (**Fig. 1**).

In developed countries or regions, there are generally fewer differences between income groups or social classes in per capita consumption of energy, proteins or fats, though some surveys show poorer groups eat more energy as saturated fats or as refined sugar. However, most national and small-sample surveys show there are marked differences in intakes of vitamins and minerals such as iron and calcium. Those who are poorest (by whatever measure) often have very low intakes of these nutrients, well below reference levels, which indicates a high risk of poor health outcomes (**Table 4**). Smoking complicates this picture: those on low incomes who smoke have lower micronutrient intakes than those who do not smoke, which is partly an income effect (they cannot afford to buy enough appropriate food) but also a direct effect of smoking (smokers have different dietary patterns – in particular, lower fruit intakes – whatever their income). Those on lower incomes are more likely to be smokers.

Socioeconomic status not only affects how much money people have to spend on food; it also increasingly affects their social and physical environment, which has implications for food. In many countries, geographical socioeconomic polarization means that poorer people tend to live in low-quality housing, with limited domestic equipment, in residential areas with few, if any, shopping facilities and insufficient public transport. Food shops selling a wider range of better-quality goods, often at cheaper prices than small local shops, tend to be located where the wealthier live, or to be only accessible by car. Car ownership and housing tenure are becoming good indicators of health; part of that relationship is mediated by economic and physical access to sufficient, healthy food.

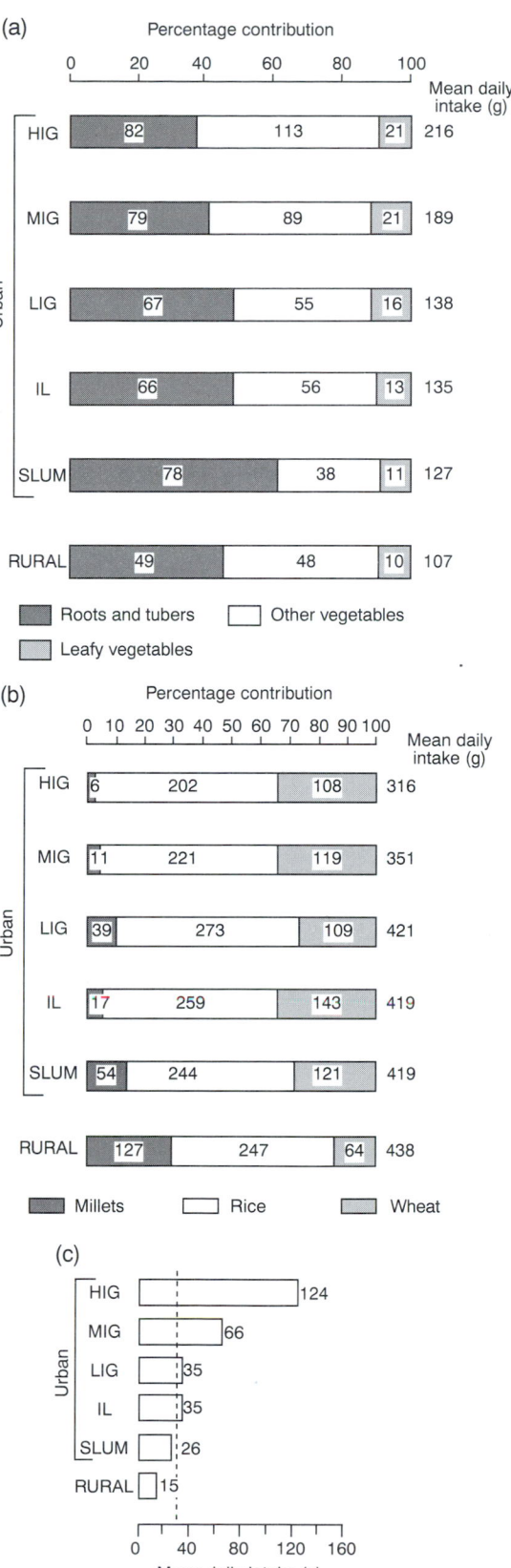

Figure 1 Average intake of foodstuffs in different urban and rural groups in India. (a) Vegetables (recommended daily intake 150 g); (b) millets and cereals (recommended daily intake 460 g); (c) fruit (recommended daily intake 30 g). Numbers in each bar indicate mean intake (g per day). HIG, high-income group; IL, industrial labourers; LIG, low-income group; MIG, middle-income group. Taken from: *Nutrition News* (1988) Vols 9/5–6 and (1989) Vol 10/1. National Institute of Nutrition, Hyderabad, India.

Table 4 British women: mean daily energy and nutrient intakes (7-day weighed intake)

Nutrient	All women (n = 1110)	Unemployed (n = 57)	Benefit recipients (n = 153)	Social classes IV and V (n = 222)	Lone mothers (n = 76)
Energy (kal)	1680	1640	1560	1580	1580
Energy (MJ)	7.0	6.8	6.5	6.6	6.6
Protein (g)	62.0	56.5	55.6	57.3	56.3
Fat (g)	73.5	71.9	67.7	69.6	69.9
Fibre (g)	18.6	17.7	16.8	16.9	16.1
Iron (mg)	12.3	10.4	11.8	11.6	11.5
Calcium (mg)	730	642	636	660	605
Zinc (mg)	8.4	7.5	7.4	7.7	7.5
Folate (μg)	219	190	192	196	199
Vitamin A (μg)[a]	1488	1003	1328	1217	1206
Vitamin C (mg)	73.1	72.1	55.4	55.8	55.8
Vitamin E (mg)	8.6	7.1	7.5	8.2	7.3

Data from Gregory J, Foster K, Tyler H and Wiseman M (1990) *The Dietary and Nutritional Survey of British Adults*. London: HMSO. Crown copyright is reproduced with permission of the Controller of Her Majesty's Stationery Office.
[a]Retinol equivalent.

These general findings have been examined in individual countries. For example, analyses of national survey data sets in the USA or Australia show weak relationships between nutrients and income. Educational status or household size were more predictive of low intakes. At subnational (state) level, however, the relationship between nutrients and income is more evident, as in several European countries. A different approach from national surveys looks at usage of food banks (free food provision). In many developed countries the numbers using food banks as a main food source has increased rapidly in the 1990s. Participants tend to be welfare recipients or unemployed, often with dependent children, from female headed households, and proportionately more likely to be ethnic minorities. All of these indicate lower socioeconomic status. However, studies of black African, black Caribbean or black British households in the UK, or black American, black African households in the USA, have shown their members more likely to eat a varied, 'healthy' diet (higher micronutrients, lower proportion of energy from fat) than their white counterparts, whatever the income level. South Asian households in the UK are less homogeneous in income and diet; some eat more pulses, whole cereals and vegetables than white counterparts, but many also have high fat and saturated fat intakes.

Many studies have shown nutrient intakes to be low, dietary patterns less healthy and dental caries more common in children from lower socioeconomic status households. Nonetheless, there is also evidence that parents, especially mothers, go without food or eat less healthily to ensure their children have enough and the best to eat in poorer households. Indeed, this is true throughout the world: parents try to buffer their children from the worst consequences of low socioeconomic status. Evidence that boys are always fed better than girls is equivocal, even for south Asia.

Socioeconomic Differences in Growth and Nutritional Status

Variations, both within and between populations, in body size at a given age and in the rate of maturation are partly genetic and partly environmental in origin. The most important determinants of birthweight and child growth – adequacy of the diet, quality of the environment and access to health services – are also core elements of the standard of living. As a result, indices of child growth and birthweight have long been recognized as sensitive indicators of social inequality.

In most countries, women from poorer families produce infants of lower birthweights (with lower chances of survival) than do women from better-off families (**Table 5**). Some of this socioeconomic differential reflects the size of the mothers; women are often smaller in poorer families. However, differences in birthweight also reflect what Hytten calls a 'comprehensive pattern of deprivation': a poorer quality diet, low pregnancy weight gain, mothers being underweight at conception, absence of or poor quality of prenatal care, poor housing, and behaviours such as smoking, alcohol and drug use.

Height in children and adults is positively associated with socioeconomic status throughout the world. **Fig. 2** shows the range of boys' heights from richer and poorer families in a number of countries. Social class differences in boys' heights varied from very little in Scandinavia to around 12 cm in the Indian samples. A number of studies have shown that when

Table 5 Male birthweights in different socioeconomic groups

Country/population	Mean birthweight	
	Well-off (kg)	Poor (kg)
Tehran, Iran	3.43	3.27
Shiraz, Iran	3.18	3.02
Lebanon	3.50	3.40
Delhi, India	3.16	2.74
Campinas, Brazil	3.41[a]	3.18[a]
Baltimore, USA		
black	2.97[a]	2.91[a]
white	3.27[a]	3.13[a]

From Eveleth PB (1986) Population differences in growth, environmental and genetic factors. In: Falkner and Tanner (1986).

indicators of social position are expressed on a continuous or graded scale, the relationship with height is monotonic: i.e. height increases with an increase in social position. This observation appears to be true even between groups from narrowly defined social strata, as shown by data from a single slum in Bangladesh (**Table 6**). A range of in-depth studies in developing countries of the relationship between socioeconomic status and height of children has consistently shown height responsive to individual socioeconomic indicators, whether of asset wealth or income itself, or proxy indicators such as land-holding, grain yields, parental education or occupation (**Table 7**).

A similar relationship can be shown in developed countries. For example, in the US National Health and Nutrition Examination Survey, child height increased monotonically in relation to increments in both household income and parental education (the data were controlled for race). In Britain, the National Child Health and Development Study showed that the difference in height at age 7 years between children born in social classes I and II and those in class V averaged 3.3 cm; at age 16 years the difference was 4.4 cm, in both instances controlling for confounding variables. In recent years, social class gradients in height, weight and age of peak height velocity and menarche have begun to attenuate in a few rich countries (Sweden, Norway, Finland and Hong Kong). This seems to be because secular trends in growth have been faster among children from lower social classes, and probably indicate generally high living standards rather than growth in a 'classless' society.

Social class gradients in attained adult height are also well documented. In British adults, and in Swedes born up to the mid 1950s, for instance, average heights of manual and nonmanual classes differ by about 3 cm for men, 2 cm for women. These averages may mask the effects of upward mobility: those who move up a class tend to be taller than those who stay within the same social class. In both Swedish and British populations, attained adult height has been shown to be related to economic conditions during childhood, independent of parental height

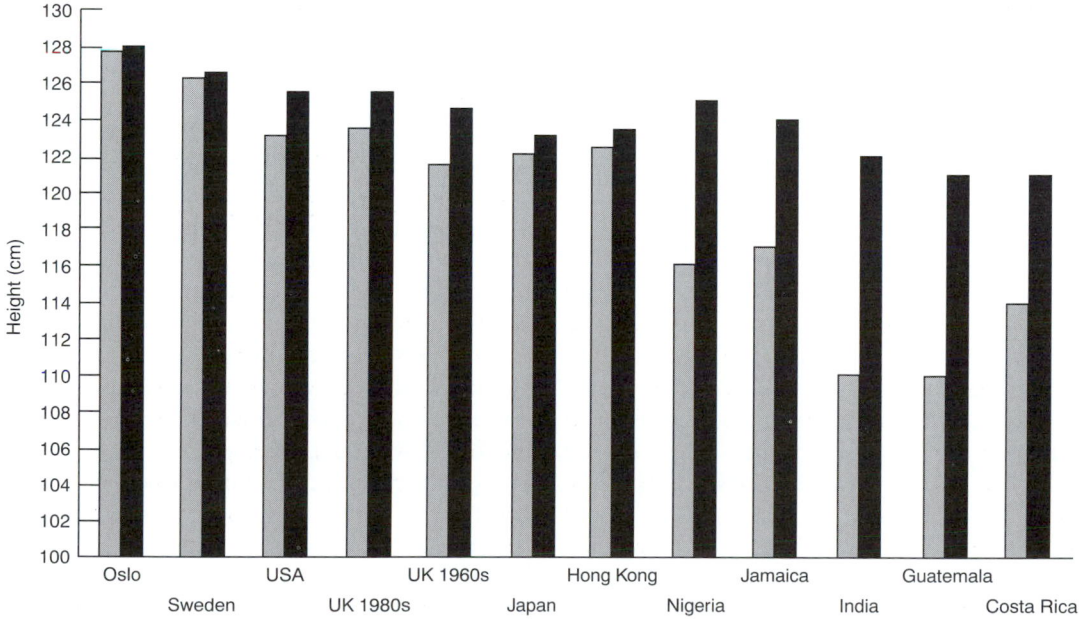

Figure 2 Median heights of boys aged 7.5 years of high (solid bars) or low (shaded bars) socioeconomic status in various populations. From Eveleth PB and Tanner JM (1990) *Worldwide Variation in Human Growth*, 2nd edn, p 199. Cambridge University Press. (With permission.)

Table 6 Adult and child anthropometric status by livelihood group in a Bangladeshi slum

Variable	Landlords/traders	Petty traders	Labourers (male labour)	Labourers (female/child labour)	Statistical significance (P)
Children <5 years					
n	50	85	109	69	
Weight/age as % of NCHS median: mean (SD)	77.9 (9.8)	77.8 (8.9)	75.0 (9.9)	69.7 (11.1)	0.001
Height/age as % of NCHS median: mean (SD)	91.4 (3.8)	90.7 (3.6)	89.9 (6.5)	87.9 (6.5)	0.001
Weight/height as % of NCHS median: mean (SD)	92.3 (9.7)	92.9 (7.8)	91.5 (10.1)	87.4 (9.2)	0.001
Adults – men					
n	34	55	70	40	
BMI: mean (SD)	20.4 (2.4)	19.1 (2.8)	18.8 (2.2)	17.5 (1.6)	0.001
Adults – nonpregnant women					
n	31	47	67	41	
BMI: mean (SD)	20.1 (3.3)	19.0 (2.3)	18.7 (2.3)	17.3 (1.4)	0.001

Data from Pryer J (1990) Socio-economic and environmental aspects of undernutrition and ill-health in an urban slum in Bangladesh. PhD Thesis, University of London.
BMI, body mass index; NCHS, National Center for Health Statistics; SD, standard deviation.

and birthweight. Environmental influences exhibit an intergenerational as well as intragenerational effect on attained adult height.

In addition to the relationships described above, there is also consistent evidence of an association between temporal changes in socioeconomic status and height or physical maturation, both at the population and individual levels. For example, positive associations have been found between increased gross national product and average stature in France, decline in menarcheal age in Norway, and between per capita income and height in Italian conscripts, and survivorship to adulthood. At the individual level, a Polish study showed statural gains of sons over their fathers were significantly greater among fathers who had progressed socioeconomically compared with their parents. Reversals in the secular trend in height or menarcheal age have been shown to coincide with periods of economic decline, such as occurred in Norway, Germany and France during World War II, and in three periods in Moscow (during the civil war following the October Revolution, during mass collectivization, and during the late 1930s and World War II).

Turning to indicators of 'thinness' – weight for height in children and body mass index (weight in kg divided by height in metres squared) in adults – there is no evidence of a consistent monotonic associ-

ation between 'thinness' and social class or livelihood worldwide. In many low-income countries there is evidence of positive associations between indicators of socioeconomic status and both child weight for height and adult body mass index (BMI) (**Tables 6–8**). However, for countries undergoing the epidemiological transition, the situation appears more complex. For example, national surveys in Brazil conducted during 1974 and 1989 indicated that, at the population level, the frequency of underweight had declined while obesity had increased. In both 1974 and 1989, inverse, monotonic social gradients in underweight were evident both in adults (BMI) and children (weight for age), and the reduction was relatively uniform across the social strata. However, among adults, while increases in the prevalence of obesity (assessed as BMI) were observed for each social stratum, the proportionate increase was greatest for the poorest families. The relationship between measures of income and obesity over time was also not straightforward. For men, the social gradient in obesity was attenuated. Among women, the highest prevalence of obesity was no longer among the richest but in the middle income group, and the greatest increases in prevalence had occurred among the poorest women. In China, where the epidemiological transition has been very rapid, national surveys in 1989 and 1991 indicated an increase in adult

Table 7 Reported significant associations between household socioeconomic and demographic characteristics, and indices of anthropometric status, in children

	ZHA or Ht	ZWA or Wt	ZWH	AC	SF
High caste	M	M			
Land	M,H	J,M	M	M	
Livestock	A,B	A,B		A	
Income	A,J	A,J,G	J	A	A
Grain yield	M	M		M	
House type	L,K,I	K,I,L,H			
Sanitation	I	I			
Water supply	I	I			
Father's occupation	C,E,B	E,B,H		B	
Father's education	M	M		M	B[a]
Mother's education	M,L	M		M	
Mother's age	C	G	M		
Birth order[b]	J,F,C,O,N	G,N			
Number of siblings[b]	J[c],C	I,G,N[c],H			
Family size[b] or parity[b]	I,D	I,D			

Adapted from Strickland SS and Tuffrey VR (1997).
[a]Not distinguished by sex of parent.
[b]Negative association.
[c]Children from medium-size families smallest.
AC, mid-upper arm circumference; Ht, height; SF, skinfold thickness; Wt, weight; ZHA, ZWA, ZWH, standard deviation scores of height for age, weight for age and weight for height, compared with NCHS references.
Key to locations: A, Bangladesh; B, Bolivia; C, Britain; D, England; E, Brazil; F, Czechoslovakia; G, Colombia; H, Costa Rica; I, Gambia; J, Guatemala; K, India; L, Jamaica; M, Nepal; N, Nigeria; O, USA.

Table 8 Reported significant associations between household socioeconomic characteristics and indices of anthropometric status in adults

	Height	Weight	BMI	SF
House type	C	C		
Land ownership	F	C,F	C,F	
Income	A	A[a]	D	A[a]
Livelihood		E	E	
Assets	F	F	F	
Socioeconomic index			B	

Adapted from Strickland SS and Tuffrey VR (1997).
[a]Negative association.
BMI, body mass index; SF, skinfold thickness.
Key to locations: A, USA; B, Congo; C, India; D, Brazil; E, Bangladesh; F, Nepal.

underweight among the lowest income groups at the same time as an increase in obesity among the middle-income and rich groups.

The association between socioeconomic status and weight for height among children is also not consistent. Studies in Britain, Sweden and Australia found no clear social class gradients in overweight or obesity in primary school children, although a class gradient in overweight and obesity was found among both boys and girls aged 11–16 years, but not 5–10 years, in Perth, Australia. However, strong and persistent inverse social class gradients in weight for height and obesity by early adulthood have been reported for Britain, the USA, Sweden, Italy and Australia. Furthermore, childhood to adult cohort studies in the UK and Sweden indicate a strong inverse social class gradient between social conditions in childhood and obesity in young adulthood. These socioeconomic differentials in obesity continue in adulthood, though the associations are more likely to be strong in women than in men.

The relationship between socioeconomic status and indicators of 'thinness' in developed countries probably depends on a number of factors, which include not only dietary patterns, but also physical activity in work and leisure, consciousness of and attitudes to body size and shape, as well as diet-related health issues.

The Future

Socioeconomic differentials seem to be increasing in a number of countries, whether in developed, developing or 'transitional' economies. Several agencies use child and adult anthropometric indices as indicators of socioeconomic status, and to monitor the effects of social change. Longitudinal data from Sri Lanka and Nepal suggest adult anthropometric indices may be more reliable than children's, as children are often buffered against seasonal nutritional stress by physiological and social support mechanisms. The Nepal data also indicate that adult body size does influence fitness, productivity and reproductive performance. However, these disadvantages do not necessarily translate into equivalent socioeconomic disadvantage for the whole household. The 'circle' is neither necessarily 'vicious' nor resistant to social and biological mitigating effects.

See also: **Dietary Guidelines**: International Perspectives. **Dietary Intake Measurement**: Methodology; Validation. **Dietary Surveys**: Surveys of National Food Intake; Surveys of Food Intake in Groups and Individuals. **Nutrient Requirements**: International Perspectives. **Nutritional Status**: Dietary Assessment; Anthropometric Assessment. **Nutritional Surveillance**: In Industrialized and Developing Countries. **Urban Nutrition**: Overview. **World Health Organization**: Role.

Further Reading

Barker DJP (1994) *Mothers, Babies and Diseases in Later Life*. London: BMJ Publishing.

Burnett J (1989) *Plenty and Want: A Social History of Food in England from 1815 to the Present Day*, 3rd edn. London: Routledge.

Davey Smith G, Blane D and Bartley M (1994) Explanations for socio-economic differentials in mortality: evidence from Britain and elsewhere. *European Journal of Public Health*. 4:131–144.

Dorling D (1997) *Death in Britain: How Local Mortality Rates Have Changed: 1950s–1990s*. York: Joseph Rowntree Foundation.

Dowler E, Barlösius E, Feichtinger E and Köhler B (1997) Poverty, food and nutrition. In: Köhler B, Feichtinger E, Barlösius E and Dowler E (eds) *Poverty and Food in Welfare Societies*, pp 17–30. Berlin: Edition Sigma.

Drèze J and Sen A, eds (1990) *The Political Economy of Hunger*, vol. 1. *Entitlement and Wellbeing*. Oxford: Clarendon Press.

Falkner F and Tanner JM (1986) *Human Growth. A Comprehensive Treatise*, vol. 3. *Methodology, Ecological, Genetic and Nutritional Effects on Growth*, 2nd edn. New York: Plenum.

Gribble JN and Preston SH, eds (1993) *The Epidemiological Transition. Policy and Planning Implications for Developing Countries*. Washington: National Academy Press.

Hobscraft JN, McDonald JW and Rutstein SO (1984) Socio-economic factors in infant and child mortality: a cross-national comparison. *Population Studies* 38:193–223.

Köhler B, Feichtinger E, Barlösius E and Dowler E, eds (1997) *Poverty and Food in Welfare Societies*. Berlin: Edition Sigma.

Popkin BM (1994) The nutrition transition in low-income countries: an emerging crisis. *Nutrition Reviews* 52(9):285–298.

Riches G, ed. (1997) *First World Hunger: Food Security and Welfare Politics*. Basingstoke: Macmillan.

Shetty PS and McPherson K, eds (1997) *Diet, Nutrition and Chronic Disease: Lessons from Contrasting Worlds*. Chichester: Wiley.

Strickland SS and Tuffrey VR (1997) *Form and Function. A Study of Nutrition, Adaptation and Social Inequality in Three Gurung Villages of the Nepal Himalayas*. London: Smith-Gordon.

Wheeler EF (1991) Intra-household food and nutrient allocation. *Nutrition Research Reviews* 4:69–81.

SODIUM

Physiology

A R Michell, Animal Health Trust, Centre for Small Animal Studies, Lanwades Park, Kentford, UK

Physiological, Clinical and Nutritional Importance of Sodium

Despite the fact that the body contains more calcium and potassium, sodium is arguably the most important cation because it dictates the volume of extracellular fluid (ECF) and its concentration affects osmotic concentration of both ECF and intracellular fluid (ICF). Abnormalities of ECF sodium concentration cause movement of water into or out of cells, thus altering the osmotic concentration of ICF in parallel and causing swelling or shrinkage of cells. The main impact of this is on the brain because its cells are rigidly enclosed by the cranium.

Sodium depletion is mainly caused by enteric, renal or adrenal disease, and sodium retention is caused by renal disease; healthy kidneys are well able to excrete excess dietary salt. However, chronic ingestion of excess salt, whether or not it increases ECF volume, is a predisposing or exacerbating factor in hypertension. Until the 1980s, knowledge of the regulation of body sodium mainly concerned defences against depletion, while in the 1990s there has been a rapid growth in knowledge of the mechanisms which excrete excess sodium. This seems appropriate since most species, especially humans, dogs and laboratory rats, are exposed to dietary sodium intakes well above their nutritional requirement.

The nutritional requirement is a reflection of obligatory losses (maintenance) and the needs of growth, pregnancy and lactation. Abnormal losses owing to disease, or in animals such as humans and horses which sweat extensively, raise the requirement. The impact of equine sweating is different from that in humans. Human sweat always contains sodium at concentrations well below plasma levels (and when aldosterone secretion is raised, levels of sweat sodium fall very low); horse sweat is hypertonic but this helps to offset the osmotic effect of the increased respiratory water loss during exertion, i.e. it may be a defence against hypernatraemia, rather than a potential cause of sodium depletion.

Consideration of the physiology of sodium thus includes its distribution in the body, regulation of total content and concentration, causes of and responses to depletion or excess, and their nutritional implications.

Distribution

Sodium behaves physiologically as a cation, i.e. a positively charged ion; its distribution and effects are fairly independent of the negative ions (anions) which originally accompanied its ingestion though they may affect its absorption and excretion. Most sodium is in ECF (**Table 1**), kept there by the sodium pump, an enzyme system, Na^+/K^+-exchanging ATPase, which uses substantial amounts of energy (adenosine triphosphate; ATP) in maintaining a low intracellular sodium concentration and a high intracellular potassium (K^+) concentration. Sodium transport is a central issue in the physiology of sodium for a number of reasons:

1. It helps to maintain the ionic environment of ICF and the volume of ECF.
2. It prevents cell swelling (the Na^+ efflux exceeds the K^+ influx).
3. It establishes gradients which, in various tissues, allow transport of other cations in exchange, other anions in parallel or organic solutes – these are often cotransported with sodium down concentration gradients which are secondary to the low sodium environment created by the pump.
4. It establishes the membrane voltages on which

excitability and secretory activities frequently depend.
5. The energy expenditure of the pump is a substantial portion of total metabolic activity and contributes to thermogenesis.
6. Sodium transport is not only a key factor in the retention and loss of sodium in the kidney, gut, salivary and sweat glands but also influences the excretion or retention of many other solutes. Thus, for example, diuretics intended to promote sodium excretion may also cause unintentional losses of potassium and magnesium. Similarly, when renal sodium excretion increases appropriately in response to ingestion of excess salt, there may also be unwanted losses of calcium and in postmenopausal women these may contribute to loss of bone mineral.

Bone also contains substantial quantities of sodium but, as yet, its significance is unknown since it does not appear to be mobilized during sodium depletion. Gut fluids contain considerable amounts of sodium, mostly secretory rather than dietary, and mostly reabsorbed in more distal regions of the intestine.

Extracellular Sodium

Of the extracellular fluid, most is in interstitial fluid (ISF) in the tissue spaces, providing the transport medium between capillaries and cells. The sodium concentration in plasma is slightly above that in ISF because plasma contains more proteins, notably albumin, which do not readily escape into ISF across the capillary membranes, and the effect of their negative charges is to hold more positively charged ions, notably sodium, in circulation (Gibbs–Donnan equilibrium).

The main effects of excess ECF volume are seen as expanded ISF, visible clinically as oedema (or ascites when fluid accumulates in the abdomen rather than the tissue spaces). Mild oedema is merely a cosmetic problem in itself but pulmonary or cerebral oedema, or severe ascites, are potentially serious forms. Oedema can result from excess ingestion or retention of sodium (overall expansion of ECF) or 'leakage' from plasma to ISF, with plasma volume continuously replenished by renal sodium retention. Such maldistribution of ECF occurs if plasma albumin is very low (renal leakage, hepatic impairment or severe malnutrition), or with excessive capillary blood pressure (venous blockage, inactivity, heart failure, or arteriolar dilation, e.g. from heat or allergy), capillary damage, or lymphatic blockage. The latter prevents the removal of proteins which have leaked into ISF. Accumulation of protein in ISF undermines

Table 1 Summary of sodium (Na) distribution and requirements

Typical plasma Na concentration (mmol l^{-1})	145 (130–160)
Typical body Na content (mmol kg^{-1})	50–55
Typical proportion (%) of total Na	
ICF	10
ECF	50
Bone	40
Maintenance requirement in mammals (mmol per kg per day)	
Sheep	0.1
Cattle and goats	0.3–0.7
Pigs	0.6
Rats	0.6
Dogs	0.2–0.5
Humans	?<0.6

1 mmol = 23 mg Na^+, 58.5 mg NaCl.

the osmotic gradient which normally favours uptake of water at the venous end of the capillary, where the pressure is lower. Since oedema involves the expansion of a larger compartment (ISF) from a smaller one (plasma) it is only possible as long as the latter is replenished; hence the kidney, while seldom the primary cause of oedema, is always the enabling cause; the use of diuretics is therefore appropriate in the treatment of nonrenal as well as renal causes of oedema.

The main effect of inadequate ECF volume is to reduce plasma volume and thus to compromise cardiovascular function, in extreme cases by causing circulatory shock.

Regulation of ECF Sodium

In a mature, nonpregnant, nonlactating, healthy animal, sodium excretion matches sodium intake and is often used to estimate it, although this is not reliable, especially when intake is low. Dietary sodium is readily available, i.e. readily absorbed; thus the traditional view of sodium regulation emphasizes renal regulation of urinary Na^+ loss. This oversimplifies the more subtle interplay seen, for example, in herbivorous animals, where salt appetite may contribute to regulation by intensifying during sodium depletion. Moreover, in many herbivores the faeces, rather than urine, may be the major route of sodium excretion and the gut may therefore be an important regulator of sodium balance. Indeed, it is interesting that sodium transport mechanisms in the small intestine show considerable similarities to those of the proximal part of the renal tubules (e.g. linked transport of Na^+, glucose and amino acids) whereas the colon, like the distal nephron, responds to the salt-retaining (and potassium-shedding) hormone of the adrenal cortex, aldosterone.

Provided that the adrenal gland is healthy, urinary and faecal sodium loss can be reduced virtually to zero. Sweat loss can also be very low, although with severe exertion in hot climates the volume of sweat may exceed the ability of aldosterone to reduce its sodium concentration and net loss of sodium can occur. Aldosterone also reduces salivary sodium (and raises [K^+]).

There are two components to the regulation of ECF sodium: the total amount of sodium retained and its concentration. The former is regulated by mechanisms which directly affect sodium, whereas the latter is essentially regulated via water balance. Thus whatever sodium is retained in ECF is 'clothed' with the appropriate amount of water to maintain the normal plasma sodium concentration within narrow limits; deviations of less than 1% (hard to measure in the laboratory) trigger corrective responses. Thus a raised plasma sodium concentration (e.g. after water loss) stimulates both thirst and renal water conservation; antidiuretic hormone (ADH) from the posterior pituitary reduces urine output through its effect on the renal collecting ducts. Even one of these mechanisms can defend body water; thus diabetes insipidus (inadequate production or effect of ADH) does not cause severe dehydration but polydipsia (increased fluid intake; 'thirst' is a sensation).

Excess salt intake does not raise plasma sodium concentration (hypernatraemia) if water is available and the patient can drink; the excess sodium is diluted. The resulting increase in ECF volume then stimulates increased sodium excretion. Sodium also enables ECF to hold water against the osmotic 'pull' of the solutes in ICF and sodium thus functions as the 'osmotic skeleton' of ECF; it is the main determinant of its volume.

Plasma sodium concentration is therefore only indirectly related to sodium balance. When ECF volume, notably circulating volume, is severely reduced, this stimulus, rather than Na^+ concentration, becomes the main drive for thirst and ADH secretion. Until ECF volume is restored, water is retained (to protect ECF volume) even though this undermines the protection of ECF Na^+ concentration and, as a result, plasma sodium falls. Thus, during sodium depletion, contraction of ECF volume precedes significant reductions of plasma Na^+ which is therefore a poor index of sodium status.

Sodium-retaining Hormones

Sodium depletion, by reducing plasma volume and renal perfusion, stimulates the production of renin (from the kidneys) which generates angiotensin in circulation. This hormone is a vasoconstrictor (so protects blood pressure), stimulates thirst (so helps to restore ECF volume) and, above all, stimulates sodium retention both directly (renally) and indirectly (by stimulating adrenal secretion of aldosterone); it thus reduces the sodium concentration of urine, faeces, saliva and sweat, but not milk.

Indices of aldosterone secretion (reduced sodium or potassium concentration in urine, faeces, etc.) are often taken as evidence of sodium depletion or inadequate sodium intake, but the following points apply:

1. Aldosterone secretion is also stimulated directly by hyperkalaemia (elevated plasma K^+) and promotes potassium excretion.

2. Such interpretations involve a subjective judgement concerning adequate or excessive sodium intake. Because physiologists and clinicians were traditionally more concerned with sodium depletion as well as its consequences and the defences against it, elevated aldosterone secretion was readily seen as a warning signal. However, if sodium intakes associated with increased aldosterone have no other harmful effects, and especially if excess sodium intakes cause concern, low levels of aldosterone secretion might equally indicate excessive salt intake.

While sodium reabsorption in the distal nephron, influenced by aldosterone, is particularly important because it can produce sodium-free urine and promote potassium loss, the great majority of renal sodium reabsorption occurs elsewhere; about 25% in the loop of Henle and most in the proximal tubule. The loop is also a main site of magnesium reabsorption, hence the tendency for loop diuretics to cause hypomagnesaemia.

The factors controlling proximal reabsorption are incompletely understood but their effect is clear: proximal reabsorption of sodium increases or decreases according to the need to enhance or diminish plasma volume. Since the fluid in the proximal tubule is similar to plasma, having been formed from it by glomerular filtration, it has the ideal composition for this purpose.

Natriuretic Hormones

Excretion of excess sodium involves not only suppression of salt-retention mechanisms but also activation of sodium-shedding (natriuretic) mechanisms. Two types of hormones are involved: atrial natriuretic peptide (ANP), produced by the cardiac atria when they are overstretched (reduction of ECF volume being an appropriate response to cardiac overload), and active sodium transport inhibitors (ASTIs), probably produced within the brain. These were probably the original molecules associated with the receptors binding cardiac glycoside drugs and are therefore also called 'endogenous digitalis-like inhibitors' (EDLIs); their exact identity remains uncertain. Atrial natriuretic peptide has various effects which essentially oppose those of the salt retention induced by aldosterone: it increases sodium excretion, lowers arterial pressure and promotes movement of ECF towards the interstitial compartment.

Other hormones (e.g. sex steroids, parathyroid hormone, calcitonin, thyroid hormone, prolactin) affect renal sodium retention or loss but are not thought to regulate it.

Adequate, Inadequate and Excess Sodium

It is unlikely that adult daily maintenance requirement exceeds 0.6 mmol per kg body weight and could well be below this in many mammals. Newborn, growing, pregnant or lactating animals have increased requirements. The appropriate sodium intake for humans remains controversial with some cultures managing on less than 1 mmol per day, while Western intakes may be in the range 200–300 mmol per day, more where processed foods are heavily consumed. There has been insufficient awareness among physicians and human nutritionists of just how high such intakes are, compared with requirements in other animals. Granted that humans are bipeds with a stressful lifestyle quite different from those of animals, there is no real evidence that human obligatory losses or sodium requirements are significantly greater. Rather, there is an ingrained tradition of regarding sodium intake as a benign pleasure, involving a harmless and healthy dietary constituent. The main warnings against this view come from the fact that hypertension is virtually unknown in low-salt cultures and that they do not even have an age-related rise in 'normal' blood pressure. Moreover, there are numerous studies which, when rigorously analysed, indicate that human arterial pressure and salt intake are positively correlated; sufficiently to anticipate reductions in the prevalence of hypertension in response to manageable reductions in dietary sodium. Unfortunately, such reductions are handicapped by inadequate food labelling and the fact that most sodium is added by the processor rather than the consumer.

Because obligatory losses of sodium are so low, dietary sodium depletion is hard to induce and sodium deficiency usually results from losses caused by renal, adrenal or enteric disease; renal disease may cause either retention or loss of sodium. Globally, both in humans and animals, the most common cause of sodium deficits is acute diarrhoea. Fortunately, sufficient gut usually remains unaffected for uptake of sodium and water to be stimulated by suitably formulated oral rehydration solutions. These essentially restore ECF volume (and acid–base balance), allowing natural defences to over-come the underlying cause of the diarrhoea. Despite some species variations, such solutions usually work best if their glucose : sodium ratio (in mmol l^{-1}) is close to unity and they are virtually isotonic (i.e. they have a similar osmotic concentration to ECF; hypertonic solutions draw water into the gut). The function of glucose in these solutions is to promote sodium uptake; its nutritional contribution is trivial. Anions such as citrate, acetate, propionate, bicarbonate and amino acids (e.g. glycine and alanine) may further enhance the uptake of sodium and therefore water. These sodium cotransport mechanisms are very similar to those of the proximal renal tubule. More recently, nutritional oral rehydration solutions which provide calories and glutamine (to sustain the form and function of enteric villi) have been successfully used in calves.

Sodium is thus central to the management of two of the most widespread clinical problems; hypertension (in humans) and diarrhoea. Indeed, the World Health Organization (WHO) regards the discovery of oral rehydration, which depends on restoration of enteric sodium uptake, as the main life-saving development in twentieth century medicine. This powerful clinical application rests on a simple physiological observation concerning an elementary but vital dietary constituent.

See also: **Electrolytes**: Water-Electrolyte Balance; Acid-Base Balance. **Energy**: Energy Requirements; Energy Balance; Measurement of Energy Intake and Expenditure. **Energy Metabolism:** Tricarboxylic Acid Cycle and Oxidative Phosphorylation. **Hypertension**: Physiology; Nutritional Management; Interrelationships Between Hypertension and Diabetes. **Potassium**: Physiology, Dietary Sources and Requirements. **Renal Function and Disorders**: Nutritional Management of Renal Disorders.

Further Reading

Avery ME and Snyder JD (1990) Oral therapy for acute diarrhea. *New England Journal of Medicine* 323:891–894.

Brooks HW, White DG, Wagstaff AJ and Michell AR (1997) Evaluation of a glutamine-containing oral rehydration solution for the treatment of calf diarrhoea. *Veterinary Journal* 153:163–170.

Denton DA (1982) *The Hunger for Salt.* Berlin: Springer-Verlag.

El-Dahr SS and Chevalier RL (1990) Special needs of the newborn infant in fluid therapy. *Pediatric Clinics of North America* 37:323–335.

Field M, Rao MC and Chang EB (1989) Intestinal electrolyte transport and diarrheal disease. *New England Journal of Medicine* 321:800–806, 879–883.

Hirschhorn N and Grenough WB (1991) Progress in oral rehydration therapy. *Scientific American* 264:16–22.

Law MR, Frost CD and Wald NJ (1991) By how much does dietary salt lower blood pressure? *British Medical Journal* 302:811–815; 815–818; 819–824.

Maxwell MH, Kleenan CR and Narins RG (1987) *Clinical Disorders of Fluid and Electrolyte Metabolism,* 4th edn. New York: McGraw-Hill.

Michell AR (1989) Physiological aspects of mammalian sodium requirement. *Nutrition Research Reviews* 2:149–160.

Michell AR (1991) Regulation of salt and water balance. *Journal of Small Animal Practice* 32:135–145.

Michell AR (1995) *The Clinical Biology of Sodium.*

Rutlen DL, Christensen G, Helgesen KG and Ilebekk A (1990) Influence of atrial natriuretic factor on intravascular volume displacement in pigs. *American Journal of Physiology* 259:H1595–1600.

Sodium chloride *see* **Salt**: Epidemiology.

Spirits *see* **Alcohol**: Absorption, Metabolism and Physiological Effects; Disease Risk and Beneficial Effects; Effects of Consumption on Diet and Nutritional Status.

Starch *see* **Carbohydrates**: Chemistry and Classification (Including Dietary Fibre); Regulation of Carbohydrate Metabolism; Requirements and Dietary Importance; Resistant Starch and Oligosaccharides.

STARVATION AND FASTING

Biochemical Aspects

J Bines, Royal Children's Hospital, Parkville, Victoria, Australia

During the course of a normal 24 h day the body's essential cellular and organ functions remain homeostatic despite intermittent nutrient intake and changing metabolic demand. A highly sophisticated and integrated system provides the metabolic adaptation for these normal changes in substrate provision and utilization. A basic knowledge of the normal metabolic response in the feeding-fasting cycle is pivotal to the understanding of the changes that occur during periods of prolonged fasting and starvation. In this review of the biochemical aspects of the metabolic response to fasting and starvation, the term 'fasting' is defined as the total absence of nutrient intake, while 'starvation' is defined as a prolonged period of inadequate food intake.

During a period of prolonged fasting the body undergoes the following sequence of changes: (1) depletion of fuel stores; (2) metabolic adaptation; (3) decompensation and death. The extent and rate of progression through these steps depends on the amount of fuel stores at initiation of the fast, the severity and duration of nutritional deprivation, and the presence or absence of significant catabolic stress such as injury, sepsis or cancer (**Table 1**).

Metabolic Changes

Energy requirements

Energy is essential to the body for many important functions. These include the maintenance of cellular integrity and function, new tissue synthesis, thermoregulation and physical activity. The energy requirements of an individual vary with age, sex, body composition, physical activity and stress. In the normal adult at rest approximately 75% of energy requirements reflect the energy needs of major organs (brain 20%, skeletal muscle 18–22%, abdominal muscles 25%, heart 11%). However, during normal daily life the total energy requirement and the proportion of energy needed by different tissues may vary. For example, with exercise the energy requirement of skeletal muscles increases, and during a meal the

Table 1 The clinical features of starvation and fasting

	'Uncomplicated' protein–energy malnutrition (marasmus)	'Hypoalbuminaemic' malnutrition (kwashiorkor)	'Stressed' malnutrition (mixed)
Aetiology	Decreased energy intake	Decreased protein intake plus stress	Decreased energy and protein intakes plus stress
Metabolic adaptation			
Weight loss	Slow (months to years)	Intermediate (weeks to months)	Rapid (weeks)
Resting energy expenditure	Decreased	Decreased or increased	Increased
Nitrogen loss	Minimal	Increased	Increased
Water, sodium	Initial loss	Retention	Retention
Hormonal	Early small increase in: catecholamines glucagon cortisol growth hormone then slow decrease Decreased insulin	Increase in: catecholamines glucagon cortisol growth hormone	Increase in: catecholamines glucagon cortisol growth hormone
Laboratory parameters			
Albumin	Normal–slowly decreased	Decreased	Decreased
Transferrin	Normal–slowly decreased	Decreased	Decreased
Total lymphocyte count	Normal–slowly decreased	Decreased	Decreased
Skin hypersensitivity	Decreased	Decreased	Decreased

abdominal organs require more energy for the process of digestion and absorption. Children require additional energy for growth.

Energy production

The body derives its energy from the metabolism of carbohydrate, fat and protein provided exogenously in the fed state and endogenously in the postabsorptive state. A mixture of metabolic fuels including glucose, triacylglycerols, ketone bodies, nonesterified fatty acids and amino acids are present in the circulation. The proportion of these energy substrates in the blood at any one time depends on the fed or fasting state of the individual, the extent of fuel stores and the body's recent and current metabolic demand. In a normal, nonobese 70 kg adult there are approximately 500 MJ (120 000 kcal) contained in adipose tissue, 100 MJ (24,000 kcal) stored in muscle and visceral proteins, and 4.2 MJ (1000 kcal) stored as liver and muscle glycogen. During a normal day only half of the total energy requirement is met by carbohydrate metabolism. At this rate glycogen stores would be exhausted after 1–2 days of fasting. However, glycogen stores are maintained for a longer period owing to the production of glucose from gluconeogenesis (**Fig. 1**).

Carbohydrate metabolism   Glucose plays a key role in body metabolism. It is the preferred metabolic fuel for many tissues and is an essential fuel for the retina, red blood cells, the renal medulla and the brain under normal conditions. In the fed state glucose is derived from the digestion and absorption of carbohydrates provided in the meal. Exogenous fats and proteins absorbed in excess of requirements may also be metabolized to glucose for use as energy or converted to glycogen or fat for storage. To produce energy from glucose, three metabolic pathways are involved (**Fig. 2**). Glucose is first oxidized to form pyruvate via the glycolytic pathway. Pyruvate then enters the Krebs cycle and is completely oxidized to form NADH + H, FADH$_2$ and carbon dioxide. The

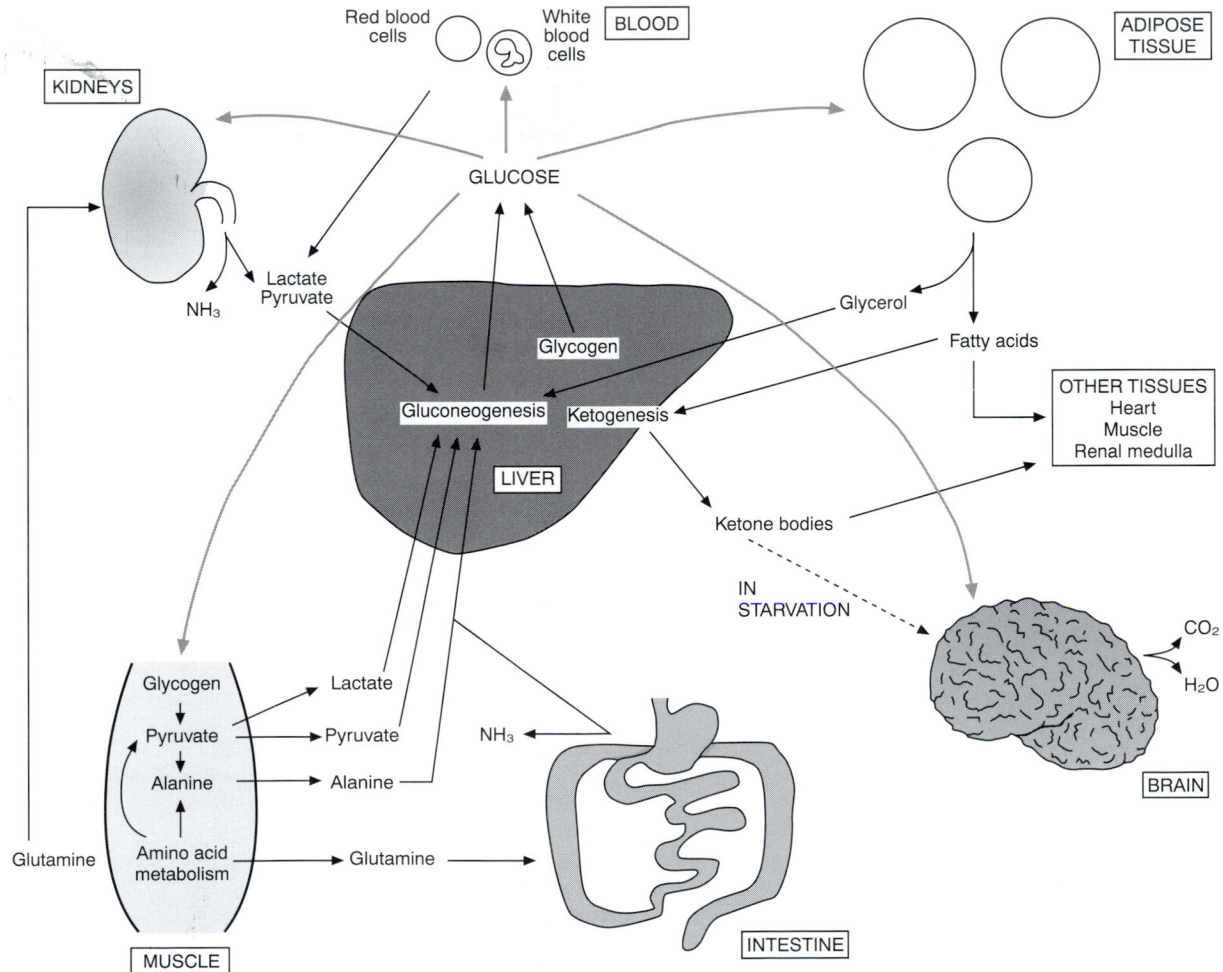

Figure 1   The production, transport and metabolism of energy substrates in the postabsorptive state.

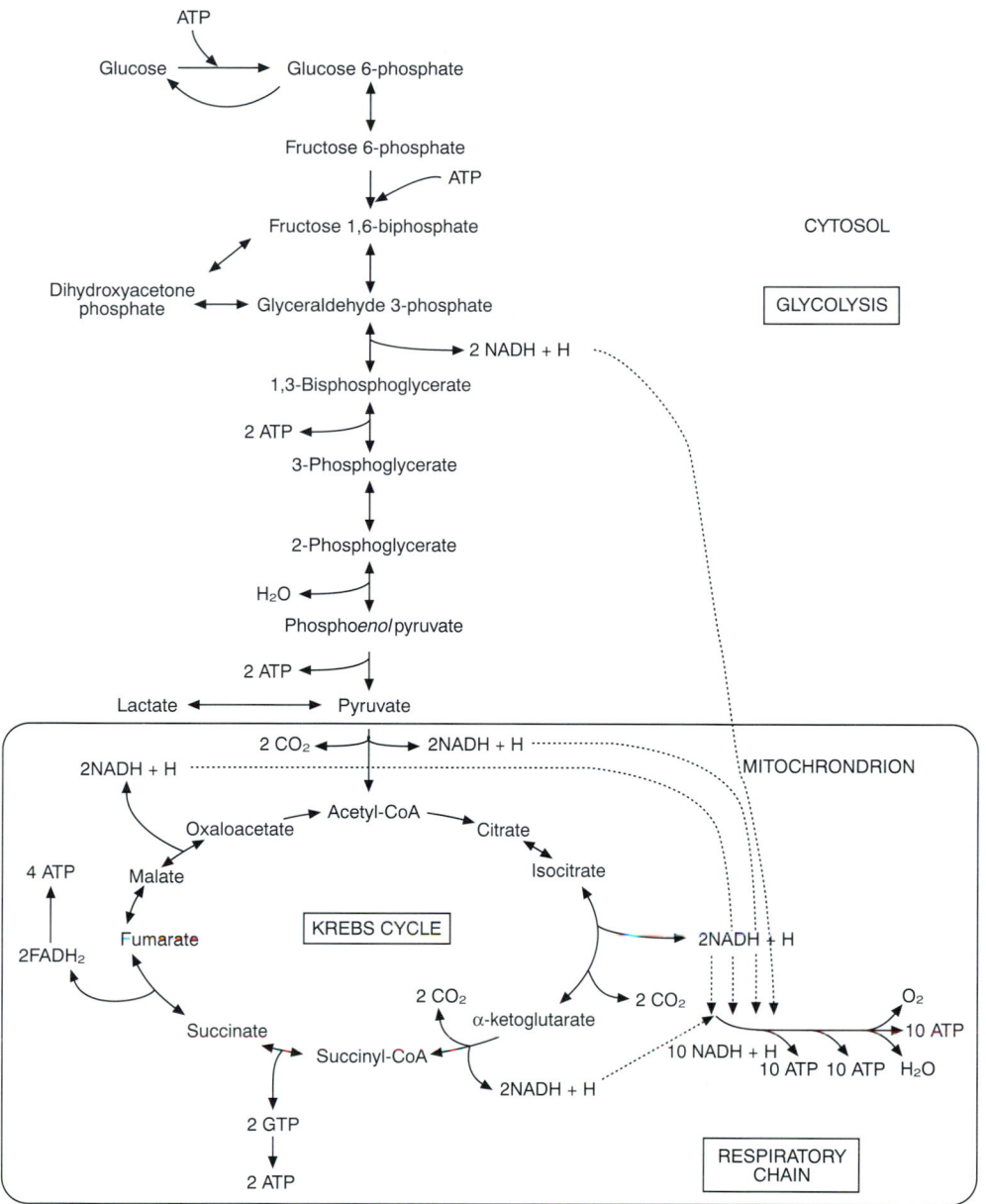

Figure 2 The production of energy from glucose via the glycolytic pathway, the Krebs cycle and the respiratory chain.

NADH + H transports hydrogen to the respiratory chain where it is used to reduce oxygen to water. The net yield of energy from the metabolism of 1 molecule of glucose is 38 molecules of ATP.

Because of the strict glucose requirements of the brain the circulating blood glucose pool is tightly controlled at around 16 g. Three important mechanisms are responsible for this regulation.

1. Insulin enhances glucose uptake into muscle and fat and stimulates glycogen synthesis. It also inhibits lipolysis, glycogenolysis and gluconeogenesis. High insulin levels will decrease blood glucose levels. Conversely, low insulin levels will cause a rise in blood glucose level by decreased inhibition of glycogenolysis and reduced peripheral uptake of glucose.

2. Glucagon increases liver glycogen breakdown, gluconeogenesis and ketogenesis from fatty acids. It also stimulates lipolysis from adipocytes in extrahepatic tissue. The net result of glucagon activity is an increase in blood glucose concentration which helps to maintain blood glucose levels despite the effect of insulin.

3. Neuroendocrine response to glucose deprivation in the brain rapidly increases glucose release from liver glycogen.

The fed state is characterized by increased blood concentrations of glucose, amino acids and fat. Insulin secretion is stimulated while glucagon levels remain unchanged or are decreased. As a result there is increased glucose uptake into tissues and enhanced glycogen, protein and triacylglycerol synthesis. Glucagon balances this effect by stimulating glycogen breakdown to maintain blood glucose levels. By this mechanism blood glucose levels are controlled during periods of surplus carbohydrate ingestion and excess glucose is stored as glycogen or fat.

Glycogen is a complex hydrated polymer of glucose arranged in a highly branched, spherical form. It allows glucose to be stored in large amounts without causing osmotic shifts. The terminal glucose molecules within this branching structure are accessible to the enzymes mediating glycogen breakdown to allow the rapid release of glucose in times of stress. The glycogen molecule expands in size after a carbohydrate-rich meal to approximately 40 nm in diameter and shrinks to 10 nm in diameter or less between meals. An adult man receiving a normal carbohydrate-containing diet has approximately 70 g of liver glycogen and 200 g of muscle glycogen. The enzyme required for glycogen breakdown to glucose, glucose-6-phosphatase, is present only in the liver. Muscle glycogen is metabolized by anaerobic glycolysis to form pyruvate and lactate. Lactate is then transported to the liver where it acts as a precursor for gluconeogenesis. This is called the Cori cycle (**Fig. 3**). The Cori cycle contributes to about 40% of the normal plasma glucose turnover. It has the advantage of providing energy (net 3 molecules of ATP) without the loss of glucose molecules. The energy required for the resynthesis of glucose in the liver is derived from fatty acid oxidation. The total body glycogen stores can meet the needs of the brain for about 3 days. After this period alternative sources of metabolic fuel must be found.

Protein metabolism Body nitrogen resides in two main compartments. About half of the body's nitrogen is contained in extracellular tissues such as collagen. The nitrogen present within these tissues is relatively fixed and does not change significantly with starvation. The nitrogen turnover within this compartment can be assessed by the measurement of hydroxyproline excretion. The remaining nitrogen is present in the lean muscle mass, comprising skeletal and visceral muscle. The proteins within these tissues are constantly being broken down and resynthesized at a rate of 3–3.5 g per kg per day in a young adult. Measurement of urinary 3-methylhistidine excretion and creatinine excretion can be used to estimate the fractional catabolic rate of skeletal muscle.

In the fed state amino acids digested and absorbed in excess of the body's immediate requirements for incorporation into proteins or other molecules, are either oxidized for energy, or metabolized to glycogen or fat. When metabolized for energy, protein provides approximately 17 kJ g^{-1} (4 kcal g^{-1}).

Prolonged fasting results in a depletion of liver and muscle glycogen stores. In this clinical setting the conversion of amino acids to glucose contributes to the glucose requirements of the brain. The transition to metabolism of amino acids as an energy source is mediated by an alteration in the balance of insulin and glucagon. The breakdown of tissue protein to provide glucose results in a sustained loss of body nitrogen of approximately 12 g per day. Experimentally, this loss of body nitrogen can be prevented by the administration of glucose. As a result of muscle protein breakdown, amino acids – predominantly alanine and glutamine – are released into the circulation. However, the amount of alanine released exceeds the alanine content of the muscle protein; about one-third of the alanine released from muscle

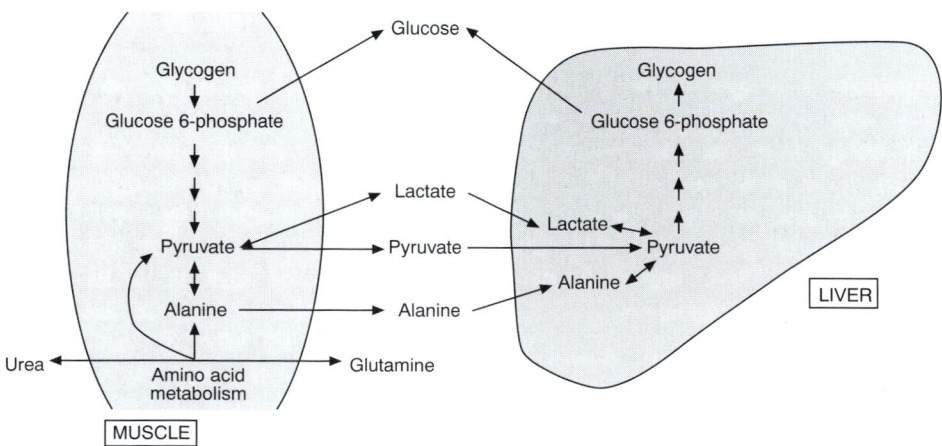

Figure 3 The metabolism of muscle glycogen and protein to form glucose involving the Cori cycle (lactate to glucose) and the glucose–alanine cycle.

originates from muscle protein, while the remaining two-thirds is derived from pyruvate. Pyruvate is formed by the metabolism of muscle glycogen or by the transamination of other amino acids contained within the muscle protein. Alanine is transported to the liver where it is rapidly taken up and converted to glucose: this is known as the glucose–alanine cycle (see Fig. 3). Despite the increased release of alanine from muscle, plasma alanine levels fall in early fasting. This results from the rapid uptake and conversion of alanine by the liver.

Fat metabolism Fat is an efficient store of energy providing approximately 38 kJ g^{-1} (9 kcal g^{-1}). Fat is predominantly stored as triacylglycerols within adipocytes. The amount of fat stores may vary substantially between individuals. In the fed state insulin stimulates triacylglycerol synthesis. During fasting, triacylglycerol is converted to fatty acids and glycerol (**Fig. 4**). Within days, glycerol and palmitate release increases by 2–3 times fed levels. This release is regulated by hormone-sensitive lipase. Owing to the absence of glycerol kinase in white adipose tissue, glycerol cannot be completely metabolized within the adipocytes and is transported to the liver where it is

converted to glucose by gluconeogenesis. The fatty acids either are released from the adipocytes to be oxidized by the liver or other tissues, or may be reesterified with glycerol 3-phosphate and reenter the cycle to form triacylglycerol (Fig. 4). The energy cost of reesterification of fatty acids in starvation may account for 2–3% of the resting energy expenditure.

Fatty acids delivered to the liver may be oxidized or reesterified into triacylglycerols. Fatty acid oxidation is stimulated by the activation of carnitine/acyl carnitine translocase acyltransferase, which effects the transport of long-chain fatty acids into the mitochondria. Most of the acety-CoA produced from fatty acid oxidation is metabolized to acetoacetate which in turn may be converted to β-hydroxybutyrate and acetone. These products are known as ketone bodies. Although ketone bodies are produced in small quantities in the fed state they are generally metabolized by the liver and are not released into the circulation. During fasting the rate of production of acetoacetate and β-hydroxybutyrate significantly increases. These metabolites are released into the circulation and can be used by the brain and other tissues as an alternative energy source.

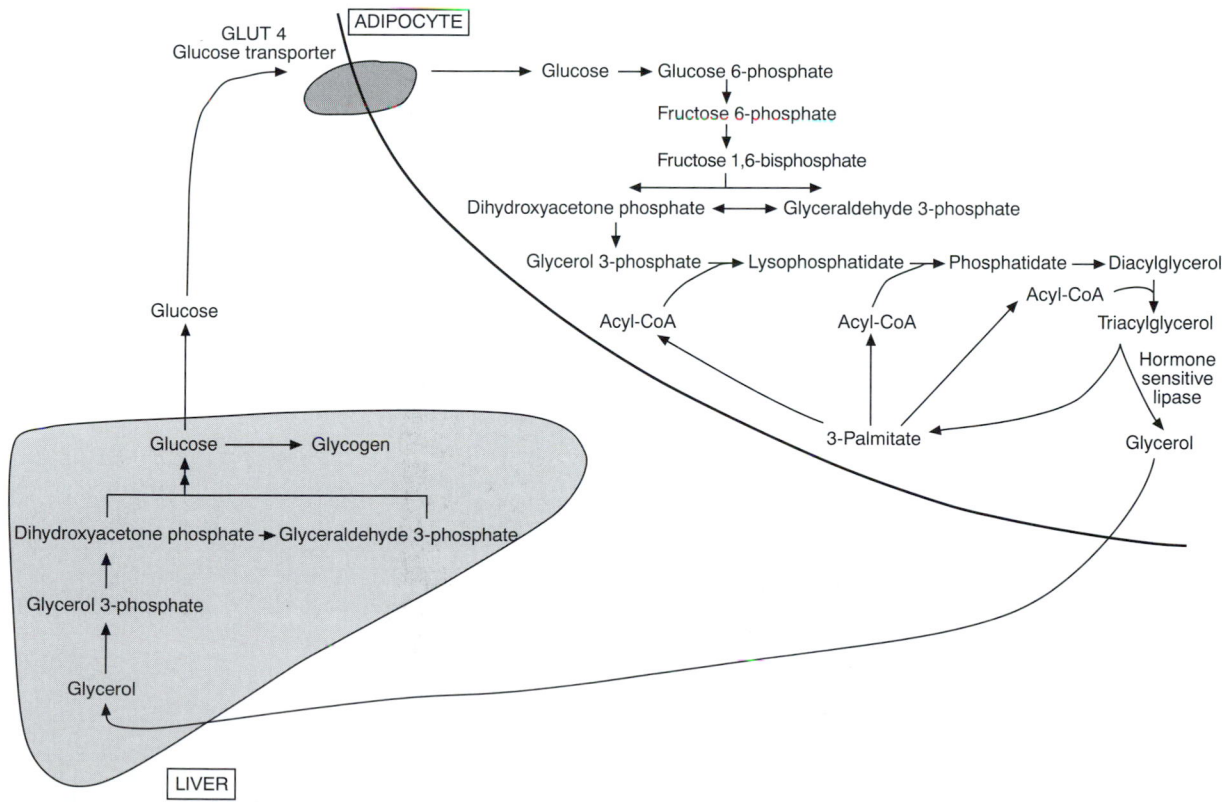

Figure 4 The triacylglycerol-fatty acid cycle.

Metabolic Adaptation

Postabsorptive state

The postabsorptive state commences when the last nutrient is absorbed from the previous meal and continues until the next meal or for approximately 12 hours during a normal overnight fast. Metabolically it is the period when there is a transition from exogenous energy consumption to reliance on endogenous energy sources. The release from the liver of approximately 200–250 g of glucose per day or 8–10 g per hour balances the rate of glucose utilization of the brain and other tissues. During an overnight fast a significant proportion of the glucose requirements are met by the breakdown of liver glycogen. The remaining glucose is formed from non-carbohydrate sources: glycerol (from triacylglycerols), pyruvate and lactate (from muscle).

Prolonged fasting

In a normal adult, resting energy expenditure is proportional to lean body mass. Prolonged fasting is associated with a loss of lean body mass and in a reduction in resting energy expenditure. Fourteen to 21 days after commencing a starvation diet there is a 15% reduction in resting energy expenditure. However, at this time there is only a 5% reduction in lean body mass. Clearly another mechanism contributes to the decreased resting energy expenditure observed in early starvation.

A number of hormonal changes occur as a response to starvation that may alter resting energy expenditure. Decreased activity of $5'$-monodeiodinase in the liver and peripheral tissues resulting in a reduction in the conversion of thyroxine (T_4) to the metabolically active form, triiodothyronine (T_3), has been observed within hours to days in patients on a starvation diet. This effect is modified by both the carbohydrate intake and the total energy content of the diet. However, the mechanism linking low circulating T_3 levels to decreased resting energy expenditure in starvation is not well understood. Catecholamine secretion and turnover is decreased in uncomplicated starvation. This is clinically recognized as a reduction of core temperature, heart rate and blood pressure of patients on starvation diets. Another factor contributing to the reduced resting energy expenditure observed in patients on starvation diets may be reduced activity of the sodium-potassium pump. The activity of this pump is influenced by circulating T_3, catecholamines and insulin, all known to have altered levels in starvation. There is some evidence to suggest that in prolonged starvation increased intracellular sodium and decreased intracellular potassium levels are linked to decreased pumping of sodium from cells.

With increasing duration of the fast and depletion of liver and muscle glycogen stores the conversion of amino acids to glucose contributes to the glucose requirements of the brain. The transition to metabolism of amino acids as an energy source is mediated by a change in balance of insulin and glucagon. Insulin levels fall while glucagon levels tend to be maintained or even slightly increased. Blood levels of the branched-chain amino acids double after 3–5 days of fasting but fall again if fasting is prolonged. These amino acids help to support gluconeogenesis until fat metabolism has adapted fully. During early fasting the muscle releases alanine and glutamine. The glucose–alanine cycle provides glucose to the muscle in exchange for alanine provided to the liver as a precursor for gluconeogenesis (see Fig. 3). Glutamine released from the muscle during fasting is preferentially taken up by the intestine where it is used as an energy source and by the kidney where it is used for renal ammonia production. Although the metabolism of amino acids to glucose is a very important metabolic adaptation to fasting, it only provides about 45 g glucose per day. This amount alone is insufficient to meet the glucose requirements of the brain and must be supplemented by energy produced from fat metabolism.

The mobilization of triacylglycerol stores to provide energy is regulated by a number of factors. Lipolysis is stimulated by glucagon and adrenocorticotrophic hormone (ACTH) during starvation. This effect is mediated by cyclic AMP-dependent protein kinase which stimulates hormone-sensitive lipase and inhibits acetyl-CoA carboxylase (**Fig. 5**). In prolonged starvation cortisol increases hormone-sensitive lipase synthesis. Insulin levels fall by 35% within 24 h of fasting. This is associated with a 50–80% increase in the rate of lipolysis. Low circulating insulin levels cause a reduction in the uptake of glucose into adipocytes by altering the function of the GLUT 4 glucose transporter. Adequate amounts of glycerol 3-phosphate are therefore unavailable for the reesterification of fatty acids produced from triacylglycerol breakdown. Nonesterified fatty acids are released into the circulation and free fatty acid concentrations increase from 0.5–0.8 mmol l^{-1} to 1.2–1.6 mmol l^{-1} within the first few days of fasting. Fatty acids circulate bound to albumin and can be oxidized in the liver or other tissues to produce energy. The switch to using ketone bodies as an energy source by the brain appears to be primarily controlled by the blood concentration of ketone bodies rather than a hormonal effect. Ketone body production by the liver peaks after 3–4 days of fasting.

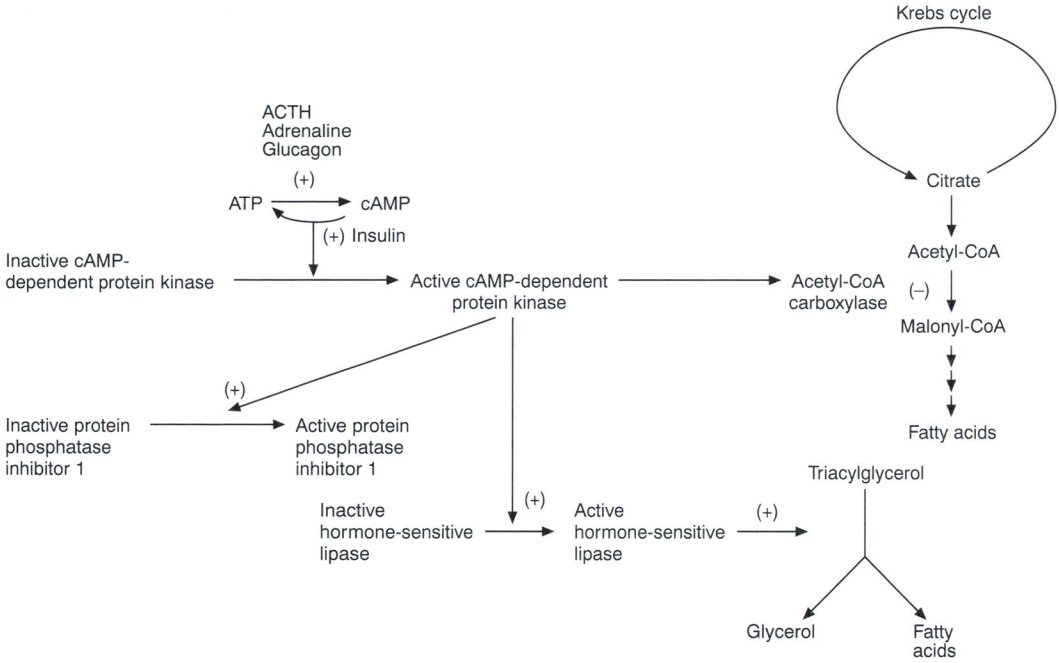

Figure 5 Lipolysis is stimulated by the action of glucagon, ACTH and adrenaline. This effect is mediated by cAMP-dependent protein kinase.

However, blood ketone body levels continue to rise rapidly for the first 7–10 days before stabilizing at around 6–8 mM at 2–3 weeks. The continued rise in blood ketone body levels despite the achievement of maximal liver production early in fasting is due to decreased renal excretion of ketone bodies and increasing muscle fatty acid oxidation.

As fatty acid oxidation and ketone body formation increase there is a reduction in glucose production and oxidation. This may be mediated by inhibition of the pyruvate dehydrogenase complex activity. After a 3-week fast positron emission tomography scans have shown a marked reduction in glucose metabolism throughout the brain. Glucose uptake of the brain is more than halved after a fast of 5 weeks.

After a period of fasting longer than 2 weeks there is a shift to conserve muscle protein and reduce body protein turnover. Urinary nitrogen losses decrease to .4–6 g per day and about half of this is excreted as ammonia required to buffer acid produced by ketoacids. This transition appears to be directly or indirectly dependent on increasing blood ketone body concentration. With prolonged fasting, muscles change from ketone body production to fatty acid oxidation. This may potentially conserve branched-chain amino acids, which may in turn limit proteolysis. There is some evidence to suggest that leucine can stimulate protein synthesis. A small increase in insulin in response to high circulating levels of ketone bodies may also influence protein metabolism.

With increasing ketone body production the liver reduces the rate of gluconeogenesis. The kidney becomes the major gluconeogenic organ and produces half of the body's glucose requirements. Glutamine is the predominant substrate for kidney gluconeogenesis and the nitrogen product of this process provides the ammonia needed to buffer ketoacids in the urine.

Death will occur when there is a failure to replenish fuel stores and insufficient available energy to maintain essential bodily functions. As fat is the predominant source of energy the time until death in uncomplicated fasting will depend on the size of the fat stores. In a normal adult fat stores will be sufficient to sustain life for approximately 60–70 days. The extent of protein loss is also linked to survival. A loss of more than half of the lean body mass compartment (about half of total body protein) is predictive of death.

See also: **Adaptation**: Overview of Adaptive Responses to Malnutrition. **Amino Acids**: Metabolism. **Carbohydrates**: Regulation of Carbohydrate Metabolism. **Energy**: Energy Balance. **Fatty Acids**: Metabolism. **Malnutrition**: Definition, Classification and Epidemiology; Primary Malnutrition; Secondary Malnutrition.

Further Reading

Cahill GF (1970) Starvation in man. *New England Journal of Medicine* **282**:668–675.

Denton RM and McCormack JG (1995) Fuel selection at the level of the mitochondria in mammalian tissues. *Proceedings of the Nutrition Society* **54**:11–22.

Hoffe LJ (1994) Starvation. In: Shils ME, Olson JA and Shike M (eds) *Modern Nutrition in Health and Disease*, vol. 2, chap. 56, pp 927–949. Philadelphia: Lea & Febiger.

Keys A, Brozek J, Henschel A *et al.* (1950) *The Biology of Human Starvation*. Minneapolis: University of Minnesota Press.

Klein S, Sakurai Y, Romijn JA and Carroll RM (1993) Progressive alterations in lipid and glucose metabolism during short-term fasting in young adult men. *American Journal of Physiology* **265**:E801–806.

Love AHG (1986) Metabolic response to malnutrition: its relevance to enteral feeding. *Gut* **27**:9–13.

MacDonald IA and Webber J (1995) Feeding, fasting and starvation: factors affecting fuel utilization. *Proceedings of the Nutrition Society* **54**:267–274.

Randle PJ (1995) Metabolic fuel selection: general integration at the whole body level. *Proceedings of the Nutrition Society* **54**(1):317–327.

Robinson AM and Williamson DH (1980) Physiological roles of ketones as substrates and signals in mammalian tissues. *Physiological Reviews* **60**:143–187.

Shulman GL and Landau BR (1992) Pathways of glycogen repletion. *Physiological Reviews* **72**:1019–1035.

Smith R and Williamson DH (1996) Biochemical background. In: Weatherall DJ, Ledingham JEG and Warrell DA (eds) *Oxford Textbook of Medicine*, vol. 1, pp 1271–1278 Oxford: Oxford Medical.

Snell K (1980) Muscle alanine synthesis and hepatic gluconeogenesis. *Biochemical Society Transactions* **8**:205–213.

STEATORRHOEA

Nutritional Management

A Burke and **J L Rombeau**, University of Pennsylvania, Philadelphia, Pennsylvania, USA

Steatorrhoea is the presence of excess fat in the faeces, defined as more than 7 g per 24 h when 100 g of fat is ingested in the diet. It is a symptom rather than a disease. In this article we review the pathophysiology of steatorrhoea and some of the clinical conditions commonly associated with it. We review the approach to diagnosing the underlying cause and the rationale to the treatment of steatorrhoea and how it is tailored to the different underlying diseases. We discuss the principles of nutrition support and pharmacological interventions in steatorrhoea. Prognosis is dependent on the underlying pathology.

Aetiology

The normal absorption of lipids is complex. It commences with the digestion of triacylglycerols to glycerol and fatty acids by lingual and gastric lipases. Both of these enzymes are resistant to acid digestion in the stomach are inactivated by physiological concentrations of bile acids in the small intestinal lumen. Pancreatic lipase is protected from acid digestion in the duodenum by the concomitant secretion of bicarbonate by the pancreas. Approximately 300 000 IU of lipase activity are secreted postprandially by the normal pancreas. Pancreatic lipase digests fats into fatty acid and monoacylglycerols. This process is aided by the dispersion of dietary fat into micelles by bile acids. Micelles provide a shuttle for the lipids from the bulk water phase across the unstirred water layer to the region adjacent to the cell surface, where they are absorbed by passive translocation. They are resynthesized into complex lipids in the smooth endoplasmic reticulum and are complexed with proteins in the rough endoplasmic reticulum within the enterocyte. The resultant chylomicrons are extruded into the lymphatics. Steatorrhoea is caused by a defect in any of these metabolic steps (**Fig. 1**).

The causes of steatorrhoea are grouped under the headings of exocrine pancreatic deficiency, small bowel defects, bile salt deficiency and 'miscellaneous'. Chronic pancreatitis, cystic fibrosis, coeliac disease, short bowel syndrome and bile salt deficiency are the commonest disorders associated with steatorrhoea (**Table 1**). Steatorrhoea is a pathophysiological process and not a specific disease *per se*, therefore its true prevalence is not known (**Table 2**).

Clinical Features

Between 50% and 100% of patients with steatorrhoea have weight loss and 80–97% have diarrhoea. Typically, but not necessarily, the stool is

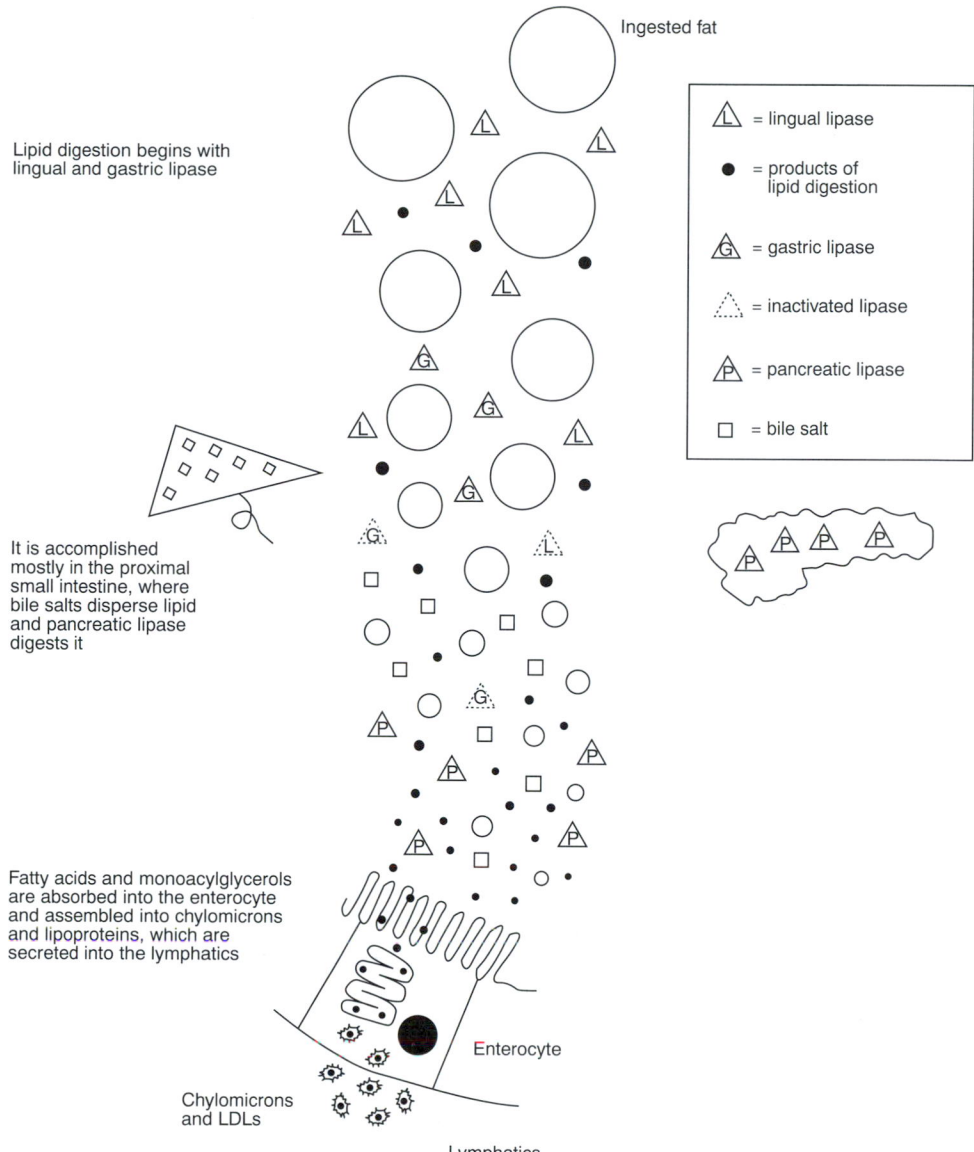

Figure 1 Normal lipid digestion and absorption.

bulky. Malodorous diarrhoea and excessive flatus occur when there is associated carbohydrate malabsorption. Less commonly the stool has a foamy or oily appearance. This occurs with the higher faecal fat content seen more often with steatorrhoea of pancreatic origin. Manifestations of fat-soluble vitamin deficiency, such as osteomalacia with vitamin D deficiency or neurological disturbance with vitamin E deficiency, may occur with long-standing steatorrhoea. Dermatitis from vitamin A deficiency is uncommon in the USA and coagulopathy from vitamin K deficiency is rare as intestinal flora make vitamin K. Low serum levels of fat-soluble vitamins in the absence of deficiency-induced symptoms is a more common event.

Nutritional Management

The treatment of steatorrhoea varies with the underlying disease and so diagnosis of the aetiology is important. Steatorrhoea of nonpancreatic origin is usually associated with generalized malabsorption, which must also be taken into account in prescribing nutrition-metabolic treatments.

Initial evaluations

First it is necessary to establish the diagnosis of steatorrhoea. The patient is placed on a 100 g fat diet commencing 48 h before the start of a 72 h faecal fat collection. A quantitative measurement of faecal fat is made. The presence of more than 20 g fat in 24 h

Table 1 Conditions associated with steatorrhoea and corresponding intervention

	Treatment of underlying disease	Fat restriction	Nutritional support[b]	Pancreatic insufficiency
Intramural small bowel disease				
Gluten enteropathy (coeliac sprue, nontropical sprue)	X			
Dermatitis herpetiformis[a]	X			
Tropical sprue	X		X	
Whipple's disease	X		X	
Nongranulomatous jejunitis			X	
Abetalipoproteinaemia		X	X	
Amyloidosis (primary or secondary)			X	
Eosinophilic gastroenteritis			X	
Food allergy[a]	X			
Small bowel resection (minor or massive)[a]		X	X[c]	
Intestinal lymphangiectasis		X	X	
Metastatic carcinoma			X	
Metastatic carcinoid diseases			X	
IBD			X	
Intestinal lymphoma			X	
Tuberculosis enteritis			X	
Radiation enteritis			X	
Insufficient intraluminal pancreatic enzyme activity				
Chronic pancreatitis		X	X[c]	X
Pancreatic carcinoma			X[c]	X
Pancreatic resection			X[c]	X
Cystic fibrosis				
Children[a]			X[c]	X
Adults		X	X[c]	X
Pancreatic duct/ampulla of Vater obstruction (stones, parasites)[a]			X[c]	X
Insufficient intraluminal bile acid activity[a]				
Biliary obstruction with/without jaundice		X	X	
Bacterial overgrowth syndrome secondary to stasis/diverticula		X	X	
Cholecystocolonic fistula		X	X	
Biliary resection and Crohn's disease		X	X	
Severe parenchymal liver disease		X	X	
Cholestatic liver disease		X	X	
Binding agents (cholestyramine)		X	X	
Parasitosis				
Giardiasis	X			
Stronglyoidiasis	X		X	
Capillarias	X		X	
Hookworm	X		X	
Coccidioidomycosis	X		X	
Schistosomiasis	X		X	

From Marotta and Floch (1989). With permission.

suggests exocrine pancreatic insufficiency. The Sudan stain is a useful qualitative test for the presence of steatorrhoea.

Clinical history provides important information as to the aetiology of the steatorrhoea. A patient with long-standing excessive alcohol intake and chronic abdominal pain is likely to have chronic pancreatitis. The child with recurrent respiratory infections may have cystic fibrosis. The patient with several bowel resections for Crohn's disease may have bile salt deficiency or short bowel syndrome. Patients with pancreatic steatorrhoea are more likely to have oily stools. Patients with intestinal steatorrhoea are more likely to have foul-smelling stools with flatulence, fatigue, malaise, anaemia, low serum albumin levels and other findings of generalized malabsorption. Symptoms of malnutrition are more common than steatorrhoea in elderly patients with coeliac disease,

Table 1 Continued

	Treatment of underlying disease	Fat restriction	Nutritional support[b]	Pancreatic insufficiency
Immunoglobulin deficiencies			X	
Drug-induced (colchicine, neomycin, methotrexate, phenindione)			X	
Multiple defects (unclear)				
Zollinger–Ellison syndrome	X		X	
Scleroderma			X	
Postgastrectomy			X	
Mast cell disease			X	
Diabetes mellitus			X	
Endocrinopathies	X		X	
Acquired immune deficiency syndrome (AIDS)			X	
Malabsorption in the elderly	X	X	X	
Thyrotoxicosis	X		X	

From Marotta and Floch (1989).
[a]These conditions are more common.
[b]Nutritional support may be needed only until treatment of underlying disease is effective.
[c]Recommend use of medium-chain triacylglycerols.

Table 2 Prevalence of steatorrhoea in various clinical conditions

Aetiology	Prevalence of steatorrhoea	Reference
Chronic pancreatitis	25–30%	A
Cystic fibrosis	90%	B
Coeliac disease (symptomatic, untreated)	almost 100%	C
Crohn's disease	30–40%	D
Short bowel syndrome	>90%	
AIDS	up to 50%	E

A Bank S (1986) Chronic pancreatitis: Clinical features and medical management. *American Journal of Gastroenterology* **18**:153–167.
B FitzSimmons SC, Burkhart GA, Borowitz D, Grand RJ, Hammerstrom T, Durie PR, Lloyd-Still JD and Lowenfels AB (1997) High dose pancreatic enzyme supplements and fibrosing colonopathy in children with cystic fibrosis. *New England Journal of Medicine* **336**:1283–1289.
C Green PA and Wollaeger EE (1960) The clinical behaviour of sprue in the United States. *Gastroenterology* **38**:399–418.
D Gerson CD, Cohen N and Janowitz HD (1973) Small intestine absorptive function in regional enteritis. *Gastroenterology* **64**:907–912.
E Koch J, Garcia-Shelton YL, Neal EA, Chan MF, Weaver KE and Cello JP (1996) Steatorrhea: a common manifestation in patients with HIV/AIDS. *Nutrition* **12**:507–510.

who make up to 30% of newly diagnosed cases. The sites and causes of lipid malabsorption and steatorrhoea are shown in **Fig. 2**.

Further investigations

If the patient's clinical picture suggests a possible small bowel source for the aetiology of steatorrhoea, an upper gastrointestinal (GI) endoscopy with small bowel biopsy should be performed. This may miss patchy lesions such as lymphoma, lymphangiectasia or radiation enteritis. Under these circumstances, a small bowel radiograph may be more useful. Although frequently used to measure jejunal absorption, the D-xylose test has a false positive and false negative rate of 20–30% (and a higher false negative rate in renal impairment), which limits its utility. A Schilling test is useful to test terminal ileal function, especially if bile salt depletion is suspected. If pancreatic insufficiency is suspected a Secretin test should be performed. An oblique radiograph of the abdomen or an abdominal computerized tomography (CT) scan can confirm pancreatic calcification and an endoscopic retrograde cholangio-pancreatico-gram (ERCP) may demonstrate the beaded shaped ducts of chronic pancreatitis (the commonest cause of pancreatic insufficiency in humans). Measurement of serum trypsinogen level is useful in patients with severe steatorrhoea. It is decreased in patients with steatorrhoea of pancreatic origin, but not in steatorrhoea of nonpancreatic origin. Serum trypsinogen levels are normal in patients with chronic pancreatitis without steatorrhoea.

General Principles of Nutrition Support in Steatorrhoea

The first principle of nutritional support is to feed into the bowel if possible. If the GI tract can be used safely and efficaciously, it is the preferred site for nutrient delivery.

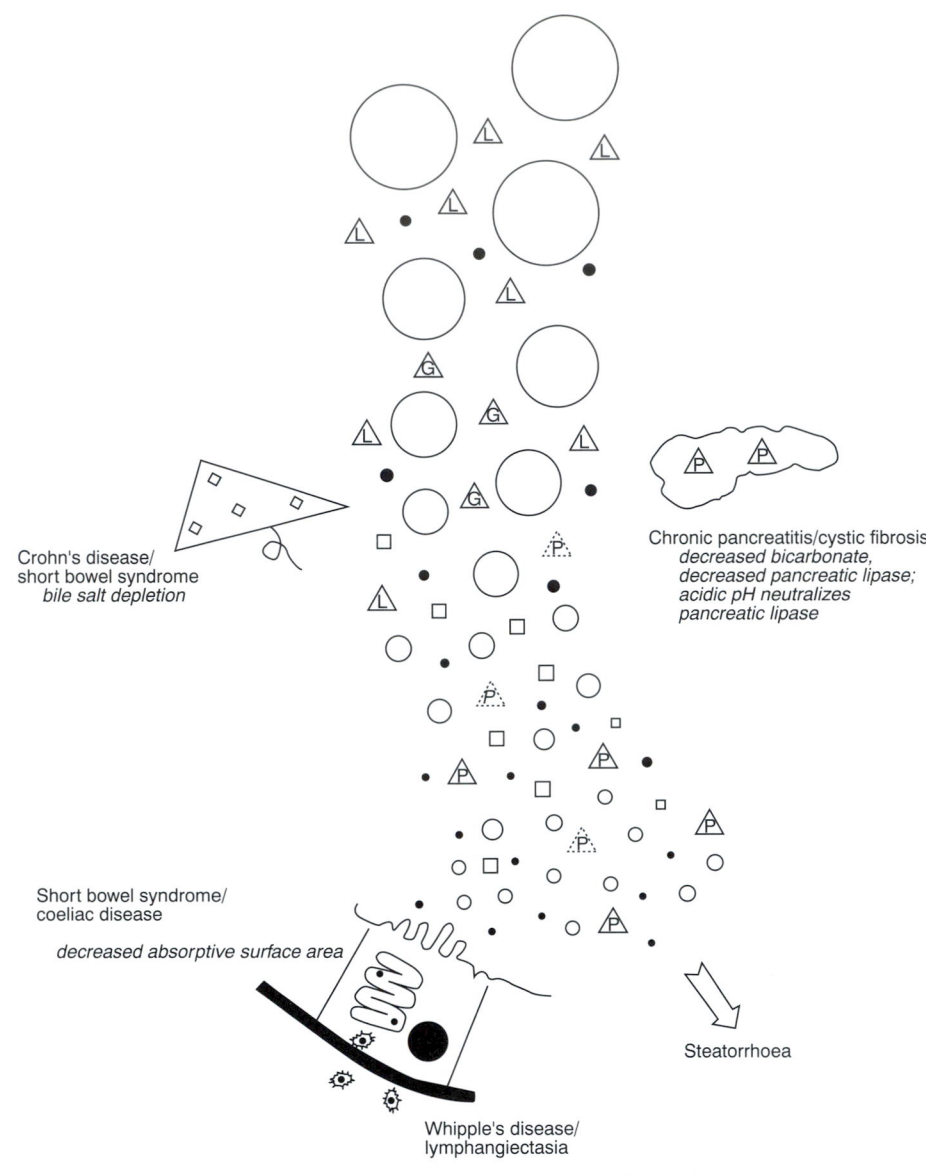

Crohn's disease/
short bowel syndrome
bile salt depletion

Chronic pancreatitis/cystic fibrosis
*decreased bicarbonate,
decreased pancreatic lipase;
acidic pH neutralizes
pancreatic lipase*

Short bowel syndrome/
coeliac disease

decreased absorptive surface area

Steatorrhoea

Whipple's disease/
lymphangiectasia

decreased transfer to lymphatics

Figure 2 Sites and causes of lipid malabsorption and steatorrhoea. Key as in Fig. 1.

Owing to inefficient digestion and absorption, patients with steatorrhoea often consume large amounts of energy to achieve their daily requirements. Many patients with steatorrhoea restrict their fat intake to minimize symptoms. As fat is the most energetically dense substrate, $38 \, kJ \, g^{-1}$ ($9 \, kcal \, g^{-1}$) compared with $17 \, kJ \, g^{-1}$ ($4 \, kcal \, g^{-1}$) for carbohydrate and protein, maintaining an adequate energy intake can be difficult when a low-fat diet is consumed. The assistance of a dietitian is invaluable. In many hospitals, the dietitian is the only individual with formal training in nutrition.

All diets need to contain at least some long-chain fatty acids to provide the two essential fatty acids. These are linoleic acid ($C_{18:2 \, n-6}$) and α-linolenic acid ($C_{18:3 \, n-3}$), of which the daily requirements are approximately 2.5–5 g of linoleic and 2–3 g of α-linolenic acid per day. Safflower oil contains 70% linoleic acid.

Medium-chain triacylglycerols (C_6–C_{12}) are more easily digested by pancreatic and mucosal lipases than long-chain triacylglycerols, do not require micelle formation for absorption and are absorbed directly into the portal vein instead of the lymphatics (important in lymphangiectasia). They provide a good source of energy and may help solubilize and aid absorption of fat-soluble vitamins. Unfortunately the use of medium-chain triacylglycerols is limited by their impalatability, expense and cathartic effect at high doses. A recent report challenges the use of medium-chain triacylglycerols by showing that typical laboratory methods to measure faecal fats fail to extract medium-chain triacylglycerols and so underestimate their concentration. Although the investigators confirmed that medium-chain triacylglycerols were better absorbed than long-chain fatty acids, when pancreatic enzyme supplements were used, faecal losses of medium- and long-chain fatty acids were the same.

Attention should be paid to fat-soluble vitamin intake (vitamins A, D, E and K) and to levels of trace elements and divalent cations, particularly calcium, zinc and magnesium. Dietary divalent cations can from insoluble soaps with intraluminal fatty acids and thus be unavailable for absorption. Decreased bone mineral density is common with malabsorption and may be due in part to low vitamin D levels. Vitamin A and E levels are also reduced (**Table 3**).

Steatorrhoea of pancreatic origin

Chronic pancreatitis is the commonest cause of steatorrhoea in adults and it is most often the result of chronic alcohol abuse. Steatorrhoea occurs when more than 90% of the exocrine pancreas is damaged. The patient may have debilitating abdominal pain, increased narcotic use leading to anorexia, diabetes mellitus (which often precedes the onset of steatorrhoea), or abdominal surgery performed to palliate pancreatic pain or other adverse sequelae of chronic pancreatitis. Alcohol should be completely avoided. Adequate energy intake is the most important aspect of dietary therapy and diet should be adjusted for the individual patient. The low-fat (< 25% of energy), high-protein diet recommended by Marrota and Floch provides a starting point. Pancreatic enzyme supplements are prescribed to improve fat absorption and are the first line therapy for abdominal pain in patients with chronic pancreatitis. The normal human pancreas secretes 300 000 units of lipolytic activity 4–6 h postprandially. Most pancreatic enzyme supplements contain 5000–8000 units per capsule. 30 000 IU of porcine lipase will usually decrease steatorrhoea by more than 50%, but most patients continue to secrete more than 10 g fat per 24 h. Typical recommendations are to take 4–6 capsules with meals and 2–3 capsules with snacks. Increasing the number of capsules beyond this amount leads to decreasing patient compliance. Bicarbonate secretion is also impaired in chronic pancreatitis. The duodenal contents tend to maintain a pH of <4, at which pancreatic lipase is inactivated. In one report, only 8% of ingested lipase was recovered from the duodenum of adults with pancreatic insufficiency. Enteric coated preparations designed to release their enzymes above a particular pH partly overcome this problem. H_2 blockers and proton pump inhibitors decrease gastric acid production, raise duodenal pH and slightly improve the efficacy of pancreatic enzyme supplements. Up to 25% of chronic pancreatitis patients have small bowel microbial overgrowth, particularly if they are on chronic narcotics or have had GI surgery. A course

Table 3 Micronutrient supplementation in steatorrhoea

Micronutrient	Route	Dosage per day
Fat-soluble vitamins		
A (water-soluble capsules)	PO	USP 25 000–50 000 units maintenance; 100 000–200 000 units for severe deficiency
D	PO	50 000 units, increase as needed to raise serum calcium to normal
E	PO	100–200 iu per kg per day α-tocopherol
K	PO	USP 4–12 mg menadione
	IV	Vitamin K_1 (Mephyton) 10 mg ampoule slowly over 10 min for acute bleeding episodes only
Water-soluble vitamins		
B_{12}	IM/IV	100 μg daily for first 2 weeks or 1000 μg loading dose; then 100 μg monthly
Folic acid	PO	5 mg daily for 1 month, 1 mg per day maintenance
Other B vitamins, C		As indicated
Minerals		
Calcium	PO	1200–1500 mg elemental
Magnesium	PO	1–4 g magnesium gluconate
Potassium	PO	Maximum 150 mEq (5850 mg)
Zinc	PO	As indicated
Iron	PO	As indicated

From Marotta and Floch (1989). With permission.
PO, orally; IV, intravenously; IM/IV, intramuscularly/intravenously.

of antibiotics may be necessary to improve diarrhoea and reduce steatorrhoea in these patients. Dietary fibre partly interferes with lipid absorption by trapping pancreatic lipase, bile salts and lipid or by increasing the viscosity of intestinal contents and the thickness of the unstirred water layer. If steatorrhoea remains despite optimizing enzyme supplements and antisecretory therapy, it may be necessary to decrease the intake of dietary fibre.

Cystic fibrosis

Pancreatic insufficiency occurs in 95% of cystic fibrosis patients with the $\Delta 508$ genotype but is uncommon in other genotypes. Abnormalities in intestinal mucus and bile salt metabolism compound the problem. Recurrent respiratory infections lead to anorexia and increased metabolic requirements. $\Delta 508$ homozygote patients have higher resting metabolic rates, exceeding 121% predicted compared with controls or cystic fibrosis patients with other genotypes. This difference in metabolic rate remains after correcting for differences in pulmonary function. Relative underweight (weight loss corrected for height) correlates inversely with survival, especially in those with severe pulmonary symptoms. Exercise capacity, while clearly related to pulmonary function, is also independently influenced by nutritional status. This is possibly due to deleterious effects of malnutrition on respiratory muscle mass. Malnutrition and decreased respiratory function, once begun, tend to be relentless. Temporary nocturnal nasogastric drip feeding can offset the acute decline in body weight associated with respiratory infection. Children with cystic fibrosis thrive and maintain normal growth velocity when adequate nutrition is maintained. This usually includes a diet of normal to high fat content and adequate pancreatic enzyme supplementation with acid suppression. Even if steatorrhoea cannot be fully controlled, fat intake should not be reduced at the expense of energy intake. At a constant coefficient of fat absorption, increasing the amount of dietary fat increases the amount of fat excreted, but will also increase the total amount of fat and energy absorbed. Attention should also be directed to ensuring adequate protein intake. Young children have high protein requirements and poorly controlled steatorrhoea leads to increased faecal nitrogen losses. Near normalization of faecal fat excretion can be achieved in most cystic fibrosis patients with the combination of pancreatic enzyme supplementation and omeprazole. Low-fat diets lead to growth failure due to inadequate energy intake.

Overzealous use of pancreatic enzyme supplements in cystic fibrosis has been associated with the development of colonic strictures. The relative risk of fibrosing colopathy in patients taking <24 000 IU lipase : 24 001–50 000 IU lipase : > 50 000 IU lipase was 1 : 10.9 : 199.5. The mechanism for this is unclear. In one report, bowel wall thickness, as determined by ultrasound, was increased in cystic fibrosis patients compared with normal controls and was independent of dose of pancreatic supplements. Conflicting reports implicate and exonerate various products and formulation of pancreatic enzyme supplements. At present, there is no direct evidence that pancreatic enzyme supplements play a major role in the pathogenesis of fibrosing colopathy.

Owing to their physical properties, it has been hypothesized that taurine-conjugated bile salts might improve lipid absorption compared with glycine-conjugated bile salts. Taurine-conjugated bile salts are more water-soluble and less toxic than their glycine-conjugated counterparts. They remain in solution in the acidic duodenal environment and are not absorbed in the proximal jejunum, thus maintaining micelle structure along more of the length of the small bowel. Taurine supplementation at a dose of 30 mg per kg per day improved fat absorption in two studies. However, weight gains were modest and of borderline significance ($P<0.1$) in one and absent in the other. Other studies have failed to show improvement in fat absorption and despite earlier enthusiasm there seems to be little role for taurine in improving nutritional status in cystic fibrosis.

Coeliac disease

Coeliac disease produces subtotal villous atrophy and loss of mucosal surface area which leads to malabsorption of all macronutrients. Gluten, including wheat, rye, barley and oat products, should be eliminated permanently from the diet. Steroids or cyclosporin A are rarely required. Once the mucosa has recovered, further dietary modifications are not necessary.

Short bowel syndrome

Short bowel syndrome consists of severe diarrhoea, weight loss and malnutrition owing to massive loss of the absorptive capacity of the gut. It is most commonly caused by removal of more than half of the small intestine, but it may also be due to surgical bypass or intrinsic disease of the gut. Surgical resections of the small intestine for Crohn's disease is the most common cause of short bowel syndrome, followed by mesenteric vascular insufficiency, radiation or trauma. In children, congenital defects may also cause short bowel syndrome. Loss of more than 50% of the bowel leads to long-term malabsorption. In the intact bowel, most absorption occurs in the jejunum. Following jejunal resection the ileum adapts to increase its absorption, although it does not acquire the enterohumeral regulatory function of the jejunum. Following resection of the terminal ileum, the jejunum is unable to adapt to absorb bile salts or vitamin B_{12}, and greater steatorrhoea occurs than with equivalent lengths of jejunal resection. Significant bile salt loss begins if more than 25 cm of terminal ileum is resected.

The presence of the colon influences the manifestations and management of the condition. The colon influences small bowel motility and the caecal brake prolongs intestinal transit and improves absorption. Colonic fermentation of undigested carbohydrate produces short-chain fatty acids which in turn increase water sodium absorption. However, following ileal resection, large amounts of bile salts enter the colon and produce a cathartic diarrhoea. In the first 1–3 months following massive small bowel resection, the bowel undergoes hypertrophy, elongation and hyperplasia, leading to increase in villous height, crypt depth and number of enterocytes per unit length of bowel. This is followed by gradual adaptation of the remaining gut which continues over a period of 1–2 years. Parenteral nutrition is essential to provide adequate nutrient intake as well as to replace massive water and electrolyte losses during the initial treatment of short bowel syndrome. It is useful to measure the electrolyte content as well as the volume of the stomal output to assist in the maintenance of water and electrolyte balance. Oral supplementation should be commenced early as this stimulates bowel growth and adaptation, even though it will provide little effective nutrition in the initial postoperative period. There is no advantage to using expensive elemental diets. Polymeric supplements via nasogastric tube or tube gastrostomy is preferred. Total parenteral nutrition in the absence of enteral feeding leads to mucosal atrophy. H_2 blockers should be given to control gastric hypersecretion. Codeine, loperamide or diphenoxylate sodium are given to reduce diarrhoea and slow intestinal transit. As absorption improves, oral intake is increased and parenteral nutrition decreased. To increase energy density, there is a tendency to use high-fat diets in patients with short bowel syndrome. However, a recent study suggests that this may not be the best approach, particularly in patients with an intact colon. In these patients, bacterial digestion of dietary carbohydrates produces short-chain fatty acids which are absorbed by the colon, providing an additional 1900 kJ (450 kcal). In patients with a high jejunostomy, altering the fat content of the diet while maintaining its energy value did not seem to have any significant effect on their symptoms or nutrition,

and in these patients a more balanced approach to dietary composition may be appropriate. Close monitoring of nutritional status is essential as both over- and underfeeding need to be avoided. Patients with less than 100 cm of jejunum remaining, or less than 50 cm of jejunum but with an intact colon, are likely to require some level of long-term parenteral nutrition.

Bile salt malabsorption

Bile salt malabsorption occurs with loss of terminal ileal function, most commonly with Crohn's disease, but it also occurs following gastric surgery, cholecystectomy, and is associated with diabetes mellitus and cystic fibrosis. Diarrhoea is watery due to the cathartic effect of bile salts entering the colon. Cholestyramine, although unpalatable, chelates bile salt and reduces the magnitude of diarrhoea. If bile salt malabsorption is severe, the bile salt pool becomes depleted and fat malabsorption develops. A low-fat diet reduces the diarrhoea by decreasing the amount of lipid entering the colon, restores normal bowel flora, and improves the absorption of sodium, potassium and other minerals by decreasing the interference of lipid in the intestinal water layer of the small intestine. Attention should be directed to the intake of fat-soluble vitamins and essential fatty acids, which can be supplemented parenterally when necessary. In patients with severe bile salt depletion, replacement with cholylsarcosine, a derivative of cholic acid, shows promise but no clinical trials have been published to date.

Steatorrhoea in AIDS

Malnutrition, malabsorption and diarrhoea are common in AIDS patients. One study of 45 AIDS patients with unexplained diarrhoea or weight loss, despite adequate energy intake, demonstrated steatorrhoea in 22 (49%). Opportunistic infection of the gut, CD4 count or AIDS-defining illness did not predict the presence of this steatorrhoea, which is idiopathic in many cases. Measurements of stool ova and parasites, culture and sensitivity studies together with faecal leucocyte and acid-fast stains, with a small bowel biopsy if necessary, should be performed to rule out infectious aetiologies. A diet containing 85% of the fat content as medium-chain triacylglycerols decreases stool fat and nitrogen content and increases fat absorption compared with diets with long-chain triacylglycerols. No difference in body weight was noted over the 12 day experimental period. Bile salt and vitamin B_{12} malabsorption and abnormal intestinal absorption and permeability have been demonstrated in AIDS patients and may contribute to diarrhoea and malnutrition. In one case report, a dramatic response was seen following the administration of cholestyramine.

Nutritional Supplements

When the above dietary measures are insufficient to maintain nutritional status, enteral or parenteral supplements are necessary. If additional nutritional needs are modest nocturnal feeding via nasogastric tube or gastrostomy is usually sufficient. Parenteral nutrition is rarely required except for those with short bowel syndrome. Oral intake should be encouraged in these patients and parenteral nutrition is prescribed as needed. Close monitoring of body weight, muscle and fat stores as well as vitamin and mineral levels are necessary.

Antidiarrhoeal therapy

Patients often complain bitterly of steatorrhoea. When pancreatic enzyme supplements are ineffective, antidiarrhoeal agents may slow transit time and allow for increased absorption. Codeine, loperamide and diphenoxylate hydrochloride (lomotil) are the most commonly used. They provide little benefit to patients with chronic pancreatitis who are taking large amounts of nacrotics for pain, but they are useful for patients with short bowel syndrome. Octreotide is a very effective antimotility agent but needs to be used with caution. It decreases pancreatic secretion and can inhibit gut adaptation. Its use should probably be reserved for patients with short bowel syndrome of several years' duration where further gut adaptation is not expected.

Prognosis

The prognosis of steatorrhoea depends very much on the underlying diagnosis. Patients with chronic pancreatitis can usually be maintained on oral diets, while those with short bowel syndrome may require lifelong parenteral supplementation. Patients with coeliac disease who are compliant with a gluten-free diet have a normal life expectancy whereas cystic fibrosis patients can expect an inexorable decline in pulmonary function – the commonest cause for death in this group.

Conclusions

The key principle to the nutritional management of steatorrhoea is to diagnose and treat the underlying cause if possible. Evaluation should be directed by the clinical history. A multifaceted approach with enzyme supplements, acid suppression, bile salt manipulation and nutritional support may be necessary to maintain adequate nutritional status. Fat restriction is not always appropriate. Attention should be paid to ensure adequate intake of fat-soluble vitamins and essential fatty acids. Diarrhoea and fat malabsorption may persist even in the presence of optimal management of steatorrhoea. Once adequate nutritional status is achieved and maintained, the prognosis depends on the natural history of the underlying disease.

See also: **Coeliac Disease**: Aetiology and Nutritional Management. **Cystic Fibrosis**: Dietary Aspects and Nutritional Management. **Gastrointestinal Tract**: Structure and Function of the Small Intestine. **HIV Disease**: Nutritional Management. **Malabsorption Syndromes**: Nutritional Management. **Nutritional Support**: Enteral Feeding; Parenteral Nutrition. **Therapeutic Dietetics**: Short Bowel Syndrome.

Further Reading

Berger DL and Malt RA (1996) Management of the short gut syndrome. *Advances in Surgery* 29:43–57.

Caliari S, Benini L, Sembenini C, Gregori B, Carnielli V and Vantini I (1996) Medium-chain triglyceride absorption in patients with pancreatic insufficiency. *Scandinavian Journal of Gastroenterology* 31:90–94.

FitzSimmons SC, Burkhart GA, Borowitz D, Grand RJ, Hammerstrom T, Durie PR, Lloyd-Still JD and Lowenfels AB (1997) High dose pancreatic enzyme supplements and fibrosing colonopathy in children with cystic fibrosis. *New England Journal of Medicine* 336:1283–1289.

Heijerman HGM (1992) New modalities in the treatment of exocrine pancreatic insufficiency in cystic fibrosis. *Netherlands Journal of Medicine* 41:105–109.

Ladefoged K, Hessov I and Jarnum S (1996) Nutrition in short-bowel syndrome. *Scandinavian Journal of Gastroenterology* 31:122–131.

Marotta RB and Floch MH (1989) Dietary therapy of steatorrhoea. *Gastroenterology Clinics of North America* 18(3):485–511.

Nordgaard I, Stenbaek Hansen B and Brobech Mortensen P (1994) Colon as a digestive organ in patients with short bowel. *Lancet* 343:373–376.

Olsen WA (1973) Medical intelligence, current concepts. A practical approach to diagnosis of disorders of intestinal absorption. *New England Journal of Medicine* 23:1358–1361.

Rombeau JE and Caldwell MD (eds) (1993) *Clinical Nutrition: Parenteral Nutrition*, 2nd edn. Philadelphia: WB Saunders.

Rombeau JE and Rolandelli RH (eds) (1997) *Clinical Nutrition: Enteral Nutrition and Tube Feeding*, 3rd edn. Philadelphia: WB Saunders.

Toskes PP (1995) Medical management of chronic pancreatitis. *Scandinavian Journal of Gastroenterology* 30:74–80.

> **Stomach** *see* **Gastrointestinal Tract**: Structure and Function of the Stomach.

STROKE

Nutritional Management

S McLaren, University of Kingston, Kingston upon Thames, Surrey, UK

Stroke is a syndrome that is sudden in onset, featuring signs of cerebral dysfunction of more than 24 h duration which are vascular in origin. In first strokes, thromboembolic infarction is the underlying pathophysiological event in approximately 80% of cases. Of the remainder, 10% have been attributed to primary intracerebral haemorrhage, 5% to subarachnoid haemorrhage and 5% to uncertain types. Stroke is common, the incidence rising with age. In the UK combined incidence figures for males and females are 0.08 per thousand population less than 45 years of age, rising to 20.30 per thousand it over 85 years. Resulting neurological and functional impairments vary in range, combination and severity. These can include altered consciousness, motor paralysis, and somatosensory, auditory, olfactory and visual loss. Impairments of memory, speech, language and continence can also occur.

The challenge of nutritional management is apparent in the scope of issues presented. These include the physical, psychological and social impact of stroke on appetite and food ingestion, as well as pre-stroke nutritional status. Potential effects of injury, immobilization and infective complications on energy and nitrogen requirements must be considered. In individuals in whom oral feeding cannot be established, intravenous hydration and artificial nutritional support by the enteral route may be necessary. Finally, the presence of disorders such as diabetes mellitus and hypertension, which are known risk factors for stroke, can require dietary modifications as part of the overall plan of treatment. Effective nutritional management of stroke requires a multidisciplinary approach in which the skills and knowledge of physician, dietitian, nurse, speech therapist, physiotherapist and occupational therapist are effectively and efficiently integrated to the benefit of the patient.

Stroke: Risks of Protein–Energy Malnutrition

A number of factors may interact to impair the nutritional status of individuals who have suffered a stroke. These include factors which have led to a deterioration in pre-stroke nutritional status, direct physical and psychosocial effects of stroke on the consumption of food and fluids following hospital admission, and organizational factors which can hinder efficient, effective meal delivery and consumption in institutional settings.

Pre-stroke nutritional status

The prevalence of protein–energy malnutrition at the time of hospital admission following stroke has been reported at 15%, on the evidence of anthropometric and biochemical indicators of nutritional status. Specifically, a low serum albumin concentration has been found to be a significant predictor of post-stroke functional impairment, morbidity and mortality. Risk factors for malnutrition identified at the time of hospital admission have included increasing age, dementia and inadequate dental status. These findings are consistent with those found in wider surveys of elderly populations where risk factors for protein–energy malnutrition also included social isolation, bereavement, poverty, physical disability, inadequate facilities for preparing and cooking food, and the impact of multiple medications on appetite. The significance of a low serum albumin concentration in predicting clinical outcomes has been noted in other geriatric populations, where it may be more a reflection of disease severity than an indicator of nutritional status.

Post-stroke eating problems

Neurological and functional impairments can result in eating problems following stroke. These have been associated with an inadequate consumption of food and fluids and a deterioration in body mass index, triceps skinfold thickness, midarm muscle circumference and serum protein concentrations during the acute phase of recovery. Specific problems contributing to this have included anorexia, impaired lip closure leading to oral repulsion of food and fluids, dysphagia, an inability to manipulate utensils linked to loss of motor skills in eating, and difficulties in maintaining an upright posture to aid food ingestion at mealtimes. The presence of visual field and/or perceptual deficits can result in an inability to see or perceive the contents of a meal tray, while aphasia, dysphasia or dysarthria can hinder or prevent the expression of dietary preferences. Loss of concentration and short-term memory impairment are common sequelae to stroke and can make it difficult for individuals to sustain the sequence of activities necessary to complete a meal, or even to remember to eat and drink.

Organizational factors

A number of organizational factors can hinder dietary provision and consumption in institutional settings where dependent elderly people are recovering from a range of disorders including stroke. These include an inadequate mealtime environment, marked by poor lighting, noise, sterile decor, temperature extremes and lack of facilities for socializing. Lack of manpower or involvement of untrained personnel in dietary selection, meal delivery and supervision may result in the delivery of a meal which is inappropriate in relation to texture, portion size and post-stroke swallowing capacity, or inadequate assistance in relation to the level of physical dependency. The provision of effective nutritional care requires a concerted approach by health professionals in developing evidence-based standards and guidelines for nutritional screening, assessment and all stages in the provision of dietary support which are linked to clinical audit.

Management of Psychosocial and Physical Problems Impairing Food Consumption

Following acute stroke, early screening and assessment are essential to identify individuals who are capable of ingesting sufficient food via the oral route without risks of aspiration, and those who require artificial nutritional support owing to the severity of dysphagia or cognitive and functional impairments. In individuals who are capable of taking food orally, the provision of support for psychosocial and physical problems is a vital aspect of nutritional management.

Psychosocial problems

In the acute phase following stroke, 25–30% of patients develop clinical signs of depression, 30% are anxious, and a similar proportion report loss of confidence as a major psychological problem. Depression may result from an interaction of several factors including left frontal lobe damage, reactions to physical loss and impaired performance of activities of daily living. Comparatively little is known of interactions between depression, anorexia and nutritional status in the early stages of recovery following stroke in individuals with and without physical eating problems. However, patterns of behavioural disturbance characterized by verbal expressions of depressed mood, anorexia and insomnia have been identified and associated with weight loss. Anxiety-evoking experiences relating to being fed, or choking in the presence of dysphagia, may also result in avoidance or withdrawal from eating. General approaches to the treatment of post-stroke depression can involve the use of antidepressant drugs and behavioural and psychotherapeutic techniques. Specifically, the exercise of therapeutic skills in communication, assisting eating and providing emotional support are vital in alleviating mealtime anxiety and increasing interest in food.

The enjoyment of eating as a social activity can be affected adversely by post-stroke depression and impairments of speech, language, lip closure and manual dexterity. Severely disabled individuals who are relearning swallowing techniques initially require a quiet environment with privacy. As swallowing and other difficulties abate, social integration at mealtimes can be achieved in conjunction with sensitive assistance.

Communication problems

The aphasia/dysphasia prevalent in 20–30% of acute strokes and anarthria/dysarthria in 40% result in difficulty in expressing thoughts in language or a total inability to do so (expressive motor aphasia/dysphasia) as well as difficulty in comprehending language (receptive aphasia/dysphasia) or producing speech (anarthria/dysarthria). Expressive aphasia, also known as Broca's aphasia, results from strokes affecting the prefrontal gyrus, while Werricke's receptive aphasia results from lesions of the central sulcus. In contrast, dysarthria results from neurological damage affecting the neuromuscular systems which control the mechanisms of speech production. Since these systems are also concerned with swallowing, it is common to find difficulty with swallowing (dysphagia) present in dysarthric individuals.

The communication problems result in inabilities/difficulties in expressing meal preferences (aphasia/dysarthria), reading a menu or writing preferences down (aphasia can occur in conjunction with dyslexia and dysgraphia). In contrast, receptive aphasia can impair the ability to comprehend instructions at mealtimes and thus affects compliance with rehabilitative advice. If paralysis, visual field and perceptual deficits are combined with expressive dysphasia and dysarthria, then nonverbal communication can also be limited, resulting in an inability to denote assent or dissent by nodding the head or to use gestures to convey meaning or point to food items/utensils. Early involvement of speech therapists is vital to enable individuals to regain lost functions in speech and language. In selected patients use of visual material, i.e. charts or pictures of food items and symbols, can be helpful. Use of short sentences, normal volume speech, avoidance of jargon and patience in allowing individuals to respond to questions are also helpful in general communication.

Impairments of arm movement and posture

Stroke can affect one or many of the areas and neural mechanisms controlling voluntary movement and posture. These include the motor cortex and associated pathways, cerebellum, basal ganglia and brainstem. The impact on eating skills can be considerable, since weakness or paralysis affecting the arm occurs in 80% of strokes. Loss of coordination, spatial impairment, abnormal muscle tone and sensory loss may also occur. Common problems resulting from this are difficulties manipulating cutlery, lifting/loading utensils, cutting food, inserting food in the mouth, drinking from a cup, or discerning the spatial relationships between objects.

If one arm is unaffected, then some degree of compensation is possible, particularly if this is dominant. Use of the unaffected hand is important in detecting temperatures of food and liquids where sensation is impaired. An occupational therapy assessment is necessary to identify appropriate aids to feeding. Lightweight plastic cups with moulded handles and cutlery with built up indented handles may be useful, while plateguards and nonslip mats can be provided. Where upper limb impairment is severe, individuals may require continuous assistance with food preparation and ingestion.

Postural impairment following stroke can result in an inability to maintain an upright sitting position for effective food preparation, insertion, chewing and swallowing. A physiotherapy assessment can identify the most effective postural techniques to counteract abnormal muscle tone (spasticity) and appropriate aids to seated balance. The latter can include moulded seating, tilting chairs with table attachment and limb stabilizers.

Visual field loss and visual neglect

It has been estimated that 30–60% of individuals who sustain an acute stroke suffer from visual field loss due to partial or complete hemianopia. Neurological damage affecting the parietal or temporal lobes and involving the sensory pathway between the optic chiasma and visual cortex underlies this problem. The impact of loss in up to half the visual field is that food items on a meal tray may not be seen and therefore may remain uneaten. Compensatory interventions include instruction in scanning the visual field, or placing items within it for those who are unable to do this. Consistent placement of items on a meal tray and verbal identification of contents using a clock system is also helpful.

Neurological damage affecting the visual cortex of the occipital lobe, common following right hemisphere strokes, can result in neglect of half the visual space. A classic feature of this problem is failing to eat food on the left side of a plate. Affected individuals need reminding to focus on food items in the neglected space; placing a coloured marker on one side of the plate can be helpful. This problem may occur in conjunction with visual field loss.

Attention span, short-term memory

Impairment of attention span and short-term memory of a few minutes duration are common following stroke. Attention deficits result in an inability either to focus on immediate events or to establish a new focus unless a current stimulus is removed. As a consequence, an activity which requires a sequence of steps, such as eating a meal with two or three courses, cannot be completed. Lack of concentration is also unhelpful in relearning eating patterns. Removing or minimizing distractions at mealtimes, simplifying the complexity of information necessary to regain eating skills and providing verbal, written or auditory alarms as reminders to eat are important in overcoming this problem.

Swallowing

Difficulty in swallowing (dysphagia) affects approximately 25–45% of the stroke population. Variable in severity, it is characterized by sensory and/or motor loss affecting one or more of the stages of swallowing, i.e. oral preparation, oral transport, pharyngeal transport and reflex swallowing (**Table 1**). The effects of stroke on oesophageal peristalsis are not fully known. Typical features of dysphagia can include oral repulsion of food/fluids, impaction and retention of food in the cheek cavity, choking or regurgitation of food/fluids through the nose and mouth. Swallowing and gag reflexes may be absent.

Table 1 Stages of swallowing: effects of stroke

Stage	Effects of stroke
1. Oral preparation Duration variable Lip closure forms anterior seal Comminution of food by mandibular, maxillary teeth; chewing of food Salivation evoked by parasympathetic nervous system Bolus formation controlled by tongue Sensory feedback from oral mucosa on volume and consistency determine timing of bolus ejection	Inadequate lip seal causes leakage of food/fluid chewing slower, food impacts in oral sulci Hyposecretion of saliva Paralysis of tongue impairs bolus formation Sensory loss leads to impaired bolus lateralization
2. Oral transport Duration 1 s Bolus of 5–15 cm³ separated, moved to tongue midline Oral cavity sealed, mandible raised, pressure exerted by tongue against palate propels bolus to posterior oral cavity	Slowed transport Bolus localization, separation and formation impaired; can lead to food retention in oral cavity Lack of fine motor coordination may lead to loss of liquid bolus control; risk of aspiration Abnormal positioning of bolus; diminished tongue elevation; inadequate bolus propulsion
3. Pharyngeal transport/reflex swallowing Duration 0.5–0.6 s Bolus impacts on sensory receptors in tissues of soft palate, pharynx, tongue, fauces Swallowing reflex stimulated; elevation/closure of velopharyngeal mechanism, elevation of larynx, closure of vocal cords, pharyngeal peristalsis, relaxation of oesophageal sphincter Respiration transiently ceases as bolus enters oesophagus; breathing resumed; soft palate returned to resting position	Events may occur in abnormal sequence/timing Impaired sensation, delay/absent swallowing reflex Velopharyngeal closure impaired; food regurgitated through nose/mouth Incomplete laryngeal elevation/vocal cord adduction Swallowing reflex delay/absence leading to coughing, aspiration
4. Oesophageal transport Duration 8–20 s Peristalsis moves bolus to stomach	Effects of stroke little investigated Ageing results in slight impairment of peristaltic amplitude

Complications resulting from dysphagia can be life-threatening, i.e. aspiration of food/fluid into the respiratory tract, pulmonary infection and dehydration. Longer hospital stay, strong inverse correlations with functional capacity and an increased mortality have been associated with the presence of dysphagia. Early identification of the problem is therefore vital, encompassing bedside assessment, videofluoroscopy and, if necessary, oesophagoscopy.

Bedside assessment encompasses the medical history relating to onset of swallowing problems: oral sensory and motor testing; laryngeal and pharyngeal assessment; presence/absence of swallowing, cough and gag reflexes; cognitive and language function; and alertness, attention span and ability to follow instructions. Aspiration of food or fluid into the respiratory tract is not always accompanied by choking; it may be silent, or indicated by voice changes (wet, hoarse, gurgling) and breathlessness. Loss of swallowing and protective gag reflexes or the presence of features of dysphagia or aspiration when attempting to swallow a teaspoon of clear fluid at an initial screen are indications that nil should be given by mouth. Further detailed investigation is then necessary.

Bedside assessment is limited in its ability to detect some cases of oropharyngeal dysphagia and individuals who are aspirating food, fluids or saliva into the respiratory tract. Videofluoroscopy provides a more detailed radiological assessment of swallowing which can detect functional impairments resulting in aspiration, evaluate the optimal head/neck position during swallowing, and determine the impact of food textures on the process. Where an oral diet can be attempted, modification of food textures can ensure an adequate intake is tolerated, reducing aspiration risk (**Table 2**). Compensatory therapeutic techniques, summarized in **Table 3**, may also benefit different stages of swallowing.

Nutrient Requirements

A variety of approaches to the estimation of energy requirements can be used. Predictive equations can

Table 2 Food textures suitable for different levels of dysphagia

Dysphagia severity		Designation	Food textures omitted	Food textures allowed
I	Severely impaired oral preparatory stage Reduced pharyngeal peristalsis Reduced swallowing reflex[a]	Patients unable to chew solids or swallow thin liquids safely	Coarse, hard or brittle textures *Unsuitable foods:* fruits, nuts, raw vegetables, sticky foods, all foods requiring bolus formation or controlled oral manipulation No thin liquids	Thick, homogeneous, smooth textures or semisolids; cold liquids thickened with commercial agent *Suitable foods:* poached eggs, soft puddings, thick vegetable/fruit purée
II	Moderately impaired oral preparation Reduced pharyngeal peristalsis	Patients who cannot swallow thin liquids and have minimum tolerance of chewed food	Coarse, hard, brittle textures No thin liquids	Thick, homogeneous purées, semisolids *Suitable foods:* cold thickened beverages, eggs, yogurt, cottage cheese, custards, puréed vegetables, fruits, tender meats
III	Mild impairment of oral preparation Mild chewing problems	Patients who can tolerate soft foods and liquids	Coarse, hard, brittle textures *Unsuitable foods:* nuts, minced meat, raw, stringy, crisp vegetables	Soft foods, not puréed or blended *Suitable foods:* soft bread, eggs, cottage cheese, casseroled small meat pieces, macaroni, hot/cold thick puddings
IV	Mild oral preparation impairment Can chew soft textures	Patients who can tolerate soft food textures and liquids	Coarse, fibrous, hard foods *Unsuitable foods:* nuts, deep fried or raw, crisp foods	Soft foods not requiring grinding or chopping *Suitable foods:* soft, toasted bread, cold cereals, milk, pasta, eggs, cooked, canned or over-ripe fruit, fine moist meats, tender vegetables, soft desserts

Adapted from Martin (1991).
[a]Videofluoroscopy screening essential for safety.

provide an estimate of resting energy expenditure based on body weight, height, age and sex. Modifications to equations can be applied which incorporate activity and injury factors. Additional requirements for tissue repletion should be considered in malnourished individuals. Estimation of resting energy expenditure by indirect calorimetry using a portable metabolic monitor provides more accurate estimates derived from the repiratory quotient. Values obtained do not consider periods of activity, pyrexia, pain or energy increments necessary for nutritional repletion. Further corrections are therefore necessary.

Following stroke a number of factors may affect energy requirements. Inactivity caused by paralysis will reduce energy expenditure, but the presence of pulmonary infection, a common complication of stroke, will increase it (a 1°C rise in core temperature raises energy expenditure by 13%). The impact of the cerebral injury on post-stroke metabolism, notably on resting energy expenditure at different levels of stroke severity, has not been fully investigated. Evidence for metabolic injury responses based on hormonal profiles and changes in blood glucose concentration in the acute phase is limited. Hyperglycaemia is common following stroke and has been associated with an increased morbidity and mortality. Hyperglycaemia can be attributed to overt or latent diabetes mellitus, stress responses, and effects of glucose intolerance in elderly subjects. Elevated plasma cortisol and catecholamine concentrations representing a transient stress response have been reported in the first 72 h following stroke.

Nitrogen requirements following stroke can be

Table 3 Impaired swallowing: therapeutic interventions

Stage of swallowing	Interventions
Oral preparation	Exercises to improve labial/mandibular closure, tongue elevation and lateralization (speech therapy) Lowering of palatal vault using prosthesis to improve bolus formation Compensate motor/sensory losses by positioning food on, and tilting head towards unaffected side Improvement of bolus localization by cold, thick, non-acid liquids
Oral transport	As above Posterior positioning of food on the tongue Use of straw positioned posteriorly to improve liquid swallows
Pharyngeal transport/reflex swallowing	Limit size of bolus; improve clearance by following each food swallow with dry swallow Thick, smooth homogeneous food textures require less peristaltic action Palatal training device may help to trigger swallowing reflex and reduce aspiration Posture upright, head stable in midline, slight forward flexion to protect airway Synchronize inspiration, breath holding, swallowing, expiration; cough on expiration to clear food debris Adduction exercises to assist laryngeal closure if impaired (speech therapist)
Oesophageal transport	Remain sitting in upright posture for 30 min after meal to prevent regurgitation/aspiration

estimated using reference ranges based on body weight, or using nitrogen balance studies. The chronic disorders diabetes mellitus and hypertension are common in the stroke population, which is predominantly elderly. Both disorders require dietary manipulation.

Fluid balance requirements also require careful assessment, since dehydration is a serious risk in individuals with dysphagia and physical disabilities which impair fluid consumption. Oral intake of fluid is contraindicated where the swallowing and gag reflex are lost and swallowing is impaired. Intravenous fluid replacement therapy is then necessary, usually short term. Fluid requirements can be calculated on the basis of 35 ml per kg body weight daily, but sepsis and fever can increase needs. Fluid intake and output in conjunction with insensible losses should be monitored on a daily basis together with the symptoms of dehydration, i.e. thirst, dry mucous membranes and loss of skin turgor.

Artificial Nutritional Support

The presence of severe dysphagia, cognitive and complex physical impairments may render oral feeding unsafe or insufficient to meet nutritional requirements. If the gastrointestinal tract is functional, the options for delivering enteral nutritional support are either via a fine-bore nasogastric tube or via a catheter inserted by percutaneous endoscopic gas-

trostomy (PEG). Decisions concerning the choice of route are influenced by the anticipated duration of dysphagia, and benefits versus risks. Impact on nutritional status, rehabilitation, quality of life, safety, tolerance, flexibility, ease of use, costs of insertion, removal and maintenance are all important considerations. In the majority of cases dysphagia resolves within the acute phase of stroke, i.e. approximately 3 weeks. For relatively short time periods, enteral feeding by fine-bore nasogastric catheter is usually undertaken. This can be preferable because of the technical simplicity of intubation, maintenance and removal, low cost and ease of use. Discomfort and risks of aspiration, accidental endotracheal intubation and displacement or perforation of the oesophagus are the potential complications, most of which are uncommon, although aspiration may occur in up to 10% of patients.

For feeding over longer time periods, a PEG tube inserted under local anaesthetic offers greater comfort, toleration, ease of use and reported improvements in nutritional status. However costs are greater, and this more invasive procedure carries a technique-related fatality of 1–2%. Minor complications include stomal sepsis, leaking and outlet blockage. Peritonitis, perforation, gastrointestinal bleeding and intestinal obstruction can occur, but are rare. Most enterostomy catheters are made from non-acid-hardening polyurethane or silicone and can be left in situ for up to 6 months. No consensus exists concerning the time period within which gastrostomy feeding should be initiated following stroke, but it should be considered where dysphagia is likely to persist beyond 14 days, and earlier for those intolerant of nasogastric tube feeding. In a small number of cases, enteral nutrition may be contraindicated following stroke owing to gastrointestinal bleeding resulting from severe stress ulceration. Rarely, non-stroke-related contraindications may also be present, i.e. gastrointestinal failure, ascites, Crohn's disease, bleeding and clotting disorders.

Evaluation of Nutritional Support

It is vital that nutritional status is monitored in the acute phase of recovery and that dietary intakes are readjusted accordingly. Appropriate dietary, anthropometric and clinical assessments which can be performed on a weekly basis are discussed (See: **Nutritional Status**: Dietary Assessment; Anthropometric Assessment). Other important components of monitoring include recovery of physical functions related to independence in eating including swallowing capacity and the complications of enteral support techniques. Providing effective nutritional management following stroke requires the coordination of the professional skills of doctor, nurse, speech therapist, dietitian, occupational therapist and physiotherapist, ideally within the context of a nutrition support team. Dynamic leadership and clear accountability, lines of communication and referral policies are essential for the team to deliver effective support. Follow-up services in the community are also necessary to prevent deterioration in nutritional status in the later stages of rehabilitation.

See also: **Diabetes Mellitus**: Dietary Management. **Energy**: Energy Requirements; Energy Balance; Measurement of Energy Intake and Expenditure. **Hypertension**: Nutritional Management. **Malnutrition**: Secondary Malnutrition. **Nutritional Status**: Dietary Assessment; Anthropometric Assessment. **Older People**: Nutritional Requirements; Nutritional Management of Geriatric Patients. **Protein**: Requirements and Role in Diet.

Further Reading

Aptaker RL, Roth EJ, Reichhardt G, Duerden ME and Levy CE (1994) Serum albumin level as a predictor of geriatric stroke rehabilitation outcome. *Archives of Physical and Medical Rehabilitation* 75:80–84.

Axelsson K, Asplund K, Norberg A and Alafusoff L (1988) Nutritional status in patients with acute stroke. *Acta Medica Scandinavica* 22:217–224.

Barer DH (1989) The natural history, and functional consequences of dysphagia after hemispheric stroke. *Journal of Neurology, Neurosurgery and Psychiatry* 52:236–241.

Logemann J (1983) *Evaluation and Treatment of Swallowing Disorders*. San Diego: College Hill Press.

Logemann J (1990) Factors affecting ability to resume oral nutrition in the oropharyngeal dysphagic individual. *Dysphagia* 4:202–208.

Malmgren R, Bamford J, Waterlow C, Sandercock P and Slattery J (1989) Projecting the number of patients with first ever strokes and patients newly handicapped by stroke in England and Wales. *British Medical Journal* 298:656–660.

Martin AW (1991) Dietary management of swallowing disorders. *Dysphagia* 6:129–134. Springer-Verlag.

Miller RM and Groher ME (1984) *Dysphagia, Diagnosis and Management*. Boston: Butterworth.

Morley JE, Glick Z and Rubenstein LZ (1995) *Geriatric Nutrition: A Comprehensive Review*, 2nd edn. New York: Raven Press.

O'Mahoney D and McIntyre AS (1995) Artificial feeding for elderly patients after stroke. *Age and Ageing* 24:533–535.

O'Neill PA, Davies I, Fullerton K and Bennett D (1991) Stress hormone and glucose response following acute stroke in the elderly. *Stroke* 22(7):842–847.

Splaingard ML, Hutchins B, Sulton LD and Chandhum G (1988) Aspiration in rehabilitation patients: videofluoroscopy vs bedside clinical assessments. *Archives of Physical and Medical Rehabilitation* 69:637–640.

Wade DT, Langton Hewer R, Skilbeck CE and David RM (1985) *Stroke: A Critical Approach to Diagnosis, Treatment and Management*. London: Chapman & Hall.

Wanklyn P, Cox N and Belfield P (1995) Outcome in patients who require a gastrostomy after stroke. *Age and Ageing* 24:510–514.

SUCROSE

Contents
Nutritional Role, Absorption and Metabolism
Dietary Sucrose and Disease

Nutritional Role, Absorption and Metabolism

J Brand-Miller, Department of Biochemistry, University of Sydney, New South Wales, Australia

Sucrose plays a unique role in human diets. It satisfies our instinctual desire for sweetness and contributes an average of 10% of the energy in modern Western diets. Sucrose has many functional roles in foods which extend beyond its sweetness, including preservative, textural and flavour modifying qualities. Unfortunately, sucrose has a 'bad reputation', especially in respect of dental caries. In the past, refined sucrose was suggested to cause diabetes, overweight, heart disease, micronutrient deficiencies and even hyperactivity in children. But within the last decade a wealth of new research on sugars in the diet has shown most of these assumptions to be false. We now know that refined sucrose consumption is much lower than we originally estimated (45–65 g per day instead of 125 g per day in industrialized countries), that intake of sugars correlates inversely with the fat content of the diet (the higher the sugar intake, the lower the fat), and that high-sucrose diets are associated with *lower* body weight. In addition, new research shows that moderate intake of sugars is associated with the highest intakes of micronutrients and that sucrose-containing foods do not raise the plasma glucose level any more than most starchy foods. While dental caries is still associated with high sucrose consumption in nonindustrialized countries, there is no relationship in developed nations. The intake of fluoride, frequency of food intake and dental hygiene are more important factors influencing the incidence of dental caries in these countries.

What is Sucrose?

Sucrose is a pleasant tasting substance that contributes most of the sweetness in our diet. It has played a role in human diets ever since primates began evolving on a diet of fruit and berries in the tropical forests of Africa 50 million years ago. Sucrose is chemically classified as a carbohydrate and a simple sugar, specifically a disaccharide composed of glucose and fructose (**Fig. 1**). Its proper scientific name is β-D-fructofuranosyl-α-D-glucopyranoside. The natural sweetness of fruit and honey comes from mixtures of sucrose, glucose and fructose. The mild sweetness of milk comes from another disaccharide, lactose, composed of glucose and galactose.

Because sweetness comes from a mixture of sugars (not just sucrose) in many sources, we use different terms to define the original source, e.g. naturally occurring sugars, refined sugars, added sugars, concentrated sugars, intrinsic sugars and extrinsic sugars. Refined sucrose is also known as table sugar, cane sugar or beet sugar. Unfortunately, the term 'sugar' means different things to different people, and the literature can be confusing. In this article, as in everyday language, the word 'sugar' refers to refined sucrose, unless otherwise indicated.

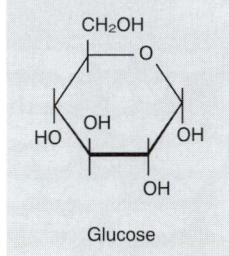
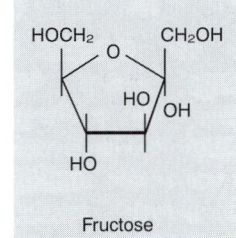

Figure 1 The chemical structure of glucose, fructose and sucrose.

The Role of Sucrose in the Diet

Historical perspective

Sugar cane and sugar beet have a naturally high content of sucrose and have been commercially exploited as a concentrated sources of sucrose since 1600 AD. Sugar cane was first cultivated in Papua New Guinea 10 000 years ago, and the practice spread gradually to Egypt (2300 years ago), Arabia (1300 years ago) and Japan (1100 years ago). Sugar beet was first grown in Europe 500 years ago. Prior to this, refined sucrose was still a rare and expensive commodity and honey was much cheaper. When the industrial revolution began 200 years ago, sucrose consumption increased dramatically, replacing honey as the major source of concentrated sweetness. Intake of refined sucrose peaked in about 1900 and consumption has remained, with minor variations, much the same over the past century. Since 1970 high-fructose corn syrup solids (glucose–fructose syrups made from hydrolysed corn starch) have partially replaced refined sucrose in manufactured products, particularly in the USA.

Instinctual liking for sweetness

The appreciation of the sensation of sweetness runs deep in the human psyche. In literature and mythology sweetness is linked with pleasure and goodness and in everyday language we use terms associated with sweetness to describe those we love (sweetie pie, honeybun). Our first food, breast milk, is sweet – in fact it is the sweetest of all mammalian milks. Newborn human infants drink more of a sweet solution than of plain water or of a salty, acidic or bitter solution. It is not a learned taste: everyone could be said to be born with a 'sweet tooth'. The reason for this sweet preference is not known. We could speculate that the brain's dependence on glucose as its sole source of fuel has coevolved in an environment where glucose or its precursor was not evenly distributed throughout the food supply. Perhaps those early primates who were able to detect sweetness best were most likely to survive.

Hunter-gatherers of the past relished honey and other sources of concentrated sweetness such as maple syrup, dried fruit and honey ants (**Table 1**). Wild honey was so highly prized that we went to great lengths to obtain it. Australian Aboriginals would attach a tiny feather to a bee and follow it all the way back to its hive. The Wild Men (Veddas) of Sri Lanka esteemed honey so highly that they regularly risked their lives to obtain it.

The contribution of sucrose to energy intake

The contribution of macronutrients and individual sugars to total energy intakes in industrialized nations is shown in **Table 2**. Sucrose is at the top of the league table for sugars, contributions coming from both the naturally occurring sources of sweetness such as fruit and vegetables and also from refined sucrose. Sucrose, like all carbohydrates, is burned (oxidized) in the body to yield energy, specifically $16 \, kJ \, g^{-1}$. This is only half the energy yield of a gram of fat ($37 \, kJ \, g^{-1}$) and much less than

Table 1 Sources of sweetness in human diets

- Honey
- Manna
- Honey ants
- Grape sugar
- Dates
- Maple sugar
- Sorghum
- Corn syrup solids
- High-fructose corn syrup solids
- Sugar beets
- Sugar cane
- Sugar alcohols (e.g. sorbitol)
- Intense sweetners (e.g. saccharin)

Table 2 The contribution of different types of carbohydrate and sucrose to energy intake in industrialized nations

Macronutrients	% energy (adults)	Men (g per day)	Women (g per day)	Children (g per day)
Carbohydrate	45			
Starch	21–23			
Total sugars	21–24			
Added (refined) sugars	9–11	60–70	40–50	40–50
Naturally occurring sugars	11–16	60–80	60–75	60–70
Individual sugars				
Sucrose	9–10			
Glucose	4–5			
Fructose	4–5			
Lactose	2–4			
Maltose	<0.3			

that of alcohol (29 kJ g^{-1}). Other carbohydrates such as starch, glucose and fructose have the same energy content per gram as sucrose. The new 'intense' sweeteners such as aspartame contribute virtually no energy, hence their use in 'low joule' products.

In Western countries, total carbohydrate intake amounts to about 200–280 g per day for the average man and woman, or about 45% of all the food energy eaten (protein contributes 15–20%, fat 35–40%). About half of our carbohydrate is in the form of starch (100–140 g per day), the other half representing a mixture of sugars, with sucrose predominating (Table 2). A decade ago, the only figures we had for consumption of refined sucrose were derived from apparent consumption statistics (production plus imports minus export, wastage and nonfood usage). These statistics suggested that the average intake was around 50 kg per head per year or 125 g per day for every man, woman and child, equivalent to 25% of total energy intake. Only recently have we been able to estimate accurately intake of refined or added sugars (most of which is refined sucrose but includes small amounts of honey, molasses, high-fructose corn syrup solids, etc). These more direct estimates show daily intakes of 40–50 g in women and 60–70 g in men in developed countries. Children ingest 40–50 g per day refined sugars. Thus apparent consumption or per capita calculations overestimated consumption by as much as three times. Refined sugars today contribute about 10% of total energy in industrialized nations in Europe, North America and Australasia. Japan is an exception with intakes of only 10–20 g per day. Intakes of refined sucrose in nonindustrialized countries are also small, averaging 1–20 g per day.

Some countries have made a distinction between the sugars that are consumed with intact cell wall structure (intrinsic sugars) and those which have been released from nature's original packaging (extrinsic sugars). In this classification, the sugars in an orange are intrinsic sugars while those in orange juice are extrinsic. The lactose in milk is also extrinsic because it is not inside a cell wall. The belief is that nonmilk extrinsic sugars are less desirable because they will be absorbed more quickly into the bloodstream and that the fibre and micronutrient content of the food or diet will be lower. However, recent research has shown that many of these assumptions are incorrect.

Functional roles of sucrose in foods

Refined sucrose is added to foods for more than just its sweetness. The difficulties inherent in producing low-joule products using intense sweeteners attest to this. For example, sucrose contributes to the bulk and texture of cakes and cookies and it provides viscosity and mouth feel in liquids such as soft drinks and fruit juices. Sucrose is also a powerful preservative and contributes the long storage life of jams and confectionery. In frozen products like ice cream, sucrose has multiple functions: it acts as an emulsifier, preventing the separation of the water and fat phases; it lowers the freezing point, thereby making the product more liquid and 'creamier' at the temperature eaten. The presence of sucrose retards the crystallization of the lactose in dairy foods and milk chocolate (tiny crystals of lactose feel like sand on the tongue). In canned fruit, sucrose syrups are used to prevent mushiness caused by the osmotic movement of sugar out of the fruit and into the surrounding fluid. Because sucrose masks unpleasant flavours, sugar syrups are used as carriers for drugs and medicines, especially for young children who cannot swallow tablet formulations. In products like yogurt and coffee it masks the acidity or bitterness and balances the sugar–acid ratio in fruit juices and cordials. Lastly, sucrose is a substrate for fermentation. It is added as food for the yeast in bread-making and beer-making. But it is converted to alcohol and other products in the process and therefore not consumed as sucrose. For all these reasons, when manufacturers design a low joule–low sugar product, they find that many substances need to be added to perform all the roles that sucrose did alone.

Patterns of Consumption

Honey versus sucrose

In preindustrial times, honey was the main source of concentrated sweetness in the diets of many peoples. There are no precise figures for historical consumption because honey was part of either a hunter-gatherer or subsistence economy. Until recently historians and food writers have proposed that it was a scarce commodity available only to a wealthy few. However, a reappraisal of the evidence in the Stone Age, Antiquity, the Middle Ages and early Modern times suggests that ordinary people ate much larger quantities of honey than has previously been acknowledged. The Ancient Egyptians, for example, made frequent use of honey in their spiced breads, cakes and pastries, and for priming beer and wine. In Roman times, half the recipes in a famous cookery book call for honey, and in Ancient Greece, those who died some distance from home were sometimes preserved in honey. These details give an impression of plenty. Even the poorest people could own a beehive because bees often made their homes in a hollow log or a broken pot. Wealthy landowners might own dozens of beautifully constructed beehives and employ a beekeeper. During medieval times we know that honey was sold in large volumes (gallons and even barrels), units unlikely to be used for a scarce commodity. It was present in sufficient abundance to make mead a common alcoholic drink made from honey.

It is therefore possible that intakes of honey at various times during history may well have rivalled our current consumption of refined sugar. There are implications therefore for the role of sugar in modern diets. Refined sugar may not have displaced more nutrient-rich items from our present-day diets but only the nutritionally comparable food, honey.

Changes in sucrose consumption

It is a much more straightforward business to enquire about sugar (refined sucrose) consumption than honey consumption in preindustrial times. All sugar supplies, in Europe, came from imports, so customs records constitute a readily accessible record of national consumption. In the 1520s, the Dissolution of the Monasteries reduced demand for beeswax for church candles and brought about a small decrease in the production of honey. Almost simultaneous with this came an increase in the supply of refined sucrose, imported from the new European colonies. Sugar was still considerably more expensive than honey, but this combination of events gained it a more complete following among the wealthy. Cookery books were used exclusively by the well-to-do at this time and clearly illustrate that, for this section of society, sugar had, by the 1550s, usurped honey's place in the diet.

It was not until the early 1700s, however, when the supply of sugar boomed, its price fell, and coffee, tea and chocolate entered the British diet, that ordinary people finally began to buy significant amounts, and the per capita consumption reached 1.8 kg per year. The changeover from honey to sugar occurred more gradually in rural areas than in the cities. From this point sugar consumption rose inexorably, while honey consumption declined. Beekeeping ceased to be the general custom that it had been in former years – there was no longer a hive in every garden. By the beginning of this century the availability of refined sugar reached about 50 kg per head per year in most industrialized nations. Surprisingly, it did not continue to increase but remained at approximately this level or declined throughout the next 100 years. The 'steady state' suggests that the market and the taste buds have reached saturation.

Added versus naturally occurring sugars

Recent studies also show that the intake of naturally occurring sugars from fruits and vegetables (including juices) is about 40–80 g per day, roughly equivalent to the intake of refined sugars. Thus all sugars contribute about 20–22% total energy intake in developed countries, or about half of all the carbohydrate eaten.

The sugar–fat seesaw

In industrialized nations the intake of sugar varies from person to person, but there is a consistent relationship between sugars and fat intake. As refined sugar intake rises, fat falls, and vice versa. As the total sugars intake rises, most of the increase is due to refined sugars (refined sucrose, corn syrup solids, etc). This relationship has important implications. The proportion of individuals achieving dietary guidelines for lower intakes of total and saturated fats is much higher among subgroups with higher intakes of total sugars and refined sucrose. In the past, we believed that sugar and fat went 'hand-in-hand' in foods and that a diet high in sugar was likely to be high in fat as well. But it turns out that the reverse is true: a high-sugar diet is more likely to be low in fat. It seems that very few people achieve a low-fat diet without also increasing sugars intake. Perhaps humans, consciously or not, strive to eat calories in their most concentrated energy-dense form.

One of the most important implications of these findings is that recommendations to reduce *both* sugar and fat may be counterproductive. A reduction in fat intake is certainly more likely to result in desirable changes in body weight, blood lipids, insulin sensitivity and cardiovascular risk factors. Trying to reduce sugar intake as well may not only compromise the effort to reduce fat, but reduce the palatability of the diet and hence long-term compliance with a low-fat diet.

Effect on micronutrient intake

Refined sucrose and other added sugars are regarded by many people as undesirable because they are 'empty calories' (energy without micronutrients). It was reasoned that sucrose would 'dilute' the micronutrient (vitamin, mineral) content of the diet and that high sugar intake would increase the likelihood of micronutrient deficiencies. When these assumptions were tested, diets containing moderate amounts of added sugars were found to be *no less* nutritious than diets low in sugar. This has been shown to be the case in both adults and children. Very high consumption of refined sugars is associated with low micronutrient intake, but so too is very low intake of sugars. Moderate consumption of sugars is associated with the highest intake of micronutrients.

One of the reasons for this unexpected result is the sugar–fat seesaw, i.e. low-sugar diets are higher in fat, which is essentially a poor source of micronutrients too. Another reason is that sweetened breakfast cereals and dairy products such as flavoured milk, yogurts and ice cream are a good source of micronutrients. Fruit juice drinks are a source of vitamin C as well as sugars. Thus refined sucrose aids the consumption of some nutritious but fairly unpalatable or bland foods.

Digestion and Absorption of Sucrose

Digestion

In the mouth, food is mixed with saliva and masticated. The physical matrix that encases the sucrose, e.g. the plant cell wall, is partially disrupted in the process. Mixing occurs very effectively in the stomach and sucrose is dispersed throughout the gastric contents. Peristaltic movements drive the semifluid material, called chyme, through the pyloric sphincter into the duodenum. The rate of stomach emptying varies as a function of the volume and acidity of the stomach contents as well as the osmolality of the chyme in the small intestine. Solutions that are acidic and hyperosmotic are emptied more slowly. Thus an acidic, high-sucrose food such as sweetened yogurt will be emptied relatively slowly.

Once in the small intestine, sucrose is too large to cross the epithelial cell membrane and must therefore be hydrolysed for absorption to take place. The enzyme responsible for sucrose digestion is an α-glucosidase called sucrase, located in the microvillous brush border lining the small intestine (**Fig. 2**). It digests some of the breakdown products of starch digestion as well as sucrose. Sucrose in foods is also easily hydrolysed under weakly acidic conditions at room temperature such that considerable hydrolysis occurs even before ingestion, e.g. in soft drinks. Hydrolysis is accelerated by heating so that much of the sucrose used in food is actually swallowed as an equimolar mixture of glucose and fructose. Conditions in the stomach are also likely to hydrolyse sucrose, further increasing the monosaccharide concentration in the chyme.

Hydrolysis within the brush border is extremely rapid and the rate-limiting step is not digestion, but the transport of monosaccharides across the enterocyte. Sucrase, however, is located physically close to the monosaccharide cotransporter systems in the microvillus membrane.

Absorption of glucose and fructose

The glucose product of sucrose digestion is transported across the epithelial cell membrane more rapidly than is free glucose, a phenomenon that may be related to specific glucose transporters that are not dependent on sodium. The fructose released by sucrose digestion is absorbed more slowly across the brush border membrane by a process called facilitated diffusion (carrier-mediated). Fructose appears to be absorbed better when ingested with glucose (separately or combined in sucrose) than it is by itself. This explains why 100 g fructose gives rise to osmotic diarrhoea whereas 250 g sucrose does not. The absorption of free fructose is incomplete when intakes exceed about 35 g per day.

Once inside the epithelial cell, glucose and fructose are presumed to traverse the enterocyte by diffusion. The basal-lateral membrane acts as a barrier preventing the free movement of monosaccharides into and out of the enterocyte. Movement across the

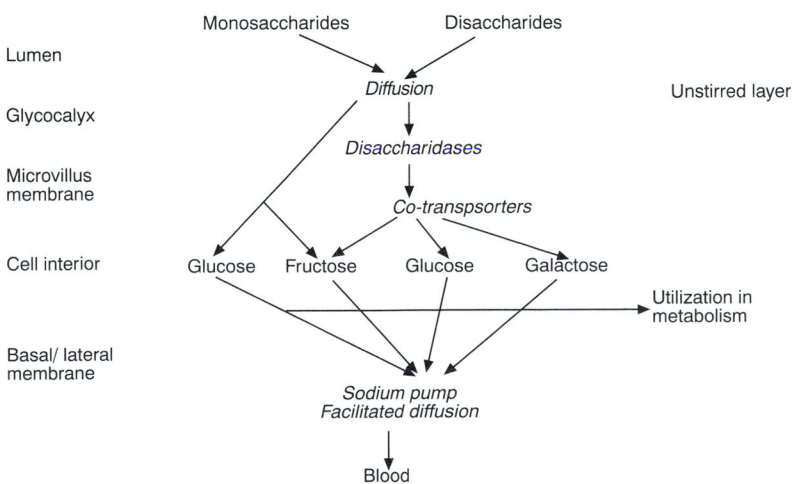

Figure 2 Disaccharidases such as sucrase are located on the luminal side of the brush border membrane of the small intestine. From Southgate (1995; p 207).

membrane appears to be energy-dependent but sodium-independent.

Metabolism of glucose

From the epithelial cell, the monosaccharides pass into the portal circulation and to the liver where some of the glucose and virtually all the fructose is removed. The remainder of the glucose passes into the systemic circulation, entering the peripheral tissues by mass action and/or under the influence of the hormone insulin.

Metabolism of fructose

When fructose reaches the liver, most is removed from the bloodstream and converted to glucose, lipid or lactate. Some fructose is converted in the liver to fructose-1-phosphate, which is spilt into two C_3 products, glyceraldehyde and dihydroxacetone phosphate. The latter is an intermediate for both the glycolytic and gluconeogenic pathways. The glyceraldehyde is phosphorylated and recombines with dihydroxyacetone phosphate to produce fructose-diphosphate and ultimately glycogen. The major metabolic effect of fructose is to increase the production of pyruvate and lactate. This has the effect of depressing fatty acid oxidation and increasing the esterification and the synthesis of very low-density lipoprotein (VLDL). There is only a small rise in plasma glucose (and insulin) levels because gluconeogenesis is strongly inhibited. A rise in plasma lactate is seen after fructose consumption.

Metabolic Sequelae

Consumption of sucrose (and other carbohydrates such as starch) produces a range of metabolic and hormonal responses, all of which serve to limit the rise in plasma glucose levels to within acceptable levels. Blood glucose levels above 10 mM will result in glycosuria (glucose in the urine), a waste of valuable energy, and levels below 3–4 mM will impair brain function. Insulin plays an important role in bringing blood glucose levels back to normal after a meal. It does that by promoting glucose uptake in the liver and muscle cells and inhibiting gluconeogenesis in the liver. Dietary carbohydrate, including sucrose has four main metabolic fates: (1) oxidation in tissues, mainly as glucose molecules; (2) storage as glycogen in liver and muscle cells; (3) storage as triacylglycerol (TAG), mainly in the liver; and (4) conversion of glucose into C_3 storage as precursors in the liver where they are used as substrates for gluconeogenesis. The latter is a futile cycle, but it seems that large amounts of glucose undergo this transformation.

During the 4 h after a typical meal, the amount of ingested carbohydrate far exceeds the amount of glucose that can be oxidized in the cells. As a result, most of the dietary glucose is stored as glycogen in liver and skeletal muscles and is subsequently released and oxidized within the next 12 h.

Insulin stimulates glucose oxidation by enhancing glucose transport into insulin-sensitive cells. Inside the mitochondria, insulin stimulates glycolysis at several steps and activates pyruvate dehydogenase complex, the port of entry of glucose-derived acetyl-CoA into the tricarboxylic acid (TCA) cycle (**Fig. 3**). Insulin also inhibits lipolysis in adipose tissue, thereby lowering plasma free fatty acid levels (FFA) and reducing lipid oxidation in the muscle cells. The inhibition of fat oxidation is directly related to reduced plasma FFA and mirrors the stimulation of glucose oxidation.

The body's glycogen reserves are small (250–500 g in a 50–70 kg adult human), although the capacity to store more can be developed by exercise, training and diet. A normal diet provides about 200–280 g carbohydrate a day. Thus within any 24 h period, there is total oxidation of absorbed dietary carbohydrate, including sucrose. Other metabolic pathways for disposal of dietary carbohydrate, such as conversion into TAG or nonessential amino acids, are not quantitatively important.

Plasma glucose and insulin responses

After a meal containing sucrose, the plasma glucose rises reaching a peak within 15–30 min and returns to baseline within 2 h. The classification of carbohydrates as sugars or starches does not predict the magnitude of this response. In the past it was assumed that refined sucrose caused a more rapid rise in blood glucose levels than starchy foods or naturally occurring sources of sugars like fruit. This view has been shown to be incorrect. Most starchy foods, including potatoes, bread and many packaged breakfast cereals, are digested and absorbed rapidly and the blood glucose response is almost as high as that seen with an equivalent load of pure glucose. Foods containing refined sucrose, such as soft drinks and ice cream, have been shown to give moderate rises in blood glucose. Furthermore, the glycaemic response to foods containing refined sugars is similar to that of foods containing naturally occurring sugars.

The 'glycaemic index' approach has been used to classify foods according to their ability to raise the level of glucose in the blood. Foods are tested in equivalent carbohydrate portions according to standardized methodology. On a scale where glucose = 100, the glycaemic index of refined sucrose (= 65) is

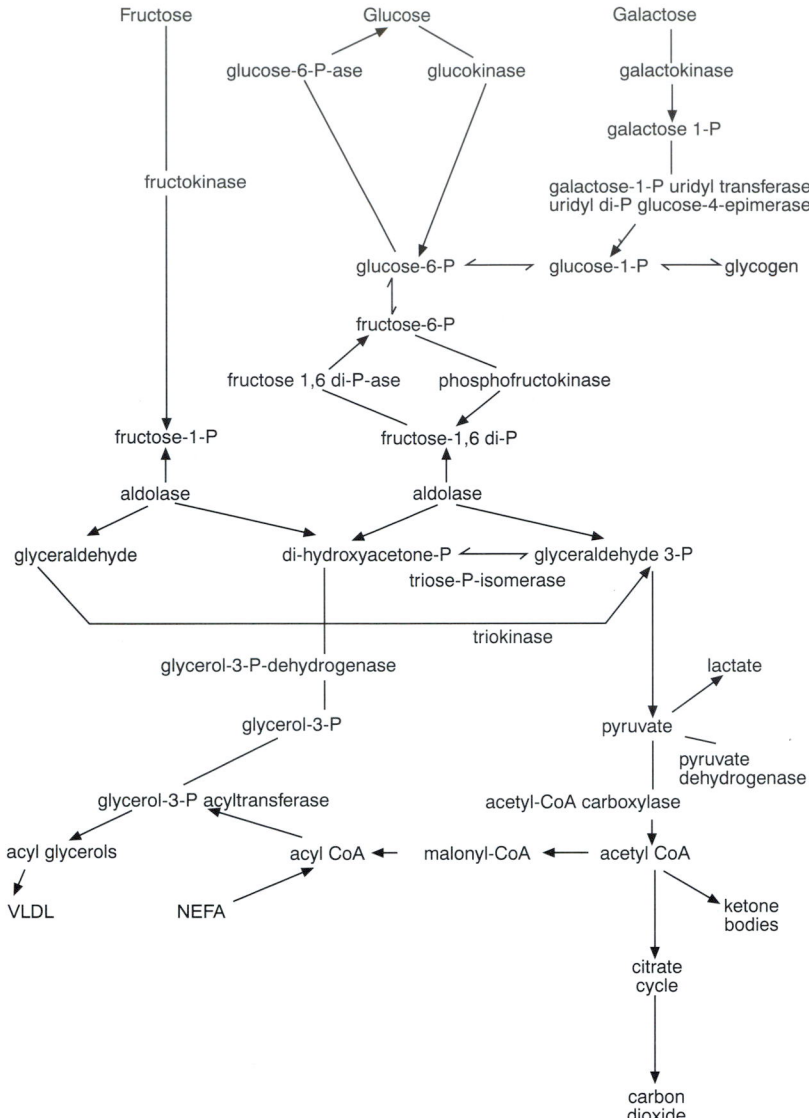

Figure 3 The monosaccharide products of sucrose digestion are metabolized to carbon dioxide and water via the tricarboxylic acid (TCA) cycle. From Southgate (1995).

similar to that of white bread (= 70). **Table 3** shows the glycaemic index of a range of common foods. Refined sucrose elicits an insulin response commensurate with its glycaemic response, i.e. it does not stimulate inappropriately high insulin secretion.

See also: **Carbohydrates**: Chemistry and Classification (Including Dietary Fibre); Regulation of Carbohydrate Metabolism; Requirements and Dietary Importance. **Dental Disease**: Aetiology and Epidemiology. **Diabetes Mellitus**: Classification and Chemical Pathology; Dietary Management. **Fructose**: Absorption and Metabolism. **Glucose**: Chemistry, Dietary Sources and Glycaemic Index; Metabolism and Maintenance of Blood Glucose Level.

Further Reading

Allsop K and Brand Miller JC (1996) Honey revisited: a reappraisal of honey in pre-industrial diets. *British Journal of Nutrition* 75:513–520.

Baghurst KI, Baghurst PA and Record SJ (1992) Demographic and nutritional profiles of people consuming varying levels of added sugars. *Nutrition Research* 12:1455–1465.

Bolton-Smith C and Woodward M (1994) Dietary composition and fat to sugar ratios in relation to obesity. *International Journal of Obesity* 18:820–828.

Brand Miller J, Pang E and Broomhead L (1995) The glycemic index of foods containing sugars: comparison of foods with naturally occurring versus added sugars. *British Journal of Nutrition* 73:613–623.

Table 3 Glycaemic index of foods (glucose = 100)

Food	Index	Food	Index	Food	Index
Breakfast cereals		Sao	70	Peach	
Kellogg's AllBran™	30	Watercracker	78	canned in juice	30
Kellogg's Cocopops™	77			fresh	28
Kellogg's Cornflakes	77	**Sweet biscuits**		Pear (av)	36
Kellogg's Mini Wheats™	58	Arrowroot	69	Pineapple	66
Museli		Morning coffee	79	Plum	24
toasted*	43	Oatmeal	55	Raisins	64
untoasted	56	Shredded wheatmeal	62	Rockmelon	65
Kellogg's Nutrigrain™	66	Shortbread (commercial)	64	Sultanas	56
Porridge (av)	50			Watermelon	72
Puffed Wheat	80	**Cakes**			
Rice bran	19	Apple muffin	44	**Dairy foods**	
Kellogg's Rice Bubbles™	89	Banana cake	47	Milk	
Kellogg's Special K™	54	Sponge cake	46	whole (av)	27
Kellogg's Sultana Bran™	54	Waffles	76	skim	32
Kellogg's Sustain™	68			chocolate flavour	34
Uncle Toby's Vita Brits™	61	**Vegetables**		custard (made with	43
Sanitarium Weetbix™	69	Beetroot	64	powder)	
		Carrots	49	Ice cream (av)	61
Grains/Paste		Parsnip	97	low-fat	50
Buckwheat	54	Peas (green)	48	Yoghurt (flavoured, low-fat)	33
Bulgur wheat	48	Potato			
Rice		baked (av)	85	**Beverages**	
Calrose (white)	83	new (av)	62	Apple juice	41
Doongara/basmati	59	pontiac	56	Cordial (diluted)	66
Calrose (brown)	76	French fries	75	Fanta™	68
		Pumpkin	75	Lucozade™	95
Noodles (instant)	47	Sweet corn	48	Orange juice	53
Pasta		Sweet potato	48		
egg fettucine	32	Swede	72	**Snack and convenience**	
ravioli (meat)	39	Yam	51	**foods**	
spaghetti (av)	41			Corn chips	72
vermicelli	35	**Legumes**		Fish fingers	38
Taco shells	68	Baked beans (av)	48	Peanuts	14
		Broad beans (av)	79	Popcorn	55
Bread		Butter beans (av)	31	Potato crisps	57
Bagel	72	Chickpeas (av)	33	Sausages	28
Croissant*	67	Haricot beans (av)	38	Soup	
Crumpet	69	Kidney beans (av)	27	lentil	44
Fruit loaf (white)	47	Lentils (av)	28	pea	66
Kibbled barley bread (av)	45	Soya beans (av)	18	tomato	38
Mixed grain bread (av)	45				
Oat bran bread (av)	44	**Fruit**		**Confectionery**	
Pita bread	57	Apple (av)	36	Chocolate	49
Rye bread		Apricot (dried)	31	Jelly beans	80
kernel, e.g. pumpernickel	50	Banana (av)	53	Life Savers™	70
flour, e.g. blackbread	76	Cherries	23	Mars™ bars	68
White bread (av)	70	Grapefruit	25	Muesli bars	61
Wholemeal bread (av)	77	Grapes	43		
		Kiwifruit	58	**Sugars**	
Crackers/crispbread		Mango	51	Honey	58
Jatz	55	Orange (av)	43	Fructose	20
Kavli	71	Papaya (paw paw)	56	Glucose	100
Puffed crispbread	81			Lactose	57
Ryvita	69			Maltose	105
				Sucrose	65

COMA (1989) *Dietary sugars and human disease*. Report of the Panel on Dietary Sugars, Report on Health and Social Subjects no. 37. London: HMSO.

Davis EA (1995) Functionality of sugars: physicochemical interactions in foods. *American Journal of Clinical Nutrition* 62:170S–177S.

Gibney M, Sigman-Grant M, Stanton JL and Keast DR (1995) Consumption of sugars. *American Journal of Clinical Nutrition* 62(supplement):178S–194S.

Gibson SA (1993) Consumption and sources of sugars in the diets of British schoolchildren: are high-sugar diets nutritionally inferior? 6:355–371.

Glinnsmann WH, Irausquin H and Park Y (1986) *Evaluation of health aspects of sugars contained in carbohydrate sweeteners*. Report of the Sugars Task Force 1986. Washington: US Food and Drug Administration.

Jenkins DJA, Wolever TMS, Taylor RH, Barker H, Fielden H, Baldwin J, Bowling AC, Newman HC, Jenkins AL and Goff DV (1981) Glycemic index of foods: a physiological basis for carbohydrate exchange. *American Journal of Clinical Nutrition* 34:362–366.

Southgate D (1995) Digestion and metabolism of sugars. *American Journal of Clinical Nutrition* 62:203S–211S.

Truswell AS (1994) Food carbohydrates and plasma lipids – an update. *American Journal of Clinical Nutrition* 59:710S–718S.

Wolever TMS and Brand Miller JC (1995). Sugars and blood glucose control. *American Journal of Clinical Nutrition* 62:212S–227S.

Dietary Sucrose and Disease

I Macdonald, University of London, UK

The disaccharide sucrose, consisting of a molecule of glucose and one of fructose, was first seriously considered to be a factor in the causation of disease in the early 1970s, when it was linked with diseases whose incidence and consequent mortality suddenly increased at that time, such as obesity, cardiovascular disease, diabetes and dental caries. The link was based almost entirely on association, with little support from experimental evidence. In the intervening years scientific evidence has accumulated to test whether the association is a cause and effect relationship. The overall evidence for the role of sucrose in the aetiology of these noncommunicable diseases is considered below.

Body Weight

The capacity of the body to store carbohydrate is, unlike fat, very limited and little of the carbohydrate in the diet is converted to body fat. As the carbohydrate stores of the body are limited and only capable of covering oxidation for a few days at most, there must be a tight metabolic control of carbohydrate balance (*See:* **Carbohydrates:** Regulation of Carbohydrate Metabolism). This efficiency of maintaining carbohydrate balance despite large changes in carbohydrate intake suggests that there is some kind of carbohydrate autoregulation in that, to an extent, carbohydrate controls its own oxidation. On the other hand, as any excess of dietary carbohydrate is oxidized, this will lead to fat accumulation, because of the reduction in fat oxidation for energy.

It has also been postulated that carbohydrates inhibit food intake, perhaps by mechanisms that are responsible for maintaining stable glycogen levels, and that changes in these glycogen stores provide the primary feedback to regulate appetite, although this is by no means proved. It is known that in the hierarchy of suppressing energy intake proteins are the most effective, followed by carbohydrate, with fat having a low satiating effect.

Another factor that militates against dietary carbohydrate being a major source of depot fat is postprandial thermogenesis. Fat causes the least diet-induced thermogenesis compared with the other macronutrients, with protein having the most and carbohydrate in between. Short-term studies have shown that different carbohydrates have different thermogenic effects: sucrose and fructose are more thermogenic than glucose. There seems to be no difference in the degree of thermogenesis of polysaccharides of varying chain length.

Satiety has a taste and olfaction component, and it has been suggested that sugar is unique in its effects on appetite because of its desirable taste, and that this may overrule other satiety mechanisms that regulate the control that normally follows the ingestion of other carbohydrates. It is postulated that this pleasant taste will lead to an increase in food intake. There is no evidence that sweetness alone, either in beverages or food, stimulates increased food intake. The sensation of sweetness, as such, does not seem to result in an increase in the amount of food eaten.

Many studies have shown that in an *ad libitum* diet, a high sucrose intake is accompanied by a low fat intake and vice versa.

There is considerable evidence that, at least in short-term studies, human subjects consume more energy and gain more body weight when they have access to a high-fat diet compared with one low in fat and high in carbohydrate. A joint report by the Food and Agriculture Organization (FAO) and the World Health Organization (WHO) stated that a diet providing at least 55% of energy from a variety of carbohydrate sources, as compared with a high-fat diet, reduces the likelihood that body fat accumulation will occur, and that this effect may, in part, be due to the low energy density of foods high in complex carbohydrates. It also stated that there are no data to suggest that different types of carbohydrates differentially affect total energy intake.

Turning to the therapeutic aspects of carbohydrates, especially sucrose, in the treatment of overweight and obesity, it has been reported that an *ad libitum* diet low in fat and high in carbohydrate, containing sucrose, is superior to a fixed-energy mixed diet for maintaining weight after a major weight loss. It has also been reported that a high sucrose content in a hypoenergetic, low-fat diet did not adversely affect weight loss, metabolism, plasma lipids or emotion.

Cardiovascular Disease

The original concept that sucrose was a factor in the aetiology of cardiovascular disease, in particular coronary heart disease, was primarily based on the positive association of the sucrose consumption of a country and its incidence of coronary heart disease (CHD). However, countries such as Cuba, Venezuela, Colombia, Costa Rica and Honduras have a very high consumption of sucrose and low rates of CHD. Furthermore, in the USA between the 1920s and the 1960s the per capita consumption of sucrose remained constant, a period during which there was a marked rise in mortality from CHD.

Turning to studies of individuals, the elevation of plasma triacylglycerol concentrations in response to the ingestion of large amounts of sucrose and fructose has been recognized for some time. This response is probably due to the fructose moiety of sucrose which, when consumed in large quantities, leads to increased levels of very low-density lipoprotein (VLDL) in the plasma. This increase in VLDL is considered to be transient.

The current dietary advice worldwide is to reduce fat intake and replace it with up to 55% of food energy from carbohydrate. The plasma concentration of high-density lipoprotein (HDL) cholesterol, the apparently protective lipoprotein, is inversely related to the plasma triacylglycerol level, so if this response to dietary carbohydrate – especially sucrose – is marked, then increasing the carbohydrate intake would not be good advice.

Some people, especially those with central obesity, hypertriacylglycerolaemia, hyperinsulinaemia and hypertension ('syndrome X'), have a marked increase in plasma lipid levels in response to sucrose ingestion, and it would be prudent for them to reduce their intake of carbohydrate, especially sucrose.

The FAO/WHO report on carbohydrates stated that there is no evidence of a causal role of sucrose in the aetiology of CHD, supporting the conclusion of the UK Committee on Medical Aspects of Food Policy (COMA) which stated that the present evidence does not support any direct link between sugar consumption and the risk of CHD.

Little is known of the role of carbohydrates, including sucrose, in other cardiovascular diseases such as stroke, hypertension and peripheral vascular disease. Some studies, mainly in animals, have shown that very high levels of sucrose in the diet can cause a slight rise in systolic blood pressure. This could be due to the reduction in urinary sodium excretion or to an increase in sympathetic nervous activity, both of which occur after the ingestion of sucrose. However, there is no evidence as yet that the current consumption of sucrose in humans has any adverse effect on blood pressure.

Diabetes Mellitus

Since the main feature of diabetes mellitus is a raised level of glucose in the blood, it seemed logical to consider dietary sugar as likely cause, especially in non-insulin-dependent diabetes mellitus (NIDDM). Numerous epidemiological and experimental studies have considered this relationship, and the evidence from both these approaches appears to exclude sugar consumption *per se* as a factor in the development of NIDDM.

High-carbohydrate, low-fat diets as currently recommended do, in the short term, raise plasma insulin concentrations – as well as plasma triacylglycerol levels – and this has been interpreted as indicating an increase in insulin resistance, as is found in NIDDM. However, it is probable that the beneficial effect of a high-carbohydrate diet on body weight, etc., outweighs any possible consequence of an increase in insulin resistance.

Therapy

Recommendations for an increase in carbohydrate and a reduction in fat in the diet have also been applied to those with diabetes. The belief that meals containing sugars result in higher blood levels of glucose than do meals containing equivalent amounts of starch still persists, even though it has been shown that cooked starches, such as bread, rice and potato, result in blood glucose levels similar to the response of an equivalent intake of glucose, and frequently elicit a response greater than that observed with an equivalent intake of sucrose. There are also indications that an increase in carbohydrate-rich foodstuffs can contribute to an improved metabolic profile in diabetes.

Despite this, the long-standing restriction on sucrose in the diet of diabetic patients remained unchanged until the rationale behind this ban was questioned, and it is now considered that the harmful effects of sucrose have been probably been exaggerated. Though sucrose is now permitted in the diet of diabetic patients, these individuals are still advised to limit their sugar intake to amounts lower than those consumed by the rest of the population.

Sucrose ingestion does, however, produce a greater blood glucose response than do some starchy foods such as beans, which produce a low blood glucose profile. Adding 30–50 g of sucrose per day to the diet of a person with insulin-dependent diabetes mellitus or NIDDM does not seem to have an effect on blood glucose or insulin, provided that the replacement is isoenergetic with starch. Because consuming a high-carbohydrate, low-fat diet can be difficult, the addition of sucrose may have psychological consequences that can make it easier to follow correct dietary advice.

Reactive hypoglycaemia

Reactive hypoglycaemia is a rare syndrome in which the blood glucose level falls below the fasting level and is accompanied by symptoms such as tremor and lightheadedness. There is no evidence that sucrose ingestion is more likely to result in hypoglycaemia than is glucose ingestion. In fact, in one study of subjects with reactive hypoglycaemia, sucrose elicited a flatter glucose response and produced symptoms in 30% of subjects, whereas with glucose 100% of subjects had symptoms.

Dental Caries

Dental caries is a disease characterized by progressive demineralization of the enamel and dentine of the teeth, with a characteristic pattern of decay which may lead to the loss of part of the tooth. Carbohydrates (including starches) and sucrose in particular are important caries-promoting components of food, and many studies have confirmed that sucrose is a risk factor for caries. Attempts to study the relationship between sucrose consumption and caries are complicated because:

1. Sucrose is consumed in different physical forms and with different dietary patterns.
2. Estimates of the amount of sucrose consumed tend to be unreliable.
3. Caries takes several years to develop, and consumption patterns may change.

4. Caries is influenced by many other factors such as oral hygiene, fluoride use, education, etc.

Sucrose is not the sole factor in the causation of caries. Oral bacteria, such as *Streptococcus mutans*, are essential. They congregate in large masses, known as dental plaque, where they hydrolyse the starches and metabolize the sugars to form mainly acid, which demineralizes the hard tissue underneath. The presence of food residues in the mouth after the food or drink has been swallowed provides the plaque bacteria with soluble, nutritious substances to enhance their activities. It is worth noting that sugars do not give rise to dangerous levels of acid in the mouth when plaque is absent or is present in only thin amounts.

Saliva has an important role in the development of caries, as a protective fluid. Saliva dilutes the substrate needed by the bacteria and neutralizes the acid end product of bacterial fermentation. It is also involved in the remineralization process, and it is possible that the presence of calcium and phosphate in saliva may inhibit demineralization.

Other factors affecting cariogenesis include minerals and trace elements in the mouth, in particular fluoride. The presence of fluoride in the saliva, plaque or dental enamel helps to remineralize the tooth after each demineralizing attack.

Turning to the pattern of consumption of sucrose or sucrose-containing foods, it seems that the more often foods and drinks containing sucrose are consumed, the greater the potential risk to teeth. Not only is there an increase in acidity at each exposure, but a short interval between fermentable carbohydrate ingestion does not allow the remineralization process to take place. Constant nibbling or sipping sugared drinks throughout the day is considered harmful to the teeth.

There seems to be a loose correlation between the amount of sugar consumed and the extent of caries. This is probably due to the many variables other than sucrose in the aetiology of caries. In the USA and in most industrialized European countries there has been a marked decline in the incidence of caries, despite little change in sugar consumption over the same period. However, in developing countries the prevalence of caries is still related to the increasing consumption of fermentable carbohydrates.

Though sugar is unquestionably a risk factor for caries, it seems that a successful way to reduce the incidence of caries lies not in persuading the population or individual to reduce sugar intake, which may fall on deaf ears, but in tackling another factor in the complicated background in the aetiology of caries. A highly successful approach has been to increase the fluoride exposure of the teeth, either through the water supply or toothpaste, and this appears to have been responsible, at least in part, for the fall in incidence of caries seen in many countries, despite little or no fall in sucrose consumption.

The FAO/WHO report on food-based dietary guidelines accepted that the frequent consumption of sugar and other fermentable carbohydrates throughout the day increases the cariogenic risk potential of the diet, especially in the absence of oral hygienic practices. It stated that sugar intake plays a minor role in caries prevention where fluoridation and hygienic measures have been taken.

Many fruits not only provide sucrose, but are also acidic; although 'an apple a day' may 'keep the doctor away', it will not keep the dentist away!

Influence on Behaviour

Many functional disorders such as childhood overactivity, juvenile delinquency and violent behaviour have been laid at the door of reactive hypoglycaemia, and this in turn was felt to occur more often after the ingestion of sucrose than after other carbohydrates. The assumption was that simple carbohydrates are more quickly digested and absorbed than complex carbohydrates, leading to a greater increase in blood glucose concentration and consequently a greater output of insulin, with the result that the blood glucose concentration then falls to very low levels. However, the blood glucose response after ingestion is now known to be no less (and indeed may be greater) for many food carbohydrates compared with sucrose, owing to the fructose moiety in sucrose which does not *per se* stimulate insulin release. Clinical reactive hypoglycaemia is an uncommon condition.

More than 13 reputable studies, representing over 400 subjects, have looked into the effects of sugar on undesirable behaviour, notably in children. The results do not support the view that refined sucrose affects hyperactivity, the attention span or cognitive performance in children. On the contrary, there are studies that suggest that sucrose might have a sedative effect. For example, babies given a sucrose solution prior to heel prick to obtain blood cried only half as much as those given water only. In another study on infants undergoing circumcision, those given a pacifier moistened with sucrose cried less than those not given sucrose. More recently a study has been reported showing that sucrose has an analgesic effect in infants with intestinal colic. Whether these calming effects of sucrose are present in older children and adults is not known. These effects may be explained by the observation that sugars,

especially glucose, can affect the levels in the brain of the neurotransmitter serotonin, an effect not seen if protein is consumed with the carbohydrate.

There is evidence that glucose is involved in memory storage in both experimental animals and humans, an effect best demonstrated in elderly subjects. Whether sucrose has any such effect is unknown, although fructose at high doses has been shown to improve memory.

Other Disorders

Kidney stones

After the ingestion of sugars and amino acids there is increased excretion of calcium and magnesium in the urine, an effect not unique to any specific sugar, and there is some epidemiological and experimental evidence linking kidney stones with nutritional factors, including sugars. Though most persons would not be affected, the consumption of high levels of sugars in individuals susceptible to renal stones would be inadvisable.

Nutrient deficiencies

It is obvious that sucrose, as a highly refined carbohydrate, can be used with other purified macronutrients to manufacture foods that are low in essential nutrients, and that excessive consumption of such 'empty calorie' foods may give rise to nutrient deficiencies. A report from the USA by the Food and Drug Administration found no persuasive evidence that sugars, as they are commonly used and consumed: (1) have unique properties or uses relative to the production of 'empty calorie' diets; (2) are identified as a significant cause of nutrient deficiencies in the USA; or (3) have compromised the food supply so that foods for nutritionally well-balanced meals are no longer freely available in the marketplace. It is perhaps worth noting that there is no evidence that sucrose interferes with the bioavailability of vitamins, minerals or trace nutrients.

Cancer

Nutritional factors, especially obesity, are recognized as contributing to cancer risk. In 1989 a UK government report stated that there was no evidence for a specific role for sugars in the development of breast cancer and little evidence of a direct contribution of dietary sugars to overall cancer risk. More recently, an FAO/WHO Expert Consultation Report stated that dietary carbohydrates do not have a known role in the aetiology of lung, breast, stomach, prostate, pancreas, oesophagus, liver or cervical cancers. Colorectal cancers are not in that list, possibly because there is some debate on whether epidemiological associations between sucrose and colorectal cancer are in fact cause and effect.

Dietary Goals and Guidelines

There have been several official publications and reports on dietary goals and recommendations for sucrose. At the international level the FAO/WHO report on food-based dietary guidelines did not propose any specific limit for sugar consumption since the putative relationship of sugar consumption to obesity is offset by the inverse relationship seen between sugar and fat intake. The interim FAO/WHO report on carbohydrates in human nutrition recommended that excessive intakes of sugars which compromise micronutrient density should be avoided. It also stated that there was no involvement of sucrose, other sugars and starch in the aetiology of diseases related to life style.

In the UK, the COMA report on dietary sugars and human disease made no recommendation on levels of consumption, whereas the COMA report on dietary reference values advised that the population's average daily intake of 'nonmilk extrinsic sugars' should not exceed 60 g or 10% of total dietary energy.

The most recent dietary guidelines published by the US Department of Agriculture clarified the distinction between complex carbohydrates and sugars, and while stating that diets high in sugar do not cause hyperactivity or diabetes, recommended a diet moderate in sugars.

See also: **Adipose Tissue**: Structure, Function and Metabolism of Adipose Tissue. **Behaviour**: Dietary Effects on Mood and Behaviour. **Cancer**: Epidemiology and Associations Between Diet and Cancer. **Carbohydrates**: Regulation of Carbohydrate Metabolism. **Coronary Heart Disease**: Aetiology; Prevention. **Dental Disease**: Aetiology and Epidemiology. **Diabetes Mellitus**: Aetiology and Epidemiology; Dietary Management. **Fructose**: Absorption and Metabolism. **Hyperactivity**: Dietary Issues. **Obesity**: Definition, Aetiology and Assessment; Early Obesity and Prognosis. **Sucrose**: Nutritional Role, Absorption and Metabolism.

Further Reading

Blaak EE and Saris WHM (1995) Health aspects of various digestible carbohydrates. *Nutrition Research* 15:1547–1573.

FAO/WHO (1996) *Preparation and Use of Food-based Dietary Guidelines*. FAO/WHO Consultation WHO/NUT/96.6. Geneva: WHO.

FAO/WHO (1997) *Carbohydrates in Human Nutrition*. Interim report of a joint FAO/WHO Expert Consultation. Geneva: WHO.

Frayn KN and Kingman SM (1995) Dietary sugars and lipid metabolism in humans. *American Journal of Clinical Nutrition* 62:250S–263S.

Glinsmann WH, Irausquin H and Park YK (1986) Evaluation of health aspects of sugars contained in carbohydrate sweeteners. *Journal of Nutrition* 116(11S):S1–S216.

Kandelman D (1997) Sugar, alternative sweeteners and meal frequency in relation to caries prevention: new perspectives. *British Journal of Nutrition* 77:S121–S128.

Konig KG and Navia JM (1995) Nutritional role of sugars in oral health. *American Journal of Clinical Nutrition* 62:275S–283S.

Navia JM (1994) Carbohydrates and dental health. *American Journal of Clinical Nutrition* 59:719S–727S.

UK Department of Health (1989) *Dietary Sugars and Human Disease*. Report 37. London: HMSO.

US Department of Agriculture (1996) *Dietary Guidelines for Americans*. Washington: USDA.

Vessby B (1994) Dietary carbohydrates in diabetes. *American Journal of Clinical Nutrition* 59:742S–746S.

Wolever TMS and Miller JB (1995) Sugars and blood glucose control. *American Journal of Clinical Nutrition* 62:212S–227S.

Sugar *see* **Carbohydrates**: Chemistry and Classification (Including Dietary Fibre); Regulation of Carbohydrate Metabolism; Requirements and Dietary Importance. **Galactose**: Absorption and Metabolism. **Glucose**: Chemistry, Dietary Sources and Glycaemic Index; Metabolism and Maintenance of Blood Glucose Level; Glucose Tolerance. **Sucrose**: Nutritional Role, Absorption and Metabolism; Dietary Sucrose and Disease.

SURGERY

Contents
Perioperative Feeding
Long-term Nutritional Management of Patients

Perioperative Feeding

S A Hill, Southampton General Hospital,
Southampton, UK

A surgical procedure constitutes a physical insult to the patient and induces stress. As a result, hormonal changes induce a catabolic state which is designed to maintain adequate delivery of nutrients to essential organs and tissue in need of repair. Protein breakdown and a negative nitrogen balance prevail unless adequate energy and protein are provided exogenously. The nutritional status of the surgical patient and its role in determining outcome have been of interest since 1936 when Studley showed that patients with a preoperative weight loss of greater than 20% had an 8-fold increase in mortality following emergency surgery compared with their better-nourished counterparts. More recently, interest in the hypercatabolic state in critically ill surgical patients has led to important discoveries concerning gut function and its relationship to nutrient provision, and recent work has focused on the role of enteral, rather than parenteral, nutrition in perioperative nutritional support. Despite a clear association between malnutrition and a high risk of surgical morbidity and mortality, there is still controversy over the benefits of perioperative feeding.

Preoperative Assessment

Patients most likely to benefit from perioperative nutritional support are those who are malnourished at presentation for major surgery. The definition of malnourishment is central to the discussion of who requires perioperative feeding. Despite many suggested clinical indices of nutritional status, no single measure selectively and specifically identifies all malnourished patients.

Clinical assessment

A full clinical history and examination plus a diet history must be taken. It has been suggested that clinical assessment is better than any single index of nutritional status, correctly identifying 75% of malnourished patients. Other studies refute this, showing that clinical judgment alone will correctly identify 80% of well-nourished individuals but only 40% of those nutritionally depleted.

Age

Extremes of age present different nutritional problems. Children have differing nutritional requirements, especially during growth spurts. The elderly, with coexisting disease, late presentation and inadequate, unbalanced oral intake, should all be suspected of malnutrition.

Weight

The present and the usual weights of the patient should be recorded. Unfortunately, few patients can give an accurate premorbid weight, which makes estimate of relative weight loss inaccurate. Current obesity, the presence of ascites or dehydration may also mislead. The time over which weight loss occurred is important. A recent weight loss exceeding 4.5% over 1 month is predictive of a high rate of surgical mortality. Despite its shortcomings, weight loss is predictive of postoperative surgical complications

Anthropometric assessment

Measurements are taken from the nondominant upper arm: triceps skinfold thickness (TST) and mid-arm circumference (MAC). From these two measures, mid-arm muscle circumference (MAMC) can be calculated. The TST provides an accurate estimation of total body fat and MAMC reflects total body protein. Anthropometric measures are useful for baseline and long-term assessment of nutritional status, but are relatively insensitive to short-term changes such as those following surgery.

Biochemical markers

Plasma proteins such as albumin, prealbumin, transferrin and retinol-binding protein are often used as nutritional markers since hepatic production is related to substrate availability. However, plasma protein levels are also influenced by fluid shifts between body compartments. Plasma albumin is easily measured but reflects not only changes in synthesis but also in degradation, excretion and transvascular transfer as well as exogenous administration. Albumin is more a marker of metabolic stress than nutrition as hepatic synthesis of albumin falls in favour of increased acute-phase protein synthesis. Despite these limitations, low albumin levels do correlate with an increased incidence of postoperative morbidity and mortality. Hypoalbuminaemic (albumin < 35 g l^{-1}) patients have a 4-fold increase in morbidity and a 6-fold increase in mortality following surgery. Severely hypoalbuminaemic patients with albumin levels below 20 g l^{-1} have a mortality rate greater than 60%.

Prealbumin has a shorter half-life (36 h) than albumin (21 days) and is not affected by exogenous albumin administration; its short half-life makes it ideal for following short-term changes in nutritional state. Transferrin has a shorter half-life than albumin (7 days) but levels are influenced by factors other than nutrition such as iron deficiency or iron overload. A transferrin level below 2.2 g l^{-1} is associated with a higher complication rate and mortality increases 2.5-fold if levels are below 1.7 g l^{-1}. Reduced plasma levels of retinol-binding protein are associated with an increased incidence of surgical morbidity and mortality.

Urinary markers are not very specific to nutritional status although 3-methylhistidine is relatively specific to skeletal muscle breakdown. Urinary urea is influenced by many disease states and is a poor guide to extent of protein breakdown. Although creatine/height index reflects muscle protein turnover and total muscle mass there is no clear association with either postoperative morbidity or mortality.

Immunologic markers

Both total lymphocyte count (TLC) and delayed hypersensitivity have been shown to reflect nutritional status of surgical patients. Lymphocytopenia below 1200 mm^{-3} and anergy to skin testing are both associated with increased surgical morbidity and mortality. The incidence of sepsis is increased 4-fold and mortality 6-fold in patients with preoperative anergy.

Patients who are malnourished and subsequently reverse their anergic state with perioperative nutritional support have a much lower incidence of postoperative complications than those who fail to do so. However, neither TLC nor anergy are very specific markers, being influenced by many factors other than nutrition.

Multivariate indices

A number of scoring systems have been suggested for assessment of nutritional status, none of which is universally adopted. If all the commonly used markers are assessed then 86% of all surgical patients have at least one abnormal value, yet not all are clinically malnourished. The components of multivariate scoring systems usually incorporate one measure from each of the main categories detailed in **Table 1**. Logistic regression models identifying nutritional variables which independently predict poor surgical outcome have been developed for specific surgical conditions but are not necessarily applicable to all surgical patients.

Technically advanced measures

Methods that can be used at the bedside include indirect calorimetry, bioelectrical impedance and measures of muscle function. Of these, indirect calorimetry is of particular use in the critical care setting where the resting energy expenditure of the ventilated patient may be measured in order to assess energy requirements. Muscle function tests deserve special mention, since the force-frequency relationship of the electrically stimulated adductor pollicis appears to follow changes in nutritional status.

Although it is generally accepted that malnutrition is associated with increased surgical morbidity and mortality, the absence of a simple, linear measure of nutrition makes it difficult both to determine when

Table 1 Measurements used to assess nutritional status

Anthropometric	Immunologic	Biochemical	
Height	Total lymphocyte count	1.	Plasma proteins:
Weight	Delayed hypersensitivity reaction		albumin
Mid-arm circumference			prealbumin
Triceps skinfold thickness			transferrin
			retinol-binding protein
		2.	Urinary products:
			urinary urea
			creatine–height index
			3-methylhistidine

Table 2 Deleterious effects of malnutrition and how these may be reduced by perioperative feeding

Effects of malnutrition	Beneficial effects of optimal perioperative feeding
Impaired humoral immunity	Reduced infection rate
Impaired cell-mediated immunity	Improved immune function
Reduced inflammatory response	
Reduced fibroplasia	Improved wound strength
	Improved wound healing
Negative nitrogen balance	Improved nitrogen balance
Muscle bulk reduced	Minimized weight loss
Reduced muscle metabolism	
Reduced gut function	Preservation of gut function
Impaired respiratory muscle function	Improved sense of wellbeing by patient
Reduced cardiac mass and contractility	
Reduction in CNS transmitter formation	

CNS, central nervous system.

'significant' malnutrition is present and to follow improvement in nutrition perioperatively.

The Role and Nature of Perioperative Support

Malnutrition weakens the body's defence and repair systems in several ways resulting in an increase in postoperative complications and a slower recovery. An optimal feeding regimen in the perioperative period can reverse many of the deleterious effects of malnutrition resulting in a reduction in infective complications and improved wound strength (**Table 2**). As a result hospital stay may be reduced with additional cost-saving. However, for maximum benefit, the nutritional strategy must be planned preoperatively with a multidisciplinary feeding team, addressing route of feeding, composition of feed and timing of feeding.

Routes for perioperative nutrition

Patients may be fed either enterally or parenterally or by a combination of both routes (**Table 3**). Parenteral

Table 3 Routes available for perioperative feeding

Oral
Sip feeds

Enteral
Nasogastric, fine-bore feeding tube
Percutaneous gastrostomy
Percutaneous jejunostomy
Nasojejunal feeding tube
Surgical gastrostomy
Surgical jejunostomy

Parenteral
Peripheral, for supplementary or total parenteral nutrition
Central, for total parenteral nutrition

nutrition may be delivered through either a peripheral or a central venous catheter. Early experience with the peripheral route highlighted several problems, particularly the high incidence of thrombophlebitis but also the need for intravenous feed preparations with lower osmolality and consequently an inadequate energy content. This led to the central route being adopted for delivery of total parenteral nutrition (TPN), and most reported studies comparing TPN with enteral feeding have used the central venous route for delivery. More recently, with the development of less thrombogenic catheter material there has been a resurgence of interest in the peripheral route for TPN, and it has been recommended as the route of choice when no long-term indication for TPN exists.

Many studies have shown that energy intake goals are reached more frequently with TPN, delivered by the central route, or with a combination of enteral plus parenteral feeding, than with enteral feeding alone.

A recent development is the more widespread use of percutaneous and operative tube gastrostomies and jejunostomies. The introduction of percutaneous endoscopic gastrostomy (PEG) has provided a safe, bedside technique for gastrostomy placement. Tube jejunostomies are now being placed at the time of operation in patients undergoing abdominal surgery for both gastrointestinal tract resections and hepatic transplantation. Both approaches provide enteral nutrition where previously this was thought inappropriate. Studies have shown that enteral feeding can be started within 24 h of surgery proximal to an anastomosis without any increase in anastomotic leak. The jejunal route is often more successful than the gastric; early, transient, gastric stasis frequently follows gastrointestinal surgery but jejunal absorption is not impaired despite absence of bowel sounds. Tube jejunostomies are less problematic than nasojejunal tubes, in particular with a lower rate of reflux back into the stomach provided they are positioned beyond the ligament of Treitz. Ideally jejunostomies should be placed at the time of operation, but may be placed percutaneously under fluoroscopic control. Nasojejunal tubes may be placed at the time of operation or endoscopically, and the position should be confirmed radiologically; positioning is much less reliable than for percutaneous methods and nasojejunal tubes are prone to blockage if used for longer than a few days.

There is continuing controversy over the role of TPN compared with enteral nutrition following major abdominal surgery involving anastomoses. This is despite numerous studies that show the benefits of early enteral feeding. The gastrointestinal tract is pivotal in the development of sepsis and the septic inflammatory response syndrome (SIRS) in critically ill surgical patients, and the protection offered against bacterial translocation and sepsis by early enteral feeding is clear. However, it must be said that there is still some dispute over the true physiologic significance of bacterial translocation in humans. The advantages and disadvantages of enteral compared with parenteral routes are outlined in **Table 4**.

Although some degree of enteral feeding may be tolerated postoperatively there are often intermittent episodes of apparent intolerance with increased residual volumes and excessive diarrhoea. In order to ensure adequate energy and nitrogen delivery, particularly in critically ill surgical patients, enteral and parenteral feeding may be combined. The peripheral route for parenteral feeding is of particular importance when such mixed strategies of feeding are adopted, ensuring adequate energy intake with minimum risk while gut function returns to normal. Peripheral parenteral feeding should be the route of choice if supplementary or total intravenous nutrition is needed for periods of less than 10 days.

Content of feed

Feed, whether for enteral or parenteral use, must provide adequate energy and replace nitrogen losses. The nutritional state of the patient preoperatively must also be taken into account.

Energy needs Most calculations of the energy requirements of surgical patients are based on the Harris–Benedict equations for basal energy expenditure (BEE) in kilocalories for males and females:

$$BEE \text{ (male)} = 66 + 13.8W + 5H - 6.8A$$
$$BEE \text{ (female)} = 655 + 9.5W + 1.8H - 4.7A$$

where W is the weight in kilograms, H is the height in centimetres and A is age in years, giving a value of 25–35 kcal kg^{-1} (105–147 kJ kg^{-1}) per 24 h. Critically ill surgical patients require in the order of 1.2–1.5 times BEE. This energy can largely be provided by carbohydrate and fat.

Carbohydrate, glucose In the metabolically stressed patient glucose demands increase; gluconeogenesis ensues with increased glucose flux and mild hyper-

Table 4 Advantages and disadvantages of parenteral nutrition compared with enteral feeding

Enteral	Parenteral
Advantages	
Preserves gut mucosa	Reliable delivery of nutrients
Increases gut blood flow	Reduces incidence of postoperative complications
Reduces incidence bacterial translocation	
Reduces incidence of sepsis	
Reduces incidence of infection	
Inexpensive	
Avoids catheter-related complications	
Disadvantages	
Increases incidence of gastrointestinal disturbances	Catheter-related complications:
Less reliable delivery of daily nutrients	infective[a]
Increased diarrhoea	thrombotic
Aspiration risk	insertion-related[a]
	Costly to make
	Medical insertion of line necessary
	Gut mucosal atrophy
	Immunosuppression
	Metabolic complications

[a]More frequently associated with central than peripherally inserted catheters.

glycaemia. A glucose infusion of 5 mg per kg per min (about 7 g per kg per day) will both suppress protein catabolism and provide adequate energy intake. If higher infusion rates are used, then glucose utilization becomes inefficient. A minimum glucose intake of 2 g per kg per day will supply the central nervous system with adequate fuel and prevent acidosis and ketosis. The remainder of the energy requirement can be provided by fats.

Fats Dietary fat is in the form of triacylglycerols. Aerobic metabolism of fat provides $38.9 \, \text{kJ} \, \text{g}^{-1}$ ($9.3 \, \text{kcal} \, \text{g}^{-1}$) whereas glucose provides $17.2 \, \text{kJ} \, \text{g}^{-1}$ ($4.1 \, \text{kcal} \, \text{g}^{-1}$). Fat cannot be used as sole energy source but is an efficient source in combination with glucose. Standard enteral feeds have a glucose to fat ratio supplying $4.2 \, \text{kJ} \, \text{ml}^{-1}$ ($1 \, \text{kcal} \, \text{ml}^{-1}$) of feed; other formulae provide a greater proportion of energy as fat, $6.3 \, \text{kJ} \, \text{ml}^{-1}$ ($1.5 \, \text{kcal} \, \text{ml}^{-1}$), to reduce the volume of feed needed to meet energy requirements. Lipid emulsions for parenteral use are isotonic and can be used peripherally, unlike hypertonic glucose solutions.

The type of fatty acids used to provide energy may also be important. The triacylglycerols found in commonly used lipid emulsions are mainly long-chain triacylglycerols (LCTs) with 16–18 carbon atoms. Medium-chain triacylglycerols (MCTs) with 8–10 carbons, found in coconut oil, are more soluble and more rapidly cleared from the circulation. Recent work suggests that improved nitrogen balance and reduced weight loss can be achieved in postoperative surgical patients fed parenterally with a 1 : 1 ratio of LCT to MCT.

Lipid emulsions also provide essential fatty acids, particularly linoleic acid, which are intimately associated with immunomodulation through arachidonic acid, an n-6 polyunsaturated fatty acid (PUFA), and its metabolites. Fish oil contains n-3 PUFAs rather than n-6 PUFAs found in vegetable oil; n-3 PUFAs appear to enhance cellular immune function by altering macrophage eicosanoid production. This may be of benefit to the critically ill surgical patient, where amplification of macrophage-derived factors appears to be involved in SIRS which in turn may lead to multiorgan failure.

There are disadvantages associated with parenteral lipid administration. Parenteral fat emulsions produce protein-free lipid particles which may form abnormal lipoprotein particles. These may be associated with pulmonary damage and worsening hypoxia which may be of importance in the critically ill patient. Excessive fat administration may be associated with hepatic dysfunction and fatty deposition in the liver.

Protein Protein breakdown of muscle induces a negative nitrogen balance, weakness and reduced immune responsiveness. The nitrogen requirement of postoperative patients can be estimated from urinary losses, in the absence of renal failure:

$$\text{Total daily nitrogen losses (g)} = 1.25 \times \text{UUN} + 2$$

where UUN is 24 h urinary urea nitrogen; this is generally 12–18 g per 24 h. When calculating protein requirements, 6.25 g of protein is equivalent to 1 g nitrogen.

Enteral formulae may have an elemental or polymeric composition; the former type contains predigested nutrients which, theoretically, should be more readily absorbed by the small bowel. Such elemental preparations have a higher osmolality which may lead to diarrhoea and intolerance if introduced too rapidly. Elemental feeds are often used for jejunal feeding, although no difference in nitrogen balance or other markers of nutrition has been found when compared with polymeric enteral feed.

Both enteral feeds and TPN enriched with essential branched-chain amino acids (BCAA) – leucine, isoleucine and valine – have been shown to improve nitrogen balance in patients with hepatic encephalopathy. The BCAA differ from other amino acids in that they can be metabolized in muscle. Enrichment of parenteral feeds with 45% BCAA improves nitrogen balance, increases absolute lymphocyte count, increases plasma transferrin levels and reverses skin anergy. Despite such demonstrable improvements in markers of nutritional status there is little evidence of any accompanying difference in surgical morbidity or mortality. Thus, apart from hepatic dysfunction, there is little evidence to recommend BCAA-enriched feeds.

The amino acid glutamine has received a great deal of attention. Although nonessential in health, glutamine is conditionally essential in stress and illness. Glutamine is the most abundant amino acid in the body, making up 60% of the free amino acid pool in skeletal muscle. The gastrointestinal tract is the principal organ of glutamine utilization and extracts 12–13% of circulating glutamine and 50–70% of enterally supplied glutamine. Glutamine deficiency is associated with mucosal atrophy and loss of function. In surgical stress glutamine uptake by the gastrointestinal tract increases but if sepsis intervenes, glutamine uptake and utilization fall and, in the rat model, bacterial translocation increases. These changes appear to be cytokine-mediated. Compared with standard TPN, glutamine-supplemented TPN is associated with increased jejunal mucosal weight, less villous atrophy and enhancement of gut immune function. Glutamine is not usually included in TPN as it is relatively unstable, but dipeptide and acetylated forms may soon be commercially available. Patients given enteral glutamine supplementation preoperatively for 10 days had reduced infective complications and length of stay. However, little patient data are available and the clinical role of glutamine has yet to be established.

Vitamins, trace elements, growth factors Minimum daily requirements for vitamins and trace elements should be met, paying particular attention to the fat-soluble vitamins and those whose absorption enterally may be affected by the site of surgery, e.g. vitamin B_{12}.

Of recent interest has been the use of growth factors to enhance wound healing. Growth hormone (GH) stimulates hepatic synthesis and secretion of the somatomedin insulin-like growth factor I (IGF-I) which has an anabolic action. When GH is given during TPN, fat is mobilized and oxidized in preference to glucose which enhances the protein-sparing effect of TPN. This may be beneficial in the critically ill patient where delivery of adequate nutrients does not necessarily ensure adequate cellular uptake. Other growth factors produced locally and systemically can influence wound strength and rate of healing. The use of such growth factors in combination with various perioperative feeding regimens has yet to be established.

Timing of feeding

Preoperative feeding Many patients present with gastrointestinal tract emergencies; only in the case of incapacitating malnutrition would the need for preoperative feeding delay surgery. There have been few sufficiently large, randomized, controlled trials of preoperative feeding of malnourished patients awaiting major surgery. Compared with a standard hospital diet, 2–3 days of preoperative, centrally delivered TPN has no influence on morbidity or mortality. The Veterans Affairs Total Parenteral Nutrition Cooperative Study failed to show any reduction in surgical morbidity or mortality following 7–10 days of preoperative feeding. Other studies have indicated that 7–10 days of preoperative TPN can reduce the incidence of major postoperative complications such as intraabdominal abscess, peritonitis, anastomotic leakage and ileus. There is some evidence that if more attention is paid to encouraging oral intake of energy, nitrogen and vitamins then the apparent benefit of TPN preoperatively disappears, apart from a lower wound infection rate. The role of preoperative enteral feeding has yet to be thoroughly investigated.

Postoperative feeding The immediate postoperative period is often characterized by fasting due to nausea, vomiting and abdominal distension, all of which prevent adequate oral intake. For most patients this period lasts fewer than 10 days and will be accompanied by weight loss but few serious complications. Where it is anticipated that the period of fasting will exceed 7–10 days, postoperative nutrition is essential and should be planned preoperatively. Wherever possible enteral feed should be used; contraindications to this route are summarized in **Table 5**.

Early feeding is now considered beneficial and should begin within 24 h of surgery, even in the presence of an anastomosis. Enteral feed must be introduced within 72 h to maintain intestinal mucosal weight, thickness and nitrogen content. Early intolerance of enteral feeding is not uncommon, particularly if an elemental formula with a high osmolality is used. Full-strength feed should be introduced at a low, constant rate (20–25 ml h^{-1}), avoiding bolus feeds and increased gradually by 25 ml h^{-1} every 6 h until full requirements are met. Adequate means of decompression as well as feeding should be provided. Minor gastrointestinal symptoms are more common with enteral feeding than with TPN and are the major reason for failure of enteral feeding. The incidence of diarrhoea in critically ill patients appears to be no higher in those enterally than parenterally fed. Other minor problems are cramping abdominal pains and abdominal distension, which often settle if feeding rate is reduced and bolus feeding changed to continuous. Despite these minor complications, the incidence of sepsis and the overall complication rate following surgery is lower for enteral than central parenteral feeding even when allowance is made for catheter-related sepsis. Complications associated with nutritional support should be borne in mind (**Table 6**).

The duration of postoperative nutritional support will necessarily depend on individual patient requirements. When markers for acute stress are falling and

Table 5 Contraindications to enteral feeding

Absolute contraindications
1.	Complete mechanical intestinal obstruction
2.	Short bowel syndrome
3.	Acute, severe pancreatitis
4.	High-output fistula

Relative contraindications
1.	Gastric stasis; jejunal feeding may be successful
2.	Ileus, where energy goals not met; consider supplementing with parenteral feed
3.	Persistent diarrhoea; consider reintroduction of feed at lower rate or using elemental formula

Table 6 Complications of enteral tubes versus central parenteral catheters in nutritional support

Enteral	Parenteral
Related to insertion	
Tube misplacement into lungs:	Pneumothorax
pneumonia	Haemothorax
empyema	Hydrothorax/mediastinum
hydrothorax	Arterial haemorrhage
pneumothorax	Haematoma
Tube coiling in mouth or oesophagus: aspiration risk	Air embolism
	Cardiac arrhythmias
	Brachial plexus damage
Later complications	
Aspiration pneumonia	Air embolism
nasal/oesophageal erosions	Catheter migration, atrial perforation and tamponade
Sinusitis	Catheter-related sepsis
Perforation/malposition; peritonitis	Subclavian vein thrombosis
Abdominal cramps	Acalculous cholecystitis
Abdominal distension	Metabolic abnormalities
Diarrhoea	

albumin levels are improving, when sepsis has settled, gastrointestinal symptoms have abated and there is no reason to suspect gut dysfunction, then an oral diet may be introduced gradually. The place of sip feeding is receiving increased attention and the use of energy supplements in this form may be useful.

Nutrition for Specific Surgical Conditions

There are certain groups of patients who will always require nutritional support in the perioperative period. In the following conditions long-term feeding is not anticipated.

Malignancies of the upper gastrointestinal tract

Patients with upper gastrointestinal tract carcinoma have a higher incidence of malnutrition than those with carcinomas of the lower gastrointestinal tract. The introduction of preoperative TPN for 7 or more days reduces the incidence of septic complications from 100% to 16.7% in malnourished patients with gastric carcinoma, although with no difference in mortality. At least 60% of patients with carcinoma of the oesophagus are significantly malnourished at the time of presentation; patients with more than 8.5% weight loss have a 90% incidence of negative nitrogen balance. Until recently such patients would have been fed parenterally. Increasingly, gastrostomies and jejunostomies are being used: both provide adequate nutrition and complication rates are low. The use of high protein–energy enteral nutrition in such patients is associated with improvements in immune function and a reduction in postoperative sepsis.

Inflammatory bowel disease

Chronic malnutrition is more common in Crohn's disease than in ulcerative colitis. Up to 33% patients presenting for surgery are malnourished with depletion of protein, energy, trace elements, electrolytes and vitamins. Total parenteral nutrition is used in the management of severe episodes and in cases of enteric fistulas. In less severe cases tube feeding with an elemental diet may be as effective as TPN in normalizing nitrogen balance. Patients who receive TPN for 5 or more days preoperatively have significantly fewer postoperative complications than those who receive no additional nutritional support. Surgical intervention is often an emergency procedure and nutritional support will be needed postoperatively.

Acute pancreatitis

Severe, acute pancreatitis is accompanied by extreme metabolic stress and a rapid decline in nutritional status. Surgery is often required in critically ill patients to remove necrotic tissue which induces a shock-like syndrome. In such severe cases, TPN is required and should be introduced as early as possible in the clinical course to limit nitrogen loss and provide adequate energy. Total parenteral nutrition has been shown to reduce pancreatic secretory activity and so reduce autolysis. The optimum feeding regimen is still controversial, particularly the use of fat emulsions. It seems likely that persistent hyperlipidaemia is related to the disease process rather than the use of lipid in feeding regimens and is indicative of a poor prognosis. Pancreatic secretory activity is also reduced if amino acids are given either parenterally or enterally into the duodenum. The role of enteral feeding in acute pancreatitis is unclear although successful enteral feeding through tube jejunostomy has been reported.

Enterocutaneous fistula

The incidence of malnutrition in patients with enterocutaneous fistula presenting for surgery is high, varying from 20% to 70% depending on the site of the fistula. The number of procedures eventually required differs for individual patients and nutritional support is essential in optimizing fistula closure. Total parenteral nutrition is used in cases where the fistula is high in the gastrointestinal tract, since enteral feeding often worsens fluid loss through the fistula. Both nitrogen and fluid balance must be carefully managed, with essential fatty acids, trace elements and vitamin supplements being given as early as possible. Nutritional support reduces fistula output, reduces mortality and will promote spontaneous closure of up to 80% of enterocutaneous fistulas.

Liver resection, liver failure and transplantation

The use of enteral nutrition, containing 50% lipid as MCTs and amino acids enriched with BCAAs, for 7 days prior to and after hepatectomy for hepatocellular carcinoma reduces postoperative morbidity, especially infective complications, but not mortality. Severe hepatic dysfunction is associated with an alteration in the amino acid content of plasma. Increased muscle breakdown leads to an increase in the aromatic amino acids and a reduction in BCAAs. Patients with chronic liver failure are cachectic and malnourished, and adequate supplies of protein and energy must be provided perioperatively without precipitating encephalopathy. A significant proportion of protein intake, should consist of BCAAs, which reduce the perioperative risk of encephalopathy. Both enteral and parenteral routes have been used successfully postoperatively in transplant recipients. Tube jejunostomy or nasojejunal tubes are placed at the time of surgery and feeding starts within 18 h of return from theatre. Despite the use of immunosuppressive treatment, the incidence of infection is low (5%). Gut function appears well preserved whether the enteral or parenteral route is chosen, and the majority of patients tolerate oral intake within 10 days of surgery.

See also: **Cancer**: Epidemiology of Colorectal Cancer. **Colonic Diseases and Disorders**: Nutritional Management. **Liver Disorders**: Nutritional Management. **Nutritional Support**: Enteral Feeding; Parenteral Nutrition. **Protein**: Synthesis and Turnover. **Surgery**: Long-term Nutritional Management of Patients.

Further Reading

Campos ACL and Maguid MM (1992) A critical appraisal of the usefulness of perioperative nutritional support. *American Journal of Clinical Nutrition* 55:117–130.

Chwals WJ (1992) Metabolism and nutrition in pediatric surgical patients. *Surgical Clinics of North America* 72(6):1237–1266.

Herndon DN, Nguyen TT and Gilpin DA (1993) Growth factors: local and systemic. *Archives of Surgery* 128:1227–1234.

Kelly KG (1993) Advances in perioperative nutritional support. *Medical Clinics of North America* 77(2):465–475.

King's Fund Centre (1992) *A Positive Approach to Nutrition as Treatment.* London: King's Fund Centre.

Meguid MM, Campos AC and Hammond WG (1990) Nutritional support in surgical practice: Part I. *American Journal of Surgery* 159:345–358.

Meguid MM, Campos AC and Hammond WG (1990) Nutritional support in surgical practice: Part II. *American Journal of Surgery* 159:427–443.

Rollandelli RH and Ullrich JR (1994) Nutritional support in the frail elderly surgical patient. *Surgical Clinics of North America* 74(1):79–92.

Saunders C, Nishikawa R and Wolfe B (1993) Surgical nutrition: a review. *Journal of the Royal College of Surgeons of Edinburgh* 38:195–204.

Long-term Nutritional Management of Patients

D Wilmore, Harvard Medical School, Boston, Massachusetts, USA

Patients with severe and prolonged catabolic illnesses – usually related to an accidental injury or a complication following a major operation – require extended hospitalization, and frequently suffer from long-term inflammation or infection. It is important that nutrition is integrated into the overall care of this type of patient, for treatment is often complicated by the use of multiple antibiotics, cardiotonic drugs, ventilator support and frequent and repeated operations. If patients do not receive adequate nutritional support, they rapidly lose significant amounts of weight, and this tissue loss is associated with a decrease in immunological responses, poor wound healing, skeletal muscle weakness and a prolonged convalescence.

The Metabolic Response to Injury

General features

The catabolic responses that occur following injury are related to the extent of the trauma – the greater the injury, the more extensive the responses. Classically, injury responses have been categorized according to the time when events occurred following the accident. The early events were classified as the 'ebb' period, and this was associated with features of the injury response that occurred during the period of shock, hypotension or low blood flow. With stabilization and resuscitation, the patient's circulatory status improves and the individual's physiological and biochemical responses evolves into the hypermetabolic or 'flow' phase of injury (**Table 1**). However, when prompt care is provided by an experienced field emergency unit, resuscitation is often started within minutes of the injury, and thus blood loss is attenuated and tissue oxygenation is assured. Under these conditions, the 'ebb' or hypometabolic phase is minimal, and the patient almost immediately moves into the hypermetabolic phase characterized by increased oxygen consumption and a hyperdynamic circulation.

Specific responses

Negative nitrogen balance Following major injury or infection, there is increased loss of nitrogen from the body, reflecting the increased net breakdown of body protein. The increased urinary nitrogen excretion is characterized primarily by accelerated ureagenesis and is related to the extent of injury or infection, but modified by the patient's gender,

Table 2 Estimates of nitrogen loss following catabolic illness (first 10 days, *ad lib.* feedings)

Precipitating factor	Cumulative nitrogen loss (G)
Injury	
Major burn	170
Multiple injury	150
Peritonitis	136
Simple fracture	115
Major operation	50
Minor operation	24
Infection	
Typhoid fever (untreated)	116
Pneumonia (untreated)	59
Tularaemia (treated)	52
Q fever (treated)	40
Sandfly fever (untreated)	16

Adapted from Wilmore (1977).

nutritional status and age (**Table 2**). Nitrogen balance (the value calculated by subtracting all measured nitrogen losses from nitrogen intake) is negative, especially during the early part of the hypermetabolic or flow phase of injury, even in the face of forced feedings.

Nitrogen equilibrium in normal individuals is a balance between rates of protein synthesis and degradation. Negative nitrogen balance occurs if the breakdown rate of protein increases and exceeds the rate of protein synthesis or if the breakdown rate remains the same and the rate of synthesis decreases. Using isotopically labelled amino acids, these flux rates have been quantified. Protein synthesis is diminished in normal subjects when food is restricted or prolonged bed rest is imposed. In contrast, protein breakdown is accelerated in injured or septic patients. Feeding stressed individuals after the initial period of stress enhances the protein synthetic rate to match the accelerated breakdown rate and therefore nitrogen equilibrium or balance can be achieved (**Table 3**).

Table 1 Alterations that occur following injury

'Ebb' phase	'Flow' phase
Blood glucose concentration elevated	Blood glucose concentration normal or slightly elevated
Normal glucose production	Increased glucose production
Free fatty acids elevated	Free fatty acids normal or slightly elevated – flux increased
Insulin concentration low	Insulin concentration normal or elevated
Catecholamines and glucagon elevated	Catecholamines high normal, or elevated; glucagon elevated
Blood lactate elevated	Blood lactate normal
Oxygen consumption depressed	Blood lactate normal
Cardiac output below normal	Cardiac output increased
Core temperature below normal	Core temperature elevated

Table 3 Alterations in rates of protein synthesis and catabolism that may affect hospitalized patients

	Synthesis	Catabolism
Normal:		
starvation	↓	0
fed, bed rest	↓	0
Elective surgical procedure	↓	0
Injury/sepsis:		
IV dextrose	↑↑	↑↑↑
fed	↑↑↑	↑↑↑

Key: ↓, decrease; ↑, increase; 0, no change; IV, intravenous.
Adapted from Wilmore (1977).

Muscle is the source of this extensive catabolism; amino acids are released following degradation of the actin and myosin proteins to support the visceral organs and immunological tissue of the body and presumably provide substrate for the healing wound. Alanine and glutamine constitute the major proportion of the amino acid nitrogen released from muscle. Glutamine is utilized for acid-based homeostasis, supports the proliferative response of immunological tissue and the gastrointestinal tract, is a major gluconeogenic precursor and serves as substrate for glutathione biosynthesis in the liver. Alanine also serves as an important gluconeogenic precursor (**Fig. 1**). While other amino acids may be synthesized in the liver from these nitrogen donors, the net effect is to enhance ureagenesis.

Both in the fed and underfed state, visceral tissue is supported by the accelerated breakdown of skeletal muscle. Thus, the carcase feeds the viscera and the area of inflammation in an effort to support self-repair.

Alterations in glucose metabolism   Hyperglycaemia and insulin resistance are common after injury. Accelerated gluconeogenesis occurs and is coupled with a comparable increase in glucose clearance, although some organs (e.g. skeletal muscles) demonstrate a high degree of insulin resistance.

A variety of studies have been performed to determine the sites of utilization of the glucose produced by the liver. In one investigation, net glucose flux across uninjured extremities was low, suggesting that fat, not glucose, was the primary fuel for resting skeletal muscle in the postabsorptive state. However, increased glucose uptake occurred across the injured extremity which also released large quantities of lactate, representing as much as 80% of the glucose consumed. The glucose metabolized by the central nervous system in the injured patient is approximately normal (120 g per day), whereas the rate of glucose consumed by the kidneys is approximately twice normal (75 g per day) (**Fig. 2**). Thus, a constant amount of glucose is provided for the healing wound

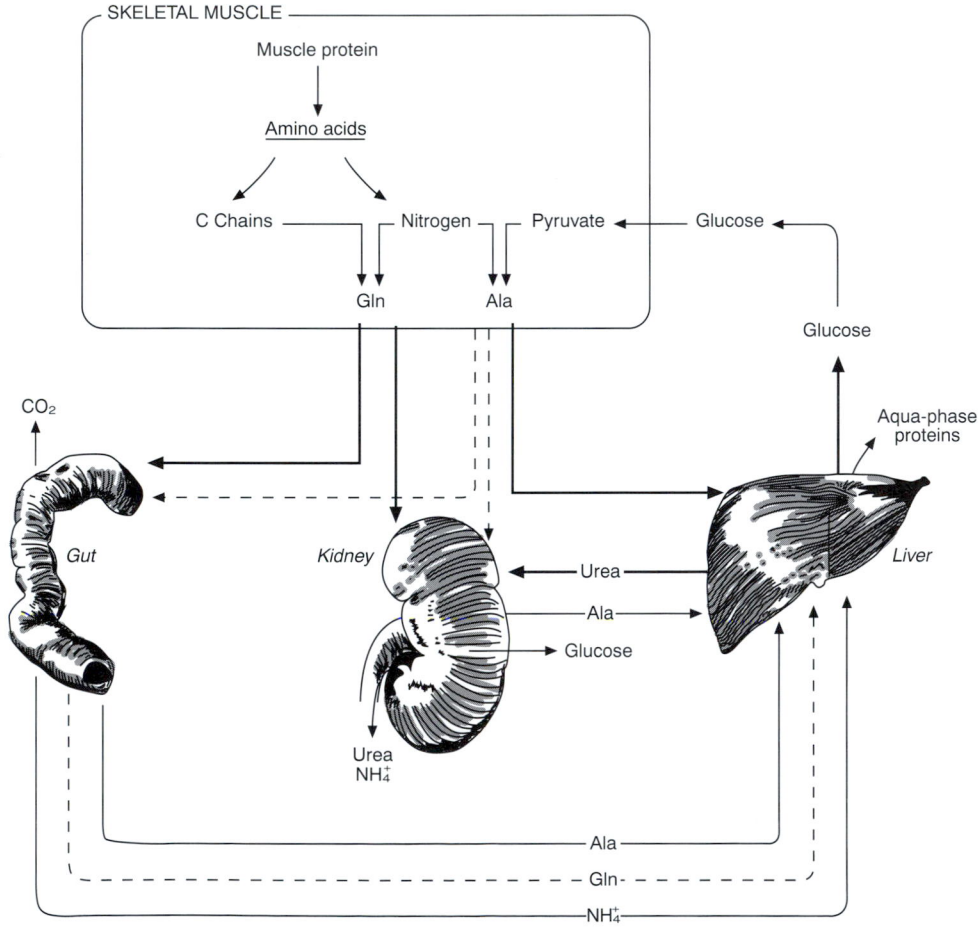

Figure 1   The pathways for the handling of amino acids following trauma or infection. Glutamine (Gln) and alanine (Ala) are the principal amino acids involved in the intraorgan transport of nitrogen and carbon. The formation of NH_4^+ by the kidney and urea by the liver represents 'obligatory' losses of nitrogen from the body during these catabolic states.

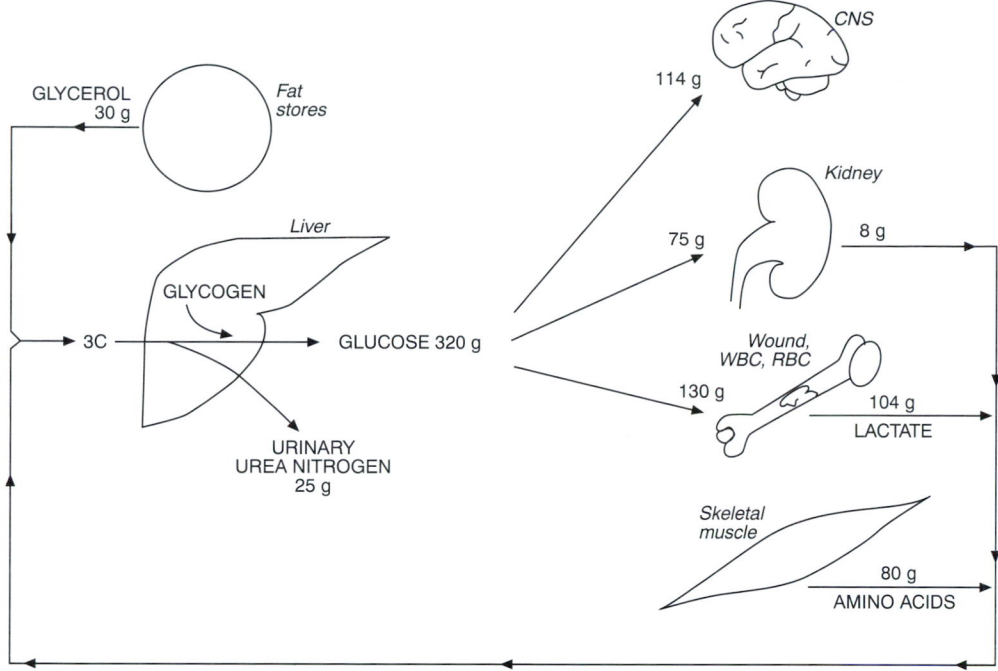

Figure 2 Injury and infection are associated with increased hepatic gluconeogenesis. The figure shows the 24 h flux of six-carbon and three-carbon units following severe injury. The wound converts the glucose to lactate which is recycled to the liver and reconverted to glucose (e.g. the Cori cycle). Glucose oxidized by the brain and kidney is replaced by amino acids arising from skeletal muscle and glycerol arising from adipose tissue. CNS, central nervous system; RBC, red blood cell; WBC, white blood cell.

and other essential organs. Precursors such as lactate which arise from aerobic glycolysis within the wound, and amino acids from skeletal muscle, support this process and ensure that the necessary substrate is available for gluconeogenesis until recovery occurs.

The hypermetabolic response With the onset of the flow phase, the whole-body metabolic rate rises, and this elevation is proportional to the degree of injury (**Fig. 3**). In patients with a long-bone fracture this increase may be minor (15–20%), but in individuals with more extensive injuries, severe infection or flame burns this hypermetabolic state creates a major drain on the body's energy stores. For example, patients with large thermal injuries have measured resting metabolic requirements 50–100% above normal, and this increased energy demand may be maintained for 30–50 days after injury.

The hypermetabolism is associated with an increase in central temperature, which appears reset 1–2°C above normal. Calculation of the contribution of the hyperthermia to the hypermetabolic response fails to account for a large portion of the increased energy demands due to thermoregulatory drives, particularly in individuals with large thermal injuries. Other studies have demonstrated that the hypermetabolic response can be reduced in part by caring

for the patient in a warm environment or, in the case of a burn patient, by wrapping the wound with dressings to prevent evaporative water loss.

The hyperdynamic circulatory state To support the heightened metabolism, cardiac output rises during the flow phase. Augmented blood flow is necessary to maintain wound perfusion which is markedly increased, but also supports the increased demands of visceral organs. Control of wound circulation is similar to that in other critical tissues (heart, brain, working skeletal muscle), in which blood flow varies as a function of local metabolic conditions rather than being controlled by integrated central vasoregulatory reflexes. This implies that as long as blood pressure is maintained, wound perfusion is ensured. Simultaneously, the increased catecholamines enhance cardiac output to support the increased perfusion.

Response mediators

The available evidence suggests that signals from the injury site reach the central nervous system (CNS) and initiate a classic 'stress' response. These signals are nervous afferent messages and hormonal signals.

Kehlet utilized neural blockade to prevent afferent information from reaching the CNS in patients undergoing elective operations. This led to

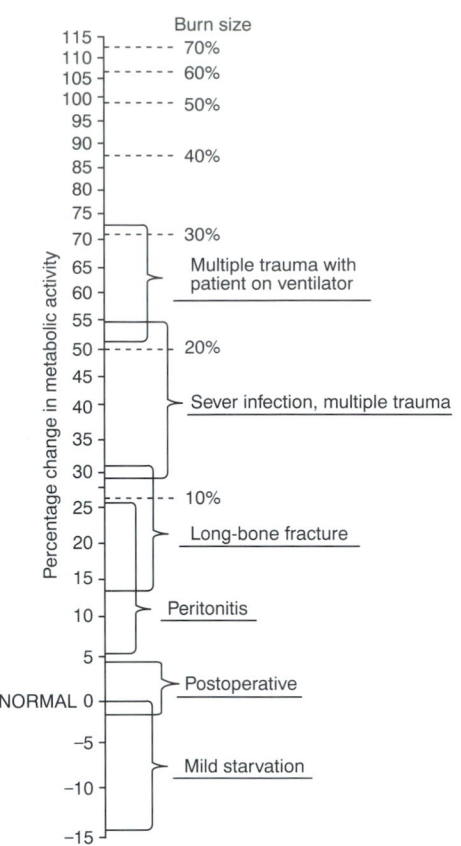

Figure 3 The percentage change in metabolic activity (basal metabolic rate) following trauma, infection and burn injury.

measurable reduction in nitrogen losses in these patients and, when coupled with laparoscopic procedures, has greatly reduced the injury responses to elective operations. In addition to afferent nervous signals, circulating factors also initiate the metabolic response to injury, and a variety of factors were proposed. However, it was not until cytokines were discovered that it was realized that tumour necrosis factor (TNF), interleukin 1 (IL-1), IL-6 and other factors could serve as humoral mediators arising in the wound, at other sites of inflammation or elsewhere in the body.

In addition, attention has turned to the role of cytokines at the tissue level, such as the liver and the CNS. Interleukins 1 and 6 have been detected in the cerebrospinal fluid of head-injured patients, IL-1 may be able to cross the blood–brain barrier, and TNF receptors are present in the murine brain. Finally, it has been demonstrated that chronic CNS exposure to IL-1 produces catabolism in experimental animals. This evidence led investigators to conclude that injury evoked by a wide variety of stimuli resulted in a reasonably similar set of CNS and organ responses. However, the neuroendocrine response represented a final common pathway

directed at maintaining homeostasis and protecting against potentially harmful events. Infusion of the counterregulatory hormones glucagon, glucocorticoids and catecholamines into normal human volunteers in concentrations comparable to those in injured patients resulted in metabolic alterations similar to those observed in septic or injured patients. The nitrogen loss seen with this combination of hormones was modest, however, and was not associated with net skeletal muscle protein breakdown. It has been demonstrated that by using somatostatin to block insulin secretions, as observed in the ebb phase of injury, a triple hormone infusion resulted in much larger nitrogen losses.

Although the relative contributions of cytokines and the counterregulatory hormones to the injury responses are unclear, these mediators appear to have both additive and synergistic effects when they act together.

Thus, afferent nervous and circulating signals generally arising from the injury site reach the brain and other tissues to initiate the injury responses. The central nervous system serves to integrate and amplify these signals.

Nutrient Requirements

The guidelines for providing safe nutritional support for the critically ill have evolved since the 1970s. At that time there was great enthusiasm for providing large amounts of energy and protein to sick patients (hyperalimentation). However, this approach has been tempered and now lower quantities of energy and protein are given.

Current recommendations support the use of enteral feedings whenever possible. This may be facilitated by the placement of a feeding jejunostomy at the time of initial laparotomy following the injury. Alternatively, the percutaneous placement of a gastrostomy tube can be performed at a later and more convenient time. A special gastrostomy tube with an extension into the jejunum can be utilized for feeding early after injury, and this device is well tolerated in many patients. If the enteral feedings are not tolerated, then intravenous nutrition should be provided. In general, the first step in planning nutritional support is to determine the energy requirements. This can be estimated by first determining the basal metabolic rate of the individual in the noninjured state and then increasing this amount by an estimated percentage based on the extent of injury (Fig. 3). Alternatively, oxygen consumption can be measured and the energy requirements based on this determination. Daily requirements are generally in the range 125–

190 kJ kg^{-1} (30–45 kcal kg^{-1}), and this energy is usually given as 50–60% carbohydrate, 20–30% fat and 20% protein. Protein requirements are 1.5–2.0 g kg^{-1} per day in patients with normal renal and liver function.

Nutrition should be initiated after satisfactory resuscitation and/or operative recovery has been achieved. Both tube feeding and intravenous infusions of nutritional solutions should be started gradually. Gastrostomy and jejunostomy feedings are advanced gradually over a period of 2–4 days, and then only as tolerated by the patients. Intravenous feedings can usually be increased more rapidly, with hyperglycaemia being the rate-limiting indicator of tolerance.

Overfeeding is one of the major complications to be avoided, and since the determination of energy requirements is often imprecise, the novice often pushes for more, not less, energy to be infused. Studies have demonstrated that overfeeding is associated with increased weight gain which is only fat and water. Moreover, marked hyperglycaemia may occur, accompanied by an osmotic diuresis and acute volume loss characterized by hypotension and seizures. Severe hepatic dysfunction is a longer-term sequela of overfeeding. If large carbohydrate loads are administered, the increased rate of carbon dioxide production may prevent the patient being weaned from a ventilator. Thus, the general recommendation for dextrose administration is that it should not exceed 4–5 mg kg^{-1} min^{-1} (400–500 g per day in a 70 kg individual). The blood glucose concentration should be maintained at 5.5–11 mmol l^{-1} (100–200 mg dl^{-1}) and, if necessary, insulin should be provided to maintain this concentration.

Commercially available tube feedings provide usual vitamin and trace element requirements, and an intravenous vitamin and trace element package is also available for the patient requiring intravenous support. Supplemental zinc (and possibly other trace elements such as selenium) should be given to patients with burns, large wounds or significant gastrointestinal fluid losses. For example, about 12 mg of zinc is lost per litre of small bowel fluid lost. Many clinicians also provide supplemental antioxidant nutrients (e.g. vitamins C and E, β-carotene, glutamine) via the enteral route during severe catabolic stress. Randomized trials of this approach are forthcoming. Plasma glucose, electrolytes (including magnesium) and triacylglycerol levels must be serially monitored, and renal, hepatic and pulmonary function should be tested at appropriate intervals to evaluate the metabolic response to the specialized feeding. The nutrient mix should be adjusted as needed to avoid metabolic complications.

The Role of Nutritional Support

There is a long clinical history demonstrating that improvement in the care of the catabolic patient is coupled with an increase in nutritional intake. This is best observed when reviewing burn mortality in the second half of the twentieth century. For patients aged 20–50 years, the LD_{50} (the size of burn at which 50% of patients survive and 50% die) has increased from 45% total body surface (during the years 1942–52) to about 70% in the 1990s. Moreover, a report has suggested that an anabolic factor such as growth hormone can enhance survival even further, with mortality rates of 12% in a high-risk burn population (an LD_{50} calculated as about 95%).

Given this perspective, most physicians support their patients with adequate macronutrients and micronutrients, adjusted for specific organ failure. It is not known how soon after a major insult (e.g. traumatic injury or a specific complication which may occur following elective surgery) the nutritional support should be instituted. The standard of practice is that some type of nutritional support should be started by at least 7–10 days after injury in the patient who was previously well nourished. In patients with nutritional depletion, intervention should be sooner.

A variety of markers have been advocated by some as indicating the adequacy of nutritional therapy. Thus, clinicians have followed serum albumin, retinol-binding protein and transferrin levels, nitrogen balance and body compositional changes. There is no compelling evidence that alteration in these surrogate markers guarantees an improvement in clinical outcome. Other studies have compared the complication rates associated with parenteral nutrition versus enteral nutrition, and it is clear that cost and morbidity are reduced with enteral feedings. However, no study has compared enteral feedings with simple *ad lib.* nutrition taken by the patient. Special nutrient formulations are being marketed with the claim that the composition is beneficial for a specific disease process. These formulae include large doses of glutamine, arginine, n-3 fatty acids and increased vitamins. The data are inadequate to endorse any specific approach, but some investigations suggest promise in this area.

Studies have demonstrated that present methods of nutritional support enhance body fat and water gain, but do little to support the erosion of lean body mass. In an effort to reverse this loss of structural and functional tissue, anabolic factors have been administered: the agent that has received the most attention to date has been growth hormone (GH). This substance, now made by recombinant technology, enhances protein synthesis, causes retention of minerals, and oxidizes adipose tissue as a primary fuel. In one study, depleted patients received feedings to achieve weight gain, with some receiving GH and others not. The control group gained about 3 kg of body weight, which was primarily fat and water. The treatment group gained about 4.5 kg; much was protein and its associated water (**Fig. 4**). Other studies have demonstrated that such nitrogen retention is associated with maintenance of muscle strength in the postoperative period. In addition, GH accelerates wound healing which shortens hospitalization and may reduce mortality in patients with major burn injury.

Care of Specific Patient Groups

The injured patient

Blunt and penetrating injuries to the torso may disable the gastrointestinal tract and require some type of nutritional intervention. If a laparotomy is performed, a feeding jejunostomy can be placed and a commercially prepared formula administered. If this type of access is contraindicated or unavailable, then insertion of a nasojejunal tube should be considered. Either type of feeding bypasses the stomach, which is prone to ileus and poor emptying in the early post-injury period. Isotonic formulae are started slowly (15 ml h^{-1}) via the tube and administered at a constant rate by a feeding pump. If abdominal pain, distension or diarrhoea are not evident, the feeding is advanced by an additional 5 ml every 6 h. If feeding intolerance is noted, the feeds are stopped for 6 h,

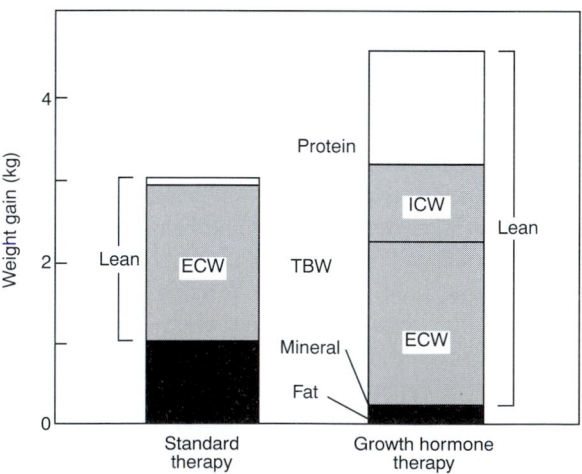

Figure 4 The anabolic response to 3 weeks of nutritional repletion with or without growth hormone. Patients receiving standard therapy gained predominantly water and fat. Treated patients gained significantly more protein, with an appropriate expansion of water. ECW, extracellular water; ICW, intracellular water; TBW, total body water.

then restarted at an infusion rate which was previously tolerated by the patient.

Daily requirements for the trauma patient are in the range 125–168 kJ kg^{-1} (30–40 kcal kg^{-1}) for energy and 1.5–2.0 g kg^{-1} for protein. If this cannot be delivered by the enteral route, then intravenous (IV) nutrition is indicated. This therapy is initiated after haemodynamic stability has been achieved; about half the total nutrient requirement is given the first day, and if it is tolerated, the total nutritional requirement is infused over the next 24 h. The patient is constantly monitored for hyperglycaemia, glucosuria, electrolyte imbalance, hypertriacylglycerolaemia and fluid overload. Formula adjustments are made to accommodate altered biochemical or physiological derangements and insulin is added to the formula if hyperglycaemia occurs. As bowel function increases, tube or enteral feedings can be started and gradually advanced and the IV nutrient infusion gradually diminished.

Patients with sepsis and multiorgan failure

Patients with sepsis and multiorgan failure are usually ventilated and cared for in an intensive care unit. Enteral feeding is rarely possible in the early course of the illness because of persistent ileus and hence intravenous nutrition is indicated. The general rule is not to cause further physiological perturbation with the feeding, so giving 105–145 kJ kg^{-1} (25–35 kcal kg^{-1}) with 1.5 g kg^{-1} protein daily is usually adequate. If anuric renal failure is present, the solutions should be concentrated and restricted in volume to 1.0–1.25 l per day. By using concentrated glucose (50% or 70%), amino acids and a highly concentrated lipid emulsion, approximately 5.5–6.3 MJ (1300–1500 kcal) can be provided in the restricted volume. With dialysis the administration of both fluid and macronutrients can be liberalized. However, in the face of elevated blood urea nitrogen or ammonia concentrations (as seen in hepatic failure), protein should be restricted to provide only 20–30 g per day, depending on the clinical status of the individual.

Burns patients

Burns patients have extraordinarily high energy needs which may be as much as 14.7–16.8 MJ (3500–4000 kcal) per day, equivalent to 168–210 kJ kg^{-1} (40–50 kcal kg^{-1}) per day. The daily protein requirement is usually 2.0–2.5 g kg^{-1} and vitamin and mineral requirements may also be greater than normal   (See: **Burns Patients:** Nutritional Management). Burns patients can usually be fed by nasogastric or nasojejunal tubes, with or without parenteral supplementation. Operations are frequent (every 2–3 days), and the tube feeding is usually stopped for 6–8 h during the perioperative period. Because fluid requirements are high (3–7 l per day) owing to the increased evaporative water loss across the burn wound, some parenteral support is usually necessary. It is possible to supplement these patients with intravenous formulae that are isotonic or slightly hypertonic solutions because of the large fluid volume utilized.

As the burn wound is healed and closed with skin grafts, the energy requirements return towards normal. The supplemental intravenous feedings are often stopped and the patient supported with tube feedings until enteral intake is possible.

Short bowel syndrome

Massive intestinal resection is necessary following abdominal trauma, bowel infarction due to vascular accident of the mesenteric vessels, extensive inflammatory bowel disease and congenital abnormalities. Loss of absorptive surface area results in chronic malabsorption and undernutrition, creating a chronic catabolic state.

Central venous nutrition should not be considered in the *immediate* postoperative period until cardiovascular stability is achieved and the bloodstream is cleared of infection. When this is achieved a new single-lumen percutaneous central venous catheter should be placed, and every effort made to maintain sterility of this access site.

As the patient recovers from the operative procedure (and the attendant complications), the individual may be able to take oral fluid and food. Initially, oral intake should be highly controlled – only small volumes (600–1000 ml per 24 h) of isotonic fluids (salt- and glucose-containing solutions such as Gatorade, Pedialyte or other oral electrolyte solutions) should be given in small, frequent amounts along with small meals and snacks of complex carbohydrates and proteins to supply 2.5–4.2 MJ (600–1000 kcal) per day. Foods such as oatmeal, rice, baked potatoes and pasta should form the basis of the patient's diet. Whole food is *never* sacrificed for administration of a liquid formula diet unless precluded by severe nausea. Small amounts of the trophic amino acid glutamine (5–10 g) dissolved in water can be started at this time and given 2–3 times a day.

As the patient's intake gradually increases, other drugs can be given, which may reduce net stool output. These agents include drugs that inhibit gastric acid secretion; antiperistaltic drugs such as co-phenotrope (Lomotil), tincture of opium and codeine; bile salt binders; and somatostatin analogues which are antisecretory agents. Inhibition of gastric acid output may be desirable, particularly in the face of gastric hypersecretion which is thought to occur in as many as a third of patients following massive bowel resection.

Shortly before discharge, a more permanent central venous line should be placed and the patient and family should be thoroughly instructed on all aspects of catheter care and IV infusion before discharge. If the patient has an 'ostomy' and a portion of unused colon, plans should be made to anastomose all bowel remnants and place all available surface area in continuity with the luminal contents. This operation should be planned early (1–3 months) after resection, if possible, especially in the individual with a high-output ostomy.

In the immediate postoperative period, referral to a gastrointestinal rehabilitation unit will facilitate this educational process concerning intake of appropriate food and maintaining adequate hydration in order to maximize bowel compensation, particularly if specific nutrients and growth factors are administered.

In one study examining the effects of trophic substances on the bowel, 47 patients with short bowel syndrome who had received intravenous nutrition for an average of 6 years received glutamine, growth hormone and diet to induce bowel compensation. The glutamine and growth hormone were specific agents trophic to the gastrointestinal tract, and the diet was a high-carbohydrate, low-fat diet designed to optimize nutrient absorption. At the time of discharge, 60% of the group were free of intravenous support. One year after, 40% of the 47 patients remained off total parenteral nutrition (TPN), another 40% had reduced their TPN requirement and the remainder were unchanged. Thus, it appears that the administration of trophic substances can increase bowel compensation and increase enteral nutrient absorption, making long-term TPN unnecessary in many patients.

See also: **Body Composition**: Determination and Physiological Significance. **Burns Patients**: Nutritional Management. **Colonic Diseases and Disorders**: Nutritional Management. **Cytokines**: Nutritional Aspects. **Infection**: Nutritional Interactions; Nutritional Management. **Nutritional Support**: Enteral Feeding; Parenteral Nutrition. **Protein**: Requirements and Role in Diet; Synthesis and Turnover.

Further Reading

Aulick LH and Wilmore DW (1983) Hypermetabolism in trauma. In: Girardier L and Stock MJ (eds) *Mammalian Thermogenesis*, p. 259. London: Chapman & Hall.

Bessey PQ and Lowe KA (1993) Early hormonal changes effect the catabolic responses to trauma. *Annals of Surgery* 218:476–489.

Bessey PQ, Watters JM, Aoki TT and Wilmore DW (1984) Combined hormonal infusion simulates the metabolic response to injury. *Annals of Surgery*, **200**:264.

Byrne TA, Presinger RL, Young LS, Ziegler TR and Wilmore DW (1995) A new treatment for patients with the short bowel syndrome. *Annals of Surgery*, **222**:243–255.

Carthertson D and Tilstone WJ (1969) Metabolism during the post injury period. *Advances in Clinical Chemistry* **12**:1.

Dinnarello CA and Wolff S (1993) The role of interleukin-1 in disease. *New England Journal & Medicine* **328**:106–113.

Egdahl RH and Hume DM (1959) The importance of the brain in the endocrine response to injury. *Annals of Surgery* **150**:697.

Herndon DN, Barrow RE, Kunkel KR *et al.* (1990) Effects of recombinant human growth on donor site healing in severely burned children. *Annals of Surgery* 211:424–431.

Hill AG, Jacobson L, Gonzalez J, Rounds J, Maizoub J and Wilmore DW (1996) Chronic central nervous system exposure to interleukin-1 causes catabolism in the rat. *American Journal of Physiology* **271**:R1142–1148.

Kehlet H (1987) Modification of responses to surgery and anesthesia by neural blockade. In: Cousins MJ and Bridenbaugh PO (eds) *Neural Blockade in Clinical Anesthesia and Management of Pain*, p 145. Philadelphia: JB Lippincott.

Knox J, Demling R, Wilmore DW *et al.* (1995) Increased survival after major burn injury: the effect of growth hormone therapy in adults. *Journal of Trauma* **39**:526–530.

Watters JM, Bessey PQ, Dinarello CA, Wolff SM and Wilmore DW (1986) Both inflammatory and endocrine mediators stimulate host responses to sepsis. *Archives of Surgery* **121**:179–190.

Wilmore DW (1977) *The Metabolic Management of the Critically Ill*. New York: Plenum.

Wilmore DW, Mason AD, Johnson DW and Pruitt BA (1975) Effect of ambient temperature on heat production and heat loss in burn patients. *Journal of Applied Physiology* **38**:593–597.

T

Tea *see* **Caffeine**: Chemistry and Physiological Effects.

Teeth *see* **Dental Disease**: Aetiology and Epidemiology.

THERAPEUTIC DIETETICS

Contents
Lung Diseases
Intensive Care Management
Short Bowel Syndrome

Lung Diseases

A MacDonald, Birmingham Children's Hospital, Birmingham, UK

Nutritional support in respiratory disorders has received increased attention over recent years. Malnutrition and weight loss are commonly reported in patients with chronic obstructive pulmonary disease and the nutritional problems, together with its aetiology is well defined in cystic fibrosis. Novel diet therapies, such as exclusion of food allergens and reduction of salt intake, have been tried as possible treatments for asthma.

Chronic Obstructive Pulmonary Disease

Chronic obstructive pulmonary disease (COPD) is a term used to describe a variety of obstructive lung diseases, such as chronic bronchitis, emphysema, asthma, bronchiectasis and combinations of these. The prevalence is higher in the UK than in other countries; each year about 30 million working days are lost and 30 000 people die from COPD. Although mortality rises steeply with age, approximately a quarter of the deaths occur before retirement age.

Chronic bronchitis

Definition and aetiology Chronic bronchitis is defined as a daily cough with sputum for at least 3 months of the year, for 2 or more consecutive years. It develops in response to long-term irritants on the bronchial mucosa. Important irritants include cigarette smoke, dust, smoke and fumes; other causes include respiratory infection, particularly in infancy, and exposure to dampness, sudden changes in temperature and fog.

Prevalence In the UK bronchitis affects 10% of older people, and it is more common in industrial countries.

Clinical features The disease progresses over many years from a troublesome cough producing a little clear sputum to marked wheezing, severe breathlessness leading to poor exercise tolerance, and copious and purulent sputum.

Pathology There is hypertrophy of the mucus-secreting glands and an increase in the number of goblet cells in the bronchi and bronchioles with a consequent decrease in ciliated cells. There is, therefore, less efficient transport of the increased mucus in the airways. Mucosal oedema and permanent structural damage of the airway wall reduces the calibre of the air passages.

Prognosis Bronchitis is a slowly progressive disorder unless the precipitating factors are avoided and it is treated.

Emphysema

Diagnosis and aetiology Emphysema means 'inflation' in the sense of abnormal distension with air. Although usually confined to a pathological process in the lungs, emphysema is also used to describe simple overinflation of normal lung and the abnormal process of air in body tissues other than the lungs. Causes of emphysema include cigarette smoking and exposure to heavy metals such as cadmium; 5% of cases of early presenting cases are caused by the autosomal recessive disorder, α_1-antitrypsin deficiency.

Prevalence The prevalence increases with age. Emphysema affects almost 5% of older people and is more common in industrialized countries.

Clinical features Symptoms include intense dyspnoea with purse-lip breathing and overinflation of the chest.

Pathology There are two types of emphysema: panacinar and centrilobular.

Panacinar emphysema   A generalized destruction of the alveolar walls occurs. As a consequence, the elastic network of the normal lung is badly disorganized and the lung becomes floppy, leading to a severe degree of airways obstruction, particularly during expansion.

Centrilobular or centriacinar emphysema   Distension and damage affect the respiratory bronchioles; the more distal alveolar ducts and alveoli tend to be well preserved. This is very common and not necessarily associated with disability.

Prognosis   The prognosis is variable. Progression is slow providing the disease is treated.

Bronchiectasis

Definition and aetiology   Bronchiectasis is the abnormal dilatation of the bronchi. The most common cause is damage to the bronchial tree after an infection such as whooping cough or severe pneumonia. However, other causes include bronchopulmonary aspergillosis, bronchial obstruction due to an inhaled foreign body such as a peanut, external gland compression and bronchial tumours, congenital anomaly and ciliary dyskinesia. It is common in patients with cystic fibrosis and immunoglobulin A deficiency.

Prevalence   The prevalence is unknown, but it has been suggested that bronchiectasis may affect 1 in 1000 of the population. Although it usually starts in childhood it can affect people of any age.

Clinical features   There is considerable variation in the severity of bronchiectasis, but the disease is characterized by a chronic cough and copious sputum. In dry bronchiectasis, sputum may only be produced during a chest infection. Exacerbations of infection are common and may be associated with haemoptysis. Other clinical features include halitosis, coarse lung crackles, bronchospasm and finger clubbing.

Pathology   Bronchiectasis may be localized to just part of a lung if there is a local cause. It is usually patchy in distribution. The wall of the bronchus is thin and dilated. It has much reduced elastin and commonly heavy inflammatory cell infiltration. The lung supplied by the bronchiectatic airways may show patchy consolidation and scarring and be reduced in volume.

Prognosis   The prognosis is related to severity. The disease can be controlled by effective treatment and the vast majority of people have a life expectancy that is nearly normal. The outlook is much less certain in those with extensive lung destruction or airways obstructions.

Nutritional management in COPD

Malnutrition is an important clinical problem in a subpopulation of patients with COPD. It was first reported in COPD as early as 1955. Studies suggest malnutrition occurs in 27–71% of patients, increasing with the severity of airways obstruction. In one of the larger studies examining patients with stable COPD, one-quarter of 779 men were less than 90% of their ideal body weight. However, in patients who need hospital admission malnutrition approaches or exceeds 50%.

Malnutrition has a considerable impact on both morbidity and mortality. Reduced respiratory muscle mass and function as well as increased susceptibility to infection are recognized as deleterious consequences of malnutrition in patients with or without lung disease. In a necropsy study, diaphragm muscle mass was reduced by 43% in malnourished patients whose weights were 71% of ideal body weight.

There is also evidence to suggest that malnutrition may adversely affect muscle aerobic capacity and exercise tolerance in patients with stable COPD. Furthermore, it has been demonstrated when a patient with COPD begins to lose weight progressively, the average reported life expectancy is only 2.9 years, and considerably less in malnourished patients who have survived an episode of acute respiratory failure during an exacerbation of their disease. However, it is not certain whether this implies a causal relationship or whether low weight is a marker for more severely impaired lung function.

Reasons for malnutrition

The cause of progressive weight loss in patients with COPD is not well understood, but the following factors have been implicated.

Increased resting energy expenditure   The relationship between resting energy expenditure (REE), lung function, oxygen cost of breathing and malnutrition in COPD has been the focus of much attention in recent years. Results of studies on REE are conflicting. In two early studies of malnourished patients with COPD, one described 10 patients whose REE was 113% of that predicted, and the other described 7 patients with an REE of 115% of predicted expenditure. In contrast, two later studies found REE to be only 94% and 104% of predicted values in stable, fasted COPD patients. It has therefore been hypothesized that if patients with COPD are not hypermetabolic, then malnutrition is related more to impaired gas exchange (as evidenced by a low diffusing capacity of carbon monoxide) than to airflow obstruction. The impaired gas exchange results from loss of the pulmonary capillary bed, and may well result in an inability to augment cardiac output in response to the stress of even minimal effort, leading to lack of oxygen delivery to the tissues and nutritional depletion. An alternative hypothesis is that malnutrition is precipitated by acute illnesses leading to a combination of anorexia and hypercatabolism causing significant weight loss.

Reduced energy intake Many studies have examined the energy intake of malnourished COPD patients and have shown this to be either similar to well-nourished patients with COPD or higher than the respective dietary recommendations. Most of these studies have been conducted on stable patients, however, several factors may adversely affect energy and nutrient intake. These include anorexia due to acute infection; chronic sputum production and frequent coughing, which may alter desire for and taste of food; shortness of breath and fatigue which can interfere with the ability to prepare and ingest adequate meals; and side effects of medications including nausea, vomiting, diarrhoea, dry mouth and gastric irritation, which may limit dietary intake.

Nutritional support

Several controlled studies have evaluated the effect of nutritional support in COPD in both outpatients and inpatients, and the outcomes were related to the overall energy intake achieved. Weight gain was only achieved by substantially increasing energy intake by more than 30% above the usual intake, amounting to more than 190 kJ kg^{-1} (45 kcal kg^{-1}) per day. Moreover, improvement in muscle function or exercise tolerance occurred only with concomitant weight gain. In one of these controlled studies oral supplementation was given for 3 months to ambulatory malnourished patients with chronic obstructive lung disease. Daily energy intake increased by 48% above the usual intake and corresponded to 197 kJ kg^{-1} (47 kcal kg^{-1}) on average. The authors reported a mean weight gain of 4.2 kg, an increase in maximal respiratory pressures and in handgrip and sternomastoid strength, and a decrease in sternomastoid muscle fatiguability; similar improvements were not observed in a control group. However, these improvements were not maintained when oral supplementation was discontinued. In a further study, six malnourished patients received an additional 4.2 MJ (1000 kcal) via a nasogastric tube

for 16 days, whereas a control group of four received only an additional 420 kJ (100 kcal). A weight gain of 2.4 kg, and improvements in respiratory muscle strength and endurance were seen in the fed patients but not in the control groups. Other studies have not been able to demonstrate improvements in weight gain or muscle performance, but equally have been less successful in increasing energy intake.

Type of nutritional support If the patient with COPD is less than 90% of the ideal body weight for height, nutritional support should be considered. This can be difficult in COPD but it can be provided on three levels.

Normal high-energy, high-protein diet For many patients with COPD, adequate nutritional support may be provided by advising them to eact larger portions, frequent snacks and food fortification using high-energy and high-protein foods such as milk, yoghurt, butter and cream. Drinks of low nutritional value such as tea, fruit squash and clear soup should be discouraged. For some patients who lack vitality, use of readily prepared microwave dinners with a rest prior to mealtime may be helpful. A daily multivitamin and mineral supplement may be indicated.

Food supplements High-energy, high-protein supplements (**Table 1**) can be used to augment a patient's dietary intake. They are available in the form of milky sweet and savoury drinks, fortified fruit juices, milk shake powder, glucose polymer powders and liquids, and puddings. Patients and carers need to be given full instructions regarding their use in order to optimize this form of nutritional supplementation. Unfortunately, many studies have found in COPD that use of these supplements led to reduction in usual energy intake, and cause symptoms such as bloating, nausea and early satiety.

Tube feeding Overnight tube feeding should be considered in patients with COPD when oral methods of maintaining nutritional status have failed. The composition of tube feeds for patients with COPD has received some attention. Carbon dioxide production ($V\text{CO}_2$) is higher when carbohydrates are the main energy source and lower when fat is mainly oxidized. However, patients with COPD who are in a stable clinical state usually appear to tolerate carbohydrates without difficulty. Respiratory failure has not been reported in studies in patients with COPD receiving nutritional support with enteral feeds and nutritional supplements containing up to 54% carbohydrate, but further work

Table 1 Proprietary dietary supplements

Brand name	Form	Energy content
Fortified milk drinks		
Fortisip (Nutricia)	Liquid	300 kcal per 200 ml (1260 kJ)
Ensure Plus (Ross)	Liquid	300 kcal per 200 ml (1260 kJ)
Entera (Fresenius)	Liquid	300 kcal per 200 ml (1260 kJ)
Fresubin (Fresenius)	Liquid	200 kcal per 200 ml (840 kJ)
Milk shake powders		
Scandishake (SHS)	Powder	1 sachet + 240 ml milk = 600 kcal (2520 kJ)
Fortified fruit juices		
Fortijuice (Nutricia)	Liquid	250 kcal per 200 ml (1050 kJ)
Enlive (Ross)	Liquid	300 kcal per 240 ml (1260 kJ)
Provide (Fresenius)	Liquid	150 kcal per 250 ml (630 kJ)
Glucose drinks		
Calsip (Fresenius)	Liquid	200 kcal per 200 ml (840 kJ)
Hycal (Smith Kline)	Liquid	243 kcal per 171 ml (1021 kJ)
Liquid Polycal (Nutricia)	Liquid	500 kcal per 200 ml (2100 kJ)
Liquid Maxijul (SHS)	Liquid	400 kcal per 200 ml (1680 kJ)
Glucose polymer powders		
Super Soluble Maxijul (SHS)	Powder	384 kcal per 100 g (1613 kJ)
Polycal (Nutricia)	Powder	380 kcal per 100 g (1596 kJ)
Polycose (Abbott)	Powder	380 kcal per 100 g (1596 kJ)
Caloreen (Clintec)	Powder	400 kcal per 100 g (1680 kJ)

is needed to determine the optimal and safest feeding regimens for these patients.

Feeding patients on artificial ventilation

The artificial ventilator may be used to control the breathing pattern of patients who have acute breathing problems, e.g. respiratory failure with worsening blood gas concentrations. If the patient is able to be enterally fed, the composition of feed has a profound effect on gas exchanges, especially CO_2 production and therefore respiratory quotient (the ratio of CO_2 produced to O_2 consumed). As CO_2 production is greater during carbohydrate metabolism, a diet high in carbohydrate requires increased ventilation to eliminate the excess CO_2, whereas high-fat feeds reduce CO_2 production and are therefore potentially beneficial. Overfeeding negates any beneficial response to high-fat feeds, as the conversion of energy to fat involves a disproportionately large production of CO_2.

Cystic Fibrosis

Definition and aetiology

In cystic fibrosis (CF) there is widespread dysfunction of exocrine glands, which causes chronic pulmonary disease, pancreatic enzyme deficiency, intestinal obstruction in the neonate (distal intestinal obstruction syndrome), liver disease, infertility (especially in males) and abnormally high concentrations of electrolytes in the sweat. It is the most common inherited disease in white populations. A gene located on chromosome 7 (at $\Delta F508$ in 78% of UK patients) codes for the protein called cystic fibrosis transmembrane regulator (CFTR) which is defective in CF. This protein acts as a cyclic AMP-activated chloride channel blocker.

Incidence

Cystic fibrosis affects 1 in 2500 births in white populations, 1 in 20 000 in Afro-Caribbean populations and 1 in 1 000 000 births in Asians. It is almost unknown in Japan, China and black Africa.

Clinical features

Most children with CF present with malabsorption and failure to thrive, accompanied by recurrent or persistent chest infections. In the lungs viscid mucus in the smaller airways predisposes to chronic infection, particularly with *Staphylococcus aureus* and *Haemophilus influenzae*, and subsequently with *Pseudomonas* species. This leads to damage of the bronchial wall, bronchiectasis and abscess formation.

About 90% of CF patients have pancreatic insufficiency, requiring pancreatic enzyme supplements. Untreated patients pass frequent, large, pale, offensive, greasy stools. Ten to fifteen per cent of babies present with a meconium ileus resulting from the blockage of the terminal ileum by highly proteinaceous meconium at birth. Distal intestinal obstruction syndrome may occur later in childhood or adult life. In addition to these symptoms a number of other complications may occur in CF (**Table 2**).

Chemical pathology

The protein CFTR regulates the chloride channel in the cell at its luminal surface and its absence or dysfunction results in an abnormally high concentration of sodium in sweat and in a low water content in the mucus produced by airways, pancreas and intestine. In the lung, this leads to ciliary dysfunction and to repeated infection and colonization with bacteria, resulting in a vicious cycle of bacterial colonization, 'lung inflammation' and scarring, causing severe bronchiectasis which progressively destroys lung function.

Table 2 Complications of cystic fibrosis

Respiratory
   Pneumothorax
   Asthma, wheezing
   Haemoptysis
   Nasal polyps
   Respiratory failure
   Core pulmonale
   Allergic bronchopulmonary aspergillosis

Gastrointestinal
   Meconium ileus
   Rectal prolapse
   Distal intestinal obstruction syndrome
   Abdominal distension
   Colonic strictures
   Intussusception
   Gastrooesophageal reflux
   Biliary cirrhosis
   Hepatomegaly
   Portal hypertension
   Cholelithiasis
   Cholecystitis
   Obstructive jaundice
   Pancreatitis

Other
   Diabetes
   Male infertility
   Amyloidosis
   Arthropathy
   Salt depletion
   Growth failure, weight loss, failure to thrive
   Delayed puberty
   Osteopenia

Nutritional management

Nutritional intervention in CF is associated with better growth, improvement or stabilization of pulmonary function, and possibly improved survival. It is known in CF that malnutrition has many adverse effects on pulmonary function including decreased ventilatory drive, impaired pulmonary muscle function, decreased exercise tolerance and altered pulmonary immune response.

Reasons for malnutrition The nutritional problems in cystic fibrosis are multifactorial and include increases in intestinal losses, energy requirements and urinary glucose losses. One or more factors almost invariably coexist in combination with an inadequate energy intake. Malabsorption in CF occurs mainly as a result of maldigestion secondary to pancreatic insufficiency, which is rarely normal despite improved pancreatic enzyme preparations. In addition, abnormal bile salt metabolism, liver disease, mucosal absorptive abnormalities and short bowel syndrome, after intestinal resection in the neonatal period, may all contribute. It has been estimated that stool energy losses account for 10% of gross energy intake in CF, three times higher than normal.

Although patients with moderate lung disease may have a comparable total daily energy expenditure to controls, resting energy expenditure has been shown to be increased by 9–30%. This is related to the increased work of breathing, lung infection and inflammation, enteral feeding, and drugs such as salbutamol. Diabetes, if undiagnosed or inadequately controlled, may increase energy losses owing to glycosuria. Further substantial nutrient losses may occur in the sputum; these have been estimated as up to 1–5% of gross energy intake and up to 14% of total nitrogen losses. In addition, dietary assessments indicate that patients with CF have poor appetites and rarely achieve the 'normal' recommended energy intake (**Table 3**).

Nutritional support Nutritional requirements will vary according to the clinical state as well as the age, sex and activity of the individual, and it is impossible to give universal recommendations. Although it is commonly recommended to advocate an energy intake of 120–150% of estimated average requirements, it is better to assess and monitor energy intake and equate this to the nutritional status of the patient. If weight gain or growth is poor, the usual energy intake is increased by a further 20–30% of total intake. Of the total energy, it is recommended that 35–40% is supplied from fat, 15% from protein and 45–50% from carbohydrate.

Table 3 Factors associated with low dietary energy intake in cystic fibrosis

- Poor appetite
    respiratory infection
    abdominal pain, vomiting and oesophagitis
    side effects of medications, including nausea,
    vomiting, diarrhoea

- Behavioural feeding problems and eating disorders
    as a consequence of pressure to eat a high-
    energy, high-protein diet
    inappropriate concepts of body image

- Dislike of fatty or high-energy foods

- Poor use of dietary supplements
    used as meal replacements rather than as a
    supplement to meals
    may displace energy and nutrients provided by
    other foods so net energy intake does not
    improve
    excessive use may cause bloating, nausea and
    diarrhoea

- Lack of financial resources

- Consumer pressure and health promotions to eat high-
    fibre, low-sugar foods
    foods purchased for rest of family may be low-fat
    and low-sugar and are given to CF child for
    convenience
    13% of adult patients restrict fat as a
    consequence of health promotion messages

Nutritional support is provided on three levels according to the appetite and nutritional status of the patient.

High-energy, high-protein diet   A diet that encourages energy and protein-concentrated foods is advocated. Foods such as full-cream milk, cheese, meat, full-cream yoghurt, milk puddings, cakes and biscuits are encouraged. Frequent snacks are as important as regular meals, and it has been shown that overall energy intake is improved by 16% when the frequency is increased from three to four meals daily, and a further 7% when meals extend from four to five daily. However, it is necessary to establish good mealtime routines early, and not permit children to substitute sweets and chocolate for savoury food at mealtimes or unsatisfactory eating habits may develop which may be difficult to change in the future.

Dietary supplements   Although almost half of adult patients take dietary supplements (see Table 1), there are few published data to demonstrate their efficacy in CF. One recent study was unable to show any improvement in height and weight z scores when up to 30% of energy requirements were supplied by a supplement for 3 months. Dietary supplements should therefore be reserved for weight loss, any decline in height z score, if intake of a range of nutrients does not meet dietary reference values, or during acute chest infections. In order to avoid reducing the intake of normal food, the quantity recommended is age-dependent (**Table 4**).

Enteral nutrition   Only 5% of paediatric patients are likely to need enteral feeding. This should be considered if a child is persistently less than 85% expected weight for height, or has failed to gain weight over a 3–6 month period. Enteral feeding is associated with improvements in body fat, height, lean body mass, muscle mass, increased total body nitrogen, improved strength and development of secondary sexual characteristics. To produce lasting benefit, numerous studies have demonstrated that enteral feeding should be continued long-term. The choice of route used is influenced by the duration of feeding and by the preference of the patient and family.

It is common practice to give enteral feeding for 8–10 h overnight, with at least 40–50% of the estimated energy requirement given via the feed. Most patients tolerate an energy-dense polymeric feed providing at least $6.3 \, \text{kJ ml}^{-1}$ ($1.5 \, \text{kcal ml}^{-1}$) with additional pancreatic enzymes. However, there is some support for the use of chemically defined elemental or short-chain peptide feeds; these are generally low in fat and are administered without the use of pancreatic enzymes, although there is little evidence in favour of this practice and it would be disputed by some.

Vitamin and mineral supplements   Low serum concentrations of vitamin A are reported in CF, particularly when compliance with vitamin supplements is poor. Documented clinical features include night blindness, conjunctival and corneal xerosis, dry, thickened skin, and abnormalities of bronchial mucosal epithelialization. Routine additional vitamin

Table 4 Recommended dosage of dietary supplements in cystic fibrosis

Age (years)	Daily dosage of energy	
	(kcal)	(kJ)
1–2	200	840
3–5	400	1680
6–11	600	2520
>12	800	3360

From MacDonald (1994).

A supplements are given. However, this topic does warrant further study, as CF patients receiving vitamin A supplements are known to have a hepatic reserve nearly 3.5 times greater than that of normal controls, despite low serum concentrations, and there is concern this may lead to hepatic toxicity.

Reduced bone mineral density is repeatedly reported in adults with cystic fibrosis. The cause of this is likely to be multifactorial but is probably not related to abnormal bone mineral and vitamin D metabolism, although 25-hydroxyvitamin D levels have been reported to be low in adult patients. Possible contributory factors include low body mass index, disease severity, inadequate calcium intake, delayed puberty, and widespread use of systemic or inhaled steroids. Routine vitamin D (but not calcium) supplements are recommended for patients with pancreatic insufficiency.

Blood levels of vitamin E are nearly always low unless supplements are given. In older patients, undetectable serum concentrations of vitamin E have been noted in association with neurological syndromes. Symptoms include progressive ophthalmoplegia, unsteadiness on walking, loss of reflexes, tremor and ataxia.

Some CF centres recommend routine salt supplements to all CF infants on normal infant formula which is low in sodium, and during hot weather. Anorexia and poor growth may result from chronic salt depletion. Significant hyponatraemia may be accompanied by vomiting.

Pancreatic enzymes Approximately 90% of patients with cystic fibrosis require pancreatic enzymes to reduce steatorrhoea. These enzymes are derived from animal pancreatic extracts; they are presented in powder, tablet or capsule form and contain a combination of lipase, protease and amylase. In addition to enzyme content, many factors affect the bioavailability of pancreatic enzymes including enzyme source, manufacturing process, stability, enteric coating of acid-resistant tablets, formulation as microspheres or microtablets, and particle size. For children, the lower-strength enteric-coated microspheres are commonly used (Creon: Solvay; Pancrease: Cilag). These enzymes have been found to achieve 90% fat absorption if administered in appropriate dosages and are more effective than the original pancreatic powder.

Prognosis

Survival among patients with CF has steadily improved since the 1960s. Over a third of cystic fibrosis patients are now over the age of 15 years, and the CF population in the UK is increasing by 120–140 patients a year. It has been predicted that the median survival will be at least 40 years for children born in the 1990s.

Asthma

Definition and aetiology

Asthma is defined as reversible partial obstruction to airflow in the intrathoracic airways. It is caused by the smooth muscle surrounding the bronchi having an abnormally increased reaction to stimuli, which is thought to have an inflammatory basis. Specific bronchial stimuli include inhaled allergents, e.g. house-dust mite and pollen, cat, fur occupational allergens and drugs such as aspirin. Nonspecific bronchial stimuli include viral infections, cold, air, exercise, emotional stress and inhaled pollutants.

Prevalence

The incidence of asthma appears to be increasing and it is estimated that 10–15% of individuals will experience wheezing at some time in their lives. It is most common in children and it is twice as common in boys as in girls, but by adolescence equal numbers are affected.

Clinical features

Asthma usually presents as attacks of wheezing, which commonly occur following exercise and viral infections, and on exposure to cold air. Less severe symptoms are nocturnal coughing and wheezing. A cough producing small amounts of yellowish sputum or bronchial plugs is common. Some patients present with breathlessness alone or in cor pulmonale.

Pathology

A combination of a genetic predisposition and environmental influences (e.g. house-dust mite) results in chronic inflammation of the bronchial mucosa and airway hyperactivity. Exposure of the sensitized airway to a number of trigger factors results in bronchoconstriction, mucosal oedema and excessive mucus production which in turn lead to airway narrowing and the clinical features of asthma.

Dietetic management

Food intolerance There is some suggestion that intolerance to foods may act as a trigger for some cases of asthma. Common food allergens identified include milk, eggs, nuts, orange squash, wheat and red wine. The additives sulfur dioxide, tartrazine, sodium benzoate and salicylates have been implicated, although in the case of sulfur dioxide its ability to cause asthma depends on the nature of the food it is added to, the level of residual sulfur dioxide in the food and the sensitivity of the patient. Foods such as nuts, cola drinks, ice and foods cooked in oil have been found to cause symptoms more frequently in Asian children.

The incidence of food intolerance in asthma, although disputed, is thought to be small. In a study of 300 patients with asthma aged between 7 months to 80 years, only 11 patients were found to have reactions to food following placebo-controlled, double-blind challenges, and 5 of these had other reactions instead of asthma. In a further study, only 5 out of 54 teenagers with chronic asthma had a deterioration of lung function when given a double-blind oral provocation challenge with acetylsalicylic acid.

Both immediate and delayed onset symptoms have been reported in asthma. The use of diagnostic diets is difficult. This is partly because of the variability of asthma, delayed reactions, effect of other precipitating triggers and dangers of inducing an asthma attack during food challenges. A simple exclusion diet excluding foods implicated on history is perhaps the most useful diagnostic diet. Because of the inherent problems with asthma, strict elimination or oligoallergenic diets are rarely used.

Dietary sodium It has been suggested that a high salt intake may act as a trigger for asthma. A correlation between regional mortality from asthma and purchase of table salt per person has been reported in England and Wales. Experimental data have been reported to show that changes in dietary sodium intake can influence levels of airway reactivity or peak flow levels in patients with asthma. Other epidemiological studies have also suggested association between a higher dietary sodium intake and a higher prevalence of self-reported wheeze in adults and children. However, not all of the evidence supports this hypothesis. At least three epidemiological surveys and two experimental studies found no evidence of an association between sodium intake and asthma.

Prognosis

Asthma is responsible in the UK for 10–20% of all acute medical admissions to paediatric wards in children aged 1–14 years. There are 20–30 deaths from asthma in children each year and the overall mortality rate in the UK is more than 2000 per year.

See also: **Cystic Fibrosis**: Dietary Aspects and Nutritional Management. **Dietetics**: The Role of Dietetics in Health Care. **Energy**: Measurement of Energy Intake and Expenditure. **Nutritional Support**: Enteral Feeding. **Sodium**: Physiology. **Vitamin Supplementation**: Role.

Further Reading

Britton J, Pavord I, Richards K *et al.* (1994) Dietary sodium and the risk of airway hyper-reactivity in a random adult population. *Thorax* **49**:875–880.

Burney PGJ (1987) A diet rich in sodium may potentiate asthma: epidemiological evidence for a new hypothesis. *Chest* **91** (supplement):143–148S.

Couriel J (1997) Respiratory disorders. In: Lissauer T and Clayden G (eds) *Illustrated Textbook of Paediatrics*, pp 157–171. London: Mosby.

Crompton GK and Haslett C (1995) Diseases of the respiratory system. In: Edwards CRW, Bouchier IAD, Haslett C and Chilvers ER (eds) *Davidson's Principles and Practice of Medicine*, pp 313–404. Edinburgh: Churchill Livingstone.

Goldstein SA, Thomashow BM, Kvetan V, Askanazi J, Kinney JM and Elwyn DH (1988) Nitrogen and energy relationships in malnourished patients with emphysema. *American Review of Respiratory Disease* **138**:634–644.

Hind CRK and Walshaw MJ (1996) Chest disease. In: Axford J (ed.) *Medicine*, Chap. 7.1–7.9. Oxford: Blackwell.

Hodge L, Yan KY and Loblay RL (1996) Assessment of food chemical intolerance in adult asthmatic subjects. *Thorax* **51**:805–809.

Liebermann D and Heimer D (1991) Effect of dietary sodium on the severity of bronchial asthma. *Thorax* **47**:360–362.

MacDonald A (1994) Cystic fibrosis. In: Shaw V and Lawson M (eds) *Clinical Paediatric Dietetics*, pp. 110–124. Oxford: Blackwell.

Manaher S and Burke F (1996) Pulmonary disease. In: Morrison G and Hark L (eds) *Medical Nutrition and Disease*, pp 279–287. Oxford: Blackwell.

Openbrier DR, Irwin MM, Dauber JH, Owens G and Rogers RM (1984) Factors affecting nutritional status and the impact of nutritional support in patients with emphysema. *Chest* **85**:67–95.

Salamoni F, Roulet M, Gudinchet F, Pilet M, Thieband D and Burckhardt P (1996) Bone mineral content in cystic fibrosis patients: correlation with fat free mass. *Archives of Disease in Childhood* **74**:314–318.

Vandenbergh E, Van de Woestijne KP and Gyselen A (1967) Weight changes in the terminal stages of chronic obstructive pulmonary disease. *American Review of Respiratory Disease* **95**:556–565.

Walters S, Britton J and Hodson ME (1994) Hospital care for adults with cystic fibrosis; an overview and comparison between special cystic fibrosis clinics and general clinics using a patient questionnaire. *Thorax* **49**:300–306.

Intensive Care Management

Susan McAreavey and **Patricia Queen Samour,**
Nutrition Services, Beth Israel Deaconess Medical
Center, Boston, Massachusetts, USA

Copyright © 1998 Academic Press

Therapeutic dietetics is the provision of nutritional therapy to prevent and/or treat malnutrition, including both macro- and micronutrient deficiencies. In the context of the intensive care unit (ICU) other management goals include promoting positive nitrogen balance for wound healing, correcting fluid, metabolic or electrolyte imbalances, and improving patient outcomes. To meet these needs, an understanding of the metabolic response to injury is imperative as this will affect the nutrition support regimen. Factors such as the type of nutrition support (enteral and parenteral), initiation, route (e.g. gastric, jejunal) and rate must be seriously evaluated and changes made as the patient's status changes. Each patient requires an individualized nutrition assessment with ongoing nutritional management throughout their stay in the ICU.

The provision of adequate amounts of energy and protein is critical to patient outcome in order to maintain lean body mass and support wound healing. Nutritional goals can be achieved by the early initiation of nutrition support, preferably enterally if the gut is adequately perfused. If goals are unattainable by enteral support alone, a combination of parenteral and enteral may be used or the parenteral route can be used until gut function improves.

Patients in the ICU present many challenges to the dietetics practitioner as these patients are often physiologically stressed owing to the metabolic response to injury and their metabolic status can change radically during their course of treatment.

Malnutrition

Malnutrition is a common problem in the critically ill patient which may be present on admission or develop in the ICU. Malnutrition may develop quickly secondary to hypermetabolism and hypercatabolism commonly seen in the ICU patient. Without adequate exogenous energy and protein, energy is obtained from excessive protein breakdown of both muscle and visceral protein, and gluconeogenesis. Malnutrition has many detrimental effects on the major body systems including respiratory, cardiac and gastrointestinal (GI) tract. Patients who are malnourished are at a higher risk of developing infections and experiencing delayed wound healing. They also have a higher incidence of mortality and morbidity and a longer length of stay in the ICU than non-malnourished patients.

Metabolic Response to Trauma, Injury or Sepsis

It is critical to nutrition management to understand how the metabolic response to injury affects substrate utilization, initiation and route of nutrition support. The metabolic response to injury may be initiated by a number of stimuli such as sepsis, inflammation, shock, thermal injury and trauma. The magnitude of the response depends upon the type, severity and duration of the injury. This response to injury is commonly called the ebb and flow phases (**Table 1**).

The ebb (shock) phase usually lasts 24–48 h and is characterized by hypovolaemic shock, decreased tissue perfusion, hypometabolism and tissue hypoxia. The flow phase has two responses: the acute and adaptive phases. The acute phase develops after the patient is fluid resuscitated and haemodynamically stable. There is also an increased energy

Table 1 Metabolic response to injury or critical illness

Ebb phase (hypovolaemic shock)	Flow phase – acute (catabolism predominates)	Flow phase – adaptive (anabolism predominates)
↓ Tissue perfusion	↑ Glucocorticoids	Hormone response gradually diminishes
↓ Metabolic rate	↑ Glucogen	↓ Hypermetabolic rate
↓ Oxygen consumption	↑ Catecholamines	Potential for restoration of body protein
↓ Blood pressure	Release of cytokines	Wound healing
↓ Body temperature	Production of acute-phase proteins	
	↑ Excretion of nitrogen	
	↑ Oxygen consumption	
	Impaired utilization of fuels	

Source: Pendley et al. (1994). Used with permission of Ross Products Division, Abbott Laboratories, Columbus, OH. From Enteral Nutrition Support in Critical Care. © 1994 Ross Products Division, Abbott Laboratories.

expenditure and catabolism. The acute flow phase will subside within 7–10 days unless there is further injury or trauma which would prolong hypermetabolism. The adaptive flow phase occurs when the hormonal response is diminished with a resultant decrease in hypermetabolism.

During the ebb phase, management is focused on haemodynamic stability and not on nutrition. Once haemodynamic stability is achieved, nutrition support should be implemented as quickly as possible. Once adequate nutrient intake is provided, tissue repair and restoration of body stores is possible.

Effects of Stress on Substrate Utilization

Knowledge of the metabolic response to injury as it affects nutrient metabolism and body composition is essential for nutrition management. In this stress situation, hypermetabolism results in an increased mobilization of stored substrates including carbohydrate, protein and free fatty acids. Each substrate plays a key role in the response to stress. Glucose is an important fuel for the healing process as well as for metabolism of the central nervous system and the immune system. Glucose is initially provided from glycolysis (use of glycogen) followed by gluconeogenesis (glucose production from fat and amino acids). The resultant rise in circulating glucose results in an increased insulin secretion. Hyperglycaemia is common in the ICU patient owing to insulin resistance and excessive glucose production via gluconeogenesis. Protein is needed for gluconeogenesis, synthesis of acute-phase proteins, thermogenesis and tissue repair. Protein catabolism is initiated by glucagon, catecholamines and cortisol during the injury response. Protein, broken down into its constituent amino acids, is preferentially mobilized from peripheral muscle initially, sparing visceral protein stores. Fatty acids and glycerol are mobilized by catecholamine-stimulated lipolysis. These mobilized fatty acids are used to provide energy for cardiac and skeletal muscle, liver and other tissues.

Starvation Metabolism Versus Stress Metabolism

Starvation metabolism is similar to stress metabolism in that in early starvation the primary fuel sources are stored glycogen and glucose synthesized by gluconeogenesis. As starvation continues, an adaptive response occurs in which fatty acids, ketones and glycerol become primary fuel sources, sparing protein stores. The result is decreased catabolism. In stress metabolism, ketone production is decreased compared to starvation. Catabolism ensues and

results in rapid depletion of fat and protein stores. Protein synthesis is increased in the stress response with the increased production of acute-phase proteins and in the process of tissue repair to support healing. Unfortunately, the rate of catabolism most often exceeds this, resulting in depleted muscle and visceral protein stores. A normal healthy adult may withstand a week of (non-intensive care) stress without protein and energy intake. The ICU patient will use their storage fuels more quickly owing to the intense catabolism. Eventually, in such a patient, decreased protein synthesis, organ dysfunction, impaired immune response, sepsis, and eventually death, will result.

Nutrition Assessment

Critically ill ICU patients require ongoing nutritional assessment and management. Assessment should begin on admission to the unit and include screening for pre-existing malnutrition. Patients with past medical histories of alcoholism, liver disease, renal failure, cardiac failure, cancer, AIDS or inflammatory bowel disease are at a higher risk for being malnourished on admission. Evaluation of weight history prior to admission is important as fluid overload and peripheral oedema are common in the ICU. This information should be obtained from the patient's care-givers when possible. A recent unintentional weight loss of >10% usual body weight (UBW) may be indicative of pre-existing malnutrition. Hepatic secretory proteins such as albumin, transferrin, retinol binding protein and prealbumin are laboratory indicators of malnutrition. Use of these parameters is of limited value in the ICU as factors such as fluid status, hepatic dysfunction, infection and inflammation affect their reliability. Preinjury biochemical data are more useful in screening for baseline nutritional status.

Nutrient Requirements

Energy

Assessment of energy needs in the ICU patient is another challenge for the dietetic practitioner. Owing to the hypermetabolism associated with stress and injury, energy needs are elevated to a variable degree depending on the severity of the injury. It is important, however, to avoid both over- and underfeeding. Over-feeding may result in hyperglycaemia, hepatic steatosis, immunosuppression, impaired liver function and increased resting energy expenditure (REE). Under-feeding may lead to progressive weight loss, impaired wound healing, infection, protein malnutrition, organ failure and death.

Two common methods of determining energy needs in the ICU setting are by (1) factorial methods, and (2) indirect calorimetry. Factorial methods utilize predictive equations. The Harris–Benedict equation is commonly used to predict REE, based on age, weight, height and sex (**Table 2**). Typically, a stress factor is added to account for the increased metabolic demands of stress and injury. This method of estimating energy needs may overestimate the actual energy expenditure of the ICU patient owing to such variables as decreased work of breathing with mechanical ventilation, sedation, and the use of paralytic agents which decrease metabolic rate. Other predictive equations, specifically designed for critically ill ICU patients, are available; these include factors for sepsis, trauma and mechanical ventilation. Energy needs of the critically ill can usually be met by providing energy in the range of 100–125 kJ (25–30 kcal) per kg body weight. Increased energy needs are found in patients with severe stress, sepsis or burns.

Indirect calorimetry is the other frequently used method of determining energy needs. This method is more accurate than factorial methods. It measures oxygen consumption and carbon dioxide production to determine REE. Indirect calorimetry is indicated for patients with altered body composition, inappropriate response to conventional nutrition support, difficulty weaning from ventilator support, postoperative organ transplantation and sepsis.

Energy sources A mixed fuel diet is recommended in meeting the energy needs of the critical care patient; they should consist of 30–70% energy from carbohydrate, 15–20% from protein and 15–30% from fat. The primary fuel during critical illness is glucose. Hyperglycaemia is common in the stressed patient. As elevated glucose levels can affect immunological function, glycaemic control is important. The excessive provision of parenteral carbohydrate is associated with hepatic steatosis and lipogenesis, as well as increased carbon dioxide production which can compromise respiratory function and exacerbate hyperglycaemia. To reduce the risk of these complications parenteral administration of 4–5 mg per kg per minute should not be exceeded. Protein needs will be described in detail below. Fat should provide the balance of energy needs and an adequate intake of linoleic acid is needed to prevent an essential fatty acid deficiency (4% of total energy). Diets high in n-6 polyunsaturated fatty acids (PUFA) are immunosuppressive. A lower rate of n-6 to n-3 (e.g. fish oil) may be appropriate when excessive inflammation is present and an enhanced immune response is desired. Medium-chain triglyceride (MCT) oil contains fats of chain lengths of from 6 to 12 carbons. They are advantageous in oral–enteral feeding of the stressed and septic patient, as there is no need for pancreatic lipase and bile salts for digestion. MCTs are also beneficial in hyperlipidaemia.

Most parenteral fat solutions are composed of long-chain fatty acids (LCFA), i.e. those greater than 16 carbons in length, these may be immunosuppressive when infused over short periods of time. Continuous infusion of the fat emulsion over 12–24 h may be more desirable. Enteral products contain a combination of n-6 and n-3 fatty acids and the amount varies depending on the product. Many formulae also contain varying amounts of MCT oil. Although there are no established requirements for n-3 fatty acids in the ICU patient, their use is under clinical investigation as immune-enhancing and anti-inflammatory agents.

Protein

Protein needs of the normal healthy adult can be met with 0.8 g per kg body weight. With critical illness these needs increase to 1.5–2.0 g per kg body weight, depending on the severity of the injury. Providing levels above this amount does not improve uptake and utilization, and excessive amounts of protein may lead to ureagenesis. A recommended intake of 1.5 g per kg body weight during the catabolic phase should be provided to match losses. Protein may be increased during the flow-adaptive phase when restoration of lean body mass is possible. Protein needs may be estimated by measuring 24-hour urinary excretion of nitrogen. Total nitrogen excretion also includes nitrogen lost in faeces, skin and the

Table 2 Harris–Benedict equation for estimating energy expenditure (REE) (In Nutrition Support: Theory and Therapeutics. Eds Shikora et al)

| Males: | $REE = 66.5 + 13.8W + 5.0H - 6.8A$ |
| Females: | $REE = 655.1 + 9.6W + 1.8H - 4.7A$ |

Stress factor	Adjustments for REE (%)
Mild starvation	0.85–1.00
Postoperative (no complications)	1.00–1.05
Peritonitis	1.05–1.25
Cancer	1.10–1.45
Severe head injury	1.30–1.50
Multiple trauma	1.25–1.75
Severe infection	1.50–1.75
Thermal injury	1.25–2.00

W, weight in kg; H height in cm; A, age in years. The stress factors have been subsequently added to compensate for the increased energy expenditure of illness.

respiratory tract. Additional losses must be taken into consideration if there is fistula output, wound drainage, dialysis, diarrhoea or gastric output.

Patients with renal and/or hepatic failure may not tolerate protein in the range of 1.5–2.0 g per kg body weight. However, restricting protein in these patients may lead to further protein depletion. Close monitoring of biochemical data and tolerance to protein intake is an essential component of nutritional management of these metabolically compromised high-risk patients.

Use of specialized amino acids such as branched-chain amino acids (BCAA), glutamine and arginine may be beneficial in the critically ill patient. BCAA supplemented parenteral and enteral nutrition formulae may result in improved nitrogen retention and hepatic protein synthesis, and decreased protein degradation. Glutamine is the preferred fuel for the gut enterocyte, a building block for nucleotides, and a source of glutathione which protects the enterocyte as an antioxidant. Glutamine protects and helps heal the gut, especially during critical illness, and may reduce the duration of the infection and the length of stay in the ICU. Additional research is needed in this area as to the benefits of glutamine and the amounts needed as a supplement to parenteral and enteral feeding. The use of arginine is also controversial and additional clinical research is needed with this specialized amino acid. Arginine has been shown to exhibit a trophic effect on the thymus and enhances the responsiveness of macrophages and lymphocytes to antigens. While supplementation may improve host immunity in the critically ill patient, a minimal effective dose has not been established.

Vitamins and minerals

Vitamins and minerals are essential to maintaining normal metabolic processes and may become deficient in critical illness. The exact requirements for micronutrients for the critically ill patient are unknown. Deficiencies of micronutrients are unusual when individuals are fed adequately and have normal metabolism. However, with critical illness both intake and normal metabolism are altered. Critically ill patients have greater requirements and may have abnormal losses of micronutrients. Both enteral and parenteral solutions/formulations have sufficient amounts to maintain serum levels of most patients, but for the critically ill it may be insufficient.

Potassium, magnesium, zinc, and phosphorus should be provided at levels that will maintain normal serum levels. Zinc is important in enzymatic reactions within the body and a deficiency may result

Table 3 Suggested daily mineral supplementation for the critically ill

Mineral	RDA	Recommendation for the critically ill patient
Iron	10 mg	–
Zinc	12–15 mg	50 mg
Copper	2–3 mg	–
Chromium	0.05–0.2 mg	–
Selenium	55–70 μg	100 μg
Manganese	0.15–0.8 mg	25–50 mg
Molybdenum	0.15–0.5 mg	0.2–0.5 mg

Data compiled from multiple sources. Table taken from Shikora SA and Blackburn GL (eds) (1997) *Nutrition Support: Theory and Therapeutics*. New York: Chapman & Hall.

in impaired wound healing. Zinc, copper and selenium are crucial for normal metabolism and may also serve as antioxidants. See **Table 3** for suggested daily mineral supplementation for critically ill.

Supplemental vitamins A and C are suggested in critical illness as they aid in wound healing. There has also been a recent increase in the use of antioxidants such as vitamins E and C in the critically ill. However, further research is needed in this area. See **Table 4** for suggested daily vitamin supplements for critically ill.

Table 4 Suggested daily vitamin supplementation for the critically ill

Vitamin	RDA	Recommendation for the critically ill patient
Fat-soluble vitamins		
A	1000 iu	2500–10 000 iu
D	400 iu	400 iu
E	12–15 iu	400 iu
K	1 μg kg^{-1}	1 mg
Water-soluble vitamins		
B$_1$ (thiamin)	1–1.5 mg	10 mg
B$_2$ (riboflavin)	1.1–1.8 mg	10 mg
B$_6$ (pyridoxine)	1.6–2.2 mg	20 mg
B$_{12}$	2–3 μg	20 mg
Niacin	14–20 mg	200 mg
Pantothenic acid	4–10 mg	100 mg
Biotin	80–100 μg	5 mg
Folic acid	180–200 μg	2 mg
C (ascorbic acid)	45–60 mg	1000 mg

Data compiled from multiple sources. Table taken from Shikora SA and Blackburn GL (eds) (1997) *Nutrition Support: Theory and Therapeutics*. New York: Chapman & Hall.

Initiation and Mode of Nutrition Support

Early nutrition support is recommended in critical illness to avoid the malnutrition associated with hypermetabolism and hypercatabolism. Prior to initiating nutrition support, the patient must be hemodynamically stable (at the beginning of the acute flow phase; see Table 1). The patient must also have stable vital functions, an acid–base balance within physiological range, and adequate perfusion of tissues.

Parenteral access through a central line can be used early in the ICU patient to provide nutrients until the GI tract can be used. Parenteral support should be used in patients with pancreatic dysfunction or a nonfunctioning GI tract such as short bowel syndrome or severe malabsorption. Parenteral support does have associated GI and metabolic complications. Potential GI complications include fatty liver, cholestasis and gut atrophy. A comprehensive assessment and rapid transition to enteral formula when possible will help reduce these complications. Potential metabolic complications are also a concern; these include hyper/hypoglycaemia, electrolyte abnormalities, hypertriglyceridemia, prerenal azotaemia and hyper/hypovolaemia. Close monitoring of biochemical indices, fluid balance and electrolyte status may help minimize complications associated with parenteral feeding.

Patients in the ICU should be transferred from parenteral to enteral nutrition as early as possible. However, gastric ileus is common in critical illness and may result in poor tolerance to gastric feeding. Narcotics which are commonly used in the ICU setting also decrease gastric motility and cause difficulty in advancing gastric feeding. Nasojejunal placement or jejunostomy feeding tube are optimal in the ICU. As the jejunum recovers more quickly postoperatively, this type of feeding route allows for the early initiation of enteral feeding. If enteral nutrition support will be of a chronic nature, then other tube sites and/or types of feeding tubes can be used (e.g. gastrostomy).

Relative Benefits of Enteral Support

There are numerous benefits of using enteral nutrition when feeding the critically ill patient. Enteral feeding helps to maintain gut integrity and reduce the risk of infections. Enteral nutrition is more physiological than parenteral nutrition and stimulates nutritive blood flow and gut trophic factors. Early enteral feeding may reduce the hypermetabolic response to injury. Enteral support is far less expensive than parenteral support.

The contraindications to initiating enteral nutrition include mesenteric ischaemic, septic or cardiogenic shock, bowel obstruction (unless feeding below the obstruction is possible), and a small bowel resection greater than 90%. Early enteral feeding is feasible when feeding postpylorically beyond the ligament of Trietz. Initiation of feeding with a low-fat elemental formula is possible within 24 h of surgery or upon admission to the ICU in nonsurgical patients. All enteral feeding should be initiated at a low flow rate and advanced slowly. Feeding tolerance and advancement of feeding should be evaluated according the ICU guidelines. Beginning feeding at $10 \, cm^3$ per hour with an elemental or predigested formula and advancing daily by increments of $10 \, cm^3$ per hour is a common practice. Once the patient has reached the established goal rate, transition may be made to a standard polymeric formula. Standard polymeric formulae may be used initially if there is adequate GI tract perfusion, bowel sounds, and sufficient pancreatic function to ensure digestion of nutrients.

Formula Selection

There are three major types of enteral formulae used in the critical care setting (**Table 5**). These are: standard polymeric, predigested (elemental and/or peptide-based) and disease-specific. Standard polymeric formulae are usually $1.0 \, kcal \, ml^{-1}$, but higher concentrations are available commercially. Product selection should be based on the energy needs of the patient, the amount of fluid available for enteral nutrition, and the requirement for micro- and macronutrients to provide 100% of established needs.

Standard polymeric formulae require pancreatic enzymes for digestion. These formulae vary in their amount of protein and fibre, in particular. High-protein formulae with more than 20% of energy from protein are typically needed in the ICU patient. The rationale for giving fibre-containing formulae to a patient is to maintain normal bowel function. Enteral products containing insoluble and soluble fibre are usually well tolerated in patients.

Soluble fibre can be fermented by colonic bacteria, enhancing bacterial growth and the production of short-chain fatty acids. Short-chain fatty acids are the fuel for the colonocyte; its role in the ICU patient requires further research.

Predigested formulae include elemental formulae that contain free amino acids and/or peptides. Critically ill patients may not tolerate standard polymeric formulae owing to malabsorption, diarrhoea, GI atrophy or organ dysfunction. ICU patients may benefit from formulae containing di- or tripeptides versus free amino acids or intact proteins. Numerous

Table 5 Adult oral and enteral formulae (for product information, contact a local sales representative or contact the manufacturer directly – see listing of manufacturers at foot of table)

Formula	Manufacturer	Formula	Manufacturer
Standard polymeric formulae (approximately 1.0–1.2 kcal ml^{-1} and 14–16% of total energy as protein, intact macronutrients, usually lactose-free, low osmolality)		**Predigested/elemental formulae** (approximately 1.0–1.5 kcal ml^{-1} and 8–17% of total energy as protein; nutrients are partially or fully hydrolysed, lactose-free, high osmolality)	
Attain	Sherwood Medical	Accupep HPF	Sherwood Medical
Ensure	Ross	Alitraq	Ross
Isocal	Mead Johnson	Crucial	Nestlé
Isosource	Novartis	Criticare HN	Mead Johnson
Nutrilan	Elan	Immun-Aid	McGaw
Nutrition	Nutrition Medical	L-Emental	Nutrition Medical
Nutren 1.0	Nestlé	L-Emental Plus	Nutrition Medical
Resource	Novartis	Peptamen	Nestlé
Osmolite	Ross	Peptamen VHP	Nestlé
		Perative	Ross
High-nitrogen polymeric formulae (approximately 1.0–2.0 kcal ml^{-1} and >15% of total energy as protein, intact macronutrients, lactose-free, low-to-moderate osmolality)		ProPeptide	Nutrition Medical
		ProPeptide VHN	Nutrition Medical
		Reabilan	Nestlé
		Reabilan HN	Nestlé
		Sandosource Peptide	Novartis
Boost	Mead Johnson	Vital HN	Ross
Ensure High Protein	Ross	Tolerex	Novartis
Ensure Plus HN	Ross	TraumaCal	Mead Johnson
Isocal HN	Mead Johnson	Vivonex Plus	Novartis
Isolan	Elan	Vivonex T.E.N.	Novartis
Isosource HN	Novartis		
Isotein HN	Novartis	**Milk-based formulae** (designed as oral supplements, lactose-containing)	
Nitrolan	Elan		
Osmolite HN	Ross	Carnation Instant Breakfast	Nestlé
Promote	Ross	Meritene Powder	Novartis
Replete	Nestlé	Sustacal Nutritional Powder	Mead Johnson
Sustacal	Mead Johnson	Sustagen	Mead Johnson
High-nitrogen polymeric formulae with fibre (approximately 1.0–2.0 kcal ml^{-1} and >15% of total energy as protein, intact macronutrients, lactose-free, contain fibre from natural food sources of soya polysaccharide, osmolality varies)		**Specialty formulae** (designed to meet specialized nutrient demands of specific disease states or medical conditions)	
		Half-strength	
Fibersource HN	Novartis	Entrition 0.5	Nestlé
Isosource VHN	Novartis	Introlan	Elan
Promote with Fiber	Ross	Introlite	Ross
Protain XL	Sherwood Medical	Pre-Attain	Sherwood Medical
Replete with Fiber	Nestlé		
		Low carbohydrate-high fat	
		Isosource 1.5 Calorie	Novartis
		Nutrivent	Nestlé
		Pulmocare	Ross
		Respalor	Mead Johnson

Elan Pharma Nutrition Division, (formerly O'Brien/KMI), 2 Thurber Blvd, Smithfield, RI 02917, USA; (+1) 800-237-3535.
McGaw, Inc., 2525 McGaw Ave, PO Box 19791, Irvine. CA 92713-9791, USA; (+1) 800-854-6851.
Mead Johnson Europe, c/o BMS Pharmaceutical Group, LaGrande Arche, 92044 Paris La Defense Cedex, France; (+33) 1 40 90 66 47.
Mead Johnson Nutritional Group, 2400 West Lloyd Expressway, Evansville, IN 47721-0001, USA; (+1) 800-457-3550.
Nestlé Clinical Nutrition Co, 3 Parkway North, Suite 500, PO Box 760, Deerfield, IL 60015-0760, USA; (+1) 800-422-2752.
Novartis Nutrition Corp., 5320 West 23rd St, PO Box 370, Minneapolis, MN 55440, USA; (+1) 800-999-9978.
Nutrition Medical, 308 12th Ave S, Buffalo, MN 55313, USA; (+1) 800-569-7828.
Ross Laboratories, 625 Cleveland Ave, Columbus, OH 43215, USA; (+1) 800-551-5838.
Sherwood Medical, 1915 Olive St, St Louis, MO 63103, USA; (+1) 800-428-4400.

studies substantiate an improved absorption and retention of nitrogen with peptide-based formulae.

There are numerous commercially available enteral products designed for specific diseases or conditions. These include renal disease, hepatic disease, respiratory compromise and immune system enhancement. Enteral formulae developed for renal impairment contain balanced amino acids from high biological value protein with modified electrolytes. In the ICU patient, restricting protein is not advisable as it may result in further catabolism, immune system impairment and poor patient outcome. If necessary, short-term dialysis may be warranted.

The development of hepatic formulae was based on the assumption that patients with hepatic dysfunction could not metabolize certain amino acids, leading to elevated plasma amino acids crossing the blood–brain barrier and resulting in encephalopathy. It was hypothesized that feeding patients with formulae enriched with branched-chain amino acids and devoid of aromatic amino acids could correct encephalopathy. These hepatic formulae also contain minimal electrolytes which could exacerbate ascites and renal failure. Although they have advantages in the short term, they have poor protein quality. As liver function improves, transition should be made to a standard high-protein polymeric formula. The need for specific formulae for patients with pulmonary compromise (e.g. low-carbohydrate, high-fat contents) is met with reservation. By feeding a lower total amount of energy as suggested in critical illness, the need for such specialized products is averted, and less carbohydrate administration will automatically correspond to less carbon dioxide produced. Immune-enhancing formulae containing RNA, nucleotides, arginine, fish oils and structured lipids are available; these are being evaluated in patients who are immunosuppressed post trauma. Several studies have shown a reduction in postoperative complications such as infection and organ failure and a reduced length of overall hospital stay.

Monitoring tolerance to enteral formulae in the ICU is as important as the selection of the product. GI complications include delayed gastric emptying, abdominal distension and constipation. Careful selection of formula and placement of feeding tube, monitoring tolerance and progression to established goal rates can ensure optimal nutrition and minimize complications. Potential metabolic complications include hyper/hypglycaemia, hypertonic dehydration, overhydration and electrolyte abnormalities. Close monitoring of laboratory data, intake and output balance and daily weighing will allow for prevention – and timely treatment – of potential problems.

See also: **Amino Acids**: Chemistry and Classification; Metabolism. **Ascorbic Acid**: Physiology, Dietary Sources and Requirements. **Dietary Fibre (Fiber)**: Physiological Effects and Effects on Absorption. **Energy**: Measurement of Energy Intake and Expenditure. **Fatty Acids**: Health Effects of n-6 Polyunsaturated Fatty Acids; Health Effects of n-3 Polyunsaturated Fatty Acids. **Magnesium**: Physiology, Dietary Sources and Requirements. **Malnutrition**: Definition, Classification and Epidemiology; Primary Malnutrition; Secondary Malnutrition. **Nutritional Status**: Dietary Assessment. **Phosphorus**: Physiology, Dietary Sources and Requirements. **Potassium**: Physiology, Dietary Sources and Requirements. **Protein**: Requirements and Role in Diet. **Retinol**: Physiology. **Zinc**: Physiology.

Further Reading

Babineau TJ, Pomposelli T, Forse RA and Blackburn GL (1994) Lipids. *Nutrition in Critical Care*. St Louis: CV Mosby.

Bower RH, Cerra FB, Bershadsky B, Licari JJ, Hoyt DB, Jensen GL, Van Buren CT, Rothkopf MM, Daly JM and Adelsberg BR (1995) Early enteral administration of a formula (Impact) supplemented with arginine, nucleotides, and fish oil in intensive care unit patients: results of a multicenter, prospective, randomized, clinical trial. *Critical Care Medicine* 23:652–659.

Cerra F, Benitez MR, Blackburn GL, Irwin RS, Jeejeebhoy L, Shronts E, Wolf RR and Zaloga GP (1997) Applied nutrition in ICU patients: a consensus statement of the American College of Chest Physicians. *Chest* 111:769–778.

Donald P, Miller E and Shirmer B (1994) Repletion of nutritional parameters in surgical patients receiving peptide versus amino acid elemental feedings. *Nutrition Research* 14:13–17.

Gottschlich MM, Matarese LE and Shronts EP (eds) (1993) *Nutrition Support Dietitians Core Curriculum*, 2nd edn. Baltimore: American Society of Parenteral and Enteral Nutrition.

Kinsella JE, Lokesh B, Broughton S and Whelan J (1990) Dietary polyunsaturated fatty acids and eicosaniods: potential effects on the modulation of inflammatory and immune cells: an overview. *Nutrition* 6:24–44.

Pendley FC, Geckle RK and Campbell SM (1994) In: Gussler JD (ed.) *Enteral Nutrition Support in Critical Care, A Practical Reference for Clinicans*, Abbott Laboratories, Ohio: Ross Products Division.

Porter C and Cohen NH (1996) Indirect calorimetry in critically ill patients: role of the clinical dietitian in interpreting results. *Journal of the American Dietetic Association* 96:49–57.

Shikora SA (1997) Nutritional support for critically ill. In: Shikora SA and Blackburn GL (eds) *Nutrition Support: Theory and Practice*, pp 464–480. New York: Chapman & Hall.

Shou J (1994) Glutamine. In: Zaloga G (ed.) *Nutrition in Critical Care*. St Louis: CV Mosby.

Stack JA, Babineau TJ and Bistrian BR (1996) Assessment of nutritional status in clinical practice. *Gastroentologist* 4 (supplement 1): S8–S15.

Ziegler F, Olliver JM, Cynober L, *et al.* (1990) Efficiency of enteral nitrogen support in surgical patients: small peptides versus nondegraded proteins. *Gut* 31:1277–1283.

Short Bowel Syndrome

L Howard, Albany Medical College, Albany, New York, USA

M Malone, Albany College of Pharmacy, Albany, New York, USA

The nutritional management of the short bowel syndrome patient can be a significant therapeutic challenge. Prior to discussing the issues involved in the therapy of these patients it is important to define this syndrome, its aetiology, prevalence, pathophysiology, clinical manifestations and diagnosis.

Definition

Short bowel syndrome describes a patient who has lost sufficient bowel absorbing surface such that malabsorption of a range of nutrients leads to malnutrition. The loss of bowel can result from gastrointestinal disease or trauma, usually associated with extensive surgical resection or bowel bypass. The loss always involves the small intestine and may also involve part or all of the large intestine and/or stomach.

Short-bowel-related malnutrition usually presents as weight loss, diarrhoea, dehydration and specific mineral and vitamin deficiency syndromes.

Aetiology

Table 1 lists common adult and paediatric causes of short bowel syndrome. Prior to the availability of total parenteral nutrition, few patients survived massive bowel resection. Parenteral nutrition allows the patient to meet their massive fluid and electrolyte losses and to maintain their protein and energy status while their remaining bowel slowly adapts. There is always an uncertainty as to how complete the adaptation will be, and whether the patient will be able to survive without artificial nutrition. In the 1980s, the commonest aetiologies of the short bowel syndrome were Crohn's disease or mesenteric thrombosis in adults and necrotizing enterocolitis or intestinal atresia in children. This reflected in part the diagnoses in which physicians were prepared to gamble that patients could recover from a massive bowel resection and lead a near-normal life. The recent availability of long-term intravenous nutrition at home has changed the medical perspective as to which patients can benefit from massive bowel resection and still experience meaningful survival. For this reason, in most medically advanced countries cancer of the gastrointestinal tract is now the commonest cause of short bowel syndrome.

Prevalence

Although the true prevalence of the short bowel syndrome is not known, some information exists about the number of patients going home on parenteral nutrition in the United States and Western European countries and for most of these patients gastrointestinal failure due to resection or extensive disease of the small bowel is the primary problem.

In 1992, using Medicare data and information from the North American Home Parenteral Nutrition Registry, it was estimated that this therapy was used in 120 per million population in the USA. This was significantly higher than the treatment rate quoted in the UK and Europe in the same period. Prevalence data of HPN per million population were 5 in the UK, 1.7–2.6 in France, Holland, Belgium and Italy and 13.9 in Denmark. The commonest underlying diagnosis for US patients was cancer, accounting for 40% of all patients in whom home parenteral nutrition was initiated. As shown in **Table 2**, this represents a shift from a preponderance of patients with Crohn's disease and mesenteric

Table 1 Causes of the short bowel syndrome

Adults	Children
Crohn's disease	Necrotizing enterocolitis
Mesenteric infarction	Intestinal atresia
Radiation enteritis	Midgut volvulus
Malignancy	Gastroschisis
Trauma	Aganglionosis
Jejunal ileal bypass	Trauma

Table 2 Changes in underlying diagnosis of patients receiving home parenteral nutrition

Year	Crohn's disease and ischaemic bowel disease	Neoplasm
1978[a]	63%	17%
1985–91[b]	17%	40%

[a]358 patients: NY Academy of Medicine TPN Registry.
[b]5393 patients: North American HPEN Patient Registry.

infarction in the late 1970s to a greater current use in cancer patients. The same shift has occurred in a number of European countries and may reflect more universal agreement that home parenteral nutrition is relatively safe and is cost-effective if it leads to dehospitalization, even when life expectancy is short.

Pathophysiology

A number of factors influence the severity of symptoms following intestinal resection. These include the extent and site of the small bowel resected, the presence or absence of the ileocaecal valve, the preservation of colon and/or stomach, the health of the remaining bowel and the amount of time elapsed since the resection allowing for full adaption.

Extent and site of the small bowel resected

In a normal adult the small bowel consists of approximately 30 cm of duodenum, 300 cm of jejunum and 200 cm of ileum. Jejunal resections are better tolerated than ileal resections, but unfortunately it is more common for disease to involve the ileum. Retained ileum is able to adapt to jejunal functions by absorbing a higher percentage of fluid, electrolytes, calories and protein; it also provides specialized functions not duplicated in the jejunum. These specialized functions are active bile salt and vitamin B_{12} absorption. Passive bile salt absorption occurs throughout the small bowel, but active bile salt absorption is confined to the ileum and is quantitatively the most important. Ileal resection disrupts the bile salt enterohepatic cycle and although the liver compensates by increasing bile salt production, if more than half (100 cm) the ileum is missing the intraluminal bile salt concentration cannot be sustained. This results in impairment of the formation of complex micelles and the absorption of fat. Along with fat malabsorption there is also malabsorption of fat-soluble vitamins (vitamins A, D, E and K) and divalent cations (calcium, magnesium, zinc and copper). Malabsorbed fat reaching the colon is converted by colonic bacteria to cathartic hydroxylated fatty acids and this leads to many large, pale, loose stools and much offensive gas, the so-called syndrome of steatorrhoea. More modest ileal resections (< 100 cm) are compatible with a normal lumenal bile salt concentration and normal fat absorption, but a large amount of these bile salts escape into the colon where they are also deconjugated to cathartic substances, inducing so-called cholerrhoeic diarrhoea.

Vitamin B_{12} and intrinsic factor receptors are present only in the terminal ileum. Receptor adherence allows vitamin B_{12} to enter the enterocyte, and pass on into the portal circulation bound to its transport protein, transcobalamin II. This complex is either taken up by the liver, where vitamin B_{12} is stored, or passed on to target tissues.

In a recent study, 25% of patients (103) who following surgery had 150 cm or less of residual small bowel required long-term parenteral nutrition. This was most often true of patients with an end jejunostomy and a remaining small bowel of less than 115 cm, a jejuno-ileal anastomosis with less than 35 cm of small bowel and a jejuno-colic anastomosis with less than 60 cm.

Presence of the ileocaecal valve

This valve makes a very important contribution to small bowel absorption. The valve exerts a slowing effect on gastric emptying and small bowel transit, increasing the length of time available for nutrient absorption. It also acts as a barrier to retrograde bacterial colonization and the breakdown of fat and bile salts to cathartic substances.

In short-bowel patients who have lost the ileocaecal valve attempts have been made to slow bowel transit by either fashioning an artificial valve through circumferential resection of 1 cm of outer longitudinal muscle, allowing circular muscle to prolapse into the lumen, or by reversing a segment of small bowel. Neither procedure has met with great success.

Preservation of the colon and/or stomach

The colon can contribute significantly to water, electrolyte and energy conservation in short-bowel patients. The colon normally receives 1–2 l of chyme per day and absorbs 95% of the fluid. The colon can absorb as much as 3–4 l of fluid in a short-bowel patient, however, absorption may be offset by the unabsorbed fat or bile salts stimulating colon secretion. Bacteria in the colon can ferment complex polysaccharides such as dietary fibre to short-chain fatty acids (acetate, propionate and butyrate), which are actively absorbed. Butyrate particularly serves as a fuel for the colonocyte. The colon can also conserve small amounts of nitrogen.

Small bowel resection leads to temporary hypergastrinaemia. Gastrin has desirable trophic effects on the upper small bowel but the increased acid secretion can reduce duodenal pH, inactivating pancreatic enzymes and adversely affecting lumenal digestion. Histamine₂ receptor antagonists (H_2RA) blockers have been shown to inhibit excess acid production, thus reducing small bowel fluid output. These medications do not block gastrin output so the gastrin trophic benefit is retained. Partial or complete gastrectomy is associated with the dumping syndrome and this further compromises short bowel

Table 3   Nutritional and metabolic consequences of the short bowel syndrome

Timescale	Problem	Result
Acute – first few days	Net loss of bowel fluid	Dehydration Hypovolaemia Prerenal azotaemia
	Net loss of bowel electrolytes	Na, K, Cl, HCO_3 imbalance
Subacute – first few weeks	Energy malabsorption Protein malabsorption Water-soluble vitamin deficiency	Weight loss Hypoproteinaemia Thiamin deficiency Folate deficiency
	Divalent cation malabsorption	Ca, Mg, Zn, Cu deficiency
Chronic – months to years	Fat-soluble vitamin depletion Vitamin B_{12} and iron deficiency Trace element deficiency Nephrolithiasis Cholelithiasis Osteopenic bone disease	Vitamin A, D, E, K deficiency Anaemia, neuropathy Cu, Cr, Se, Mo deficiency Calcium oxalate stones Cholesterol gallstones Compression fractures

absorption. Gastrectomy can also lead to iron and vitamin B_{12} malabsorption.

Health of the remaining small bowel

Many disease processes which lead to small bowel resection also involve the remaining small bowel, further compromising absorption and adaption. This is particularly characteristic of the recurrent inflammation of Crohn's disease or the smoldering fibrosis of radiation enteritis.

Time interval between resection and maximal bowel adaption

If the nutritional status of the patient is well maintained by appropriate enteral and parenteral management, then complete bowel adaption is usually achieved in 3 to 12 months.

Clinical Manifestations and Diagnosis

Table 3 outlines the nutritional and metabolic consequences of the short bowel syndrome. The earliest problems relate to fluid and electrolyte depletion. A normal bowel absorbs a net 2–3 l of fluid per day, but a short bowel may excrete a net of 2–3 l per day or more, necessitating intravenous replacement. This net loss of small bowel fluid is associated with electrolyte losses which acutely lead to monovalent cation or anion imbalance. As shown in **Table 4**, gastrointestinal (GI) losses of these minerals vary with the

Table 4   Enteric fluid volumes and their sodium, potassium, chloride and bicarbonate content[a]

	Fluid volume (l per day)[b]	Na (mmol l^{-1})	K[c] (mmol l^{-1})	Cl (mmol l^{-1})	HCO_3[d] (mmol l^{-1})
Oral intake	2–3				
Enteric secretions					
Saliva	1–2	10	30	10	30
Gastric juice	2	60	9	90	0
Bile	2–3	150	10	90	70
Small bowel	1	100	5	100	20
Colon	Variable	40	100	15	60

[a]Enteric secretions are also rich in divalent cations (Ca, Mg, Zn, Cu), and their loss is increased by steatorrhoea, a high bowel fistula, or prolonged suction.
[b]Of the 9 l per day of oral enteric fluid presented to the upper small bowel, normally 50% is absorbed in the jejunum, 40% in the ileum, and 10% in the colon. In short-bowel patients, the colon can absorb greater amounts, up to 3 l per day.
[c]Potassium losses are small except in secretions distal to the ileocaecal valve. The colon ion exchange is partly controlled by aldosterone and therefore Na depletion increases K loss in the stool.
[d]Bicarbonate losses must be replaced in parenteral solutions as acetate or lactate because of potential precipitation of bicarbonate with ingredients such as calcium.

amount and level of remaining bowel. The loss of bicarbonate or chloride also determines whether the patient has a subtraction alkalosis or acidosis.

While clinical recognition of acute fluid depletion is not difficult, more modest chronic dehydration requires careful measurement of urine output over several days. A urine volume of less than 15 ml per kg per day, or 1 l per day in a 70 kg person, implies borderline dehydration. Such patients have to maintain a high urine concentration specific gravity (>1025) and are at risk over time of developing kidney dysfunction.

Compared with the acute weight loss of negative fluid balance, the weight loss of protein and energy malabsorption occurs gradually over weeks or months and is associated eventually with cachexia, depigmentation and thinning of the hair and dependent oedema. Water-soluble vitamin deficiency, particularly of thiamin and folate, can also occur at this point together with depletion of divalent cations (Ca, Mg, Zn, Cu).

After several months, or even years, short-bowel patients can develop deficiencies of fat-soluble vitamins, iron and vitamin B_{12}. **Table 5** summarizes the enteral and parenteral requirements for essential fatty acids, minerals and vitamins and lists their metabolic function, the clinical signs of deficiency and their laboratory assessment, showing normal and deficient values.

Short-bowel patients are at high risk for kidney stones, gallstones and osteopenic bone disease. Kidney stones are most common in patients with small bowel resection but where the colon is retained and is anastomosed to the remaining small intestine. This reflects the fact that unabsorbed fatty acids complex with divalent cations, particularly lumenal calcium. In the normal bowel dietary oxalate forms insoluble complexes with lumenal calcium. With steatorrhoea, less calcium is available, so oxalates stay as soluble oxalic acid which is readily absorbed in the colon. Such patients may absorb three times the normal amount of dietary oxalate; this has to be excreted renally and leads to an increased incidence of calculi formulation. Kidney stones are especially likely to form if the patient has a low urine output and is depleted in other urine crystal solubilizers such as magnesium and citrate.

Gallstones also occur commonly in short-bowel patients, because interruption of the bile salt enterohepatic cycle depletes the bile salt pool and impairs solubilization of biliary cholesterol.

Bone mineral loss in short-bowel patients reflects several factors, particularly calcium and vitamin D depletion and increased bone mineral mobilization to replace excessive GI losses of fixed base ($NaHCO_3$).

Management of the Short Bowel Syndrome

In the immediate postoperative phase, most patients are managed by parenteral nutrition to provide baseline nutrient and fluid requirements and replacement of abnormal GI losses. This requires daily weighings and careful input and output measurements. GI losses are frequently quite modest (<2 l per day) until the patient starts to take fluid and food by mouth. **Table 6** gives the fluid input and output of a 42 year-old man with massive bowel resection and a high jejunostomy secondary to resection for strictures and fistulas from Crohn's disease.

Daily baseline fluid, energy and protein (amino acid) requirements are 35 ml kg^{-1}, 120 J kg^{-1} (30 cal kg^{-1}) and 0.8 g kg^{-1}, respectively. Parenteral essential fatty acid, mineral and vitamin requirements are summarized in Table 5. Replacement of abnormal GI losses depends on the amount and type of fluid being lost, as shown in Table 4. Since some of this loss represents oral fluid intake, only net GI fluid loss needs to be replaced. However it should be emphasized that oral intake usually contains only small amounts of electrolytes, whereas the stimulated GI secretion contains significant electrolytes and therefore the electrolyte replacement needs to be more generous than that in net GI fluid loss. Sometimes it is necessary to measure these ostomy mineral losses to ensure correct replacement. GI losses also contain significant amounts of divalent cations, so these also require replacement in the parenteral formula. Fluid balance is assured if the patient's urine output is 1.5–2 l and their daily weight stays relatively constant. If the patient is protein–energy depleted and extra amounts are provided to restore normal body composition, then a gain of 1 kg per week can be expected. However, the clinician must always question whether any weight gain reflects fluid overload since it is easy for patients, particularly older subjects, to develop congestive heart failure.

In the early phases of short bowel syndrome, it is common practice to reduce abnormal GI losses by prescribing H_2RA's to treat the excessive gastric acid output, and anticholinergic agents (diphenoxylate, loperamide or tincture of opium) to reduce hypermotility.

Despite the loss of specific transport processes and altered GI hormones and secretions, full adaptive changes in the remaining small bowel only occur once the patient starts oral feeding. The initial dietary recommendation for short-bowel patients is to eat small, frequent meals of low-lactose, low-osmolar food (avoiding simple sugars), with most energy

Table 5   Clinical and laboratory assessment of essential fatty acids, minerals and vitamins

Nutrient	Adults		Clinical assessment		Laboratory assessment	
	Daily enteral requirements	Daily parenteral requirements	Metabolic function	Deficiency	Normal	Deficient
Essential fatty acids	1–2% of total calorie intake	2–4 g	Components of all lipid membranes, precursor of prostaglandins	Scaly dermatitis	Triene : tetraene ratio <0.4 plasma or red cell membrane	Triene : tetraene ratio >0.7
Calcium	800–1200 mg	5–15 mmol	Body content 600 g; bone crystal (99%), blood clotting, nerve and muscle excitability	Osteomalacia, tetany	2.2–2.7 mmol l^{-1} (8.6–10.8 mg dl^{-1})	<2.2 mmol l^{-1} (8.6 mg dl^{-1}) if serum albumin normal
Phosphorus	800–1200 mg	20–45 mmol	Body content 600 g; bone crystal (85%), ~P bonds, chief intracellular anion	Osteomalacia, haemolytic anaemia, ↓ HbO_2, dissociation, ↓ phagocystosis	0.8–1.5 mmol l^{-1} (2.5–4.5 mg dl^{-1}) serum	<0.8 mmol l^{-1} (2.5 mg dl^{-1}); severe if <0.3 mmol l^{-1} (1.0 mg dl^{-1})
Sulfur	No available data		Body content 175 g; occurs in methionine, cysteine, thiamine, insulin, chondroitin sulfate, etc.	Unknown	No value available	No value available
Potassium	2–5 g	50–100 mmol	Body content 160 g; main intracellular cation	Muscular weakness, cardiac irritability, metabolic alkalosis	3.5–5.0 mmol l^{-1} (3.5–5.0 mEq l^{-1}) serum	<3.5 mmol l^{-1} (3.5 mEq l^{-1}); severe if <2.5 mmol l^{-1} (2.5 mEq l^{-1})
Sodium	1–3 g	50–100 mmol	Body content 100 g; main extracellular cation	↓ Circulating blood volume, ↓ BP, ↓ urine output	135–145 mmol l^{-1} (135–145 mEq l^{-1}) serum	<130 mmol l^{-1} (130 mEq l^{-1} except if H_2O retention is primary problem
Chloride	2–5 g	150–180 mmol	Body content 79 g; main extracellular cation	Metabolic alkalosis	98–106 mmol l^{-1} (98–106 mEq l^{-1}) serum	<85 mmol l^{-1} (85 mEq l^{-1})

Table 5 Continued

Nutrient	Adults		Clinical assessment		Laboratory assessment	
	Daily enteral requirements	Daily parenteral requirements	Metabolic function	Deficiency	Normal	Deficient
Magnesium	300 mg	5–10 mmol	Body content 25 g; cofactor for many enzymes including phosphorylases, phosphotransferases (Na$^+$/K$^+$-exchanging ATPase, vitamin D hydroxylases)	Tetany, muscle weakness secondary to hypokalaemia and hypocalcaemia	0.5–1.0 mmol l^{-1} (1.3–2.5 mg dl^{-1}) serum	<0.4 mmol l^{-1} (1.0 mg dl^{-1})
Iron	10 mg	1–2 mg	Body content 4 g; haeme compounds, cytochrome enzymes, iron stores	Microcytic, hypochromic anaemia, ↓ immunocompetence	Serum iron >10 mmol l^{-1} (60 mg dl^{-1}); TIBC 45 mmol l^{-1} (250 mg dl^{-1}); plasma ferritin >30 mg dl^{-1}	Serum iron <9 mmol l^{-1} (50 μg dl^{-1}); TIBC >54 mmol l^{-1} (300 μg dl^{-1}); plasma ferritin <20 mg dl^{-1}
Zinc	15 mg	3–12 mg	Body content 2 g; cofactor for many enzymes including dehydrogenase, carboxypeptidase	Growth retardation and hypogonadism; impaired immunocompetence	11–18 mmol l^{-1} (70–120 μg dl^{-1}) plasma	<8 mmol l^{-1} (50 mg dl^{-1}) if serum albumin normal
Copper	2–3 mg	0.3–0.5 mg	Body content 100 mg; cofactor for lysyl oxidase (collagen synthesis), cytochrome oxidase, tyrosinase	Anaemia and neutropenia scorbutic-like osteopenia in children	14–20 mmol l^{-1} (90–130 μg dl^{-1}) plasma	<8 mmol l^{-1} (50 μg dl^{-1})
Iodine	0.15 mg	0.15 mg	Body content 30 mg; component of thyroid hormones	Cretinism/myxoedema	300–850 mmol l^{-1} (4–11 μg dl^{-1})	<300 mmol l^{-1} (4 μg dl^{-1}) if thyroxine (T_4) binding protein normal
Manganese	2–5 mg	2–5 mg	Body content 20 mg; cofactor for lipid, cholesterol, mucopolysaccharide synthesis	Abnormal clotting not corrected by vitamin K	100–180 mmol l^{-1} (6–10 μg dl^{-1}) whole blood	<90 mmol l^{-1} (4 μg dl^{-1})

Continued

Table 5   Continued

| Nutrient | Adults | | Clinical assessment | | Laboratory assessment | |
	Daily enteral requirements	Daily parenteral requirements	Metabolic function	Deficiency	Normal	Deficient
Chromium	50–200 μg	15 μg	Body content 6 mg; part of insulin receptor mechanism	Glucose intolerance	35–75 mmol l^{-1} (2–4 μg ml^{-1}) plasma	<20 mmol l^{-1} (1 μg ml^{-1})
Molybdenum	0.15–0.5 mg	0.01–0.5 mg	Body content 5 mg; cofactor for xanthine oxidase	Confusional state secondary to increased methionine	5–20 mmol l^{-1} (0.5–2 μg ml^{-1}) plasma	<5 mmol l^{-1} (0.5 μg ml^{-1})
Selenium	0.05–0.3 mg	0.05–0.1 mg	Cofactor for glutathione peroxidase	Muscle weakness, haemolytic anaemia	0.3 mmol l^{-1} (0.02 μg ml^{-1}) whole blood	<0.02 mmol l^{-1} (0.15 mg dl^{-1})
Cobalt	3 μg	5 μg	Body content 80 μg; metallo-cofactor for cobalamin (vitamin B$_{12}$)	Unknown in man	35–85 mmol l^{-1} (2–5 μg ml^{-1}) plasma	<35 mmol l^{-1} (2 μg ml^{-1})
Ascorbic acid	35 mg	100 mg	Microsomal electron transport, tryosine, tryptophan, and dopamine synthesis, steroid synthesis, hydroxylation of collagen proline and lysine residues; folic acid metabolism	Scurvy, perifollicular haemorrhages, bleeding gums, osteopenia, and subperiosteal haemorrhages; defective wound healing	(a) 28–60 mmol l^{-1} (0.5–1.0 mg dl^{-1}) serum 850–1700 mmol l^{-1} (b) (15–30 mg dl^{-1}) leucocytes	(a) <6 mmol l^{-1} (0.1 mg dl^{-1}) (b) <400 mmol l^{-1} (7 mg dl^{-1})
Thiamin	1–1.5 mg	3.0 mg	Cofactor (TPP) for transketolase, pyruvate and ketoglutarate decarboxylase, oxidation of branched-chain ketoacids	High output cardiac failure, polyneuritis	(a) 8–15 IU ETK (b) <10% TPP effect	(a) <8 IU (b) >20% TPP effect
Riboflavin	1.3–1.6 mg	3.6 mg	Converted to electron acceptors and donators, flavin mononucleotide (FMN) and flavin adenine dinucleotide (FAD)	Cheilosis, glossitis seborrhoeic dermatitis	<1.2 EGR activation coefficient	>1.2 EGR activation coefficient

Table 5 Continued

| Nutrient | Adults | | Clinical assessment | | Laboratory assessment | |
	Daily enteral requirements	Daily parenteral requirements	Metabolic function	Deficiency	Normal	Deficient
Niacin	13–18 mg	40 mg	Converted to electron acceptors and donors, nicotinamide dinucleotides (NAD, NADP)	Pellagra; pigmented dermatitis, ulceration of mucous membranes, CNS depression	Niacin, 30–70 mmol l^{-1} (4–9 μg ml^{-1}); 2-pyridone/N'methyl ratio >2.0 whole blood	<24 mmol l^{-1} (3 μg ml^{-1}) <2.0
Biotin	100–200 μg	60 μg	Cofactor for carboxylation enzymes where CO_2 is added, such as pyruvate → oxaloacetate, acetyl-coA → malonyl-CoA	Alopecia, seborrhoeic dermatitis, neuritis	800–2000 mmol l^{-1} (200–500 μg ml^{-1}) serum	<800 mmol l^{-1} (200 μg ml^{-1})
Pantothenic acid	5 mg	15 mg	Converted to coenzyme A	Irritability, burning paraesthesias	700–1800 mmol l^{-1} (150–400 μg ml^{-1}) serum	<700 mmol l^{-1} (150 μg ml^{-1})
Pyridoxine	2 mg	4 mg	Cofactor (PLP) for many enzymes including transaminases, phosphorylases, amino oxidases	Glossitis, polyneuritis seizures, microcytic hypochromic anaemia	EGOT Index <1.5	EGOT index >1.5
Folic acid	400 μg	400 μg	Cofactor for purine and pyrimidine synthesis and metabolism of serine, histidine, homocysteine and ethanolamine	Megaloblastic defect of red blood cells and mucous membranes	(a) 7–20 mmol l^{-1} (3–9 μg ml^{-1}) serum (b) 400–1400 mmol l^{-1} (150–600 μg ml^{-1}) RBC	(a) <7 mmol l^{-1} (3 μg ml^{-1}) (b) <200 mmol l^{-1} (100 μg ml^{-1})
Cobalamin	3 μg	5 μg	Methyl B_{12} involved in methyl donor reactions; 5' deoxyadenosyl B_{12} involved in carboxylation reactions	Megaloblastic defect of red blood cells and mucous membranes, central and peripheral neuropathy	150–650 mmol l^{-1} (200–900 μg ml^{-1}) serum	<100 mmol l^{-1} (150 μg ml^{-1})
Vitamin A	4000 IU	3300 IU	Light-sensitive pigment in retina, epithelial maintenance (retinoic acid)	Night blindness and xerophthalmia, testicular atrophy keratosis of skin	0.7–2.0 mmol l^{-1} (20–60 μg dl^{-1}) serum	<0.7 mmol l^{-1} (20 μg ml^{-1})

Continued

Table 5 Continued

Nutrient	Adults		Clinical assessment		Laboratory assessment	
	Daily enteral requirements	Daily parenteral requirements	Metabolic function	Deficiency	Normal	Deficient
Vitamin D	200 IU	200 IU	Calcium, phosphorus and possibly magnesium absorption from intestine, calcium deposition and mobilization from bone	Osteomalacia (rickets in growing children), muscle weakness	25–200 mmol l^{-1} (10–80 µg ml^{-1}) serum	<13 mmol l^{-1} (5 µg ml^{-1})
Vitamin E	8 mg	10–15 mg	Prevents peroxidation of polyunsaturated lipids	Haemolytic anaemia of newborn, dystrophic changes of retina and posterior column nuclei	0.2–0.3 mmol l^{-1} (0.8–1.2 mg dl^{-1}) serum 10% haemolysis	<0.01 mmol l^{-1} (0.5 mg dl^{-1}) >20% haemolysis
Vitamin K	70–140 µg	200 µg	Involved in synthesis of clotting factors II, VII, IX and X	Bleeding tendency presenting as epistaxis ecchymosis; gastrointestinal, urinary or CNS haemorrhage	Prothrombin time <1 s prolonged over control	PT > 2 s prolonged

Abbreviations: TIBC, total iron binding capacity; ETK, erythrocyte transketolase; TPP, thiamine pyrophosphate; EGR, erythrocyte glutathione reductase; EGOT, erythrocyte glutamic oxaloacelate transaminase; RBC, red blood cells; PLP, pyridoxal phosphate; NAD, nicotinamide adenine dinucleotide; NADP, nicotinamide adenine dinucleotide phosphate; CoA, coenzyme A.

Table 6 24-h fluid balance in a man with a high jejunostomy requiring parenteral replacement

Input	(ml)	Output	(ml)
Food	1000	Insensible	500
Drink	2000	Sweat	1000
Intravenous	4000	Ostomy	4000
		Urine	1500
Total	7000		7000

coming from complex carbohydrate. The tolerance for dietary fat depends in part on the type of short bowel syndrome. Patients with an end-jejunostomy tolerate high-fat diets without greater loss of fluid or monovalent electrolytes. They do, however, lose more divalent cations in their GI secretions. If the patient has an ileum in continuity with the residual jejunum and/or colon, then the amount of dietary fat is an issue because unabsorbed fatty acids induce active salt and water secretion, in addition to binding lumenal divalent cations, making fluid and mineral balance more negative.

Parenteral nutrition, especially in infants, tends to cause cholestasis which may progress to cirrhosis and liver failure. Oral feeding is one important measure for preventing this serious complication, perhaps in part because food stimulates cholecystokinin and bile secretion. Some authorities have recommended ursodeoxycholate (8–10 mg per kg per day) to prevent bile sludge and improve bile secretion in short-bowel patients. This reduces the risk of gallstones by improving cholesterol solubilization. However, taken orally ursodeoxycholate tends to aggravate diarrhoea in short-bowel patients. This diarrhoea may be partly circumvented by an intravenous formulation, already available in several European countries and soon to be released in the USA.

Another important reason for encouraging short-bowel patients to take food by mouth is the growing evidence that enteral nutrition somehow protects patients from infectious complications. Animal studies have shown decreased translocation of gut bacteria to mesenteric lymph nodes and the lungs and a reduction of stress hypercatabolism. These phenomena have not been substantiated in humans; however enteral feeding may prevent bacterial overgrowth and decrease the risk of aspiration pneumonia. An oral diet also provides nutrients not present in standard parenteral nutrition solutions and present only in low concentration in most synthetic tube enteral formulae. These nutrients are not the classical essential nutrients because they can be synthesized endogenously, but they appear to become 'conditionally essential' in severely depleted patients.

These nutrients and their purported metabolic functions are summarized in **Table 7**. Preliminary data also suggests that bowel growth factors such as growth hormone and epidermal growth factor may promote short bowel adaption.

Tube enteral nutrition may also have a part to play in supporting the short-bowel patient. Enteral formulae delivered into the stomach or, if necessary, into the upper jejunum can support patients who are almost in balance but cannot quite sustain themselves on oral intake alone. Such patients often tolerate overnight tube feeding using a slow constant infusion. If the patient can become independent of parenteral nutrition, their treatment has fewer risks and is far less expensive. The adaption to tube enteral feeding is often slow, taking several months, during which time some parenteral support is frequently necessary. This approach is especially appropriate for children who may have a proximal motility disorder from *in utero* bowel obstruction, in addition to their short bowel syndrome due to atresia, gastroschisis or aganglionosis. Such infants often vomit with bolus oral feeding and become reluctant to take food by mouth. Under these circumstances, enteral tube feeding can support GI adaption and alleviate concerns about the development of parenteral nutrition cholestasis. It allows the child slowly to develop an interest in eating, avoiding a psychological aversion to forced oral feeding. Many short-bowel patients will not tolerate the high osmolarity of monomeric formulae and do better with peptide and oligosaccharide-based formulae.

Psychosocial Support for Patients and Their Families

If the patient experiences rapid bowel adaption, as may occur in weeks if their short bowel includes some ileum, an ileocaecal valve and total colon, then patient and family distress rapidly subsides. If, on the other hand, the patient is discharged with an ostomy and is indefinitely dependent on parenteral and/or enteral feeding lines, their distress is likely to be ongoing and overwhelming.

Experience and patient questionnaires have shown that patients and families do better if certain core issues are addressed. These can be summarized as follows.

1. Since most of the day-to-day management falls on patients and their families, it becomes very important that they actively participate in all their own management decisions.
2. Important benefits are derived from contact with other patients and their families. This is helpful in sorting out of social, financial and medical issues.

Table 7 Conditionally essential nutrients

Nutrient	Metabolic function	Supporting experimental data	
		Animal studies	Human studies
Glutamine	Fuel for enterocytes and immunocytes. Preserves hepatic glutathione	Improves gut morphology and ↑ glucose absorption, ↓ bacterial translocation	Parenteral supplement: ↓ infections and hospital LOS[a] in BMT[b] patients
Nucleotides	Derivatives (cAMP, cGMP) serve as mediators for many metabolic processes	↑ immune competence and intestinal and hepatic regeneration following injury	In critically ill adults ↓ infections and hospital LOS
Arginine	Via nitric oxide enhances lymphocyte cytotoxicity. Substrate for polyamine synthesis. Via release of HGH[c] promotes protein synthesis	Supplements ↑ survival from burns, trauma, sepsis. Antitumour effect	↑ T helper cells in patients with cancer surgery; ↓ hospital LOS; ↑ wound healing
Branched-chain amino acids	Level in muscle regulates muscle-protein breakdown; ↓ in catabolic patients, especially those with liver disease	Supplements reduce muscle protein breakdown; ↑ nitrogen balance	Supplements ↓ hepatic encephalopathy; ↑ nitrogen balance in septic patients but effect on survival not demonstrated
Sulfur-containing amino acids [Methionine ↓ S-adenosyl methionine (SAM) ↓ Homocysteine ↓ Cysteine → Glutathione Taurine, Carnitine]	Glutathione, chief cytoplasmic free radical scavenger. Taurine conjugates bile salts. Carnitine transports fatty acids into mitochondria for β-oxidation. SAM donates methyl group to choline and creatine	↓ choline affects cell wall fluidity. Glutathione depletion ↑ free radical cell damage. Depletion is reversed with SAM	Trans-sulfuration products depleted in long-term parenteral nutrition patients. SAM supplementation ↓ cholestasis
Short-chain fatty acids	Derived by bacterial breakdown from soluble fibres such as pectin. Fuel for enterocytes, particularly colonocytes	Stimulates bowel epithelial growth and ↑ strength of colonic anastomoses	↓ pouchitis and bypassed bowel enteritis
n-3 fatty acids	Promote production of prostaglandins and leukotrienes of n-3 series (PGE$_3$ LTB$_5$, etc.) and reduce production from n-6 series (PGE$_2$ LTB$_4$, etc.) which are pro-inflammatory	↓ autoimmune disease; ↓ platelet adhesiveness	↓ hospital LOS in critically ill adults; ↓ BP; ↓ IgA nephritis; ↓ rheumatoid arthritis; ↓ platelet abnormalities in type I diabetes

[a]LOS, length of stay.
[b]BMT, bone marrow transplant.
[c]HGH, human growth hormone.

3. Patients, especially in a long-term undertaking, need access to a knowledgeable Nutrition Support Physician who can recognize complications such as micronutrient depletion syndromes.
4. Patients need help with restraining medical costs so private insurance lifetime benefits are conserved as long as possible. This is particularly important if they are able to continue working. They need assurance that health planners are aware of their financial costs (> $100 000 per

year on home parenteral nutrition) and are working to reduce cost without forfeiting quality.

5. Most patients want to stay abreast of new research findings pertinent to their condition.

Many large home parenteral and enteral nutrition support programmes have local patient and family support groups. In addition there are national organizations which support short-bowel patients such as the Oley Foundation for Home Parenteral and Enteral Nutrition in North America and PINNT (Patients on Intravenous and Nasogastric Nutrition Therapy) in the UK.

Role of Small Bowel Transplantation

Many patients and their families live with the hope that small bowel transplantation will provide a long-term solution to the malabsorption of extreme short bowel syndrome. Although there is growing success with small bowel transplantation, the GI tract is a highly immunogenic organ and requires a large amount of post-transplant immunosuppression to prevent graft rejection or graft versus host disease. The large amount of immunosuppressive drugs puts the patient at risk for chronic viral infections such as cytomegalovirus (CMV) and lymphoproliferative cancers. Because of these serious complications survival following small bowel transplant, with or without the liver or other visceral organs, is about 50% at 2 years. As shown in **Fig. 1**, this compares poorly with home parenteral nutrition survival rates of 70–90%, depending on the underlying diagnosis. Research efforts are underway to develop and evaluate the chimaeric state (two genetic cell populations) in bowel transplant recipients by conducting simultaneous bowel and bone marrow transplantation. The chimaeric state could dramatically decrease the need for post-transplant immunosuppression. Preliminary results have not been promising. Studies also are underway to try and develop a CMV vaccine. At present transplants are largely confined to short-bowel patients with severe parenteral nutrition associated liver failure or patients who have run out of sites for central venous catheter access.

An important question for transplantation scientists is how many potential candidates are there for this therapy once transplantation solves its current difficulties? This number depends on the criteria set for transplantation recipients. In the USA there were 40 000 home parenteral nutrition patients in 1992. As discussed earlier in this article, many of these patients had diagnoses with a short life expectancy and many others stayed on home parenteral nutrition therapy for less than a year. If transplant recipient criteria are 55 years or younger, a benign diagnosis,

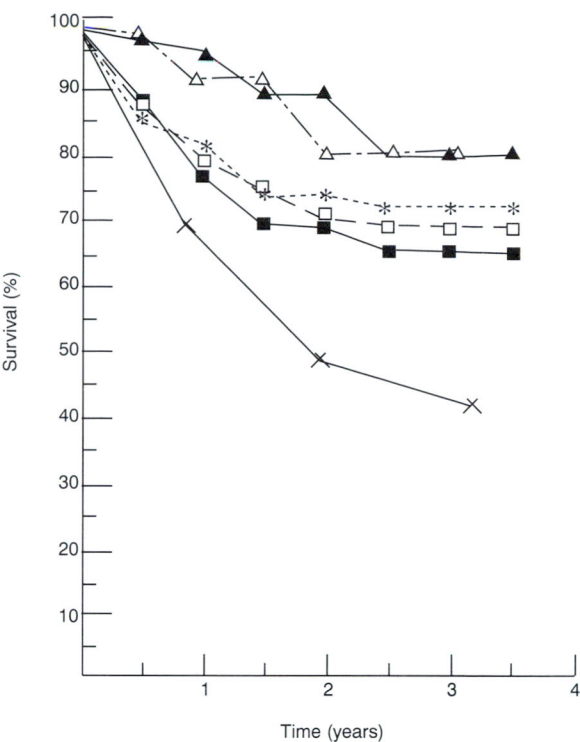

Figure 1 Survival on home parenteral nutrition for short-bowel patients with a variety of benign disorders compared with survival following small bowel transplantation. Points are derived by life table analysis from data published by the Oley Foundation, Albany, New York, USA and from Todo et al. *Ann Surg* 1995. Note that in the early post-transplant period 1 in 4 survivors must continue parenteral nutrition. Key: △, congenital bowel disease; ▲, Crohn's disease; *, ischaemic bowel disease; □, motility disorders; ■, radiation enteritis; ×, transplantation.

such as those shown in Fig. 1, and 3 years at least on home parenteral nutrition, which suggests that further bowel adaption and graduating to just enteral dependence is unlikely, then there will be about 500–1000 small bowel transplant candidates per year. This could justify 20–30 small-bowel transplant centres in the USA.

Successful small bowel transplantation would most likely be cost saving compared with long-term home parenteral nutrition for short-bowel patients; however, it would probably not be less hazardous or more cost-effective than home tube enteral nutrition.

See also: **Cobalamins**: Physiology, Dietary Sources and Requirements. **Electrolytes**: Water-Electrolyte Balance. **Gastrointestinal Tract**: Structure and Function of the Small Intestine. **Nutritional Support**: Parenteral Nutrition; In the Home Setting. **Steatorrhoea**: Nutritional Management.

Further Reading

Byrne TA, Persinger RL, Young LS, Ziegler TR and Wilmore DW (1995) A new treatment for patients with short bowel syndrome: growth hormone, glutamine and modified diet. *Annals of Surgery* 222:243–255.

Carbonnel F, Cosnes J, Chevret S, Beaugerie L, Ngo Y, Malafosse M, Parc R, Le Quintrec Y and Gendre JP (1996) The role of anatomic factors in nutritional autonomy after extensive small bowel resection. *Journal of Parenteral and Enteral Nutrition* 20:275–280.

Grant JP, Chapman G and Russell MK (1996) Malabsorption associated with surgical procedures and its treatment. *Nutrition in Clinical Practice* 11:43–52.

Howard L, Ament M, Fleming CR, Shike M and Steiger E (1995) Current use and clinical outcome of home parenteral and enteral nutrition therapies in the United States. *Gastroenterology* 109:355–365.

Ovesen L, Chu R and Howard L (1983) The influence of dietary fat on jejunostomy output in patients with severe short bowel syndrome. *American Journal of Clinical Nutrition* 38(2):270–277.

Powell Tuck J (1994) Management of gut failure: a physicians view. *Lancet* 344:1061–1064.

Purdum PP and Kirby DF (1991) Short bowel syndrome: a review of the role of nutrition support. *Journal of Parenteral and Enteral Nutrition* 15:93–101.

Quigley EMM, Marsh MN, Shaffer JL and Martin RS (1993) Hepatobiliary complications of TPN. *Gastroenterology* 104:286–301.

Scolapio JS, Camilleri M, Fleming CR, Oenning LV, Burton DD, Sebo JJ, Batts KP and Kelly DG (1997) Effect of growth hormone, glutamine and diet on adaption in short bowel syndrome. A randomized controlled study. *Gastroenterology* 113:1074–1081.

Todo S, Reyes J, Furukawa H, Abu-Elmagd K, Lee RG, Tzakis A, Rao AS and Starzi TE (1995) Outcome analysis of 71 clinical intestinal transplantations. *Annals of Surgery* 222:270–282.

THIAMIN

Contents
Physiology
Beriberi

Physiology

A E Cathcart and **D I Thurnham**, University of Ulster, Coleraine, Northern Ireland, UK

Absorption, Transport and Storage

A well-nourished human adult body contains approximately 30 mg of thiamin, around 80–90% as thiamin diphosphate (TDP), 10% as thiamin triphosphate (TTP), with a small amount of thiamin monophosphate (TMP) and thiamin. The structure of thiamin is shown in **Fig. 1**. A continuous supply of thiamin is required to satisfy the body's relatively high turnover rate.

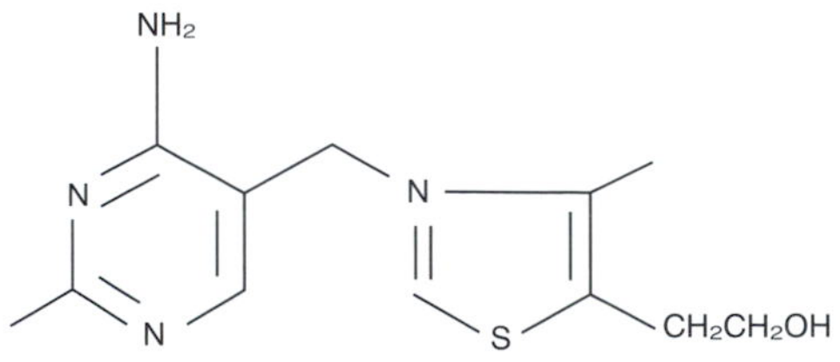

Figure 1 The chemical structure of thiamin.

In food, thiamin occurs mainly as phosphates and these are broken down in the gut by phosphatases to give free thiamin for absorption. Absorption is usually limited to a maximum of 8–15 mg daily. The absorption mechanism is saturated at relatively low concentrations of thiamin, and increasing doses of thiamin from 2.5 mg to 50 mg have little effect on plasma concentrations as it is excreted in well-nourished individuals.

The active absorption of usual dietary amounts is greatest in the jejunum and ileum, acting at low thiamin concentrations via a saturable active carrier-mediated process, thereby accumulating thiamin against a concentration gradient. At thiamin concentrations of 2 μM (0.46 mg l^{-1}) or more, passive diffusion is significant. The mechanism of thiamin entry into the mucosa is not fully understood; the carrier-mediated system is dependent either on thiamin phosphorylation-dephosphorylation coupling or on some metabolic energetic mechanism, possibly activation by sodium ions. The mechanism of thiamin exit on the serosal side is dependent on Na$^+$ and on normal function of ATPase on this side of the cell. Transport into the red blood cells seems to be by a process of facilitated diffusion. Thiamin is taken up by most of the tissues in a similar manner to that detailed above. In alcoholics, thiamin absorption is often depressed owing to impaired active transport from mucosal cells into the circulation, and may be accompanied by other nutrient-deficient states, e.g. folate deficiency.

As with most water-soluble vitamins, thiamin is not stored in the body in large amounts or for any period of time in any tissues. The liver is the main storage organ (0.20–0.76 mg per 100 g), with smaller amounts in the normal heart (0.28–0.79 mg per 100 g), kidney (0.24–0.58 mg per 100 g), and brain (0.14–0.44 mg per 100 g). Although the muscle content is low compared with that of the organs listed, it makes up 40% of total body thiamin owing to its size.

Metabolism and Excretion

Upon absorption by the intestine, thiamin is phosphorylated to the phosphate ester, thiamin monophosphate, by intestinal epithelial cells. On reaching the bloodstream, TMP is converted to the metabolically active diphosphate ester by adenosine triphosphate (ATP) which acts as a phosphate donor. Thiamin diphosphate is therefore often referred to as thiamine pyrophosphate (TPP). The TDP ester is transported across the blood–brain barrier, where a portion is phosphorylated to TTP by the enzyme thiamin pyrophosphokinase. However, TDP is the predominant form in all tissues including those in the brain. Thiamin triphosphate may be further hydrolysed to TDP, the essential cofactor for carbohydrate metabolism. In the other tissues, thiamin is quickly converted to TDP and to a lesser extent TTP and TMP.

Thiamin together with TMP circulate in the plasma bound to albumin. When the binding capacity of plasma albumin is exceeded, or thiamin is in excess of tissue needs and storage, it is rapidly excreted in the urine. The three phosphate esters are hydrolysed by their respective phosphatases to yield free thiamin which is then rapidly excreted or metabolized. The factor regulating this process in opposition to phosphorylation of thiamin is as yet unknown. In addition to free thiamin, small amounts of TDP, thiochrome and thiamin disulfide are also excreted. Thus, there is a relationship between tissue needs and urinary excretion, with urinary excretion after a test dose being one measure of the adequacy of thiamin stores. Thiamin is actively secreted into milk by the lactating mother and is not lost in faeces.

Metabolic Function and Essentiality

Metabolic function

Thiamin is an organic molecule containing a pyrimidine and a thiazole nucleus. The active form of thiamin in the body is TDP which acts as a coenzyme/cofactor in the oxidative phosphorylation of α-ketoacids and in the transketolase reactions. These two reaction pathways are involved in glucose metabolism (**Fig. 2**), so that thiamin is mainly required for energy metabolism. Requirements are proportional to the intake of dietary energy when the energy source is carbohydrate. When diets are low in carbohydrate and a high proportion of energy is supplied by fat, a thiamin-sparing effect is exerted, and the thiamin requirement is reduced. Thiamin, as TTP, may have a part to play in nerve cell transmissions.

Oxidative decarboxylation of α-ketoacids to aldehydes The decarboxylation and oxidation of pyruvate gives acetyl-S-Coenzyme A, which then enters the tricarboxylic acid (Krebs) cycle where further oxidation yields carbon dioxide and water. This oxidative decarboxylation is accomplished by a multienzyme pyruvate dehydrogenase complex (PDHC), comprising three enzymes, a TDP-dependent pyruvate decarboxylase, a lipoic acid-bound dihydrolipoyl transacetylase and a dihydrolipoyl dehydrogenase (an FAD-dependent enzyme) which reoxidizes the reduced lipoic acid. An analogous series of reactions involving the α-ketoglutarate dehydrogenase complex (α-KGDHC) catalyses the conversion of α-ketoglutarate to succinyl-S-CoA in the tricarboxylic acid (TCA) cycle. The decarboxylation of the three branched-chain α-ketoacids derived from the deamination of leucine, isoleucine and valine, namely α-ketoisocaproic acid, α-keto-β-methylvaleric acid and α-ketoisovaleric acid, is achieved by a multienzyme complex similar to those described above.

The entry of pyruvate into the TCA cycle by oxidative decarboxylation via the PDHC is regulated by the phosphorylation and dephosphorylation of the complex by a phosphatase which activates the enzyme and a protein kinase which inactivates it. The activity of the α-KGDHC is claimed not to be regulated by this mechanism.

Transketolase reactions Here the transketolase TDP reacts with the appropriate ketosugars to break the carbon-to-carbon bond between C2 and C3 to form a TDP-glycoaldehyde intermediate which is transferred to a suitable acceptor aldehyde in the pentose or hexose monophosphate shunt (HMPS)

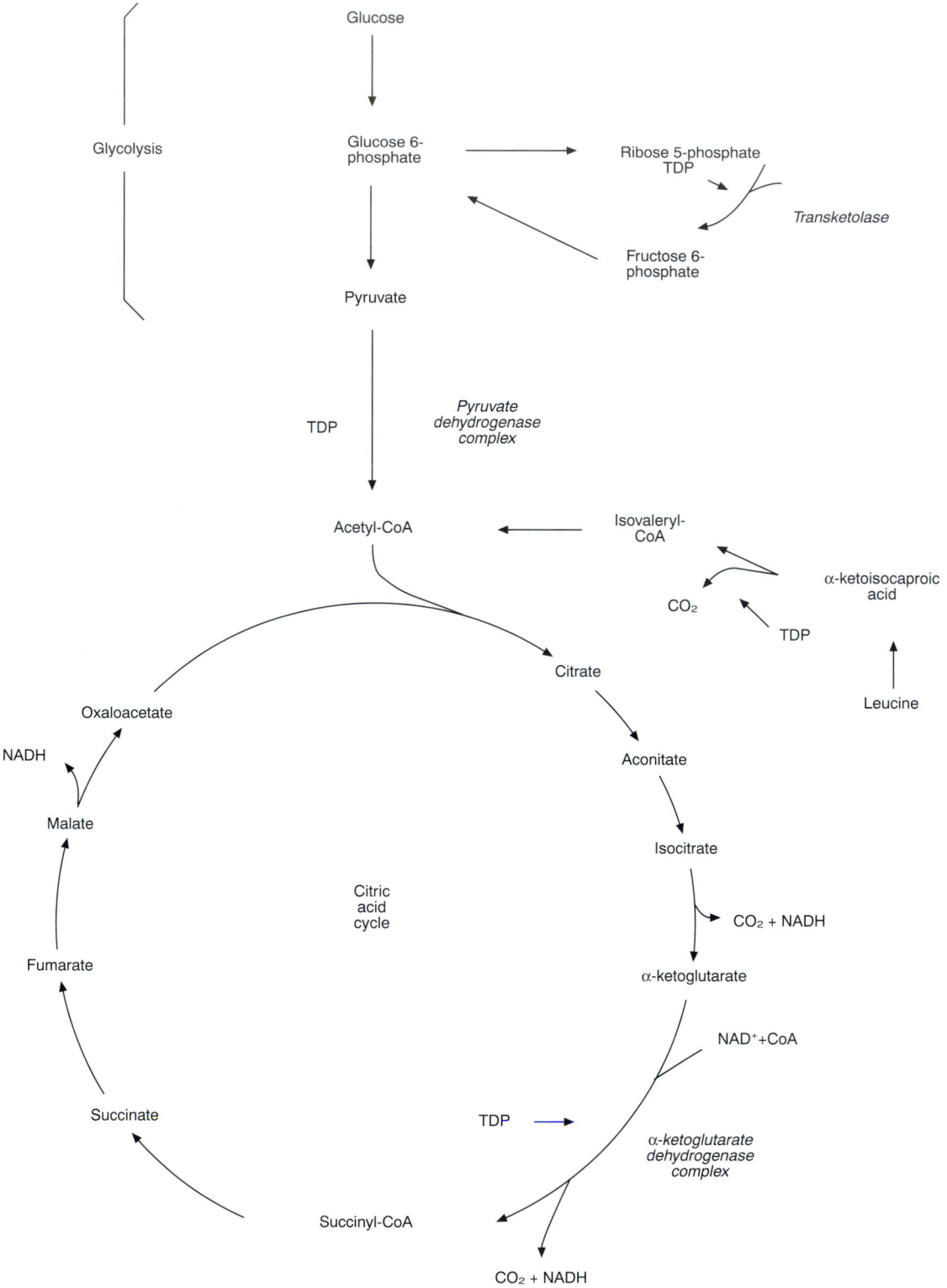

Figure 2   The major metabolic pathways involving thiamin diphosphate (TPD).

pathway for the oxidation of glucose. Glycolysis is the main pathway for the oxidation of glucose and this second metabolic pathway for glucose is important, not so much for energy production (as is the TCA cycle), as for the production of pentoses for RNA and DNA synthesis and NADPH for the biosynthesis of fatty acids and other products, while also supplying intermediate sugars for glycolysis.

Other functions Polyneuritis, which is so often a feature of thiamin deficiency, is evidence of a specific function in neural tissues, and the existence of TTP in brain and other neural tissues suggests a direct role for thiamin in neural excitation. It has been repeatedly demonstrated that the stimulation of nerves or treatment with certain neuroactive drugs results in a decrease in the level of TDP and particularly TTP in the nerve, concomitant with an increase in free TMP in the surrounding fluid. It has been postulated that TTP plays an essential role in nerve transmission involving a gating mechanism for Na^+ and K^+ transport via (Na^+-K^+)-ATPase. This is supported by the fact that nerves contain a constant and significant level of TTP (10%) and also that patients with Leigh disease (subacute necrotizing encephalomyelopathy) have a deficiency of TTP (but normal TDP), and this is accompanied by severe neurological involvement. The presence of an inhibitor of TTP synthesis from TDP is thought to be the contributing factor here.

Thiamin has also been shown to bear a relationship to the levels and function of various neurotransmitters namely the serotonergic, adrenergic and cholinergic systems. Whether, or to what extent, changes in these systems are responsible for the neurologic symptoms of thiamin deficiency remains to be established.

Essentiality

A deficiency of thiamin in the body may manifest in a variety of ways. Beriberi is the traditional thiamin deficiency disease, and its occurrence in communities of Asia and the Far East, where highly milled rice is the staple cereal, led to the discovery of thiamin and indeed to the first experiments in nutrition. Beriberi is characterized by involvement of the nervous and cardiac systems, with one or other system being predominantly affected: the cardiac system in wet beriberi and the nervous system in dry beriberi (*See:* **Thiamin:** Beriberi). In addition to beriberi, the decreased activity of cerebral thiamin-dependent enzymes results in a wide spectrum of acquired and inherited disorders including congenital lactic acidosis, intermittent ataxia of childhood, Leigh disease and the Wernicke–Korsakoff syndrome. Recent evidence also suggests that thiamin neurochemistry is

disrupted in Alzheimer's disease. The role of thiamin deficiency in Wernicke–Korsakoff syndrome is well established. This syndrome and Alzheimer's disease are both associated with marked loss of cholinergic neurons in the nucleus basalis and with memory loss, suggesting that alterations of thiamin-dependent enzymes and/or disrupted neurotransmissions could also be implicated in the pathophysiology of Alzheimer's disease.

Assessment of Thiamin Status

Promising indices of thiamin status

Erythrocyte transketolase assay The erythrocyte transketolase (TKL) assay is regarded as a major advance in the measurement of thiamin status, as it is the first technique that is as sensitive in deficiency as it is in normality, and is a measure of functional vitamin status as the erythrocytes are among the first tissues to be affected by thiamin deficiency. The transketolase enzyme is dependent on the coenzyme TDP, this thiamin dependency forming the basis of this test.

Firstly, the basal (absolute holo-) TKL activity is measured, i.e. the amount representing the endogenous enzyme activity which is dependent on the amount of coenzyme in the erythrocytes (and therefore on thiamin nutrition). Secondly, the enzyme activity with excess coenzyme added *in vitro* is determined and represents the maximum potential enzyme activity, i.e. stimulated activity. The comparison of basal and stimulated activity indicates the degree of saturation of the enzyme with coenzyme, and is expressed either as the activity coefficient (AC) or as the percentage stimulation or TPP effect (TPPE).

$$AC = \frac{\text{stimulated enzyme activity}}{\text{basal enzyme activity}}$$

Percentage stimulation or TPPE (%)

$$= \frac{\text{stimulated activity} - \text{basal activity}}{\text{basal activity}} \times 100$$

Generally, the higher the AC or TPPE the greater the degree of deficiency. Activity coefficients of 1–1.14, are normal; values of 1.14–1.25 indicate marginal deficiency, and values of 1.25 or more indicate severe deficiency.

Several workers have compared the TKL test with results obtained by urinary excretion, and good agreement is reported when using fresh samples. However, the TKL assay does have problems, for apo-TKL (i.e. the TKL enzyme with no TDP coenzyme) is unstable both *in vivo* and *in vitro*, making comparison and interpretation between laboratories difficult, as well as reducing the apparent degree of thiamin deficiency in states of chronic thiamin deficiency. The basal activity also depends on the average age of the erythrocyte, with young red cells having higher TKL activity than older ones. The instability of the TKL apoenzyme makes its use in field studies limited and strict experimental protocols are essential. The ratio of basal to stimulated activity is used to assess thiamin status because of the great intersubject variability in basal activity, and it is assumed that stimulated activity (i.e. maximum potential activity) is not affected by deficiency. The apoenzyme level is directly affected by vitamin status, by certain diseases and by the administration of certain hormones or drugs which may confound the interpretation. In prolonged experimental thiamin deficiency, there is a reduction in apoenzyme level. Both basal and stimulated erythrocyte TKL activities tend to fall with no change in the TPPE or AC. In such cases basal enzyme activity should also be considered as the TPPE may suggest normal thiamin nutriture and mask an actual deficiency. Furthermore, in population studies it is frequently reported that TKL results do not correlate well with dietary intakes of thiamin. A recent study of British teenagers found that although thiamin intakes appeared largely adequate when compared with current UK recommendations, there was no statistically significant relationship between intake and either of the methods used to assess status, namely total erythrocyte thiamin, and basal or stimulated transketolase activities; status results were actually indicative of deficiency in the group. This suggests strongly a need for the reevaluation of thiamin status indices, dietary thiamin availability and the thiamin requirement in this group.

High-performance liquid chromatography Red blood cell thiamin measurement using high-performance liquid chromatography has been reported to produce the same results as measuring basal TKL activity, and its limitation is the relatively small (20%) decrease in red cell thiamin, even in beriberi. However, no statistically significant relationship has been reported between either of the status indices used. Red cell thiamin concentrations or basal TKL activity are reported to parallel the fall in liver, kidney and muscle in deficiency states.

Less reliable indices of thiamin status

A number of less reliable indices exist for the measurement of thiamin status. The measurement of *urinary thiamin excretion* by both microbiological and fluorescent (thiochrome) methods have technical problems and are not particularly sensitive in the deficient state. Urinary thiamin levels do not adequately reflect body stores but provide an index of the dietary intake, levels responding particularly to excessive thiamin intakes. A *thiamin load test* has also been used as an index of status. After the parenteral administration of 5 mg of thiamin, its excretion is measured and subjects excreting less than 20 μg during the following 4 h are deficient. Actual *thiamin concentrations in blood* (serum, red blood cells and whole blood) have been investigated; when measured by older methods these are insensitive indices, as relatively modest declines are observed even in cases of frank beriberi.

Thiamin requirements

The UK dietary reference value (DRV) for thiamin is expressed per energy intake because of its essential role in energy metabolism. The reference nutrient intake (RNI) while allowing for variance, is 0.4 mg per 1000 kcal (4.2 MJ), and it is recommended that the intake should not fall below 0.4 mg per day in people on very low-energy diets. There is no specific DRV for thiamin in pregnancy or lactation, as there is no evidence for increased needs for thiamin in normal pregnancy when expressed per unit of energy. Furthermore, recommended energy intakes are increased by 1.9–2.4 MJ (450–570 kcal) per day for lactation, which should meet the losses of thiamin in milk.

The daily allowance of thiamin recommended by the Food and Nutrition Board of the USA is 0.5 mg per 1000 kcal (4.2 MJ); a minimum intake of 1 mg per day is recommended for the elderly, even if they consume less than 2000 kcal (8.4 MJ) per day (since it has been suggested that thiamin may be used less efficiently in older persons), and a minimum of 0.8 mg is recommended for other adults, with an increase of 0.6 mg per 1000 kcal (4.2 MJ) in pregnancy and lactation.

The thiamin requirement is related to metabolic rate and is greatest when carbohydrate is the energy source. As thiamin is not stored in the body in any appreciable amount, a disturbance affecting the gastrointestinal tract or an increase in metabolic rate (e.g. in pregnancy, lactation, childhood, hard physical labour and fever) may necessitate an increased thiamin intake. Beriberi has been associated with malaria and pyrexias, and has been shown to occur during the preharvest season in developing countries when the energy requirements are high and food reserves from the previous year's crop are almost depleted, so that elevated energy requirement may not be met by the diet.

Women are less affected by beriberi than are men even when they consume the same type of food, but there is no consistent indication that the sexes have different needs. Differences between the sexes in factors that may affect thiamin status need investigation, e.g. the amount of food eaten, levels of illness or infection, and energy requirements. The use of oral contraceptives has no influence on thiamin status.

Dietary Sources and High Intakes

Thiamin is widely distributed in raw foodstuffs. Thiamin is present in greatest amounts in brewer's yeast, germ and aleuron layer of ripe wheat, and in egg yolk and mammalian liver, and in smaller amounts in milk, green vegetables, potatoes and meat. Particularly rich sources are organ meats, wholegrain and enriched cereals and bread, legumes, nuts and meat. Poor sources are polished rice, sugar, alcohol, fat and refined foods.

The thiamin content of rice as grown and as eaten may vary widely, being altered by milling and cooking methods. The intake of highly milled rice was the first aetiological factor identified in the development of beriberi, and its use led to the discovery of thiamin. Up to 80% of the original thiamin in the grain can be lost in milling and washing prior to cooking, and in boiling. Thiamin is water-soluble and the rate of destruction increases with water and alkali.

Thiamin already present in the diet can be made unavailable by the enzyme thiaminase, found in raw fish (eaten as such), or by heat-stable antithiamines, found in fish and tea. Such antagonists can aggravate thiamin deficiency in the diet, especially in pregnant and lactating women and their offspring.

In maple syrup urine disease (MSUD), also called branched-chain ketoaciduria, where the branched-chain α-ketoacids derived from the three amino acids are not decarboxylated but are excreted in the urine, patients are not thiamin-deficient but may illustrate a dependency and a response to large doses of thiamin or TDP. High intakes of thiamin administered orally are nontoxic; the rapidly saturable thiamin absorption mechanism limits the amount taken up from a single dose to 2.5 mg, and thiamin in excess of plasma protein binding is excreted, restricting the amount of thiamin entering and remaining in the body. However, there are a few reports of toxicity from large and frequent doses of parenterally administered thiamin, and of cases of contact dermatitis in persons handling the vitamin.

See also: **Carbohydrates**: Requirements and Dietary Importance. **Glucose**: Metabolism and Maintenance of Blood Glucose Level. **Lactation**: Dietary Requirements. **Pregnancy**: Nutrient Requirements. **Thiamin**: Beriberi.

Further Reading

Bailey AL, Finglas PM, Wright AJA and Southon S (1994) Thiamin intake, erythrocyte transketolase (EC 2.2.1.1) activity and total thiamin in adolescents. *British Journal of Nutrition* 72:111–125.

Brin M, Tai M, Ostashever AS and Kalinsky H (1960) The effect of thiamin deficiency on the activity of erythrocyte hemolysate transketolase. *Journal of Nutrition* 71:273–281.

Cooper JR, Itokawa Y and Pincus JH (1969) Thiamin triphosphate deficiency in subacute necrotizing encephalomyelopathy. *Science* 164:74–75.

Department of Health (1991) Thiamin. *Dietary Reference Values for Food Energy and Nutrients for the United Kingdom*, pp 90–93. London: HMSO.

Gibson RS (1990) *Principles of Nutritional Assessment*. Oxford University Press.

Gubler CJ (1984) Thiamin. *Handbook of Vitamins*, 2nd edn, pp 245–297. New York: Marcel Dekker.

Heroux M, Rao VLR, Lavoie J, Richardson JS and Butterworth RF (1996) Alterations of thiamin phosphorylation and of thiamin dependent enzymes in Alzheimer's disease. *Metabolic Brain Disease* 11:81–88.

Mastrogiacomo F, Bettendorf L, Grisar T and Kish SJ (1996) Brain thiamine, its phosphate esters, and its metabolising enzymes in Alzheimer's disease. *Annals of Neurology* 39:585–591.

Marcus R and Coulston AM (1985) Water soluble vitamins. The vitamin B complex and ascorbic acid. *Goodman and Gilman's The Pharmacological Basis of Therapeutics*, 7th edn, pp 1551–1555. New York: Macmillan.

Rindi G and Ventura U (1972) Thiamine intestinal transport. *Physiological Reviews* 52:821–827.

Sauberlich HE, Herman YF, Stevens CO and Herman RH (1979) Thiamin requirements of the adult human. *American Journal of Clinical Nutrition* 32:2337–2248.

Beriberi

A E Cathcart and **D I Thurnham**, University of Ulster, Coleraine, Northern Ireland, UK

Aetiology

Beriberi is caused by a deficiency of the water-soluble B vitamin, thiamin. Thiamin plays an essential role in carbohydrate metabolism. It is present in the body in the active coenzyme forms with little being stored. In experiments withdrawal of thiamin is quickly followed by biochemical and clinical abnormalities. Humans are thus dependent on a constant supply in the diet to meet their daily requirements.

In the late nineteenth and early twentieth centuries beriberi was endemic in countries of Asia and the Far East, where highly milled rice was the staple cereal. Widespread beriberi dates from the introduction of steam-powered rice mills in the late nineteenth century. This was exaggerated by the socioeconomic conditions at the time, when large sections of the community lived in closed or controlled communities with restricted eating habits, e.g. Chinese immigrant miners received rice for wages in Malaya. Beriberi cases were observed 3–4 months after the introduction of a new mill. Morbidity and mortality were so great that a Dutch medical team was sent to Java in the late 1800s to investigate the cause of this disease. Many theories evolved on the aetiology of beriberi, e.g. infection, intoxication and various nutritional theories. Much progress was made in a relatively short period of time, and in 1900 Ejikman and Grijns discovered that rice bran, or 'polishings', prevented and cured polyneuritis in chickens. By 1926 this curative and preventative substance was isolated from rice bran by Jansen and Donath in Java and later by Williams. In 1936, it was given the name thiamine, now known internationally as thiamin. This discovery lead to the almost total eradication of beriberi as a primary health-care problem in these previously endemic areas through a number of measures, described later in this article.

Within the cereal grain, the germ and bran portions contain most of the thiamin, thus the intake is related closely to milling practices. Rice which is parboiled prior to milling retains most of the thiamin (~180 µg per 100 g), whereas highly milled rice is particularly low in thiamin (60 µg per 100 g). In India beriberi was only endemic in coastal regions where rice was raw milled, but in other parts of India, Pakistan and Sri Lanka parboiling prevented beriberi. Although usually associated with rice diets, beriberi has been seen in association with the consumption of other cereals, e.g. highly milled wheat by fishermen in Newfoundland and Labrador (1930s) and British troops in the Third Indian Division beseiged by Turks at Kut-el-Amara (1916); millet consumption in The Gambia. Beriberi should not be linked specifically with rice but rather with impoverished or restricted diets in which the cereal is refined and is virtually the sole food item.

The discovery that the milling of rice and the subsequent removal of thiamin was an aetiological factor was of great value in the prevention of beriberi. The lack of adequate dietary intake alone does not solve the aetiological puzzle, since the absence of thiamin does not necessarily cause neuritis in animals unless carbohydrate is given, and in humans a fall in the ratio of thiamin to carbohydrate and protein in the diet is also a causal factor with beriberi occurring when the proportion of thiamin (in mg) per 1000 calories (4200 J) falls below 0.3. This relationship is based on the essential role of thiamin in carbohydrate metabolism in the body. However, any factor leading to an increased demand for thiamin by the body may be classed as aetiological, and these are numerous.

Endemic beriberi has shown a seasonal incidence, often increasing in the pre-harvest farming months, possibly because of the increased physical exertion required at this time. With increased muscular work, the thiamin requirement will be increased when the principal energy source is carbohydrate, and carbohydrate intake is high in the diets of developing countries. There may be increased rice consumption to meet these increased requirements, exacerbating possible subclinical thiamin deficiency, or as is typical of harvest time in such countries, the previous year's harvest reserves may be almost depleted so that the extra requirement is not met. Young men are most affected by beriberi, possibly because they may work hardest at this time of year and/or possibly have the highest intake of carbohydrates.

Beriberi onset is often associated with a nonspecific fever bout, relating to the pyretic effect of disease on metabolic requirements. Other factors such as rapid growth, hyperthyroidism, pregnancy and lactation, may also exacerbate a pre-existing subclinical thiamin deficiency. There may also be increased requirements of thiamin as in diarrhoea or malabsorption, e.g. in pyloric stenosis, dysentery or steatorrhoea, and these may lead to deficiency even with apparently adequate dietary intakes. Beriberi has been reported in the West among HIV-infected patients resulting possibly from increased metabolic rate, gastrointestinal disturbances and/or low intakes. In addition, in Western countries, thiamin deficiency is most common among chronic alcoholics through defective intake and absorption of thiamin, together with the high carbohydrate intake leading to increased requirements and thus relative deficiency. Alcoholism has also been associated with outbreaks of thiamin deficiency in developing countries (see below). Thiamin deficiency may present as occidental beriberi heart disease, Wernicke's disease or Korsakoff's psychosis.

Prevalence

Beriberi was a major health problem in many Asian countries in the late nineteenth and early twentieth centuries. When the aetiology was attributed to milled rice consumption many reports described a spectacular reduction of beriberi in China, Japan, the Philippines, Malaysia, Singapore, Indonesia and Burma, and in areas of India where beriberi was endemic among people consuming highly milled rice. The dramatic reduction in incidence in Japan after this time is seen clearly from **Table 1**. Beriberi remains endemic in some southeast Asian countries, e.g. in areas of Thailand, China, Burma and Vietnam.

Although the incidence of beriberi in endemic areas has decreased, beriberi has not completely disappeared; however the pattern of incidence has changed. In recent years, the reappearance of widespread thiamin deficiency has been reported in Japan, The Gambia and South Africa. While thiamin deficiency appears to be related to alcohol intake in Durban (1987), among the !Kung San tribe in Namibia (1987) and in 'palm wine tappers' in The Gambia (1952), this was not the case in the Gambian community outbreak of 1988 or in Japan in 1980, where the increased consumption of imported milled rice and refined food intake, respectively, were suggested as major aetiological factors. This link between milled rice intake and beriberi in Africa was recognized in 1954, when it was commented of rice importation into The Gambia that it is 'unfortunately usually highly milled grain and increases the risk of beriberi in this predominently cereal-eating community'. In The Gambia, importation of milled rice has risen steadily since the 1970s and in the village where beriberi occurred milled rice provides a larger proportion of total cereal energy at the time of year of the outbreak (1988) than at any other time of the year. However, steamed millet products make up the remaining cereal energy and during the rainy season, after prolonged storage of millet, the thiamin content of these products are comparable to that of boiled imported rice.

In 1992–93 an epidemic outbreak of peripheral neuropathy occurred in Cuba affecting some 50 862 people. Clinical features of Strachan's syndrome and beriberi were observed, with thiamin deficiency suggested as one possible aetiological factor. Multivitamin supplements given to the whole population curbed the epidemic.

A sudden unexplained death syndrome (SUDS) has been partially related to thiamin deficiency. Although the appearance of SUDS dates back to 1915 among Philippinos in Manila and in the Hawaiian Islands and Chinese and Japanese in later years, there has been a recent surge in interest because of recent outbreaks among Thai construction workers in Singapore (91% of whom are from the northeast provinces of Thailand where thiamin deficiency is epidemic or endemic) and among southeast Asian refugees in the USA. SUDS is characterized by sudden and unexplained death in sleep with no premonitory signs.

Clinical and Biochemical Manifestations

Beriberi is a state in which usually both cardiac and nervous functions are disturbed. It is believed that the more serious the nervous lesion, the greater is the muscular pain and the less likely is the development of the more threatening and acute fulminating beriberi. The heart is saved from extreme insufficiency by the patient being forced to take complete rest at an early stage in the attack.

The three cardinal signs of beriberi include oedema and neurological and cardiovascular symptoms. Endemic beriberi in adults is usually described as either wet or dry, according to the presence or absence of oedema. **Fig. 1** shows typical beriberi patients. The forms of beriberi in humans can be categorized into five main types:

1. wet (subacute, cardiac) beriberi;
2. acute (fulminant) beriberi;
3. dry (chronic, atrophic, polyneuropathy) beriberi;
4. infantile beriberi; and
5. occidental beriberi.

Early clinical symptoms are common to both wet and dry beriberi. There is mild anorexia and an ill-defined malaise which is associated with heaviness of the legs and may cause difficulty in walking. There may be slight oedema of the legs and face and the patient may complain of precordial pain and palpitations. The pulse is usually full and the rate may be increased. The calf muscles are tender to pressure exertion and there may be complaints of 'pins and needles' and leg numbness. The tendon jerks are sluggish but sometimes exaggerated. Anaesthesia of the skin, especially over the tibia is common. All these symptoms may persist for months or even years

Table 1 Number of deaths and death rates of beriberi in selected years in Japan

Year	Total number	Death rate per 100 000 population
1900	7 180	15
1910	9 598	19
1920	14 239	25
1930	15 419	24
1940	7 179	10
1950	3 955	5
1959	447	0.5

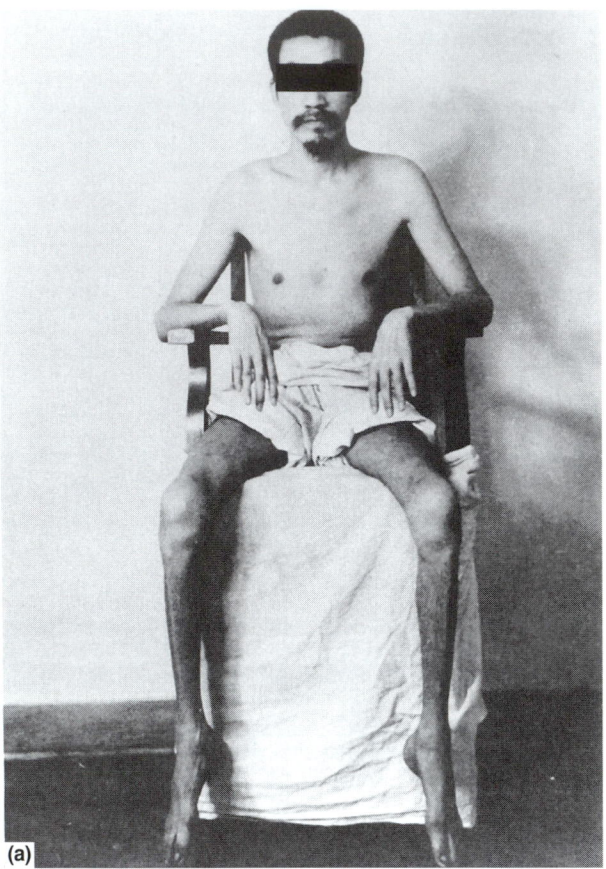

Figure 1 (a) Wrist drop and foot drop in a Chinese patient with dry beriberi. Reprinted with permission from Recheigl M, *CRC Handbook Series in Nutrition and Food, Vol. III, Section E: Nutritional Disorders*. Copyright CRC Press, Boca Raton Florida. © 1978.

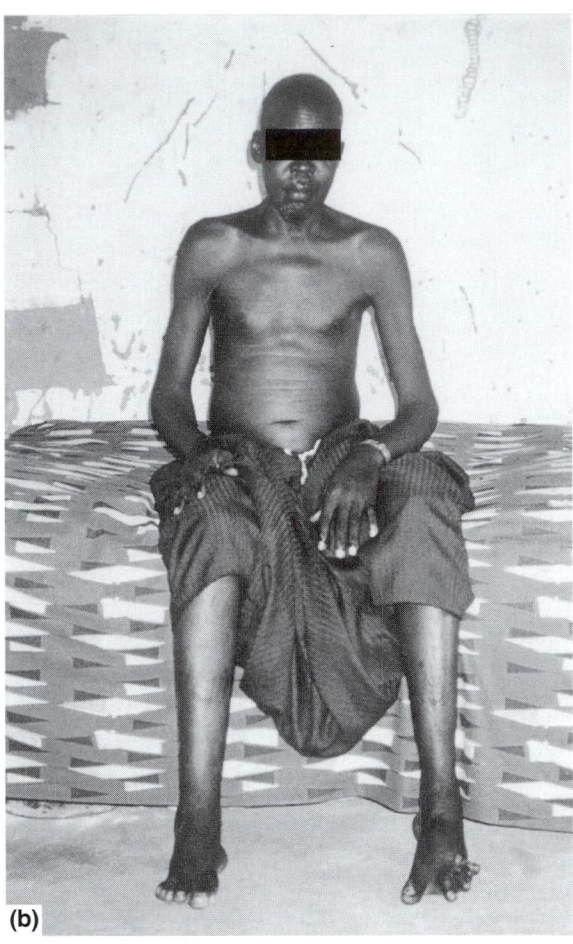

Figure 1 (b) Facial, abdominal and leg beriberi in a Gambian patient with suspected wet beriberi. Initially this man was treated unsuccessfully for heart failure, but later responded dramatically to 100 mg of thiamin per day. Unfortunately the patient died after changing to a treatment prescribed by the local medicine man.

and may develop into either wet or dry beriberi at any stage.

The clinical features associated with each type of endemic beriberi are listed in **Tables 2–5**. It should be stressed that although a number of symptoms have been described for each type of beriberi, none is pathognomonic; the disease is variable with every possible blend of the three sets of cardinal symptoms encountered, so that no one or two signs can be relied on to reveal all cases of beriberi.

Occidental beriberi heart disease may develop in chronic alcoholics with cardiac failure characterized by general oedema, pulmonary congestion and dyspnoea. The myocardium is damaged by either direct action of alcohol or thiamin deficiency. There are no signs of a high cardiac output synonymous with chronic beriberi. Sudden circulatory collapse with lactic acidosis, although less frequent, has been reported and is often overlooked in clinical investigation.

Deficiency of thiamin in the body impairs the activities of the enzymes that require, as a cofactor, thiamin diphosphate (TDP), the active form of thiamin in the body. TDP-requiring enzymes are involved in the oxidative phosphorylation of α-keto acids and in transketolase reactions, two reaction pathways involved in glucose metabolism. The concentration of pyruvic acid in the blood may rise to several times the normal value in severe beriberi since its conversion to acetyl-S-CoA is blocked by TDP deficiency, which will supress pyruvate dehydrogenase activity. Thiamin excretion is decreased and may be as low as 0–14 μg in 24 h.

Pathophysiology

Most pathological and anatomical knowledge of beriberi is based on studies carried out at the turn of the twentieth century, when beriberi was endemic in Asia and the Far East. The pathological manifestations associated with beriberi are listed in **Table 6**.

Table 2 Clinical manifestations of mild and subacute wet beriberi

Anorexia is common

Associated with a nonspecific bout of fever which may increase thiamin requirements

Nervous manifestations including alterations of tendon reflexes

Calf muscles have both a sensation of fullness, tightening or muscular ischaemia and hardening. This hardening is of value in detecting beriberi in early stages. Later pitting oedema is a more useful sign

Cardiovascular system signs and symptoms are prominent and important, ranging from breathlessness on exertion and palpitations to those found in the acute fulminant form (see Table 3)

Oedema appears to be related to physical activity, usually appearing at the end of a day's work. Oedema is due to some degree of congestive heart failure in some cases

Tachycardia is always present in well-developed cases, as is heart enlargement

Modified from Recheigl M. *CRC Handbook Series in Nutrition and Food, Vol. III, Section E: Nutritional Disorders*. Copyright CRC Press, Boca Raton Florida. © 1978.

Table 3 Clinical manifestations of acute fulminant wet beriberi

The whole picture is dominated by insufficiency of the heart and vessels and the course is usually fatal

Vomiting is common usually indicating the onset of acute symptoms

Tachycardia exists

Pulse is full, regular, even and weak at 120–150 beats per minute (a very high frequency is seldom seen)

Wave-like motion are seen over the heart

On percussion, heart is enlarged in all directions but mostly to the left

Systolic pressure is normal at first, finally falling to below 100, often reaching 80 or 70 at death

Enlarged and tender liver and epigastric region, spontaneously painful

Little lung disturbance with only mild tympany on percussion

Respiration is rough and whistling, without rales which will develop later as the condition worsens

Death is terrible. Patient is severely dyspnoeic, there are violent heart palpitations, intense pericordial agony and restlessness, intense thirst with drinking initiating vomiting, there is an anxious look on the face, cyanosis is more marked on inspiration and the patient dies usually fully conscious

Modified from Recheigl M. *CRC Handbook Series in Nutrition and Food, Vol. III, Section E: Nutritional Disorders*. Copyright CRC Press, Boca Raton Florida. © 1978.

Table 4 Clinical manifestations of dry beriberi

Generally seen in older adults only

A chronic condition of muscular atrophy and polyneuritis

Weak, wasted and painful muscles make walking difficult and at a more advanced stage, feeding and dressing are almost impossible. Patient may become bedridden, cachetic and very susceptible to infection

Sensory nerve disturbances are evident from hypoaesthesia, with paraesthesia as an early sign and with kinaesthesia in severe cases possibly giving rise to Rombergism. Anaesthesia may become almost complete

Motor nerve disturbances are evident from flaccid paralysis of extensor muscles resulting in 'wrist drop' and 'foot drop', the flexor muscles are also affected but less seriously

Achilles tendon reflexes are usually hypoactive with the patellar reflex affected later

Modified from Recheigl M. *CRC Handbook Series in Nutrition and Food, Vol. III, Section E: Nutritional Disorders*. Copyright CRC Press, Boca Raton Florida. © 1978.

Table 5 Clinical manifestations of infantile beriberi

Occurs between 2 and 3 months of age in breast fed infants whose mothers are thiamin deficient

Infant is pale, oedematous and ill-tempered

Gastrointestinal disturbances are evident through loss of appetite, vomiting of milk, diarrhoea and green faeces

Hoarseness and often blepharoptosis are present

Cardiovascular system manifestations are similar to those in adult beriberi, but with higher tachycardia. Dilation of the right ventricle, accelerated cardiac rhythm and a marked accentuation of the second pulmonary sound. Diastolic pressure is decreased. Sudden development of an acute fulminating type of beriberi may result possibly due to a slight infection

Liver and spleen are enlarged and palpable owing to congestion caused by cardiovascular impairment

Cerebral rather than peripheral nerves are paralysed. Hypoactivity of the Achilles tendon and patellar reflexes

In advanced beriberi the facial expression is apathic, the infant becomes incapable of fixing the head, body positioning and grasping power are weak

In severe cases, convulsion followed by a comatous state leads to cerebral infantile beriberi

There has been little addition to this knowledge. These studies were carried out when beriberi was not viewed as a deficiency disease, so that it is possible that the pathologists may have been somewhat biased as to what they thought they ought to see in relation to aetiology. As with clinical signs of beriberi, the pathology of each case varies in the extent of nervous and cardiac system involvement. The

Table 6 Pathological manifestations of beriberi

Generally there is anasarca, hypercardium, hydrothorax, ascites, hydrops in all serous cavities and anasarca and hydrops in all cavities

Cardiac findings:
  Fatty degeneration of the heart, of varying severity
  Dilatation of heart, most often right side
  Hypertrophy of both ventricles, most often the left ventricle only

Hyperaemia and oedema of the lungs

General venous congestion with cloudy swelling and fatty degeneration of the cellular elements of the liver and kidneys

Spleen is usually enlarged, and the intestines show venous hyperaemia with frequent small haemorrhages in the mucous membrane

Nervous system findings:
  Brain: usually hyperaemia of the membranes, oedema of the pia, and hyperaemia of the brain. Increased fluid in ventricles, oedema and anaemia of brain substance
  Vagus degeneration of the cranial nerves
  Spinal cord: hyperaemia of membranes, and serous effusions in peridural and subarachnoid spaces. Atrophy and partial loss of ganglion cells of the anterior horn
  Peripheral nerves: severe degeneration and atrophy
  Swelling and constriction of the medullary sheath, degeneration into droplets, invasion of fatty granular cells,
  complete absorption of medulla and axis cylinder so that only the empty sheath of Schwann remains
  Degeneration or loss of nerve fibres

Degeneration of muscle fibres comparable to that of nerves

Modified from Recheigl M. *CRC Handbook Series in Nutrition and Food, Vol. III, Section E: Nutritional Disorders.* Copyright CRC Press, Boca Raton Florida. © 1978.

pathological anatomy of beriberi involves changes in the nervous system including peripheral nerves and cord, changes in the heart including hypertrophy, dilatation, and fragmentations of the muscle fibres, and anasarca, oedema and effusions.

The underlying pathogenic mechanism of thiamin deficiency is unknown. As outlined below, the role of thiamin in carbohydrate metabolism is thought to be involved. Since the brain, nervous tissue and heart muscle use glucose in large amounts as a primary source of energy, carbohydrate metabolism is especially deranged in these tissues in thiamin deficiency. However, the non-cofactor role of thiamin in nerve conduction should not be ruled out.

A deficiency of thiamin is associated with elevated blood levels of pyruvate since the conversion of pyruvate to acetyl-S-CoA requires the action of the TDP-dependent enzyme, pyruvate dehydrogenase. Pyruvate is not converted to acetyl-S-CoA as is required for efficient glucose metabolism. In wet beriberi, the accumulation of pyruvate and lactate dilate the peripheral blood vessels, especially in the muscles, as in normal subjects during exercise. In beriberi, this vasodilation may be extreme and lead to capillary leakage. The cardiac output is increased to maintain the circulation, adding a burden on the already impaired heart muscle. As the disease progresses, the heart dilates and congestive heart failure accentuates the oedema, i.e. high output heart failure, and sudden death may result from myocardial failure.

Recently, a hypothesis for the pathophysiological link between heart failure, vasodilation and lactic acidosis has been made, suggesting that cellular ATP depletion and endogenous adenosine release play a role. The biochemical lesion here is acetyl-S-CoA deficiency as outlined below. Intracellular AMP accumulates as a consequence of ATP depletion, causing enhanced adenosine production by cytosolic-5'-nucleotidase. The adenosine is released extracellularly by a nucleoside transporter in the cell wall, this endogenous release being directly proportional to cystolic AMP accumulation. Adenosine infusion in conscious humans leads to systemic vasodilation, tachycardia, flushing, headache, restlesness, precordial agony, palpitation, fear and an urge to breath deeply. Acetyl-S-CoA deficiency, as a result of thiamin deficiency, will lead to ATP depletion since an adequate supply of acetyl-S-CoA into the citric acid cycle is necessary for the production of the thermodynamic driving force for the process of oxidative phosphorylation of ADP to produce ATP.

The lactic acidosis can be explained by the fact that cellular ATP depletion is an important stimulus for glycolysis. This stimulation will cause an increased pyruvate production while the metabolic block existing at the level of pyruvate dehydrogenase, the thiamin-dependent enzyme, causes decreased utilization and pyruvate accumulation. The enzyme lactate dehydrogenase will equilibrate pyruvate and lactate, increasing lactate levels and causing lactic acidosis.

Management

Beriberi is treated by the immediate administration of thiamin together with the institution of a good diet. Generally, there is a dramatic improvement within a few hours following intramuscular or intravenous administration of 50–100 mg of thiamin hydrochloride to a beriberi patient. In adult beriberi, oral treatment with 50 mg of thiamin given three times daily should continue for some days, the dose later being reduced to a maintenance level of 5–10 mg per day. Within a few hours the wet beriberi patient has responded; breathing is easier, the pulse rate slower, extremities cooler and rapid diuresis begins to dispose of oedema. In dry beriberi, no such spectacular improvement is likely to be seen. The patient is generally undernourished and with the provision of a good mixed diet slow improvement is expected. The usual physiotherapeutic treatment of polyneuropathy should be carried out, a diet rich in thiamin and with the minimum of carbohydrate and fluid should be given, and the possibility of other vitamin deficiencies should be borne in mind. Nicotinic acid, riboflavin and pyridoxine may be given and signs of vitamin B_{12} deficiency investigated. Heart failure may be treated with bed rest. The underlying cause of the thiamin deficiency should be investigated and treated. Chronic alcoholics should be treated for alcohol addiction, and patients in whom deficiency is secondary to disease of the stomach, duodenum or intestine, or to endogenous depression, need appropriate treatment. Glucose administration may precipitate heart failure in a state of marginal thiamin deficiency. All patients requiring glucose should receive prophylactically 100 mg of thiamin added to the first few litres of intravenous fluid.

Specific doses of thiamin are recommended for the treatment of thiamin deficiency of varying severities and in certain groups. In severe cardiac beriberi 10–20 mg of thiamin intramuscularly should be given several times each day. In severe heart failure or when convulsions or coma occur in infants, 25–50 mg thiamin should be administered intravenously and very slowly followed by intramuscular daily doses. In critically ill adults, 50–100 mg should be given slowly intravenously, with the same amount intramuscularly for the next few days. After improvement, oral therapy must be instituted and thiamin should continue 5–10 mg three times per day until maximum improvement has occurred. Neuritis of pregnancy should receive 5–10 mg per day parenterally if vomiting is severe.

Prevention

Endemic beriberi in Asia and the Far East has declined greatly since the discovery that the disease was caused by a lack of thiamin, and that this was mainly attributed to the consumption of highly milled rice. Since this time there have been improvements in socioeconomic factors in these areas with concomitant changes in diet, food distribution and lifestyle factors. In 1958, the Joint FAO/WHO Expert Committee on Nutrition listed methods for the prevention of beriberi, and through the review of these suggested techniques by the Nutrition Commitee for Asia and the Far East, and by their implementation, beriberi has almost been eradicated as a primary health-care problem. Reasons for the decline in beriberi are obscure as no single preventative measure has been applied effectively over a wide area. Generally, beriberi can be prevented by increasing the intake of thiamin, this being achievable through a number of measures as outlined below.

A general dietary improvement may increase the thiamin intake but this is not easy in countries where poverty, ignorance and scarcity of food are the norm. A dietary change from rice to wheat was forced upon the Japanese population through a general rice shortage. Improved socioeconomic conditions, and the consequent intake of a better diet, occurred in Japan, Taiwan and Malaysia and in larger cities where beriberi was common at that time. Changing from milled rice to either hand-pounded, undermilled or parboiled rice would increase thiamin content and thus intake. There is no evidence that this option has been successful in the fight against beriberi since these procedures are difficult to promote. Hand pounding is tedious and rice eaters are conservative, preferring a certain type of rice. Rice enrichment is another useful option but has been difficult to implement since there are many small mills processing home-grown rice. Fortified rice was available in Japan but only to the armed forces, and in other Asian countries rice enrichment was not pursued vigorously at all. It is believed that the distribution of synthetic thiamin to the population, as in Japan, is the most effective method in beriberi prevention, especially in infants. This is not suprising, as dietary and other lifestyle patterns are, as always, difficult if not impossible to alter even in the event of enormous morbidity and mortality from a preventable disease.

See also: **Carbohydrates**: Requirements and Dietary Importance. **Energy**: Energy Requirements. **Thiamin**: Physiology.

Further Reading

Bakker SJL and Leunissen KML (1995) Hypothesis on cellular ATP depletion and adenosine release as causes of heart failure and vasodilation in cardiovascular beriberi. *Medical Hypothesis* 45:265–267.

Cathcart AE (1998) *Monitoring seasoual changes in factors affecting thiamin status in a Gambian village.* PhD thesis, University of Ulster.

Davidson R and Eastwood MA (1986) *Human Nutrition and Dietetics*, 8th edn. Edinburgh: Churchill Livingstone.

Kawai C, Wakabayashi A, Matsumura T and Yui Y (1980) Reappearance of beriberi heart disease in Japan. *American Journal of Medicine* 69:383–386.

Kril JJ (1996) Neuropathology of thiamin deficiency disorders. *Metabolic Brain Disease* 11:9–17.

Liu S, Zhang K and Riley M (1995) Thiamine deficiency is associated with ethnicity in a subtropical area of China. *Asia Pacific Journal of Nutrition* 1:1–6.

Loue S, Okello D and Kawuma M (1996) Beriberi and thiamin deficiency in HIV infection. *AIDS* 10:931–932.

Naidoo DP (1987) Beriberi heart disease in Durban. *South African Medical Journal* 72:241–244.

Padua AB and Juliano BO (1974) Effect of parboiling on thiamin, protein and fat of rice. *Journal of Science and Food Agriculture* 25:697–701.

Platt BS (1958) Epidemiology and clinical features of endemic beriberi. Proceedings of a conference on beriberi, endemic goitre and hypervitaminosis A. *Proceedings of the Federation of the American Societies of Experimental Biology* 17(supplement 2):3–20.

Platt BS and Grant MW (1954) Food consumption in The Gambia. In: *Malnutrition in African Mothers, Infants and Young Children*. Report of the Second Inter-African Conference on Nutrition held under the Auspices of the Commission for Technical Co-operation in Africa South of the Sahara (CCTA), Fajara, The Gambia, 19–27 November 1952. London: HMSO.

Roman GC (1994) An epidemic in Cuba of optic neuropathy, sensorineural deafness, peripheral sensory neuropathy and dorsolateral myelonneuropathy. *Journal of Neurological Sciences* 127:11–28.

Shimazonono N and Katsura E (eds) (1965) *Beriberi and Thiamin*. Kyoto: Vitamin B Research Committee of Japan.

Tang CM, Wells JC, Rolfe M and Cham K (1989) Outbreak of beriberi in The Gambia. *Lancet* ii:206–207.

Tanphaichitr V, Lerdvuthisopon N, Dhanamitta S and Valyasevi A (1990) Thiamin status in Northeastern Thais. *Internal Medicine* 6:43–46.

Thurnham DI (1978) *Handbook Series on Nutrition and Food*, pp. 3–14. Boca Raton: CRC Press.

van der Westhuyzen J, Davis RE, Icke GC and Jenkins T (1987) Thiamin status and biochemical indices of malnutrition and alcoholism in settled communities of !Kung San. *Journal of Tropical Medicine and Hygiene* 90:283–289.

Walters JH and Smith DA (1952) Oedematous beriberi in palm wine tappers. *West African Medical Journal* 1:21–28.

Williams RR (1961) *Towards the Conquest of Beriberi*. Cambridge, MA: Havard University Press.

Wong ML, Ong CN, Tan TC, Phua KH, Goh LG, Lee HP, Chawalit S and Orapun M (1992) Sudden unexplained death syndrome. *Tropical and Geographical Medicine* 44:S1–S19.

THIRST

Physiology

J Leiper, Department of Biomedical Sciences, University Medical School, Aberdeen, Scotland, UK

Role of Thirst in Water Balance

Approximately 70% of the lean body mass of an individual is composed of water. About two-thirds of the total body water (TBW) volume is held within the cells of the body (intracellular pool), while the remaining one-third (extracellular pool) is divided between the circulating blood plasma (intravascular pool) and the fluid-filled spaces between the cells (interstitial pool). The volume and distribution of the body fluids are mainly determined by the amounts of body water and sodium. In humans, total body water content is regulated daily to within about 0.2% of lean body mass in normal, temperate conditions by factors which control input and output. The kidneys regulate water excretion in excess of the evaporative loss and the faecal and obligatory urine losses. Water intake occurs in the form of food and drink, with the sensation of thirst underpinning drinking behavior.

Perception of Thirst

Thirst is a sensation which is best described as the desire to drink. The reason for drinking may not be directly involved with a physiological need for water intake, but can be prompted by habit, ritual, taste, nutrients, craving for alcohol, caffeine or other drugs in a beverage, or a desire to consume a fluid which will give a warming or cooling sensation. Much of the perception of thirst is a learned or conditioned process, with signals such as dryness of the mouth or throat initiating drinking, while a feeling of fullness of the stomach can stop ingestion before a fluid deficit has been restored. Although it is true that thirst in humans is a poor indicator of acute hydration status and that daily fluid intake is normally in excess of obligatory water loss, the preservation of total body water volume under a variety of environmental and nutritional stresses is remarkably robust and is mainly due to the drive to drink which the sensation of thirst chronically provokes.

Assessment of Thirst

In humans two main techniques have been used to identify the perception of thirst and its alleviation by drinking. The first method is to monitor the volume of drink voluntarily ingested by an individual within an allotted time period, and to compare the amount drunk with the volume of fluid required to restore a given water deficit or other imbalance of the body water pools. The other method is to assess the individual's perceived rating of thirst by asking them to record on a visual analogue scale their responses to

a series of questions which are thought to relate to the sensation of thirst (**Fig. 1**). The questionnaire technique has the advantages that it allows a series of measurements to be made before, during and following the period of drinking, and appears to give an indication of the relative strength of a given stimulus. Although in many studies both methods are used to gauge the sensation of thirst and the responses have been correlated to a number of physiological parameters that are known to influence the drive to drink, it is widely recognized that at present there is no consistently reliable measure of the thirst sensation.

The Physiological Regulation of Thirst

As thirst is the major factor controlling water intake, the physiological regulation of thirst is associated with the need to maintain a relatively stable volume

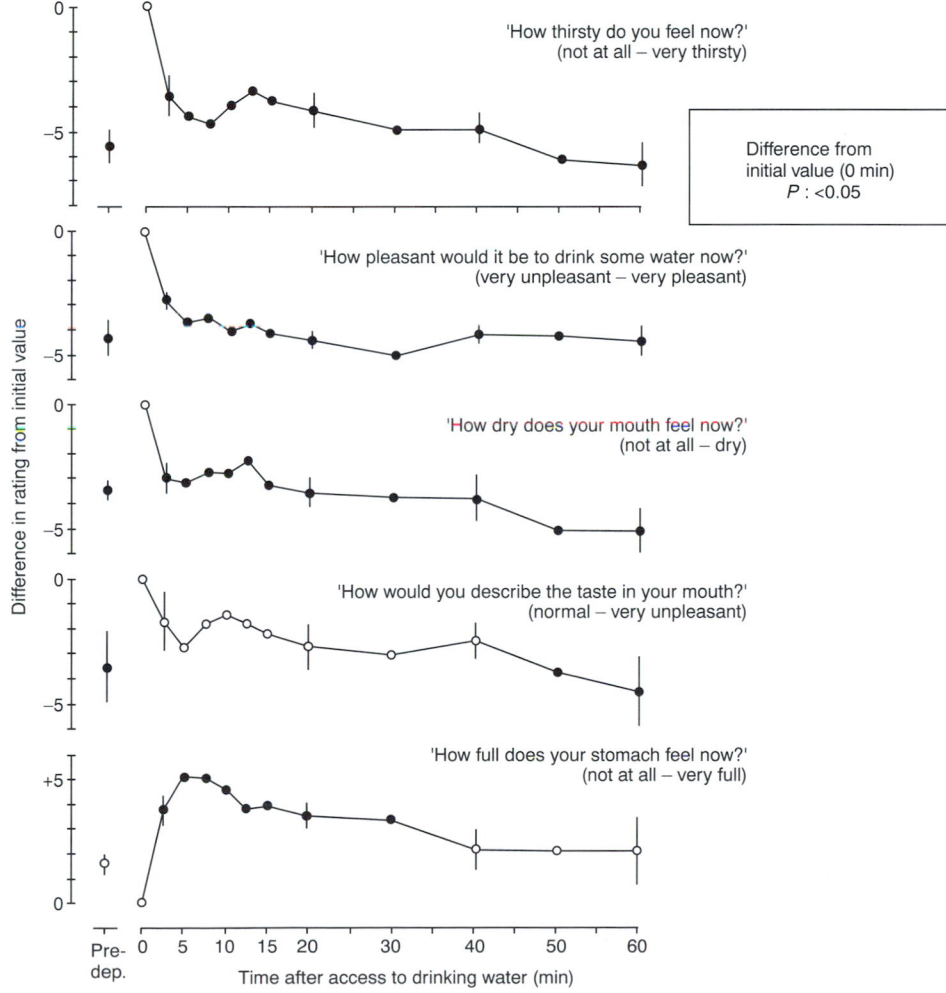

Figure 1 Subjective responses to a series of five questions assessed by visual analogue scale ratings from individuals deprived of water for 24 h. Questions were asked before and during a 60 min rehydration period. The data are shown as differences (in cm) from initial values and significant differences are indicated by filled symbols. Redrawn with permission from Rolls BJ, Wood RJ, Rolls ET, Lind H, Lind W and Ledingham JGG (1980) Thirst following water deprivation in humans. *American Journal of Physiology* **239**:R476–482.

of total body water. Although water is lost from the body continually, albeit usually in relatively small amounts, and hence the body is almost always developing a water deficit, water intake is intermittent. The amount of fluid usually ingested is in excess of that required to replace the losses incurred since the last water intake. The factors which initiate, maintain and end the drinking response are various and are not fully understood. However, as the regulation of the volume and composition of the various water pools of the body plays an essential role in controlling the perception of thirst, an understanding of the homeostatic mechanisms involved has given us the best insight we have into the complexities of the perception of thirst.

The total volume, distribution and composition of body fluids must be regulated within narrow limits for normal cellular function to be maintained. Body water is passively distributed between the extracellular and intracellular pools according to osmotic, oncotic and hydrostatic forces, as shown in **Fig. 2**. Sodium and chloride are the two most abundant osmotically active components of the extracellular fluid and are therefore important in maintaining its volume. Potassium, phosphate and protein fulfil a similar role in regulating the intracellular fluid volume. The distribution of water between the intravascular and extravascular pools is dependent on the balance of hydrostatic and oncotic pressures across the capillaries and postcapillary venules.

Variation in the water-to-solute ratio of a body fluid pool result in changes in the tonicity and hence effective osmolality of the fluid. As the various body water pools are in dynamic equilibrium with each other (Fig. 2) there is a tendency for adjustments to occur throughout the body as water moves from regions of low solute concentration to those of higher solute concentration. Since changes in plasma osmolality are relatively easy to monitor, there is a tendency to equate change in the circulation as the effector of fluid balance control. It is, however, important to remember that any alteration in one body pool will affect the others and that receptors which initiate responses affecting water balance may reside at sites far removed from the circulation.

Loss of water from the body or an increase in the circulating solute concentration causes an increase in the osmolality primarily of the extracellular fluid. Water then moves into the extracellular space from the cells, resulting in a reduction in cell volume. Changes in plasma osmolality are therefore thought to be signalled to the effector mechanisms by changes in the cell volume of specific specialized cells, collectively termed osmoreceptors. As the main solute determining the tonicity of the extracellular fluid is sodium, there has been some debate as to whether the receptor cells detect changes in osmolality or changes in sodium ion content. The evidence suggests that at least the majority of receptors respond to osmolality rather than to sodium concentration. These osmoreceptors have a regulatory role not only in the perception of thirst, but also in the maintenance of the circulating levels of hormones that regulate the excretion of water and solute by the kidneys (**Fig. 3**). As increases in the extracellular osmolality effectively decrease the volume of the cells in the body, this form of dehydration is termed cellular dehydration.

Alteration in the volume of the extracellular fluid pool without change in its osmolality also affects the fluid balance hormone concentrations and the sensation of thirst. Changes in the volume of blood in the circulation affect the blood and capillary pressures and atrial filling pressure. The effect on capillary pressure will tend to redistribute body water and help to adjust the circulating fluid volume, and the change in venous return to the heart will alter the cardiopulmonary and arterial stretch receptor (baroreceptor) activity. The level of afferent activity from these baroreceptors directly affects both the sensation of thirst and the secretion of some fluid balance hormones. Additionally, modifications to the arterial blood pressure can directly affect renal perfusion, which together with baroreceptor activity to the kidneys regulates the renin–angiotensin system (**Fig. 4**). Although the effect on the kidneys can influence the perception of thirst, the main renal response is to regulate water and solute excretion in the urine. A decrease in the volume of the extracellular pool with no concomitant change in plasma osmolality is termed extracellular dehydration.

When humans are given access to fluids after the development of a water deficit, their drinking response usually follows a pattern of rapid ingestion of more than 50% of the total intake followed by intermittent consumption of relatively small volumes of drink over a longer period. While initiation of the

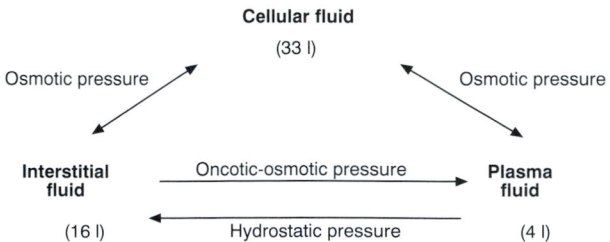

Figure 2 Diagrammatic representation of the forces which regulate the distribution of the body water pools. The volumes given are those determined in a single male subject with a lean body mass of 75.8 kg.

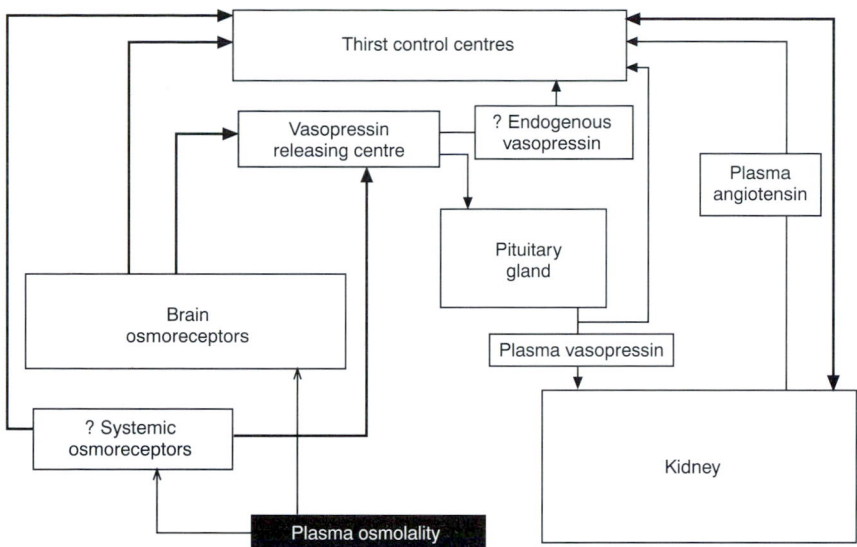

Figure 3 Schematic representation of the main factors proposed in osmotically induced regulation of the sensation of thirst and their interaction with the control of diuresis. A rise in plasma osmolality will tend to stimulate greater excitatory activity, while a decrease in osmolality will activate more inhibitory inputs. Neural pathways are indicated by ➡ and hormonal input by →.

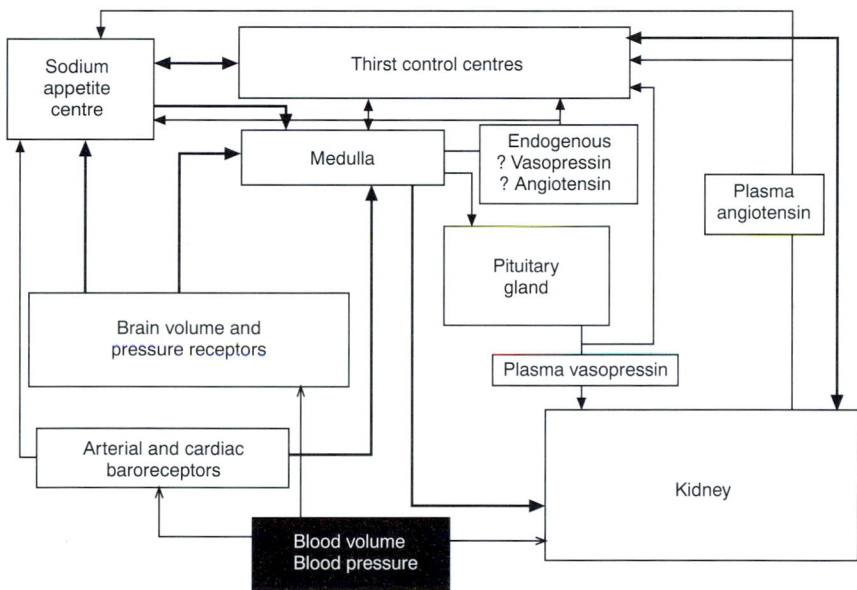

Figure 4 Schematic representation of the main factors proposed in volaemic-induced regulation of the sensation of thirst and their interaction with the control of diuresis and sodium appetite. A fall in circulating blood volume will decrease baroreceptor activity which will increase excitatory activity, while a rise in volume will have the opposite effect. Reduction in blood pressure will decrease renal perfusion which will activate the renal renin–angiotensin system. Neural pathways are indicated by ➡ and hormonal input by →.

response to drink is due mainly to osmotic or blood volume (volaemic) changes, there appear to be other mechanisms involved in the control of the continuation and satiety responses. Receptors in the mouth, oesophagus and gastrointestinal tract appear to be major factors in the acute regulation of thirst satiation: while chronic regulation of thirst is controlled mainly by the effect that the volume and solute content of ingested drinks has on restoring any fluid deficit (**Fig. 5**). There is a close relationship between eating and drinking, with about 70% of daily fluid intake normally being associated with meals (**Fig. 6**). The desire to drink while eating is probably produced by a series of responses including the mechano-chemical composition of the food before absorption, the neuroendocrine response to digestion, the movement of water into the intestine during digestion and the osmotic solute load which occurs

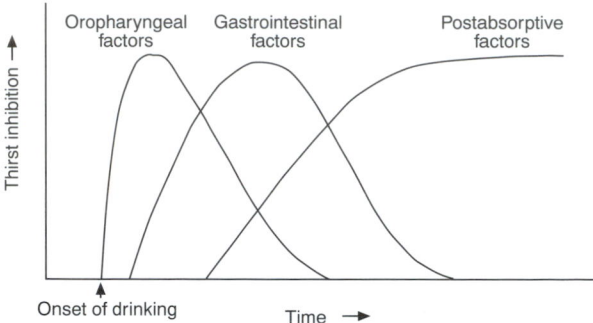

Figure 5 Schematic diagram depicting the proposed onset, duration and overlap of various inhibitory signals to continue fluid ingestion following initiation of drinking in response to a fluid deficit. Redrawn with permission from Verbalis JG (1990) Inhibitory controls of drinking: satiation of thirst. In: Ramsay DJ and Booth DA (eds) *Thirst: Physiological and Psychological Aspects*, pp 313–330. London: Springer-Verlag.

following absorption. The intake of minerals is essential to replace those lost from the body and for growth. The majority of mineral intake is supplied by the food ingested, and indications of a desire or appetite for ingesting specific minerals have been shown in animals and man. Although sodium appetite has been linked to the sensation of thirst, anatomically and functionally the controlling mechanisms are distinct and separate.

Mechanisms of Thirst Regulation

The sensation of thirst is regulated separately both by the osmotic pressure and volume of the body fluids and as such is closely related to the control mechanisms which are responsible for the secretion of the fluid balance hormones that affect water and solute reabsorption in the kidneys and play a role in blood pressure control. These hormones arginine vasopressin, atrial natriuretic peptide, oxytocin and the renin–angiotensin–aldosterone system – are central to the regulation of thirst. Regions of the brain in the hypothalamus and forebrain appear to be the main areas involved in the control of thirst and anti-diuresis, and collectively these parts of the brain have been termed the thirst control centres. Neurons which are responsive to changes in osmolality, intra-vascular volume (volaemia) and blood pressure are found within these areas of the brain, as are other receptors which are responsive to many of the fluid balance hormones. Neural pathways from the thirst control centres and the kidneys may allow some direct integration between the control of thirst and excretion, while within the brain all of the major fluid balance hormones are present as neurohormones. Afferent input from systemic receptors monitoring osmolality, circulating sodium concentration and changes in intravascular volume and pressure also have roles in controlling the feeling of thirst. Therefore, there appears to be a complex integrated

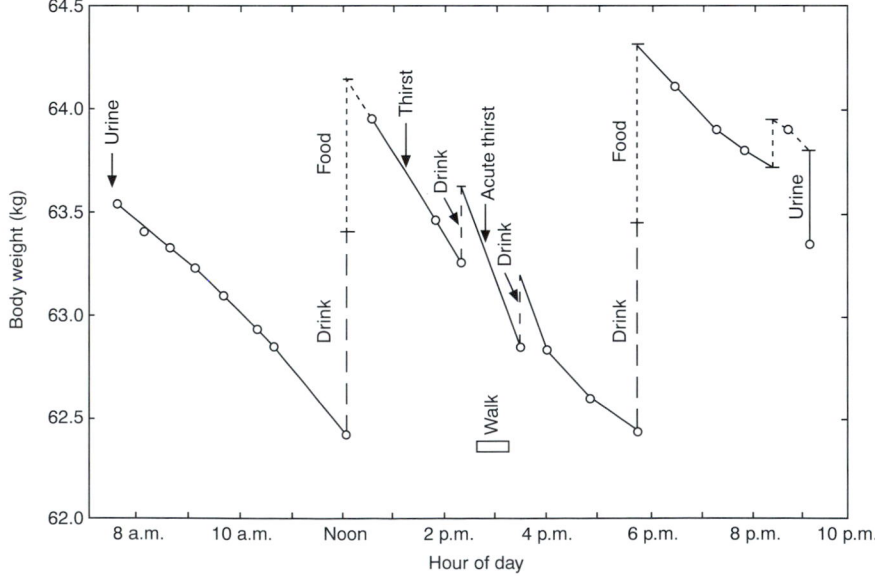

Figure 6 Changes in body weight during 13 h in the desert. The majority of the volume of drink ingested was associated with food intake. Sweat loss varied from 150 to 700 ml h^{-1}, total fluid intake was 3.05 l. At the end of the period body mass was essentially the same at the beginning and end of the day, therefore water intake and output were equal. From Adolph ED, *Physiology of Man in the Desert*. Copyright © 1947. Reprinted by permission of John Wiley & Sons Inc.

system for both monitoring the status of the body water pools and controlling intake and excretion (Figs 3 and 4). Many of the regulatory mechanisms controlling water balance appear to overlap with other stimuli that appear to subserve the same response; it is assumed that this effect is required in order to ensure that the blocking of one type of stimulus will not prevent homeostatic control.

Osmotic regulation of thirst

The osmolality of circulating plasma is normally maintained within a very narrow range between 270 and 295 mosmol kg^{-1}, with the circulating levels of the antidiuretic hormone arginine vasopressin playing a major role in its homeostatic regulation. An increase of as little as 2–3% in plasma osmolality is sufficient to produce a strong sensation of thirst and a significant increase in circulating arginine vasopressin concentration (**Fig. 7**). The osmoreceptors which monitor the tonicity of the body pools appear to reside mainly in an area of the brain which lacks a blood–brain barrier, therefore they appear to respond primarily to changes that occur in the osmolality of the blood rather than in the cerebral intersti-

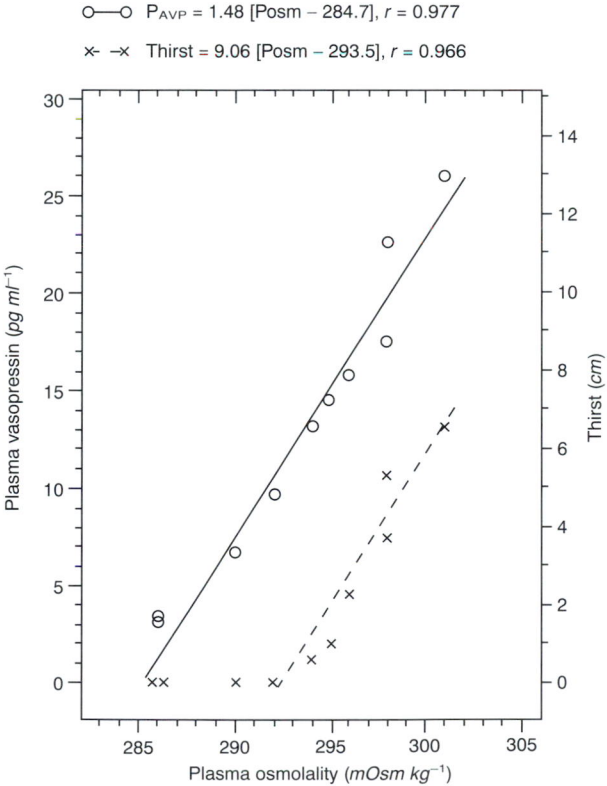

Figure 7 The relationship of plasma vasopressin (○) and thirst (×) to plasma osmolality in a volunteer during infusion of 5% saline. Redrawn with permission from Robertson GL (1984) Abnormalities of thirst regulation (Nephrology forum). *Kidney International* **25**:460–469.

tium. Although the changes in the circulating levels of arginine vasopressin and the perception of thirst appear to parallel one another, it is unlikely that the same receptors are responsible for both responses; the probability is that there are different neurons which react to the same stimulus. However, there may be some neurohormonal interaction between the osmotically activated thirst centres and the 'vasopressin releasing centre' in the brain, and arginine vasopressin responsive neurons have been detected within the thirst centres (Fig. 3).

The current theory of the osmotic control of thirst suggests that there is constant output of both inhibitory and excitatory neural activity from the respective osmoreceptors to the thirst centres and the arginine vasopressin releasing centres. Within the normal range for plasma osmolality, the inhibitory and excitatory activities in the thirst centres effectively cancel one another out and there is neither a sensation of thirst nor of satiety. However, at this level of activity there is release of a basal level of arginine vasopressin which is sufficient to maintain a state of half-maximum antidiuresis. A rise in plasma osmolality above the normal level stimulates greater excitatory output, resulting in an increase in the feeling of thirst and higher levels of circulating arginine vasopressin. Raised levels of arginine vasopressin increase the concentrating ability of the kidneys. A decrease in plasma osmolality below the normal range increases the inhibitory output, producing a feeling of satiety, and arginine vasopressin release is suppressed, thus allowing urinary dilution (Fig. 3).

Cells and fibers within the brain have been shown to contain several hormones, including angiotensin and vasopressin, within the same cell. Although neurons associated with the thirst centres can be activated *in vitro* by vasopressin, it is not clear whether peripheral or neural generated arginine vasopressin levels influence the perception of thirst.

Volaemic regulation of thirst

The receptors that initiate hypovolaemic thirst are generally thought to be the cardiovascular baroreceptors which respond to underfilling of the circulation by reducing their inhibitory nerve impulse activity to the thirst centres. However, in areas of the brain associated with the thirst centres there are different specialized neurons that are either responsive to volaemic, pressure or osmotic changes. This suggests that at least part of the response to changes in blood volume originates in the brain.

It is thought that changes in blood pressure and osmolality are monitored mainly within the brain, while variations in blood volume are principally sensed by the peripheral baroreceptors, with a degree of overlap between the different receptors. The mechanisms which respond to changes in intravascular volume and pressure do not appear to be as sensitive as those responsive to osmotic changes, for example a decrease of about 10% of the plasma volume is required to initiate hypovolaemic thirst. As fairly large variations in blood volume and pressure occur during normal daily activity, such as postural changes and physical activity, this apparent lack of sensitivity presumably prevents overactivity of the volaemic control mechanisms. As with osmotic thirst, the control of volaemic thirst is thought to be a balance between continuous inhibitory and excitatory neural activity, although in this system the basal level appears to be essentially inhibitory. Another difference in the basic control mechanism between the two systems occurs owing to the requirement for both solute, mainly sodium, and water, to restore the extracellular volume. Therefore, extracellular dehydration causes an initial thirst and a delayed increase in sodium appetite.

Reduction in the intravascular volume sufficient to lower cardiac output and arterial blood pressure decreases afferent activity from the low and high pressure cardiovascular baroreceptors to the thirst centres and increases sympathetic activity to the kidneys. As afferent input from the baroreceptors to the thirst centres is inhibitory, a decrease in activity produces a reflex increase in the perception of thirst and also appears to stimulate arginine vasopressin release directly. The increase in sympathetic activity to the kidneys directly promotes greater renal renin release. In addition, reduction in blood pressure lowers the renal perfusion pressure; this stimulates renin release both as a direct pressure effect and by decreasing the delivery of sodium to the kidneys.

Increased activation of the renin–angiotensin–aldosterone system also helps regulate hypovolaemic thirst. While circulating levels of both vasopressin and aldosterone affect water and sodium reabsorption in the kidneys and thereby control water and solute loss, angiotensin acts directly on the thirst and sodium appetite centres to stimulate their respective responses. Neurons which are stimulated by angiotensin are found in areas of the brain that lacks a blood–brain barrier, therefore circulating angiotensin has direct access to both centres. In addition, the release of neurally generated angiotensin is promoted by suitable neuron activity responding to sensory stimuli (Fig. 4).

There are thus a variety of neural and hormonal responses which interact to modulate and control both thirst and urine excretion. A number of other hormones including oxytocin, atrial natriuretic peptide, tachykinins, neuropeptide Y, thyroid hormones, corticotrophin releasing factor and steroid hormones have also been shown experimentally to affect the drinking response. Under normal conditions of water and solute loss both osmotic and volaemic dehydration occurs, so that stimuli from receptors for both systems are usually involved in the sensation of thirst. Increases in extracellular osmolality appears to be more effective than hypovolaemia in promoting the thirst and hence drinking response. Greater than 70% of the stimulus to drink appears to be generated by increased osmolality.

Mechanisms for terminating the sensation of thirst

Although undoubtedly decreasing osmolality and increasing extracellular volume promote a reduction in the perception of thirst by reactivating inhibitory neuron activity, there is usually a decrease in the perception of thirst and termination of drinking before circulating osmolality, volume and hormonal levels have returned to pre-dehydration levels. While it could be argued that receptors in the brain may be responsible for the early cessation of the perception of thirst, the majority of the evidence suggests that it is receptors in the upper gastrointestinal tract which promote the early termination of drinking. Although the nature and neural connections of these proposed receptors have not been characterized, most appear to have an inhibitory response. It has been suggested that as much of the thirst and drinking response is behavioural, an individual learns what volume of drink is required to restore a given water deficit. Termination of drinking therefore could be a learned response which anticipates a future fluid deficit or matches a known current level of dehydration. The stimuli for gauging the current level of dehydration may be the same as those which initiate the sensation of thirst.

The mere presence of liquid, particularly cold liquid, in the mouth reduces the perception of thirst. The response of receptors in the mouth and oesophagus to different chemical, tactile, pressure and temperature stimuli is thought to be part of the mechanism which influences the relative intensity of the perception of thirst. The neural activity involved in swallowing, and perhaps also signals from the oropharyngeal and gastric receptors, are thought to be effective in sensing or metering the volume of liquid ingested. Distension of the stomach tends to inhibit drinking owing to increased gastric stretch receptor activity, although this response does not always reduce the perception of thirst. Taste and other psychological factors can have a stimulatory effect on consumption of a drink which is considered to be palatable.

The continuation and termination of the acute sensation of thirst is regulated by a series of stimuli which apparently operate before all of the drink consumed has been absorbed and before disturbances in the body water pools have been corrected. A variety of receptors located from the mouth to the upper part of the small intestine, and probably neural control from the higher centres of the brain, appear to monitor and regulate the initial volume consumed. After absorption, if restoration of body water pools has not occurred, the sensation of thirst is once again initiated, presumably by the same homeostatic stimuli which initially evoked the feeling of thirst, and drinking restarts. The integration of the pre- and postabsorptive stimuli modulates the sensation of thirst and ultimately the volume of drink consumed.

Fluid Requirements

Renal reabsorption can reduce the volume of water and solute loss, and hence slow the rate of progress of a fluid deficit, but it cannot stop its development. Intake of fluid either as food or drink is required to restore a fluid deficit. Daily fluid intake is highly variable between individuals and the rate of loss is dependent on factors such as environmental temperature, physical activity, sweating rate, antidiuretic function and dietary solute load. A representative normal daily water turnover in a sedentary individual living in a temperate climate and eating a typical Western diet is about 2–3 l, and a minimum daily fluid intake of about 1.7 l is necessary to conserve fluid balance. The water content of the typical Western diet approximates to about 1 litre and metabolically derived water produces in the order of about 300 ml, which together almost offsets the daily obligatory water loss. Therefore in many situations the requirement for fluid intake can actually be very low.

There are conditions in which water loss is greater than that indicated above and replacement obviously requires a compensatory increase in daily fluid intake (Fig. 6). Urine volume is related to the solute content of the diet, with a minimum volume of about 500 ml being necessary to eliminate the daily solute load. Diets rich in protein or foods with a high sodium content require a greater obligatory urine output for excretion. The renal concentrating ability at maximum antidiuresis determines the minimum urinary water loss for a given dietary solute load. Normally there is a wide range of urinary osmolality such that the same solute load can be excreted in 500 ml of urine with an osmolality of 1400 mosmol kg^{-1} or in 23 l of urine with an osmolality of 30 mosmol kg^{-1}. This feature of renal excretion allows body water balance to be maintained while fluid intake volume is varied.

Prolonged relatively intense muscular activity, elevated ambient temperature and fever all increase the rate of evaporative sweat loss. Individual sweat rates are highly variable, but daily losses of between 10 and 15 l have been recorded. Daily faecal losses associated with a Western diet are usually between 100 and 200 ml daily; however diarrhoea, particularly infectious diarrhoea, can produce prodigious faecal water losses which are potentially fatal.

Inappropriate fluid intake can be produced following lesions or development of tumours in regions of the brain associated with the thirst centres. Diabetes insipidus promotes an increase in the volume of fluid ingested, which is caused by a lowering of the basal threshold set point for osmotic thirst. A similar, although less pronounced, lowering of the osmotic thirst threshold occurs during pregnancy. In both the young and the elderly the thirst response can be blunted and inappropriate drinking habits may occur. Psychogenic disturbances in the sensation of thirst and hence fluid intake have also been reported for a variety of clinical conditions.

See also: **Appetite**: Physiological and Neurobiological Aspects; Psychobiological and Behavioural Aspects. **Behaviour**: Dietary Effects on Mood and Behaviour. **Body Composition**: Determination and Physiological Significance. **Brain and Nervous System**: Biology, Metabolism and Nutritional Requirements. **Dehydration**: Physiological Effects and Management. **Diarrhoeal (Diarrheal) Diseases**: Nutritional Factors. **Electrolytes**: Water-Electrolyte Balance. **Gastrointestinal Tract**: Structure and Function of the Stomach; Structure and Function of the Small Intestine; Structure and Function of the Colon. **Infants**: Nutritional Requirements. **Older People**: Nutritional Requirements; Physiological Changes; Nutritionally Related Problems; Nutritional Management of Geriatric Patients. **Pregnancy**: Nutrient Requirements. **Salt**: Epidemiology. **Sodium**: Physiology.

Further Reading

Adolph ED and Associates (1947) *Physiology of Man in the Desert*. New York: Interscience.

Engell DB, Maller O, Sawka MN, Francesconi RN, Drolet L and Young AJ (1987) Thirst and fluid intake following graded hypohydration levels in humans. *Physiology and Behaviour* 40:229–236.

Johnson AK and Edwards GL (1990) Central projections of osmotic and hypovolaemic signals in homeostatic thirst. In: Ramsay DJ and Booth DA (eds) *Thirst: Physiological and Psychological Aspects*, pp 149–175. London: Springer-Verlag.

Maughan RJ (1994) Fluid and electrolyte loss and replacement in exercise. In: Harries BJ, Williams C, Stanish CW and Micheli A (eds) *Oxford Textbook of Sports Medicine*, pp 82–93. New York: Oxford University Press.

Phillips PA, Rolls BJ, Ledingham JGG and Morton JJ (1984) Body fluid changes, thirst and drinking in man during free access to water. *Physiology and Behaviour* 33:357–363.

Ramsay DJ (1989) The importance of thirst in the maintainance of fluid balance. In: Bayliss PH (ed.) *Water and Salt Homeostasis in Health and Disease*, Clinical Endocrinology and Metabolism, vol. 3, no. 2, pp 371–391. London: Baillière Tindall.

Ramsay DJ (1990) Water: distribution between compartments and its relationship to thirst. In: Ramsay DJ and Booth DA (eds) *Thirst: Physiological and Psychological Aspects*, pp 23–34. London: Springer-Verlag.

Ramsay DJ and Thrasher TN (1986) Hyperosmotic and hypovolemic thirst. In: de Caro G, Epstein AN and Massi M (eds) *The Physiology of Thirst and Sodium Appetite*, pp 83–96. New York: Plenum Press.

Robertson GL (1984) Abnormalities of thirst regulation (Nephrology forum). *Kidney International* 25:460–469.

Rolls BJ and Rolls ET (1982) *Thirst*. Cambridge: Cambridge University Press.

Rolls BJ, Wood RJ and Rolls ET (1980) Thirst: The initiation, maintenance, and termination of drinking. *Progress in Psychobiology and Physiological Psychology* 9:263–321.

Rolls BJ, Wood RJ, Rolls ET, Lind H, Lind W and Ledingham JGG (1980) Thirst following water deprivation in humans. *American Journal of Physiology* 239:R476–482.

Verbalis JG (1990) Inhibitory controls of drinking: satiation of thirst. In: Ramsay DJ and Booth DA (eds) *Thirst: Physiological and Psychological Aspects*, pp 313–330. London: Springer-Verlag.

TOCOPHEROLS

Physiology

T Sheehy and **P A Morrissey**, Department of Nutrition, University College, Cork, Ireland

Vitamin E is an essential nutrient for all higher animals, including humans. Vitamin E activity is derived from tocopherols and tocotrienols, which are lipid-soluble compounds originally synthesized by plants. There are four forms (α-, β-, γ- and δ-) of each, all of which have antioxidant properties but differing biological activities. α-Tocopherol is the most effective lipid-soluble antioxidant present in membranes and lipoproteins, and its function in these locations is to protect the unsaturated bonds of phospholipids from damage caused by free radicals. However, it is unclear whether this is the only function of the vitamin. This article will review the structure of tocopherols, their absorption, transport and storage, and their metabolic function. In addition, the major dietary sources, daily requirements and methods of assessing vitamin E status will be discussed. Finally, the possible role of increasing dietary or supplemental vitamin E intake in the prevention of chronic diseases will be considered, along with the safety of high intakes.

The structures of α-, β-, γ- and δ-tocopherol are shown in **Fig. 1**. All are derivatives of 2-methyl-6-chromanol onto which a saturated 16-carbon isoprenoid chain is attached at C2. α-Tocopherol is methylated at C5, C7 and C8 on the chromanol ring, while the other homologues (β-, γ- and δ-) have differing degrees of methylation. Tocotrienols differ from the corresponding tocopherols in that the isoprenoid side chain is unsaturated at C3′, C7′ and C11′.

The isoprenoid side chain has three centres of asymmetry, at C2, C4′, and C8′. Tocopherols and tocotrienols isolated from natural sources have the R-configuration in all three asymmetric centres and are given the prefix 2R, 4′R, 8′R-, or *RRR*-. They are more biologically active than their synthetic counterparts, which are mixtures of all eight possible stereoisomers and are given the prefix *all-rac*. *RRR*-α-tocopherol has an activity of 1 mg α-tocopherol equivalents (α-TE) per mg compound. The activities of *RRR*-β-, *RRR*-γ-, and *RRR*-δ-tocopherol are 0.5, 0.1 and 0.03 mg α-TE per mg compound, respectively. Of the tocotrienols, only *RRR*-α-tocotrienol has significant biological activity (0.3 mg α-TE per mg).

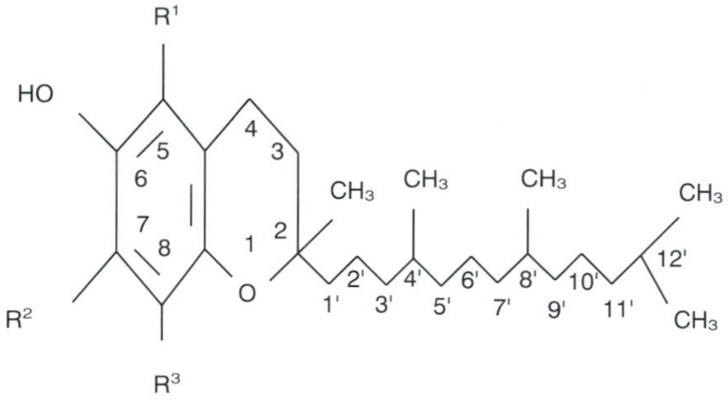

Compound	R¹	R²	R³
α-Tocopherol	CH₃	CH₃	CH₃
β-Tocopherol	CH₃	H	CH₃
γ-Tocopherol	H	CH₃	CH₃
δ-Tocopherol	H	H	CH₃

Figure 1 The four major forms of vitamin E (α-, β-, γ- and δ-tocopherol) differ by the number and position of methyl groups on the chromanol ring. In α-tocopherol, the most biologically active form, the chromanol ring is fully methylated. In β- and γ-tocopherol, the ring contains two methyl groups, while in δ-tocopherol it is methylated at one position. The corresponding tocotrienols have the same structural arrangement except for the presence of double bonds on the isoprenoid side chain at C3′, C7′ and C11′. Eight stereoisomers of vitamin E can be synthesized based on the rotational direction of the methyl groups at the 2-position on the chromanol ring and the 4′- and 8′-positions on the isoprenoid side chain.

Absorption, Transport and Storage

Many of the conditions necessary for triacylglycerol and cholesterol absorption are also needed for tocopherol absorption. The process itself is known to be incomplete, but estimates of absorption efficiency vary widely. Lipids (including tocopherols) are emulsified into smaller particles in the stomach and small intestine and then mixed with pancreatic and biliary secretions. Triacylglycerols are converted to monoacylglycerols and fatty acids by pancreatic lipase and these, together with bile salts, form micelles in which tocopherols and other hydrophobic molecules become solubilized. The principal site of tocopherol absorption in humans is believed to be the proximal small intestine. Transport across the brush border membrane appears to be by passive diffusion. There are no major differences in the absorption of α- and γ-tocopherol (the forms which predominate in the diet). However, α-tocopheryl acetate (the most common form of vitamin E supplement) must first be hydrolysed in the small intestine by pancreatic esterase.

Following absorption, tocopherols are secreted from the enterocyte in chylomicrons. These enter the general circulation via the lymphatic system and are catabolized by the action of lipoprotein lipase, which is bound to the surface of the endothelial lining of the capillary walls. In the process, some tocopherol is released to tissues, while the remainder is taken up by the liver as part of the chylomicron remnants. Subsequently, tocopherol is secreted from the liver in very low-density lipoproteins (VLDL) for delivery to tissues. Natural *RRR*-α-tocopherol is preferentially incorporated into VLDL at the expense of other stereoisomers (e.g. *SRR*-α-tocopherol) or the other (β-, γ-, δ-) homologues. This may be due to the existence of a hepatic tocopherol binding protein which recognizes the hydroxyl and methyl groups on the chromanol ring, as well as the stereochemistry of the C2 position.

Catabolism of VLDL and chylomicrons by lipoprotein lipase results in the delivery of α-tocopherol to low-density lipoprotein (LDL) and high-density lipoprotein (HDL). Several mechanisms seem to be capable of delivering tocopherols from these lipoproteins to tissues, including direct exchange, nonspecific transfer during lipoprotein hydrolysis by lipoprotein lipase, lipoprotein receptor-mediated endocytosis, and HDL-mediated delivery. The relative importance of each of these mechanisms has not been fully clarified, but tissues capable of synthesizing lipoprotein lipase (e.g. adipose tissue, muscle) may obtain their tocopherol by the lipoprotein lipase mechanism, whereas adrenal glands may rely more on the LDL receptor mechanism, and erythrocytes may depend on direct transfer of tocopherol from the lipoproteins.

The highest concentrations of α-tocopherol in the body are in the adipose tissues and adrenal glands. Adipose tissue is also the major store of the vitamin, followed by liver and skeletal muscle. The rate of uptake and turnover of α-tocopherol by different tissues varies greatly. Uptake is most rapid into lungs, liver, spleen, kidney and red cells (in rats, $t_{1/2}$ < 15 days) and slowest in brain, adipose tissue and spinal cord ($t_{1/2}$ > 30 days). Likewise, depletion of α-tocopherol from plasma and liver during times of dietary deficiency is rapid, whereas adipose tissue, brain, spinal cord and neural tissue are much more difficult to deplete. Little is known about the factors that govern the levels and turnover of tocopherols in individual tissues.

Metabolism and Excretion

Apart from oxidation and reduction, α-tocopherol metabolism in the body appears to be limited. The primary oxidation product of α-tocopherol may be α-tocopherol quinone, which can be reduced to a hydroquinone by quinone reductase. Two catabolites of α-tocopherol which have been identified *in vivo* are 2-(3-hydroxy-3-methyl-5-carboxypentyl)-3,5,6-

trimethyl-1,4-benzoquinone and its γ-lactone (Simon's metabolites). These compounds are excreted in the urine, chiefly in the form of glucuronides.

The principal route of tocopherol elimination from the body is via the faeces. Faecal tocopherol arises from incomplete absorption, secretion from mucosal cells, desquamation and biliary excretion. However, the vitamin is not secreted in pancreatic or intestinal juice. The extent of faecal excretion of α-tocopherol may vary from 10 to 75% of the administered dose. When large doses are administered, a considerable amount is secreted in bile, which may account for the relative safety of vitamin E compared with vitamins A and D. Urinary excretion of α-tocopherol represents about 1% of the administered dose. Skin may make a small contribution to α-tocopherol elimination by desquamation.

Metabolic Function and Essentiality

Tocopherols function as lipid-soluble antioxidants which protect membranes and lipoproteins against damage caused by lipid oxidation. However, because the wide array of deficiency symptoms observed in different species is difficult to explain by way of a simple antioxidant hypothesis, this has led to suggestions that tocopherols may also have more specific roles, such as in nucleic acid and mitochondrial metabolism and in the maintenance of membrane integrity. At this time, however, conclusive evidence for non-antioxidant functions is lacking.

Tocopherols and Prevention of Lipid Oxidation

Lipid oxidation is a process which may occur during normal aerobic cellular metabolism and during the metabolism of drugs. In the process, polyunsaturated fatty acids (PUFA), such as those in cellular and subcellular membranes, give up loosely bound hydrogen atoms from an allylic CH_2 group to highly reactive free radicals and are converted to fatty acid radicals (i) (**Fig. 2**). The fatty acid radical usually rearranges to a conjugated diene and takes up molecular oxygen, producing a peroxyl radical (ii), and this compound attacks a second PUFA, resulting in the formation of a hydroperoxide and a second fatty acid radical (iii). A chain reaction may then ensue (iv). The hydroperoxides which are continuously produced as a part of the process may split in the presence of iron or copper to peroxyl or alkoxyl radicals (v), which serve to accelerate the chain reaction, or they may break down to aldehydes, ketones, alkanes and other products (vi). Some of these compounds

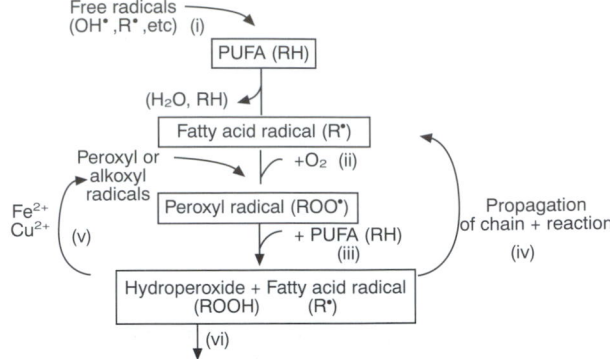

Aldehydes, ketones, acids, alkanes, epoxides, polymers, etc.

Figure 2 Oxidation of polyunsaturated fatty acids. Reaction of a free radical with a polyunsaturated fatty acid results in the formation of a fatty acid radical. After rearrangement and uptake of oxygen, the resultant peroxyl radical attacks another PUFA, producing a second fatty acid radical and a hydroperoxide. Iron- or copper-catalysed breakdown of hydroperoxides to peroxyl or alkoxyl radicals increases the rate of oxidation. Eventually, undesirable breakdown products such as aldehydes, ketones, alkanes and acids accumulate.

may bind to and disrupt cellular macromolecules such as DNA and proteins, while others have chemotactic properties which may induce inflammatory reactions.

Lipid oxidation may be prevented or retarded in several ways. Living animals possess elaborate enzymatic systems which minimize the amount of free radicals arising during the course of normal metabolism. These enzymes include glutathione peroxidase, catalase, superoxide dismutase and glutathione reductase. Second, free iron or copper concentrations in plasma and tissues are maintained at extremely low levels by complexing the metals to proteins such as transferrin, ferritin, caeruloplasmin and albumin. This helps to minimize transition metal-catalysed decomposition of hydroperoxides. Third, in the event that a chain reaction does occur, chain-breaking antioxidants can quench the reaction.

α-Tocopherol accounts for most of the lipid-soluble chain-breaking antioxidant activity in mammalian tissues and plasma. It donates its phenolic H atom to peroxyl radicals, and in the process becomes an α-tocopheroxyl radical. However, this radical is relatively stable because the unpaired electron on the oxygen atom is delocalized throughout the aromatic ring structure. Under normal conditions it does not react with membrane PUFA, and so propagation of the chain reaction is inhibited. The usual fate of the tocopheroxyl radical is either reaction with a second peroxyl or other radical to form a nonradical product, or else regeneration to α-tocopherol.

Membranes usually contain less than one α-tocopherol molecule per 1000–2000 phospholipids, and yet α-tocopherol is extremely effective in protecting membrane phospholipids against oxidative damage. The hydrophobicity of the isoprenoid side chain helps to fix α-tocopherol in the most fluid part of the membrane, close to the PUFA at risk of oxidative damage. In addition, α-tocopherol scavenges peroxyl radicals about 10 000 times faster than they can react with PUFA. The length of the side chain also plays a critical role in the overall effectiveness of α-tocopherol because it positions the phenolic OH group at the membrane surface, allowing any α-tocopheroxyl radicals formed to be converted back to α-tocopherol. The mechanism of α-tocopherol regeneration in microsomes and mitochondria appears to be enzymatic, arising from NADPH-, NADH- and succinate-dependent electron transport (enhanced by ubiquinol), while in membranes and lipoproteins, ascorbate and reduced thiols (glutathione and dihydrolipoate) regenerate α-tocopherol by a nonenzymatic mechanism.

Assessment of Vitamin E Status

Assessment of vitamin E status can be based on the measurement of static or functional indices. Static measurements include the determination of vitamin E in plasma or serum, platelets and red blood cells. The normal lower limit of serum vitamin E for children over 12 and adults is 11.6 μmol l^{-1}; for children aged 6 months to 12 years, the lower limit is approximately 7–9.3 μmol l^{-1}, and for newborn and young infants it may be even lower because of the low levels of circulating lipoproteins. Because of the close correlation which exists between them, vitamin E concentrations in serum are usually expressed relative to serum lipids. The threshold for clinical deficiency in older children and adults is approximately <0.8 mg total vitamin E per g total lipid, while for children aged 1–12 years the threshold is <0.6 mg g^{-1}. Platelet α-tocopherol concentration was proposed as a measure of vitamin E status on the grounds that it is sensitive to changes in dietary α-tocopherol intake and does not passively reflect plasma lipid changes. However, more blood is required and extraction procedures are more complex, which limits its usefulness for routine assessment. Red cell α-tocopherol concentrations are not widely used as vitamin E status indicators because of the influence of plasma lipids and haematocrit changes.

Functional tests include the determination of erythrocyte haemolysis and erythrocyte malondialdehyde production *in vitro*. These tests may be useful in experimental situations but they need to be harmonized so that interlaboratory variability is minimized. Another *in vitro* technique, LDL susceptibility to oxidation, does not reflect plasma α-tocopherol concentrations in unsupplemented individuals. Pentane and ethane are hydrocarbon products of the breakdown of lipid hydroperoxides and their levels in expired air respond to changes in vitamin E status. Measurement of breath pentane or ethane is noninvasive, but the technique is unlikely to be routine for some time because of technical constraints. In reality, all of these tests measure oxidative susceptibility (of cells, lipoproteins or the whole body) rather than vitamin E status *per se*.

Requirements and Groups at Risk of Deficiency

Requirements

The dietary requirement for vitamin E depends to some extent on the intake of other nutrients. The main determinant is the content and composition of dietary PUFA. In addition, vitamin E has important nutritional and metabolic interrelationships with selenium, sulfur amino acids, β-carotene, vitamin C and transition metals.

In the UK, the vitamin E requirement is regarded as the intake that maintains serum tocopherol : cholesterol ratios above 2.25 μmol mmol^{-1}. In a representative sample of UK adults in which the 2.5th and 97.5th centiles of vitamin E intake were 3.5–19.5 (median 9.3) mg α-TE per day (males) and 2.5–15.2 (median 6.7) mg α-TE per day (females), only 0.7% of subjects had serum tocopherol : cholesterol ratios below 2.25 μmol mmol^{-1}. The Panel on Dietary Reference Values therefore concluded that these ranges of intake were safe and adequate. Reference Nutrient Intakes (RNIs) were not set because of the dependence of vitamin E requirements on dietary PUFA, coupled with the wide range of PUFA intakes in the UK.

The US RDAs were derived after considering evidence that the average consumption of α-tocopherol in the diet was between 9.5 and 13.4 IU (i.e. 6.4–9.0 mg *RRR*-α-tocopherol) per day. The RDA for adult males is 15 IU (equivalent to 15 mg of *all-rac* α-tocopheryl acetate or 10 mg *RRR*-α-tocopherol), while that for adult females is 12 IU (i.e. 8 mg *RRR*-α-tocopherol). Because of the absence of clinical or biochemical evidence of inadequate vitamin E status in the general population, this level of intake was judged to be adequate. However, some experts have argued that this RDA provides little or no safety margin for individuals whose requirements deviate from normal. Indeed, one of the main difficulties in setting an RDA for vitamin E is the lack of easily recognizable pathological symptoms when consumption is inadequate, so that deficiencies in the general population could go unnoticed. A further argument for increasing the RDA is the fact that about one-fifth of the vitamin E intake is derived from fats and oils. If the general population heeds dietary advice to reduce total fat intake while increasing polyunsaturated fatty acids as a proportion of total fat, then intake of vitamin E may fail to keep pace with the increased requirements. There is also a view that the criterion upon which the RDA for vitamin E ought to be based should be the amount needed for optimal protection of cells and tissues against oxidative damage.

Groups at risk of vitamin E deficiency

Premature infants are especially at risk of vitamin E deficiency, probably because the placenta does not transfer α-tocopherol to the fetus in adequate amounts. This susceptibility to deficiency results in erythrocyte fragility and haemolytic anaemia, which is reversible by vitamin E therapy. Vitamin E has also been used, with mixed results, in the treatment of other conditions associated with prematurity, including retinopathy of prematurity, bronchopulmonary dysplasia and periventricular haemorrhage.

Dietary vitamin E deficiency rarely occurs in older infants, children and adults in developed and most developing countries because of the widespread distribution of the vitamin in the food supply. In these subjects, the most common cause of vitamin E deficiency is malabsorption due to disorders of the gastrointestinal tract or liver which interfere with the digestion or absorption of lipid. These conditions include a β-lipoproteinaemia and other disorders of β-lipoprotein secretion, chronic cholestatic hepatobiliary diseases, cystic fibrosis and other causes of pancreatic insufficiency, and short bowel syndrome. There is also an extremely rare disorder in which primary vitamin E deficiency occurs in the absence of lipid malabsorption, possibly on account of an inborn error of metabolism affecting hepatic α-tocopherol binding protein. Patients on total parenteral nutrition (TPN) without adequate vitamin E supplementation are also prone to vitamin E deficiency. The clinical features of vitamin E deficiency include spinocerebellar ataxia, loss of deep tendon reflexes, a wide-based, unsteady gait, intention tremor, skeletal myopathy, pigmented retinopathy, restriction of upward gaze (ophthalmoplegia), loss of position, pain, vibratory or touch sensations, and visual field loss.

Dietary Sources and High Intakes

Dietary sources

Vitamin E activity in plants is influenced by species, variety and stage of maturity as well as by harvesting, processing and storage conditions. In animal foods, the content of vitamin E can be increased by dietary supplementation. Since tocopherols and tocotrienols occur in varying proportions in most foods, it is more convenient to express the vitamin E content as α-tocopherol equivalents (α-TE) to account for their different biological activities.

Margarines, mayonnaises, salad dressing and cooking oils are important dietary sources of vitamin E. Wheatgerm, sunflower, cottonseed and safflower oils typically contain about 1700, 500, 400 and 350 mg α-TE kg^{-1}, respectively. Hard margarines range from 100–250 mg α-TE kg^{-1}, while soft spreads generally contain about 50–100 mg α-TE kg^{-1}. Cereals are moderate sources of vitamin E, providing between 6 mg α-TE kg^{-1} (barley) and 23 mg α-TE kg^{-1} (rye). However, some breakfast cereals are fortified with α-tocopheryl acetate, and these make an important contribution to vitamin E intake. Fresh fruit and vegetables generally contain about 1–10 mg α-TE kg^{-1}, while the vitamin E concentration of nuts ranges from 7 mg α-TE kg^{-1} in coconuts to 450 mg α-TE kg^{-1} in almonds.

The concentration of vitamin E in animal products is usually low but they may be significant sources because of their high consumption. Meats contain approximately 1–5 mg α-TE kg^{-1}, while the vitamin E content of fish is slightly higher. Whole eggs contain about 5–10 mg α-TE kg^{-1}, with about 2–5 times higher levels being present in the yolk. Whole milk contains about 4 mg α-TE kg^{-1}. However, skim milk contains little vitamin E because of the removal of the fat. Butter and lard provide about 10–30 mg α-TE kg^{-1}.

Pharmacological uses of tocopherols

As free radicals have been implicated in many diseases, such as coronary heart disease (CHD), cancer and inflammatory conditions, a protective role for α-tocopherol has been suggested. In many cases, the evidence from cell culture, animal and human studies supports this idea, but it is important to recognize that conclusive proof will only be provided by well-designed intervention trials.

Vitamin E modulates many of the important events in atherogenesis, including the oxidative modification of LDL. In the absence of vitamin E, LDL is easily oxidized and is taken up by macrophages in the arterial intima, leading to the accumulation of lipid-laden foam cells and later, fatty streaks. Its presence in the intima may also result in the release of cytotoxic compounds which damage the endothelial layer, leading to platelet aggregation, release of growth factors, and migration and proliferation of smooth muscle cells. Increasing the α-tocopherol content of LDL by taking vitamin E supplements or by *in vitro* enrichment significantly increases LDL stability against oxidation. A major epidemiological study comparing 16 European populations with up to six-fold differences in age-specific CHD mortality showed that plasma total cholesterol and diastolic blood pressure had only a moderate direct association with CHD mortality, whereas mortality was predicted to 62% by lipid-standardized plasma vitamin E concentration, and by up to 90% by the combination of five factors: plasma lipid-standardized vitamin E, plasma total cholesterol, plasma lipid-standardized vitamin A, diastolic blood pressure, and plasma vitamin C. The 1996 Cambridge Heart Antioxidant Study, which was a double-blind, placebo-controlled trial, showed that vitamin E supplementation (400–800 IU per day for approximately 500 days) significantly reduced the rate of nonfatal myocardial infarction in patients with angiographically proven coronary atherosclerosis. It should be noted, however, that there was a slight, albeit not statistically significant, increase in cardiovascular deaths in this group, which requires further study.

Vitamin E has powerful effects in the prevention and regression of certain cancers in animal models and cell culture systems. However, not all cancers respond to vitamin E. Similarly, in humans, some epidemiological studies have suggested that vitamin E may protect against cancer (most commonly lung, oesophageal and colorectal cancer) but in many, the associations between vitamin E intake or serum α-tocopherol and cancer incidence have been weak. Whether this is due to the vitamin actually only having a weak effect or to limitations in the design of different studies is unclear.

Vitamin E deficiency impairs immune responses, while supplementation with higher than recommended dietary levels enhances humoral and cell-mediated immunity and increases the efficiency of phagocytes. Indeed, in animal studies, the vitamin E requirement for an optimal immune response appears to be several times higher than that needed to prevent frank vitamin E deficiency. The mechanism of the immunostimulatory effect of vitamin E appears to be mainly related to its antioxidant function, although other antioxidants do not produce similar actions. Vitamin E could function either by decreasing concentrations of reactive oxygen species (e.g. hydrogen peroxide), thereby preventing oxidat-

ive damage to the stimulated immune and phagocytic cells, or by modulating production of arachidonic acid metabolites, such as prostaglandins.

The release of reactive oxygen species is a characteristic feature of inflammation. These compounds (including superoxide anion, hydroxyl radical, hydrogen peroxide and singlet oxygen) may originate via the arachidonic acid cascade or during the respiratory burst which occurs during phagocytosis. Vitamin E administration significantly relieved symptoms in patients suffering from several types of acute or chronic inflammatory conditions such as acute arthritis, spondylitis ankylosans, rheumatoid arthritis and osteoarthritis. In many cases it was as effective as standard drug therapy and was associated with a lower incidence of side effects.

Safety of high intakes

Few side effects have been observed in humans, even at pharmacological intakes of up to about 3000 IU (equivalent to 3000 mg α-tocopheryl acetate) per day. Likewise, clinical studies in which 200 IU of vitamin E per day or more have been administered for periods of up to 4.5 years have consistently shown no adverse effects associated with supplementation. However, vitamin E reduces platelet adhesion, and there have been a few cases of bleeding after surgery associated with intakes of 800–1200 IU of vitamin E per day. For this reason, it is advisable to discourage vitamin E supplementation within 2 weeks on either side of surgery. In addition, high levels of vitamin E are contraindicated in individuals receiving anticoagulant therapy.

See Colour Plate 13.

See also: **Antioxidants**: Diet and Antioxidant Defence; Observational Epidemiology; Intervention Studies. **Ascorbic Acid**: Physiology, Dietary Sources and Requirements; Scurvy. **Carotenoids**: Chemistry, Sources and Physiology; Epidemiology. **Lipids**: Chemistry and Classification; Composition and Role of Phospholipids in the Body. **Lipoproteins**: Physiology.

Further Reading

Bjornebøe A, Bjornebøe G-E Aa and Drevon CA (1990) Absorption, transport and distribution of vitamin E. *Journal of Nutrition* 120:233–242.

Buettner GR (1993) The pecking order of free radicals and antioxidants: lipid peroxidation, α-tocopherol, and ascorbate. *Archives of Biochemistry and Biophysics* 300:535–543.

Burton GW, Foster DO, Perly B, Slater TF, Smith ICP and Ingold KU (1985) Biological antioxidants. *Philosophical Transactions of the Royal Society (London) B* 311:565–578.

Frei B (1994) *Natural Antioxidants in Human Health and Disease*. London: Academic Press.

Halliwell B (1996) Antioxidants in human health and disease. In: McCormick DB (ed.) *Annual Reviews in Nutrition*, vol. 16, pp 33–50. Palo Alto: Annual Reviews.

Machlin LJ (1980) *Vitamin E: A Comprehensive Treatise*. New York: Marcel Dekker.

Machlin LJ (1984) Vitamin E. In: Machlin LJ (ed.) *Handbook of Vitamins: Nutritional, Biochemical, and Clinical Aspects*, pp 99–145. New York: Marcel Dekker.

Packer L and Fuchs J (1993) *Vitamin E in Health and Disease*. New York: Marcel Dekker.

Reaven PD and Witztum J (1996) Oxidized low density lipoproteins in atherogenesis: role of dietary modifications. In: McCormick DB (ed.) *Annual Reviews in Nutrition*, vol. 16, pp 51–71. Palo Alto: Annual Reviews.

Traber MG and Sies H (1996) Vitamin E in humans: demand and delivery. In: McCormick DB (ed.) *Annual Reviews in Nutrition*, vol. 16, pp 321–347. Palo Alto: Annual Reviews.

Trace elements *see* **Chromium**: Physiology, Dietary Sources and Requirements. **Copper**: Physiology, Dietary Sources and Requirements. **Immunity**: Role of Iron and Zinc. **Iodine**: Physiology, Dietary Sources and Requirements. **Iron**: Physiology, Dietary Sources and Requirements. **Manganese**: Physiology, Dietary Sources and Requirements. **Selenium**: Physiology, Dietary Sources and Requirements. **Zinc**: Physiology.

Trans-fatty acids *see* **Fatty Acids**: Health Effects of Trans-Fatty Acids.

Tumour *see* **Cancer**: Epidemiology and Associations Between Diet and Cancer; Epidemiology of Breast Cancer; Epidemiology of Colorectal Cancer; Epidemiology of Lung Cancer; Epidemiology of Gastrointestinal Cancers other than Colorectal Cancers.

U

ULTRATRACE ELEMENTS

Physiology

F Nielsen, Grand Forks Human Nutrition Research Center, Grand Forks, ND, USA

Definition

In the earlier part of this century, scientists could qualitatively detect small amounts of several mineral elements in living organisms. In reports, these elements were described as being present in 'traces' or 'trace amounts'. It is not surprising that these elements soon became known as trace elements. Today, sophisticated analytical techniques have permitted the accurate measurement of the amount of many mineral elements, some at very low concentrations, in biological material. The trace elements found in living organisms may be essential, that is, indispensable for growth and health, or they may be nonessential, fortuitous reminders of our geochemical origins or indicators of environmental exposure. Some of the nonessential trace elements can be beneficial to health through pharmacological action. All of the trace elements are toxic when intake is excessive.

Trace elements are those elements of the periodic table that occur in animals or humans in amounts measured in mg per kg of body weight or less. The trace elements essential for health are usually required by humans in amounts measured in mg per day; these elements include copper, iron, manganese and zinc. The individual trace elements are discussed elsewhere in the encyclopaedia. Since 1980, the term 'ultratrace element' has appeared in the nutritional literature. Ultratrace elements have been defined as those elements with estimated dietary requirements usually less than 1 mg kg^{-1}, and often less than 50 μg kg^{-1} of diet for laboratory animals. For humans, the term often is used to indicate an element with an established, estimated or suspected requirement of less than 1 mg per day or generally indicated by μg per day. At least 18 elements could be considered ultratrace elements: aluminium, arsenic, boron, bromine, cadmium, chromium, fluorine, germanium, iodine, lead, lithium, molybdenum, nickel, rubidium, selenium, silicon, tin and vanadium. Emerging evidence indicates that silicon should be categorized as a trace element instead of an ultratrace element. However, knowledge about the practical importance or beneficial actions of silicon is in a state similar to that for most of the ultratrace elements; thus it is considered as one of them here. Cobalt perhaps also belongs in the ultratrace category; however, it is required only in the form of vitamin B$_{12}$ and thus is usually discussed as a vitamin.

The quality of the experimental evidence for nutritional essentiality varies widely for the ultratrace elements. The evidence for the essentiality of three elements, iodine, molybdenum and selenium, is substantial and noncontroversial; specific biochemical functions have been defined for these elements. The nutritional importance of iodine and selenium are such that they have separate entries in this encyclopaedia. Molybdenum, however, is given very little nutritional attention, apparently because a deficiency of this element has not been unequivocally identified in humans other than individuals nourished by total parenteral nutrition or with genetic defects causing disturbances in metabolic pathways involving this element. Specific biochemical functions have not been defined for the other 15 ultratrace elements listed above. Thus, their essentiality is based on circumstantial evidence, which most often is that a dietary deprivation in an animal model results in a suboptimal biological function that is preventable or reversible by an intake of physiological amounts of the element in question. Often the circumstantial evidence includes an identified essential function in a lower form of life, and biochemical actions consistent with a biological role or beneficial action in humans. The circumstantial evidence for essentiality is substantial for arsenic, boron, chromium, nickel, silicon and vanadium. The evidence for essentiality for the other elements is generally limited to a few gross observations in one or two species by one or two research groups. However, it should be noted that two of these ultratrace elements have beneficial actions when ingested in high (pharmacological) amounts: they are fluorine, which prevents tooth caries, and lithium, which is used to treat manic-depressive disorders.

Although aluminium has a separate article, and the elements cadmium, lead and nickel are discussed in the entry 'Heavy Metals, Toxicology' the focus in those entries is toxicity; thus, these elements will be included in the following discussion. Chromium, however, which also has a separate entry, will not be included.

Absorption, Transport and Storage

Homeostasis (maintenance of a steady optimal concentration of an element in the body) regulation involves the processes of absorption, storage and excretion. The relative importance of these three processes varies among the ultratrace elements. The amount absorbed from the gastrointestinal tract is often the controlling mechanism for positively charged ultratrace elements such as aluminium, nickel and tin. With these trace elements, if the body content is low, or if intake is low, the percentage of the element absorbed from the gastrointestinal tract is increased, and vice versa. Elements that exist mainly as negatively charged ions or oxyanions, such as arsenic, boron and fluoride, are usually absorbed quite freely and completely from the gastrointestinal tract. Excretion through the urine, bile, sweat and breath is, therefore, the major mechanism for controlling the amount of these ultratrace elements in an organism. By being stored at inactive sites or in an inactive form, some ultratrace elements are prevented from causing adverse reactions when present in high quantities. An example of this homeostatic process is the binding of cadmium by the cysteine-rich protein called metallothionein. Release of an ultratrace element from storage forms also can be important in preventing deficiency.

Absorption of ultratrace elements from the intestinal lumen can occur in three ways. These are described below.

Table 1 Absorption, transport and storage characteristics of the ultratrace elements

Element	Major mechanism(s) for homeostasis	Means of absorption	Percentage of ingested absorbed	Transport and storage vehicles
Aluminium	Absorption	Uncertain; some evidence for passive diffusion through the paracellular pathway; also, evidence for active absorption through processes shared with active processes of calcium; probably occurs in proximal duodenum; citrate combined with aluminum enhances absorption	Less than 1%	Transferrin carries aluminium in plasma; bone a possible storage site
Arsenic	Urinary excretion; inorganic arsenic as mostly dimethylarsinic acid and organic arsenic as mostly arsenobetaine	Inorganic arsenate becomes sequestered in or on mucosal tissue, then absorption involves a simple movement down a concentration gradient; organic arsenic absorbed mainly by simple diffusion through lipid regions of the intestinal boundary	Soluble inorganic forms, >90%; slightly soluble inorganic forms, 20–30%; inorganic forms with foods, 60–75%; methylated forms, 45–90%	Before excretion inorganic arsenic is converted into monomethyl arsonic acid and dimethylarsinic acid; arsenobetaine not biotransformed; arsenocholine transformed to arsenobetaine
Boron	Urinary excretion	Ingested boron is converted into $B(OH)_3$ and absorbed in this form, probably by passive diffusion	Greater than 90%	Boron transported through the body as undissociated $B(OH)_3$; bone a possible storage site
Bromine	Urinary excretion	Probably passive diffusion because no apparent saturable component	75–90%	None identified
Cadmium	Absorption	May share a common absorption mechanism with other metals (e.g. zinc) but mechanism is less efficient for cadmium	5%	Incorporated into metallothionein which probably is both a storage and transport vehicle
Fluorine	50% daily intake excreted in urine; about 50% daily intake stored in bone and developing teeth	Absorption by passive diffusion and inversely related to pH. Significant portion absorbed as hydrogen fluoride from stomach; absorption of fluoride also occurs throughout the small intestine	75–90%	Exists as fluoride ion in plasma; hydrogen fluoride is the form in diffusion equilibration across cell membranes. Stored in bone
Germanium	Urinary excretion	Has not been conclusively determined but most likely is by passive diffusion	Greater than 90%	None identified

Table 1 Continued

Element	Major mechanism(s) for homeostasis	Means of absorption	Percentage of ingested absorbed	Transport and storage vehicles
Lead	Absorption	Uncertain; thought to be by passive diffusion in small intestine, but evidence has been presented for an active transport, perhaps involving the system for calcium	Adults 5–15% Children 40–50%	Bone is a repository for lead
Lithium	Urinary excretion	Passive diffusion by paracellular transport via the tight junctions and pericellular spaces	Lithium chloride highly absorbed – greater than 90%	Bone can serve as a store for lithium
Molybdenum	Urinary and biliary excretion	Uncertain, possible that molybdate is moved both by diffusion and by active transport, but at high concentrations active transport is a small portion of flux; absorption occurs rapidly in stomach and continues throughout the small intestine	50–93%	Molybdate in blood loosely attached to erythrocytes and tends to bind α_2-macroglobulin. Liver and kidney retain highest amount of molybdate
Nickel	Both absorption and urinary excretion	Uncertain, evidence both for passive diffusion (perhaps as an amino acid or other low molecular weight complex) and for energy driven transport; occurs in the small intestine	<10% with food	Transported in blood principally bound to serum albumin with small amounts bound to L-histidine and α_2-macroglobulin; no organ accumulates physiological amounts of nickel
Rubidium	Excretion through kidney and intestine	Resembles potassium in its pattern of absorption; rubidium and potassium thought to share a transport system	Highly absorbed	None identified
Silicon	Both absorption and urinary excretion	Mechanisms involved in intestinal absorption have not been described	Food silicon near 50%; insoluble or poorly soluble silicates ≈1%	Silicon in plasma believed to exist as undisassociated monomeric silicic acid
Tin	Absorption	Mechanisms involved in intestinal absorption have not been described	About 3%. Percentage increases when very low amounts are ingested	None identified. Bone might be a repository
Vanadium	Absorption	Vanadate has been suggested to be absorbed through phosphate or other anion transport systems; vanadyl has been suggested to use iron transport systems. Absorption occurs in the duodenum	<10%	Converted into vanadyl-transferrin and vanadyl-ferritin; whether transferrin is the transport vehicle and ferritin is the storage vehicle for vanadium remains to be determined. Bone is a respository for excess vanadium

1. Passive diffusion – passive transport driven by a difference in concentration of the element between the two sides of the luminal membrane and the mucosa. Transmembrane movement of ions occurs through pores or channels within the membrane and is an energy-independent process. A significant amount of passive transport across the intestinal mucosa may occur through a paracellular pathway, or the transport between cells across intercellular tight junctions.
2. Facilitated diffusion – the transfer of an element across the membrane by carrier proteins embedded in the membrane. Facilitated transport resembles simple diffusion because it is not energy dependent and is driven by a difference in the ion concentration between two sides of a membrane. Facilitated transport occurs much more rapidly than simple diffusion and is saturable because of a finite number of carrier proteins.
3. Active transport – the accumulation within, or the extrusion from, a cell of an element in opposition to a concentration gradient. Active transport is saturable, is energy dependent and involves a carrier protein that usually is quite specific for an element. The mechanisms of absorption for the various ultratrace elements are given in **Table 1**; this table also lists the known transport and storage vehicles for these elements.

Metabolism and Excretion

Knowledge about chemical changes that must occur before excretion for most of the ultratrace elements is quite limited. Perhaps the best characterized is inorganic arsenic, which is methylated into monomethylarsonic acid and dimethylarsinic acid, and organic arsenic, which is converted into, or remains mostly as, arsenobetaine before being excreted in the urine. Other ultratrace elements that are known to be incorporated into biochemical metabolites for transport and/or excretion include aluminium bound to transferrin, cadmium incorporated into metallothionein, nickel as the α-2-macroglobulin nickeloplasmin or bound to albumin and L-histidine, and vanadium converted into vanadyl-transferrin and vanadyl-ferritin (see **Table 1**). A known important metabolite of molybdenum is a small nonprotein cofactor containing a pterin nucleus that is present at the active site of molybdoenzymes. More than 40% of molybdenum not attached to an enzyme in liver also exists as this cofactor bound to the mitochondrial outer membrane. This form can be transferred to an apoenzyme of xanthine oxidase or sulfite oxidase which transforms it into an active enzyme molecule. Molecules of biological importance for the

ultratrace elements are shown in **Table 2**. The ultratrace elements are excreted from the body mainly via the faeces and urine. Faecal excretion of absorbed ultratrace elements usually results from biliary excretion, but may be of nonbiliary origin (e.g. through the pancreas or intestine). Ultratrace elements may also be excreted through sweat and breath. Ultratrace elements also are removed from the body through the loss of blood (e.g. menses), skin, hair, semen, saliva and nails. Table 2 gives the major routes of excretion for the ultratrace elements.

Requirements and High Intakes

As already mentioned, the ultratrace elements other than selenium and iodine are a disparate group in terms of their possible requirement or nutritional importance for human health and wellbeing. Although molybdenum has known essential functions, it has no unequivocally identified practical nutritional importance. The other 14 ultratrace elements discussed here have been suggested to be essential based on circumstantial evidence. This evidence is presented below along with some indication of possible requirement (extrapolated from the deficient animal intakes shown in **Table 3**), and some indication as to what constitutes a high intake.

Aluminium

A dietary deficiency of aluminium in goats reportedly results in increased abortions, depressed growth, incoordination and weakness in hind legs, and decreased life expectancy. Aluminium deficiency has also been reported to depress growth in chicks. Other biochemical actions that suggest aluminium could possibly act in an essential role include the *in vitro* findings that it activates the enzyme adenylate cyclase, enhances calmodulin activity, stimulates DNA synthesis in cell cultures, and stimulates osteoblasts to form bone through activating a putative G protein-coupled cation sensing system.

If humans have a requirement for aluminium, it probably is much less than 1.0 mg per day. Aluminium toxicity apparently is not a concern for healthy individuals. Cooking foods in aluminium cookware does not lead to detrimental intakes of aluminium. High dietary ingestion of aluminium probably is not a cause of Alzheimer's disease. However, high intakes of aluminium through such sources as buffered analgesics and antacids by susceptible individuals (e.g. those with impaired kidney function including the elderly and low-birthweight infants) may lead to pathological consequences and thus should be avoided. For most healthy individuals, an

Table 2 Excretion, retention and possible biological roles of the ultratrace elements

Element	Organs of high content (typical concentration)	Major excretory route after ingestion	Molecules of biological importance	Possible biological role
Aluminium	Bone (1–12 $\mu g\ g^{-1}$) Lung (35 $\mu g\ g^{-1}$)	Urine; also significant amounts in bile	Aluminium binds to proteins, nucleotides and phospholipids; aluminium bound transferrin apparently is a transport molecule	Enzyme activator
Arsenic	Hair (0.65 $\mu g\ g^{-1}$) Nails (0.35 $\mu g\ g^{-1}$) Skin (0.10 $\mu g\ g^{-1}$)	Urine	Methylation of inorganic oxyarsenic anions occurs in organisms ranging from microbial to mammalian; methylated end products include arsenocholine, arsenobetaine, dimethylarsinic acid and methylarsonic acid; arsenite methyltransferase and monomethylarsonic acid methyltransferase use *S*-adenosylmethionine for the methyl donor	Metabolism of methionine, or involved in labile methyl metabolism; regulation of gene expression
Boron	Bone (1.6 $\mu g\ g^{-1}$) Fingernails (15 $\mu g\ g^{-1}$) Hair (1 $\mu g\ g^{-1}$) Teeth (5 $\mu g\ g^{-1}$)	Urine	Boron biochemistry essentially that of boric acid, which forms ester complexes with hydroxyl groups, preferably those adjacent and *cis*, in organic compounds. Five naturally occurring boron esters (all antibiotics) synthesized by various bacteria have been characterized	Cell membrane function or stability such that it influences the response to hormone action, transmembrane signalling or transmembrane movement of regulatory cations or anions
Bromine	Hair (3.0 $\mu g\ g^{-1}$) Liver (4.0 $\mu g\ g^{-1}$) Lung (6.0 $\mu g\ g^{-1}$) Testis (5.0 $\mu g\ g^{-1}$)	Urine	Exists as Br$^-$ ion *in vivo*, binds to proteins and amino acids	Electrolyte balance
Cadmium	Kidney (14 $\mu g\ g^{-1}$) Liver (4 $\mu g\ g^{-1}$)	Urine and gastrointestinal tract	Metallothionein, a high sulfhydryl-containing protein involved in regulating cadmium distribution	Involved in metallathionein metabolism and utilization
Fluorine	Bones (1–5 mg g^{-1}) Teeth (500 $\mu g\ g^{-1}$)	Urine	Exists as fluoride ion or hydrogen fluoride in body fluids; about 99% of body fluorine found in mineralized tissues as fluoroapatite	Role in biological mineralization
Germanium	Bone (9 $\mu g\ g^{-1}$) Liver (0.3 $\mu g\ g^{-1}$) Pancreas (0.2 $\mu g\ g^{-1}$) Testis (0.5 $\mu g\ g^{-1}$)	Urine	None identified	Role in immune function
Lead	Aorta (1–2 $\mu g\ g^{-1}$) Bone (25 $\mu g\ g^{-1}$) Kidney (1–2 $\mu g\ g^{-1}$) Liver (1–2 $\mu g\ g^{-1}$)	Urine; also significant amounts in bile	Plasma lead mostly bound to albumin; blood lead binds mostly to haemoglobin but some binds a low molecular weight protein in erythrocytes	Facilitates iron absorption and/or utilization

Table 2 Continued

Element	Organs of high content (typical concentration)	Major excretory route after ingestion	Molecules of biological importance	Possible biological role
Lithium	Adrenal gland (60 ng g^{-1}) Bone (100 ng g^{-1}) Lymph nodes (200 ng g^{-1}) Pituitary gland (135 ng g^{-1})	Urine	None identified	Regulation of some endocrine function
Molybdenum	Kidney (0.4 μg g^{-1}) Liver (0.6 μg g^{-1})	Urine; also significant amounts in bile	Molybdoenzymes of aldehyde oxidase, xanthine oxidase/dehydrogenase and sulfite oxidase in which molyldenum exists as a small nonprotein factor containing a pterin nucleus; molybdate ion (MoO$_4^{2+}$), the form that exists in blood and urine	Molybdoenzymes oxidize and detoxify various pyrimidines, purines and pteridines; catalyse the transformation of hypoxanthine to xanthine and xanthine to uric acid; and catalyse the conversion of sulfite to sulfate
Nickel	Adrenal glands (25 ng g^{-1}) Bone (33 ng g^{-1}) Kidney (10 ng g^{-1}) Thyroid (30 ng g^{-1})	Urine as low molecular weight complexes	Binding of Ni^{2-} by various ligands including amino acids (especially histidine and cysteine), proteins (especially albumin), and a macroglobulin called nickelo-plasmin important in transport and excretion. Ni^{2+} component of urease; Ni^{3+} essential for enzymatic hydrogenation, desulfurization and carboxylation reactions in mostly anaerobic microorganisms	Cofactor or structural component in specific metalloenzymes; role in a metabolic pathway involving vitamin B$_{12}$ and folic acid. Role similar to potassium; neurophysiological function
Rubidium	Brain (4 μg g^{-1}) Kidney (5 μg g^{-1}) Liver (6.5 μg g^{-1}) Testis (20 μg g^{-1})	Urine; also significant amounts excreted through intestinal tract	None identified	Role similar to potassium; neurophysiological function
Silicon	Aorta (16 μg g^{-1}) Bone (18 μg g^{-1}) Skin (4 μg g^{-1}) Tendon (12 μg g^{-1})	Urine	Silicic acid (SiOH$_4$) is the form believed to exist in plasma; magnesium orthosilicate is probably the form in urine. The bound form of silicon has never been rigorously identified	Structural role in some mucopolysaccharide or collagen; role in the initiation of calcification and in collagen formation
Tin	Bone (0.8 μg g^{-1}) Kidney (0.2 μg g^{-1}) Liver (0.4 μg g^{-1})	Urine, also significant amounts in bile	Sn^{2+} is absorbed and excreted more readily than Sn^{4+}	Role in some redox reaction
Vanadium	Bone (120 ng g^{-1}) Kidney (120 ng g^{-1}) Liver (120 ng g^{-1}) Spleen (120 ng g^{-1}) Testis (200 ng g^{-1})	Urine; also significant amount in bile	Vanadyl (VO^{2+}), vanadate (H$_2$VO$_4^-$ or VO$_3^-$) and peroxovanadyl [V–OO]$^-$; VO^{2+} complexes with proteins, especially those associated with iron (e.g. transferrin, haemoglobin)	Lower forms of life have haloperoxidases that require vanadium for activity; a similar role might exist in higher forms of life

None of the suggested biological functions or roles of any of the ultratrace elements have been conclusively or unequivocally identified in higher forms of life except for those of molybdenum.

Table 3 Human body content, and deficient, typical and rich sources of intakes of ultratrace elements

Element	Apparent deficient intake (species)	Human body content	Typical human daily dietary intake	Rich sources
Aluminium	160 μg kg^{-1} (goat)	30–50 mg	2–10 mg	Baked goods prepared with chemical leavening agents (e.g. baking powder), processed cheese, grains, vegetables, herbs, tea, antacids, buffered analgesics
Arsenic	<25 μg kg^{-1} (chicks) <35 μg kg^{-1} (goat) <15 μg kg^{-1} (hamster) <30 μg kg^{-1} (rat)	1–2 mg	12–60 μg	Shellfish, fish, grain, cereal products
Boron	<0.3 mg kg^{-1} (chick) 0.25–0.35 mg per day (human) <0.3 mg kg^{-1} (rat)	10–20 mg	0.5–3.5 mg	Food and drink of plant origin, especially noncitrus fruits, leafy vegetables, nuts, pulses, legumes, wine, cider, beer
Bromine	0.8 mg kg^{-1} (goat)	200–350 mg	2–8 mg	Grain, nuts, fish
Cadmium	<5 μg kg^{-1} (goat) <4 μg kg^{-1} (rat)	5–20 mg	10–20 μg	Shellfish, grains – especially those grown on high-cadmium soils, leafy vegetables
Fluorine	<0.3 mg kg^{-1} (goat) <0.45 mg kg^{-1} (rat)	3 g	Fluoridated areas, 1–3 mg Nonfluoridated areas, 0.3–0.6 mg	Fish, tea, fluoridated water
Germanium	0.7 mg kg^{-1} (rat)	3 mg	0.4–3.4 mg	Wheat bran, vegetables, leguminous seeds
Lead	<32 μg kg^{-1} (pig) <45 μg kg^{-1} (rat)	Children less than age 10 years, 2 mg Adults, 120 mg	15–100 μg	Seafood, plant foodstuffs grown under high-lead conditions
Lithium	<1.5 mg kg^{-1} (goat) <15 μg kg^{-1} (rat)	350 μg	200–600 μg	Eggs, meat, processed meat, fish, milk, milk products, potatoes, vegetables (content varies with geological origin)
Molybdenum	<25 μg kg^{-1} (goat) <25 μg per day (human) <30 μg kg^{-1} (rat)	10 mg	50–100 μg	Milk and milk products, dried legumes, pulses, organ meats (liver and kidney), cereals and baked goods
Nickel	<100 μg kg^{-1} (goat) <20 μg kg^{-1} (rat)	1–2 mg	70–260 μg	Chocolate, nuts, dried beans and peas, grains
Rubidium	180 μg kg^{-1} (goat)	360 mg	1–5 mg	Coffee, black tea, fruits and vegetables (especially asparagus), poultry, fish
Silicon	<2.0 mg kg^{-1} (chick) <4.5 mg kg^{-1} (rat)	2–3 g	20–50 mg	Unrefined grains of high fibre content, cereal products
Tin	<20 μg kg^{-1} (rat)	7–14 mg	1–40 mg	Canned foods
Vanadium	<10 μg kg^{-1} (goat)	100 μg	10–30 μg	Shellfish, mushrooms, parsley, dill seed, black pepper, and some prepared foods

aluminium intake of 125 mg per day should not lead to toxicological consequences.

Arsenic

Arsenic deprivation has been induced in chickens, hamsters, goats, pigs and rats. In the goat, pig and rat, the most consistent signs of deprivation were depressed growth and abnormal reproduction characterized by impaired fertility and elevated perinatal mortality. Other notable signs of deprivation in goats were depressed serum triacylglycerol concentrations and death during lactation. Myocardial damage was also present in lactating goats. Other signs of arsenic deprivation have been reported, including changes in mineral concentrations in various organs. However, listing all signs reported to be caused by arsenic deficiency may be misleading because studies with chicks, rats and hamsters have revealed that the nature and severity of the signs are affected by a number of dietary and other factors. For example, female rats fed a diet that is conducive to kidney calcification have more severe calcification when dietary arsenic is low; kidney iron was also elevated. Male rats fed the same diet do not show these changes.

Other factors that affect the response to arsenic deprivation include methionine, arginine, choline, taurine and guanidoacetic acid. In other words, the signs of arsenic deprivation were changed and generally enhanced by nutritional stressors that affected sulfur amino acid or labile methyl-group metabolism; this suggests that arsenic has a biochemical function that affects these substances. Further evidence for this suggestion is the finding that arsenic deprivation slightly increases liver S-adenosylhomocysteine (SAH) and decreases liver S-adenosylmethionine (SAM) concentrations in animal models, thus resulting in a decreased SAM/SAH ratio; SAM and SAH are involved in methyl transfer. Additionally, arsenite can induce the isolated cell production of certain proteins known as heat shock proteins. The control of production of these proteins in response to arsenite apparently is at the transcriptional level, and involves changes in the methylation of core histones. It also has been shown that arsenic can increase the methylation of the $p53$ promoter, or DNA, in human lung cells.

It has been suggested, based upon animal data, that a possible arsenic requirement for humans eating 8.37 MJ (2000 kcal) would be 12–25 µg per day; this is near the typical daily intake shown in **Table 3**. Because of mechanisms for the homeostatic regulation of arsenic (including methylation, then excretion in urine), its toxicity through oral intake is relatively low; it is actually less toxic than selenium,

an ultratrace element with a well-established nutritional value. Toxic quantities of inorganic arsenic generally are reported in milligrams. For example, reported estimated fatal acute doses of arsenic for humans range from 70 to 300 mg or about 1.0 to 4.0 mg per kg body weight. Some forms of organic arsenic are virtually nontoxic; a 10 g per kg body weight dose of arsenobetaine depressed spontaneous motility and respiration in male mice, but these symptoms disappeared within 1 h. Results of numerous epidemiological studies have suggested an association between chronic overexposure to arsenic and the incidence of some forms of cancer; however, the role of arsenic in carcinogenesis remains controversial. Arsenic does not seem to act as a primary carcinogen, and is either an inactive or extremely weak mitogen. In the USA, a standard known as a reference dose (RfD; lifetime exposure that is unlikely to cause adverse health effects) of 0.3 µg per kg body weight per day, or 21 µg per day for a 70 kg human, has been suggested for inorganic arsenic. Because of safety factors in the determination, the RfD for arsenic conflicts with the possible arsenic requirement; this conflict is similar to that for some other mineral elements including zinc. These conflicts are currently being addressed by nutritionists and toxicologists.

Boron

Listing the signs of boron deficiency for animal models is difficult because most studies have used stressors to enhance the response to changes in dietary boron. Thus, the response to boron deprivation varied as the diet changed in its content of nutrients such as calcium, phosphorus, magnesium, potassium and vitamin D. Although the nature and severity of the changes varied with dietary composition, many of the findings indicated that boron deprivation impairs calcium metabolism, brain function and energy metabolism. Recent studies also suggest that boron deprivation impairs immune function and exacerbates adjuvant-induced arthritis in rats. Feeding low boron to humans (< 0.3 mg per day) altered the metabolism of macrominerals, electrolytes and nitrogen, as well as oxidative metabolism, and produces changes in erythropoiesis and haematopoiesis. Boron deprivation also altered electroencephalograms to suggest depressed behavioural activation and mental alertness, depressed psychomotor skills and cognitive processes of attention and memory, and enhanced some effects of oestrogen therapy such as increases in concentrations of serum 17β-oestradiol and plasma copper. Other findings suggest that boron may have an essential function. *In vitro* it competitively inhibits oxidoreductase enzymes, which require pyridine or flavin nucleotides, and enzymes such as serine proteases which form transition state analogues with boronic acid or borate derivatives. Boron has an essential function in plants, in which it influences redox actions involved in cellular membrane transport. This latter finding supports the hypothesis that boron has a role in cell membrane function or stability such that it influences the response to hormone action, transmembrane signalling, or transmembrane movement of regulatory cations or anions. Another finding in support of this hypothesis is that boron influences the transport of extracellular calcium into and the release of intracellular calcium in rat platelets activated by thrombin.

An analysis of both human and animal data has resulted in the suggestion by a World Health Organization (WHO) publication that an acceptable safe range of population mean intakes of boron for adults could well be 1.0 to 13 mg per day. In other words, 1.0 mg probably covers any requirement and 13 mg will not lead to any toxicological consequences. Boron has a low order of toxicity when administered orally. Toxicity signs in animals generally occur only after dietary boron exceeds 100 μg g^{-1}. The low order of toxicity of boron for humans is shown by the use of boron as a food preservative between 1870 and 1920 without apparent harm. It was reported in 1904 that when doses equivalent to more than 0.5 g of boric acid were consumed daily, disturbances in appetite, digestion and health occurred. It was concluded in this report that this much boron per day was too much for an average person to receive regularly.

Bromine

It has been reported that a dietary deficiency of bromide results in depression of growth, fertility, haematocrit, haemoglobin and life expectancy, and increases in milk fat and spontaneous abortions in goats. Other biological actions that suggest bromine could possibly act in an essential role include the findings that bromide alleviates growth retardation caused by hyperthyroidism in mice and chicks, and insomnia exhibited by many haemodialysis patients has been associated with bromide deficit.

If humans have a requirement for bromide, based on deficient intakes for animals it is probably no more than 1.0 mg per day. Bromine ingested as the bromide ion has a low order of toxicity; thus bromine is not of toxicological concern in nutrition.

Cadmium

Deficiency of cadmium reportedly depresses growth of rats and goats. Other *in vitro* biochemical actions that suggest cadmium could possibly act as an essential element include the finding that it has transforming growth factor activity and stimulates growth of cells in soft agar.

If humans have a requirement for cadmium, based on deficient intakes for animals it is probably less than 5 μg per day. Although cadmium may be an essential element at these extremely low amounts, it is of more concern because of its toxicological properties. Cadmium has a long half-life in the body and thus high intakes can lead to accumulation, resulting in damage to some organs, especially the kidney. The toxicological aspects of cadmium have been discussed earlier   (*See:* **Heavy Metals: Toxicology**).

Fluorine

Reported unequivocal or specific signs of fluoride deficiency are almost nonexistent. A study with goats indicated that a fluoride deficiency decreases life expectancy and caused pathological histology in the kidney and endocrine organs. Most of the evidence accepted as showing a need for fluoride comes from studies in which it was orally administered in pharmacological doses. Pharmacological doses of fluoride have been shown to prevent tooth caries, improve fertility, haematopoiesis and growth in iron-deficient mice and rats, prevent phosphorus-induced nephrocalcinosis, and perhaps prevent bone loss leading to osteoporosis.

Although fluoride is not generally considered an essential element in the classical sense for humans, it still is considered a beneficial element. Because of this, in the USA, an estimated safe and adequate daily dietary intake (ESADDI) has been established for fluoride; these are (in mg): infant aged 0 to 0.5 years, 0.1–0.5, and aged 0.5 to 1 years, 0.2–1.0; children and adolescents aged 1 to 3 years, 0.5–1.5, aged 4 to 6 years, 1.0–2.5, and aged 7 years and older, 1.5–2.5; adults, 1.5–4.0. These intakes provide amounts of fluoride that will give protection against dental caries and generally not result in any consequential mottling of teeth; they should not be considered intakes that are needed to prevent a nutritional deficiency of fluoride. Chronic fluoride toxicity through excessive intake mainly through water supplies and industrial exposure has been reported in many parts of the world. Chronic toxicity resulting from the ingestion of water and food providing in excess of 2.0 mg per day is manifested by dental fluorosis or mottled enamel ranging from barely discernible with intakes not much above 2.0 mg per day to stained and pitted enamel with much higher amounts. Crippling skeletal fluorosis apparently occurs in people who ingest 10 to 25 mg per day for 7 to 20 years.

Germanium

A low germanium intake has been found to alter bone and liver mineral composition and decrease tibial DNA in rats. Germanium also reverses changes in rats caused by silicon deprivation, and is touted as having anticancer properties because some organic complexes of germanium can inhibit tumour formation in animal models.

If humans have a requirement for germanium, based on animal deprivation studies, it is probably less than 0.5 mg per day. The toxicity of germanium depends upon its form. Some organic forms of germanium are less toxic than inorganic forms. Inorganic germanium toxicity results in kidney damage. Some individuals consuming high amounts of organic germanium supplements contaminated with inorganic germanium have died from kidney failure. Although germanium has long been believed to have a low order of toxicity because of its diffusible state and rapid elimination from the body, until more knowledge is obtained about the intakes at which germanium becomes toxic, they probably should not greatly exceed those found in a typical diet. An intake of no more than 5.0 mg per day would meet any possible need for germanium and most likely will be below the level found to have toxicological consequences.

Lead

A large number of findings have come from one source which suggest that a low dietary intake of lead is disadvantageous to pigs and rats. Apparent deficiency signs found include: depressed growth; anaemia; elevated serum cholesterol, phospholipids and bile acids; disturbed iron metabolism; decreased liver glucose, triacylglycerols, LDL-cholesterol and phospholipids; increased liver cholesterol; and altered blood and liver enzymes. A beneficial action of lead (2 μg g^{-1} versus 30 ng g^{-1} diet) is that it alleviates iron deficiency signs in young rats.

If humans have a requirement for lead, it is probably less than 30 μg per day based on animal deprivation studies. Although lead may have beneficial effects at low intakes, lead toxicity is of more concern than lead deficiency. Lead is considered one of the major environmental pollutants because of the past use of lead-based paints and the combustion of fuels containing lead additives. The toxicological aspects of lead have been discussed earlier (*See:* **Heavy Metals:** Toxicology).

Lithium

Lithium deficiency reportedly results in depressed fertility, birthweight and lifespan, and altered activity of liver and blood enzymes in goats. In rats, lithium deficiency apparently depresses fertility, birthweight, litter size and weaning weight. Other *in vitro* biochemical actions suggesting that lithium could possibly act as an essential element include the stimulation of growth of some cultured cells, and having insulinomimetic action. Lithium is best known for its pharmacological properties; it is used to treat manic-depressive psychosis. Its ability to affect mental function perhaps explains the report that incidence of violent crimes is lower in areas with high-lithium drinking water.

If humans have a requirement for lithium, based on animal deprivation studies it is probably less than 25 μg per day, which is much less than the usual dietary intake (see **Table 3**). Lithium is not a particularly toxic element, but the principal disadvantage in the use of lithium for psychiatric disorders is the narrow safety margin between therapeutic and toxic doses. About 500 mg lithium per day is needed to raise serum concentrations to be effective in these disorders; this is close to the concentration where mild toxicity signs of gastrointestinal disturbances, muscular weakness, tremor, drowsiness and a dazed feeling begin to appear. Severe toxicity results in coma, muscle tremor, convulsions and even death.

Molybdenum

The evidence for the essentiality of molybdenum is substantial and conclusive. Molybdenum functions as a cofactor in enzymes that catalyse the hydroxylation of various substrates. Aldehyde oxidase oxidizes and detoxifies various pyrimidines, purines, pteridines and related compounds. Xanthine oxidase/dehydrogenase catalyses the transformation of hypoxanthine to xanthine, and xanthine to uric acid. Sulfite oxidase catalyses the transformation of sulfite to sulfate. Attempts to produce molybdenum deficiency signs in rats, chickens and humans have resulted in only limited success. Deficiency signs in animals are best obtained when the diet is supplemented with massive amounts of tungsten, an antagonist of molybdenum metabolism. Nonetheless, reported deficiency signs for goats and pigs are depressed food consumption and growth, impaired reproduction characterized by increased mortality in both mothers and offspring, and elevated copper concentrations in liver and brain. A molybdenum-responsive syndrome found in hatching chicks is characterized by a high incidence of late embryonic mortality, mandibular distortion, anophthalmia, and defects in leg bone and feather development. The incidence of this syndrome was particularly high in commercial flocks reared on diets containing high concentrations of copper, another molybdenum metabolism antagonist.

Examples of nutritional standards that have been set for molybdenum are the current US ESADDIs, which are the following (in μg): infants aged 0 to 0.5 years, 15–30, and aged 0.5 to 1.0 years, 20–40; children and adolescents aged 1 to 3 years, 25–50, aged 4 to 6 years, 30–75, aged 7 to 10 years, 50–150, and aged 11 years and older, 75–200; adults, 75–200. Data to support these estimates are scant. These values were set by using balance data, which may be questionable, and through the reasoning that usual dietary intakes are within this range and do not result in signs of deficiency or toxicity. Recent studies indicate that the requirement of molybdenum for adults is actually close to 25 μg per day. Large oral doses are necessary to overcome the homeostatic control of molybdenum; thus it is a relatively non-toxic element. Nonetheless, the upper value of the ESADDI should be used as a guide for a safe intake of molybdenum because even a moderate intake of 540 μg per day has been associated with a loss of copper in urine; most signs of molybdenum toxicity are similar or identical to those of copper deficiency.

Nickel

Based on recent studies with rats and goats, nickel deprivation depresses growth, reproductive performance and plasma glucose, and alters the distribution of other elements in the body, including calcium, iron and zinc. As with other ultratrace elements, the nature and severity of signs of nickel deprivation are affected by diet composition. For example, vitamin B_{12} status affects signs of nickel deprivation in rats, and the effects suggest that vitamin B_{12} must be present for optimal nickel function. The nickel function also may involve folic acid because an interaction between these two affected the vitamin B_{12} and folic acid-dependent pathway of methionine synthesis from homocysteine. Nickel might function as a cofactor or structural component in specific metalloenzymes in higher organisms because such enzymes have been identified in bacteria, fungi, plants and invertebrates. These nickel-containing enzymes include urease, hydrogenase, methylcoenzyme M reductase and carbon monoxide dehydrogenase. Moreover, nickel can activate numerous enzymes in vitro.

Based on animal studies, the postulated nickel dietary requirement for humans should be less than 100 μg per day; a requirement of 25–35 μg per day has been suggested. Life-threatening toxicity of nickel through oral intake is unlikely. Because of excellent homeostatic regulation, nickel salts exert their toxic action mainly by gastrointestinal irritation and not by inherent toxicity. Generally, greater than 250 μg nickel per g of diet are required to produce signs of nickel toxicity (such as depressed growth and anaemia) in animals; by weight extrapolation, a daily oral dose of 250 mg of soluble nickel should produce toxic symptoms in humans. More moderate doses of nickel, however, may have adverse effects in humans. An oral dose in water as low as 600 μg nickel as nickel sulfate, which is highly absorbed when given to fasting subjects, produced a positive skin reaction in some fasting individuals with nickel allergy. That dose is only a few times higher than the human daily requirement postulated above.

Rubidium

Rubidium deficiency in goats reportedly results in depressed food intake and life expectancy, and increased spontaneous abortions. If rubidium is required by humans, the requirement probably would be no more than a few hundred μg per day, based on animal data. Rubidium is a relatively non-toxic element and thus is not of toxicological concern from the nutritional point of view.

Silicon

Most of the signs of silicon deficiency in chickens and rats indicate aberrant metabolism of connective tissue and bone. For example, chicks fed a silicon-deficient diet exhibit structural abnormalities of the skull, depressed collagen content in bone, and long-bone abnormalities characterized by small, poorly formed joints and defective endochondral bone growth. Silicon deprivation can affect the response to other dietary manipulations. For example, rats fed a diet low in calcium and high in aluminium accumulated high amounts of aluminium in the brain; silicon supplements prevented the accumulation. Also, high dietary aluminium depressed brain zinc concentrations in thyroidectomized rats fed low dietary silicon; silicon supplements prevented the depression. This effect was not seen in nonthyroidectomized rats. Other biochemical actions suggest that silicon is an essential element. Silicon is consistently found in collagen, and in bone tissue culture has been found to be needed for maximal bone prolylhydroxylase activity. Silicon deficiency decreases ornithine aminotransferase, an enzyme in the collagen formation pathway, in rats. Finally, silicon is essential for some lower forms of life in which silica serves a structural role and possibly affects gene expression.

Postulating a silicon requirement for humans is difficult because only limited data are available. If dietary silicon is highly available, human requirements may be about 2–5 mg per day, based on animal data. However, much of the silicon found in most diets probably occurs as aluminosilicates and silica from which silicon is not readily available. Thus the recommended intake of silicon probably should be higher than the estimated requirement. On the basis of balance data, a silicon intake of 30–35 mg per day was suggested for athletes; this was 5–10 mg higher than for nonatheletes. Silicon is essentially nontoxic when taken orally. Magnesium trisilicate, an over-the-counter antacid, has been used by humans for more than 40 years without obvious deleterious effects. Other silicates are food additives used as anticaking or antifoaming agents.

Tin

A dietary deficiency of tin has been reported to depress growth, response to sound and feed efficiency; alter the mineral composition of several organs; and cause hair loss in rats. Additionally, tin has been shown to influence haem oxygenase activity and has been associated with thymus immune and homeostatic functions.

If tin is required by humans, the requirement probably would not be much more than 20 µg per day, based on animal studies. Inorganic tin is relatively nontoxic. However, the routine consumption of foods packed in unlacquerd tin-plated cans may result in excessive exposure to tin which could adversely affect the metabolism of other essential trace elements including zinc and copper. Because 50 mg per day of tin was found to affect zinc and copper metabolism, routine intakes near this amount probably should be avoided.

Vanadium

Vanadium-deprived goats were found to exhibit an increased abortion rate and depressed milk production. About 40% of kids from vanadium-deprived goats died between days 7 and 91 of life with some deaths preceded by convulsions; only 8% of kids from vanadium-supplemented goats died during the same time. Also, skeletal deformations were seen in the forelegs, and forefoot tarsal joints were thickened. In rats, vanadium deprivation increases thyroid weight and decreases growth. Other biochemical actions support the suggestion that vanadium could possibly act in an essential role. *In vitro* studies with cells and pharmacological studies with animals have shown that vanadium has insulin-mimetic properties; numerous stimulatory effects on cell proliferation and differentiation; effects on cell phosphorylation-dephosphorylation; effects on glucose and ion transport across the plasma membrane; and effects on oxidation-reduction processes. Some algae, lichens, fungi, and bacteria contain enzymes that require vanadium for activity. The enzymes include nitrogenase in bacteria, and bromoperoxidase, iodoperoxidase and chloroperoxidase in algae, lichens and fungi, respectively. The haloperoxidases catalyse the oxidation of halide ions by hydrogen peroxide, thus facilitating the formation of a carbon–halogen bond. The best known haloperoxidase in animals is thyroid peroxidase. Vanadium deprivation in rats affects the response of thyroid peroxidase to changing dietary iodine concentrations.

If vanadium is essential for humans, its requirement most likely is small. Based on animal data, a daily intake of 10 µg probably will meet any postulated vanadium requirement. Vanadium can be a relatively toxic element. Animal data indicate that long-term daily intake over 10 mg of vanadium might lead to toxicological consequences. Limited studies with humans support this contention. For example, when six subjects were fed 4.5–18 mg of vanadium daily for 6 to 10 weeks, green tongue, cramps and diarrhoea were observed at the higher doses.

Dietary Sources

The requirements for the ultratrace elements will be met if a person consumes a diet based on the US Department of Agriculture guide known as the Food Pyramid, i.e. 6–11 servings of bread, cereal, rice and pasta; 3–5 servings of vegetables; 2–4 servings of fruit; 2–3 servings of milk, yogurt and cheese, meat, poultry, fish, dry beans, eggs and nuts; and sparing consumption of fats, oils and sweets. For some areas of the world, especially in developing countries where traditional, monotonous diets are based primarily on a cereal (particularly rice) or tuber staple, the intake of several ultratrace elements (e.g. arsenic, boron, molybdenum) could be possibly low. Reported typical dietary intakes (mostly for industrialized countries) and rich sources of the ultratrace elements are shown in **Table 3**.

See also: **Aluminium**: Occurence and Toxicity. **Chromium**: Physiology, Dietary Sources and Requirements. **Cobalamins**: Physiology, Dietary Sources and Requirements. **Cofactors**: Organic Cofactors. **Dental Disease**: Aetiology and Epidemiology. **Heavy Metals**: Toxicology. **Iodine**: Physiology, Dietary Sources and Requirements. **Selenium**: Physiology, Dietary Sources and Requirements.

Further Reading

Chappell WR, Abernathy CO and Cothern CR (eds) (1994) *Arsenic. Exposure and Health*. Northwood: Science and Technology Letters.

Ciba Foundation (1986) *Silicon Biochemistry*. Chichester: John Wiley & Sons.

Editorial (1994) Health effects of boron. *Environmental Health Perspectives Supplement* **102**(supplement 7).

FAO/WHO (1996) *Trace Elements in Human Nutrition and Health*. Geneva: World Health Organization.

Frieden E (ed.) (1984) *Biochemistry of the Essential Ultratrace Elements*. New York: Plenum.

Mertz W (ed.) (1986, 1987) *Trace Elements in Human and Animal Nutrition*, vols 1 and 2. Orlando and San Diego: Academic Press.

Nielsen FH (1986) Other elements: Sb, Ba, B, Br, Cs, Ge, Rb, Ag, Sr, Sn, Ti, Zr, Be, Bi, Ga, Au, In, Nb, Sc, Te, Tl, W. In: Mertz W (ed.) *Trace Elements in Human and Animal Nutrition*, vol. 2, pp 415–463. Orlando: Academic Press.

Nielsen FH (1994) Ultratrace minerals. In: Shils ME, Olson JA and Shike M (eds) *Modern Nutrition in Health and Disease*, 8th edn, vol. 1, pp 269–286. Philadelphia: Lea & Febiger. (9th edition with updated chapter on ultratrace minerals in progress.)

Nielsen FH (1996) Other trace elements. In: Ziegler EE and Filer LJ Jr (eds) *Present Knowledge in Nutrition*, 7th edn pp 353–376. Washington DC: ILSI Press.

Sigel H and Sigel A (eds) (1995) *Metal Ions in Biological Systems*, vol. 23, Nickel and its Role in Biology. New York: Marcel Dekker.

Sigel H and Sigel A (eds) (1995) *Metal Ions in Biological Systems*, vol. 31, Vanadium and its Role in Life. New York: Marcel Dekker.

UNITED NATIONS CHILDREN'S FUND

History and Role

D Alnwick, UNICEF, New York, NY, USA

J P Greaves, Blackheath, London, UK

The United Nations Children's Fund (UNICEF) is that part of the United Nations (UN) system that has a special mandate to improve the welfare of children and women. Beginning with a restricted mandate for a limited period, the organization now has a permanent concern for the whole child throughout the world. This article describes the history of the organization, with special reference to how its approach to nutrition has evolved over the years. The article also describes its present structure, funding, role and programmes.

History

UNICEF was established for a limited period by the General Assembly of the UN in December 1946 as the United Nations International Children's Emergency Fund, to provide assistance to children in Europe and China suffering from the devastations of World War II. In 1950 its life was extended for a further 3 years, with a mandate covering all developing countries, and in 1953 the General Assembly gave it permanent status, in recognition of the chronic and continuing needs of children. Its name was changed to that by which it is known today: 'International' was dropped as being redundant, and 'Emergency' as too restrictive, but the familiar acronym was retained.

Early days

In its early days UNICEF gave priority to relief and rehabilitation, and the provision of material assistance, laying the foundations for its reputation as an efficient supply agency. UNICEF needed people 'in the field' to ensure supplies reached those for whom they were intended; this was the origin of UNICEF's network of country offices The 'specialized agencies' – the Food and Agriculture Organization of the United Nation (FAO), the World Health Organization (WHO) – provided technical advice from a Regional or Headquarters base.

In the year after it was created, the International Children's Emergency Fund (as it then was) requested FAO and the WHO Interim Commission (WHO itself not formally having been established) for technical advice on child nutrition. A joint committee of specialists in nutrition and paediatrics was established, and its advisory report provided basic information on such matters as the energy and protein needs of different age groups, the importance of breastfeeding, the negative effects of infections on nutritional status, and the consequences of deficiencies of micronutrients such as iodine, iron and vitamin A. These remain major issues in public nutrition, although there have been changes in emphasis and approach, and an increasing understanding of how to address them in operational ways that increase the likelihood of success. For UNICEF it has been a period during which the agency has developed its own technical capacity and become recognized as primarily a developmental rather than a humanitarian organization, dealing in ideas as well as supplies.

During its early years UNICEF's work on nutrition concentrated on support to direct child feeding, especially through provision of dried skim milk, which was in plentiful supply. This was sometimes coupled to the development of local dairy industries. Fortification of milk powder with vitamin A was an issue – and sometimes still is today. Later, following the common scientific perception of the day, and guided by the Protein Advisory Group (PAG) of the UN system, UNICEF shifted attention to commercial production of low-cost high-protein supplementary foods for children. Costs could not be kept so low that those for whom they were chiefly designed could afford them, and though a frequent condition for UNICEF provision of plant was that the government should subsidize the product for the poor, this commitment could not be maintained.

Applied nutrition and nutrition planning

During the 1960s UNICEF was providing support, with FAO technical inputs, to so-called 'applied nutrition programmes' (ANP), which were essentially educational programmes at local level encouraging the production and consumption of 'nutritious foods'. Emphasis was placed on horticulture and raising of small animals; kitchen, school and community gardens; and use of appropriate technology to store, preserve and prepare foods, and conserve fuel. Nutrition education was always a component and such programmes were often linked to provision of health services, such as immunization, potable water and environmental sanitation. Although some of these programmes attempted to be responsive to local needs and to mobilize local resources, insufficient attention was given in practice to these critical matters, and ANPs tended to be regarded as of peripheral significance. Nevertheless in some countries they were acknowledged to have laid the groundwork of national nutrition policies, to have provided the first practical experience of intersectoral cooperation at various levels, and to have increased recognition of the need to involve local people in community programmes.

The 1970s saw attempts to introduce nutrition strategies into regional and national development planning. The UNICEF Executive Board in 1971 declared that 'the best action was through the establishment of national food and nutrition policies'. Governments were asked to consider specific measures designed to improve nutritional conditions of mothers and children in low-income families. However this was primarily food based, and the insight of the Mixed Committee of the League of Nations, with its call in 1937 for multisectoral approaches to problems of hunger and malnutrition with a 'marriage of agriculture and medicine', seemed to have been lost. In some quarters the pendulum swung to the opposite extreme, and claims were made that malnutrition in young children was precipitated solely by infection. Many found it difficult to accept that malnutrition could result either from infection or from an inadequate diet, or often from some combination of the two. Meanwhile UNICEF continued to tackle poor child nutrition through interventions of various complementary kinds – public health, small-scale agriculture, appropriate technology, the organization of women's groups – which did not require waiting until the whole problem of poverty was solved.

During this period experience of programme delivery and coverage and better understanding of the development process led to the formulation of concepts that have had a profound effect on the operational approach to improving nutrition. One of these was the basic services concept, first publicly discussed by UNICEF's Executive Director in a statement to the World Food Conference in 1974, but accepted as policy by the Executive Board and endorsed by the General Assembly in 1976. The essence of this approach lies in promoting and responding to community initiatives, the involvement of local community or village-level workers, appropriate technology, and effective support, technical supervision and referral services. The objective is to foster self-reliance. Similar principles are behind the primary health care (PHC) approach, endorsed by the WHO/UNICEF jointly sponsored international conference on PHC in Alma Ata in 1978. The PHC strategy involves shifting the focus of attention to the primary level of health care, involving the community in its establishment and management, and recognizing the many different sectoral activities that contribute to improved health – amongst which the Declaration of Alma Ata included the 'promotion of food supply and proper nutrition'. Experience of these approaches has demonstrated the difficulty of generating community participation, and the generally inadequate attention given to training and support of village-level workers. More fundamentally, problems have been encountered in the comprehension and acceptance of the philosophy of the approaches, underlying the importance of effective communication. Often nongovernmental organizations (NGOs) are able to overcome these handicaps: the challenge then is to translate their local successes into the national scene.

Child survival and development

In 1982 UNICEF launched a new initiative, known as the Child Survival and Development Revolution (CSDR), which focused on the young child and emphasized low-cost actions appropriate for the family, but suitable for national application. Key components (all reflecting the synergism between nutrition and infection) were: the promotion of exclusive breast-feeding for the first 6 months of life, and thereafter appropriate complementary feeding; immunization against the six EPI (WHO's Expanded Programme of Immunization) diseases; oral rehydration therapy in the control of diarrhoea; and regular growth monitoring of the child (for the first 3 years of life), primarily to help the mother promote optimal growth. Sometimes referred to as the GOBI strategy, it relied heavily on mass communications and social mobilization. The component that received most support was immunization, and in 1991 the UN recognized the attainment of the 1990 goal towards universal child immunization (UCI): 80% of all infants immunized against tuberculosis, polio, diphtheria, pertussis, tetanus and measles.

UNICEF had become concerned by the erosion of breastfeeding consequent on urbanization and encouraged by aggressive marketing of breastmilk substitutes, and was actively involved with WHO and NGOs in steps that led to the adoption in 1981 by the World Health Assembly of the International Code of Marketing of Breast-milk Substitutes. In 1990 UNICEF convened with WHO, with the cosponsorship of the US Agency for International Development (USAID) and the Swedish International Development Authority (SIDA), an international conference on the Protection, Promotion and Support of Breastfeeding. This issued the Innocenti Declaration (named from its venue at the historic Spedale degli Innocenti in Florence, home of UNICEF's International Child Development Centre), which called for the reinforcement of a 'breastfeeding culture' and its vigorous defence against incursions of a 'bottle-feeding culture'.

Growth monitoring was perceived as a useful tool for promoting satisfactory growth of children, which itself represented the outcome of influences of diet and disease. Furthermore, child growth was held to be a sensitive and reliable indicator of overall development, and UNICEF advocated that nutritional status should be considered along with more conventional economic indicators in assessing situations and determining policy, in the context of its advocacy of 'structural adjustment with a human face'. Growth charts and weighing scales were widely distributed, but the approach came into some disrepute when it was recognized that too often it was perceived as an end in itself, a sort of technological fix, with little attention to how monitoring should be done and the results used. This was confirmed by a number of studies, which came to the scarcely surprising conclusion that GMP (growth monitoring and promotion) sometimes worked and sometimes (more often) did not: it depended on how it was done. Meanwhile UNICEF had invested in the development of a new electronic portable solar-powered stand-on scale, sensitive enough to weigh infants, children and adults. The scale became generally available in 1996.

Aware of the importance of communications and concerned to identify simple messages about survival and development of universal validity – though often requiring local adaptation or addition of specificity – UNICEF published with WHO and UNESCO (United Nations Educational, Scientific and Cultural Organization), 'Facts for Life: what every family and community has a right to know' about safe motherhood, timing births, breastfeeding, child growth, diarrhoea and oral rehydration, immunization, respiratory infections, malaria, basic hygiene and AIDS.

A New Strategy and Summit Goals

In 1990 the UNICEF Executive Board approved a new strategy for improving nutrition of children and women in developing countries. The strategy stemmed from the Convention on the Rights of the Child: freedom from hunger and malnutrition are recognized as basic human rights; continued malnutrition is unacceptable. The strategy proposed a methodology for the identification of appropriate actions through situation assessment and analysis, rather than through a predetermined set of technical interventions. This so-called triple-A cycle (assessment, analysis and action, followed by reassessment etc.) is applicable at household, district and national levels.

Nutrition status is seen as an outcome. Immediate determinants are dietary intake and infectious disease. Underlying influences can be grouped into three major clusters: household food security, health services coupled with a healthy environment, and care for children and women. The degree to which the three conditions necessary for good nutrition are fulfilled depends on the availability and control of human, economic and organizational resources at different levels of society: household, community, national and international. Education has an important role, against a background of political, economic, cultural and ideological factors. The conceptual framework advocated by the strategy for analysing the nutrition situation is shown in **Fig. 1**.

The strategy proposes a number of nutrition goals for the 1990s. These are shared with WHO, and were endorsed by Heads of Government at the World Summit for Children in September 1990. The goals are:

- reduction of severe and moderate malnutrition among under-fives by half of 1990 levels;
- reduction of the rate of low birthweight (less than 2.5 kg) to less than 10%;
- virtual elimination of iodine deficiency disorders (IDD);
- virtual elimination of vitamin A deficiency (VAD) and its consequences, including blindness;
- reduction of iron deficiency anaemia (IDA) in women by one-third of 1990 levels;
- empowerment of all women to exclusively breast-feed their children for 4–6 months, and to continue breastfeeding with complementary food for up to 2 years of age or beyond.

The Summit endorsed a number of other goals related to women's health and education, child health and sanitation, and basic education, all of which are relevant to the attainment of the goals for nutrition. Governments committed themselves to prepare and execute National Plans of Action to implement the Summit goals, and 2 years later 135 countries had developed their programmes.

In 1991 the first meeting on a global scale to pursue Summit goals was held in Montreal, Canada: a policy conference on overcoming micronutrient malnutrition entitled *Ending Hidden Hunger*. In 1992 the FAO/WHO International Conference on Nutrition in Rome included in its World Declaration and Plan of Action for Nutrition a commitment to the nutritional goals of the World Summit for Children.

Structure

Within the UN system UNICEF's comparative advantage relates to its field-based structure. At the end of 1995 UNICEF had programmes of cooperation with governments in 145 countries, and deployed staff in 249 locations in 131 countries. There were 76 fully established country offices headed by a Representative, more than twice the number a decade before. There are now seven regional offices supporting country operations: for Asia (Bangkok, Kathmandu), Middle East and North Africa (Amman), sub-Saharan Africa (Nairobi,

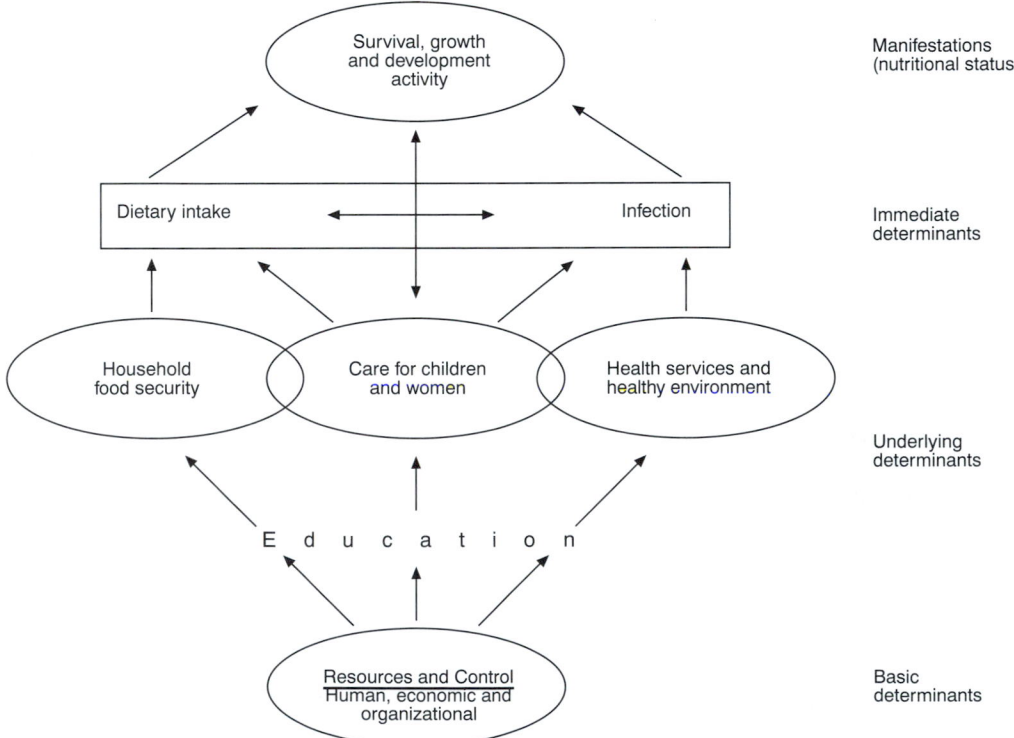

Figure 1   Determinants of child survival and development and nutritional status.

Abidjan), Latin America and the Caribbean (Bogota), and Central and Eastern Europe, Commonwealth of Independent States and the Baltics (Geneva). Headquarters functions are carried out in New York, Copenhagen (for supplies), Geneva (office for Europe), Florence (International Child Development Centre) and Tokyo (relations with Japan). Of some 7600 staff members in 1995, 80% work in the field. About 2400 of the staff are professional, international and (about 1000) national officers (recruited to serve in their own countries, alongside international colleagues). UNICEF staff are of 151 different nationalities; of the professional staff, 67% are from developing countries and 33% from industrialized countries, and 40% are women.

UNICEF is governed by an Executive Board consisting of representatives of 36 countries (reduced from 41 in 1994), serving on a rotational basis. The Board is responsible for overall policy, and for authorizing receipt and expenditure of funds. The Executive Director is appointed by the Secretary-General of the UN in consultation with the Board. All other staff are appointed by the Executive Director.

UNICEF has established a unique structure of supporting bodies in most industrialized countries. Known as National Committees for UNICEF, these are largely autonomous organizations with an important role of advocacy and fund-raising. They each have a formal relationship with UNICEF, and are responsible for fund-raising operations in their own countries, public information and development education, and promotion of UNICEF concerns, including the Convention on the Rights of the Child and follow-up of the Children's Summit. Much of their work is supported through voluntary action. In 1994 new National Committees were formed, bringing the total number officially recognized by UNICEF to 38.

Funding

UNICEF is funded entirely through voluntary donations, chiefly from governments, but also from private institutions and individuals. Total income has increased to US$1011 million in 1995 (**Fig. 2**). This sum included $163 million for emergencies. Of the total, governments and intergovernmental organizations contributed 65%. In 1995 the National Committees contributed about 30% of the overall budget.

UNICEF has developed supportive relationships with international service organizations such as Rotary International, which has contributed $85 million for the global eradication of polio, and Kiwanis International, which is raising funds

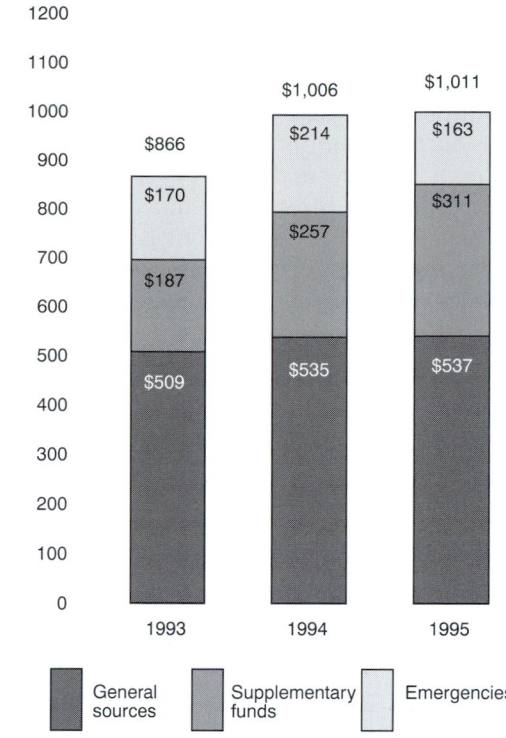

Figure 2 UNICEF Income 1993–1995 (in millions of US dollars).

towards its $75 million target for the elimination of IDD. In 1995 passengers on international flights donated $3 million to UNICEF through the 'Change for Good' programme, developed between National Committees and field offices and a number of participating airlines.

Income is divided between contributions for general resources (54% in 1995), supplementary funds (30%), and emergencies (16%) (**Fig. 3**). General

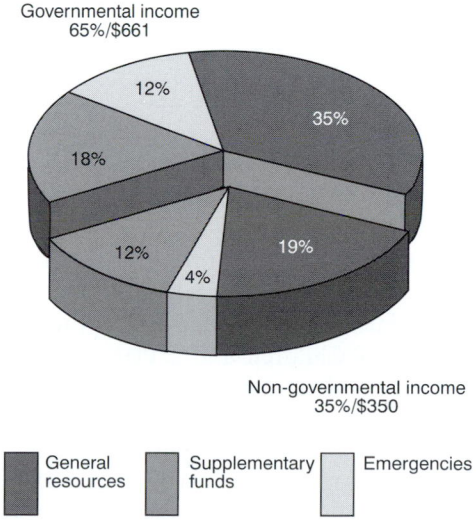

Figure 3 UNICEF Income by Sources 1995 (in millions of US dollars). Total income $1011 million.

resources are available for cooperation in country programmes approved by the Executive Board, as well as for programme support and administrative expenditures. Allocations are made to country programmes according to three criteria: annual number of deaths of children under 5 per 1000 live births, income level (GNP per caput), and the size of the child population. Thus most money is allocated to the larger, and poorer, countries. Representatives have the responsibility to negotiate with governments programmes of cooperation within these allocations. Additionally, they may negotiate further support, which the Board may approve subject to special purpose supplementary funding becoming available.

Total expenditure in 1995 was $1023 million: $804 (79%) in cash and supply assistance, $109 million in programme support, and $110 million in administrative services and other charges.

Although 163 countries made some contribution to UNICEF in 1995, only 10 contributed over $40 million from both the governmental and private sectors, providing 80% of UNICEF's total income for the year. Three countries contributed over $100 million: the USA, Sweden and the Netherlands.

Role

UNICEF's role can be appropriately summarized by the following quotations from its Mission Statement, adopted by its Executive Board in January 1996:

> UNICEF is mandated by the United Nations General Assembly to advocate for the protection of children's rights, to help meet their basic needs and to expand their opportunities to reach their full potential ... UNICEF aims, through its country programmes, to promote the equal rights of women and girls and to support their full participation in the political, social and economic development of their communities.

UNICEF pursues its advocacy and educational role at all levels and in all possible fora. The World Summit for Children at the UN in New York in September 1990 attracted 71 Heads of State and Government, and Ministers or other senior officials of 88 other countries – at that time the largest gathering of world leaders in history. The Summit adopted a World Declaration on the Survival, Protection and Development of Children and a Plan of Action for implementing the Declaration in the 1990s. Another form of UNICEF advocacy is the annual publication of The Progress of Nations, which presents league tables of how companies are reaching agreed Summit and other goals, and shows that the relationship between economic growth and social progress is not fixed. Some nations regularly achieve far more for

their children – in health, nutrition and education – than other nations with considerably higher levels of income.

UNICEF's programming role is essentially a country activity, conducted by the UNICEF Representatives and their staff, in close collaboration with officials of concerned government departments (for example, of planning, health, education, and social affairs ministries), and in consultation with representatives of other UN agencies and NGOs. The country programming process, which begins with a Situation Analysis (describing the situation of women and children in the country, and reviewing past programmes of cooperation and potential areas of future cooperation), is intended to ensure that the UNICEF country programme relates to the needs of children and women in the country, is fully integrated into the government programme, reflects government policy and programmes as well as policies established for UNICEF by its Board, and is complementary to assistance provided by other multilateral and bilateral agencies. The process involves balancing a global ethic with country priorities, but there need be no inconsistency between setting international and national goals and targets, and at the same time working to empower local partners to participate in progress towards improved nutrition. 'Bottom-up' advance need not be an alternative to 'top-down' advocacy and policy development.

UNICEF works closely with other UN agencies concerned with nutrition, particularly WHO, FAO, the World Food Programme (WFP), the International Fund for Agricultural Development (IFAD) and the World Bank. A long-standing mechanism for harmonization of policies with WHO exists in the form of a Joint Committee on Health Policy, and a formal agreement has been made more recently with the United Nations High Commissioner for Refugees (UNHCR). UNICEF is a major supporter of the Sub-Committee on Nutrition (SCN) of the UN Administrative Committee on Coordination (ACC), which consists of the Heads of all the UN agencies under the chairmanship of the Secretary-General. The SCN (which has evolved from the earlier PAG) currently has 16 UN members, and is the focal point for harmonizing policies and activities on nutrition within the UN system.

Programmes

UNICEF's programmes are in five main areas: health, nutrition, water and sanitation, education (primary school, early child development, adult literacy and nonformal education), and children in especially difficult circumstances (a euphemism covering abandoned children, street children, abused children, victims of civil strife and war). Cross-cutting concerns are the Convention on the Rights of the Child, women in development, urban basic services, environment, communications and evaluation. With regard to emergencies, UNICEF is responsive to natural and man-made disasters within the constraints of its mandate and resources, and in close cooperation with other parts of the UN system. Thus UNICEF would not normally provide food aid, this being the province of WFP, but could provide supplementary or therapeutic foods for children, health supplies, blankets and tents, fuel for heating, water purifiers, cash assistance and logistical support.

In the area of nutrition, UNICEF promotes and pursues four major strategies to address the causes of malnutrition at immediate, underlying and basic levels (see Fig. 1), as much as possible within the framework of national plans of action arising from the World Summit for Children and the International Conference on Nutrition.

The first strategy is to promote improved national nutrition policies and programmes through policy dialogue, training (popularizing the conceptual framework discussed above), and the use of improved information systems.

The second strategy is to promote community participation and empowerment through improved assessment, analysis and capacity to design and implement sustainable actions. Central features include support to community organizations and the use of growth monitoring and promotion.

Thirdly, and specifically, the protection, promotion and support of breastfeeding, which perfectly exemplifies the 'food, health, care' triad, together with appropriate and timely complementary foods and improved child feeding practices. A particular global programme launched in 1991 with WHO is the Baby Friendly Hospital Initiative, which formally recognizes maternity facilities that follow specified practices that enable mothers to make an informed choice about how to feed their babies and that helps them to establish and maintain lactation. By the end of 1995 over 4000 hospitals had received a baby-friendly plaque. By end March 1998, 13,237 hospitals in 117 countries had been declared baby-

friendly. This included 148 hospitals in 13 industrialized countries, for the baby-friendly goals apply equally in both rich and poor countries.

The fourth strategy relates to the control of the three micronutrient deficiencies (of vitamin A, iodine and iron), by a country-specific blend of short-term and long-term measures, involving dietary diversification, food fortification and nutrient supplementation. With regard to IDD, there was a general consensus that the most effective way of attaining the Summit goal of virtual elimination by the year 2000, on a sustainable basis, was through the iodization of salt. In 1993 a mid-decade goal was established for Universal Salt Iodization (USI). By the end of 1995 the goal of 90% salt iodization had been achieved by 19 nations, with 11 more passing the 70% mark.

See also: **Anaemia (Anemia)**: Iron-Deficiency Anaemia. **Food Aid**: Overview. **Food Aid Organizations**: History and Role. **Infants**: Milk-feeding and Weaning; Low-birthweight and Preterm Infants. **Iodine**: Iodine Deficiency Disorders. **Malnutrition**: Definition, Classification and Epidemiology. **Retinol**: Hypovitaminosis A.

Further Reading

Bellamy C (1996) *The State of the World's Children 1996* (containing Social Goals for 1995 and 2000). Oxford: Oxford University Press.

Bellamy C (1998) *The State of the World's Children 1998* (special focus on *nutrition*). Oxford: Oxford University Press.

Black M (1986) *The Children and the Nations. The Story of UNICEF*. New York: United Nations Children's Fund.

Black M (1996) *Children First. The Story of UNICEF, Past and Present*. Oxford: Oxford University Press.

Grant JP (1991) *The State of the World's Children 1991* (containing full texts of the Convention on the Rights of the Child, and the World Declaration and Plan of Action from the World Summit for Children). Oxford: Oxford University Press.

UNICEF (1990) *Strategy for Improved Nutrition of Children and Women in Developing Countries. A UNICEF Policy Review*. New York: United Nations Children's Fund.

UNICEF (1996) *Annual Report, 1996*. New York: United Nations Children's Fund.

UNICEF (1996) *The Progress of Nations, 1996*. New York: United Nations Children's Fund.

URBAN NUTRITION

Overview

N W Solomons, CeSSIAM, Guatemala City, Guatemala

The Historical and Modern City

Cities have existed for at least 5000 years, dating back to the time of the historical Jericho and Babylon (and even earlier, if we consider ancient Troy). As cities were generally walled until only a few centuries ago, when gunpowder and other explosives rendered stone walls of any thickness vulnerable to attack, historians presume that cities grew up as a form of collective protection. The large cities of today have grown up around ports, forts, communication hubs, ceremonial centres and seats of government.

The chances of suffering from any of the plagues of antiquity or of the Middle Ages were greatest where population density was highest. The great epidemics related to person-to-person or to point-source transmissions were the legacy of cities. It is not inconsistent that John Snow's intervention into a cholera epidemic involved the water supply of London, and that Edward Jenner found natural resistance to smallpox in the English milkmaids of the countryside while variola ravaged the eighteenth century urban populations. The image of life in the cities of the eighteenth and nineteenth centuries is not a positive one. Take as examples the teeming, dreary tenements and oppressive sweatshop working conditions of Dickens' London.

Food supply and food safety were precarious in the historical city. In the era before refrigeration, chances of spoilage were greater the further the consumer was from the point of production. Contamination from urban stockyards and slaughterhouses adversely influenced the living conditions. Moreover, those who produced food, i.e. farmers and herders in the countryside, have always had the first chance to consume it, or consumed it in a fresher state than those in the cities. Famines often occurred when a walled city's population was under siege.

Advances in transportation, refrigeration, and sewage treatment and disposal have allowed the modern city overcome some of these problems. Contemporary cities around the world, however, suffer an expansion of population and a burden of marginalized citizens that strain their resources to implement ambitious improvements regarding food and food supply. In recent centuries, wealth has been more concentrated in urban centres, but it is unevenly distributed. The metropolitan areas tend to house both the wealthiest and the poorest, with the ranks of the latter swelling more rapidly.

Demographic transition, urbanization and urban complexity

The two most important demographic trends worldwide are increasing longevity and urbanization. The decreased mortality from infectious diseases and decreased fertility along with increased literacy and increasing national wealth are the global demographic changes in these two domains. Longevity and urbanization also interact. The move from rural to urban living has accelerated since the close of World War II and the decolonization of the tropical regions of the world. An urban area is generally considered to be an aggregate of more than 20 000 persons. In 1950, the urban population of developing countries was 17%; by the year 2000, this is projected to have reached 44%. In the Americas, 75% of the population will be urban by the millennium, whereas in Africa it will be 40%.

Taken as a single metropolitan area, the Tokyo–Yokohama conurbation in Japan, with 30 million inhabitants, is the world's largest metropolis. Greater Mexico City (25 million) and greater São Paulo (21 million), both in Latin America, are the leading metropolises of the less industralized countries. In Asia, Seoul, Bombay, Calcutta, Jakarta, Delhi-New Delhi, Manila and Shanghai all have more than 10 million residents.

The process of moving from a tribal or pastoral state to settled agriculture and then on to urban life is characterized by the increasing complexity by which people satisfy their basic human needs for food and shelter. A tribe is made up of individuals in what is often a large, extended family. The demographic breakdown of a city has multiple units, beginning with the individual and the family, then aggregated into family households in neighbourhoods that belong to districts or boroughs that finally constitute the city. This, with its suburbs, makes up the greater metropolis. Interactions within classes and across the different levels of society make for intricate variations from one metropolis to the next.

Origins of urban nutrition

Nutrition as a science is a phenomenon of the twentieth century, and it has only been since the 1950s that epidemiological and community nutrition studies have benefited from biochemical laboratory support and insights from experimental animals. Current nutrition knowledge on deficiency states is mostly based on research in rural populations. This is due to the fact that poverty and nutritional deficiencies in the developing world are more prevalent in rural areas. **Table 1** provides a series of contrasting differences between situations in rural and urban settings.

Urbanization may be considered as a process which occurs in incremental stages. A given family could move from a dispersed settlement directly to the largest city of their nation. However, there are a series of other options along the way including the hamlet, the village, the town, the small city and the medium-sized city. By studying phenomena along this continuum of ever-larger aggregations of population, one can probe the question of whether any specific quanta or thresholds of size or density are associated with the expression of what we term 'urbanization.'

Diet and Dietary Change with Urbanization

Supplying a city with food is a logistical problem. An infrastructure for transport, storage and distribution must exist. The larger the city, the more complex are the issues of the supply chain and the distribution

network. If the food must be preserved, some of the recipe options of rural cuisine may be curtailed. If traditional foods do not travel or keep well, other commodities will be offered to meet energy needs. These considerations have repercussions both for the total food offering and for the ability to maintain traditional cuisine from rural origins.

It is generally conceded that diets differ between the urban and rural populations. In an affluent society, diversity may be on the side of the rural population which has access to their own produce, including garden items, as well as to the items of processed foods. In less affluent societies, rural populations are largely subsistence farmers with a traditional diet composed of a limited number of staple foods; it is in the cities that domestically produced specialty items and imported foodstuffs are more likely to offer increased variety. As such, dietary patterns will change when rural families migrate to the city. The diet will generally combine elements of the traditional rural fare with new elements from the urban culture. The income of migrants tends to increase with longer duration of residence in the city, providing more disposable funds to permit diversification of their diets.

Nutrition transition is a concept that has critical relevance to urban nutrition. Popkin defines nutrition transition as 'the rapid shift in the structure of diet in low-income countries and the coexisting problems of under- and overnutrition'. He adds that 'an increasing proportion of people [in low-income nations] consume the types of diets associated with

Table 1 Rural/urban contrasts

	Urban	Rural
Population density	High	Low
Occupational pursuits	Diverse	Agricultural
Political visibility	High	Low
Economic status	Dependent on employment state	Dependent on weather, prices
Social mobility	Possible	Difficult
Social class distribution	Balanced	Many peasants, few landlords
Transportation	Organized transit system	Hitchhiking, beasts of burden
Density of automobiles	High	Low
Environmental pollution	Industrial, automotive	Pesticide, herbicide
Premium on literacy	High	Low
Reliance on processed and stabilized foodstuffs	High	Low
Participation in monetary economy	High	Low

From Solomons (1987).

chronic diseases'. A high prevalence of chronic disease is related to longevity; longer life enables degenerative processes to become expressed. Specific individual susceptibility is finally determined in the balance between noxious exposures and protective behaviours. The choice of foods acts in two ways; some components seem to be damaging to health and others seem to be protective. Fat, especially saturated fat of animal origin, is implicated in the aetiology of cardiovascular disease, certain neoplasms and obesity. The percentage of energy derived from fat in foods in the city is usually higher than that in rural areas. Life-style factors including smoking, occupational hazards and the lack of physical exercise operate in tandem with diet change in the city to predispose to chronic disease incidence.

Urban agriculture

Urban agriculture, using marginal lands within the confines of the metropolitan area, can save up to 20% on outlays of cash for food for poor families at the expense of 1–2 days of labour per week. The type of plants that are grown in urban settings are largely foods that contribute micronutrients, and much less likely to be the staples that provide the bulk of energy and protein. For reasons of sanitation and zoonotic diseases, as well as waste disposal, domestic livestock in the cities are a much more remote option, although aquaculture with treated waste waters could provide fish, crustaceans and molluscs as a step towards meeting the protein needs of urban populations.

Street foods

Roads and highways may be a phenomenon of rural communication but the street is an urban entity. Street foods are defined by the Food and Agricultural Organization as 'ready to eat foods and beverages prepared and/or sold by vendors, especially in streets and other similar public places'. With urban life has come the opportunity – and at times the necessity – to consume one or more meals in the day away from one's home. One-quarter or more of daily energy intake is often consumed outside of poor urban homes by adult workers and high-school children. Cafeterias and restaurants serve the more affluent looking for a meal outside the household, while for low-income populations, their need is fulfilled by street foods.

The main concerns about street foods have been issues of sanitation and microbiology. The dietetics, anthropology and economics have remained more obscure. As Atkinson has said with respect to street foods: 'safety has to be assessed not by middle-class standards but in relation to other food sources and the environmental conditions in the homes of those buying these foods'. Positive aspects are the accessibility of these foods to the poor and the economic empowerment that street foods represent for the vendors. Scrutiny of street food by municipal authorities may arise from the fact that it is an unregulated, informal activity from which taxes or licensure revenues cannot be collected. Street food is a convenient scapegoat for politicians and bureaucrats when explaining local epidemics that may relate to other failings of the municipal investment in infrastructure.

Nutritional Status and its Change with Urbanization

The World Bank defines food security as 'access of all people at all times to enough food for an active healthy life.' Without entering into the minutiae of dietary balance and micronutrient status, the guarantee of food security is of primary importance for all populations. In low-income nations, economic stagnation, structural adjustment and cutbacks in public services have both induced the rural poor to migrate to cities and produced greater poverty in the cities. Subsidies for the poor were once a popular policy, but constraints and structural adjustment have made this strategy for improved food accessibility more modest and rare.

Urban life also brings changes in household and family structure. With the transition from extended families living in compounds in the countryside, city life gives rise to nuclear or one-parent families or elderly people living away from other generations; the loss of traditional patterns can lead to discrimination in allocation within the unit while isolation produces exposure to food insecurity. Being urban and poor confronts individuals and populations with a series of issues that impinge on their diet and nutriture.

In general, differences in food preferences are observed between urban and rural populations, with a lesser proportion of energy coming from the traditional staples in urban cuisine. More prestigious staples such as rice or wheat are sought instead of coarser staples such as maize, sorghum, millet or cassava, which might have been the main fare in rural areas. The types of stoves and fuels used in cooking in towns and cities may also lead to changes in dietary habits, as well as the increasing amount of food consumed away from home.

Viteri reviewed nutritional adequacy in urban populations. His overall conclusion was that weights and heights are higher and micronutrient status is better in the cities. However, in modern times, wealth and the wealthy are concentrated in cities. Whereas the countryside may be made up largely of the poor, the cities have various proportions of the affluent, the middle-class and the poor, and blended samples from all three strata may give an unrealistic picture of general nutritional standards.

Undernutrition

From Dhaka, Bangladesh to Port Moresby, Papua New Guinea come reports that document high prevalences of undernutrition among the urban poor. Interest in deficiencies of micronutrients (rather than macronutrients) now predominates. In the slums of Dhaka, for instance, vitamin A deficiency is found even among breast-fed infants. Iron deficiency anaemia is a condition that traditionally has not respected social class; thus it is not surprising that urban residence provides little protection against ferropenic anaemia.

Traditionally, iodine deficiency disorders are considered to be more prominent in more remote and isolated populations than in urban ones. This may be explained, in part, by the predominant location of the great cities in lowland or coastal locations, closer to iodine exposure from marine sources. When cities are both inland and in highland locations, this rural-to-urban gradient may not obtain. In a national survey in Guatemala, higher goitre rates were found in urban areas than in rural ones. Also in Guatemala, riboflavin nutriture was slightly superior in rural children than in urban ones. The processing and storage conditions of cow's milk may be the differential factor; milk and dairy products are the major source of this nutrient, and in rural areas they may be fresher, with less destruction of the vitamin.

Overnutrition

The concept of nutrition transition articulates a theory of increased exposure to the noxious influences of foods. These are generally believed to derive from imbalances with excess intakes of certain nutrients. Too much total energy, too much energy from fat, too much cholesterol, too much refined carbohydrates and too much iron comprise the litany of excesses considered to combine with environmental and genetic factors to promote chronic diseases. Consumption of more processed foods can result in lower intakes of potassium and higher intakes of sodium than was the fare in rural areas. Urban residence, compared with rural living, is felt to predispose to greater risks of these dietary excesses, conducive to chronic disease. Among areas of concern for the detriments of overnutrition are China, Singapore, Brazil and Mexico, especially in their urban areas.

Short stature is the result of growth failure in early life. It is now realized that being short is a risk factor for obesity. Sedentary life style and energy-dense foods, both possible consequences of city life, characterize the association of urbanization, dietary excess and body overload with stored energy, atherogenic lipids, sodium and oxidants such as iron.

Overconsumption and overnutrition, moreover, may not be uniform within families as the proportion of meals eaten in the home declines, and activity rates may differ markedly across different generations. Heterogeneity of body composition exists within families. As demonstrated in Jakarta, paradoxical mixtures can occur frequently in poor urban homes by which the body habitus of one generation contrasts with that of the next: obese parents and underweight children or vice versa.

Specific Urban Populations and Circumstances

Consideration of the underlying concepts of complexity and heterogeneity leads us to examine specific age-groups and ecological niches within metropolitan areas.

Urban infants

The duration and pattern of breast-feeding may be influenced by changing life styles and availability of alternatives to breast milk. The current worldwide tendency is toward a shorter and lower intensity of breast-feeding. The need for mothers to work as well as the availability (and advertising) of substitute formulae contribute to the decrease in breast-feeding. This is of concern because alternative feeding practices can alter infant nutrition. There is also the danger of more frequent infections from contamination of the weaning foods.

As infants grow into toddlers, the existence of sewer systems, indoor plumbing and concrete paving may reduce the transmission of geohelminths such as hookworms, roundworms and whipworms. To the extent that these three parasites produce nutritional deterioration, the effects will be less where the conditions impede faecal–oral transmission. Better sanitation infrastructure *per se* does not guarantee lower rates of all transmissible diseases; for instance, food-borne infections can become more common in urban settings as maternal work outside the home results in longer intervals between preparation and consumption of meals, with food maintained under less than ideal storage conditions.

Street children

Street children are a phenomenon that is only found in cities. They have been the subjects of more lore and speculation than of actual understanding. On the whole, the nutritional science community has eschewed inquiry into the status of this subsegment of the urban population. It is important to differentiate children who live *in* the street from those who live *of* the street. Those who are in the street make it not only their workplace but their home, often living in age-peer bands away from their families. Those who live of the street merely find a livelihood from one or more of the various options: begging, stealing and prostitution, as well as guarding and washing cars, shining shoes, and entertaining as jugglers, magicians or fire-eaters. Children living *in* the street are often orphans or runaways; however, most street children in a study in Jakarta were very much a part of a family and many attended school, at least part of the time (i.e. they lived *of* the street); they considered scavenged food of low status and preferred to beg or purchase their fare; and compared with urban children living conventionally, street children had better nutritional status and more disposable income.

Urban elderly

Urbanization may be a factor in the transition from the extended family pattern of traditional rural society to the nuclear family (mother, father and offspring) with the risk of widespread disintegration into single-parent households. The welfare of the older population becomes a concern in this transition. The possibilities for a continued vigorous and productive life style may be more limited for the elderly in cities as the urban job market may be restricted to the young adult population, whereas those on the land or of the land may continue to exercise their agricultural pursuits until disability or death intervenes. Maintaining an active life style, furthermore, may be a retardant to disability. Thus, food security may be a concern for the elderly among the urban poor, one that may be precarious for the oldest generation.

Urban pollution

Contamination and pollution of the environment is characteristic of any habitat in which humans are found, be it rural or urban. The range, variety and nature of noxious agents differs. Pollution can result from the system of providing food, and general pollution of the environment can influence the nutritional status of the population. Pollution in the urban area takes many forms, including noise, particulate and gaseous emissions, and chemical and microbiological contaminants.

Urban refuse, whether in municipal landfills or in informal dumping sites, provides for a precarious

Table 2 Opportunities in urban nutrition research

Basic description of diet and nutrition in selected townships and metropolises

Rural–urban comparisons

Role of family and household relationships

Influence of rural-to-urban migration on nutritional status and dietary status

Universality of dietary factors for degenerative diseases

Contributions of urban agriculture to the urban food supply

occupation of scavenging and recycling. The nutritional health of the subsegment of urban dwellers engaged in this activity, and the effects of direct toxic exposures, are concerns yet to be well described.

Conclusions

Because of the progressive shift of the world's population from rural residence and nomadic and pastoral pursuits, to towns, cities and metropolises, public health nutrition and the epidemiology of nutrition must focus more on what has been termed 'urban nutrition'. The essential complexity of providing for human needs in densely populated settings has repercussions for the resulting nutriture of the urban populations. Street foods, street children, urban pollution, and diet and life styles can foster or be associated with undernutrition in some circumstances and overnutrition in others.

Our understanding of nutritional conditions in rural areas may not be relevant to the problem of urban populations, and far more research is needed to gain insight into urban nutrition (**Table 2**).

See also: **Body Composition**: Determination and Physiological Significance. **Catering**: Nutritional Aspects. **Community Nutrition**: Definition and Approaches. **Coronary Heart Disease**: Aetiology. **Dental Disease**: Aetiology and Epidemiology. **Diabetes Mellitus**: Aetiology and Epidemiology. **Dietary Guidelines**: International Perspectives. **Epidemiological Studies**: Role and Interpretation. **Fertility**: Body Fat, Menarche and Fertility. **Fetal Origins of Disease**: Fetal Development and Later Disease. **Food Choice**: Factors Influencing Food Choice. **Food Processing**: Nutritional Influences. **Fruits and Vegetables**: Nutritional Value. **Infants**: Milk-feeding and Weaning. **Insulin Resistance**: Aetiology and Association with Disease. **Nutrient Requirements**: International Perspectives. **Nutrition Policies**: In Developing Countries. **Nutritional Surveillance**: In Industrialized and Developing Countries. **Obesity**: Definition, Aetiology and

Assessment. **Older People**: Nutritional Management of Geriatric Patients. **Parasitism**: Effects on Growth and Nutritional Status. **Phytochemicals**: Epidemiological Factors. **Population, Development and Nutrition**: Overview. **Religious Customs**: Influence on Diet. **Socioeconomic Status**: Relationship with Diet and Nutritional Status. **United Nations Children's Fund**: History and Role. **World Health Organization**: Role.

Further Reading

Albala C and Vio F (1995) Epidemiological transition in Latin America: the case of Chile. *Public Health* 109:431–442.

Atkinson SJ (1995) Approaches and actors in urban food security in developing countries. *Habitat International* 19:151–163.

Campos H, Mata L, Siles X, Vives M, Ordovas JM and Schaefer EJ (1992) Prevalence of cardiovascular risk factors in rural and urban Costa Rica. *Circulation* 85:648–658.

Delisle H (1989) *Urban Food Consumption Patterns in Developing Countries: Some Issues and Challenges.* Rome: Food & Agriculteral Organization.

Food & Agriculture Organization (1989) *Street Foods.* Food and Nutrition Paper no. 46. Rome: FAO.

Gross R (1987) Urbanization and nutrition from the thermodynamic and cybernetic point of view. In: Gross R and Solomons NW (eds) *Tropical Urban Nutrition*, pp. 31–60. GTZ Special Publication no. 197. Eschborn: German Agency for Technical Cooperation.

Gross R, Landfried B and Herman S (1996) Height and weight as a reflection of the nutritional situation of school-aged children working and living in the streets of Jakarta. *Social Sciences in Medicine* 43:453–458.

Krause VM, Tucker KL, Kuhnlein HV, Lopez-Palacios CY, Ruz M and Solomons NW (1992) Rural-urban variation in limed maize use and tortilla consumption by women in Guatemala. *Ecology of Food and Nutrition* 28:279–288.

Phillips DR (1993) Urbanization and human health. *Parasitology* 103:S97–S107.

Popkin BM (1995) The nutrition transition in low-income countries: an emerging crisis. *Nutrition Reviews* 52:285–298.

Popkin BM and Bisgrove EZ (1988) Urbanization and nutrition in low-income countries. *Food and Nutrition Bulletin* 10:3–23.

Solomons NW (1987) Urban nutrition in the tropics: a neglected subject of scientific inquiry. In: Gross R and Solomons NW (eds) *Tropical Urban Nutrition*, pp 15–30. GTZ Special Publication, no. 197. Eschborn: German Agency for Technical Cooperation.

Solomons NW and Gross R (1995) Urban nutrition in developing countries. *Nutrition Reviews* 53:90–95.

Viteri FE (1987) Nutrition-related health consequences of urbanization. *Food and Nutrition Bulletin* 9:33–49.

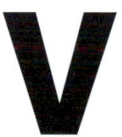

Vegan diets *see* **Vegetarian Diets**: Practice.

Vegetables *see* **Fruits and Vegetables**: Nutritional Value.

VEGETARIAN DIETS

Contents
Practice
Nutritional Adequacy

Practice

S Reddy, Leatherhead Food Research Association, Leatherhead, Surrey, UK

Classification of Vegetarian Diets

A vegetarian is defined as 'one who abstains from the use of flesh, fish or fowl as food, with or without the addition of eggs and dairy produce, and whose diet includes roots, vegetables, cereals, seeds and fruit and nuts'. Vegetarianism in practice is heterogeneous and encompasses a range of dietary habits. Vegetarianism and meat eating should not be thought of as mutually exclusive diet categories but as either end of an eating dimension. It is usually adopted gradually, firstly by avoiding red meat, followed by excluding poultry and then fish. Some vegetarians progress on to become vegans, excluding all animal foods, even honey, from their diet. The degree of vegetarianism largely depends on the reasons for which it has been adopted. **Table 1** lists the classification of vegetarian diets.

Reasons for Vegetarianism

Although popular vegetarianism is a relatively recent phenomenon in the West, it has been practised for centuries in Asia by Hindus and Buddhists for religious reasons. Pythagoras was one of the earlier advocates of vegetarianism in the West. Abstinence from meat has been associated with asceticism throughout the world. The Seventh-Day Adventist Church and Hinduism advocate vegetarianism as it is associated with *ahimsa* (not killing), and purity of thought and mind. The Rastafarian cult also advocates a vegan–fruitarian diet. In the Netherlands and the USA, many new vegetarians are followers of the teachings of George Ohsawa, who advocated the consumption of organic foods and attempted to apply Zen Buddhist philosophy to the selection of natural unprocessed foods, which he called macrobiotics. They promoted the view that vegetarian diets are more natural and wholesome than ordinary mixed diets.

Vegetarianism in the UK has a long history of association with radical and often altruistic causes, ranging from teetotalism and food reform in the nineteenth century to environmental issues and animal welfare in the twentieth century. Ethical reasons based on the conviction that raising of animals for human exploitation is unacceptable, even if humanely done, are the fundamental basis for vegetarianism. Concerns over intensive animal farming and the conditions under which animals are kept and transported have all been important reasons for the recent growth of vegetarianism. Animal welfare and a moral objection to the killing of animals are probably the main reasons for avoidance of meat, particularly by teenage girls and the young.

Vegetarian diets are typically less expensive than meat-based diets, and this is of significance to the developing countries, where near-vegetarian diets are the norm. The ecological cost and the ethics of diverting much needed staple foods for the production of animal foods have made vegetarianism an

Table 1 Classification of vegetarian diets

Type of vegetarian diet	Foods included/excluded
Semi/demi-vegetarian	Occasional consumption of poultry and fish
Pescovegetarian	Includes fish, dairy and eggs
Lacto-ovo vegetarian	Includes dairy products and eggs but excludes all animal flesh
Lactovegetarian	Includes dairy products but excludes all animal flesh and eggs
Vegan	Excludes all animal foods: meat, dairy products, eggs, honey, etc.
Fruitarian	Includes only fruits, nuts and berries
Macrobiotic	An extreme diet progresses through 10 levels, gradually eliminating all foods of animal origin, fruit and vegetables, and at the final level includes only brown rice

economic alternative in the context of managing limited world resources.

More recently, other factors have also contributed to the increased popularity of vegetarianism. Many people have been avoiding meat following the scares over bovine spongiform encephalopathy (BSE) in cattle and *salmonella* in poultry. In practice there is probably a combination of reasons why people follow vegetarianism.

Trends in Vegetarianism

Vegetarianism is particularly popular with young women, with a higher prevalence in the southern counties of the UK, and vegetarians are more likely to be from higher social classes, with above-average educational achievement. It is apparent that many people are now claiming to consume red meat less frequently, but are continuing to eat poultry and fish. Therefore, in reality the increasing trend in reported vegetarianism may be related more to infrequent consumption of flesh foods rather than their total avoidance (see **Table 2**).

Health-related Beliefs and Lifestyle Aspects of Vegetarians

Vegetarianism is generally believed to be a healthy way of life, as the diet is characterized not only by the absence of meat but by higher consumption of health-promoting foods such as fruits, vegetables, pulses, whole-grain cereals, nuts and polyunsaturated fats. However, health and lifestyle aspects of vegetarians are inextricably linked as the change to a vegetarian diet is often accompanied by a concerted change in lifestyle and an increased awareness of health and environmental issues. Similar awareness may not be seen in populations comprising lifelong vegetarians by tradition, such as South Asians from the Indian subcontinent. Young teenagers who espouse vegetarianism are known often to be motivated by ideology, particularly animal welfare, rather than by health beliefs. However, practice of vegetarianism is generally associated with increased physical activity and adoption of yoga, meditation, etc. Vegetarians have a high health awareness, tend to be nonsmokers, and are more likely to consume nutritional supplements, factors which can all be beneficial to health.

See also: **Adolescents**: Nutritional Problems. **Anaemia (Anemia)**: Iron-Deficiency Anaemia. **Antioxidants**: Diet and Antioxidant Defence. **Calcium**: Physiology. **Cancer**: Epidemiology and Associations Between Diet and Cancer. **Cobalamins**: Physiology, Dietary Sources and Requirements. **Coronary Heart Disease**: Lipid Theory of Coronary Heart Disease; Haemostatic Factors and Coronary Heart Disease. **Dairy Products**: Nutritional Value. **Diabetes Mellitus**: Dietary Management. **Fish**: Nutritional Value. **Health Foods**: Dietary Supplements - Micronutrients. **Iron**: Physiology, Dietary Sources and Requirements. **Meat, Poultry and Meat Products**: Nutritional Value. **Phytochemicals**: Classification and Occurrence; Epidemiological Factors. **Religious Customs**: Influence on Diet. **Vegetarian Diets**: Nutritional Adequacy. **Zinc**: Physiology.

Further Reading

Lewis S (1994) An opinion on the global impact of meat consumption. *American Journal of Clinical Niutrition* 59 (supplement):1099S–1102S.
Sanders TAB and Reddy S (1994) Nutritional implications of a meatless diet. *Proceedings of the Nutrition Society* 53:297–307.
Shickle D, Lewis PA, Charry M and Farrow S (1989) Differences in health, knowledge and attitudes between vegetarians and meat eaters in a random population sample. *Journal of the Royal Society of Health* 82:18–20.
Vegetarian Society (1997) Vegetarian Society Statistics Information Sheet, Altrincham, Cheshire.
Whorten JC (1994) Historical development of vegetarianism. *American Journal of Clinical Niutrition* 59 (supplement):1103S–1109S.

Table 2 Trends in vegetarianism – summary of Realeat Polls 1984–1997 showing the percentage of the UK population practising vegetarianism or avoiding red meat

Year	Vegetarian (%)	Avoiding red meat (%)
1984	2.1	1.9
1985	2.6	2.6
1986	2.7	3.1
1987	3.0	3.6
1988	3.0	5.5
1990	3.7	6.3
1993	4.3	6.5
1995	4.5	7.3
1997	5.4	8.9

Nutritional Adequacy

S Reddy, Leatherhead Food Research Association, Leatherhead, Surrey, UK

The quality of any diet depends on what foods are included, whereas vegetarian diets are defined on the basis of the foods that are excluded. It is generally accepted that vegetarian and vegan diets, but not fruitarian diets, can be nutritionally adequate and tend to be congruous with the current dietary recommendations. However, there remains the crucial issue of whether the micronutrients supplied exclusively by fish and meat (vitamins A, D and B_{12} iron, calcium and zinc) can be supplied in adequate amounts and in a utilizable form by foods of plant origin.

Nutrient Intakes

Despite the absence of meat from the diet, vegan and vegetarian diets are unremarkable with regard to their macronutrient composition. Energy intakes in both vegans and vegetarians tend to be similar to those in nonvegetarians, except in children under the age of 5, where they tend to be lower owing to the bulky nature of the diet. Sugar intakes are similar in vegans and vegetarians compared with nonvegetarians, but starch intakes are slightly greater.

Protein intakes in vegetarians are generally lower; the proportion of energy derived from protein is about 12%. Plant foods typically may not contain all the essential amino acids as in reference protein such as egg protein. However, in practice, the limiting amino acids of individual foods in vegetarian diets is of little concern, provided a mixed diet is consumed. For example, the protein quality of a combination of a cereal and pulses such as baked beans on toast is close to that of animal protein. This is achieved by the shortfall of the limiting amino acid in cereals being moderated by its levels in pulses.

The proportion of energy derived from fat is only slightly lower in vegetarian diets and is typically in the region of 30–37% of dietary energy. Saturated fat intakes tend to be marginally lower in vegetarians and depend on the extent to which dairy foods are consumed, particularly cheese, while intakes in vegans are markedly lower than in nonvegetarians. Polyunsaturated fatty acid intakes are considerably greater in vegetarians and vegans.

The intakes of several nutrients, notably vitamins B_1, folate, vitamin C, β-carotene and vitamin E tend to be higher than in nonvegetarians. However, intakes of vitamin B_{12} and available iron and calcium may be marginal. One major difference between vegetarians and omnivores is the preference of vegetarians for unrefined foods, particularly whole-grain cereals. Besides ensuring an adequate intake of most of the vitamins, with the notable exception of vitamin B_{12}, these foods provide large amounts of dietary fibre. Consequently, vegetarian diets, especially vegan diets, contain more dietary fibre than those of nonvegetarians, which has led to concern regarding its effect on mineral absorption, especially iron, zinc and calcium.

The specific nutritional questions of concern regarding vegetarianism are: firstly, whether the nutrients that are normally provided by food of animal origin can be replaced, and secondly, whether vegetarian diets can support normal growth and development. In a mixed nonvegetarian diet, animal foods form important sources of iron, vitamin B_{12}, calcium, vitamin D and zinc, which may be compromised in a vegetarian diet.

Iron

Although iron is ubiquitous, its availability from foods of plant origin is low compared with that from meat. Consequently, vegetarians are more prone to iron deficiency than meat eaters. Those at most risk are adolescent girls, women in their reproductive years, infants and toddlers. Iron intakes are relatively high in vegetarians and vegans, but iron stores in the body, as indicated by serum ferritin concentrations, are low in vegetarians compared with meat eaters. This has a number of implications; firstly, it means that low iron status during pregnancy may increase the risk of premature birth and low birthweight. Infants born to vegetarian mothers will be born with lower iron stores and, if they are breast-fed for a prolonged period, they are more likely to develop iron deficiency anaemia. High consumption of fruits and vegetables, and use of nutritional supplements by vegetarians, which enhance their intake of vitamin C, may ameliorate the deleterious effects of dietary fibre on bioavailability of non-haem iron.

Vitamin B_{12}

Animal foods are the only natural source of dietary vitamin B_{12}. Combined deficiencies of vitamin B_{12} and folate can lead to megaloblastic anaemia, where the red blood cells are immature and large in size. An increased incidence has been found in Asian vegetarians. Severe vitamin B_{12} deficiency has also been reported in Western vegans and vegetarians, but they tend to present with neurological signs of deficiency because of their high intake of folate which masks the megaloblastic anaemia. There is clearly a need for both vegans and vegetarians to be vigilant in avoiding vitamin B_{12} deficiency and consider supplementing their diet or consuming processed foods that are fortified with the vitamin.

Calcium and vitamin D

Calcium intakes in lactovegetarians tend to be similar or greater than in nonvegetarians, but lower in vegans owing to the absence of milk products from the diet. Risks to calcium nutriture among vegans arise because of their low calcium intakes and the presence of several inhibitors of calcium absorption such as oxalic acid, phytates, dietary fibre, etc., in plant foods. Consumption of unleavened breads such as chapattis, and brown rice is believed to be responsible for causing rickets and osteomalacia, particularly in Asian vegetarians. Leavening of bread with yeast destroys phytic acid and thus ameliorates its effect. Rickets is generally not a problem in other vegetarians and vegans because leavened bread is normally consumed.

Calcium nutritional status is rarely compromised if vitamin D status is satisfactory. Unlike in Asians, rickets and osteomalacia are uncommon in vegans, possibly because of adequate exposure to sunlight. Also most vegetable margarines, which are acceptable to many vegans are fortified with vitamin D. The lack of vitamin D in the vegetarian diet may not be of significance for vegetarians with healthy, outdoor lifestyles, but the housebound might need to augment their intakes by consuming foods fortified with vitamin D. Vitamin D deficiency rickets have been reported in children fed on vegan diets and in infants who have been breast-fed for prolonged periods and have not had their diets supplemented with vitamin D.

Zinc

Vegetarians and vegans have been shown to have lower levels of plasma zinc compared with nonvegetarians, even though zinc intakes were similar to or greater than those of nonvegetarians. These lower levels have been attributed to their higher intakes of dietary fibre and other modifiers of zinc absorption, such as phytic acid. However, it is uncertain whether the lower levels of zinc are of clinical significance.

Growth and development

The growth and development of vegetarian children appears to be virtually indistinguishable from that of nonvegetarian children. However, lower rates of growth, particularly in the first five years of life, have been reported in children reared on vegan and macrobiotic vegetarian diets. Despite these lower rates of growth in the first few years of life, catch-up growth occurs by the age of about 10 years. Height is normal but there is a tendency for these children to be lighter in weight for height than nonvegetarian children. The lower rates of growth in children under 5 can be attributed to their lower energy intakes. Problems of dietary inadequacy are more likely to occur in children than in adults, as their requirements relative to body weight are greater and they are unable to exert the same degree of control over

what they eat. Severe malnutrition has been reported in children fed inappropriate vegan diets. However, children can be successfully reared on vegan diets, provided considerable care is taken to avoid the major hazards of excessively bulky diets and of vitamin B_{12} and vitamin D deficiencies. Vegetarian diets that contain reasonable amounts of milk products and eggs are less likely to be inadequate.

It is generally accepted that both vegetarian and vegan diets can be nutritionally adequate and do not pose any hazard to health provided they are balanced and sensible and include a variety of foods. Problems of nutrient adequacy arise only when vegetarian diets are monotonous and extremely restricted, especially if avoidances are extensive and exclude many foods, not only animal foods. Furthermore, high intakes of dietary fibre, complex carbohydrates and antioxidants that are characteristic of vegetarian diets can offer some advantages to health.

Health of Vegetarians

Clinical studies on the general health of vegetarians and vegans have failed to show that they are less healthy than nonvegetarians. Several studies have shown that all-cause mortality in vegetarians is lower than in the general population. However, interpretation of studies on vegetarians is fraught with many problems. Vegetarians often differ from the general population in other respects, besides diet. For example, many are nonsmokers and teetotallers and tend to exercise frequently. Vegetarians, and particularly vegans, tend to be lighter in weight than nonvegetarians, and this is related to a lower proportion of body fat. Moreover, a majority of the studies are based on volunteers and, therefore are susceptible to 'volunteer bias'. The evidence of a difference in all-cause mortality between vegetarians and nonvegetarians is so far equivocal. Even if a vegetarian diet accounts for the lower mortality, it is still not certain that it is the avoidance of meat that is having an effect, rather than the protection afforded by other aspects of the diet such as higher consumption of fruit and vegetables.

Osteoporosis

Differences in the prevalence of osteoporosis between vegetarians and nonvegetarians are not well documented. Bone densities in vegetarians and non-vegetarians were found to be similar, but certain aspects of vegetarian lifestyle can be protective against bone loss. Lower protein intakes in vegetarians, effect of phytoestrogens from plant foods such as soya on oestrogen metabolism, and higher levels of physical activity are all known to prevent demineralization and bone loss.

Diabetes mellitus

Diabetes mellitus is only half as likely to be the underlying cause of death among Seventh-Day Adventist vegetarian men compared with nonvegetarian men, but this does not hold true in women. There may be a lower incidence of non-insulin-dependent diabetes (NIDDMs) in vegetarians because they tend to be leaner than nonvegetarians, and hyperinsulinism associated with obesity and lowered tissue sensitivity to insulin may not be present. Other aspects of vegetarian diets, such as high intake of complex carbohydrates, dietary fibre and generally low energy density of the diet, could resulting in improved glucose tolerance, and increased insulin sensitivity may explain the lower incidence of NIDDMs in vegetarians.

Coronary heart disease

The view that high red meat consumption is associated with increased risk of coronary heart disease is a commonly held one. Indeed, a study of Seventh-Day Adventists found that the rate of coronary heart disease (CHD) increased with increasing meat intake. Mortality and morbidity from CHD are generally lower in vegetarians than in nonvegetarians, especially in men, and it is likely that vegetarianism might confer some protection against ischaemic heart disease. In contrast, vegetarianism does not seem to confer the same protection to South Asians of Indian origin, in whom both mortality and morbidity from CHD is higher. However, the extent to which lifestyle factors other than diet such as smoking habits and exercise, contribute to the lower susceptibility to CHD is difficult to quantify. CHD is notoriously multifactorial in nature and therefore it is necessary to consider the effect of vegetarianism on the risk factors to coronary heart disease.

The fat intake of vegans is devoid of cholesterol and is low in saturated fat but the saturated fat intake of vegetarians will depend almost entirely upon the amount of dairy products and eggs they consume. Plasma cholesterol concentrations of vegans are much lower than those of either vegetarians or nonvegetarians, and are similar to the levels seen in populations where atherosclerosis is rare, while those of vegetarians are similar to or intermediate between those of vegans and nonvegetarians. The differences in total plasma cholesterol are mainly a consequence of lower low-density lipoprotein (LDL) cholesterol concentrations, although lower levels of the high-density lipoprotein (HDL) cholesterol (which is protective against CHD) have been reported in South Asian vegetarians.

Lower levels of certain blood-clotting factors (II, V, VII and X) and higher levels of anti thrombin III and fibrinolytic activity have been reported in vegans and vegetarians. These findings are of significance as high levels of LDL cholesterol and clotting factor VII are independent risk factors for coronary disease. Most studies have found that blood pressure levels tend to be lower in vegetarians, but this may be related to the lower body weights generally observed in vegetarians. The addition of meat to a vegetarian diet does not lead to an increase in blood pressure, but a change to a vegetarian diet appears to lower blood pressure modestly. This may be attributable to an increased K : Na ratio of the vegetarian diet.

Some of the modifiable risk factors of CHD other than diet, such as social support within the groups, their nonsmoking status, physically active lifestyles, their relatively low body weights, lower blood pressure, decreased risk of NIDDM and healthy blood lipid profiles, may be involved in lowering the risk of coronary disease in vegetarians. The evidence so far suggests that vegans should be less prone to both atherosclerosis and coronary heart disease than meat eaters or lacto-ovo vegetarians.

Cancer

Breast cancer Differences between vegetarians and nonvegetarians in breast cancer incidence and mortality are inconsistent, although cross-country comparisons indicate that breast cancer rates are lower in countries that consume vegetarian diets. Relatively higher intakes of phytoestrogens, particularly from soya, have been shown to be protective against breast cancer, and most vegetarians do consume soya products as a substitute for meat. The best correlations with breast cancer are with total and saturated fatty acid consumption; the consumption of animal fat does not correlate with cancer risk. Elevated plasma levels of oestradiol are believed to be associated with increased risk of breast cancer and some studies have shown that vegetarians have lower plasma oestradiol concentrations. In vegetarians, menarche occurs at a later and menopause at an earlier age. All the above factors argue in favour of a decreased risk of breast cancer among vegetarians, but there is no clear evidence that the absence of meat in the diet is protective against breast cancer.

Colon cancer In Western countries, cancers of the large bowel are up to 10 times those of many Far Eastern and developing nations, and it has been suggested that 90% of the variation in rates among countries may be due to diet. Dietary fat, particularly from animal sources, is known to increase the risk of colon cancer and the higher intake of fibre may be protective against colon cancer and indeed other diseases of the large bowel. A lower incidence of gallstones and asymptomatic diverticular disease has been reported in British vegetarians compared with the general population. Seventh-Day Adventist vegetarians in the USA have been reported to have a significantly lower incidence of colon cancer compared with nonvegetarian Adventists.

A study in the UK reported that large bowel cancer mortality did not correlate with fibre, fat or beef intake, but was negatively associated with high intakes of vegetables high in dietary fibre derived from cellulose and uronic acid. Fibre from fruits or vegetables, but not from cereals, has been consistently associated with a lower risk of colon cancer. High concentrations of faecal steroids are associated with increased risk of colon cancer, and the faecal output of bile acids is greater in meat eaters and lowest in vegans, with lactovegetarians being intermediate. A similar trend has been observed in groups of Seventh-Day Adventists of different dietary habits. High fibre intake can result in decreased colonic degradation of primary bile acids to secondary bile acids, which are known to be carcinogenic. However, the association between vegetarianism and colon cancer is still unclear, as other religious groups, such as Mormons, irrespective of their dietary habits, have a lower incidence of colon cancer than the general population.

The research studies on the health of vegetarians have so far proved to be inconclusive, but there are strong indications that a vegetarian lifestyle can be advantageous to health, particularly with regard to some forms of cancer, hypertension and coronary heart disease, where the effects are more clearly related to diet. In general, vegetarians have lower rates of some cancers (mouth, prostate and possibly colon), but there is little evidence relating this to the absence of meat in the diet. The beneficial effects of vegetarian diet are likely to be from the inclusion of a range of plant foods containing potential cancer-preventive substances such as antioxidants and phytochemicals. A semivegetarian diet containing some lean meat with good quantities of fruit and vegetables, dietary fibre, complex carbohydrates and antioxidant nutrients might offer similar benefits, while ensuring adequate intake of iron and vitamin B_{12}.

See also: **Adolescents**: Nutritional Problems. **Anaemia (Anemia)**: Iron-Deficiency Anaemia. **Antioxidants**: Diet and Antioxidant Defence. **Calcium**: Physiology. **Cancer**: Epidemiology and Associations Between Diet and Cancer. **Cobalamins**: Physiology, Dietary Sources and Requirements. **Coronary Heart Disease**: Lipid Theory of Coronary Heart Disease; Haemostatic Factors and Coronary Heart Disease. **Dairy Products**: Nutritional Value. **Diabetes Mellitus**: Dietary Management. **Fish**: Nutritional Value. **Health Foods**: Dietary Supplements - Micronutrients. **Iron**: Physiology, Dietary Sources and Requirements. **Meat, Poultry and Meat Products**: Nutritional Value. **Phytochemicals**: Classification and Occurrence; Epidemiological Factors. **Religious Customs**: Influence on Diet. **Vegetarian Diets**: Practice. **Zinc**: Physiology.

Further Reading

Alexander D, Ball M and Mann J (1994) Nutrient intake and haematological status of vegetarians and age-sex matched omnivores. *European Journal of Clinical Nutrition* 48:538–546.

Beilin LJ (1993) Vegetarian diets, alcohol consumption, and hypertension. *Annals of the New York Academy of Sciences* 676:83–91.

Burr ML, Bates CJ, Fehily AM and St Leger AS (1981) Plasma cholesterol and blood pressure in vegetarians. *Journal of Human Nutrition* 35:437–441.

Burr ML and Butland BK (1988). Heart disease in British vegetarians. *American Journal of Clinical Nutrition* 48:830–832.

Dagnelie P, van Staveren W, Vergate F, Dingian D, van den Berg H and Hautvast J (1989) Increased risk of vitamin B_{12} and iron deficiency in infants on macrobiotic diets. *American Journal of Clinical Nutrition* 50:818–824.

Draper A, Lewis J, Malhotra W and Wheeler E (1993). The energy and nutrient intakes of different types of vegetarians: a case for supplements? *British Journal of Nutrition* 69:3–19.

Key TJA, Thorogood M, Appleby PN and Burr ML (1996) Dietary habits and mortality in 1100 vegetarians and health conscious people: results of a 17 year old follow up. *British Medical Journal* 313:775–779.

Marsh A, Sanchez T, Michelsen O, Chaffee R, Fagal S (1988). Vegetarian lifestyle and bone mineral density. *American Journal of Clinical Nutrition* 48:837–841.

Reddy S, Sanders TAB (1990). Haematological studies on premenopausal Indian and Caucasian vegetarians compared with Caucasian omnivores. *British Journal of Nutrition* 64:331–338.

Reddy S, Sanders TAB (1992). Lipoprotein risk factors in vegetarian women of Indian descent are unrelated to dietary intake. *Atheroscierosis* 95:223–229.

Reddy S, Sanders TAB, Thompson MJ (1993). Faecal steroid excretion and relation to dietary intake in Indian and white vegetarians compared with white omnivores. *Proceedings of the Nutrition Society* 52:370A.

Sanders TAB, Reddy S (1994). Vegetarian diets and children. *American Journal of Clinical Nutrition* 59:1176S–1181S.

Sanders TAB, Reddy S (1994). Nutritional implications of

a meatless diet. *Proceedings of the Nutrition Society* 53:297–307.

Snowden DA (1988). Animal product consumption and mortality because of all causes combined, coronary heart disease, stroke, diabetes, and cancer in Seventh-Day Adventists. *American Journal of Clinical Nutrition* 58:739–748.

Tesar R, Natelowitz M, Shim E, Kamwell G, Brown J (1992). Axial and peripheral bone density and nutrient intakes in postmenopausal vegetarian and omnivorous women. *American Journal of Clinical Nutrition* 56:699–704.

Thorogood M, Carter R, Benfield L, McPherson K, Mann J (1987). Plasma lipids and lipoprotein cholesterol concentrations in people with different diets in Britain. *British Medical Journal* 295:351–353.

Thorogood M (1995). The epidemiology of vegetarianism and health. *Nutrition Research Reviews* 8:179–192.

van Fassen A, Hazen M, van den Brandt P, van den Bogaard, Hemus R, Janneggt R (1993). Bile acids and pH values in total faeces and in faecal water from habitually omnivorous and vegetarian subjects. *American Journal of Clinical Nutrition* 58:917–922.

Viruses *see* **Infection**: Nutritional Interactions; Nutritional Management; Nutritional Management of Measles and Human Immunodeficiency Virus in Children.

Vitamin A *see* **Retinol**: Physiology; Hypovitaminosis A.

Vitamin B$_2$ *see* **Riboflavin**: Physiology.

VITAMIN B$_6$

Physiology

D A Bender, Department of Biochemistry and Molecular Biology, University College London, London, UK

Vitamin B$_6$ has a central role in amino acid metabolism as it is the coenzyme for a variety of reactions, including transamination and decarboxylation. It is also the coenzyme of glycogen phosphorylase, and has a role in the actions of steroid and other hormones which act by modulation of gene expression.

Severe deficiency disease has only been reported in a single outbreak in infants fed overheated formula milk. However, a significant proportion of people in developed countries have marginal vitamin B$_6$ status, and this may be associated with enhanced responsiveness to steroid hormone action, and hence may be a factor in the development of hormone-dependent cancer of the breast, uterus and prostate. A number of drugs have anti-vitamin B$_6$ metabolic activity, and prolonged use may lead to secondary development of pellagra, as a result of impaired tryptophan metabolism.

Oestrogens do not cause vitamin B$_6$ deficiency. However, there is some evidence that high doses of vitamin B$_6$ may overcome some of the side effects of oestrogenic steroids used in contraceptives and as menopausal hormone replacement therapy. At high levels of intake, such supplements may cause sensory nerve damage.

Absorption, Transport and Storage

The main form of vitamin B$_6$ in foods is pyridoxal phosphate, bound to enzymes. There is also a small amount of pyridoxamine phosphate. In plant foods a significant amount of the vitamin is present as pyridoxine. A number of plants contain relatively large amounts of pyridoxine glycosides, which are not biologically available, since they are not substrates for mammalian glycosidases. They are absorbed (passively) from the intestinal lumen and are excreted more or less quantitatively in the urine. Between 5 and 50% of the total vitamin B₆ in some foods may be present as glycosides.

Pyridoxal phosphate bound to enzymes as the Schiff base is released on digestion of the protein. The phosphorylated vitamers (compounds with the biological activity of the vitamin) are dephosphorylated by membrane-bound alkaline phosphatase in the intestinal mucosa; pyridoxal, pyridoxamine and pyridoxine are all absorbed rapidly by passive diffusion. Intestinal mucosal cells have pyridoxine kinase and pyridoxine phosphate oxidase (see **Fig. 1**), so that there is net accumulation by metabolic trapping. Much of the ingested pyridoxine is released into the portal circulation as pyridoxal, after dephosphorylation at the serosal surface.

A proportion of the vitamin B₆ in foods may be biologically unavailable, especially after heating. This is the result of the formation of pyridoxyllysine by reduction of the aldimine (Schiff base), by which pyridoxal phosphate is bound to the ε-amino groups of lysine residues in proteins. A proportion of this pyridoxyllysine may be useable, since it is a substrate for pyridoxine phosphate oxidase. However, it is also a vitamin B₆ antimetabolite, and even at relatively low concentrations can accelerate the development of deficiency in experimental animals.

Metabolism and transport

Most of the absorbed vitamin B₆ is taken up by the liver, although other tissues can also take up the unphosphorylated vitamers from the circulation. Uptake is by passive diffusion, followed by metabolic trapping as phosphate esters. Pyridoxine and pyridoxamine phosphates are oxidized to pyridoxal phosphate, as shown in Fig. 1. All tissues have pyridoxine kinase activity, but pyridoxine phosphate oxidase is found only in liver, kidney and brain.

Pyridoxine phosphate oxidase is a flavoprotein, and its activity falls markedly in riboflavin deficiency. Despite this central role of riboflavin in vitamin B₆ metabolism, blood and tissue concentrations of pyridoxal phosphate are not affected by riboflavin deficiency, and riboflavin nutrition appears to have no effect on vitamin B₆ nutritional status.

Pyridoxine phosphate oxidase is inhibited by its product, pyridoxal phosphate. This is not simple product inhibition, but involves binding at a specific inhibitor site on the enzyme. The normal intracellular concentration of free pyridoxal phosphate gives

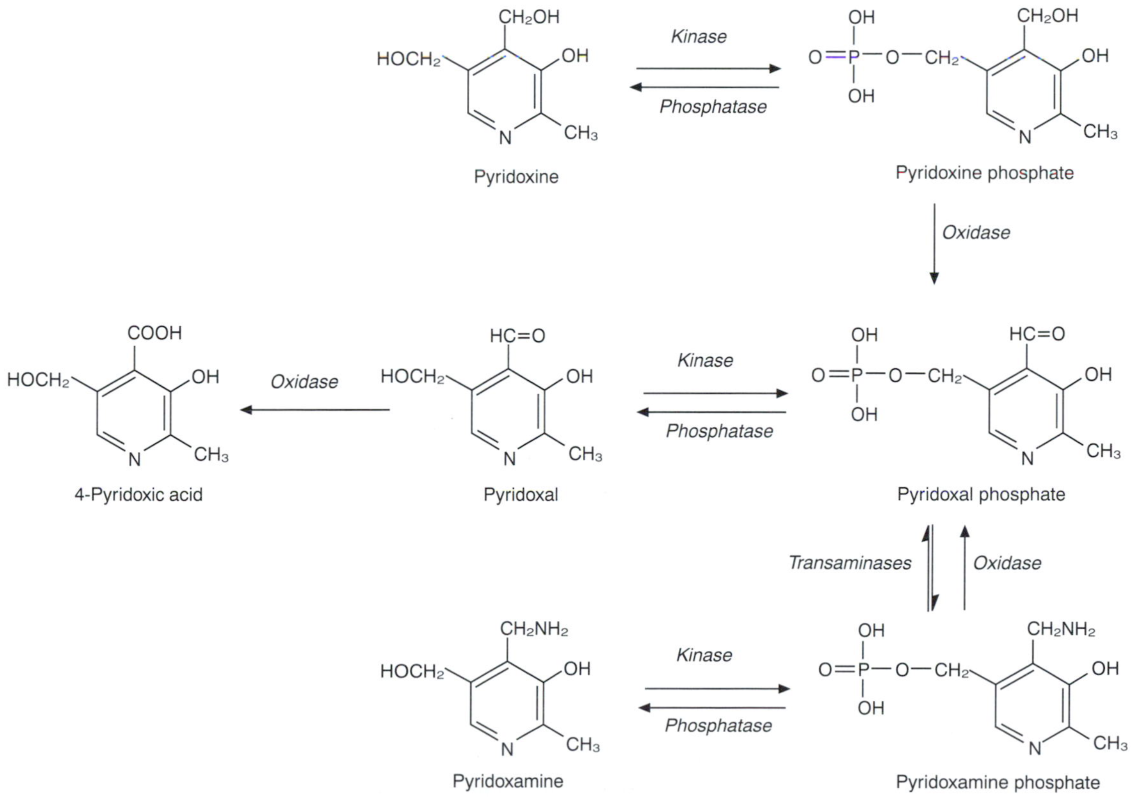

Figure 1   Metabolic interconversion of the vitamin B₆ vitamers. Pyridoxal kinase EC 2.7.1.38, pyridoxine oxidase EC 1.1.1.65, pyridoxamine phosphate oxidase 1.4.3.5, pyridoxal oxidase EC 1.1.3.12.

significant inhibition, suggesting that this may be a physiologically important mechanism in the control of tissue pyridoxal phosphate.

Pyridoxine is rapidly converted to pyridoxal phosphate in liver and other tissues. Pyridoxal phosphate does not cross cell membranes, and efflux of the vitamin from most tissues is as pyridoxal. Pyridoxal phosphate is exported from the liver specifically bound to albumin. Much of the free pyridoxal phosphate in the liver is hydrolysed to pyridoxal, which is also exported, and circulates bound to both albumin and haemoglobin in erythrocytes. Free pyridoxal remaining in the liver is rapidly oxidized to 4-pyridoxic acid, which is the main excretory product of the vitamin.

Extrahepatic tissues take up both pyridoxal and pyridoxal phosphate from the plasma. Pyridoxal phosphate is hydrolysed to pyridoxal, which can cross cell membranes, by extracellular alkaline phosphatase; it is then trapped intracellularly by phosphorylation.

Tissue concentrations of pyridoxal phosphate are controlled by the balance between phosphorylation and dephosphorylation. The activity of phosphatases acting on pyridoxal phosphate is greater than that of the kinase in most tissues. This means that pyridoxal phosphate that is not bound to enzymes will be dephosphorylated, and hence will leave the cell by diffusion. Thus there is little accumulation of pyridoxal phosphate in tissues, other than that which is bound to enzymes and therefore has a functional role.

Free pyridoxal either leaves the cells or is oxidized to 4-pyridoxic acid by aldehyde dehydrogenase, which is present in all tissues, and also by hepatic and renal aldehyde oxidase. 4-Pyridoxic acid is the main excretory product of vitamin B₆, and its excretion reflects recent intake more than the state of underlying tissue reserves of the vitamin. Small amounts of pyridoxal and pyridoxamine are also excreted in the urine, although much of the active vitamin B₆ which is filtered is reabsorbed in the kidney tubules.

Storage and body reserves

There is no specific storage of vitamin B₆ in the body; as discussed above, pyridoxal phosphate that is not bound to enzymes is rapidly dephosphorylated, oxidized to 4-pyridoxic acid and excreted.

The total body content of vitamin B₆ is of the order of 15 μmol (3.7 mg) per kg body weight. About 80% of this is in muscle, much of it associated with glycogen phosphorylase. This does not seem to function as a true reserve of the vitamin and is not released from muscle in times of deficiency.

Pyridoxal is released from muscle in starvation, as muscle glycogen reserves are exhausted, and there is less requirement for glycogen phosphorylase activity. Under these conditions it is available for redistribution to other tissues, especially liver and kidney, to meet the increased requirement for gluconeogenesis from amino acids.

Metabolic Functions of Vitamin B₆

The metabolically active vitamer is pyridoxal phosphate. This is involved in many reactions of amino acid metabolism, where the carbonyl group is the reactive moiety; in glycogen phosphorylase, where it is the phosphate group which is important in catalysis; and in the release of hormone receptors from tight nuclear binding, where again it is the carbonyl group that is important. Glycogen phosphorylase catalyses the sequential phosphorolysis of glycogen to release glucose-1-phosphate; it is thus the key enzyme in the utilization of muscle and liver glycogen reserves.

The role of pyridoxal phosphate in amino acid metabolism

Pyridoxal phosphate-dependent enzymes catalyse a number of important reactions in amino acid metabolism, including transamination to yield oxo (keto) acids, decarboxylation to yield amines, and a variety of side chain elimination and rearrangement reactions (see **Fig. 2**).

In the absence of the substrate, pyridoxal phosphate is bound to the enzyme by the formation of a Schiff base to the ε-amino group of a lysine residue. The first reaction between the substrate and the coenzyme is transfer of the aldimine linkage from this ε-amino group to the α-amino group of the substrate. The ring nitrogen of pyridoxal phosphate exerts a strong electron-withdrawing effect on the aldimine, and this leads to weakening of all three bonds about the α-carbon of the substrate; which bond is cleaved will depend on the orientation of the Schiff base relative to reactive groups of the catalytic site.

Cleavage of the α-carbon–carboxyl bond of the Schiff base leads to decarboxylation of the amino acid, followed by release of the corresponding amine and reformation of the internal Schiff base to lysine. A number of the products of the decarboxylation of amino acids are important as neurotransmitters and hormones, and as the diamines and polyamines involved in the regulation of DNA metabolism; the decarboxylation of phosphatidylserine to phosphatidylethanolamine is important in phospholipid metabolism.

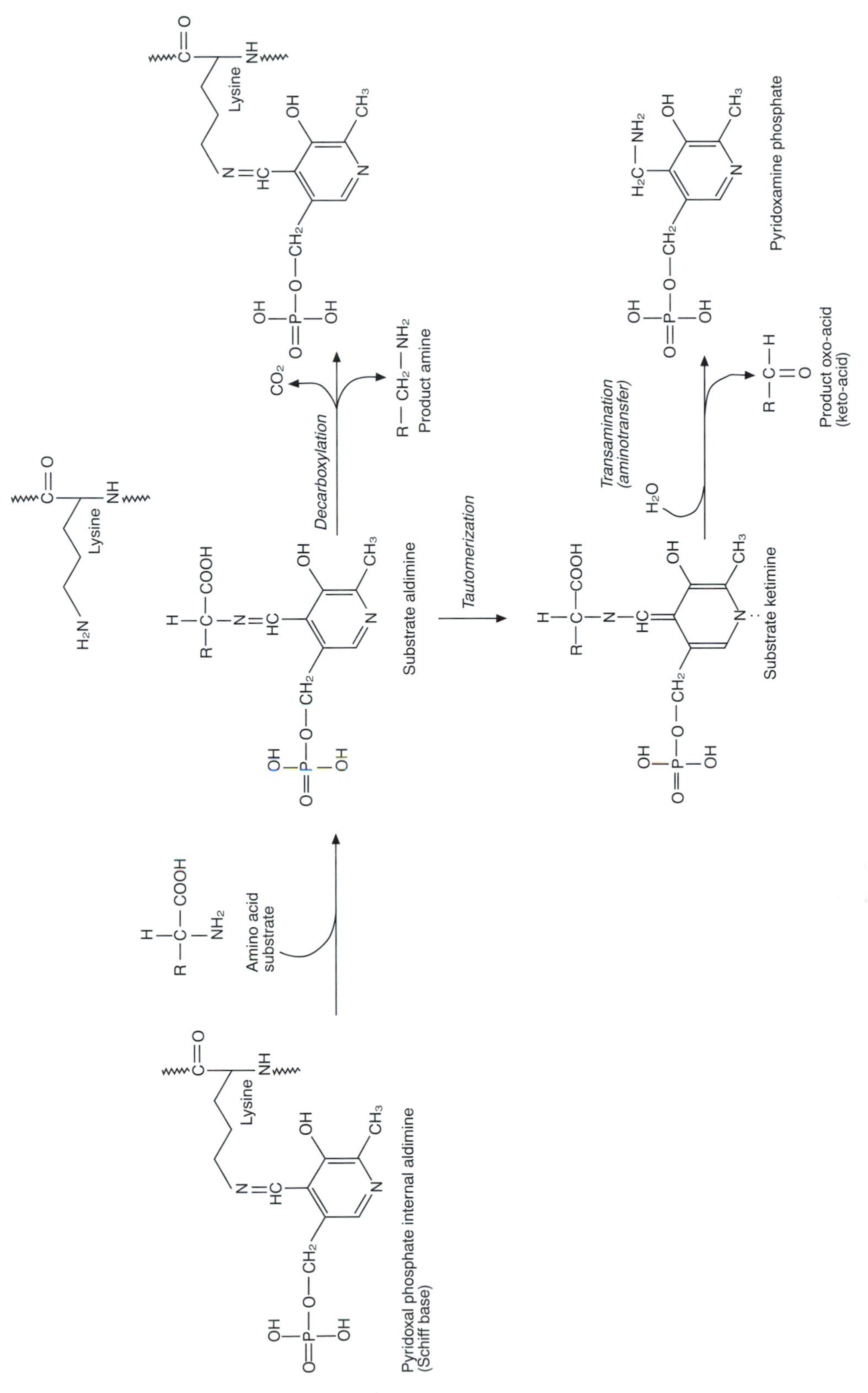

Figure 2 Reactions of amino acids in pyridoxal phosphate-dependent enzymes.

Hydrolysis of the α-carbon–amino bond of the Schiff base results in the release of the 2-oxo-acid corresponding to the amino acid substrate, and leaves pyridoxamine phosphate at the catalytic site of the enzyme. In this case there is no reformation of the internal Schiff base to the reactive lysine residue. This is the half-reaction of transamination. The process is completed by reaction of pyridoxamine phosphate with a second oxo-acid substrate, followed by the reverse of the reaction sequence shown in **Fig. 3**.

Transamination is of central importance in amino acid metabolism, providing pathways for the catabolism of all amino acids other than lysine (which does not undergo transamination). Many of these reactions are linked to the amination of 2-oxoglutarate to glutamate or glyoxylate to glycine, which are substrates for oxidative deamination, reforming the oxo-acids. Equally, transamination reactions provide a pathway for the synthesis of those amino acids for which there is an alternative source of the oxo-acid (the nonessential amino acids).

The role of pyridoxal phosphate in hormone action

Vitamin B6 has a role in the action of those hormones which act by binding to a nuclear receptor protein and modulating gene expression. Such hormones include androgens, oestrogens, progesterone, glucocorticoids, calcitriol (the active metabolite of vitamin D), retinol and retinoic acid, and the thyroid hormones. Target tissue specificity of hormone action is ensured by the presence of receptor proteins which are responsible for both nuclear uptake and the interaction with control regions of DNA.

Pyridoxal phosphate reacts with a lysine residue in the receptor protein and releases the hormone–receptor complex from tight nuclear binding. It thus acts to terminate hormone action and release receptor proteins for reutilization.

In experimental animals, vitamin B6 deficiency results in increased and prolonged nuclear uptake and retention of steroid hormones in target tissues, and there is enhanced sensitivity to low doses of hormones. In cells in culture, pyridoxal phosphate depletion results in enhanced induction of marker enzymes, while high intracellular concentrations of pyridoxal phosphate impair enzyme induction in response to the hormone.

Assessment of Vitamin B6 Status

A wide variety of methods are available for assessment of vitamin B6 status, including plasma concentrations of pyridoxal phosphate or total vitamin, urinary excretion of 4-pyridoxic acid or total vitamin B6, activation of erythrocyte transaminases, and the ability to metabolize test doses of tryptophan or methionine. **Table 1** shows the accepted criteria of adequacy for each of these methods.

Various pyridoxal-phosphate-dependent enzymes must compete with each other for the available pool of coenzyme. Thus the extent to which an enzyme is saturated with its coenzyme provides a means of assessing the adequacy of the tissue pool of coenzyme. This can be determined by measuring the activity of the enzyme before and after the activation of any apoenzyme present in the sample by incubation with added pyridoxal phosphate. Erythrocyte aspartate and alanine transaminases are commonly used; the results are expressed as either the percentage stimulation of activity by added pyridoxal phosphate, or the activation coefficient – the ratio of activity with added coenzyme to that without added coenzyme.

It seems likely that it is normal for a proportion

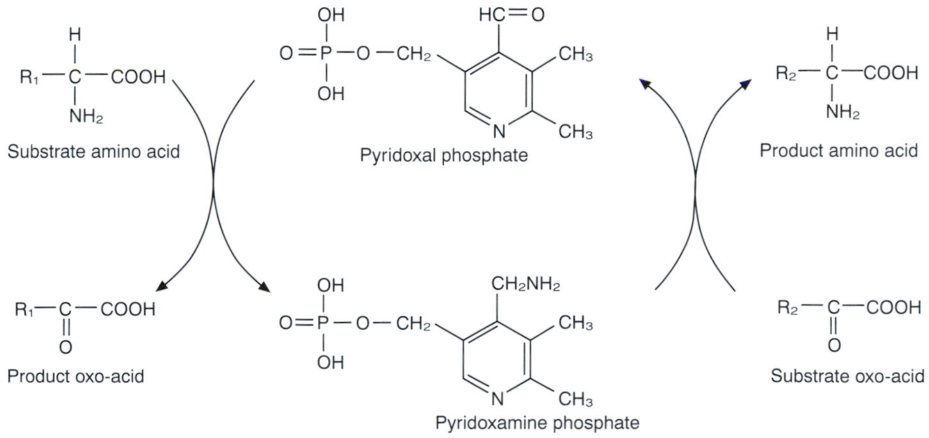

Figure 3 The reaction of transamination.

Table 1   Indices of vitamin B$_6$ nutritional status

Method	Adequate status
Plasma total vitamin B$_6$	>40 nmol (10 μg) l^{-1}
Plasma pyridoxal phosphate	>30 nmol (7.5 μg) l^{-1}
Erythrocyte alanine aminotransferase activation coefficient	<1.25
Erythrocyte aspartate aminotransferase activation coefficient	<1.80
Erythrocyte aspartate aminotransferase	>0.13 units (8.4 μkat) l^{-1}
Urine 4-pyridoxic acid	>3.0 μmol per 24 h
	>1.3 mmol per mol creatinine
Urine total vitamin B$_6$	>0.5 μmol per 24 h
	>0.2 mmol per mol creatinine
Urine xanthurenic acid after 2 g tryptophan load	<65 μmol per 24 h increase
Urine cystathionine after 3 g methionine load	<350 μmol per 24 h increase

of pyridoxal phosphate-dependent enzymes to be present as inactive apoenzyme, without coenzyme. This may be a mechanism for metabolic regulation. It is possible that increasing the intake of vitamin B$_6$, so as to ensure complete saturation of pyridoxal phosphate-dependent enzymes, may not be desirable.

The tryptophan load test

The pathway of tryptophan metabolism is shown in **Fig. 4**. Kynureninase is a pyridoxal-phosphate-depen-

dent enzyme, and in vitamin B$_6$ deficiency its activity is lower than that of tryptophan dioxygenase. This means that there is a considerable accumulation of both hydroxykynurenine and kynurenine, sufficient to permit greater metabolic flux than usual through kynurenine transaminase, resulting in increased formation of kynurenic and xanthurenic acids. Although kynurenine transaminase is also pyridoxal-phosphate-dependent, it seems to be little affected in vitamin B$_6$ deficiency; this may be because it binds

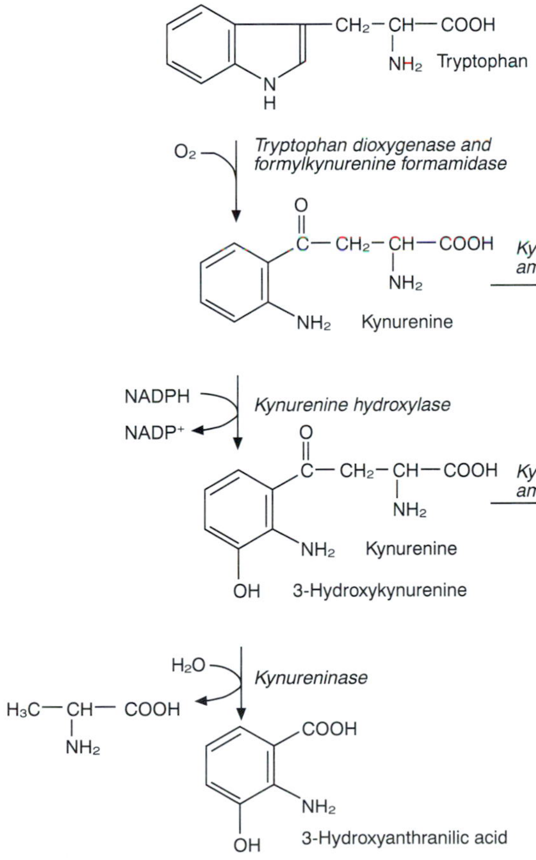

Figure 4   The tryptophan load test for vitamin B$_6$ nutritional status. Tryptophan dioxygenase EC 1.13.11.11, formylkynurenine forma-midase EC 3.5.1.9, kynurenine hydroxylase EC 1.14.13.9, kynureninase EC 3.7.1.3, kynurenine aminotransferase EC 2.6.1.7 and 2.6.1.63.

its coenzyme more tightly than does kynureninase, or because it has a slower rate of turnover.

Xanthurenic and kynurenic acids are easy to measure in urine, so that the ability to metabolize a test dose of 2 or 5 g of tryptophan has been widely adopted as a convenient and sensitive index of vitamin B_6 nutritional status. However, induction of tryptophan dioxygenase by glucocorticoid hormones will result in a greater rate of formation of kynurenine and hydroxykynurenine than the capacity of kynureninase, and will thus lead to increased formation of kynurenic and xanthurenic acids – an effect similar to that seen in vitamin B_6 deficiency. Such results may be erroneously interpreted as indicating vitamin B_6 deficiency in a variety of subjects whose problem is increased glucocorticoid secretion as a result of stress or illness, not vitamin B_6 deficiency.

Inhibition of kynureninase by oestrogen metabolites also results in accumulation of kynurenine and hydroxykynurenine, and hence increased formation of kynurenic and xanthurenic acids, again giving results which falsely suggest vitamin B_6 deficiency. In women taking oestrogens, although the tryptophan load test suggests vitamin B_6 depletion, the results of other tests of vitamin B_6 status are normal, and there is no evidence that oestrogens cause vitamin B_6 deficiency.

The methionine loading test

The metabolism of methionine, shown in **Fig. 5**, includes two pyridoxal phosphate-dependent steps, catalysed by cystathionine synthetase and cystathionase. Cystathionine synthetase is little affected by vitamin B_6 deficiency, presumably since it has a high affinity for its cofactor, and possibly also a slow rate of turnover. However, cystathionase activity falls in vitamin B_6 deficiency, and there is an increase in the tissue content of inactive apoenzyme.

The result of this is that in vitamin B_6 deficiency there is an increase in the urinary excretion of cystathionine, both after a loading dose of methionine and under basal conditions. The ability to metabolize a test dose of methionine therefore provides an additional test of vitamin B_6 nutritional status, which does not seem to be as prone to artefacts as the tryptophan load test.

Requirements

The total body pool of vitamin B_6 is of the order of 15 μmol (3.7 mg) per kg body weight. Isotope tracer studies suggest there is turnover of about 0.13% per day, and hence a minimum requirement for replacement of 0.02 μmol (5 μg) per kg body weight – some 350 μg per day for a 70 kg adult.

Most studies of vitamin B_6 requirements have followed the development of abnormalities of tryptophan and methionine metabolism during depletion, and normalization during repletion with graded intakes of the vitamin. Such studies have shown that biochemical signs of deficiency develop more rapidly when the protein intake is relatively high. Similarly, during repletion of deficient subjects, indices of nutritional status are normalized faster at low than at high levels of protein intake.

Such studies suggest a mean requirement of 13 μg of vitamin B_6 per g of dietary protein. There is no evidence that the requirements of any age group other than infants (see below), or the requirements in pregnancy and lactation, differ from 13 μg g^{-1} of dietary protein, and for all population groups Recommended Dietary Allowances (RDAs) are based on 15–16 μg g^{-1} of protein. At average adult intakes of about 100 g of protein per day, this gives an RDA of 1.5–1.6 mg of vitamin B_6. Average intakes in the UK are between 20–30 μg g^{-1} protein. Rich sources of vitamin B_6 are shown in **Table 2**.

Gross clinical deficiency of vitamin B_6 is rare. The vitamin is widely distributed in foods, and intestinal flora synthesize relatively large amounts, at least some of which is believed to be absorbed and hence available.

A number of studies have shown that between 10 and 20% of the apparently healthy population have low plasma concentrations of pyridoxal phosphate or abnormal erythrocyte transaminase activation coefficient, suggesting vitamin B_6 inadequacy or deficiency. In most studies, only one of these indices of vitamin B_6 nutritional status has been assessed. Where both have been assessed, while each shows some 10% of the population apparently inadequately provided with vitamin B_6, few of the subjects show inadequacy by both criteria.

There is a decrease in the plasma concentration of vitamin B_6 with increasing age, and some studies have shown a high prevalence of abnormal transaminase activation coefficient in elderly subjects, suggesting that the elderly may be at risk of vitamin B_6 deficiency. It is not known whether this reflects an inadequate intake, a greater requirement, or changes in the tissue distribution and metabolism of the vitamin with increasing age.

A number of drugs which react with carbonyl compounds are capable of causing vitamin B_6 depletion, including the antituberculosis drug isoniazid (iso-nicotinic acid hydrazide), penicillamine, and the anti-parkinsonian drugs Benserazide and Carbidopa. The main effect of prolonged use of these drugs is impairment of the metabolism of tryptophan as a result of reduced kynureninase activity, and the

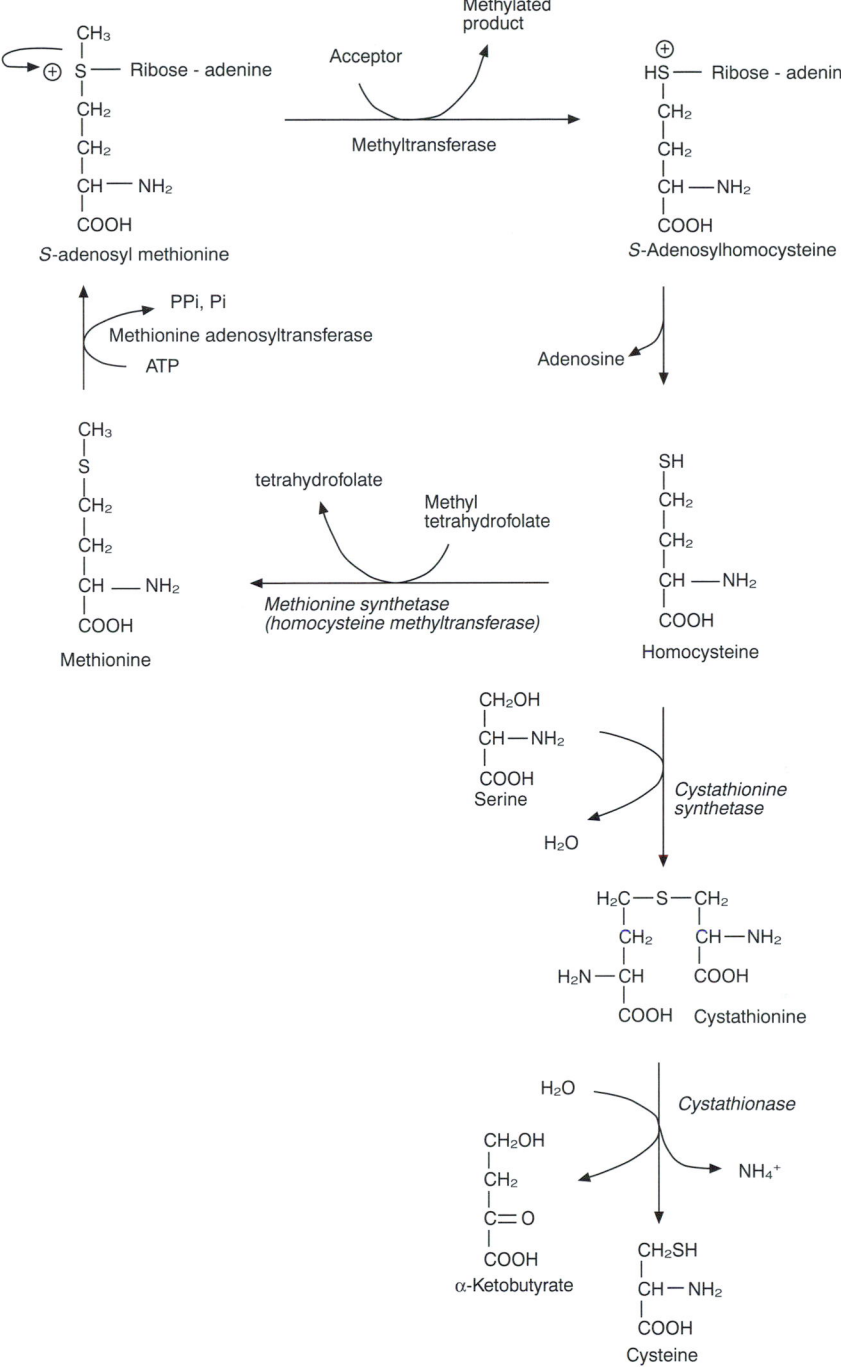

Figure 5 Methionine metabolism as a test for vitamin B$_6$ nutritional status. Methionine adenosyltransferase EC 2.5.1.6 methionine synthetase EC 2.1.1.13 (vitamin B$_{12}$-dependent), 2.1.1.5 (betaine as methyl donor), cystathionine synthetase EC 4.2.1.22, cystathionase EC 4.4.1.1.

development of the niacin deficiency disease pellagra, which responds to the administration of either vitamin B$_6$ or niacin. Isoniazid can also cause peripheral neuropathy, which responds to vitamin B$_6$, but not to niacin.

Vitamin B$_6$ requirements of infants

Estimation of the requirements of infants presents a problem, and there is a clear need for further research to achieve a realistic estimate. Human milk,

Table 2 Rich sources of vitamin B$_6$

Food	Portion (g)	mg per portion
Salmon	150	1.1
Mackerel	150	1.0
Venison	150	1.0
Bloater	150	0.9
Herring	150	0.9
Rabbit	150	0.8
Tuna	150	0.8
Liver	150	0.7
Sardines canned in oil	150	0.7
Cod	175	0.6
Crab	175	0.6
Goose	150	0.6
Mung beans (dahl)	150	0.6
Plaice	150	0.6
Potatoes	140	0.6
Avocado	130	0.5
Beef, roast	150	0.5
Kidney	150	0.5
Pork	150	0.5
Sardines canned in tomato	150	0.5
Trout	150	0.5
Turkey	150	0.5
Veal	150	0.5
Bacon joint	150	0.4
Bananas	135	0.4
Beans, red kidney	100	0.4
Beef	150	0.4
Chicken	150	0.4
Duck	150	0.4
Eel	150	0.4
Lentils	150	0.4
Brussels sprouts	75	0.3
Chestnuts	75	0.3
Halibut	150	0.3
Milk	560	0.3
Oatmeal	100	0.3
Oranges	250	0.3
Pears	150	0.3
Pilchards in tomato sauce	100	0.3
Plantain, green	85	0.3

which must be assumed to be adequate for infant nutrition, provides only some 40–100 µg l^{-1}, or 3–8 µg of vitamin B$_6$ per g of protein – very much lower than the apparent requirement for adults, although there is no reason why infants should have a lower requirement.

A first approximation of the vitamin B$_6$ needs of infants came from studies of those who convulsed as a result of gross deficiency caused by overheated infant milk formula. At intakes of 60 µg per day there was an incidence of convulsions of 0.3%. Provision of 260 µg per day prevented or cured convulsions, but 300 µg per day was required to normalize tryptophan metabolism. This is almost certainly a considerable overestimate of requirements, since pyridoxyllysine formed by heating the

vitamin with proteins has antivitamin activity, and would therefore result in a higher apparent requirement.

Based on the body content of 15 µmol (3.7 mg) of vitamin B$_6$ per kg body weight, and the rate of weight gain, the minimum requirement for infants over the first 6 months of life would appear to be 100 µg (417 nmol) per day to establish tissue reserves.

Pharmacological Uses and Toxicity of Vitamin B$_6$ Supplements

Supplements of vitamin B$_6$ ranging from 25 to 100 mg per day, and sometimes up to 2000 mg per day or higher, have been recommended for a variety of conditions, including postnatal depression, depression and other side effects associated with oral contraceptives, hyperemesis of pregnancy, the premenstrual syndrome and the carpal tunnel syndrome.

Doses of 50–200 mg of vitamin B$_6$ per day have an antiemetic effect, and the vitamin is widely used, alone or in conjunction with other antiemetics, to minimize the nausea associated with radiotherapy and to treat pregnancy sickness. There is no evidence that vitamin B$_6$ has any beneficial effect in pregnancy sickness, nor that women who suffer from morning sickness have lower vitamin B$_6$ nutritional status than other pregnant women.

Doses of vitamin B$_6$ of 100 mg per day have been reported to be beneficial in the treatment of the carpal tunnel syndrome, or what has been called tenosynovitis. However, most of the reports originate from one centre, and there appears to be little independent confirmation of the usefulness of the vitamin in this condition.

Vitamin B$_6$ and the side effects of oral contraceptives

Although oestrogens do not cause vitamin B$_6$ deficiency, the administration of vitamin B$_6$ supplements has beneficial effects on some of the side effects of both administered and endogenous oestrogens. The supplements act in two main areas: in normalizing glucose tolerance and as an antidepressant.

Mild impairment of glucose tolerance is common in pregnancy, and may indeed be severe enough to be classified as gestational diabetes mellitus, which generally resolves at parturition, although in some subjects it may persist, pregnancy having been the trigger for the development of maturity-onset diabetes. High-oestrogen oral contraceptives may also cause impaired glucose tolerance. This seems to be the result of increased tissue and blood concentrations of xanthurenic acid, because of the inhibition of kynureninase by oestrogen metabolites. Xanthurenic acid forms a complex with insulin which has little or no hormonal activity. Vitamin B$_6$ supplements may have a beneficial effect on glucose tolerance as a result of activating apokynureninase.

One of the relatively common side effects of oestrogenic oral contraceptives is depression, affecting about 6% of women in some studies. This frequently responds well to the administration of relatively large amounts of vitamin B$_6$ (generally in excess of 40 mg per day). Postnatal depression also responds to similar supplements in some studies.

Again, this does not seem to be due to correction of vitamin B$_6$ deficiency, but rather to a direct effect of pyridoxal phosphate on the metabolism of tryptophan. High concentrations of pyridoxal phosphate attenuate the response to glucocorticoid hormones; tryptophan dioxygenase is a glucocorticoid-induced enzyme, and thus its synthesis and activity will be reduced by high intakes of vitamin B$_6$. This reduces the oxidative metabolism of tryptophan, and increases the amount available for synthesis of 5-hydroxytryptamine in the brain. Increased brain 5-hydroxytryptamine synthesis has a mood-elevating effect.

Vitamin B$_6$ in the premenstrual syndrome

There are few well-controlled studies of the effects of vitamin B$_6$ in premenstrual syndrome. In general, those that have been properly controlled report little benefit from doses between 50 and 200 mg per day compared with placebo, although some studies do claim a beneficial effect. Despite the lack of evidence, vitamin B$_6$ is widely prescribed (and self-prescribed) for the treatment of the premenstrual syndrome.

Toxicity of vitamin B$_6$

Animal studies have demonstrated the development of signs of peripheral neuropathy, with ataxia, muscle weakness and loss of balance, in dogs given 200 mg pyridoxine per kg body weight for 40 to 75 days, and the development of a swaying gait and ataxia within 9 days at a dose of 300 mg kg^{-1} body weight. At a dose of 50 mg kg^{-1} body weight, there are no clinical signs of toxicity, but histologically there is a loss of myelin in dorsal nerve roots. At higher doses there is more widespread neuronal damage, with loss of myelin and degeneration of sensory fibres in peripheral nerves, the dorsal columns of the spinal cord and the descending spinal tract of the trigeminal nerve. The clinical signs of vitamin B$_6$ toxicity in animals regress after withdrawal of these massive doses, but sensory nerve conduction velocity, which decreases during the development of the neuropathy, does not recover fully. The mechanism of the neurotoxic action of vitamin B$_6$ is unknown.

The development of sensory neuropathy has been reported in patients taking 2–7 g of pyridoxine per day. Although there was residual damage in some patients, withdrawal of these extremely high doses resulted in a considerable recovery of sensory nerve function.

Other reports have suggested that intakes as low as 50 mg per day are associated with neurological damage, although these have been based on patients' reporting of symptoms rather than on detailed neurological examination.

See also: **Amino Acids**: Chemistry and Classification; Metabolism. **Glucose**: Metabolism and Maintenance of Blood Glucose Level. **Niacin**: Physiology, Dietary Sources and Requirements; Pellagra. **Pregnancy**: Safe Diet for Pregnancy. **Riboflavin**: Physiology.

Further Reading

Allgood VA and Cidlowski JA (1992) Vitamin B$_6$ modulates transcriptional activation by multiple members of the steroid hormone receptor superfamily. *Journal of Biological Chemistry* 267:3819–3824.

Bender DA (1987) Oestrogens and vitamin B$_6$ – actions and interactions. *World Review of Nutrition and Dietetics* 51:140–188.

Bender DA (1989) Vitamin B$_6$ requirements and recommendations. *European Journal of Clinical Nutrition* 43:289–309.

Bender DA (1992) Vitamin B$_6$. In: *Nutritional Biochemistry of the Vitamins*, chap. 9, pp 223–268. Cambridge: Cambridge University Press.

Bender DA and Bender AE (1997) Vitamin B$_6$. In: *Nutrition – A Reference Handbook*, chap. 20, pp 322–341. Oxford: Oxford University Press.

Dakshinamurti K (1982) Neurobiology of pyridoxine. *Advances in Nutritional Research* 4:143–179.

Fasella PM (1967) Pyridoxal phosphate. *Annual Review of Biochemistry* 36:185–210.

Ink SL and Henderson LM (1984) Vitamin B$_6$ metabolism. *Annual Review of Nutrition* 4:455–470.

Lumeng L, Lui A and Li T-K (1980) Plasma content of B$_6$ vitamers and its relationship to hepatic vitamin B$_6$ metabolism. *Journal of Clinical Investigation* 66:688–695.

Wiss O and Weber F (1964) Biochemical pathology of vitamin B$_6$ deficiency. *Vitamins and Hormones* 22:495–501.

VITAMIN K

Physiology

M Kohlmeier, University of North Carolina at Chapel Hill, Chapel Hill, NC, USA

Vitamin K is the name given to a group of substances that have been found to have antihaemorrhagic properties in birds and mammals. Vitamin K has a protective effect against bleeding because it serves as the essential cofactor for the specific carboxylation of several coagulation factors. Additional functions and activities of vitamin K continue to be discovered. Besides its long-known importance for blood coagulation, essential roles have been suggested for vitamin K in the maintenance of bone health, cell proliferation, and prevention of inappropriate calcium crystal formation (as in kidney stones, or on arterial walls or heart valves). Contrary to the common assumption, this fat-soluble vitamin will not accumulate, nor has a relevant toxicity been observed. Because there is virtually no storage, the adequacy of daily intake is very important and suboptimal status is common. There are only a few good dietary vitamin K sources, mainly dark green vegetables and a few fermented foods. The availability of dietary vitamin K depends on the presence of fat and bile during absorption in the small intestine. The contribution from intestinal flora appears to be very limited. An important factor for vitamin K status is the allocation after absorption of this scarce nutrient to various tissues, because there appears to be no effective means of redistribution. Genetic and acquired disposition critically influences this allocation. Vitamin K is an essential cofactor for the carboxylation of glutamates in more than a dozen proteins; each carboxylation reaction converts vitamin K into the inactive epoxide form. The regeneration of the vitamin K-2,3-epoxide is vital to ensure vitamin adequacy in cells. Inhibition of epoxide regeneration induces vitamin K deficiency; the resulting anticoagulation is commonly employed for medical purposes, but also for rodent pest control.

Vitamin K Sources and Disposition

Compounds with vitamin K activity

Naturally occurring compounds with vitamin K activity consist of 2-methyl-1,4-naphthoquinone and a polyisoprenoid side chain. Plants contain almost exclusively phylloquinone or vitamin K$_1$ (**Fig. 1**), which is part of the photosystem I. Bacteria contain one or more of a series of compounds with three to 13 isoprenyl units in the side chain which are collectively termed menaquinones, or vitamin K$_2$. By convention the number of isoprenyl units in the side chain is indicated as in menaquinone 7, abbreviated to MK-7.

Synthetically produced 2-methyl-1,4-naphthoquinone (menadione or vitamin K$_3$) is active when given orally because it is converted into MK-4. However, because of its potential for oxidative toxicity, it is currently used only as an additive for animal feeds.

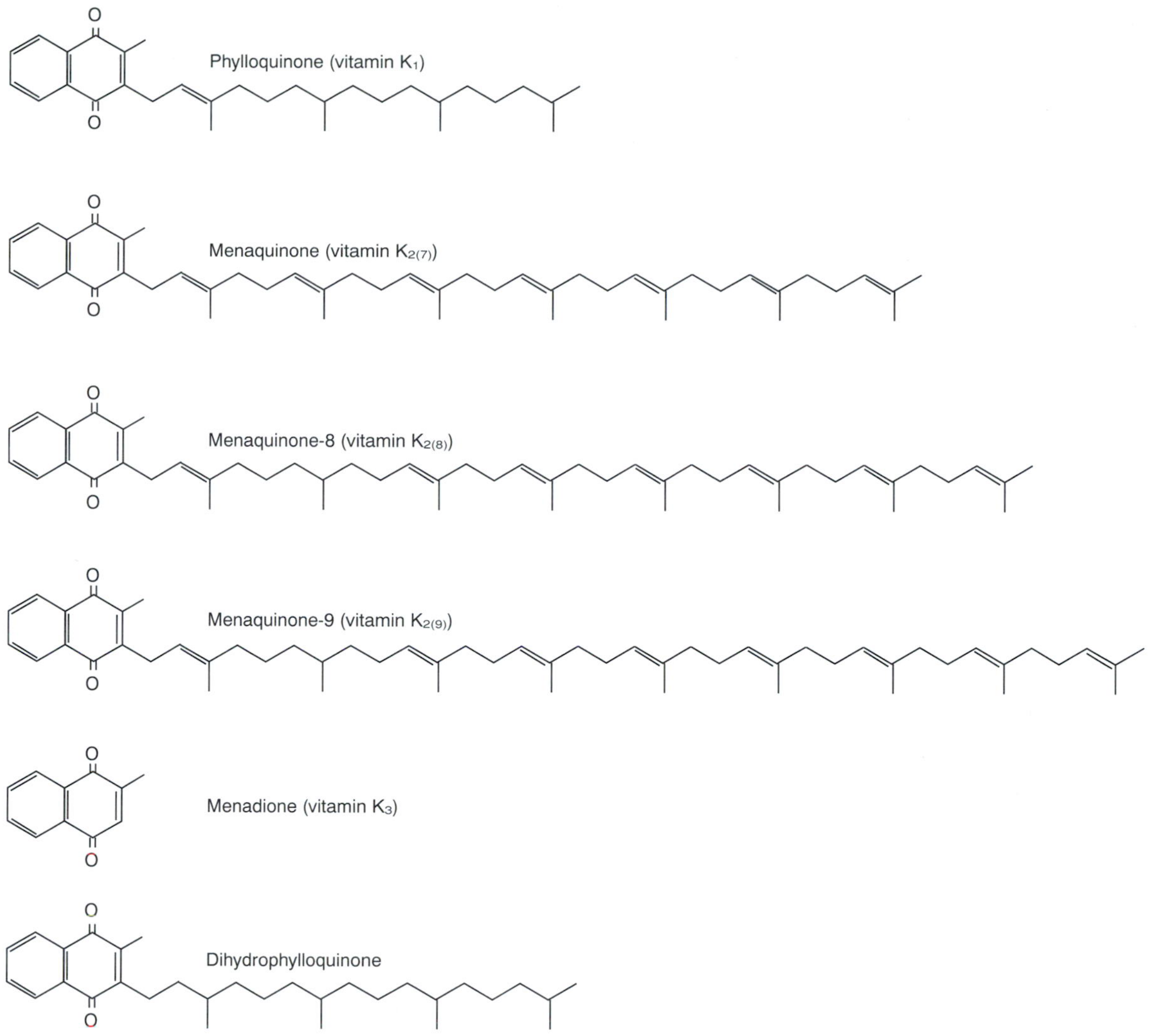

Figure 1 Vitamin K in foods and dietary supplements.

Similar concerns about potential toxicity exists in regard to other synthetic vitamin K analogues.

Intestinal absorption of dietary vitamin K

All naturally occurring forms of vitamin K in foods are highly lipophilic. Therefore vitamin K must be incorporated into mixed micelles in the duodenum before it is taken up by mucosal cells of the proximal small intestine. Since the formation of mixed micelles requires the presence of dietary fat, pancreatic lipase and bile, in their absence little of the vitamin K in a meal is absorbed. Another important determinant of vitamin K absorption is solubility. Vitamin K from oils, fermented foods and pharmaceutical preparations readily mixes with the components of micelles and is highly available. The phylloquinone in leafy vegetables, on the other hand, is tightly bound to the plant's chloroplasts and is only released by cooking or by thorough grinding or chewing.

Intestinal flora as a source of vitamin K

Most of the normal intestinal bacteria produce one or several forms of menaquinones, mostly MK-7, MK-8 and MK-9. However, only a small fraction of these appears to be absorbed from the terminal ileum and large intestine, where most of the menaquinone production takes place. These relatively small amounts appear to be sufficient to provide the minimal amounts necessary for survival, even in the complete absence of dietary vitamin K. Use of oral antibiotics often suppresses intestinal bacterial growth and thereby interferes with this endogenous source of vitamin K.

Transport and distribution to tissues

Vitamin K that has been absorbed from the proximal small intestine is secreted with chylomicrons into lymph and transported from there into blood circulation. The bulk of this vitamin K is ultimately taken up by the liver along with the chylomicron remnants, while smaller amounts are delivered to bone and other tissues. The actual tissue distribution depends on factors that influence chylomicron metabolism. Information on the vitamin K content of human tissues is still sketchy (**Table 1**). The highest phylloquinone concentration has been reported for fat in bone, intermediate concentrations for liver, heart, pancreas and bone, and concentrations below 1 μg l^{-1} in blood, muscle, lung, kidney and brain. Significant concentrations of long-chain menaquinones have been found in liver and bone. MK-4 is the main form of vitamin K in brain and kidney and is produced by side chain modification of phylloquinone and, possibly, long-chain menaquinones. Vitamin K in tissues is associated mainly with endoplasmatic reticulum and mitochondria, the majority with the latter.

Vitamin K catabolism and excretion

Once the vitamin is taken up by a particular tissue it is unlikely to leave it again in its active form. The bulk of the vitamin K taken up by the liver is converted to more polar metabolites, secreted into bile and excreted with the faeces; little intact vitamin K is found in bile. A smaller proportion of ingested vitamin K undergoes n-oxidation of the side chain and is excreted mainly as glucuronides of 2-methyl-3-(5'-carboxy-3'-methyl-2'-pentenyl)-1,4-naphthoquinone and 2-methyl-3-(3'-carboxy-3'-methylpropyl)-1,4-naphthoquinone (**Fig. 2**).

Molecular Basis of Vitamin K Action

Specific carboxylation of glutamate in proteins

Vitamin K serves as a cofactor of an enzyme that posttranslationally γ-carboxylates specific glutamate residues in a few proteins (**Table 2**). These γ-carboxylglutamate (Gla) residues confer to proteins the ability of binding calcium with high affinity and specificity. The carboxylase itself is a Gla protein. Several of the blood coagulation factors (factors II, VII, IX and X) and coagulation inhibitors (proteins C and S) contain Gla without which they cannot be activated. Protein Z is another coagulation-enhancing Gla protein, but it is less well understood. All of these coagulation-related Gla proteins are produced in the liver.

Three additional Gla proteins have been completely characterized, but have functions not related to haemostasis: bone Gla protein (BGP, osteocalcin), matrix Gla protein (MGP) and growth-arrest specific protein 6 (gas6). The function of BGP, which is produced almost exclusively in osteoblasts and odontoblasts, is still obscure; it is most likely related to the control of mineralizing activities by these cells. MGP has been shown to modulate the nucleation of calcium crystals in a variety of tissues and is essential for the prevention of arterial wall calcification. Gas6 is the specific ligand of the tyrosine–kinase receptor axl which participates in growth and differentiation modulating cell signalling. A closely related receptor with similar characteristics (dte) specifically binds protein S.

Further Gla proteins have been identified in

Table 1 Vitamin K content of adult human tissues

	Phylloquinone (nmol per kg tissue)	MK-4 (nmol per kg tissue)	MK-6 to MK-11 (nmol per kg tissue)	Total vitamin K (nmol per 70 kg body weight)
Blood (fasting)	1.8	<0.5	1.1	18
Liver	10.6	5.3	58.5	112
Pancreas	25.0	20.0	n/a	3.6
Fat in bone	64.3	n/a	59.8	22.2
Bone	5.3	n/a	9.7	53.2
Heart	9.3	0.9	n/a	3.3
Lung	1.3	0.6	n/a	<2
Muscle	n/a	n/a	n/a	n/a
Adipose tissue	n/a	n/a	n/a	n/a
Kidney	<2	6.5	n/a	<2
Brain	<2	6.0	n/a	<2

Data are from Thijssen HHW and Drittij-Reinders MJ (1996) Vitamin K status in human tissues: tissue-specific accumulation pf phylloquinone and menaquinone-4. *British Journal of Nutrition* **75**:121–127; Hodges SJ, Bejui J, Leclercq M and Delmas PD (1993) Detection and measurement of vitamins K_1 and K_2 in human cortical and trabecular bone. *Journal of Bone and Mineral Research* **8**:1005–1008.
n/a, data not available.

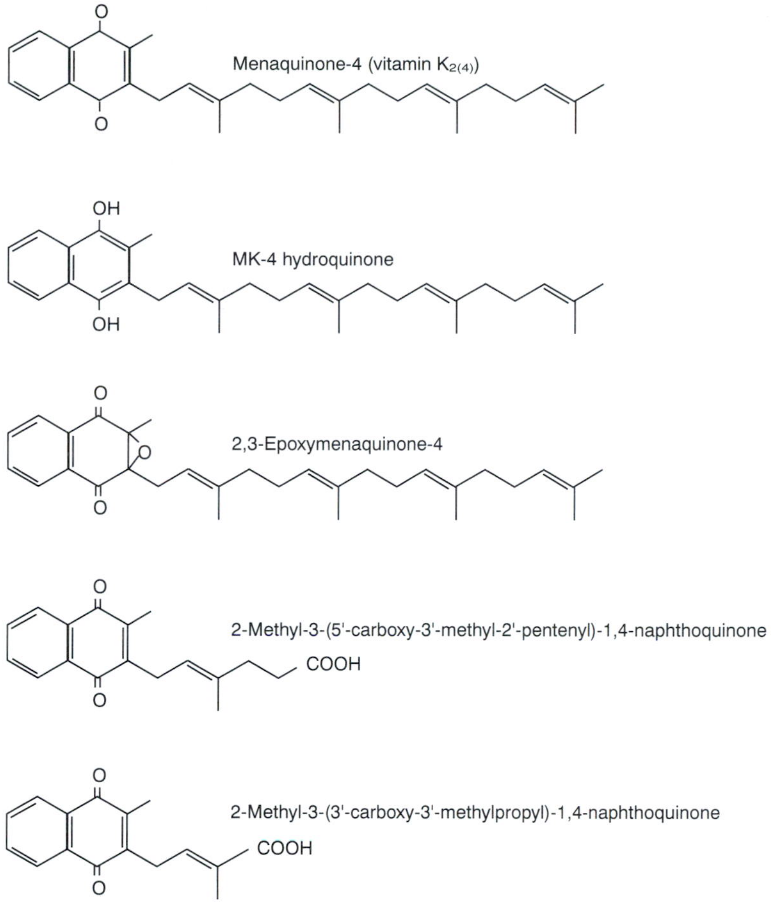

Figure 2 Vitamin K metabolites.

Table 2 Human vitamin K-dependent proteins

Name	No. of Gla residues	Function
Factor II	10	Blood coagulation cascade
Factor VII	10	Blood coagulation cascade
Factor IX	12	Blood coagulation cascade
Factor X	11	Blood coagulation cascade
Protein C	9	Inhibitor of coagulation
Protein S	11	Activator of protein C, ligand of dte receptor (growth modulation)
Protein Z	13	Enhancement of blood coagulation
gas6	5	Ligand of axl receptor (growth modulation)
Osteocalcin (bone Gla protein, BGP)	2–3	Regulation of bone mineralization (mechanism unknown)
Matrix Gla protein (MGP)	5	Modulator of calcium crystal nucleation
Vitamin K dependent carboxylase	?	Carboxylation of Gla proteins
Galactocerebroside sulfotransferase	?	Sulfatide biosynthesis in brain
n-Sulfatidase	?	Sphingolipid catabolism

various tissues and body fluids, but these have not been completely characterized. Among these nephrocalcin, a 14 kDa glycoprotein isolated from urine, atherocalcin, a 32 kDa Gla protein found in atherosclerotic plaque, and numerous other proteins detected in lung, bone, arterial wall and other tissues.

Carboxylase-independent functions of vitamin K

Vitamin K also appears to play a role in sulfatide metabolism. The activities of both galactocerebroside sulfotransferase and of n-sulfatidase in brain increase 2- to 3-fold upon addition of vitamin K to purified preparations. Vitamin K-deficient mouse pups were found to have altered sulfatide composition of brain. A warfarin-sensitive arylsulfatase (ARSE), which recently has been identified and completely sequenced, is thought to be important for normal embryonal bone and cartilage development, since mutations cause distinct abnormalities (chondrodysplasia punctata). It is not known, however, whether this enzyme actually is vitamin K-dependent, nor what its function is.

Through an as yet unknown mechanism, vitamin K has been shown to inhibit stimulated interleukin 6 (IL-6) production in cell cultures. The strongest IL-6 inhibition was found with the vitamin K catabolite 2-methyl-3-(5'-carboxy-3'-methyl-2'-pentenyl)-1,4-naphthoquinone, which does not promote carboxylase activity. These additional vitamin K functions may thus be independent of the ability to promote the carboxylation of proteins.

Regeneration of vitamin K

The active cofactor of the vitamin K-dependent carboxylase is vitamin K hydroquinone which is generated by the action of vitamin K reductase on the quinone form of vitamin K (**Fig. 3**); the quinone is the main form of vitamin K in foods. The synthesis of one γ-carboxylglutamate residue generates one molecule of vitamin K-2,3-epoxide. This inactive vitamin K metabolite may then be reduced again to the quinone form by vitamin K-2,3-epoxide reductase.

Normally, vitamin K can go through this redox cycle many times; this enables a cell to function with minimal amounts of the vitamin. Typical daily Gla synthesis is about 40 μmol, which will be produced as long as vitamin K intakes are at least 0.1 μmol per day.

Assessment of Vitamin K Status

Blood coagulation

Traditionally, blood-clotting assays have been used to monitor vitamin K activity. The most common bioassay used newly hatched chicks and determined the amount of test substance needed to maintain normal blood clotting. Blood-clotting assays are based on the fact that the coagulation factors II, VII, IX and X are vitamin-K dependent proteins which are incompletely carboxylated during vitamin K deficiency and thus have reduced activity.

Clinical blood-clotting assays such as prothrombin time can be used to monitor therapeutically induced vitamin K-deficiency for the prevention of thrombosis in high-risk patients, since these assays will detect only severe deficiencies. An additional complication comes from the fact that liver disease also impairs the production of coagulation factors and may thus interfere with the interpretation of the results. Sensitivity and specificity can be improved by measuring directly the Gla content of a particular coagulation factor in blood. One assay of this type

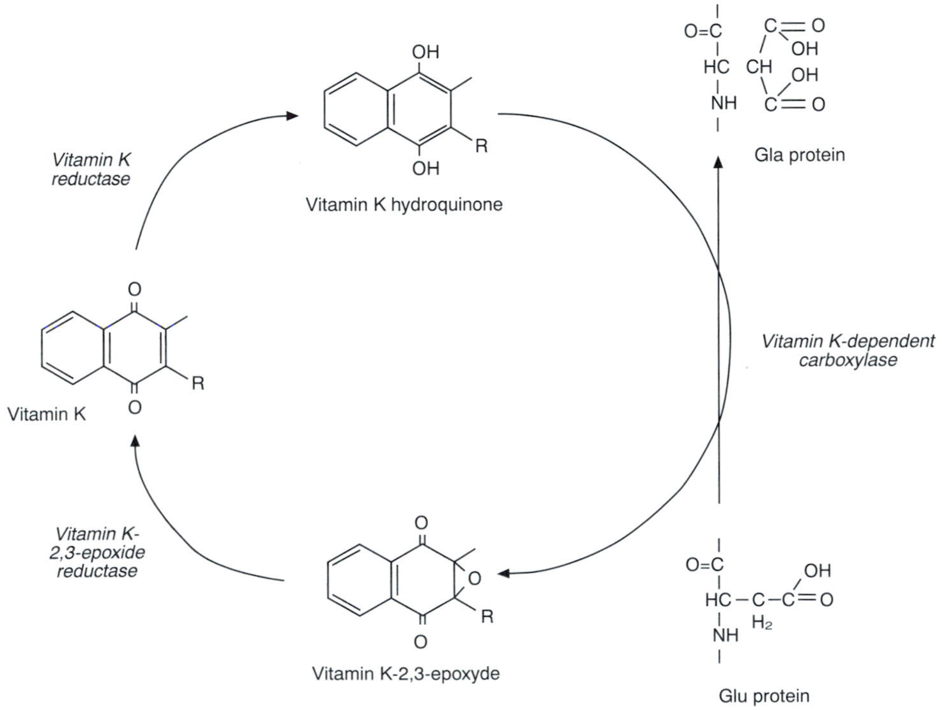

Figure 3 The vitamin K-2,3-epoxide cycle.

makes use of monoclonal antibodies that specifically detect undercarboxylated prothrombin (PIVKA II). While activity or composition of coagulation factors may indicate vitamin K status in the liver, this will not necessarily reflect availability of vitamin K to other tissues. It is important to remember that most of the menaquinones absorbed from the terminal ileum and colon are carried via the portal vein and may be retained by hepatocytes during their first pass through the liver. This largely diet-independent source will thus contribute more to the hepatic production of coagulation factors than to vitamin K function in extrahepatic tissues.

Carboxylation of extrahepatic proteins

The degree of carboxylation of BGP (osteocalcin) in plasma has been found to be a very sensitive indicator of vitamin K deficiency, even when coagulation factors were unaffected. Carboxylated BGP preferentially binds to hydroxylapatite (calcium phosphate crystals) or to the crystals of other divalent cations and can thus be removed from whole plasma. Parallel BGP measurement by immunoassay in treated and untreated samples will provide an index of Gla content that reflects vitamin K status in bone, the site of BGP synthesis. Undercarboxylated osteocalcin in serum also has been measured directly with specific monoclonal antibodies.

γ-Carboxyglutamic acid in urine

The breakdown of Gla proteins liberates free Gla, some of which is then excreted with urine. Free Gla in urine can be measured by high-performance liquid chromatography (HPLC) and fluorometry following extraction and derivatization. Switching from adequate to vitamin K-deficient diets decreases Gla excretion with urine, but the changes tend to be small unless there is severe vitamin K deficiency.

Vitamin K concentration in serum

Following ingestion of a vitamin K-rich meal blood concentrations typically increase within an hour, reach a maximum after 3–6 h and return to preprandial levels again after 12–15 h. To eliminate influences by individual meals subjects usually are asked to fast overnight for 12–14 h prior to blood sampling. Phylloquinone concentrations in blood after an overnight fast are thus influenced by recent dietary intakes, but more importantly by the rapidity of chylomicron metabolism. Apolipoprotein E polymorphism is an example of a genetic disposition that affects both chylomicron remnant clearance and vitamin K concentration. Those with the apo E isoform E-4 tend to have lower than average phylloquinone and menaquinone concentrations in fasting plasma, while those with the isoform E-2 tend to have higher concentrations. Individuals with hypertriacylglycerolaemia often have higher than average vitamin K concentrations, particularly if the hyperlipidaemia is due to delayed chylomicron clearance.

The relevance of vitamin K concentration in serum as a predictor of vitamin K status is still uncertain, since it is not clear how serum concentration relates to tissue concentrations. Nonetheless, recent evidence suggests that phylloquinone concentration in preprandial serum is a good predictor of long-term bone health; adjustment for triacylglycerol concentration does not seem to improve the predictive power.

Health Effects of Vitamin K Deficiency

Haemorrhagic disease of the newborn

The earliest and most devastating effect of vitamin K deficiency concerns infants during their first weeks of life. The vitamin K content of blood and tissues is much lower in the normal fetus and newborn than in older children and adults. In addition, vitamin K-2,3-epoxide recycling may be less efficient than later in life. This naturally low vitamin K status during intrauterine life is associated with low blood coagulability. Departure from the protective environment apparently increases a child's vulnerability and a small, but significant percentage of infants suffer from intraventricular haemorrhage. The risk is greatest in prematurely born infants (up to a third of those with less than 1500 g birthweight), in breast-fed infants and in those with gastrointestinal conditions that impair vitamin K absorption (cholestasis, diarrhoea, malabsorption syndromes, etc.). The risk of haemorrhagic events can be greatly reduced by ensuring adequate vitamin K status. For this reason most health services now either recommend or require prophylactic vitamin K administration for all newborns. A single parenteral dose (typically 1 mg intramuscularly immediately after birth) has been the most common mode of administration. Vitamin K may also be given orally; because this route is less reliable, the initial dose at birth should be repeated twice at weekly or bi-weekly intervals. Bioavailability may also be improved by the use of mixed micellar preparations containing bile constituents in addition to vitamin K.

Coagulopathy of the adult

Normal or near normal blood coagulation is usually maintained in older children and adults even in the absence of dietary vitamin K, presumably because the small amounts of bacterial menaquinones from the lower intestine are sufficient for this function. Thus, a total fast of several weeks by itself will not cause bleeding, despite the fact that vitamin K storage is minimal. However, if vitamin K production by the normal intestinal flora is reduced at the same time, as during antibiotic treatment or as a consequence of diarrhoea, significant and even dangerous bleeding may occur within days. In the absence of liver disease normal blood coagulation is restored within one or two days by the administration of vitamin K.

Bone health

At least three vitamin K-dependent proteins (BGP, MGP and protein S) are produced in bone, suggesting that vitamin K may be important for bone health. Among the elderly, bone fracture victims tend to have lower serum concentrations of phylloquinone, MK-7 and MK-8 than their peers. Prospective studies also showed that both low vitamin K concentrations and increased proportions of undercarboxylated BGP were predictive for the risk of bone fractures. Critically low bone density, which is a major cause of bone fracture in the elderly, is much more common in people with poor vitamin K status than in those with good status. Most importantly, the improvement of vitamin K status has been shown to minimize loss of bone minerals. While it remains to be seen whether supplemental vitamin K in later age actually reduces bone fracture risk, long-term vitamin K status appears to be important for bone health.

Little is known about the mechanism(s) through which vitamin K status influences bone. Bone is constantly remodelled by osteoclastic breakdown and subsequent osteoblastic rebuilding. BGP has been suggested as a mediator that links osteoclastic and osteoblastic activities; undercarboxylated BGP has been found to be ineffective for this function. As a consequence, the osteoclastic breakdown cycle may continue longer during suboptimal than during optimal vitamin K status. Another mechanism may be an inhibiting effect of vitamin K on interleukin 6 (IL-6) production. IL-6 relays the action on osteoblasts of various mediators such as parathyroid hormone (PTH) to osteoclasts (which do not have PTH receptors themselves). Vitamin K might thus dampen the catabolic effect of such hormones and limit bone mineral loss. Finally, there may be a more or less direct effect of vitamin K on PTH levels. It has recently been observed that secondary hyperparathyroidism due to renal failure is much less prevalent among patients with optimal vitamin K status compared to those with poorer vitamin K status. This is very similar to the better-investigated relationship between hyperparathyroidism and vitamin D status.

Other health risks

Evidence of particular importance of vitamin K status for the prevention of cardiovascular disease, kidney stones and other disorders is still emerging and is often controversial.

During the more advanced stages of atherosclerosis lesion development, particularly during plaque calcification, several Gla proteins are expressed, including BGP and MGP. The presence of these vitamin K-dependent proteins raises the possibility that vitamin K status has some influence on the progression of atherosclerosis. Indeed, in a group of postmenopausal women the presence of atherosclerotic calcifications of the abdominal aorta was strongly associated with marginal vitamin K status. Mice with genetically absent MGP production develop extremely severe arterial calcification a few weeks after birth; the same outcome is observed in mice treated with a vitamin K antagonist from birth. Further studies are needed to determine the preventive potential of measures that maintain optimal vitamin K status.

Calcium oxalate kidney stones were found to contain an undercarboxylated version of nephrocalcin, a mid-sized peptide secreted into urine. Urine of individuals with a history of calcium kidney stones accordingly contained a higher proportion of undercarboxylated nephrocalcin than urine of normal controls. Vitamin K antagonist (warfarin) treatment, on the other hand, did not diminish the ability of nephrocalcin to inhibit calcium oxalate crystal growth.

Alzheimer's dementia is a common affliction of the elderly whose features include a disturbance of calcium homeostasis in central neurons. Individuals with the apo E isoform E-4 are most commonly affected; about two-thirds of all patients have this genetic trait. Since this isoform is associated with lower than average vitamin K status, a causal role of the vitamin in protection against premature dementia has been suggested.

Dietary Considerations

Dietary sources and range of intakes

The major form of vitamin K in Western diets is phylloquinone, the most important source of which is green, leafy vegetables. A small serving of chard, kale or spinach contains several hundred μg of phylloquinone which is more than most people consume over several days. Broccoli and green asparagus also are excellent sources. Dark green colouring of a vegetable or fruit tends to indicate a high phylloquinone content (see **Table 3**). A few vegetable oils also contain significant amounts of phylloquinone, most importantly the oils from canola and soya beans. Hydrogenation of these oils (for the production of margarine and shortening) partially converts phylloquinone into dihydrophylloquinone, whose biological activity is unknown. Bacterial menaquinones may be found in fermented foods. *Natto*, a fermented bean dish which is commonly consumed in Japan, contains large amounts of MK-7. Some cheeses and other fermented dairy products also contain relevant quantities of menaquinones.

Habitual dietary intakes of vitamin K varies greatly between individuals and from day to day owing to the very limited number of vitamin K-rich foods. Average phylloquinone intakes of adults in the USA were found (Food and Drug Administration (FDA) total diet study) to be 60–80 µg per day. Similar intakes have been reported from the UK. Dihydrophylloquinone intakes in the US were 15–20 µg per day. Menaquinone consumption rarely exceeds 5–10 µg per day in US or European diets, but may be much higher in Japanese or other Asian diets.

Current recommendations

Average intakes of 1 µg per kg body weight are recommended by most health organizations for children and adults. This amount is sufficient to prevent bleeding in healthy people. The recommendations do not take into account, however, the newly recognized role of vitamin K for functions unrelated to blood coagulation. Thus, to maintain optimal bone health ten-fold or even higher amounts may have to be consumed. Such high intake levels can only be achieved through the regular consumption of cooked greens together with some fat, fermented foods such as natto, or dietary supplements. Since there is virtually no storage of vitamin K, the constancy of adequate intakes is likely to be more important than with most other vitamins.

Safety of very high intakes

Long-term consumption of vitamin K at levels exceeding normal intakes several hundred-fold (45 mg per day) have not caused toxic effects in humans. Reports of adverse effects of vitamin K have invariably been linked to parenterally administered preparations which always contain much larger quantities of emulsifiers and stabilizers than of vitamin K itself. Most importantly, the often suspected

Table 3 Vitamin K content of vitamin K-rich foods

	Phylloquinone concentration (µg per 100 g) (reference)		Phylloquinone content (µg) (serving size)	
Swiss chard	830	(B)	789	(1/2 cup)
Kale	724	(S)	688	(1/2 cup)
Spinach	381	(S)	362	(1/2 cup)
Broccoli	270	(B)	243	(1/2 spear)
Green asparagus	400	(B)	240	(4 spears)
Brussel sprouts	147	(S)	110	(1/2 cup)
Pistachio nut	70	(B)	29	(40 g)
Coleslaw	57	(B)	23	(1/2 cup)
Soya oil	153	(S)	23	(15 ml)
Kiwi fruit	25	(B)	19	(medium-sized fruit)
Rapeseed oil (canola)	113	(S)	17	(15 ml)
Olive oil, virgin	85	(S)	13	(15 ml)
Mayonnaise	81	(B)	12	(15 ml)
Margarine	12–118	(B)	1–12	(10 g)
	Menaquinones			
Natto	900	(S)	1350	(1 bowl)
Cheese	30	(S)	17	(60 g)

Data are from (S) Shearer MJ, Bach A and Kohlmeier M (1996) Chemistry, nutritional sources, tissue distribution and metabolism of vitamin K with special reference to bone health. *Journal of Nutrition* **126**:1181S–1186S; Shearer MJ, von Kries R and Saupe J (1992) Comparative aspects of human vitamin K metabolism and nutriture. *Journal of Nutrition Science and Vitamins* **3**(supplement 13):413–416; (B) Booth SL, Sadowski JA and Pennington JAT (1995) The phylloquinone content of foods in the US-FDA Total Diet Study. *Journal of Agriculture and Food Chemistry* **55**:823–830.

thrombosis risk when increasing vitamin K consumption from normal to very high levels has never been documented. The absence of such a thrombogenic effect is biologically plausible, since at normal vitamin K intakes the coagulation factors are fully carboxylated and an increased amount of vitamin K will not increase their activity.

Vitamin K Antagonists

Inhibition of vitamin K regeneration

Inhibitors of vitamin K-2,3-epoxide reductase interrupt the regeneration of vitamin K and thereby induce vitamin K deficiency. Potent inhibitors of vitamin regeneration include warfarin and related synthetic coumarins. Administration of these compounds inhibits carboxylation of vitamin K-dependent proteins in all tissues within hours; osteocalcin carboxylation in bone is more sensitive to this induced vitamin K deficiency than coagulation factors. Total secretion of some vitamin K-dependent proteins is also reduced by warfarin treatment, possibly as a result of selective intracellular degradation of the undercarboxylated forms. Inhibition of vitamin K regeneration is incomplete, however, since most cells also express a warfarin-insensitive epoxide reductase. This enzyme is thought to be responsible for the rapid recovery when excess vitamin K is given after warfarin treatment.

Use for pest control

Vitamin K antagonists are commonly used as rodenticides; repeated doses taken up from baits kill eventually by inducing internal bleeding. However, several naturally occurring warfarin-resistant animal strains have been identified. Accidental or intentional poisoning of humans with coumarins does occur and can be diagnosed through detection either of the drug responsible or of an abnormal accumulation of vitamin K-2,3-epoxide.

Clinical use

Medical therapy uses carefully controlled doses of compounds with anti-vitamin K activity to reduce coagulation tendency and thereby prevent thrombus formation in peripheral veins, in coronary arteries and at atrial valves. The response to a given dose depends on concurrent vitamin K intakes. A diet with a relatively constant vitamin K content greatly helps to avoid day-to-day variations of blood coagulability. Interindividual differences in response to anticoagulant treatment also have been found to be strongly influenced by individual disposition; the genetic apo E polymorphism described above appears to be a common and important modulator of vitamin K status that is associated with a lesser response in those with the apo E isoform E-2.

While both short-term and long-term anticoagulation with anti-vitamin K drugs has been shown to benefit patients in certain instances by reducing thrombosis risk, the consequences for extrahepatic tissues are still insufficiently explored. A very small percentage of patients will suffer from skin necrosis during the first days of anti-vitamin K treatment; this appears to be related to the more rapid decrease in protein C activity and the resulting imbalance of endogenous pro- and anticoagulant factors. Reduced bone mineral density in patients on long-term anti-vitamin K treatment has been observed in some studies, but not in others.

Coumarin embryopathy

Anti-vitamin K treatment during pregnancy is associated with severe risks. Coumarin-type compounds are teratogenic and appear to increase the risk of abortion and stillbirth. Upon intrauterine exposure typical abnormalities of cartilages and bones occur, probably by interfering with morphogenesis during the first 6–9 weeks of pregnancy. Similar patterns of abnormalities occur in the extremely rare genetic vitamin K epoxide reductase deficiency and in the more common genetic disorder chondrodysplasia punctata (CDPX). Embryonic exposure also may induce distinct bone abnormalities including excessive localized mineralization and nasal hypoplasia. Anti-vitamin K treatment during the second and third trimesters carries the risk of fetal haemorrhage and severe developmental disturbances. Thus, vitamin K antagonists should never be given to women who plan a pregnancy or who are already pregnant. If a pregnancy is detected, anti-vitamin K treatment must be discontinued immediately and vitamin K should be given as an antidote.

See also: **Bone**: Composition, Metabolism and Bone Growth. **Infants**: Nutritional Requirements. **Pregnancy**: Safe Diet for Pregnancy. **Renal Function and Disorders**: Nutritional Management of Renal Disorders.

Further Reading

Conly JM, Stein K, Worobetz L and Rutledge-Harding S (1994) The contribution of vitamin K_2 (menaquinones) produced by the intestinal microflora to human nutritional requirements for vitamin K. *American Journal of Gastroenterology* 89:915–923.

Jie KSG, Bots ML, Vermeer C, Witteman JCM and Grobbee DE (1995) Vitamin K intake and osteocalcin levels in women with and without aortic atherosclerosis: a population-based study. *Atherosclerosis* **116**:117–123.

Kohlmeier M, Salomon A, Saupe J and Shearer MJ (1996) Transport of vitamin K to bone in humans. *Journal of Nutrition* **126**:1192S–1196S.

Nakagawa Y, Abram V, Parks JH, Lau HSH, Kawooya JK and Coe FL (1985) Urine glycoprotein crystal growth inhibitors: evidence for a molecular abnormality in calcium oxalate nephrolithiasis. *Journal of Clinical Investigation* **76**:1455–1462.

Reddi K, Henderson B, Meghji S, Wilson M, Poole S, Hopper C, Harris M and Hodges SJ (1995) Interleukin-6 production by lipopolysaccharide-stimulated human fibroblasts is potently inhibited by naphthoquinone (vitamin K) compounds. *Cytokine* **7**:287–290.

Shearer MJ (1995) Vitamin K. *Lancet* **345**:229–234.

Sokoll LJ and Sadowski JA (1996) Comparison of biochemical indexes for assessing vitamin K nutritional status in a healthy adult population. *American Journal of Clinical Nutrition* **63**:566–573.

Suttie JW (1995) The importance of menaquinones in human nutrition. *Annual Review of Nutrition* **15**:399–417.

Vermeer C, Jie KSG and Knapen MHJ (1995) Role of vitamin K in bone metabolism. *Annual Review of Nutrition* **15**:1–22.

Von Kries R, Greer FR and Suttie JW (1993) Assessment of vitamin K status of the newborn infant. *Journal of Pediatric Gastroenterological Nutrition* **16**:231–238.

VITAMIN SUPPLEMENTATION

Role

C Kjolhede, The Mary Imogene Bassett Hospital, Cooperstown, New York, USA

Vitamin supplementation has become a regular and important part of health and nutrition care. Supplementation stands with food fortification and improved dietary intake as means of addressing vitamin deficiencies. Supplementation is very useful as prophylaxis against vitamin deficiency syndromes in premature infants and newborns, women of child-bearing age and the elderly. Multivitamins should not replace a well balanced diet, however, and if a variety of foods are eaten most healthy individuals will realize adequate amounts of vitamins from their diet. Supplementation remains an important component in the treatment of specific vitamin deficiency states and vitamin supplementation has been incorporated into several therapeutic regimens. There is little evidence, however, for some of the public's expectations of vitamin supplementation with respect to athletic performance and quality of life. Whatever the indications for vitamin supplementation, there are some important toxic effects that need to be considered when health-care providers or nutritionists recommend vitamins.

Physiological Importance of Vitamins

Vitamins are organic compounds necessary for a variety of physiological functions. The name 'vitamin' comes from the belief in the early part of the twentieth century that these were 'vital amines', essential substances. Vitamins were initially known by their clinical deficiency states. The scourges of war, famine and underdevelopment such as xerophthalmia, beriberi, scurvy and rickets later were linked to deficiencies of vitamin A, thiamin, and vitamins C and D, respectively. Modern-day society presents a number of situations where instead of war, famine and underdevelopment, we have discovered deficiencies in the haemodialysis patient, in the premature infant on total parenteral nutrition, and in the alcoholic individual. The 'vital amines' are all still required by all and by one means or another, these at-risk individuals need to take care to receive enough.

Vitamin Supplementation Versus Food Fortification Versus Dietary Sources

There are several means by which vitamin deficiencies can be treated or prevented: supplementation, food fortification and improved dietary intake. Supplementation is providing a vitamin through nondietary means. This could be in either pharmacological or dietary doses. The route could be by mouth, intramuscularly or intravenously. Food fortification is simply the use of some form of food as a vehicle for an increased concentration of the vitamin. Improved dietary intake takes advantage of the fact that certain foods contain higher concentrations of a vitamin or that the vitamin is in a more bioavailable form. These means of delivering vitamins each have advantages and disadvantages.

The advantages of supplementation are that the required nutrient can be directed at a specific individual or small group of individuals. This is the case for vitamin A supplementation of children with xerophthalmia or for vitamin K injections of newborn infants. Delivery of the supplement can be very closely controlled and individualized for different situations. Additionally, the dosing regimen of the supplement can be modified over time. For instance, the effect of vitamin D supplementation can be tailored to the individual patient suffering from kidney disease. The disadvantages of vitamin supplementation are that over the long run it is a costly means of treating or preventing deficiencies. Additionally, vitamin supplementation is dependent on both the effectiveness of a prescriber and/or delivery system and, perhaps most importantly, it depends on the compliance of the individual. No regimen will succeed in addressing the deficiency if the supplement is not ingested.

The advantage of food fortified with a vitamin as a means of delivery is that if a desirable food is selected initially, it requires no effort at compliance on the part of the individual; if the fortified food is consumed, then so too is the nutrient. In a society that on a whole consumes processed foods on a regular basis, the delivery of one or multiple vitamins becomes very simple and relatively inexpensive. Both vitamin A and vitamin D, for instance, are added to milk in the USA. The disadvantage of food fortification is that all consumers of the fortified food get the same relative amount of the vitamin irrespective of their individual needs. Thus, women of childbearing age who might benefit from increased folate intake receive the same level in various processed, fortified foods as the rest of the population. Another important consideration is that the individual or group within a population most in need of the vitamin may not consume the food fortified with that vitamin. Children from the poorest families in some developing countries who are at greatest risk for vitamin A deficiency may not receive the processed, vitamin A-fortified foods that have been promoted by their governments. Similarly in the USA, consumption of milk fortified with vitamins A and D can be limited for Black and Hispanic Americans who are lactose intolerant and thus may reject milk and dairy products.

Dietary sources theoretically should provide all the required vitamins. In reality, there are differing requirements for vitamins by gender and over the course of a lifespan and they vary according to the population's capacities to purchase and abilities to prepare foods that could provide a balanced diet. While the advantages of diet as a means for delivering vitamins seem natural and clear to many, the problems inherent in such a mechanism should be equally obvious. Diets are very difficult to modify. Dietary patterns are learned over years and thus can not be expected to change quickly. In any case, the reason for deficiencies in a given diet may be external in the first place and therefore not easily remediable. For instance, sources of vitamin C may be scarce in the extreme northern latitudes and while families may want fresh fruits all year round, the cost may be prohibitive.

In the end, the most effective methods for preventing and treating vitamin deficiencies are hybrids of all three of these means. In a particular society, the diet should be examined for vitamin sufficiency. If the diet is not sufficient, some processed foods could be fortified with vitamins that might otherwise be in short supply in the target population. Individuals in this society at specific risk could be targeted for supplementation with a vitamin and the regimen could be modified over time to meet their individual needs. In many countries of the world, this hybrid approach prevents and treats most vitamin deficiencies.

Vitamin Supplementation for Prophylaxis

There are a number of populations at risk for deficiencies of certain vitamins. Vitamin supplementation is warranted in these populations for prophylaxis against these deficiency states.

Newborn infants are at risk for haemorrhagic disease owing to low levels of vitamin K-dependent coagulation factors II, VII, IX and X. A single intramuscular injection (0.5–1.0 mg) or an oral dose (1.0–2.0 mg) of vitamin K reduces the chances for this neonatal complication. This form of vitamin K supplementation is required by law in many jurisdictions in the USA and it may be particularly important in exclusively breast-fed infants since breast milk is not a good source of vitamin K.

Premature infants have low body stores of tocopherol, vitamin E. This relative deficiency puts these infants at risk for haemolytic states and the attendant problems of anaemia and hyperbilirubinaemia. Premature infants should be supplemented with 17 mg of vitamin E per day for up to 3 months.

Vitamin D supplementation may be required for breast-fed infants since there is very little vitamin D in breast milk. Such supplementation is particularly important for those infants from certain environments and cultures who do not receive adequate exposure to sunlight. A daily supplement of 5–7.5 µg of vitamin D will provide adequate amounts of this nutrient to avoid the complication of rickets.

Elderly people are at risk for several nutrient deficiencies, not only as a result of the ageing process itself, but also because of some features of their lifestyle. Vitamin D supplementation in elderly people may be important for reasons of lack of exposure to sunlight. Elderly people are often housebound and vitamin D_3, the type of vitamin D which is formed in the skin with exposure to sunlight, is less efficiently synthesized in the older person. Vitamin B_{12} deficiency may occur in elderly people owing to malabsorption syndromes and/or atrophic gastritis, resulting in loss of intrinsic factor which is required for optimal vitamin B_{12} absorption. Oral supplementation will not be useful in these cases but 100 µg of vitamin B_{12} delivered via injection on a monthly basis will prevent any signs of deficiency.

Epidemiological studies have implicated antioxidants as important risk factors for cancer and cardiovascular disease. Specifically, foods containing vitamin A, its precursor provitamin β-carotene and vitamin E have been associated with lower rates of these chronic diseases in several studies. The limitation of these epidemiological methods is that they cannot determine cause and effect. Many of the associations may, in fact, reflect dietary intake of another agent that exists in tandem with the above-mentioned nutrients. Subsequent clinical trials of these vitamins delivered pharmacologically, albeit sometimes in dietary doses, have not demonstrated the expected protective effect against these chronic conditions. Additional clinical trials are underway.

There have been a number of reports of the effect of periconceptual folate supplementation of women on birth defects, specifically neural tube defects and cleft lip and palate. Epidemiological evidence suggested and clinical trials confirmed the important role that adequate folate nutritional status plays in the prevention of these birth defects. Mothers who have had an infant with a neural tube defect and who wish to become pregnant again should, with the advice of their physician, take 4 mg of folic acid daily (without other vitamins) at least 4 weeks before and for 3 months after becoming pregnant. All women of child-bearing age should be taking 0.4 mg (but not more than 1 mg) of folic acid per day.

Vitamin Supplementation for Deficiency States

Generalized malnutrition is usually a result of decreased dietary intake which also results in decreased vitamin intake. Isolated vitamin deficiencies rarely exist in such settings; multiple micronutrient deficiencies tend to be the rule. If macronutrient deficiency is suspected based on clinical examination and/or anthropometric indicators, micronutrient deficiencies should be assumed. In such situations, both vitamin-fortified foods and multivitamin supplementation should be considered as part of the treatment for the generalized malnutrition. Vitamin-specific clinical deficiency syndromes should be treated specifically; thus, corneal xerosis (one of the signs of vitamin A deficiency) should be treated with 200 000 IU of vitamin A initially, the next day and then in 1 week (see also below).

Individuals with malabsorption states in general, and fat malabsoption such as in cystic fibrosis more specifically, will also benefit from vitamin supplementation. The decreased absorption of the fat-soluble vitamins A, E and K are particularly important. Daily oral preparations of these vitamins can usually provide the individual with sufficient amounts to avoid significant deficiencies.

Alcoholic people suffer from nutrient deficiencies owing to a decreased appetite and a general lack of intake. Additionally, alcohol has an adverse effect on absorption and storage of various vitamins. Deficiencies in folate, thiamin, riboflavin, pyridoxine, and vitamins A, C, D and K have been noted in this population. The effect of chronic alcohol ingestion on pancreatic function has an effect on the absorption of fat-soluble vitamins. Recommendations for supplementation relate to signs and symptoms of vitamin A and K deficiency states. Assuming that no additional alcohol ingestion occurs, vitamin D levels can be restored by good dietary intake and exposure to sun. Thiamin deficiency is the suspected primary factor in the aetiology of Wernicke–Korsakoff syndrome and beriberi heart disease, both conditions found in alcoholic people, as the entities are reversed with administration of the vitamin. It is unclear whether the polyneuropathy commonly seen in alcohol abusers is due to thiamin deficiency. Alcoholic persons should be supplemented with 50 mg of thiamin daily. Standard multivitamins should be adequate supplementation for both the riboflavin and pyridoxine deficiencies seen in these people and an improved diet will correct the folic acid needs. Vitamin C deficits will be corrected with doses from 175–500 mg daily over several weeks to months.

Vitamin A stores are very low in the newborn but fortunately breast milk is a good source of vitamin A in most instances. Women from vitamin A-deficient populations, and especially those in low socioeconomic strata and of higher parity, may themselves have very marginal vitamin A stores. These lactating women should be supplemented once with 100 000 IU of vitamin A in the first month postpartum or daily with 10 000 IU of vitamin A. The vitamin A given to the mother will find its way into the breast-feeding infant, improving the nutritional status of both individuals in the process.

Vitamin A deficiency more broadly remains a problem in many lesser developed countries. Pre-school children, women of higher parity and families of lower socioeconomic strata are at particular risk. Supplementation regimens exist for biannual megadosing of vitamin A. Large, infrequent doses of vitamin A can be effective since vitamin A is a fat-soluble vitamin and can be stored in the liver. Children in areas of known or suspected vitamin A deficiency should receive 200 000 IU (100 000 IU for infants) of vitamin A by mouth every 6 months. Women in such environments can be dosed daily with 10 000 IU. Children with acute malnutrition (kwashiokor–marasmus), as one might find in a refugee camp, should be treated as if they had clinical vitamin A deficiency. They should be given 200 000 IU of vitamin A (100 000 IU for infants) initially, the next day and in 1 week.

Vitamin Supplementation as a Part of a Therapeutic Regimen

Kidney disease has an important effect on some vitamins' status. Renal disease is known to result in increased levels of vitamin A and retinol binding protein since the kidney is an important site for the metabolism of vitamin A and retinal binding protein. Supplementation with vitamin A-containing products should be approached with caution in individuals with known or suspected kidney disease. Haemodialysis, on the other hand, results in decreased levels of vitamins B_6 (pyridoxine), C and folate. These water-soluble vitamins tend to be washed out during haemodialysis and supplementation is required for individuals, who will be on long-term haemodialysis. Daily doses of 60 mg of vitamin C, 1 mg of folic acid and 10 mg of pyridoxine hydrochloride should be given to those on maintenance haemodialysis. Patients with kidney disease but not yet being dialysed should receive 5 mg of pyridoxine hydrochloride.

Niacin has been used in familial hyperlipidaemia states since the 1950s. It is still used in conjunction with other pharmacological agents to lower lipid level and it has been shown to decrease the recurrence of heart attacks. The usual daily dose is 1000–4000 mg of nicotinic acid. There are significant side effects such as flushing of the skin but these usually disappear by decreasing the dose.

There have been many claims about the efficacy of certain vitamins as curative treatment for some forms of cancer. There is no report of a rigorously designed study to substantiate these claims.

Vitamin Supplementation as a Tonic

Vitamin supplementation has occasionally been promoted for a variety of reasons including to treat the common cold, to improve athletic performance, to improve children's appetite, and generally to improve quality of life in elderly people. None of these reasons for promoting a vitamin supplement has been universally accepted and several have been scientifically refuted. For those individuals who are able to eat a variety of foods, their diet usually provides vitamins in sufficient amounts to meet normal needs; taking a low-level vitamin supplement is probably not harmful but neither has it been shown to have any substantial benefit.

Vitamin–Nutrient Interactions

Vitamin C has an important interaction with dietary iron. Nonhaem dietary sources of iron are important in many populations, particularly among vegetarians and those who cannot afford to include meat in their diet. Vitamin C (ascorbic acid) in the diet enhances the absorption of nonhaem iron. The nonhaem sources of iron in the diet supply more than 80% of the iron in the typical US diet and thus iron status may be substantially influenced by concurrent ingestion of vitamin C in either a dietary or pharmacological form.

The vitamin B_{12} content in food and in multivitamin preparations is reported to be substantially decreased by high concentrations of vitamin C. This may be of particular importance to those individuals who take megadoses of vitamin C. Surveillance for B_{12} deficiency specifically should be considered in these individuals.

The potential interaction between vitamin B_{12} and folate relates to the masking of many of the signs of B_{12} deficiency by treatment with folate. Both B_{12} and folate deficiency can present as a macrocytic anaemia. Treatment of such an anaemia with folate without due concern for the possibility of a concurrent deficiency of B_{12} may result in the amelioration of the signs of anaemia but the significant and concerning neurological effects may persist.

Vitamin Toxicity

Vitamin A supplementation to an excess has been linked to two phenomena. Vitamin A taken in high doses during the first trimester of pregnancy has been associated with increased rates of birth defects in the products of those pregnancies. This well known teratogenic effect has prompted the caution for doses not to exceed 10 000 IU per day in women who are or could be pregnant. Additionally, there are reports of bulging fontanelle, decreased appetite and vomiting among infants who were supplemented with large doses (50 000 IU) of vitamin A. This constellation of signs and symptoms is often called pseudotumor cerebri and has also been reported among older individuals who have received very large doses of vitamin A.

Toxic effects from excessive doses of vitamin D have been reported. These effects include hypercalcaemia and hypercalciuria with renal and cardiac complications in the worst cases. As little as five times the recommended daily allowance can result in toxic levels. Thus, individuals who are exposed to ample sunlight and who may be receiving vitamin D-fortified food such as milk are not only likely to be nutritionally sufficient with respect to vitamin D but should avoid taking vitamin D-containing supplements.

See also: **Alcoholism**: Effects on Nutritional Status. **Antioxidants**: Diet and Antioxidant Defence; Observational Epidemiology; Intervention Studies. **Cancer**: Epidemiology and Associations Between Diet and Cancer; Diet in Cancer Treatment. **Exercise**: Physiology of Skeletal Muscle; Diet and Exercise; Beneficial Effects. **Health Foods**: Dietary Supplements - Micronutrients. **HIV Disease**: Nutritional Management. **Infants**: Nutritional Requirements. **Lactation**: Physiology; Dietary Requirements. **Malnutrition**: Definition, Classification and Epidemiology; Primary Malnutrition; Secondary Malnutrition. **Older People**: Nutritional Requirements; Nutritional Management of Geriatric Patients. **Pregnancy**: Nutrient Requirements; Safe Diet for Pregnancy.

Further Reading

Fogelholm M (1995) Indicator of vitamin and mineral status in athletes' blood: a review. *International Journal of Sport Nutrition* 5:267–284.

Forbes GB and Woodruff CW (1985) *Pediatric Nutrition Handbook*, 2nd edn. Elk Grove Village, IL: American Academy of Paediatrics.

Hunt JR (1996) Position of the American Dietetic Association: vitamin and mineral supplementation. *Journal of the American Dietetic Association* **96**:73–77.

Mills JL and Simpson JL (1993) Prospects for prevention of neural tube defects by vitamin supplementation. *Current Opinion in Neurology and Neurosurgery* **6**:554–558.

Mitch WE and Klahr S (1988) *Nutrition and the Kidney*. Boston: Little, Brown & Co.

Shils ME, Olson JA and Shike M (1994) *Modern Nutrition in Health and Disease*, 8th edn. Philadelphia: Lea & Febiger.

Subcommittee on the Tenth Edition of the RDAs, Food and Nutrition Board, Commission on Life Sciences, National Research Council. *Recommended Dietary Allowances*, 10th edn. Washington, DC: National Academy Press.

Trowbridge FL, Harris SS, Cook J, Dunn JT, Florentino RF, Kodyar BA, Mannar MGV, Reddy V, Tontisirin K, Underwood BA and Yip R (1993) Coordinated strategies for controlling micronutrient malnutrition: a technical workshop. *Journal of Nutrition* **123**:775–787.

Willett W (1990) *Nutritional Epidemiology*. New York: Oxford University Press.

Ziegler EE and Filer LJ (1996) *Present Knowledge in Nutrition*, 7th edn. Washington, DC: ILSI Press.

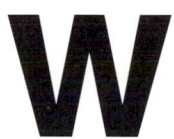

Water *see* **Thirst**: Physiology.

WEIGHT MANAGEMENT

Contents
Approaches
Weight Maintenance
Weight Cycling

Approaches

N Finer, Luton and Dunstable Hospital NHS Trust, Luton, UK

Weight loss and weight loss maintenance require a decrease in energy intake (diet), an increase in energy expenditure (exercise and physical activity), or both. Dietary management should encourage healthy eating, that is an appropriately balanced intake of macro- and micronutrients. For most obese individuals this will entail not just a decrease in total energy intake, but specifically a decrease in fat intake, together with an increase in complex carbohydrates, fruit and vegetables. A myriad diets have been popularized as a means to reducing energy intake, but few are recommended as meeting the overall nutritional needs of an obese individual, and many are so restrictive that they clearly could not be followed for more than a few weeks. Increasing exercise and physical activity has benefits beyond those that result from the relatively modest amounts of extra energy expended. These include a beneficial protection from excessive loss of lean body tissue during dieting, improved fitness and psychological health, and a greater likelihood of long-term weight maintenance. Diet and exercise are core components of behavioural treatments; such treatments, based on learning theories, also aim to help individuals become aware of the behaviours that have led to their weight gain, and to develop strategies to alter them. Weight loss can be achieved successfully with all strategies; behavioural therapies that include a strong focus on increasing exercise and activity seem to offer the best chances of long-term success.

The Concept of Desirable Weight

Body weight reflects the additive mass of the various tissues that make up the organism, and is a function of energy and nutrient balance over a prolonged period. Positive energy balance will result in weight gain (mainly from deposition of lipid in adipose tissue), while prolonged undernutrition will lead to weight loss. For most of human history, the dominant disorder of body weight has been thinness. Thinness, whether from malnutrition or disease, was associated with illness and was often a prelude to death; in societies where food supplies are scarce or seasonal, a high body weight may be seen as a desirable sign of health, and probably wealth. In contrast, in developed societies where levels of activity are low and food is plentiful, the growing prevalence of overweight and obesity has been clearly linked to illness and premature mortality. The concept of a desirable weight at which health is optimal and the risk of disease minimal has not been easy to define, largely because of the effects of many other factors such as age, sex, social status and smoking.

Dietary Management

Dietary management of obesity aims to reduce fat stores by changing eating habits to reduce energy intake below that required for weight maintenance. The term 'reducing diet' has been coined to describe such diets used to treat the obese. Since many obese individuals may eat a nutritionally inadequate (apart from energy) diet, it is important that advice on energy restriction is accompanied by the prescription of a 'healthy' diet that contains adequate protein, vitamins, calcium, trace elements and a desirable ratio of complex carbohydrate to fat. Weight loss *per se* is of no medical benefit unless it is maintained, and this will require the obese individual to adhere to a permanent change in eating habits. Many think of a 'diet' as a temporary change in eating habits (often extreme or quirky), a view encouraged by many of the diet books that hold out the promise of easy and instant success. It is essential that the concept of a long-term change in dietary habits be accepted at the start of treatment.

The energy value of weight gained or lost is approximately 31 MJ kg^{-1} (7500 kcal kg^{-1}) since it is composed approximately of 3 parts fat to 1 part lean. Thus a daily energy deficit of 2.1 MJ (500 kcal) will produce a weight loss of about 2 kg per month. For the average man or woman this represents a 20–30% reduction in energy intake, although for the obese the percentage reduction will be smaller. Thus the severely obese, for example with a body mass index (BMI) of 35 or more, will need to follow an energy-restricted diet for months rather than weeks to reverse their obesity. As weight is lost, energy requirements fall, in part because of the reduced energetic mass of the person, and also because of adaptive changes in energy expenditure. For this reason, the rate of weight loss will eventually slow and reach a plateau for any fixed level of dietary energy restriction (**Fig. 1**).

A myriad diets have been popularized and pro-moted directly to the public, reflecting every possible permutation of increasing or decreasing the major macronutrients. Fashion and commercialism have dictated many of them. **Table 1** shows the variety of diets that have been suggested, and used, for treating obesity. Many of these diets fail to focus on long-term dietary change, and the quirkiness of many makes it unlikely that they would be followed for long.

Current ideas on a reasonable reducing diet are that it should contain at least 100 g carbohydrate to prevent glycogen depletion and ketosis. High-carbohydrate diets are composed of complex carbohydrates and are thus of low energy density, which may aid management of hunger. Since high-carbohydrate diets are low in fat, they have the theoretical advantage of directly reducing the risk of cardiovascular disease. The energetic efficiency with which carbohydrate is converted and stored as fat is lower than that of dietary fat, providing a further advantage. Protein intake must be adequate to maintain lean body mass. Although there is an inevitable fall with weight loss, 0.8 g per kg per day + 1.75 g per 100 calorie deficit of protein (about 44 g daily for women and 56 g daily for men) should be consumed, and fat restricted to less than 30% of total energy. The diet should contain recommended daily intakes of vitamins, minerals and electrolytes, if necessary by supplementation; 20–30 g daily of fibre should also be consumed.

Many diets prescribe an energy intake that is based on a generalized rather than an individualized assessment of energy needs. The common prescription of 4.2–5.0 MJ (1000–1200 kcal) daily may be problematic and inappropriate. Weight loss in men will be faster and greater compared to women of equal BMI, because of the relatively greater metabolic rate per kilogram of body weight of men. The very obese, whose daily energy requirements can be as high as 12.6 MJ (3000 kcal), may lose weight at an excessive

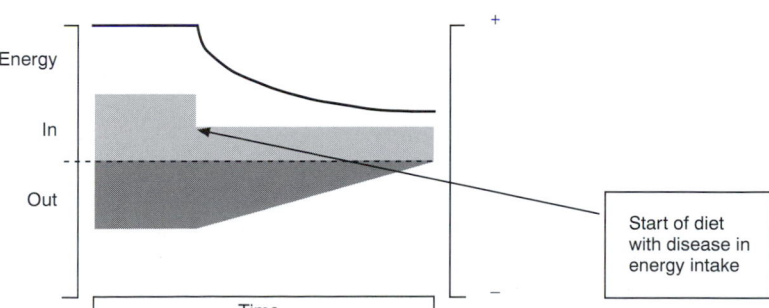

Figure 1 Fall in body weight (solid line) resulting from a fixed decrease in energy intake. Note that the rate of weight loss slows as the gap between energy expenditure (darker shading) and energy intake (lighter shading) narrows.

Table 1   Types of diet used for treating obesity

Generic name for diet	Typical dietetic modification	Popular example of diet
Starvation diet	Less than 1.2 MJ (300 kcal) per day	Grapefruit and Black Coffee
Very low-energy (protein-sparing) diets[a]	About 2 MJ (500 kcal) per day with >50 g high-quality protein; usually liquid	Cambridge Diet Modifast
Low-energy diet[a]	5–7.5 MJ (1200–1800 kcal) per day often from menus, recipes	Weight Watchers TOPS
Fixed energy deficit diet[a]	Nutritionally balanced, individually tailored to produce fixed energy deficit (e.g. 2 MJ or 500 kcal per day) based on measured or predicted energy needs	Prescribed by dietitian
High-protein diet	Over 40% protein, thus low in carbohydrate and fat	Scarsdale Medical Diet
Low-protein diet		Beverly Hills Diet
High-fat diet	Restricted carbohydrate and protein	Drinking Man's Diet
Low-fat diet[a]	Restrict fat to <20% energy	Prescribed by dietitian Pritikin Diet
High-carbohydrate diet	Effectively low fat, may be high in fibre	F-Plan Diet
Low-carbohydrate diet	Limits carbohydrate to maximum <50 g daily	Yudkin Diet
Macronutrient choice[a]	Choice from lists of macronutrients to encourage intake of foods high in complex carbohydrates	No Counting Diet
Meal replacement	Liquid formula meals of about 1.7 MJ (400 kcal) to replace 1–2 meals daily	SlimFast
Fad diets	Varied; e.g. food combining diets that require macronutrients to be eaten separately and separated by time	Hay Diet

[a]Diets considered medically reasonable under defined circumstances.

rate and develop symptoms of ketosis, postural hypotension or excessive hunger. Many obese patients fail to register or admit to the amount of food they consume, and claim that such a diet is more than their habitual intake.

One principle of energy prescription that has proved easy to administer and successful in outcome is to calculate energy requirements from standard formulae (**Table 2**), and prescribe a diet that provides a fixed energy deficit of 2.1 MJ (500 kcal). Compliance and weight loss were better with this approach than with a fixed 5 MJ (1200 kcal) diet.

A diametrically opposite approach is the use of very low-energy liquid diets. These were originally developed in the 1960s to provide a nutritionally complete intake in terms of protein, vitamins and micronutrients, but provide as little as 1.4 MJ (350 kcal) daily. The inclusion of sufficient high-quality protein was designed to prevent the excessive loss of lean body mass seen with starvation or other ketotic diets, hence the alternative term 'protein-sparing modified fast'. Appropriately selected, well-motivated patients are highly compliant with such diets, and their weight loss can be very rapid. Para-

Table 2   Formulae for estimating resting metabolic rate (RMR) for men and women. The energy expenditure over 24 h can be estimated by multiplying by a factor related to activity levels (1.3, sedentary; 1.5, moderate activity; 1.8, physically very active)

Age (years)	RMR
Men	
18–30	0.063 × weight in kg + 2.896 MJ daily
31–60	0.048 × weight in kg + 3.653 MJ daily
>60	0.049 × weight in kg + 2.459 MJ daily
Women	
18–30	0.062 × weight in kg + 2.036 MJ daily
31–60	0.034 × weight in kg + 3.538 MJ daily
>60	0.038 × weight in kg + 2.755 MJ daily

doxically, perhaps, patients seem to find it easier to mount levels of near-total restraint than more moderate restriction. It appears that withdrawing all solid or 'proper' food helps the patient to define himself or herself as 'not eating', in the same way that some quitting smokers finding easier to abstain completely from cigarettes rather than to cut down.

In the 1970s a commercial very low-energy diet formulation (the Last Chance Diet) was marketed, and was associated with a number of deaths from cardiac arrhythmia. This diet was deficient in essential amino acids and in minerals such as magnesium and potassium. It was withdrawn. In the 1980s newer, better formulated diets were commercially marketed. Concerns about their inappropriate use by already slim women, often with an eating disorder, forced governmental health agencies to issue guidelines on their use. In the USA, a task force recommended that such diets contain at least 3.3 MJ (800 kcal), be supervised by experienced physicians, and be used only by those with a BMI more than 30, for less than 16 weeks. In the UK a report from the Committee on Medical Aspects of Food Policy suggested such diets should provide a minimum of 1.7 MJ (400 kcal) and 40 g protein daily for women, and 2.1 MJ (500 kcal) and 50 g protein daily for men and tall women. They were recommended for use only by those with a BMI more than 25 and under medical supervision, for no longer than 4 weeks. The drawback of such diets is that unless they are combined with, or followed by, some other treatment (pharmacological or behavioural), weight regain, often soon and rapid, is almost universal.

More recently, low-energy liquid diets of around 3 MJ (750 kcal) daily have been popularized, often as part of an overall behaviour modification programme (see later), or in the form of sachets intended to be used as meal replacements. Both approaches have been shown to have potential for success in short-term studies lasting up to 1 year.

Exercise and Physical Activity

The term 'physical activity' refers to bodily movement produced by skeletal muscle that results in energy expenditure; it thus includes activities of daily living, as well as leisure activity from sport and exercise. The term 'exercise' refers to planned or structured bodily movements, usually undertaken in leisure time in order to improve fitness (e.g. aerobics), while 'sport' is physical activity usually in structured competitive situations (e.g. football). Physical activity at recommended levels (moderate intensity for 30 min for 5 days each week) is associated with many health benefits; these include lower all-cause mortality rates, fewer cardiovascular events such as myocardial infarction and stroke, and a lower incidence of metabolic disorders including non-insulin-dependent diabetes mellitus and osteoporosis. Levels of activity have been falling in Westernized societies largely because of a decrease in physical activity at work (from increasing mechanization) and increasingly sedentary leisure-time pursuits (such as television viewing). The Allied Dunbar National Fitness Survey of the UK showed that 70% of the population are insufficiently active, and a separate UK government survey showed that 1 in 3 adults could be classified as sedentary, i.e. taking less than half an hour of continuous moderate-intensity physical activity each week (**Fig. 2**). Both cross-sectional data and prospective studies confirm an inverse relationship between physical activity and weight gain. The finding that in many countries such as the UK, average energy intake has fallen over the time that obesity has been increasing, emphasizes the importance of inactivity as a cause of obesity. These secular changes of inactivity are most marked in children who now spend much of their leisure time watching television or in other sedentary pursuits. Health authorities in many countries now advocate an increase in physical activity as a means of preventing obesity and improving health and fitness. While there is agreement that such measures may be useful in

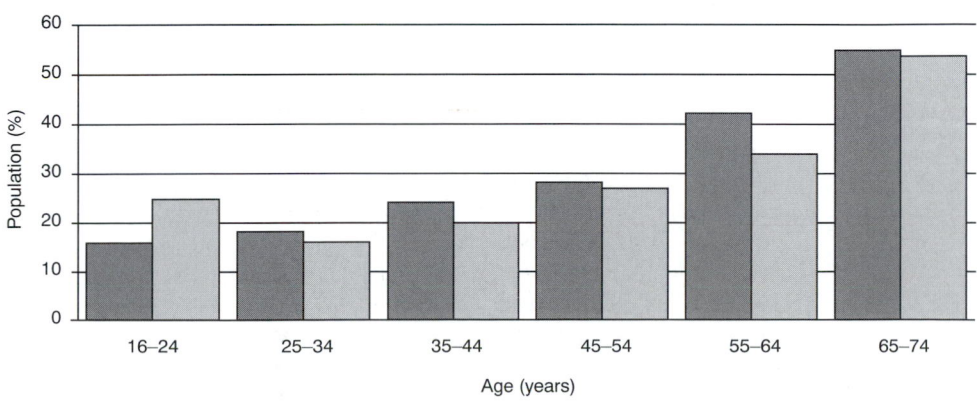

Figure 2 Percentage of adults in England by age and sex (1990–1991) with a sedentary life style; dark bars, men; light bars, women. Data from Fentem and Walker (1995).

preventing obesity, the role of exercise in treating obesity is less clear. Potential mechanisms linking exercise and activity with weight loss and weight loss maintenance are shown in **Fig. 3**. Like dietary change, increasing time spent on exercise and activity can be seen as part of a generalized behavioural change, which can be self-reinforcing.

Exercise and activity raise energy expenditure over and above the resting metabolic rate. Under some circumstances, such as prolonged vigorous exercise in trained individuals, rates of energy expenditure remain elevated for some time after the cessation of exercise. Logically, therefore, exercise should be a useful way to treat obesity. However, the amounts of exercise-induced energy expenditure are small in comparison with potential changes in energy intake.

The energy cost of activity and exercise can be expressed as a multiple of resting metabolic rate, termed a MET; the term 'physical activity level' (PAL) represents the total daily energy expenditure divided by the resting energy expenditure; it typically averages 1.5. The energy costs of walking are about 2.0 MET – for a 70 kg individual this is about 0.5 MJ h^{-1} (120 kcal h^{-1}) – while gentle running costs about 8 MET or 2 MJ h^{-1} (480 kcal h^{-1}). A moderately fit individual would only be able to maintain a level of exercise of 7 MET for about 30 min, representing an additional energy expenditure of about 1.5 MJ (360 kcal) resulting, if energy intake were maintained, in a weight loss of about 0.3 kg per week.

Energy expenditure remains above baseline for some time after exercise has stopped; this is termed 'post-exercise energy expenditure'. The effect is small and only produced by very high levels of activity, capable of achievement only by elite athletes. The mechanism for this effect is unknown. Moderate intensity exercise programmes, of the sort prescribed to the obese, are unlikely to raise energy expenditure by more than about 0.2 MJ (50 kcal) per exercise session.

Regular exercise does, however, elevate long-term energy expenditure by its effect on altering body composition. Resting metabolic rate is proportional to the fat-free mass. Exercise increases muscle development and bone mass, so directly raising metabolic rate. The purpose of weight loss is to reduce fat mass, with as little loss of fat-free mass (FFM) as possible. The loss of fat to meet the extra energy requirements of regular exercise will decrease the ratio of fat to FFM and thus indirectly favour an increase in resting metabolic rate for any given body weight. These effects are modest, and mainly only seen from the sort of high intensity achieved by athletes. Even endurance-level training over periods of up to 12 weeks increases nonexercising daily energy expenditure by less than 0.8 MJ (190 kcal).

The effects of exercise are thus quantitatively small. The relative small potential for exercise to reduce body weight is borne out by the results of trials of exercise in obesity treatment, which suggest that exercise programmes achieve weight losses of less than 0.1 kg per week, and that total weight loss averages about 3 kg. In one meta-analysis of five controlled trials of exercise without dietary restriction, mean weight loss in 95 men was 2.6 kg over 30

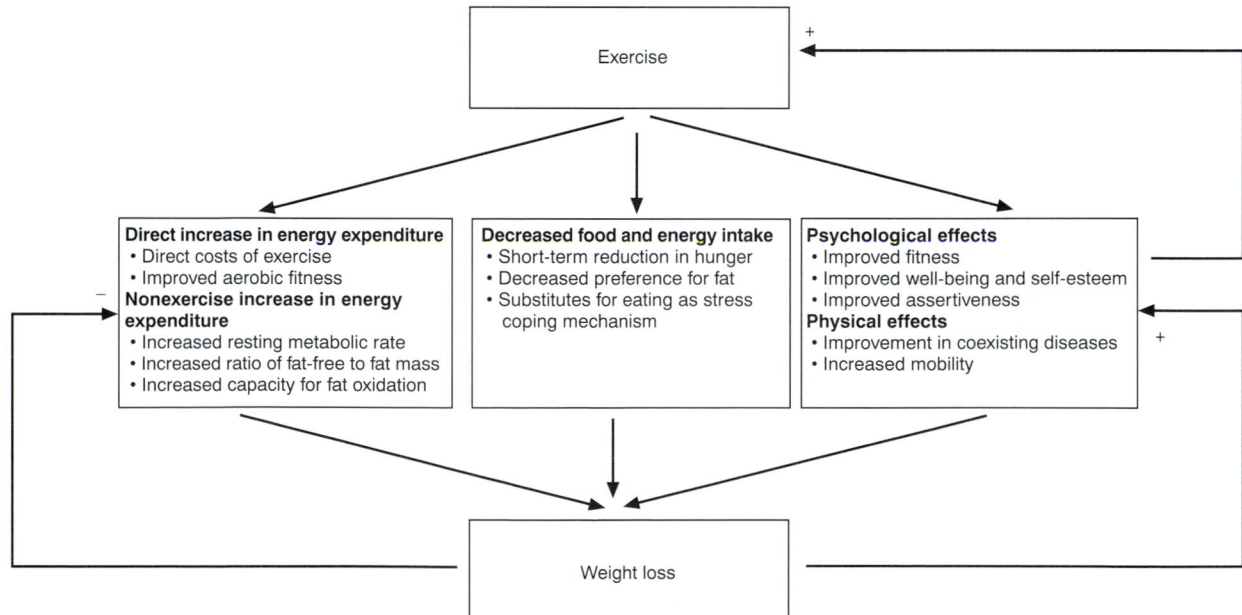

Figure 3 Mechanisms linking exercise with weight loss and weight loss maintenance.

weeks, compared with a gain of 0.4 kg in the control group.

Programmes that combine dietary and exercise interventions can be more successful, but it is often difficult to separate the effects of one from the other. In order to explore the effect of exercise on the composition of weight loss during dieting, Garrow analysed data from 21 randomized, controlled studies. All trials that combined exercise and diet and included information about weight and FFM loss were included (**Fig. 4**). A small reduction in the percentage of FFM lost is observed if exercise is included with the dietetic intervention. Thus, for example, in a woman losing 15 kg, exercise would reduce her FFM loss from 3.6 kg (24%) to 3.0 kg (20%). Similar but quantitatively greater benefits are seen in men: for a 15 kg weight loss, exercise reduced FFM loss from 3.6 kg (24%) to 2.5 kg (17%).

Activity and exercise are strong predictors for successful weight loss maintenance. A number of studies have shown that obese women who have lost weight and continue to undertake regular exercise are 3–4 times more likely to maintain their weight loss over a follow-up period of 2–3 years. The amount of exercise also correlates with the degree of success. In one study of about a hundred obese men and women who had lost about 27 kg, those with high levels of exercise were maintaining an average of 18 kg loss at 3 years, compared with 9 kg in the moderate exercise group and no weight loss in the nonexercisers. The importance of exercise and weight loss maintenance is demonstrated by a 2-year study of obese subjects treated by either diet, exercise or a combination of the two. Weight loss in the diet group at 1 year was 6.8 kg, in the exercise group 2.9 kg, and 8.9 kg in the combination treatment group. However after 2 years the groups that had included exercise were

maintaining losses of 2.2–2.7 while those on diet alone had only managed to maintain a 0.9 kg loss. Similar findings have been seen in dieters from commercial slimming groups.

Behaviour Modification

Behavioural modification is seen as the cornerstone of any treatment programme that seeks to empower and enable obese individuals to make voluntary changes in life style. Any therapy relies to a greater or lesser extent on such a principle. For example, treating hypertension should be an apparently straightforward clinical management issue, but patient noncompliance with medication is common. The skilled clinician will often include the principles of behaviour therapy in consultations to help the patient understand and put into practice the new 'life style' of taking their drugs regularly. The approach in obesity is firmly based on theories of learning, and relies on the concept that behaviours associated with weight gain and weight maintenance are to a significant extent learned and subject to modification. Such a behavioural theory is not undermined by the knowledge that genetic and environmental factors are also important in determining the predisposition to obesity. A prerequisite for successful behaviour change is that the individual must be 'ready' and motivated to change. It is common practice to assess this aspect of 'readiness' prior to enrolling patients in behavioural programmes, and a number of standardized and validated questionnaires are available. Because behavioural programmes are intensive of therapist time, patients are often treated in groups, often with manuals which allow for individual study. These groups are usually 'closed'; that is, a small group of patients start the programme simultaneously

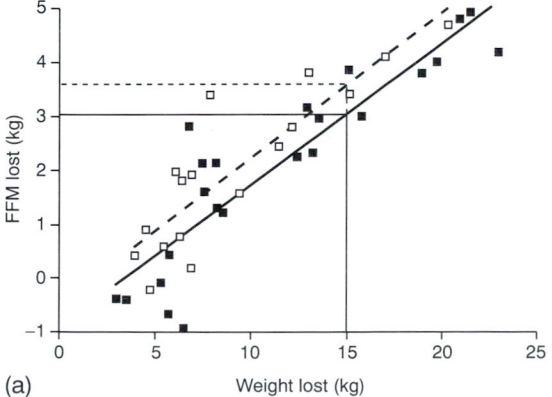
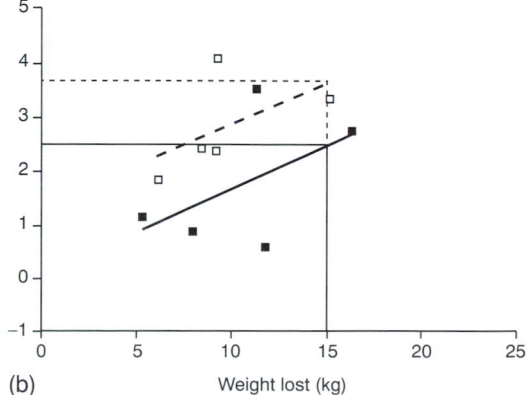

(a)   Weight lost (kg)

(b)   Weight lost (kg)

Figure 4 Relationship of total weight loss to fat-free mass loss in women (a) and men (b) undertaking a diet with exercise (solid squares, solid line) or without exercise (open squares, broken line). Data from 21 randomized controlled studies, collated by Garrow JS (1995).

Table 3   The components of a typical behaviour modification programme

Domain	Intervention strategy	Example
Self-monitoring	Food intake diaries Exercise and activity Weight change	Food diaries Activity logs Regular weighing and recording on weight charts

Nutrition	Nutrition knowledge
	
	Healthy eating
		Energy, macronutrients, understanding food
		  labelling
		Low fat, high complex carbohydrate, adequate
		  fruit and vegetable intake

Exercise and activity	Increasing daily energy-using activities Decreasing sedentariness Formal exercise	Using stairs not escalators Decrease television viewing Group workouts at sports centres
Goal setting	Realistic rates of weight loss Realistic target weight Weight maintenance	Aim for 0.5–1.0 kg weekly 10% weight loss as initial goal
Problem solving	Identifying conflicts with aims Interpersonal conflicts Stimulus control and negative feelings	Holidays, parties, restaurant meals The unhelpful relative or friend Hunger on returning home from work

Cognitive change	Modifying thoughts about and responses to
	  food cues
	Self-esteem and assertiveness training
	Preventing relapse
		Good and bad foods; food as a reward; coping
		  with 'highly desirable' foods
		Recognizing and exerting choice
		Acceptance of occasional small weight gains

and go through it together. This contrasts with many commercial diet groups, in which patients are free to join or leave at any time. More recently computer-aided interventions have been developed, but as yet results are not promising.

The components of a typical behaviour modification programme are shown in **Table 3**. For each area, patients need to learn the underlying concepts, recognize the importance to their own situation, and practise strategies to change their behaviour. The results of a large number of programmes have been published, either as audit outcome or as comparative trials. Programmes vary in duration from 12 weeks to 52 weeks (there has been a trend since the 1970s to lengthen treatment time). Drop-out rates are clearly biased by selection procedures, but are typically 10–20%. Weight loss during treatment is typically 10–15% of initial weight, at a rate of about 0.5 kg per week. In order to strengthen the impact of the intervention on weight loss, many programmes have included a period of time on very low-energy or liquid-based diets. This approach of a complete withdrawal for a time from established (abnormal) eating habits can be usefully integrated into a model of behaviour change, and is well and positively tolerated by obese patients. Although data suggest that the greater weight loss induced by very low-energy diets has little effect on the long-term results in terms of weight loss maintenance, these diets do represent a practical and pragmatic initial approach to treating

patients in a group, especially when many individuals within such a group may resist the idea that they are able to lose weight on conventional reduced-energy diets.

Research is now directed towards finding ways of improving the results of such programmes in terms of long-term weight loss maintenance. An increased focus on weight-maintaining behaviour rather than weight loss, a stronger emphasis on increasing activity and exercise, and better relapse strategies are being evaluated. Targeting the needs of specific subgroups, for example those with binge eating disorders or dysfunctional family circumstances, is another way in which behavioural therapy may be improved.

See also: **Eating Disorders**: Bulimia Nervosa. **Energy**: Measurement of Energy Intake and Expenditure. **Exercise**: Physiology of Skeletal Muscle; Diet and Exercise. **Obesity**: Definition, Aetiology and Assessment; Early Obesity and Prognosis; Fat Distribution; Treatment; Prevention; Complications of Obesity. **Starvation and Fasting**: Biochemical Aspects.

Further Reading

Activity and Health Research, Allied Dunbar National Fitness Survey (1992) *A Report on Activity Patterns and Fitness Levels: Main Findings.* London: Sports Council and Health Education Authority.

Brownell K (1997) *The Learn programme for weight control*, 7th edn. American Health Publishing.

Fentem P and Walker A (1995) Setting targets for England: challenging, measurable and achievable. In: Killoran A (ed.) *Moving On: International Perspectives on Promoting Physical Activity*. London: Health Education Authority.

Finer N ed. (1997) Obesity: a series of expert reviews. *British Medical Bulletin* 53(2):229–450.

Frost G, Masters K, King C *et al.* (1991) A new method of energy prescription to improve weight loss. *Journal of Human Nutrition and Dietetics* 4:369–373.

Thomas PR, ed. (1995) *Weighing the Options. Criteria for Evaluating Weight-management Programs*. Washington: National Academy Press.

Tremblay A, Bouchard C and Despres JP eds. (1995) Proceedings of a satellite symposium of the 7th ICO on Exercise and Obesity: Morphological, metabolic and clinical implications. *International Journal of Obesity* (supplement 4): S1–S129.

Scottish Intercollegiate Guideline Network (1996) *Obesity in Scotland*. Integrating prevention with weight management. A national clinical guideline recommended for use in Scotland. Edinburgh: SIGN

Wing RR (1997) Behavioural approaches to the treatment of obesity. In: Bray GA, Bouchard C and James WPT (eds) *Handbook of Obesity*. New York: Marcel Dekker. pp 855–873.

Weight Maintenance

S Bartlett, Johns Hopkins Bayview Medical Center, Baltimore MA, USA

Lawrence Cheskin, Johns Hopkins University School of Medicine, Baltimore, MA, USA

In 1958, Albert J. Stunkard wrote, 'Most obese persons will not stay in treatment. Of those who stay in treatment, most will not lose weight, and of those who lose weight, most will regain it'. Sadly, some 40 years later, the long-term outcome of dieting has changed only marginally. Relatively few overweight people seem able to lose weight and maintain their losses. In clinical populations, persons treated by a 5000 kJ per day (1200 kcal per day) diet and a comprehensive programme of behaviour therapy regain an average of one-third of lost weight in the year following treatment, with increasing weight gain in ensuing years. After 5 years, most dieters are heavier than they were when they initially began the diet.

Though few individuals will permanently reduce their weight to an ideal body size through a single episode of dieting, the fact remains that the health and daily activities of many individuals are remarkably compromised by their weight. An important search continues for the combination of approaches that maximize the likelihood that some degree of weight loss can be achieved and maintained. This article will summarize what is known about weight regain, relapse, and strategies that maximize the likelihood of successful long-term weight maintenance.

Weight Regain

The process of regaining lost weight is indeed a complex one incorporating biological, environmental, and psychosocial factors. Biological explanations for regain, for example the 'set-point' theory, suggest that all individuals have a predetermined weight which is largely influenced by genetic factors such as metabolism or lipoprotein lipase activity levels. For some, the 'set point' may be at a level significantly greater than cultural and medical norms. Any effort to readjust body weight triggers internal mechanisms (e.g. hunger, satiety and metabolic rate) which act in concert to return body weight to predieting levels. An alternative environmental and behavioural view is that the current abundance and variety of high-fat foods, coupled with decreasing levels of physical activity, lead to the common phenomenon of 'creeping obesity'. Psychosocial factors associated with weight regain include interpersonal conflict, poor coping skills, negative affect such as anxiety and depression, and major life stressors.

Consequences of Weight Regain

Cycles of weight loss and regain (e.g. weight cycling) are common among obese individuals. Brownell has raised concerns that such cycles may adversely affect body composition and resting metabolic rate, as well as increase the risks of morbidity and mortality. Studies of each of these issues have yielded contradictory findings. However, the National Task Force on the Prevention and Treatment of Obesity of National Institutes of Health recently reviewed studies from 1966 through 1994 and concluded that the majority of studies do not support adverse effects of weight cycling on metabolism.

There has been surprisingly little research on the psychological consequences of weight cycling. Clinical experience suggests that the adverse psychological effects may indeed be significant. Obese individuals frequently report that they feel guilty, ashamed and inadequate as a result of regaining weight, and that they are criticized for their failure by family members, coworkers, and even health-care providers. In one study, participants reported that weight regain negatively affected their self-esteem, self-confidence, general level of happiness, and satisfaction with their appearance. However, these effects may be limited to the period of time during and immediately after weight regain. Several recent studies have examined the psychological functioning of obese individuals and found only limited support for the widely held assumption that cycles of weight loss and regain are associated with long-term negative psychosocial consequences. For instance, individuals with a marked history of weight cycling do not appear to be at greater risk for depression or binge eating.

Emergence of Weight Maintenance Strategies

Without specific maintenance treatment, regain of lost weight seems likely. Wadden and colleagues treated 76 very overweight participants (mean body mass index (BMI) = 39) for one year by very low calorie-diet (VLCD), behaviour therapy (BT), or a combination of the two (VLCD + BT). No maintenance therapy was offered. At the first year following treatment, 50% of those participants in the VLCD + BT group kept off 10 kg as compared with 23% in the BT group and 14% in the VLCD group. By the 3-year follow-up, participants in both the VLCD + BT and BT groups had regained 75% of the weight lost. After the 5 years, they found that most participants in all three conditions returned to their baseline weights with no significant differences among the groups.

Participants who had regained all the lost weight were surveyed about their weight loss practices. They reported exercising, using stimulus control techniques such as hiding high-calorie foods, keeping food logs, and eating more slowly an average of only zero to two times per month. The investigators concluded that lack of weight maintenance was related, in part, to the cessation of behavioural changes that were adopted early in treatment.

Results such as these prompted obesity researchers to rethink traditional treatment methods in the 1980s. Efforts were made to understand the relapse process better. Researchers began systematically to investigate strategies to promote *weight maintenance* after weight loss.

Relapse – Return to Old Patterns

Relapse may best be viewed as a series or chain of events over time in which new behaviours are slowly unlearned and old habits return. In some cases, the relapse is brought about by exposure to a high-risk situation. A common example may be the individual who adopts a healthier lifestyle while in treatment, then returns to old patterns abruptly while on vacation away from home. In other cases, relapse is triggered over time by the gradual exposure to former cues to eat. An example of this is individuals who frequently eat in restaurants as part of their job. In the short run, they make active decisions to limit food portions, energy and fat content. Over time, however, there is a return to previous food choices. Though each instance may be rationalized ('it's my birthday so I'll have cake just this once'), the net effect is an eventual return to behaviours that previously resulted in weight gain.

Factors associated with relapse

Researchers who have extensively studied the relapse process among individuals with addictive behaviours suggest that relapse occurs when the individual is confronted with a high-risk situation, problem or emotional state, and has insufficient coping skills to deal with the situation. The following high-risk situations for relapse have been identified.

1. *Negative emotional states.* The initial lapse is precipitated by negative or unpleasant moods such as anxiety, depression, anger, frustration or boredom. In one study of obese type II diabetics in a weight loss programme, situations of emotional upset nearly always led to overeating. This appears to be the most reliable predictor of a relapse.
2. *Positive emotional states.* Here, the lapse occurs when the person is feeling good. Celebrations such as birthdays or family gatherings triggered relapse in one-third of a sample of dieters in Overeater's Anonymous.
3. *Social influence situations.* Our behaviour is often influenced by the behaviour of those around us. Direct social pressure to eat or exposure to others who are overeating may also prompt a lapse.
4. *Other triggers.* Though the majority of high-risk situations fall into the three categories above, a significant number of individuals have identified other circumstances. The need to test one's will power though exposure to certain foods or cues that stimulate eating is also an important trigger for many individuals.

However, while exposure to high-risk situations may increase the likelihood of relapse, it is mediated by the individual's ability to cope with the situation. Important cognitive variables have been identified. For example, self-efficacy is the expectation that one has control over one's behaviour in certain situations. An individual's sense of self-efficacy has been found to be a strong predictor of relapse. Individuals who perceive that they will be unable to 'resist' tempting foods and will eat excessively or inappropriately often do so. When this belief is coupled with a positive expectation of the hedonistic value of overeating, the likelihood of a dietary lapse is greatly increased.

A dichotomous, or all-or-none, thinking style has also been linked with the increased probability of relapse. Dichotomous thinking occurs when individuals establish very rigid rules for themselves about acceptable behaviours. Examples of dichotomous thoughts include 'I must never eat ice cream' or 'I must avoid all fried food all the time.' Abstinence is viewed as the standard by which behaviour is judged, and once the line has been crossed, there is no going back.

Once the individual has eaten some of the 'forbidden food' (and hence crossed the line), efforts to maintain control over eating may be abandoned ('What the heck, I've already blown it'). When coupled with a sense of guilt and discouragement, this is termed the Abstinence Violation Effect (AVE). How the individual *views* the lapse is central to whether self-efficacy regarding weight management is enhanced or reduced. If the individual attributes the lapse to internal, stable and global factors that are perceived to be uncontrollable (e.g. lack of willpower or an underlying 'addiction' to food), the AVE is enhanced. Conversely, when the cause is attributed to external, specific, and changeable factors (e.g. difficulty coping in an unanticipated high-risk situation), the AVE is reduced. Several studies have shown that the AVE is a mediating factor in the relapse process. Thus, for some, a single overeating episode or missed exercise session may be sufficient to trigger relapse.

The process of relapsing

A model incorporating situational, behavioural and attitudinal variables has been outlined to explain the process of relapse among addictive behaviours. Simply stated, relapse occurs as a process involving both behavioural and cognitive process. Coping skills are a key determinant in whether self-efficacy is enhanced or reduced, and can be used to predict long-term outcome.

This model has been extended to eating behaviours. As shown in **Fig. 1**, a positive outcome (Path 1) occurs when the individual has the necessary skills to deal with high-risk situations, leading to increased self-efficacy and long-term weight control. Conversely, when coping skills are inadequate, self-efficacy is decreased and the sense of control over weight is diminished.

Brownell (1994) has proposed that relapse occurs as a continuum of events:

> A *lapse* is a slight error slip, the first instance of backsliding. It is a discrete event like eating a forbidden food, exceeding a calorie level, or gaining weight. *Relapse* occurs when lapses string together and the person returns to his former state. When relapse is complete and there is little hope of reversing the negative trend, a *collapse* has occurred.

From the work on relapse, several important concepts have emerged.

- Relapse is a process. An understanding of points of vulnerability in the process enables targeted interventions to be developed.
- Coping skills are a central determinant of outcome. Thus, skills training is an essential component of relapse prevention efforts.

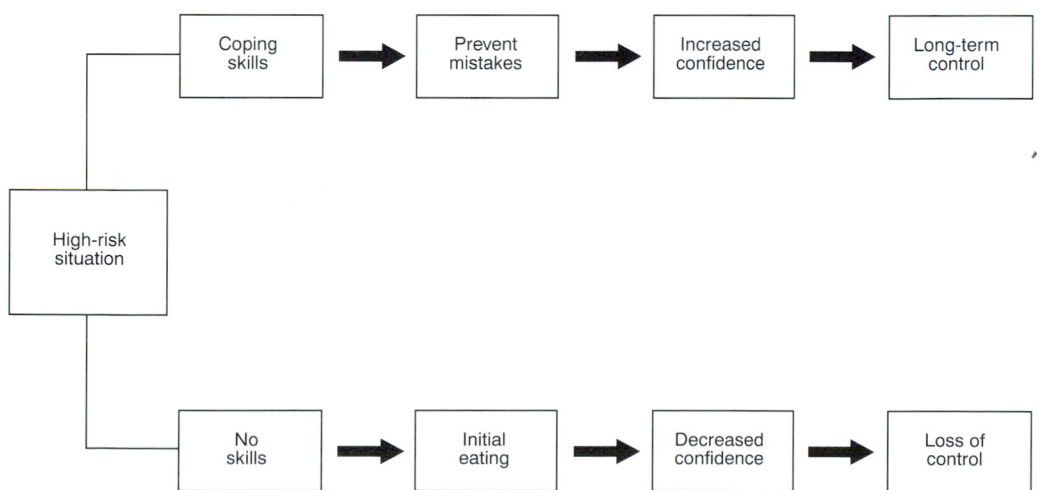

Figure 1 The process of lapse and relapse. Reprinted with permission from Brownell and Rodin (1990) *Weight Maintenance Survival Guide*, American Health Publications (adapted from the model in Marlatt and Gordon (1985)).

- Several attempts may be necessary for permanent behaviour change.
- Relapse to former behaviours does not imply that change is impossible. Rather, it suggests that if learning can occur, the likelihood of a positive outcome is enhanced. For instance, smokers successfully quit smoking on their fifth attempt, on average.

Weight Maintenance Strategies

Some individuals are able to lose large amounts of weight and sustain those losses over time. However, research has shown that maintenance is more likely to occur when individuals receive specific interventions. The following strategies have been shown to enhance long-term weight maintenance and should be routinely incorporated into the long-term care of overweight individuals.

Continued professional contact

A consistent finding among research trials has been the importance of ongoing professional contact in maintaining weight losses. Individuals who remain in contact with their treatment providers in the year following weight loss are much more likely to maintain their losses than those who discontinue treatment. It has been noted that those individuals who meet with their therapists biweekly during the year following treatment (e.g. what is generally regarded as a state-of-the-art maintenance programme), maintain 80–100% of their weight losses. Conversely, without such contact, individuals maintain only 50–60% of their losses.

Professional contact promotes ongoing awareness. The specific content of the maintenance sessions appears to be less important than the ongoing contact itself. It is likely that regular contact heightens awareness of weight, food and exercise behaviour on a regular basis. Such awareness may enhance commitment to specific goals and may bolster motivation when it begins to wane. Continued contact also fosters an ongoing focus on solutions to prevent or reverse small weight gains. Additionally, when individuals are taught how to develop and enhance their own support networks, the combination of both professional and peer support is more effective than either alone.

Exercise

Physical activity is a robust predictor of long-term weight maintenance. After the completion of a weight loss programme, exercise is a key factor in distinguishing those who maintain weight losses from those who regain. In one study, of those who maintained their losses, 92% exercised regularly, while only 34% of the regainers were physically active. Exercise combined with diet appears to be more effective in the long-term maintenance of weight loss than diet or exercise alone.

Mechanisms through which exercise may enhance weight loss or weight maintenance are elusive. Physiological effects of exercise include increased energy expenditure, sparing of lean body mass during weight loss, and a possible reversal of the metabolic decline associated with weight loss. Exercise is also beneficial to overall health because it appears to prevent, or at least retard, development of several diseases or conditions. However, the most important benefit of exercise for dieters may well be the psychological effects. Positive psychological changes associated with a regular activity programme may include changes in energy intake, decreased preference for dietary fat, along with enhanced mood, self-esteem and physical self-efficacy. It remains unclear whether this is causal relationship since those who are already motivated enough to engage in regular activity may be more likely to adopt other health-related behaviours (e.g. healthier eating practices and weight management).

Self-monitoring

Self-monitoring is the systematic observation of what one does. Self-monitoring of food, exercise and weight has been linked with enhanced weight maintenance. For example, it has been found that individuals who self-monitored and then discontinued this process during a 3-week holiday period gained significantly more weight than those who continued to monitor. In addition, individuals who self-monitor also appear to recognize small increases in weight earlier and respond appropriately.

Positive coping style

Individuals who successfully maintain their weight losses report coping strategies that differ from those who regain their weight. Maintainers are more likely to focus directly on the issue of regain and use problem-solving techniques to find solutions. On the other hand, relapsers tend to be emotion-focused and seek ways to reduce the emotional distress they are feeling. Often this self-soothing strategy involves the temporary comfort of food.

Adoption of healthier eating habits and attitudes

Successful maintainers have been queried about the specific strategies they used to avoid regain. Individuals who maintained their weight losses reported eating less overall, but notably fewer high-fat, high-sugar foods, avoiding snacks, and adopting better eating habits. In addition, they reported changing attitudes towards food and eating. Attitudinal techniques such as distinguishing hunger from cravings, modifying perfectionistic and dichotomous thoughts, and setting realistic weight and eating goals have also been shown to be important factors as well.

Pharmacotherapy and Weight Maintenance

The use of anorexiant medications in the treatment of obesity has enjoyed a resurgence in the past several years, coincident with the publication of two important studies. The first study used dexfenfluramine for 52 weeks. INDEX, as the study was known, was conducted in 24 centres in nine countries of Europe. Twenty per cent of participants lost 20% or more of their initial body weight. Plateauing of the weight loss occurred at about 6 months, with maintenance of the losses up to 12 months. The second study summarized the results of a series of National Institutes of Health (NIH)-funded studies. These randomized, controlled studies combined two agents (phentermine and d,l-fenfluramine) and provided treatment for as long as 3.5 years. Similar to the INDEX results, the combination of these medications also promoted both weight loss and long-term maintenance. In the NIH studies it was noted that when medication was withdrawn, weight was regained, and when it was reintroduced, additional weight loss occurred.

Phentermine, dl-fenfluramine and dexfenfluramine are similar in chemical structure and action to amphetamines, though notably result in less central nervous system stimulation and drug dependence. Other pharmacological agents which act in a similar fashion include phenmetrazine, diethylpropion, mazindol and phenylpropanolamine. Researchers have also investigated the use of serotonin-specific reuptake inhibitors currently used to treat depression (e.g. fluoxetine and sertraline). However, these serotonergic agents appear to produce smaller weight losses and their efficacy wanes beyond the first few months. Recently, sibutramine, a combined adrenergic and serotonergic agent has been introduced.

The value of anorexiant medications in weight maintenance is tempered by three factors. There is ongoing controversy regarding the efficacy, patient selection and safety of utilizing medications to promote weight loss and long-term weight maintenance. First, only a subset of patients achieve meaningful incremental weight loss and continued weight maintenance. Most patients experience a plateauing of

weight loss or regain after about 6 months. In addition, the mean incremental amount of weight lost is generally small as compared with placebo, though not insignificant. For example, in the INDEX study, those receiving placebo also lost a significant amount of weight (7.2 ± 0.5 kg and 10.3 ± 7.2 kg for placebo versus drug, respectively). Second, not all individuals respond to drug therapy. The INDEX study found that 20% of individuals lost no weight while taking medication. There are insufficient data to predict those who will best respond to pharmacotherapy, but those who do not lose weight within the first few weeks of administration are unlikely to respond later. Safety issues include both typical side effects, notably sleep disturbance, diarrhoea, fatigue, and dry mouth, as well as the rare though much more dangerous problems of primary pulmonary hypertension (PPH) and neurotoxicity. A recent review has suggested that the risks of PPH occurs at a rate of about 28 persons per million per year. The greatest risks are associated with the most recent use; in the 3 months following treatment a 23.1-fold increase in occurrence was reported. Neurotoxicity is also a serious risk of these medications and has been demonstrated in nonhuman primates at about 10 times the normal human dose. Cardiac valvular toxicity has recently led to the withdrawal of the fenfluramines (d, l, and dex).

Other medications such as gastrointestinal absorption inhibitors (e.g., the lipase inhibitor orlistat), satiety enhancers (e.g., CCK, chlorocitrate) and hormones (e.g., leptin) show some promise, but are not yet generally available.

Even for those agents which are known to be effective, compliance in typical medical practice may compromise the potential long-term benefit of pharmacotherapy. There is some evidence that intermittent use of anorexiants for weight maintenance is less effective than continuous use. While it has been argued that continuous use of medications to control obesity is not different from using medications to control hypertension, there are very significant behavioural concomitants of weight gain in many obese individuals. If these behavioural factors are not addressed independently of drug treatment, they are likely to reduce compliance with long-term treatment, and thus long-term efficacy. There is also evidence that dangerous side effects are much more likely to occur with long-term use.

In summary, anorexiant medications are undoubtedly of some benefit in both weight loss and weight maintenance in some obese individuals. The search continues for medications which may effectively alter nutrient absorption and energy expenditure. However, given the heterogeneous nature of obesity, it is very unlikely that any medication or combination of medications will be effective in treating all overweight individuals. As with any chronic medication, maintaining individuals on pharmacotherapy for extended periods of time requires very careful consideration. Pharmacotherapy should be reserved only for those individuals who are clearly at medical risk from their obesity (e.g. BMI > 30, or BMI > 27 in those with comorbid conditions) and those who have already failed more conservative treatment attempts. Further, the use of medication should be considered adjunctive to a comprehensive programme that includes changes in diet, exercise, and behaviour.

Outstanding Issues in Weight Maintenance Research

The basic components of a safe and effective weight loss programme have received widespread agreement. However, our understanding of optimal weight maintenance practices is in its infancy. Many questions remain unanswered. Among them:

- Does rapid weight loss (e.g. through the use of more traditionally restrictive diets) enhance or impede weight maintenance? Which individuals would benefit by a more gradual approach?
- Is ongoing vigilance to eating and exercise habits a prerequisite of weight maintenance? If so, how can undesirable side effects such as psychological fatigue be better managed or averted?
- Does the amount of weight lost influence the strategies needed to maintain the losses? If so, which strategies best facilitate the maintenance of smaller and larger weight losses?
- What is the optimal weight loss for mild, moderate, and severely obese individuals? If the optimal threshold is exceeded, is weight maintenance be compromised?
- Who will best benefit from adjunctive pharmacotherapy? When are anorexiants best initiated? Should drug therapy be continuous or incremental?

Conclusions

The challenge of obesity treatment lies not in helping individuals lose weight – rather it is the maintenance of weight loss over time that has proved so elusive. The strategies which help individuals lose weight have proved to be largely ineffective in sustaining those losses over time. Specific research has addressed the unique behaviours and attitudes faced by those seeking to sustain weight losses and has yielded some promising additions to weight management programmes. Nonetheless, current knowledge is limited to those who seek treatment in large university and hospital centres, and very little is known about individuals who successfully lose weight and keep it off on their own.

Effective maintenance strategies combine a series of behavioural, educational, and supportive measures over long periods of time. Maintenance strategies must be interwoven into every comprehensive weight loss programme from the first meeting onward. Though follow-up care need not necessarily be intensive or frequent, ongoing professional contact may be necessary to help individuals maintain weight losses over time.

See also: **Obesity**: Treatment. **Weight Management**: Weight Cycling.

Further Reading

Bray G (1993) Use and abuse of appetite-suppressant drugs in the treatment of obesity. *Annals of Internal Medicine* **119**:707–713.

Brownell KD (1994) *The LEARN Program for Weight Control*, 6th edn. Dallas, TX: American Health.

Brownell KD and Rodin J (1990) *The Weight Maintenance Survival Guide*. Dallas, TX: American Health.

Goldstein DJ and Potvin JH (1994) Long-term weight loss: the effect of pharmacologic agents. *American Journal of Clinical Nutrition* **60**:647–657.

Grilo CM, Shiffman S and Wing RR (1989) Relapse crises and coping among dieters. *Journal of Consulting and Clinical Psychology* **57**:488–495.

Grilo CM, Brownell KD and Stunkard AJ (1993) The metabolic and psychological importance of exercise in weight control. In: Stunkard AJ, and Wadden TA (eds) *Obesity: Theory and Therapy*, pp. 253–273. New York: Raven.

Guy-Grand B (1992) Clinical studies with *d*-fenfluramine. *American Journal of Clinical Nutrition* **55**:173S–176S.

Institute of Medicine (1995) *Weighing the Options: Criteria for Evaluating Weight Management Programs*. Washington: National Academy Press.

Kayman, SW, Bruvold W and Stern JS (1990) Maintenance and relapse after weight loss in women: behavioral aspects. *American Journal of Clinical Nutrition*, **52**:800–807.

Marlatt, GA and Gordon JR (eds) (1985) *Relapse Prevention: Maintenance Strategies in the Treatment of Addictive Behaviors*. New York: Guilford.

National Task Force on the Prevention and Treatment of Obesity, National Institutes of Health (1994) Weight cycling. *Journal of the American Medical Association* **272**:1196–1202.

Perri MG, Nezu AM and Veigener BJ (1992) *Improving the Long-term Management of Obesity: Theory, Research, and Clinical Guidelines*. New York: John Wiley.

Stunkard AJ (1958) The management of obesity. *New York State Journal of Medicine* 58:79–87.

Wadden TA, Sternberg JA, Letizia KA, Stunkard AJ and Foster GD (1989) Treatment of obesity by very-low-calorie diet, behaviour therapy, and their combination: A five-year perspective. *International Journal of Obesity* 13(supplement 2):39–46.

Weintraub M, Sundaresan PR, Schuster B, Moscucci M and Stein EC (1992) National Heart, Lung, and Blood Institute long-term weight control study: III. An open label study of dose adjustment of fenfluramine and phentermine. *Clinical Pharmacological Therapeutics*, 51S:581–646.

Weight Cycling

Ross Andersen and **Lawrence Cheskin**, Johns Hopkins University School of Medicine, Baltimore, MA, USA

Obesity is associated with numerous adverse health outcomes. Moreover, obesity may exacerbate many chronic diseases such as hypertension, hyperlipidaemia, osteoarthritis and musculoskeletal problems. These findings are paralleled by another alarming statistic – the increasing prevalence of obesity in both developing and developed countries. Despite an intense preoccupation with weight and dieting in the USA, it was recently reported that the percentage of overweight individuals increased between the 1976/1980 and the 1988/1991 National Health and Nutrition Examination Surveys. Current estimates place the overall prevalence of overweight (defined as a body mass index (BMI) value of ≥ 27.8 for men and ≥ 27.3 for women) at 31% of men and 35% of women. Paradoxically, 23.3% of American men and 40.1% of women were voluntarily trying to lose weight in 1990.

Unfortunately, the vast majority of dieters regain their lost weight within 5 or fewer years. The cycles of weight loss and regain have been found in some studies to be related to an increased risk of illness, mortality and feelings of helplessness in weight-fluctuating persons. The term 'weight cycling', or its lay counterpart, 'yo-yo' dieting, first emerged in the mid 1980s. Few topics in the weight and eating disorders literature have evoked as much controversy as weight cycling. Since weight regain is common after weight loss, the media has been fascinated with the concept of weight cycling and have flooded the public with equivocal reports on the topic.

Scientists have published decidedly different opinions as to whether or not weight cycling is haz-ardous as well as whether it exacerbates difficulties with long-term weight management. Although most population-based studies have reported that body weight variation increases morbidity and mortality, many of these studies have limitations which limit their generalizability. These limitations have prompted several editorials in the literature to urge caution in interpreting the hazards of weight cycling.

Definition of Weight Cycling

Weight cycling has not, unfortunately, been clearly defined. Investigators have used the terms 'weight cycling', and 'weight fluctuation' interchangeably. Both terms imply at least one cycle of weight loss and regain. Several different criteria have been used to define weight cycling in the scientific literature, for example: (1) the self-reported number of losses and regains of a set amount of weight; (2) the total number of weight cycles during a set period of time; (3) total weight lost over a lifetime; (4) difference between highest and lowest adult weight; and (5) asking patients the question 'are you a yo-yo dieter?'.

Recently, there has also been interest in weight variability. Weight variability differs from weight cycling in that variability implies a deviation from an overall trend. Hence, an individual who steadily gains weight throughout adulthood shows little variability in weight, whereas an individual who lost and regained weight several times through their adult years with an overall trend of gaining weight is demonstrating more variability. Weight variability has been described as an index derived from the number and frequency of weight fluctuations over a period of time, or more commonly the root mean square error around the overall time trend of weight (the within-person trend in weight fluctuation around the trend for weight change).

Concerns About the Hazards of Weight Cycling

Studies have raised concerns about possible hazards of weight cycling in a number of areas. These include adverse effects on metabolic processes, body fat distribution, dietary preferences, and both overall and disease-specific morbidity and mortality.

Metabolic efficiency

It has been suggested that repeated weight cycles may result in a reduction of the resting metabolic rate (RMR) which would make subsequent attempts at weight reduction more difficult. In a comparison of nonobese weight cyclers with noncyclers it was found that the weight fluctuators had lower relative RMRs expressed as RMR per kg. However, RMR was similar when expressed as RMR per day or RMR per kg fat-free mass.

A cross-sectional study of wrestlers described a direct relationship between decreased RMR and weight cycling history. Wrestlers who were repeatedly losing weight prior to wrestling meets and regaining it after the event were found to have lower resting metabolic rates than their weight-stable counterparts. In a follow-up study the RMRs of a group of 12 weight cycling wrestlers were compared with those of 13 nonwrestlers of similar weight, body composition and fitness levels. No differences in metabolic profiles were found between these two groups. As expected, when the wrestlers lost weight during the wrestling season, their RMR decreased. When they returned to their preseason weight after the competitive season, however, their metabolic rate returned to its preseason level. Competitive lightweight rowers who weight cycle throughout the competitive season have not been found to be metabolically more efficient than their noncycling counterparts.

Few studies have compared the effects of weight cycling in lean versus obese persons. Furthermore, researchers and the lay press have tried to generalize findings in competitive athletes who are constantly trying to make weight to the sedentary, obese weight cycler. It has been speculated that weight cycling may be more hazardous for lean persons who are at or below their ideal weight.

Investigators in the 1980s hypothesized that one of the reasons that weight cyclers may have a lower RMR was that they were losing metabolically active fat-free mass (FFM) when they lost weight. It was further theorized that when the weight was regained, the lost lean mass would not be fully recovered, leaving the individual metabolically compromised. This hypothesis has been disproven since it has been documented that FFM and RMR generally return to pre-dieting levels when lost weight is regained. Even repeated weight cycling has not been found to lead to a progressive decrease in the RMR. Recently it has also been shown that no relationship between total number of diets or lifetime weight loss and per cent fat or RMR is detectable.

The effects of a single weight cycle on RMR and body fat distribution has been recently examined in a group of obese women who had lost a significant amount of weight and fully regained it. Subjects in this study started the diet at 98 kg and at the end of treatment had lost 18.9 kg, of which 3.7 kg was FFM. RMR fell from 389 to 358 kJ per day during this time. Both RMR and FFM returned to baseline

levels when subjects regained all of their lost weight. Waist-to-hip ratios also remained unchanged throughout the study, suggesting that a single weight cycle did not result in excess visceral fat storage.

Body fat distribution

The question of whether weight cycling affects body fat distribution is important since android (upper body) obesity is known to be a greater risk factor for heart disease than gynoid (lower body) obesity. Reports on the relationship between weight cycling history and body fat distribution are equivocal. A moderate association (r = 0.37) between history of weight cycling and upper body obesity (high waist-to-hip ratio) has been reported. Most studies, however, have found no differences in fat distribution as a function of weight cycling history.

Preference for dietary fat

An increased preference for dietary fat may be one of the mechanisms that causes obese persons to regain weight after losing weight. The literature is equivocal, however. Some studies have reported that obese weight cyclers have an increased preference for fat and simple sugars compared with obese persons with more stable body weights. Other studies have found no relationship between fat intake and weight cycling history.

Population-based Studies

Several large population-based studies carried out since the 1950s have examined the relationship between weight cycling and weight variability and subsequent all-cause mortality. It is clear that weight reduction produces improvements in lipid and lipoprotein profiles, glucose tolerance and blood pressure. These beneficial physiological effects of weight loss would suggest that weight reduction in an obese individual should result in a reduced risk of heart attack, stroke and diabetes, and lead to increased longevity. However, the evidence to substantiate this hypothesis is scant. This may be because in these large population-based studies, there are relatively few subjects who are seriously obese.

A majority of the epidemiological investigations have reported higher death rates in subjects who have lost weight and regained it compared with those who remain weight stable or steadily gain weight. However, it is difficult to determine whether the weight loss in most population-based studies is voluntary or involuntary.

The American Cancer Society Study

The first analysis of this population examined deaths from heart disease and stroke in relation to self-reported weight loss. There was no evidence of increased survival in overweight persons (>110 of ideal body weight) who lost either 4.5–8.9 kg or ≥ 9.0 kg. One of the strengths of this study is that the investigators attempted to eliminate already unhealthy individuals from the follow-up analyses. It was not reported whether the weight loss was intentional or not.

A follow-up of the American Cancer Society Study has recently been conducted to examine the effects of weight change in overweight (BMI ≥ 27 before weight change), middle-aged women. One of the strengths of this investigation is that they examined whether or not the weight change was intentional. The lowest mortality was found in the women who intentionally lost more that 9.0 kg, whereas the highest mortality was found among the women who unintentionally lost weight.

The Honolulu Heart Study

This study examined the effects of weight change in men from self-reported weight at age 25 to the follow-up at age 45–68 years. The men were stratified into four intervals of change in BMI: < −1.13; −1.13; to +1.12; 1.13–3.75; and >3.75 BMI units. The authors reported the lowest mortality ratings in the men who had little change in BMI (i.e. −1.13 to +1.13 BMI units) in all but the second quartile of BMI at age 25. Men in the second quartile of BMI experienced the lowest mortality with small weight gains (i.e. an increase of 1.13 to 3.75 BMI units).

A subsequent analysis of the Honolulu Heart Study to examine the effects of weight loss on mortality was recently reported. After controlling for age, average weight, smoking status, cigarettes/day, alcohol consumption, physical activity, total energy intake, job classification and pre-existing disease, the men who had lost 4.5 kg had a relative risk of 1.21 when compared with those with stable weights. This increased risk was not seen in men who had never smoked.

The Framingham Heart Study

The Framingham Heart Study is an ongoing study which was established in 1948. Subjects in the study are brought in every 2 years for complete medical evaluations. In the first analysis of these data, the investigators categorized 55-year-old nonsmoking men and women into tertiles of BMI change as follows: loss of ≥ 10%, loss of 0–9%, gain of 0–9%, or gain of ≥ 10%. After controlling for baseline BMI in both men and women, it was found that minimum mortality was found in the group that gained 0–9% and the maximum mortality was seen in the group whose BMI was reduced by ≥10%.

A second study using Framingham data examined the effects of weight fluctuation on mortality. One of the strengths of this study is that several weights over a long period of time were measured. The coefficient of BMI change was found to be significantly and negatively related to mortality. Thus, weight loss increased mortality while weight gain decreased it. One of the limitations of this study is the potential bias that exists from involuntary weight loss.

The Baltimore Longitudinal Study of Aging

The Baltimore Longitudinal Study is an ongoing prospective cohort study which includes biennial complete physical exams. The relationship between weight fluctuation and mortality was studied using between three and 16 measured weights from the physical examinations. BMI was then regressed over time to obtain an overall slope of the line. After controlling for baseline BMI and weight fluctuation, it was found that increased BMI reduced mortality, while decreased BMI (weight loss) increased mortality. The authors did not control for the potential confounding effects of involuntary weight loss, cigarette smoking or alcohol consumption.

Multiple Risk Factor Intervention Trial (MRFIT)

This study examined the relationship between weight variability and mortality in high-risk middle-aged men. Categories of weight change were defined as follows: (1) 'no change', <5% change from baseline; (2) steady weight gain; or (3) steady weight loss. Weight variability was defined as the intrapersonal standard deviation of weight, calculated from clinic visits over a 6- to 7-year period. After adjusting for confounding baseline factors, the relative risk for all-cause mortality in the least variable compared with the most variable quartile was 1.64. This was the first study to report results stratified by initial body weight. Interestingly, the association between weight variability and all-cause mortality did not hold up in the heaviest quartile of men.

Animal Studies of Weight Cycling

Many of the inferences made about weight cycling have come from retrospectively examining the association between weight variation and various disease markers. Using rodents as subjects, it is possible to measure directly causal links between weight cycling, metabolic efficiency and health problems.

Early studies with rodents reported that weight cycling resulted in decreased weight loss during subsequent cycles and an increase in weight gained. A review paper which examined the weight cycling literature in animals cautioned that these studies did not have a maturity control group, and that the majority of recent studies that have used a maturity control group have not found that weight cycling affects subsequent weight loss or rates of weight regain in animals.

Early investigators of weight cycling speculated that weight cycling would result in an increase in both total and central adiposity. The majority of animal studies have not found that weight fluctuation results in excess fat accumulation or preferential visceral fat storage.

Recent studies in animals have concluded that the majority of animal data do not support the hypothesis that weight cycling results in long-term metabolic efficiency or adverse health outcomes. However, further research is needed to examine the effects of weight cycling on obese animals or those with a genetic predisposition to obesity. This would allow more clinically relevant questions to be asked.

Psychological Consequences of Weight Cycling

Dieting and weight loss are frequently associated with hopes of improved appearance and health, whereas weight regain may lead to feelings of failure and despair. There has been relatively little research on the psychological effects of weight cycling. Obese individuals report feeling ashamed, guilty and inadequate as a result of regaining lost weight. Weight cyclers tend to report significantly lower general wellbeing scores and are also less likely to report being in good or excellent health.

Recently, severe weight cyclers were compared with moderate and mild cyclers. Subjects with a severe history of weight cycling had a significantly younger age of onset of obesity and reported initiating a diet at a significantly younger age than did the mild cyclers. Interestingly, no differences were found among the three groups of weight cyclers using scales for measuring depression, tension–anxiety, fatigue, profile of mood states (POMs) or hostility–bewilderment. Mild cyclers, however, did report greater vigour than the moderate and severe cyclers. No differences in psychopathology or physical self-esteem were seen among any of the groups. However, compared with normal-weight women all three groups fell below average scores in self-esteem

In another study, low weight cyclers ($\bar{x} = 1.8$ lifetime diets) were compared with a group high weight cyclers ($\bar{x} = 7.2$ lifetime diets). No differences between groups were found on the Beck Depression Inventory, the Automatic Thoughts Questionnaire, the Hopelessness Scale or the Dysfunctional Attitude Scale. No relationship between binge eating disorder and weight cycling history has been reported. However, it has been speculated that weight cyclers who are also binge eaters would be at higher risk of adverse emotional reactions than those who are weight cyclers alone.

National Task Force on the Prevention and Treatment of Obesity

The National Institutes of Health recently addressed concerns about the hazards of weight cycling and provided guidance on the risk-to-benefit ratio of attempting weight loss. The panel of experts reviewed all of the scientific literature which examined the effects of weight change or weight fluctuation in both humans and animals. They concluded that the majority of studies do not support the hypothesis that weight cycling has adverse effects on metabolism. They also concluded that the potential hazards of weight cycling were insufficiently compelling to override the potential benefits of moderate weight loss in seriously obese patients. Finally, it was recommended that obese persons should not allow concerns about weight cycling to deter them from attempting to lose weight.

Recommendations for Future Studies on Weight Cycling

Weight cycling is clearly a very common and potentially important problem. Further work is needed to address some of the confounding design problems described above. The following still unanswered questions still need to be addressed:

1. What are the effects of voluntary as opposed to involuntary weight loss on morbidity and mortality?
2. Are there different effects of weight cycling in obese, overweight and normal-weight persons?
3. Does physical activity or lifetime physical fitness reduce weight variability?
4. Do athletes whose sport forces them to 'make weight' and thus have high weight variability show adverse health consequences?

Conclusions

The opinions of experts vary on the potential negative effects of weight cycling. Most population-based studies have found that greater weight variability is associated with a greater risk for cardiovascular disease and all-cause mortality. It is difficult to reconcile such evidence with the fact that moderate weight loss has been associated with the improvement, and in some cases the elimination, of certain chronic diseases. Given the known risks of obesity, the probable benefits of weight loss, and the possible harm of weight fluctuation in humans, we feel that treatment must continue to focus on weight loss but should place a much greater emphasis on the maintenance of weight losses. Given our present state of incomplete knowledge, it behoves those of us who treat obesity to devise treatments which minimize the risk lost weight being regained.

See also: **Cancer**: Epidemiology and Associations Between Diet and Cancer. **Coronary Heart Disease**: Lipid Theory of Coronary Heart Disease. **Fats and Oils**: Nutritional Value. **Obesity**: Fat Distribution; Prevention.

Further Reading

Bartlett SJ, Wadden TA and Vogt RA (1996) Psychosocial consequences of weight cycling. *Journal of Cons Clin Psych* 64:587–592.

Blair SN, Shaten J, Brownell K, Collins G and Lissner L (1993) Body weight change, all-cause mortality, and cause-specific mortality in the multiple risk factor intervention trial (MRFIT). *Annals of Internal Medicine* 119:749–757.

Hammond EC and Garfinkel L (1969) Coronary heart disease, stroke and aortic aneurysm: factors in the etiology. *Archives of Environmental Health* 19:167–182.

Iribarren C, Sharp DS, Burchfiel CM and Petrovitch H (1995) Association of weight loss and weight fluctuation with mortality among Japanese-American men. *New England Journal of Medicine* 333:686–692.

Jebb SA, Goldberg GR, Coward WA, Murgatroyd PR and Prentise AM (1991) Effect of weight cycling caused by intermittent dieting on metabolic rate and body composition in obese women. *International Journal of Obesity* 15:367–374.

Kheunel RH and Wadden TA (1994) Binge eating disorder, weight cycling and psychopathology. *International Journal of Eating Disorders* 15:321–329.

Lissner L, Andres R, Muller DC and Shimokata H (1990) Body weight variability in men: metabolic rate, health and longevity. *International Journal of Obesity* 14:373–383.

Lissner L, Odell PM, D'Agostino RB, Stokes J 3d, Kreger BE, Belanger AJ and Brownell KD (1991) Variability of body weight and health outcomes in the Framingham population. *New England Journal of Medicine* 324:1839–1844.

Manore MM, Berry TE, Skinner JS, Carroll SS (1991) Energy expenditure at rest and during exercise in non-obese female cyclical dieters and nondieting control subjects. *American Journal of Clinical Nutrition* 54:41–46.

Reed GW, Hill JO (1993) Weight cycling: a review of the animal literature. *Obesity Research* 1:392–402.

Steen SN, Opplinger RA, Brownell KD (1988) Metabolic effects of repeated weight loss and regain in wrestlers. *Journal of the American Medical Association* 260:47–50.

Wadden TA, Bartlett S, Letezia KA, Foster GD, Stunkard AJ (1992) Relationship of dieting history to resting metabolic rate, body composition, eating behavior, and subsequent weight loss. *American Journal of Clinical Nutrition* 56:203S–208S.

Wadden TA, Foster GD, Stunkard AJ, Conill AM (1996) Effects of weight cycling on the resting energy expenditure and body composition of obese women. *International Journal of Eating Disorders* 19:5–12.

Williamson DF, Pamuk E, Thun M, Flanders D, Byers T, Health C (1995) A prospective study of intentional weight loss and mortality in never smoking overweight white women aged 40 to 64 years. *American Journal of Epidemiology* 141:1128–1141.

Wing RR (1992) Weight cycling in humans: a review of the literature. *Annals of Behavioral Medicine* 14:113–119.

Wilson's disease *see* **Copper**: Physiology, Dietary Sources and Requirements.

Wine *see* **Alcohol**: Absorption, Metabolism and Physiological Effects; Disease Risk and Beneficial Effects; Effects of Consumption on Diet and Nutritional Status.

WORLD HEALTH ORGANIZATION

Role

J Akré, Programme of Nutrition, WHO, Geneva, Switzerland

The World Health Organization (WHO) is the intergovernmental organization within the UN system that acts as the directing and coordinating authority on international health work. It performs its functions through three principal bodies – the World Health Assembly, the Executive Board and the Secretariat. The objective of WHO, which has 191 Member States, is the attainment by all peoples of the highest possible level of health. While its headquarters is located in Geneva, Switzerland, the Organization is decentralized in six regions, each with its own regional committee and regional office. WHO's regular budget – US$842 654 000 for the biennium 1998–1999 – is augmented by voluntary contributions, which are roughly equivalent to regular budget levels. WHO works closely with and through others, including other agencies of the UN system, nongovernmental organizations, and collaborating centres around the world in numerous disciplines. In restructuring its programmes in the mid 1990s in the face of resource constraints, WHO decided to place emphasis on meeting the most pressing health needs. In seeking to prevent and overcome malnutrition, WHO promotes the tailoring of approaches to fit circumstances. While the rapidly increasing threat of noncommunicable diseases accounts for at least 40% of all deaths in developing countries and 75% in industrialized countries, many millions still cannot meet basic needs for energy and protein, are deficient in essential micronutrients, or are severely malnourished. Thus, coordinated action is called for on both fronts. Consistent with the unique normative, scientific and advisory role that WHO has played for the last half century, the Organization strives to support all its Member States in developing food and nutrition policies that will make healthy choices the easy choices for their populations.

Birth of the World Health Organization

For many thousands of years, people have exchanged remedies and diseases without really thinking of ways to work together to promote health that could go beyond purely parochial concerns. Early attempts at international cooperation in health were limited to small groups of countries, which discussed a few obviously contagious diseases such as cholera and smallpox, and strategies such as quarantine to keep them at bay. Although 11 international sanitary conferences were held in Europe between 1851 and 1903, it was not until 1907 that a worldwide international institution – the Office International d'Hygiène Publique – was founded to prepare and administer international sanitary conventions and to provide national health administrations with an opportunity for regular contacts and discussion.

The terrible epidemics which raged through Europe at the end of World War I, coupled with the mass movement of liberated prisoners of war, constituted a menace to Europe of such magnitude as to require coordinated international effort. The League of Red Cross Societies, created in 1919, attempted the task but quickly realized that intergovernmental action was essential to cope with a problem of such magnitude. As the charter of the Office International d'Hygiène Publique did not give enough power for action in individual countries, provision for necessary measures had to be made by the League of Nations, then in the process of creation.

The Geneva-based League, during its short and unhappy history between the two world wars, had been the first to invoke international health cooperation to deal with many kinds of health problems. In the same period, the Pan American Sanitary Organization, originally established in 1902, continued to work in its own geographical sphere. (In 1958 it became the Pan American Health Organization (PAHO), which serves as WHO Regional Office for the Americas (see below).)

In 1945, the United Nations (UN) Conference on International Organization, meeting in San Francisco, unanimously approved a proposal by Brazil and China to establish an autonomous international health organization within the UN system. The following year, an international conference held in New York set up an interim commission and approved the *Constitution of the World Health Organization*. This came into force on 7 April 1948, when the 26th government, out of a total of 61 signatories, formally ratified it in its national parliament. Since then, 7 April is celebrated every year as World Health Day, when attention around the globe is focused on a theme of major international public-health importance. Today, the health agency based in Geneva, Switzerland, is owned and operated by the governments of 191 countries, representing almost the entire population of the world, as reflected in its emblem (**Fig. 1**).

The Task Entrusted to WHO

WHO is defined by its constitution as the directing and coordinating authority on international health work. Its aim is 'the attainment by all peoples of the highest possible level of health', which is 'one of the fundamental rights of every human being'. The constitution lists specifically a number of responsibilities. These include the following:

- to stimulate the eradication of epidemic, endemic and other diseases;
- to promote improved nutrition, housing, sanitation, working conditions and other aspects of environmental hygiene;
- to propose international conventions and agreements in health matters;
- to promote and conduct research in the field of health;
- to develop international standards for food, biological and pharmaceutical products;
- to assist in developing an informed public opinion among all peoples on matters of health.

The agreed policy of WHO is a determined and structured effort by all countries to bring health within the reach of everyone. 'Health' is defined by WHO's constitution as a 'state of complete physical, mental and social well-being and not merely the absence of disease and infirmity'. It is seen as a shared responsibility, calling for a high degree of self-reliance from the individual, the family, the community and, of course, the nation as a whole. Because the determinants of health are so broad, the efforts of the health sector must be supported and augmented by those of many other related sectors, including agriculture, water and sanitation, finance, industry, planning, communication and education.

WHO provided the first truly global framework for setting international standards to promote and protect health. In keeping with post-war faith in the power of technology, WHO initially operated as a technical organization, fuelled by advances in biomedical research and the belief that new medical discoveries would bring spectacular improvements in health. One of its first tasks was to develop mechanisms, still in effect today, for identifying urgent research needs and then linking the world's leading specialists and research institutes in a concerted attack on the problem. Tangible results came in the form of new diagnostic tests, therapeutic drugs and vaccines. WHO also standardized the classification of diseases, terminology, nomenclature, reporting systems, research protocols, and quality and safety specifications for foods, drinking water and pharmaceutical products. Consumers the world over benefit from these standards, which are continually revised in the light of new knowledge.

As research advances produced the means for conquering one disease after another, WHO shifted its emphasis to problems of logistics. Research took on social and ethical dimensions as the Organization sought ways to extend the benefits of modern medicine to the world's populations. The early promise that sophisticated technology would bring spectacular improvements in health paled, however, against the reality of the millions of people who had no access to basic medical services. Given its constitutionally defined universal mandate and humanitarian mission, WHO began advocating changes that would eventually revolutionize the way public health was perceived. In a world that remained disease-ridden and suffering despite unprecedented technical advances, it became a matter of equity and social justice to make health progress available to all people through new approaches, new strategies and better management of resources.

High technology as an end in itself was replaced by the concept of appropriate technology, affordable and culturally acceptable to the people who would use it. To come to terms with the soaring costs of medical care in affluent countries as well as the lack of funds in developing countries, WHO placed

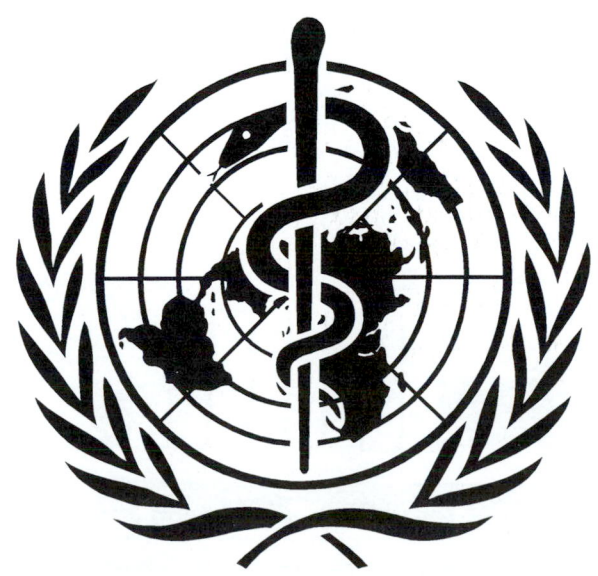

Figure 1 WHO emblem.

preventive – as opposed to curative – medicine in the forefront. The concept of primary health care, with its emphasis on individual responsibility for health and its conviction that the best help is self-help, began to take shape.

The age of technical paternalism came to a formal close in 1979 when the Member States of WHO unanimously adopted the goal of 'Health for All by the Year 2000', founded on the principles of primary health care that had been elaborated in 1978 during the International Conference on Primary Health Care at Alma-Ata (Kazakstan). Commitment to this time-limited goal guided much of the Organization's work over the next decade, though the promotion of research, particularly on disease prevention and control, continues in full force as part of WHO's global plan to push the world forward through the protection and promotion of health (see below).

Structure

WHO is a specialized agency of the UN, as provided for in the *Charter of the United Nations*. A goal-oriented organization with policies, programme and budget defined through well-developed mechanisms, WHO consists of three constituent bodies.

*   The *World Health Assembly*, which is the highest decision-making body, is held in May each year and is attended by delegations from WHO's 191 Member States and two associate members. Its main tasks are to decide on major policy matters and to approve the biennial programme budget.
*   The *Executive Board* consists of 32 persons, acting in their personal capacity, highly qualified in the field of health and designated for a 3-year term by as many Member States, which are chosen by the Health Assembly on the basis of equitable geographical distribution. The Board, which normally meets twice a year, gives effect to the decisions and policies of the Assembly, while advising it and preparing its agenda.
*   The *Secretariat* serves to carry out the decisions of the World Health Assembly and the Executive Board; it is the entire staff of WHO headed by the Director-General, who is appointed as its chief technical and administrative officer for a 5-year term by the World Health Assembly on the nomination of the Executive Board.

In general, all technical activities that are of universal applicability – such as biological and epidemiological standardization, the overall assessment of the efficacy of methods and materials, and promoting the control of disease – are the responsibility of the headquarters in Geneva (**Fig. 2**). WHO's highly decentralized structure enables it to respond directly to the needs of its membership, upon request,

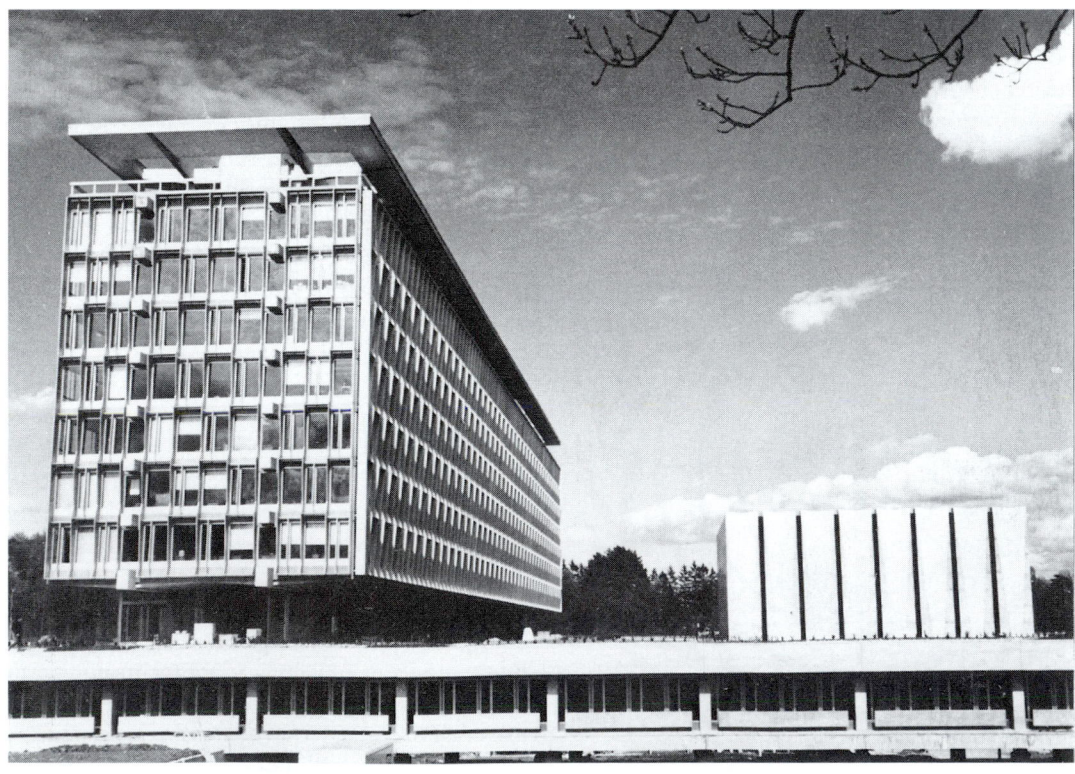

Figure 2 The headquarters of WHO in Geneva, Switzerland. Photograph by T. Farkas.

through its six regions, each consisting of a regional committee and a regional office. The regional offices, with their own directors, are responsible for formulating policies of a regional character and for monitoring regional activities. In many countries there is a resident WHO representative, who is the main intermediary for support of WHO, and who participates with the government in planning and managing national health programmes. The location of the six regional offices and the Member States covered are shown in **Fig. 3**.

Some 40% of WHO's 4300 staff members, including PAHO, work in countries all over the world, either in field programmes or as WHO representatives; 30% are in the six regional offices; and 30% at headquarters in Geneva.

WHO's normative, i.e. standard-setting, functions also include preparation and updating of the *International Classification of Diseases*, assignment of generic names for pharmaceuticals, and, since 1957, evaluating the safety for human consumption of selected food additives and contaminants in food and establishing acceptable daily intakes for these substances through the Joint FAO (Food and Agriculture Organization)/WHO Expert Committee on Food Additives.

The Committee's reports, as well as those of a similar FAO/WHO group responsible for evaluating the safety of pesticide residues, are used in the formulation of national food legislation intended to protect consumers from hazardous additives or contaminants and by the Codex Alimentarius Commission – another joint FAO/WHO body – in establishing international food standards. (Food legislation is one of the many topics regularly covered by one of WHO's half-dozen specialized international periodicals, the quarterly *International Digest of Health Legislation*.) Codex originated at a time – the early 1960s – when international efforts were being made to increase world trade by reducing tariff barriers, as well as nontariff barriers resulting from differing food regulations. Consistent with a dynamic system that is still changing to deal with ever-changing circumstances, the international community has decided to use health-related Codex standards, guidelines and recommendations as a reference in implementing relevant aspects of the trade agreements administered by the World Trade Organization (WTO) since 1995.

While the member making the largest contribution to the WHO regular budget is assessed at a maximum 25%, members making the smallest each pay 0.01%. Apart from its regular budget – US$842 654 000 for the biennium 1998–1999 – WHO receives voluntary contributions from both governmental and nongovernmental sources. In recent years the total amount of these contributions has been roughly equivalent to regular budget levels. They include contributions for fostering research in tropical diseases and human reproduction, improving community water supply, expanding immunization, preventing and controlling diarrhoeal diseases,

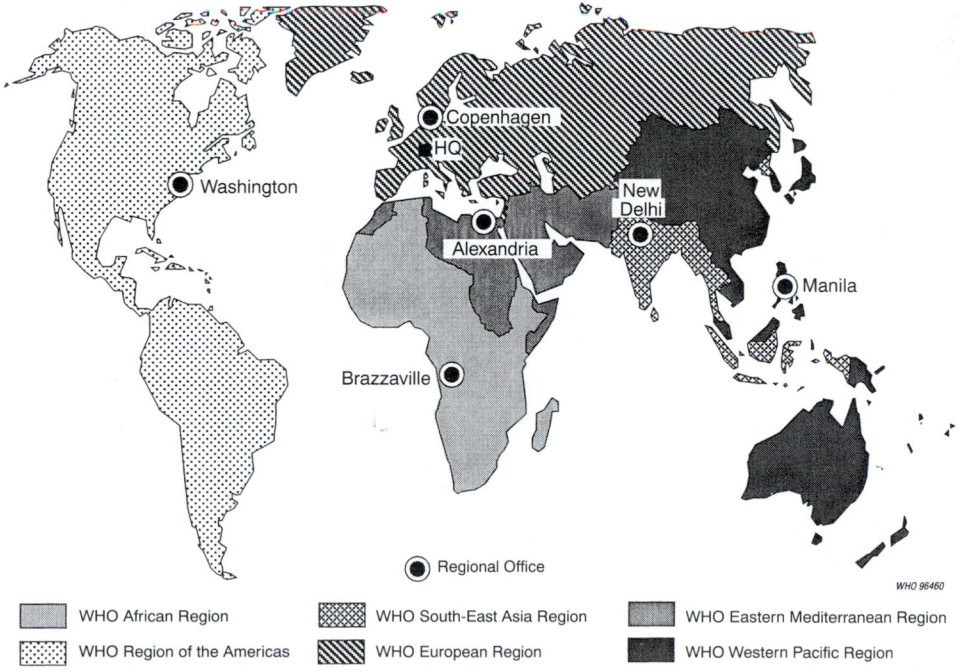

Figure 3 WHO regional offices and the areas they serve.

leprosy, malaria and yaws, and preparing a credible emergency health response to disasters and natural catastrophes.

Working with Others

From its beginning, WHO set out to work not through its small staff alone but with and through others. Many thousands of individual researchers and scientists, including Nobel laureates, have put their talents at the disposal of WHO – and their number continues to grow. The same is true of WHO collaborating centres, which have grown steadily in number and breadth of disciplines. Rather than duplicate efforts, WHO entrusts critical technical functions to established laboratories and research institutes.

From the outset, WHO was also mandated to work with other agencies within the newly created UN family of organizations. Food and nutrition work, for example, quite naturally came to involve the FAO, as did work against animal diseases and, as mentioned above, in the area of food additives, food standards, pesticide residues and contaminants. Later, WHO joined forces with the International Labour Organisation (ILO) and the United Nations Environment Programme (UNEP) in establishing the International Programme on Chemical Safety. Recognition of the increasing seriousness of the global burden of malnutrition led WHO and FAO to convene jointly, in Rome in December 1992, the International Conference on Nutrition, which was attended by over 1000 representatives of 159 Member States and the European Union. The resulting World Declaration and Plan of Action for Nutrition pledged to eliminate or substantially reduce the major forms of malnutrition and their contributing factors before the end of the decade. The Declaration's nine goals for the year 2000 and the strategy and actions of the Plan of Action serve as the platform for WHO's support to countries, especially those most in need, in five priority areas:

- assessment, prevention and management of protein–energy malnutrition;
- overcoming micronutrient malnutrition (chiefly iodine deficiency disorders, and vitamin A and iron deficiencies);
- improvements in infant and young child feeding (breast-feeding and complementary feeding);
- nutrition emergencies, particularly training in preparedness and management;
- prevention of diet-related noncommunicable diseases (including obesity, cardiovascular diseases and some cancers) and food-related communicable diseases (including diarrhoea and parasites).

The views of the United Nations Educational, Scientific and Cultural Organization (UNESCO) are regularly sought, for example on questions relating to bioethics and the health of schoolchildren. Occupational health is likewise a shared activity with the ILO, while drug dependence and abuse call for collaboration with the United Nations International Drug Control Programme. After nearly a decade of providing direct financial support and technical guidance for AIDS (acquired immunodeficiency syndrome) activities in more than 150 developing countries, in January 1996 WHO became one of the cosponsors, together with the United Nations Children's Fund (UNICEF), the United Nations Development Programme (UNDP), the United Nations Population Fund (UNFPA), UNESCO, and the World Bank, of the Joint United Nations Programme on HIV/AIDS (UNAIDS). Building on the relationship already established with the General Agreement on Tariffs and Trade (GATT), WHO works with the GATT's successor, the WTO, in connection with health-related Codex standards, guidelines and recommendations.

One of WHO's closest partners has been UNICEF, with which, for example, the early yaws and malaria campaigns were carried out. More recently, joint activities include support to countries in preventing and controlling micronutrient malnutrition and improving infant and young child feeding practices by promoting breast-feeding, and appropriate complementary feeding practices with emphasis on using locally available foods. To guide their concerted efforts in all fields, since 1948 the two agencies regularly confer on matters of joint health policy.

Collaboration was also initiated with professional, charitable and other nongovernmental organizations (NGOs) pursuing aims consonant with those of WHO. By the end of the first decade, WHO had established official relations with no fewer than 40 such bodies, ranging from the International Council of Nurses to the International Commission on Radiation Units and Measurements, and from the World Federation for Mental Health to the International Union of Nutritional Sciences. Work of vital importance for WHO's technical programmes of support for its membership has been made possible through the enthusiasm and resources of these and other valuable organizations, which have in turn benefited from the moral support and the technical information provided by WHO.

Collaboration continues unabated; examples include joint work on cancer pain relief with the International Association for the Study of Pain; efforts to ensure safe blood and blood products undertaken by WHO's Blood Safety unit together with the blood programmes of the International Federation of Red Cross and Red Crescent Societies, the International Society of Blood Transfusion, and the World Federation of Hemophilia; support for polio eradication provided through Rotary International; reinforcement of technical support to Member States for the prevention and control of iodine deficiency disorders with the help of the International Council for Control of Iodine Deficiency Disorders; and implementation of the Joint WHO/UNICEF Baby-friendly Hospital Initiative – which strives to ensure the world over a healthcare environment for new-borns where breast-feeding is the norm – with the help of La Leche League International and the International Lactation Consultant Association. The success of these joint ventures is most strikingly illustrated by the ever-lengthening list of NGOs admitted into official relations with WHO, which now numbers more than 190.

Gearing Up for the Twenty-first Century

Using pragmatic tools in pursuit of its visionary goal, WHO strives to respond to its constitutional mandate through its evolving programme of activities. These are based on the needs and priorities of activities determined by Member States themselves through the Organization's governing bodies, the World Health Assembly and the Executive Board. Changes in programme emphasis occur in response to altered political, social, economic and environmental realities.

For example, respecting the new issues and priorities of the times for WHO includes meeting the challenge implicit in redirecting the human and financial resources that, logically, should be released by the break-up of old cold-war alliances; forging new partnerships to mobilize social, political and therefore financial support for health development and international health cooperation; and opening itself up still further to all sectors of society, including NGOs and the private sector. It means grappling with the multiple consequences for health of accelerating social and demographic changes, including population growth and encroachment on forest areas and other ecological zones, ageing population structure, migration – including the mass movement of disaster-affected populations – and urbanization. It calls for dealing creatively with the impact of the indebtedness, incurred over time, that has led many countries to reduce public spending in health services, which are often regarded as being only an expenditure rather than an investment in human potential. Ironically, this last challenge comes at the very moment when WHO itself is operating within

severe financial constraints. After working with a zero-growth budget policy since 1984–1985, WHO's 1996–1997 budget suffered a drastic reduction estimated at 14% in real terms, while the number of staff worldwide dropped from just under 5400 in 1990 to 4300 in 1998. In contrast, the extraordinary changes in the political landscape during the same period saw the number of WHO Member States increase from 166 to 191.

WHO must face up to threats to human health that respect no national boundaries, such as uncontrolled dumping of toxic wastes and pollution of land, water and air, and prodigious consumption and mismanagement of natural resources. The solution of these problems hinges, to a large extent, on the degree to which WHO is able to harness the interdependence of nations and peoples as a positive force for conciliating between competing present and future needs.

In the face of changing demands, WHO is doing its utmost to preserve its inclusive approach to health and to emphasize the continuity between prevention, care, rehabilitation and health promotion for all people through the different stages of their lives. In restructuring its programmes and activities in the light of resource constraints, WHO is placing emphasis on meeting the most pressing health needs based on the following priorities:

- those which present a health emergency;
- those which affect the poorest countries and the most vulnerable groups;
- those which produce the heaviest burden of death, suffering and disability;
- those which represent a major impediment to social and economic development.

In 1995 the Executive Board and the World Health Assembly, as part of an overall global reform process, identified the need to review the basic primary healthcare principles of Alma-Ata, re-commit Member States to those principles, and renew aspects of the strategy to achieve *Health for All* in the light of changing global circumstances. Since 1978 many countries not present at Alma-Ata had attained statehood; a generation of health workers had graduated; and several key determinants of health – social, political, economic, demographic and epidemiological – had profoundly affected the health profile of populations and the level of inequalities between various subgroups. Moreover, the opportunity for improving health through multisectoral approaches, application of appropriate technology, and greater emphasis on participatory approaches all require that countries, regions and the international community look afresh at how international health policy for the next century can truly improve the long-term health status of the world's poorest countries and communities.

Food, Nutrition and World Health – Meeting the Global Challenge

Freedom from hunger and malnutrition, essential to the enjoyment of the highest attainable standard of health, is among the fundamental rights of every human being. What is more, there can be no sound social and economic development without adequate food and nutrition. This is not the same as saying that people in rich countries necessarily have a better chance of being properly nourished than do people in poor countries. There is much more to achieving healthy nutritional status than can be conveyed by such simplistic labels as 'developed' and 'developing' where countries – and most of all people – are concerned.

Even if there is some truth in the axiom 'we are what we eat', it is clear that nutritional status – a characteristic common to all that can be measured and monitored – depends on considerably more than diet. For individuals, it is best understood as the result of the complex interaction between health at any given moment, the food that is eaten, and the surrounding physical, social and economic environment. Nutritional status not only reflects the quantity of available food but also its quality, including safety, while showing to what extent the body can transform food into nutrients that will protect and promote health and permit people to function to the best advantage. Because the environment and its impact vary so greatly from individual to individual, there can be no 'standard' answer to the problem of malnutrition. Moreover, no single strategy to combat it will produce the same results in every case. The approach to preventing and overcoming malnutrition thus has to be tailored to fit the circumstances.

Nutrition and the Sweep of History

Looking back in history, one can see that a major shift is taking place in the impact on humanity of the main factors – poor diet and ill health – that have traditionally accounted for most malnutrition. Over the centuries the human species survived hand-to-mouth on whatever it could manage to hunt, gather, harvest or hoard. The diet which fuelled most of human evolution was low in fat and very low in sugar, but high in fibre and other complex carbohydrates.

In the overall context of human development, it is only recently that people in high-income countries could stop worrying about the threat of occasional hunger and increasingly indulge in preferred foods owing to radical improvements in methods of food production, processing, storage and distribution. Only in recent decades, as people benefited from greater control of infectious disease and better access to safe food, have research findings confirmed the well-founded suspicion that dietary preferences may influence the onset of several major chronic diseases, including coronary heart disease, stroke, various cancers, diabetes mellitus, gastrointestinal disorders, and various bone and joint diseases. Although many dietary factors have been investigated, those most frequently linked to such diseases figure prominently in a pattern of eating typified by the high consumption of energy-dense foods of animal origin and of foods processed or prepared with added fat, sugar and salt.

As a result, on the eve of the twenty-first century grade 2 overweight, which warrants close attention, is relatively common in industrialized and in many developing countries – up to 20% of Europeans and of Whites in the USA between 60 years of age are affected. The figure increases to 40% for women in eastern European and Mediterranean countries and Black women in the USA. Even higher prevalences are observed among American Indians, Hispanic Americans and Pacific islanders. While the prevalence of grade 2 overweight is much lower in some African and Asian countries – the range is about 3% to 17% – in South America and the Caribbean it is close to that in many European countries, about 25%. WHO estimates that major noncommunicable diseases (NCDs) are responsible for at least 40% of all deaths in developing countries and 75% in industrialized countries, where cardiovascular diseases are the first cause of mortality and cancer is the third. By the year 2020, NCDs will account for about three-quarters of all deaths in the developing world.

Meanwhile, over 800 million people still cannot meet basic needs for energy and protein, more than 2000 million people are deficient in essential micronutrients, and an estimated 174 million children under 5 years of age in developing countries are malnourished, as indicated by low weight for age, while 230 million are stunted. Malnutrition results in poor physical and cognitive development as well as lower resistance to illness. Nearly half of the estimated 11 million deaths occurring annually among children under 5 – or about 49% of young child mortality in developing countries – is associated with malnutrition.

Simultaneous Action on Two Overlapping Fronts

For these reasons, to promote healthy nutrition for

all people it is necessary to take simultaneous action on two distinct, if overlapping, fronts. On the one hand, many less-favoured nations remain handicapped by a formidable array of development constraints, including rapidly increasing population, unproductive agriculture, environmental degradation, limited health service coverage, and war and civil strife. Among the most visible – and tragic – consequences are the many millions of wasted and stunted children who do not have enough protein and energy in their diets, who suffer from cretinism and other permanent brain damage because their diets and those of their parents are deficient in iodine, or who go blind or even die for lack of vitamin A. It is in just such environments that diarrhoeal diseases resulting from contaminated food and water, frequently compounded by seasonal or chronic food shortages, take their heaviest toll in terms of malnutrition, ill health and premature death.

On the other hand, there has been a significant drop in recent years in the prevalence of infectious disease, while food availability and the quality of diets have improved for populations the world over. The result in many countries has been a sharp reduction in infant and child mortality and longer adult life expectancy. These and related factors have paved the way for a dramatic expansion of a different type of nutrition crisis: diet-related chronic disorders are now flourishing in environments where, not so long ago, infectious diseases were the greatest menace to health. Too often, one type of malnutrition is being exchanged, or – worse still – being superimposed upon another, with no net gain for human health in the process.

Labels such as 'rich' or 'poor' and 'developed' or 'developing', by themselves, provide little insight into what causes malnutrition and how it can be overcome. The fact is, wherever people reside, it is the *way they live, what they eat* and *how they interact with their environment* that determine their nutritional status. Healthy nutritional status is by no means the monopoly of rich countries, any more than malnutrition is somehow the prerogative of poor ones. Whatever the cultural influences at work in a given milieu, all governments are challenged to develop food and nutrition policies that will make healthy choices the easy choices for their populations. Consistent with the unique normative, scientific and advisory role that WHO has played for the last half century, the Organization strives to support all its 191 Member States in doing just this.

See also: **Adaptation**: Overview of Adaptive Responses to Malnutrition. **Ageing**: Biological Aspects. **Anaemia**

(Anemia): Iron-Deficiency Anaemia; Megaloblastic Anaemia. **Antioxidants**: Observational Epidemiology; Intervention Studies. **Appetite**: Physiological and Neurobiological Aspects; Psychobiological and Behavioural Aspects. **Bioavailability**: Definition and General Aspects. **Body Composition**: Determination and Physiological Significance. **Cancer**: Epidemiology and Associations Between Diet and Cancer; Epidemiology of Breast Cancer; Epidemiology of Colorectal Cancer; Epidemiology of Lung Cancer; Epidemiology of Gastrointestinal Cancers Other Than Colorectal Cancers; Diet in Cancer Treatment. **Carotenoids**: Chemistry, Sources and Physiology; Epidemiology. **Catering**: Nutritional Aspects. **Children**: Nutritional Problems of Preschool Children. **Coronary Heart Disease**: Lipid Theory of Coronary Heart Disease; Haemostatic Factors and Coronary Heart Disease; Aetiology; Prevention. **Diabetes Mellitus**: Classification and Chemical Pathology; Aetiology and Epidemiology; Dietary Management; Secondary Complications and Their Prevention. **Diarrhoeal (Diarrheal) Diseases**: Nutritional Factors. **Dietary Guidelines**: International Perspectives. **Energy**: Energy Balance; Measurement of Energy Intake and Expenditure. **Food Aid**: Overview. **Food Contaminants**: Mycotoxins - Occurrence and Toxic Effects; Pesticides. **Food Fortification**: Importance in the Diet. **Growth and Development**: Physiological Aspects. **Infants**: Nutritional Requirements; Milk-feeding and Weaning; Feeding Problems; Low-birthweight and Preterm Infants. **Iodine**: Physiology, Dietary Sources and Requirements; Iodine Deficiency Disorders. **Iron**: Physiology, Dietary Sources and Requirements. **Lactation**: Physiology; Dietary Requirements. **Malnutrition**: Definition, Classification and Epidemiology; Primary Malnutrition; Secondary Malnutrition. **Nutrient Requirements**: International Perspectives. **Nutrition Policies**: In Developed Countries; In Developing Countries. **Nutritional Status**: Dietary Assessment; Anthropometric Assessment; Biochemical Assessment; Clinical Examination. **Nutritional Surveillance**: In Industrialized and Developing Countries. **Obesity**: Definition, Aetiology and Assessment; Early Obesity and Prognosis; Fat Distribution; Treatment; Prevention; Complications of Obesity. **Osteoporosis**: Aetiology; Treatment and Prevention. **Protein**: Digestion and Bioavailability; Quality and Sources; Requirements and Role in Diet; Synthesis and Turnover; Deficiency. **Retinol**: Physiology; Hypovitaminosis A. **United Nations Children's Fund**: History and Role.

Further Reading

All of the following are available from World Health Organization, Distribution and Sales, 1211 Geneva 27, Switzerland, fax (+41–22) 791–4857. e-mail: publications@who.ch

WHO (1987) *Principles for the Safety Assessment of Food Additives and Contaminants in Food.*

WHO (1988a) *Four Decades of Achievement: Highlights of the Work of WHO.*

WHO (1988b) *A Guide to Nutritional Assessment.*

WHO (1990a) *Diet, Nutrition and the Prevention of Chronic Diseases.* World Health Organization Technical Report Series 797.

WHO (1990b) *Principles for the Toxicological Assessment of Pesticide Residues in Food.*

WHO (1991a) *Food Additives, Food Contaminants and Veterinary Drug Residues in Food.* A complete guide to reports issued by the Joint FAO/WHO Expert Committee on Food Additives.

WHO (1991b) *Joint FAO/WHO Expert Committee on Food Additives: Index of Substances Evaluated from 1st to 37th Meeting (1957–1991).*

WHO (1991c) *Strategies for Assessing the Safety of Foods Produced by Biotechnology.*

WHO (1992) *Hazard Analysis Critical Control Point Evaluations. A Guide to Identifying Hazards and Assessing Risks Associated with Food Preparation and Storage.*

WHO (1994a) *An Evaluation of Infant Growth.*

WHO (1994b) *Indicators for Assessing Iodine Deficiency Disorders and their Control through Salt Iodization.*

WHO (1994c) *Safety and Nutritional Adequacy of Irradiated Food.*

WHO (1995a) *Physical Status: the Use and Interpretation of Anthropometry.* World Health Organization Technical Report Series 854.

WHO (1995b) *Vitamin A Deficiency and its Consequences. A Field Guide to Detection and Control.*

WHO (1995c) *Global Prevalence of Vitamin A Deficiency.*

WHO (1996a) *The World Health Report 1996. Fighting Disease, Fostering Development.*

WHO (1996b) *Trace Elements in Human Nutrition and Health.*

WHO (1996c) *Indicators for Assessing Vitamin A Deficiency and their Application in Monitoring and Evaluating Intervention Programmes.*

WHO (1996d) *The International Code of Marketing of Breast-milk Substitutes.* A common review and evaluation framework.

WHO (1997a) *WHO Global Database on Child Growth and Malnutrition.*

WHO (1998a) *Obesity: Preventing and Managing the Global Epidemic.*

WHO (1998b) *Safe Vitamin A Dosage During Pregnancy and Lactation.*

WHO (1998c) *Preparation and Use of Food-based Dietary Guidelines.*

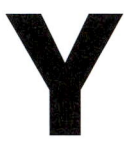

Yogurt *see* **Dairy Products**: Nutritional Value. **Functional Foods**: Definition and Potential for Nutritional Role. **Probiotics and Prebiotics**: Definition and Role.

Z

ZINC

Physiology

N W Solomons, CeSSIAM, Guatemala City, Guatemala

The element zinc was first shown to be an essential nutrient for bread mould (*Aspergillus niger*) by the French scientist, Raulin, in 1869. It was not until the twentieth century, however, that the ramifications of its essentiality for higher species were understood, first with the demonstration of its essentiality in laboratory rodents in the 1930s, followed by the discovery of deficiency syndromes in livestock in the 1950s. In the same decade, secondary (conditioned) zinc deficiency in alcoholic cirrhosis was documented, and in the 1960s, endemic zinc deficiency at the community level based on dietary factors was described.

Absorption, Transport, Distribution, Storage and Excretion of Zinc

Absorption

The maximal fractional absorption of zinc in humans is 40% from an aqueous solution, with absorption in the presence of food ranging from 1% to 40%. Zinc is absorbed by two different mechanisms. One is passive diffusion down a concentration gradient, from a higher concentration in the inner lumen of the intestinal tract to a lower concentration in the circulation; the other is an active, energy-dependent pump, linked to ATP and the action of an ATPase. Zinc can be transported across the membrane of the intestinal cell in its soluble, ionic, divalent $Zn(II)$ state, or bound to an amino acid or other small molecule that is being taken up into the cell. As in the case of iron, the extent of zinc uptake into the body is regulated in a homeostatic fashion, depending upon the adequacy of zinc status. The intestine of a zinc-sufficient individual takes up the metal with less efficiency than that of a zinc-deficient one.

Zinc in foods is enmeshed in a matrix of the organic structure of the plant and animal tissues, incorporated into proteins or chelated to binding surfaces. All the processes of intraalimentary tract dissociation and digestion bear on making zinc more available for eventual absorption. Dietary factors effecting the inhibition of absorption include binding substances and complexing agents such as phytate, dietary fibre, oxalate and polyphenols (tannins). Foods of plant origin such as soya products, wholegrains and legumes, leafy vegetables, coffee and tea contain the aforementioned inhibitors. Competitive interactions exist between zinc and other cations. Iron interferes with zinc uptake when the iron/zinc ratio exceeds 2 : 1. Calcium also inhibits zinc uptake, most probably by a similar nutrient competition mechanism; this fact has implications for zinc consumed in meals with milk, cheese and dairy products. Enhancement of dietary zinc absorption is generally considered only to be the consequence of minimizing the inhibitors to the lowest level. In food, enhancers of zinc absorption have been detected only once, in a specific variety of red wine (Zinfandel); taken with a meal, this wine increased the amount of zinc absorbed.

Transport

Recently absorbed zinc enters the portal circulation and is carried by albumin to the liver and beyond. Forty per cent of zinc in the circulation is tightly bound, incorporated into α_2-macroglobulin, a zinc metalloprotein. The remaining 60% is more loosely bound to albumin and chelated with free amino acids or small peptides, and is believed to be the nutritionally relevant transport fraction. The amount of zinc in the circulation at any given time represents 0.1% of total-body zinc.

Each meal cycle results in a decrement in circulating zinc, possibly as a result of the resynthesis of pancreatic proteases and the formation of pancreatic juice in anticipation of the next meal. Over the course of the day, a 30% decline compared with early morning fasting levels is established. In short-term fasting, in contrast, there is a transient *increase* in circulating levels of zinc, related most probably to its release from muscle. Hormonal influences also affect zinc concentration in the circulation: oestrogens lower zinc levels. The cytokine mediators of the acute-phase response to injury, infection or inflammation produce a profound decrement of up to 60% in plasma zinc, sequestering the entire loosely bound fraction in liver. A teleological explanation that zinc is assisting in the rapid hepatic production of acute-phase proteins has been proffered for this redistribution.

Distribution and storage

The best estimate of the total-body zinc for an adult human being is 2–3 g. For a 70 kg man, this would be 0.04% of the total mass. The highest concentrations of zinc are found in the pancreas and the gonads, but 57% of the zinc in the body is in skeletal muscle and 30% is in the skeleton, with 6% in integumentary tissues. Unlike iron, no 'storage pool' or 'nutritional reserves' of zinc are recognized. Zinc deposited in bone cannot be mobilized for nutritional purposes, and zinc in skeletal muscle is resistant to depletion even in situations of restricted zinc intake. Hence, the organism is relatively dependent upon a constant renewed supply of the metal to replenish the amounts normally lost daily.

Classical radioisotopic studies showed that zinc in the body turnover has a short half-life and long half-life component, but more complex, multiple-pool models have recently been advanced. The zinc that enters what has been termed the 'active nutritional pool' is managed by the liver, which contains 5% of body zinc. This is part of a 'rapidly exchangeable pool' which probably also involves the plasma and pancreas within its axis. The newly absorbed zinc serves to replace losses in adults; in children and in persons recovering from undernutrition, it is also required for participation in growth and to occupy sites in newly formed tissue, in addition to replacement of losses.

Excretion

Excretion into the faecal stream via pancreatic and intestinal secretions is not tightly regulated. The amount of zinc that enters the intestinal lumen appears to vary with the composition of the meal. Zinc shows an enteropancreatic circulation; that is, zinc enters the gut as part of meal-stimulated release of pancreatic juice only to be absorbed, in part, further down the intestine. Zinc that reaches the colon is only minimally absorbed thereafter. The faecal content is a combination of zinc that has not been absorbed from the food and zinc that has not been reabsorbed from endogenous secretions. Excretion of zinc via the intestine is also regulated in a homeostatic way. At the extremes of nutritional status, there is enhanced zinc secretion to promote its loss or decreased excretion to promote its conservation.

Daily losses of zinc in urine represent only about one-tenth or less of that lost via the faecal route. The kidney reabsorbs most of the zinc presented to it, allowing about 0.5 mg to pass into the urine. When zinc status is low, urinary excretion is also low and does not rise to normal until the body pool is expanded to normal.

Other sources of zinc loss, amounting to 1–2 mg daily, are those from the turnover of integumentary tissues, skin, hair and nails. Semen is rich in zinc, and up to 1 mg is contained in an ejaculum. Women lose some zinc within the red cells making up their menstrual periods.

Lactation represents a special form of zinc excretion. As zinc has no nutritional reserves, its supply to breast milk in nursing mothers is interesting. Zinc in milk is only poorly correlated with the maternal circulating zinc levels. A mechanism other than pure filtration by the breast must be responsible for the uptake of zinc from the maternal supply into mammary secretions. A Finnish study showed that 40 mg of zinc daily – but not 20 mg – increased the content of the element in breast milk; more zinc in milk, however, was not associated with more zinc in the circulation of the infants. In fact, the more rapidly growing infants had the *lowest* plasma zinc concentrations. A curious disorder in which the mammary gland does not incorporate zinc into the milk has been identified; offspring of such mothers are at risk of early-life zinc deficiency.

Metabolic Function and Essentiality of Zinc

Chemical characteristics

Zinc is an element in the transition metal series, number 30 in the periodic table of elements, with an atomic weight of 65.37. Zinc exists in an ionic form exclusively as a divalent cation. It has no redox potential either for being oxidized or reduced. It has a small ionic radius which gives it a strong electrostatic charge. It exhibits flexible coordination geometry and demonstrates rapid ligand exchange. In nature there are five stable isotopes with distinct relative abundances (rounded off, and in descending order): ^{64}Zn (49%); ^{66}Zn (29%); ^{68}Zn (19%); ^{67}Zn (4%); ^{70}Zn (1%). Two radioisotopes have been used as tracers in biological studies: ^{65}Zn and ^{69m}Zn.

Zinc metalloenzymes

Zinc exercises part of its physiological role as a component of zinc metalloenzymes. The first to be characterized was carbonic anhydrase. Alcohol dehydrogenase was the second. The number of enzymes in which zinc is claimed to be a tightly coordinated, essential constituent for the structural conformation, catalytic function or both (i.e. a metalloenzyme) ranges from 200 to 700. The enzymes containing zinc include all classes. Pancreatic proteases such as carboxypeptidases contain zinc. Many of the enzymes involved in transcription and translation of the genetic message and in the synthesis of nucleotide bases are zinc metalloenzymes.

Zinc fingers

A pervasive role for zinc's regulation of both genetic and protein–protein interactions has emerged in the advent of our understanding of the 'zinc finger' motif of regulatory proteins. This is a clustered sequence along a peptide chain with four cysteine residues alternating with other amino acids (or with cysteine and histidine residues); it allows zinc to form a tetrahedral complex, providing structural rigidity to the protein. The knuckling of the protein strand around this complex provides the origin of the term 'zinc finger'. Zinc finger domains are found in regulatory proteins. Some of the proteins are transcription factors in the nucleus that are sensitive to hormonal messengers such as retinoic acid or vitamin D_3. Zinc fingers are found in cytosolic proteins as well, suggesting a role for zinc in protein–protein interaction or cellular translocation of proteins and organelles.

Ionic zinc

After divalent cations such as calcium and magnesium, zinc is the most common divalent ion in the cytoplasm of cells. There is evidence that ionic zinc plays a role in membrane stabilization and in the assembly of polyribosomes. Soluble zinc may also be important in the regulation of gene expression, specifically of metallothioneine (MT), in which zinc inhibits the expression of MT. A subcellular mechanism involves (1) a metal regulatory element as part of the promoter of the regulatory gene for MT expression on the DNA strand of the chromosome; and (2) a metal-binding transcription factor which is sensitive to – and binds – zinc in the cell cytosol and nucleus. This function may be more generalized than just the regulation of zinc. There is evidence for regulation of the expression of other genes by heavy metals, notably zinc, in systems related to the transcription of certain acute-phase proteins.

Manifestations of zinc deficiency

Zinc deficiency has a range of manifestations, depending upon the severity of the restriction of the nutrient. What could be termed 'mild' zinc deficiency would not be detected on clinical examination. It represents functions that are being limited by a less than adequate availability of zinc, probably at the level of the rapidly exchangeable intra- and extracellular pools. Growth retardation and delayed development of children is one manifestation. Zinc deficiency is associated with a decrease in nitrogen retention, and this is an early occurrence in depletion of the nutrient. Teratogenesis is worth mentioning in the context of mild human zinc deficiency. The adverse effects of experimental maternal deficiency of zinc on embryonic and fetal development and on the birthing process have been well defined in rodent and small ruminant models. It has been suggested that up to half of the idiopathic anatomical birth defects in human newborns worldwide, including those of the neural tube, could be the result of marginal zinc status of the mothers.

Severe deficiency leads to anatomical and physiological 'lesions' that can be documented in a review of symptoms and an examination of the patient for physical signs. The growth effects are more profound, and frank failure to thrive may be manifest in infants and toddlers. Zinc deficiency has dermatological manifestations ranging from mild, generalized drying to a specific hyperkeratosis in the areas of pressure and stress points such as over elbow and knee joints and in the perioral area. Atrophic changes of the gastrointestinal mucosa occur and diarrhoea or loose stools may be present. Neurological and mental status examinations may reveal seizures in zinc-deficient infants. Anorexia, often associated with reports of disturbed taste and smell, is reported. Constitutional manifestations of irritability, depression, apathy and emotional lability are seen in advanced zinc deficiency. Sperm counts and sex hormone levels will be low in men, resulting in problems of libido and fertility. Immunosuppression of various parts of the host defence system can also be seen on laboratory evaluation.

Assessment of Zinc Status

Zinc status can be assessed at two levels: that of the individual patient, and that of population; both have important implications. The former assessment is relevant to clinical practice and its purpose is to assist in making a specific diagnosis for the patient in question; the latter is relevant to epidemiology and public health, and is intended to provide information about environmental (including dietary) influences at the community level, or for planning a corrective intervention, or both. The requirements for indicators in these two situations are quite distinct.

The first step in assessment of zinc status is to recognize the situations in which zinc deficiency can occur. For individual patients, clinicians must keep in mind a roster of diseases and conditions that favour zinc depletion (see below) and be attuned to the possibility of deficiency. In epidemiological and public health surveys, certain environmental and dietary situations predispose to deficiency, such as the zinc content of the soil, inhibiting substances in the diet, or communicable or genetic diseases endemic to the population.

In a general sense, the question of how much zinc is present in the body is central, but this cannot be measured directly in the living individual. When applicable, total body neutron activation can provide a signal related to the body's content. Alternatively, an isotopic dilution and/or total-body content of a nutrient. This assessment is feasible to perform for zinc; however, the use of radioisotopes represents a mild biohazard to the subject and the environment; and using stable isotope tracers of zinc involves tedious and laborious procedures. In the clinical setting, a combination of biochemical and laboratory tests and physical examination is used; the assessment strategy at the population level involves biochemical tests and functional indicators.

Zinc depletion is a type II deficiency. It shares with nitrogen, potassium, sodium, magnesium and chloride the characteristics that (1) there are no true stores of the nutrient; (2) the organism will not tolerate desaturation of tissues and will activate conservation mechanisms early on in any restriction; and (3) in young organisms, cessation of growth is an adaptive mechanism to reduce demand for the nutrient. This has profound implications for the conventional strategy of nutritional assessment, which is to assay body fluids and tissues for the nutrient.

With respect to indirect markers of status, serum or plasma zinc is the traditional index. Levels in the circulation will fall in deficiency, but zinc levels show false positive depressions with a number of conditions such as medication use and infections, while false negative results derive from haemolysis of samples, external contamination and improper sampling techniques. Measuring zinc in all circulating cellular elements (including red cells, all classes of white cells and platelets), in saliva, in cerumen, in hair, in nails, in buccal mucosa and in urine has been explored. All have severe limitations in validity and reliability with respect to individual status, although each might have legitimate application on a population survey basis.

Functional tests are an alternative that conforms to the type II nature of the deficiency of zinc. The activity of specific metalloenzymes is an approach that has reasonable potential. Another approach is to assess the state of regulatory conservation of the nutrient. Increased efficiency of absorption or decreased fractional urinary excretion of a zinc load represent evidence for zinc deficiency. Tests of dark adaptation, taste acuity and olfactory acuity represent a battery of neurological probes related to the dysfunction caused by deficiency. Tests of immunological function such as cellular immunity or specific B cell counts could be responsive to zinc depletion and repletion. In the child, growth patterns could be indicative of zinc status. The aforementioned functional indices, however, are relatively nonspecific, occurring in many conditions other than zinc deficiency. The most effective use of these tests would be in conjunction with a therapeutic trial with oral zinc administration. The advances in understanding of molecular regulation of zinc and zinc's role in regulation will enable more specific functional tests to be devised. These include tests of metallothionein regulation via mRNA, and cellular uptake of zinc under near-physiological conditions in the culture milieu.

Occurrence of zinc deficiency

Five generic mechanisms for the development of a nutrient deficiency have been identified: reduced intake; impaired uptake; increased losses; impaired utilization; and increased requirements. Based on one or a combination of these mechanisms, certain clinical situations predispose to overt zinc depletion. These include acrodermatitis enteropathica; anorexia nervosa and bulimia; unsupplemented total parenteral alimentation; malabsorptive syndromes such as cystic fibrosis, coeliac disease, short bowel syndrome and inflammatory bowel disease; alcoholic and posthepatitic cirrhosis; sickle-cell disease and other haemoglobinopathies; chronic renal disease; and chronic debilitating diseases such as haematological malignancies and solid tumours.

Zinc Nutritional Requirements

In theory, the daily zinc requirements of an individual should be the amount needed to replace that day's loss, or for replacement, growth and new tissue accretion in the growing child. In the special cases of pregnancy and injury, the requirements include the growth of the products of conception and that needed for tissue repair, respectively. During lactation, zinc lost in the milk is accounted for in the requirements. Taking into consideration the selection

Table 1 Recommended dietary allowances for zinc

	Age (years)	Zinc (mg per day)
Infants	0.0–1.0	5.0
Children	1–10	10.0
Males	11–50	15.0
	51+	15.0
Females	11–50	12.0
	51+	12.0
Pregnant		
1st trimester		15.0
2nd trimester		15.0
3rd trimester		15.0
Lactating		
1st semester		19.0
2nd semester		16.0

Data from National Research Council (1989).

of diet and the specific efficiency of zinc uptake from that fare, the daily intake requirement of an individual would be the amount of zinc in foods and beverages that would permit uptake of the given amount of zinc to be replaced (and deposited). Because of both dietary factors and genetic variability, these requirements vary widely even between individuals of the same age group and gender.

There is a subtle, but important, distinction between 'requirement' and 'recommended intake'. Whereas daily requirement is based on amounts gained and lost by the body, the recommended daily intake is that to be consumed to permit for the uptake into the body of the amount needed to replace losses or provide for growth. Two tables of recommended intakes are shown here: the recommended dietary allowances for the USA (**Table 1**), and the World Health recommendations (**Table 2**). The former provides recommendations for *individuals*, and the latter for *populations*. As a practical matter, the amount of zinc recommended for consumption varies less than individual energy requirements across age groups. This means that very different dietary zinc densities (**Table 3**) would be needed to satisfy the recommended intakes of various family members. This presents practical problems, as families generally share the same meal.

Dietary Sources and High Intakes of Zinc

As zinc is an essential nutrient for both plants and animals, it is widely distributed in human diets. Breast milk zinc concentrations range from 2 mg to 3 mg per litre. Milk zinc content varies with the

Table 2 Lower limits (mg per day) of the safe ranges of population mean intakes of dietary zinc to meet the requirements for Zn^{basal}_{Plmin} and $Zn^{normative}_{Plmin}$ from diets differing in zinc bioavailability[a]

Age range (years)	Sex	Assumed weight (kg)	A. High availability		B. Moderate availability		C. Low availability	
			Zn^{basal}_{Plmin}	$Zn^{normative}_{Plmin}$	Zn^{basal}_{Plmin}	$Zn^{normative}_{Plmin}$	Zn^{basal}_{Plmin}	$Zn^{normative}_{Plmin}$
0–0.25	F	5	1.2[b]	–	3.1[c]	–	7.1[d]	–
0–0.25	M	5	1.3[b]	–	3.4[c]		8.0[d]	
0.25–0.5	M&F	7	0.7[b]	–	1.9[c]		4.7[d]	
0.5–1	M&F	9	0.8[b]	–	–	–	–	–
0.5–1	M&F	9	2.2[e]	3.3[e]	3.4	5.6	8.0	11.1
1–3	M&F	12	2.1	3.3	3.4	5.5	7.9	11.0
3–6	M&F	17	2.5	3.9	3.9	6.5	9.2	12.9
6–10	M&F	25	2.9	4.5	4.6	7.5	10.7	15.0
10–12	F	37	3.3	5.0	5.1	8.4	12.0	16.8
12–15	F	48	4.0	6.1	6.3	10.3	14.7	20.6
15–18	F	55	4.0	6.2	6.3	10.2	14.6	20.6
18–60+	F	55	2.5	4.0	4.0	6.5	9.4	13.1
10–12	M	35	3.6	5.6	5.7	9.3	13.4	18.7
12–15	M	48	4.7	7.3	7.4	12.1	17.4	24.3
15–18	M	64	5.1	7.8	8.1	13.1	18.7	26.2
18–60+	M	65	3.6	5.6	5.7	9.4	13.4	18.7

[a]Unless otherwise specified, the CV of usual dietary zinc intakes is assumed to be 25%.
[b]Breast-fed infants receiving maternal milk only; assumed CV of intake 12.5%; assumed availability 80%.
[c]Formula-fed infants; category B availability for whey-adjusted milk formulae and for infants partly breast-fed or given low-phylate feeds supplemented with other liquid milks; assumed CV 12.5%.
[d]Formula-fed infants: category C availability applicable to phylate-rich, vegetable protein-based formulae with or without wholegrain cereals; CV 12.5%.
[e]Not applicable to infants consuming breast milk only.
From World Health Organization (1995) with permission.

Table 3 Classification of dietary zinc sources based on nutrient-energy density

Zinc category (mg per 1000 kcal)	Foods
Very poor (0–2)	Fats, oils, butter, cream cheese, sweets, chocolate, soft drinks, alcoholic drinks, sugars, jams and preserves
Poor (1–5)	Fish, fruits, refined cereal products, pastries, biscuits, cakes, puddings, tubers, plantains, sausage, french fries
Rich (4–12)	Wholegrains, pork, poultry, milk, low-fat cheese, yogurt, eggs, nuts
Very rich (12–882)	Lamb, leafy and root vegetables, crustacea, beef kidney, liver and heart, molluscs

From Solomons and Shrimpton (1983) with permission.

duration of lactation, among different nursing mothers at the same stages of lactations, and across geographical groups. The consumption of zinc from typical daily intakes of breast milk are lower than those recommended for infants, but an extraordinarily high efficiency of absorption allows adequate amounts to enter the infant's body.

The highest concentrations of zinc (up to 1 mg g^{-1}) are found in Atlantic oysters. Species of herring are second. Other fish and seafoods are rich in this metal. The densities of zinc in red meat and cereal grains are comparable, but red meat lacks any substances that would inhibit the absorption of the nutrient. The body has a high tolerance for intakes of zinc in excess of requirements, as these can generally be eliminated from the body. High oral intakes from supplements produce a metallic taste in the mouth and can produce gastric irritations and erosions. Prolonged intakes of 100 mg or more will inhibit the absorption of copper, and can produce copper deficiency anaemia.

Putative benefits for intakes of zinc in excess of requirements has been claimed for a number of diseases in which a primary zinc deficiency is not the basis. Of the conditions for which zinc has been recommended, its use as a decoppering agent in Wilson's disease is confirmed. Legitimate evidence of its efficacy in acne, peptic ulcer disease, and as a lozenge for the symptoms of the common cold can be documented. However, owing to their irritant and toxic properties, supplements containing more than twice the recommended daily intake should be used with caution. Moreover, there may be adverse interactions with excess zinc that have yet to be characterized. Professor Robert Cousins has stated: 'The concern is that nutrient imbalances and interactions caused by selective supplementation may produce toxicity not encountered with usual dietary practices'.

See also: **Adolescents**: Dietary Habits and Nutrient Requirements. **Alcohol**: Effects of Alcohol Consumption on Diet and Nutritional Status. **Children**: Nutritional Requirements of School Children. **Coeliac Disease**: Aetiology and Nutritional Management. **Cystic Fibrosis**: Dietary Aspects and Nutritional Management. **Dehydration**: Physiological Effects and Management. **Dietary Fibre (Fiber)**: Physiological Effects and Effects on Absorption. **Drugs**: Drug-Nutrient Interactions. **Food Processing**: Nutritional Influences. **Growth and Development**: Physiological Aspects. **Heavy Metals**: Toxicology. **HIV Disease**: Nutritional Management. **Immunity**: Role of Iron and Zinc. **Infants**: Nutritional Requirements. **Infection**: Nutritional Interactions. **Lactation**: Physiology. **Liver Disorders**: Nutritional Management. **Malnutrition**: Primary Malnutrition. **Nutritional Status**: Biochemical Assessment. **Nutritional Support**: Enteral Feeding; Parenteral Nutrition. **Older People**: Nutritional Requirements. **Parasitism**: Effects on Growth and Nutritional Status. **World Health Organization**: Role.

Further Reading

Cousins RJ (1996) Zinc. In: Filer JL and Ziegler E (eds) *Present Knowledge in Nutrition*, 7th edn, chap. 29, pp 296–306. Washington: ILSI Press.

Golden MHN (1994) Growth failure. Type I and type II nutrients. *SCN News* 12:10–14.

Herbert V (1968) The vitamins. In: Goodhart RS and Shils ME (eds) *Modern Nutrition in Health and Disease*, 5th edn, pp 221–244. Philadelphia: Lea & Febiger.

National Research Council (1989) *Recommended Dietary Allowances*, 9th edn. Washington: National Academy Press.

Solomons NW (1986) Competitive interaction of iron and zinc in the diet: consequences for human nutrition. *Journal of Nutrition* 116:927–935.

Solomons NW (1988) Zinc and copper. In: Shils ME and Young VR (eds) *Modern Nutrition in Health and Disease*, 7th edn, chap. 9, pp 238–262. Philadelphia: Lea & Febiger.

Solomons NW and Cousins RJ (1984) Zinc. In: Solomons NW and Rosenberg IH (eds) *Absorption and Malabsorption of Mineral Nutrients*, pp 125–197. New York: Alan R. Liss.

Solomons NW and Shrimpton R (1983) Zinc. In: Warren

K and Mahmoud AF (eds) *Tropical and Geographic Medicine*, pp 1059–1063. New York: McGraw-Hill.

Walsh CT, Sandstead HH, Prasad AS, Newberne PM and Fraker PJ (1994) Zinc: health effects and research pri-orities for the 1990s. *Environmental Health Perspectives* 102 (supplement 2): 5–46.

World Health Organization (1995) *Trace Elements in Human Health and Nutrition*. Geneva: WHO.

APPENDIX I

Food and Drug Administration Pesticide Program

Residue Monitoring 1995

This is the ninth annual report summarizing the results of the Food and Drug Administration's (FDA) pesticide residue monitoring program. The 8 previous reports, which were published in the *Journal of the Association of Official Analytical Chemists/Journal of AOAC International*, presented results from Fiscal Years (FY) 1987 through 1994. This current report includes findings obtained during FY95 (October 1, 1994 through September 30, 1995) under regulatory and incidence/level monitoring. Selected Total Diet Study findings for 1995 are also presented. Results in this and earlier reports continue to demonstrate that levels of pesticide residues in the U.S. food supply are well below established safety standards.

FDA Monitoring Program

Three federal government agencies share responsibility for the regulation of pesticides [1]. The Environmental Protection Agency (EPA) registers (i.e., approves) the use of pesticides and sets tolerances (the maximum amount of a residue that is permitted in or on a food) if use of that particular pesticide may result in residues in or on food [2]. Except for meat, poultry, and certain egg products, for which the Food Safety and Inspection Service (FSIS) of the U.S. Department of Agriculture (USDA) is responsible, FDA is charged with enforcing tolerances in imported foods and in domestically produced foods shipped in interstate commerce. FDA also acquires incidence/level data on particular commodity/pesticide combinations and carries out its market basket survey, the Total Diet Study. For 5 years, USDA's Agricultural Marketing Service (AMS), through contracts with participating states, has carried out a residue testing program directed primarily at raw agricultural products. FSIS and AMS report their pesticide residue data independently.

Regulatory Monitoring

Under this approach to pesticide residue monitoring, FDA samples individual lots of domestically produced and imported foods and analyzes them for pesticide residues to enforce the tolerances set by EPA. Domestic samples are collected as close as possible to the point of production in the distribution system; import samples are collected at the point of entry into U.S. commerce. Emphasis is on the raw agricultural product, which is analyzed as the unwashed, whole (unpeeled), raw commodity. Processed foods are also included. If illegal residues (above EPA tolerance or no tolerance for that particular food/pesticide combination) are found in domestic samples, FDA can invoke various sanctions, such as a seizure or injunction. For imports, shipments may be stopped at the port of entry when illegal residues are found. "Automatic detention" may be invoked for imports based on the finding of 1 violative shipment if there is reason to believe that the same situation will exist in future lots during the same shipping season for a specific shipper, grower, geographic area, or country.

Domestic and import food samples collected are classified as either "surveillance" or "compliance". Most samples collected by FDA are the surveillance type; that is, there is no prior knowledge or evidence that a specific food shipment contains illegal pesticide residues. Compliance samples are taken as follow-up to the finding of an illegal residue or when other evidence indicates that a pesticide residue problem may exist.

Factors considered by FDA in planning the types and numbers of samples to collect include review of recently generated state and FDA residue data, regional intelligence on pesticide use, dietary importance of the food, information on the amount of domestic food that enters interstate commerce and of imported food, chemical characteristics and toxicity of the pesticide, and production volume/pesticide usage patterns.

Analytical Methods   To analyze the large numbers of samples whose pesticide treatment history is usually unknown, FDA uses analytical methods capable of simultaneously determining a number of pesticide residues. These multiresidue methods (MRMs) can determine about half of the approximately 400 pesticides with EPA tolerances, and many others that have no tolerances. The most commonly used MRMs can also detect many metabolites, impurities, and alteration products of pesticides [3].

Single residue methods (SRMs) or selective MRMs are used to determine some pesticide residues in foods [3]. An SRM usually determines 1 pesticide; a selective MRM measures a relatively small number of chemically related pesticides. These types of methods are usually more resource-intensive per residue. Therefore, they are much less cost effective than MRMs.

The lower limit of residue measurement in FDA's determination of a specific pesticide is usually well below tolerance levels, which generally range from 0.1 to 50 parts per million (ppm). Residues present at 0.01 ppm and above are usually measurable; however, for individual pesticides, this limit may range from 0.005 to 1 ppm. In this report, the term "trace" is used to indicate residues detected, but at levels below the limit of quantitation (LQ).

FDA/State Cooperation   Personnel in FDA field offices interact with their counterparts in many states to increase FDA's effectiveness in pesticide residue monitoring. In most cases, work-sharing agreements (Memoranda of Understanding) have been established between FDA and various state agencies.

FDA also acquires and uses state-generated pesticide residue data to complement its own and other federally sponsored residue programs. For many years, FDA has supported, through a contract with Mississippi State University (MSU), the "Foodcontam" database, which is a compilation of state-collected residue data.

Animal Feeds   In addition to monitoring foods for human consumption, FDA also samples and analyzes domestic and imported feeds for pesticide residues. FDA's Center for Veterinary Medicine (CVM) directs this portion of the Agency's monitoring via its Feed Contaminants Compliance Program. Although animal feeds containing violative pesticide residues may present a potential hazard to a number of different categories of animals (e.g., laboratory animals, pets, wildlife, etc.), the major focus of CVM's monitoring is on feeds for livestock and poultry, animals that ultimately become, or produce, foods for human consumption.

CVM also reviews pesticide residue data supplied by various states under "Feedcon", a database operated by MSU under the auspices of the Association of American Feed Control Officials. These data are reviewed periodically by CVM so that potential problems arising from pesticide residues in foods of animal origin may be identified.

International Activities   FDA obtains information on foreign pesticide usage via contract with Landell Mills (Bath, England). Each year, FDA receives pesticide usage data for about 40 countries that export food to the United States. These data can be used by FDA to target its pesticide residue monitoring toward specific pesticide/commodity/country combinations.

In addition to the foreign pesticide usage data obtained through the commercial contract, under provisions of the Pesticide Monitoring Improvements Act, FDA receives information from foreign governments on pesticides used on their food exports to the United States. FDA makes this information available to FDA Districts for use in their planning of monitoring of imported foods.

As part of the exchange of information on pesticides, FDA provides foreign countries with updates on U.S. pesticide usage. FDA also supplies foreign countries annually with reports on FDA's regulatory monitoring coverage and the findings in foods imported from their respective countries, as well as a personal computer database in which coverage and findings are summarized by country/commodity/pesticide combination.

Under the auspices of the North American Free Trade Agreement (NAFTA), the United States, Mexico, and Canada have established a NAFTA Technical Working Group on Pesticides (TWG). The NAFTA Pesticide TWG now serves as the focal point for all pesticide issues that arise among the 3 NAFTA countries. The TWG reports directly to the NAFTA Sanitary and Phytosanitary Committee.

One of the major goals of the TWG is to ensure that pesticide registrations and tolerances/maximum residue limits in the 3 countries are harmonized to the extent practical, while strengthening protection of public health and the environment. A number of projects have been undertaken by the TWG to identify differing residue limits in the NAFTA countries and to determine what steps might be taken to harmonize the limits. While this is a difficult process, the TWG envisions eventual movement toward a "North America" pesticide registration and tolerance system so that citizens of all 3 countries can be assured of the safety and legality of foods produced in any 1 of the NAFTA countries.

The NAFTA TWG is cochaired by EPA, Health Canada, and Mexico's Ministry of Health (representing the Comision Intersecretarial para el Control del Proceso y Uso de Plaguicidas, Fertilizantes y Sustancias Toxicas). FDA is an active participant on the TWG and is assisting by providing expertise on enforcement monitoring programs and residue data to support harmonization activities. FDA's activities on the TWG complement its ongoing bilateral cooperation with its counterparts in Mexico and Canada.

Incidence/Level Monitoring

A complementary approach to regulatory monitoring, incidence/level monitoring is used to increase FDA's knowledge about particular pesticide/commodity combinations by analyzing certain foods to determine the presence and levels of selected pesticides. In 1995, a survey of triazine herbicides in various commodities was carried out and a statistically based monitoring survey that had been initiated in 1994 was completed.

The latter focused on domestic and imported fresh apples and processed rice. This is the second FDA survey of this type; the first covered domestic and imported pears and tomatoes [4]. These statistically based surveys were initiated to determine whether FDA data acquired under regulatory monitoring are statistically representative of the overall residue situation for a particular pesticide, commodity, or place of origin. In FDA's surveillance sampling for pesticide residues, sampling bias may be incurred by weighting sampling toward such factors as commodity or place of origin with a past history of violations or large volume of import shipments. In addition, the total number of samples of a given commodity analyzed for a particular pesticide each year may not be sufficient to draw specific conclusions about the residue situation for the whole volume of that commodity in commerce. Therefore, the objective of these statistically based surveys is to determine whether violation rates, frequency of occurrence of residues, and residue levels obtained from such a sampling regimen differ from those obtained through FDA's traditional surveillance approach.

Apples and rice were chosen as the second set of test commodities because they are widely consumed year round and have significant domestic and import components. Fresh apples and all types of processed rice (white, brown, glutinous, fragrant, parboiled, converted, etc., but not wild or brewer's rice) were included in the study. The same general procedures were followed in the apples/rice study as in the pears/tomatoes study [4]. Samples were collected throughout the United States by FDA inspectors, except for domestic rice. These samples were collected by USDA Federal Grain Inspection Service personnel, who are routinely present at the mills that process domestic rice. Most of the mills are located in those few states in which rice growing is a major agricultural industry.

Analyses were performed by the Buffalo (apples) and Minneapolis (rice) District Laboratories. The goal was to collect and analyze about 800 domestic and 800 import apple samples and about 575 domestic and 800 import rice samples.

Total Diet Study

The Total Diet Study is another major element of FDA's pesticide residue monitoring program [5]. In its previous annual pesticide reports, FDA provided Total Diet Study findings for 1987–1994 [6]. In addition, more detailed information, including estimated dietary intakes of pesticide residues covering June 1984–April 1986 [7] and July 1986–April 1991 [8], has been published. In September 1991, FDA implemented revisions to the Total Diet Study that were formulated in 1990 [9]. These revisions primarily consisted of collection and analysis of an updated and expanded number (to 261) of food items, addition of 6 age/sex groups (for a total of 14), and revised analytical coverage. Details of the recent revision are presented elsewhere [10,11].

In conducting the Total Diet Study, FDA personnel purchase foods from supermarkets or grocery stores 4 times per year, once from each of 4 geographic regions of the country. The 261 foods that comprise each market basket represent over 3500 different foods reported in USDA food consumption surveys; for example, apple pie represents all fruit pies and fruit pastries. Each collection is a composite of like foods purchased in 3 cities in a given region. The foods are prepared table-ready and then analyzed for pesticide residues (as well as radionuclides, industrial chemicals, toxic elements, trace and macro elements, vitamin B_6, and folic acid). The levels of pesticides found are used in conjunction with USDA food consumption data to estimate the dietary intakes of the pesticide residues.

Results and Discussion

Regulatory Monitoring

In 1995, 10,615 samples (10,133 surveillance and 482 compliance) were analyzed under regulatory monitoring. Of these, 5198 were domestic and 5417 were imports.

Figure I.1 shows the percentage of the 5101 domestic surveillance samples by commodity group with no residues found, nonviolative residues found, and violative residues found. (A violative residue is defined in this report as a residue which exceeds a tolerance or a residue at a level of regulatory significance for which no tolerance has been established in the sampled food.) As in earlier years, fruits and vegetables accounted for the largest proportion of the commodities analyzed in 1995; those 2 commodity groups comprised 59% of the total number of domestic surveillance samples. In 1995, no violative residues were found in nearly 99% of all domestic surveillance samples (the same percentage as in the past several years).

Appendix A contains more detailed data on domestic surveillance monitoring findings by commodity, including the total number of samples analyzed, the percent samples with no residues found, and the percent violative samples. Of the 5101 domestic surveillance samples, 64% had no detectable residues, less than 1% had over-tolerance residues, and less than 1% had residues of pesticides for which there was no tolerance for that particular pesticide/commodity combination. In the largest commodity groups, fruits and vegetables, 40 and 63% of the samples, respectively, had no residues detected. Less than 2% of the

fruit samples and about 2% of the vegetable samples contained violative residues (Figure I.1). In the milk/dairy products/eggs group, 93% of the samples had no residues detected and no violative residues were found. Within the category Other were 61 samples of baby foods/formula, nearly 3 times the number of samples of baby foods/formula collected and analyzed in 1994. This included 29 vegetable, 13 cereal, 13 fruit/fruit juice, 4 formula, 1 custard/fruit pudding, and 1 teething biscuit samples. None of the samples had violative residues.

The findings by commodity group for the 5032 import surveillance samples are shown in Figure I.2. Fruits and vegetables accounted for 85% of these samples. Overall, no violative residues were found in nearly 97% of the import surveillance samples (97% in 1993 and 96% in 1994).

Appendix B contains detailed data on the import surveillance samples. Of the 5032 samples analyzed, 66% had no residues detected, less than 1% had over-tolerance residues, and 3% had residues for which there was no tolerance for that particular pesticide/commodity combination. Fruits and vegetables had 57 and 67%, respectively, with no residues detected. The fruit group had less than 1% with over-tolerance residues and the vegetable group had 1% with over-tolerance residues; each group had 3% no-tolerance residues. No residues were found in 88% of the dairy products/eggs group and 85% of

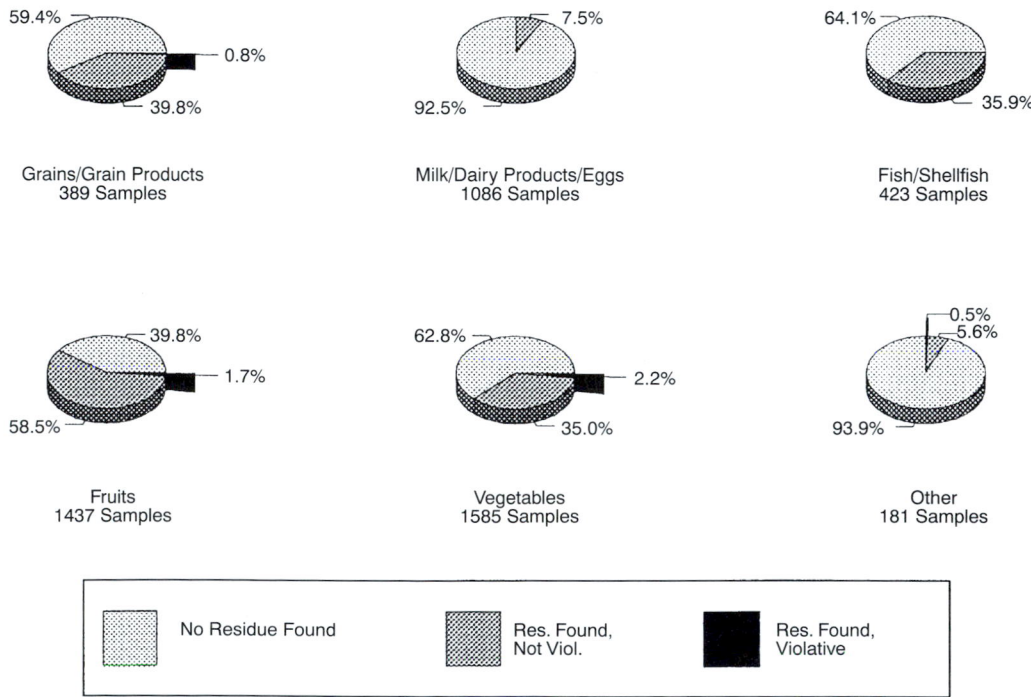

Figure I.1 Summary of results (domestic) by commodity group of 1995 sample analyses for pesticide residues (surveillance samples only).

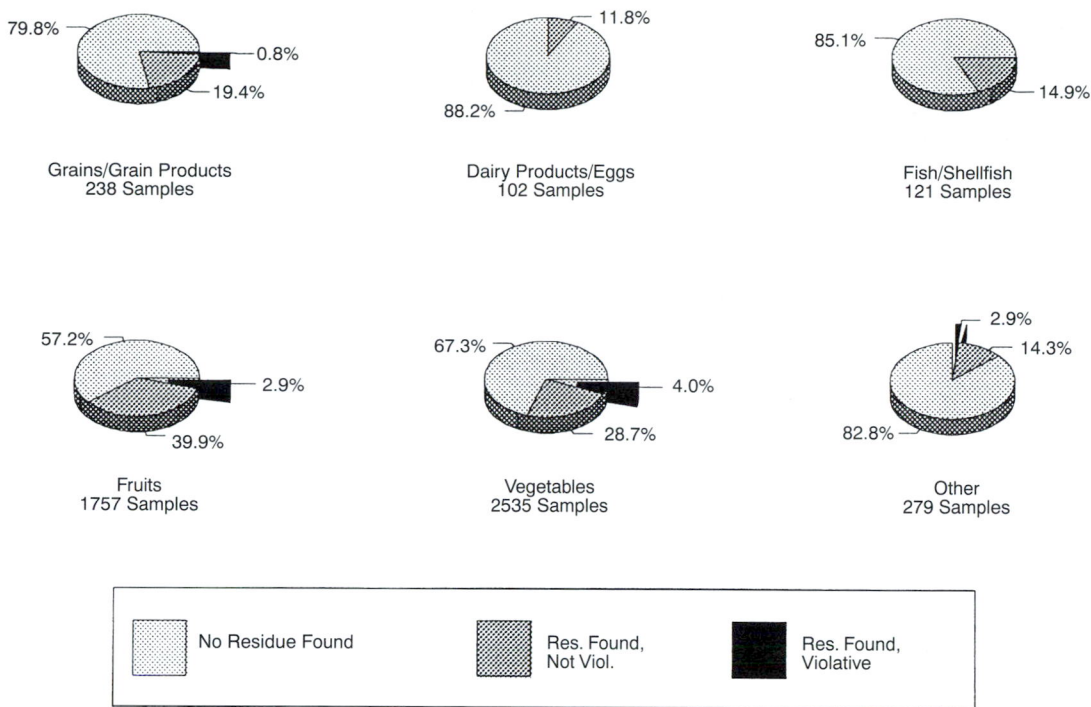

Figure I.2 Summary of results (import) by commodity group of 1995 sample analyses for pesticide residues (surveillance samples only).

the fish/shellfish group, and no violative residues were found in either of those groups.

Pesticide monitoring data collected under FDA's regulatory monitoring approach in 1995 are available to the public as a computer database. This database summarizes FDA 1995 regulatory monitoring coverage and findings by country/commodity/pesticide combination. The database also includes the monitoring data by individual sample from which the summary information was compiled. Information on purchase of this database as well as those for 1992, 1993, and 1994 is provided at the end of this report.

Geographic Coverage

Domestic. In 1995, domestic surveillance samples were collected from all 50 states and Puerto Rico. The largest numbers of samples were collected from the states in which agriculture is a major industry.

Import. Samples representing food shipments from 94 countries were collected. Table I.1 lists the numbers of samples collected and the countries from which they originated. Mexico, as usual, was the source of the largest number of samples. This large number reflects the volume and diversity of commodities imported from that country, especially during the winter months.

Pesticide Coverage Table I.2 lists the 345 pesticides that were detectable by the methods used; the 92 pesticides that were actually found are indicated.

FDA conducts ongoing research to expand the pesticide coverage of its monitoring program. This research includes testing the behavior of new or previously untested pesticides through existing analytical methods, and development of new methods to cover pesticides that cannot be determined by methods currently used by FDA. The research encompasses both U.S.-registered pesticides and foreign-use pesticides that are not registered in the United States. The list of pesticides detectable for 1995 (Table I.2) reflects the addition of a number of pesticides for which new methods had been developed and pesticides whose recovery through the analytical methods used was demonstrated as a result of ongoing research.

Surveillance/Compliance Violation Rate Comparison In 1995, 97 domestic and 385 import compliance samples were collected and analyzed (Table I.3). Because compliance samples are collected when a pesticide residue problem is known or suspected, violation rates are expectedly higher than those for surveillance samples: 12% for domestic (10% in 1994) and 11% for imports (18% in 1994). The corresponding violation rates for surveillance samples

Table I.1 Foreign countries and number of samples[a] collected and analyzed in 1995

Country	No. of samples	Country	No. of samples	Country	No. of samples
Mexico	1723	Greece	81	Hong Kong	23
Chile	467	Turkey	79	Philippines	23
The Netherlands	370	Ecuador	72	United Kingdom	21
Canada	253	Taiwan	55	Germany	17
Italy	218	Argentina	51	Denmark	16
Thailand	198	New Zealand	48	Pakistan	16
China, People's		Jamaica	47	Poland	16
Rep. of	184	Japan	47	South Africa	16
Guatemala	174	Belgium	46	Lebanon	15
Costa Rica	139	Panama	43	Australia	14
India	137	Colombia	42	Czech Republic	14
Spain	126	France	40	Egypt	13
Peru	85	Indonesia	31	Haiti	12
Israel	83	Brazil	30	Morocco	12
Dominican	91	Honduras	29	Venezuela	12
Republic		Korea, Rep. of	25	Unspecified	15

Ten or fewer samples collected from the following:

Austria	Hungary	Slovakia
Bahamas	Iceland	Slovenia
Belize	Ivory Coast	Sri Lanka
Bermuda	Kenya	St. Vincent
Bolivia	Macedonia	Surinam
Bosnia-Hercegovina	Malaysia	Sweden
Bulgaria	Martinique	Switzerland
Croatia	Moldavia	Syria
Cyprus	Netherlands Antilles	Tanzania
Dominica	Nicaragua	Trinidad & Tobago
El Salvador	Nigeria	Tunisia
Estonia	Norway	Turks & Caicos Islands
Ethiopia	Papua New Guinea	United Arab Emirates
Faeroe Islands	Portugal	Uruguay
Fiji	Russia	Vietnam, Rep. of
Ghana	Singapore	Zambia

[a]Surveillance plus compliance samples.

were 1.3% for domestic and 3.2% for imports (Figure I.3).

Most of the 1995 compliance samples were collected as follow-up to violative surveillance samples. These included follow-up samples from the same shipment as the violative surveillance sample, follow-up samples of the same commodity from the same grower or shipper, and audit samples from shipments presented for entry into the United States with a certificate of analysis (i.e., shipments subject to automatic detention).

Foodcontam Data In 1995, 11 states participated in the Foodcontam project. A wide variety of commodities was reflected in the 9394 samples reported by the 10 states whose data were available. Table I.4 lists the 10 states, the number of samples for each, and the number and percentage of samples with posi-

tive and "significant" findings. In this instance, a significant finding indicates a residue that exceeds federal or state regulatory limits, is not covered by a tolerance for the particular chemical/commodity combination, or denotes some unusual finding(s). For the 9394 samples reported, 0.8% were classified as significant.

Animal Feeds In 1995, 556 domestic feed samples (532 surveillance and 24 compliance) and 69 import feed samples (65 surveillance and 4 compliance) were collected and analyzed by FDA. Of the 532 domestic surveillance samples, 301 (57%) had no pesticide residues detected and 2 (<1%) contained violative residues (Table I.5). The latter involved 2 corn samples with chlorpyrifos-methyl residues. Of the 65 import surveillance samples, 29 (45%) had no pesticide residues detected and 1 (2%), a sample of

Table I.2 Pesticides detectable by the methods used and pesticides found (*) in 1995 regulatory monitoring[a,b]

Acephate*	Cadusafos	Cyhexatin*	Diphenylamine*
Acetochlor	Captafol	Cypermethrin*	Dipropetryn
Acrinathrin	Captan*	Cyprazine	Disulfoton
Alachlor*	Carbaryl*	Cyproconazole	Diuron
Aldicarb*	Carbofuran*	Daminozide	Edifenphos
Aldrin	Carbon tetrachloride	DCPA*	Endosulfan*
Allethrin	Carbophenothion*	DDT*	Endrin*
Allidochlor	Carbosulfan	Deltamethrin	EPN
Alpha-cypermethrin	Carboxin	Deltamethrin, trans	EPTC
Ametryn	Chlorbenside	Demeton*	Esfenvalerate*
Aminocarb	Chlorbromuron	Desmetryn	Etaconazole
Amitraz*	Chlorbufam	Dialifor	Ethalfluralin
Anilazine	Chlordane*	Di-allate	Ethephon*
Aramite	Chlordecone	N,N-Diallyl	Ethiofencarb
Atrazine	Chlordimeform*	dichloroacetamide	Ethion*
Azinphos-ethyl	Chlorethoxyfos	Diazinon*	Ethofumesate
Azinphos-methyl*	Chlorfenvinphos	Dichlobenil	Ethoprop
Bendiocarb	Chlorflurecol methyl	Dichlofenthion	Ethoxyquin*
Benfluralin	ester	Dichlofluanid	Ethylenebisdithio-
Benodanil	Chlorimuron ethyl ester	Dichlone*	carbamates*[d]
Benomyl/carbendazim*[c]	Chlornitrofen	4-(Dichloroacetyl)-1-oxa-	Ethylene dibromide
Benoxacor	Chlorobenzilate	4-azapiro[4.5]decane	Ethylene dichloride
Bensulide	Chloroform	Dichlorvos*	Etridiazole
Benzoylprop-ethyl	3-Chloro-5-methyl-4-	Diclobutrazol	Etrimfos
BHC*	nitro-1H-pyrazole	Diclofop-methyl	Famphur
Bifenox	Chloroneb	Dicloran*	Fenamiphos*
Bifenthrin*	Chloropropylate	Dicofol*	Fenarimol*
Binapacryl	Chlorothalonil*	Dicrotophos	Fenbuconazole
S-Bioallethrin	Chloroxuron	Dieldrin*	Fenfuram
Biphenyl	Chlorpropham*	Diethatyl-ethyl	Fenitrothion*
Bitertanol*	Chlorpyrifos*	Dilan	Fenobucarb
Bromacil	Chlorpyrifos-methyl*	Dimethachlor	Fenoxaprop ethyl
Bromophos	Chlorthiophos	Dimethametryn	ester
Bromophos-ethyl	Clomazone	Dimethipin	Fenoxycarb
Bromopropylate*	Coumaphos	Dimethoate*	Fenpropathrin
Bromoxynil	Crotoxyphos	Dinitramine	Fenpropimorph
Bufencarb	Crufomate	Dinobuton	Fenson
Bulan	Cyanazine	Dinocap	Fensulfothion
Bupirimate	Cyanofenphos	Dioxabenzofos	Fenthion
Butachlor	Cyanophos	Dioxacarb	Fenuron
Butocarboxim	Cycloate	Dioxathion	Fenvalerate*
Butralin	Cyfluthrin	Diphenamid	Fipronil

Continued

Pesticide	No. of samples with quantifiable residues	Residue found, range	ppm median
malathion	149	0.01–7.7	0.09
chlorpyrifos-methyl	39	0.01–1.1	0.11
diazinon	23	0.01–0.81	0.06
chlorpyrifos	10	0.01–0.08	0.03
pirimiphos-methyl	9	0.01–9.9	0.05
others	24	0.01–41	0.19

feather meal (for poultry) from Canada, contained diphenylamine. No tolerance for chlorpyrifos-methyl on corn or for diphenylamine on poultry has been set. Thus, these samples were considered to have exceeded regulatory standards.

In the 231 domestic surveillance feed samples in which 1 or more pesticides were detected, a total of 346 residues were detected (254 quantifiable and 92 trace). Malathion, chlorpyrifos-methyl, and diazinon were the most frequently found residues. The findings in samples with quantifiable residues were as follows:

Table I.2   Continued

Flamprop-M-isopropyl	Methomyl*	Phorate*	Sulfur dioxide*
Flamprop-methyl	Methoprotryne	Phosalone*	Sulphenone
Fluazifop butyl ester	Methoxychlor*	Phosmet*	Sulprofos
Fluchloralin	Methylene chloride	Phosphamidon*	TCMTB
Flucythrinate	Metobromuron	Phosphine	Tebuconazole
Flusilazole	Metolachlor	Piperonyl butoxide	Tebupirimfos
Fluvalinate	Metolcarb	Piperophos	Tecnazene
Folpet*	Metoxuron	Pirimicarb	TEPP
Fonofos*	Metribuzin	Pirimiphos-ethyl	Terbacil
Formetanate	Mevinphos*	Pirimiphos-methyl*	Terbufos
hydrochloride*	Mirex*	Pretilachlor	Terbumeton
Formothion	Monocrotophos*	Probenazole	Terbuthylazine
Fuberidazole	Monolinuron	Prochloraz	Terbutryn
Furilazole	Monuron	Procyazine	Tetradifon*
Gardona*	Myclobutanil*	Procymidone*	Tetraiodoethylene
Heptachlor*	Naled	Prodiamine	Tetrasul
Heptenophos	Napropamide	Profenofos*	Thiabendazole*
Hexachlorobenzene*	Neburon	Profluralin	Thiobencarb
Hexaconazole	Nitralin	Prolan	Thiodicarb
Hexazinone	Nitrapyrin	Promecarb	Thiometon
Imazalil*	Nitrofen	Prometryn	Thionazin
Imazamethabenz	Nitrofluorfen	Pronamide	Thiophanate-methyl
methyl ester	Nitrothal-isopropyl	Propachlor	Tolylfluanid
Iprobenfos	Norflurazon	Propanil	Toxaphene
Iprodione*	Nuarimol	Propargite*	Tralomethrin
Isazofos	Octhilinone	Propazine	Traloxydim
Isocarbamid	Ofurace	Propetamphos	Triadimefon*
Isofenphos	Omethoate*	Propham	Triadimenol*
Isoprocarb	Ovex	Propiconazole	Tri-allate
Isopropalin	Oxadiazon	Propoxur	Triazamate
Isoprothiolane	Oxadixyl	Prothiofos*	Triazophos
Lactofen	Oxamyl*	Prothoate	Tribufos
Lambda-cyhalothrin	Oxydemeton-methyl*	Pyrazon	Trichlorfon
Leptophos	Oxyfluorfen	Pyrazophos	Tricyclazole
Lindane*	Oxythioquinox	Pyrethrins	Tridiphane
Linuron*	Paclobutrazol	Pyridaphenthion	Trietazine
Malathion*	Paraquat	Quinalphos	Triflumizole
Mecarbam	Parathion*	Quintozene*	Trifluralin*
Mephosfolan	Parathion-methyl*	Quizalofop ethyl ester	Triflusulfuron methyl
Merphos*	Pebulate	Ronnel	ester
Metalaxyl*	Penconazole	Schradan	Trimethacarb
Metasystox thiol	Pendimethalin	Secbumeton	Vamidothion sulfone
Metazachlor	Permethrin*	Simazine*	Vernolate
Methabenzthiazuron	Perthane	Simetryn	Vinclozolin*
Methamidophos*	Phenothrin	Strobane	XMC
Methidathion*	Phenthoate	Sulfallate	
Methiocarb*	Phenylphenol, ortho-*	Sulfotep*	

aThe list of pesticides detectable is expressed in terms of the parent pesticide. However, monitoring coverage and findings may have included metabolites, impurities, and alteration products.

bSome of these pesticides are no longer manufactured or registered for use in the United States.

cThe analytical methodology determines carbendazim, which may result from use of benomyl or carbendazim.

dSuch as maneb.

Summary: Regulatory Monitoring

In summary, no residues were found in 64% of domestic surveillance samples and 66% of import surveillance samples (Figure I.4) analyzed under FDA's regulatory monitoring approach in 1995. Less than 1% of domestic and import surveillance samples had residue levels that were over tolerance and less than 1% of domestic and 3% of import surveillance samples had residues for which there was no tolerance. The findings for 1995 demonstrate that pesticide residue levels in foods are generally well below EPA tolerances, corroborating results presented in earlier reports [6].

Table I.3 Compliance samples by commodity group in 1995

Commodity group	Total no. of samples	Samples with no residues found, %	Samples violative, %
Domestic			
Grains and grain products	3	33	0
Milk/Eggs	5	100	0
Fish	5	80	0
Fruits	23	48	0
Vegetables	56	48	21
Other	5	80	0
Total	97	54	12
Import			
Grains and grain products	49	63	0
Cheese	3	100	0
Fish/shellfish	17	41	0
Fruits	71	68	18
Vegetables	196	52	14
Other	49	86	6
Total	385	61	11

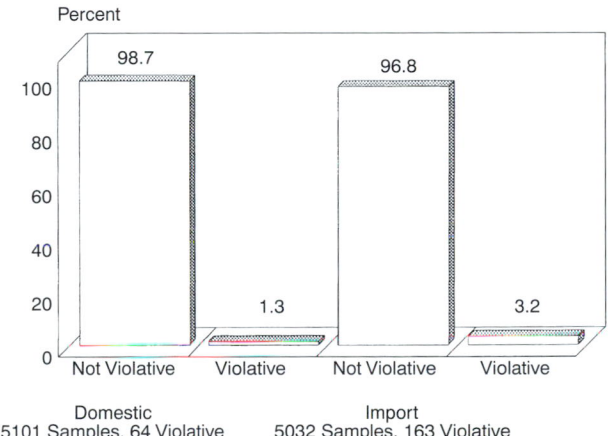

Figure I.3 Domestic and import surveillance sample violation rates for 1995.

Domestic — 5101 Samples, 64 Violative
Import — 5032 Samples, 163 Violative

Incidence/Level Monitoring

Statistically Based Survey The statistically based monitoring survey of domestic and imported fresh apples and processed rice that was begun in 1994 was completed in 1995. The original goal had been to collect 1600 samples of apples (800 domestic and 800 import). Actually, 769 domestic and 1062 import samples were collected and analyzed. For rice, 575 domestic and 800 import samples had been the goal; 598 domestic and 612 import samples were actually collected and analyzed. (These numbers are not included in the counts under Fruits and Grains and Grain Products in Appendixes A and B.) The results of the survey are being evaluated and will be submitted for publication in the scientific literature.

Table I.4 Summary of foodcontam findings for 1995[a]

State	Total samples	No. positive	Positive, %	No. significant	Significant, %
Arkansas	351	14	4.0	2	0.6
California	4694	1164	24.8	40	0.9
Georgia	540	128	23.7	7	1.3
Indiana	158	93	58.9	0	—
North Carolina	688	215	31.3	9	1.3
New York	965	321	33.3	14	1.5
Oregon	277	39	14.1	0	—
Pennsylvania	582	124	21.3	5	0.9
Virginia	703	88	12.5	2	0.3
Wisconsin	538	7	1.3	0	—
Total	9394	2193	23.3	79	0.8

[a]Data from Florida not available.

Table I.5   Summary of findings in domestic surveillance feed samples in 1995

Type of feed	Total no. of samples	Samples with no residues found		Violative samples	
		No.	%	No.	%
Whole/ground grains	167	98	59	2	1
Plant by-products	120	76	63	0	—
Mixed feed rations	116	35	30	0	—
Animal by-products	104	74	71	0	—
Hay & hay products	25	18	72	0	—
Total	532	301	57	2	<1

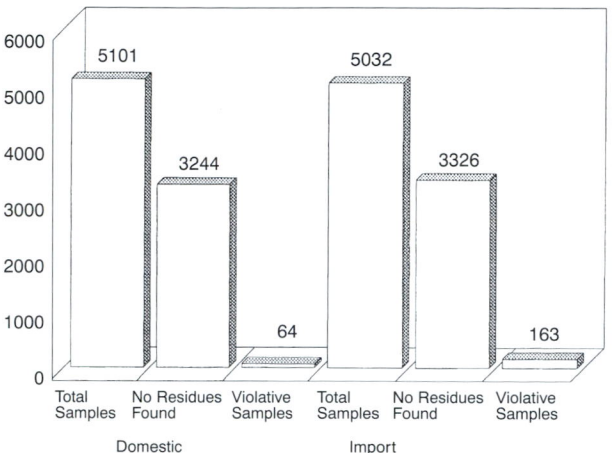

Figure I.4   Comparison of results for domestic and import surveillance samples in 1995.

Table I.6   Commodity targeted monitoring of domestic and imported foods for triazine herbicides conducted in 1995

Commodity	Number of samples analyzed	
	Domestic	Import
Apples	9	16
Bananas	2	23
Cherries	25	—
Corn	10	15
Corn, whole grain	—	1
Grapefruit	8	4
Grapes	5	20
Olives	—	25
Oranges	20	5
Pears	6	19
Plums	7	13
Total	92	140

Triazine Herbicides   The triazines are one of the most widely used classes of herbicides, and EPA has established tolerances for them on many commodities. Interest in triazines has increased recently because of potential leaching of the herbicides and their degradation products into ground and surface water. Residues of these chemicals have rarely been detected in foods, although FDA has routinely looked for the parent compounds.

Recently, FDA's Atlanta District Laboratory developed a method capable of determining 19 triazine herbicides and 4 metabolites [12]. Average recoveries ranged from 81 to 106% for the parent herbicides and 60 to 88% for the metabolites. The method was validated by the Minneapolis District Laboratory [13] and used to analyze a number of food samples in 1995. This new method was used to analyze 232 samples (92 domestic samples from 9 states and 140 import samples from 19 countries) (Table I.6). Residues were found in 5 domestic samples, all of simazine in oranges. Four samples had trace amounts and 1 sample had 0.04 ppm (LQ, 0.02 ppm). None were violative. No triazine residues were detected in the import samples.

Summary: Incidence/Level Monitoring

Under this approach, a statistically based monitoring survey of domestic and imported apples and processed rice was completed in 1995. A survey of triazine herbicides in various commodities was carried out. Few residues were found, and none were violative.

Total Diet Study

The Total Diet Study is unique in that it determines pesticide residues in foods that have been prepared as they would be consumed [5]. Of the nearly 300 chemicals that can be determined by the analytical methods used, 86 pesticide and pesticide-related chemicals were found in the foods analyzed in the 3 collections reported here. To measure the low levels of pesticides found in the Total Diet Study foods, the analytical methods used are modified to permit measurement at levels 5–10 times lower than those normally used in regulatory monitoring. In general, residues present at or above 1 part per billion can be measured.

Table I.7 lists the 17 most frequently found residues, the total number of findings, and the percent

Table I.7 Frequency of occurrence of pesticide residues found in total diet study foods in 1995[a]

Pesticide[b]	Total no. of findings	Occurrence, %
DDT	192	25
Malathion	141	18
Chlorpyrifos-methyl	130	17
Chlorpyrifos	97	12
Dieldrin	92	12
Endosulfan	81	10
Chlorpropham	44	6
Methamidophos	40	5
Carbaryl[c]	39	5
Iprodione	31	4
Thiabendazole[d]	29	4
Dimethoate	28	4
Permethrin	25	3
Hexachlorobenzene	24	3
BHC	22	3
Dicloran	21	3
Diazinon	21	3

[a]Based on 3 market baskets analyzed in 1995 consisting of 783 items.
[b]Isomers, metabolites, and related compounds are not listed separately; they are covered under the "parent" pesticide from which they arise.
[c]Reflects overall incidence; however, only 95 selected foods per market basket (i.e., 285 items total) were analyzed for N-methylcarbamates.
[d]Reflects overall incidence; however, only 67 selected foods per market basket (i.e., 201 items total) were analyzed for the benzimidazole fungicides (thiabendazole and benomyl).

occurrence in the 783 food items analyzed in 1995. DDT, an environmentally persistent chemical whose U.S. registration was higher than it has been in the past several years. This may not be an indicator of an increasing trend in DDT findings in Total Diet Study foods; however, the occurrence will be investigated. Malathion, which is used on a wide variety of crops both pre- and postharvest, was the next most frequently found residue. The levels of these 2 pesticides, as well as the others listed in Table I.7, were well below regulatory limits.

Information obtained through the Total Diet Study is used to estimate dietary intakes of pesticides; these intakes are then compared with established standards. Food consumption data to be used in estimating dietary intakes for the revised food list have not been finalized. Therefore, dietary intake information for the market baskets collected during this period is not presented.

For several years, FDA has collected and analyzed a number of baby foods in addition to those covered under the Total Diet Study. Between 1991 and 1995, this adjunct to the Total Diet Study included 23 different food items (14 fruit juices or fruits, 4 fruit des-

serts, 4 grain products, and 1 vegetable). (These numbers are not included in the analyses reported in Table I.7.) Table I.8 lists the 16 most frequently found pesticide residues in those 23 foods in 1991–1995. Carbaryl, the residue found most frequently, is an insecticide with tolerances on many fruits and grains. Dimethoate, the next most frequently found residue, also has tolerances on a number of fruits.

Summary: Total Diet Study

In 1995, the types of pesticide residues found and their frequency of occurrence in the Total Diet Study were generally consistent with those given in previous FDA reports [6]. The pesticide residue levels found were well below regulatory standards. An adjunct survey of baby foods in 1991–1995 also provided evidence of only small amounts of pesticide residues in those foods.

Summary

A total of 10,615 samples of domestically produced food and imported food from 94 countries was

Table I.8 Frequency of occurrence of pesticide residues found in selected baby foods in 1991–1995[a]

Pesticide[b]	Total no. of findings	Occurrence, %
Carbaryl[c]	77	28
Dimethoate	71	26
Iprodione	45	16
Omethoate	39	14
Malathion	36	13
Chlorpyrifos	35	13
Endosulfan	29	11
Chlorpyrifos-methyl	26	9
Thiabendazole[d]	23	8
Permethrin	22	8
Parathion	20	7
Dicloran	14	5
Propargite[e]	10	4
Acephate	9	3
Dieldrin	8	3
Benomyl[d]	7	3

[a]Based on 12 collections consisting of 276 items.
[b]Isomers, metabolites, and related compounds are not listed separately; they are covered under the "parent" pesticide from which they arise.
[c]Reflects overall incidence; however, only 17 selected foods per collection (i.e., 204 items total) were analyzed for N-methylcarbamates.
[d]Reflects overall incidence; however, only 16 selected items (i.e., 192 items total) were analyzed for the benzimidazole fungicides (thiabendazole and benomyl).
[e]Reflects overall incidence; however, only 16 selected foods per collection (i.e., 192 items total) were analyzed for this sulfur-containing compound.

analyzed for pesticide residues in 1995. Of these, 10,133 were surveillance samples, which are collected when there is no evidence of a pesticide problem. No residues were found in 64% of the domestic surveillance samples and 66% of the import surveillance samples. The higher violation rates in the 482 compliance samples reflect the fact that they are collected and analyzed when a pesticide problem is suspected. In addition, a survey of triazine herbicides was carried out and a statistically based monitoring survey of fresh apples and processed rice that had been initiated in 1994 was completed. Most of the Total Diet Study findings for 1995 were generally similar to those found in earlier periods.

This report was compiled through the efforts of the following FDA personnel: Norma J. Yess, Young H. Lee, Byron O. Bohannon (Division of Programs and Enforcement Policy), and Bernadette M. McMahon and Charles H. Parfitt (Division of Pesticides and Industrial Chemicals), Office of Plant and Dairy Foods and Beverages; Sharon A. Macuci (Division of Information Resources Management), Office of Management Systems, Washington, DC; Rodney L. Bong, Minneapolis District, Minneapolis, MN; and Sheila K. Egan and James L. Daft, Kansas City District, Kansas City, MO.

FDA pesticide monitoring data collected under the regulatory monitoring approach in 1995 are available for purchase on personal computer diskettes from the National Technical Information Service (NTIS), 5285 Port Royal Road, Springfield, VA 22161 (telephone 703-487-4650); order number PB96-503156. The databases for 1992, 1993, and 1994 are also available from NTIS. The order numbers are: 1992, PB94-500899; 1993, PB94-501681; and 1994, PB95-503132.

References

1. Yess, N.J. (1995) U.S. Food and Drug Administration monitoring of pesticide residues in foods. *Pestic. Outlook* 6, 28–31.
2. *Code of Federal Regulations* (1996) Title 40, U.S. Government Printing Office, Washington, DC, Parts 180, 185, and 186.
3. *Pesticide Analytical Manual* (1968 and revisions) Vols I (3rd Ed., 1994) and II (1971), Food and Drug Administration, Washington, DC (available from National Technical Information Service, Springfield, VA 22161).
4. Roy, R.R., Albert, R.H., Wilson, P., Laski, R.R., Roberts, J.I., Hoffmann, T.J., Bong, R.L., Bohannon, B.O., & Yess, N.J. (1995) U.S. Food and Drug Administration pesticide program: incidence/level monitoring of domestic and imported pears and tomatoes. *J. AOAC Int.* 78, 930–940.
5. Pennington, J.A.T., Capar, S.G., Parfitt, C.H., & Edwards, C.W. (1996) History of the Food and Drug Administration's Total Diet Study (Part II), 1987–1993. *J. AOAC Int.* 79, 163–170.
6. Food and Drug Administration (1995) Food and Drug Administration pesticide program – residue monitoring – 1994. *J. AOAC Int.* 78, 117A–143A (and earlier reports in the series).
7. Gunderson, E.L. (1995) Dietary intakes of pesticides, selected elements, and other chemicals: FDA Total Diet Study, June 1984–April 1986. *J. AOAC Int.* 78, 910–921.
8. Gunderson, E.L. (1995) FDA Total Diet Study, July 1986–April 1991, dietary intakes of pesticides, selected elements, and other chemicals. *J. AOAC Int.* 78, 1353–1363.
9. Pennington, J.A.T. (1992) Total Diet Studies: the identification of core foods in the United States food supply. *Food Addit. Contam.* 9, 253–264.
10. Pennington, J.A.T. (1992) The 1990 revision of the FDA Total Diet Study. *J. Nutr. Educ.* 24, 173–178.
11. Pennington, J.A.T. (1992) Appendices for the 1990 revision of the Food and Drug Administration's Total Diet Study. PB92-176239/AS, National Technical Information Service, Springfield, VA 22161.
12. Pardue, J.R. (1995) Multiresidue method for the chromatographic determination of triazine herbicides and their metabolites in raw agricultural products. *J. AOAC Int.* 78, 856–862.
13. Bong, R., Kramer, J., Heaney, L., & Murphy, L. (1995) Validation of a multiresidue method for triazine herbicides in various food commodities. *Lab. Inf. Bull.* 3998, Food and Drug Administration, Rockville, MD.

Appendix A

Analysis of Domestic Surveillance Samples by Commodity Group in 1995

Commodity Group	Total no. of samples	Samples with no residues found, %	Samples violative, %	
			Over tolerance	No tolerance
A. Grains and Grain Products				
Corn & corn products	53	81	0	0
Oats	18	67	0	0
Rice & rice products	56	86	0	0
Soybeans	38	82	0	0
Wheat	146	38	1	0
Cereal products	23	87	0	0
Other grains & grain products	55	38	2	0
Total	389	59	<1	0
B. Milk/Dairy Products/Eggs				
Cheese & cheese products	66	68	0	0
Eggs	259	98	0	0
Milk/cream & milk products	761	93	0	0
Total	1086	93	0	0
C. Fish/Shellfish				
Fish	295	53	0	0
Shellfish	128	90	0	0
Total	423	64	0	0
D. Fruits				
Blueberries	64	61	0	17
Cranberries	20	10	0	0
Grapes	52	52	0	0
Raspberries	33	24	0	0
Strawberries	107	15	1	2
Other berries	8	75	0	0
Grapefruit	22	27	0	0
Lemons	28	57	0	0
Oranges	171	6	0	0
Other citrus fruits	6	33	0	0
Apples	189	46	0	0
Pears	69	32	7	0
Apricots	28	25	4	0
Cherries	64	17	0	0
Nectarines	26	8	0	0
Olives	12	100	0	0
Peaches	200	20	<1	<1
Other pit fruits	11	73	0	0
Cantaloupe	45	62	0	2
Honeydew	14	57	0	0
Watermelon	73	86	0	0
Apple juice	110	76	0	<1
Other fruit juices	22	82	0	0
Fruit jams/jellies/pastes/toppings	11	36	0	0
Other fruits	52	88	0	2
Total	1437	40	<1	1

Continued

Appendix A Continued

Commodity Group	Total no. of samples	Samples with no residues found, %	Samples violative, % Over tolerance	No tolerance
E. Vegetables				
Corn	105	90	0	0
Green/snow/sugar/sweet peas	84	86	0	0
String beans	100	67	0	0
Other beans & peas	32	91	0	0
Cucumbers	41	61	0	2
Eggplant	17	71	0	12
Peppers, hot	12	83	0	0
Peppers, sweet	40	58	0	0
Squash	33	58	0	3
Tomatoes	100	56	0	0
Other fruits used as vegetables	10	100	0	0
Broccoli	23	74	0	0
Cabbage	65	83	0	0
Cauliflower	20	90	0	0
Celery	30	30	0	3
Collards	18	67	0	6
Endive/escarole	11	91	0	45
Kale	11	45	0	9
Lettuce, head	115	37	<1	0
Mustard greens	12	17	0	0
Romaine	85	35	4	1
Spinach	37	32	0	5
Other leaf/stem vegetables	48	60	0	19
Mushrooms/truffles & products	15	100	0	0
Carrots	130	57	2	0
Onions/leeks/scallions/shallots	28	89	0	0
Potatoes	239	56	0	2
Radishes	15	73	0	0
Red beets	15	100	0	0
Sweet potatoes/yams	25	64	0	0
Other root/tuber vegetables	9	89	0	0
Vegetables, dried or paste	45	89	0	0
Other vegetables/vegetable products	15	67	0	0
Total	1585	63	<1	2
F. Other				
Peanuts	50	94	0	0
Other nuts	17	100	0	0
Vegetable oils	13	100	0	0
Honey & other sweeteners	17	88	0	0
Baby foods/formula	61	97	0	0
Other food products	23	83	0	4
Total	181	94	0	<1
A–F Total	5101	64	<1	<1

Appendix B

Analysis of Import Surveillance Samples by Commodity Group in 1995

Commodity Group	Total no. of samples	Samples with no residues found, %	Samples violative, % Over tolerance	Samples violative, % No tolerance
A. Grains and Grain Products				
Rice, basmati	22	77	0	5
Rice, jasmine	34	91	0	0
Other rice & rice products	23	91	0	0
Wheat & wheat products	21	71	0	0
Other grains & grain products	16	100	0	0
Bakery products	21	86	0	5
Breakfast/snack foods	12	67	0	0
Macaroni	43	79	0	0
Spaghetti	18	72	0	0
Other pasta products	28	61	0	0
Total	238	80	0	<1
B. Dairy Products/Eggs				
Cheese & cheese products	75	93	0	0
Eggs	27	74	0	0
Total	102	88	0	0
C. Fish/Shellfish				
Fish	99	83	0	0
Shellfish	22	95	0	0
Total	121	85	0	0
D. Fruits				
Blackberries	30	40	0	3
Blueberries	38	97	0	0
Grapes	202	31	0	1
Raspberries	53	36	0	9
Strawberries	67	18	0	10
Other berries	20	55	0	0
Clementines	11	82	0	0
Limes	18	67	0	0
Oranges	30	70	0	7
Tangerines	12	58	0	0
Other citrus fruits	14	100	0	0
Apples	48	50	0	8
Pears	69	48	0	1
Apricots	10	50	0	0
Cherries	19	47	0	0
Nectarines	16	50	0	0
Olives	77	92	0	1
Peaches	52	48	0	4
Plums	31	55	0	0
Other pit fruits	13	100	0	0
Bananas	228	34	<1	0
Kiwi fruit	20	75	0	0
Mangoes	69	96	0	0
Papayas	81	72	0	9
Pineapples	65	75	5	0
Plantains	18	89	0	0
Other tropical fruits	56	89	0	7

Continued

Appendix B Continued

Commodity Group	Total no. of samples	Samples with no residues found, %	Samples violative, % Over tolerance	No tolerance
Cantaloupe	82	40	5	2
Honeydew	53	6	0	6
Watermelon	28	50	0	0
Other vine fruits	17	82	0	0
Apple juice	19	68	0	11
Other fruit juices	52	94	0	0
Fruit jams/jellies/toppings	41	90	0	0
Fruits, dried or paste	90	90	0	0
Other fruits & fruit products	8	88	0	0
Total	1757	57	<1	3
E. Vegetables				
Corn	45	100	0	0
Green/snow/sugar/sweet peas	90	51	0	12[a]
Mung beans	11	91	0	0
String beans	78	47	3	8
Other beans, peas, & corn	63	81	0	5
Cucumbers	96	49	0	4
Eggplant	23	48	0	0
Okra	33	73	0	9
Peppers, hot	261	46	3[a]	5
Peppers, sweet	295	76	0	1
Squash/pumpkins	110	35	0	4
Tomatoes	332	59	0	0
Other fruits used as vegetables	30	87	0	10
Artichokes	26	96	0	0
Asparagus	101	63	12	1
Bamboo shoots	20	100	0	0
Broccoli	53	70	0	0
Cabbage	16	63	0	0
Celery	20	20	0	0
Chicory	16	94	0	6
Endive/escarole	45	98	0	0
Lettuce, head	40	38	3	8
Radicchio	59	98	0	2
Romaine	44	50	7	3
Spinach	22	36	5	0
Other leaf/stem vegetables	67	64	1	10
Mushrooms/truffles, whole	47	96	0	2
Mushrooms/truffles, pieces & products	51	96	0	2
Carrots	46	67	0	0
Cassava	18	100	0	0
Onions	27	89	0	0
Potatoes	22	95	0	0
Radishes	13	62	0	0
Shallots/scallions/leeks	23	91	0	0
Sweet potatoes/yams	14	100	0	0
Water chestnuts	46	100	0	0
Other root/tuber vegetables	42	86	0	0
Vegetables, dried or paste	140	83	0	6
Vegetables with sauce	22	77	0	9
Other vegetables & vegetable products	28	82	0	0
Total	2535	67	1[a]	3[a]

Continued

Appendix B Continued

Commodity Group	Total no. of samples	Samples with no residues found, %	Samples violative, %	
			Over tolerance	No tolerance
F. Other				
Spices	14	75	0	0
Cashews	42	62	0	7
Peanuts	20	85	0	0
Other nuts & nut products	35	89	0	3
Edible seeds	24	75	0	17
Vegetable oils, crude	14	100	0	0
Vegetable oils, refined	15	100	0	0
Beverage bases	13	100	0	0
Bottled water, mineral/spring	19	100	0	0
Honey & other sweeteners	25	76	0	0
Other food products	58	79	0	0
Total	279	83	0	3
A–F Total	5032	66	<1[a]	3[a]

[a]Includes samples that have both residue(s) over tolerance and residue(s) with no tolerance.

APPENDIX II

Tables and Charts

From: Shils, Maurice E., Olson, James A., and Shilke, Moshe., eds. (1994) *Modern Nutrition in Health and Disease*, eighth edition, **2**. Philadelphia: Lea & Febiger. Reproduced with permission.

Table II.1   Conversion factors between traditional and SI units

Factors for converting nutrients expressed in metric or milleequivalent units into International System (SI) units.

1.   Definitions
   a.   Equivalent weight (EW) = atomic weight of element/valence of ionic form. Example with magnesium: atomic wt = 24, valence = 2+; therefore EW = 12
   b.   Quantity of an electrolyte in milliequivalents per liter (mEq/1) = mg of electrolyte/L/EW. Example: 48 mg of magnesium/L/12 = 4 mEq/L
   c.   Quantity of an electrolyte in mg/dl = (mEq/L × EW)/10
   d.   To convert mg/dl (= mg%) of an electrolyte to mEq/L mg/dl × 10/EW = mEq/L
   e.   1 mol = 1 molecular or atomic weight of element or compound in grams (GMWt). In solutions this is usually expressed as moles per liter; i.e., 1/mol/L = 1 M; 1 mM (mmol) = 1 mol × 10^{-3}; 1 μM ((μmol) = 1 mol × 10^{-6}; 1 nM (nmol) = 1 mol × 10^{-9}
   f.   (1)   To convert mEq/L of an electrolyte or other ions in solution to mmol/L: mEq/L divided by valence = mmol/L; e.g., (a) 2 mEq/L of magnesium (Mg^{2+}) = 2/2 = 1 mmol/L; e.g., (b) 140 mEq Na^+/L = 140/L = 140 mmol/L
      (2)   To convert mg/dl to mmol/L: (mg/dl × 10/EW) divided by valence = mmol/L; e.g., 2 mg/dl of magnesium = (2 × 10/12) divided by 2 = 0.83 mmol/L
      (3)   For organic substances: mmol/L = wt in mg/L/MW (in mg)
2.   SI units for expressing clinical laboratory data
   These units are now widely used and are increasingly required for publication of scientific data in physical, biologic, and biomedical publications. Extensive SI conversion tables have been published together with an explanation of the rationale for their use and technical aspects of usage. [1–3]
   a.   The base units of interest in physical quantities used in clinical chemistry are:

	Quantity	Base Unit
	mass	kilogram
	time	second
	amount	mole
	length	meter

   A derived unit for energy is the kjoule (kJ) 4.18 kJ = 1 kcal
   1 MJ = 239 kcal
   b.   Prefixes and symbols for decimal multiples and submultiples include:

Factor	Prefix	Symbol	Factor	Prefix	Symbol
10^8	giga	G	10^{-3}	milli	m
10^6	mega	M	10^{-8}	micro	u
10^3	kilo	k	10^{-8}	nano	n
10^2	hecto	h	10^{-12}	pico	p
10^1	deka	da	10^{-15}	femto	f
10^{-1}	deci	d	10^{-18}	atto	a
10^{-2}	centi	c			

Continued

Table II.1   Continued

3.   Conversion factors for selected compounds of nutrition interest*

Component	(1) Present Unit	(2) Conversion Factor	(3) SI Unit Symbol	(4) Mass Conversion Factor
Albumin (s)	g/dl	10	g/L	—
Aluminum (s)	μg/L	37.04	nmol/L	μg/27 = mol
Amino acids	(see ref. 3, p. 119 for individual amino acids)			
Amino acid nitrogen (p)	mg/dl	0.714	mmol/L	mg/14 = mmol
Ascorbic acid (p)	mg/dl	56.78	μmol/L	mg/176 = mmol
Calcium (s)	mg/dl	0.250	mmol/L	mg/40 = mmol
Calcium (s)	mEq/dl	0.500	mmol/L	mEq/2 = mmol
β-Carotenet (s)	μ/dl	0.0186	μmol/L	μg/536.85 umol
Chloride (s)	mEq/L	1.00	mmol/L	mEq = mmol
Cholesterol (p)	mg/dl	0.0258	mmol/L	mg/386.5 = mmol
Copper (s)	μg/dl	0.157	μmol/L	μg/63.5 = umol
Cyanocobalamin (B_{12})	pg/ml	0.738	pmol/L	pg/1355 = pmol
Ethanol (p)	mg/dl	0.217	mmol/L	mg/46 = mmol
Folic acid	ng/ml	2.265	nmol/L	ng/441.4 = nmol
Glucose (p)	mg/dl	0.0555	mmol/L	mg/180.2 = mmol
Iron (s)	μg/dl	0.179	μmol/L	μg/55.9 = μmol
Phosphate (p) (as phosphorus)	mg/dl	0.323	mmol/L	mg/31 = mmol
Potassium (s)	mEq/L	1.000	mmol/L	mEq = mmol
Potassium	mg/dl	0.256	mmol/L	mg/39.1 = mmol
Magnesium (s)	mg/dl	0.411	mmol/L	mg/24.3 = mmol
Pyridoxal (B)	ng/ml	5.981	nmol/L	ng/167 = nmol
Retinol† (p,s)	μg/dl	0.0349	μmol/L	μg 286 = μmol
Riboflavin (s)	μg/dl	26.57	nmol/L	μg/376 = nmol
Sodium (s)	mEq/L	1.00	mmol/L	mEq = mmol
Thiamin HCl (U)	μg/24 hr	0.00298	μmol/d	μg/337 = μmol
α-Tocopherol (p)	mg/dl	23.22	μmol/L	μg/431 = μmol
Vitamin D_3	μg/dl	26.01	nmol/L	μg/384 = μmol
Calcidiol	ng/ml	2.498	nmol/L	ng/400 = nmol
Zinc (s)	μg/dl	0.153	μmol/L	μg/65.4 = μmol

*To convert metric or equivalent unit per unit volume (column 1) to S.I. units per liter (column 3), multiply by the conversion factor in column 2, p = plasma; s = serum; B = blood; U = urine.
†See Appendix Table II.2 for detailed conversion figures for retinol and carotene.

REFERENCES

1. Young, D.S. (1987) *Ann. Intern. Med.*, **108** 114.
2. Lundberg, G.D. (1986) Iberson, C., Radulescu, G. *JAMA*, **255** 2329.
3. Mansen, E.R. (1987) *J. Am. Diet. Assoc.*, **87** 358.

Table II.2   Factors and formulas used in interconverting units of vitamin A and carotenoids

Factors
  1 nmol retinol = 286.42 ng
  1 nmol retinoic acid = 300.42 ng
  1 nmol β-carotene = 538.85 ng
1 μg retinol equivalent (μg RE)
  = 1 μg all-*trans* retinol
  = 3.49 nmol all-*trans* retinol
  = 6 μg all-*trans* β-carotene
  = 11.18 nmol all-*trans* β-carotene
  = 12 μg other all-*trans* provitamin A carotenoids
  = 3.33 IU_a (the international unit of all-*trans* retinol)
  = 10 IU_c (the international unit of all-*trans* β-carotene)

Table II.2   Continued

1 IU_a
  = 0.3 μg all-*trans* retinol
  = 0.3 μg RE
  = 1.05 nmol all-*trans* retinol
  = 1.8 μg all-*trans* β-carotene
  = 3.35 nmol all-*trans* β-carotene
  = 3 IU_c
  = 3.6 μg other all-*trans* provitamin A carotenoids
1 IU_c
  = 0.6 μg all-*trans* β-carotene
  = 1.12 nmol all-*trans* β-carotene
  = 0.1 μg RE
  = 0.33 IU_a
  = 1.2 μg other all-*trans* provitamin A carotenoids

Continued

Continued

Table II.2   Continued

Formulas and Examples: All-*trans* configurations of retinol and carotenoids are assumed

1. $\mu g\ RE = \mu g$ retinol $+ \mu g$ β-carotene/6
   A diet contains 500 μg retinol and 1800 μg β-carotene. Then,
   $$\mu g\ RE = 500 + 1800/6 = 800\ \mu g\ RE$$

2. $\mu g\ RE = IU_a/3.33 + IU_c/10$
   A diet contains 1667 IU_a of retinol and 3000 IU_c of β-carotene. Then,
   $$\mu g\ RE = 1667/3.33 + 3000/10 = 800\ \mu g\ RE$$

3. $\mu g\ RE = \mu g$ β-carotene/6 $+ \mu g$ other provitamin A carotenoids/12
   A serving of sweet potato contains 2400 μg of β-carotene and 480 μg of other provitamin A carotenoids. Then,
   $$\mu g\ RE = 2400/6 + 480/12 = 440\ \mu g\ RE$$

4. $$\%\ \mu g\ RE\ as\ retinol = \left[1.5 - \frac{0.15\ total\ IU}{total\ RE}\right] \times 100$$

   $$\%\ \mu g\ RE\ as\ carotenoids = \left[\frac{0.15\ total\ IU}{total\ RE} - 0.5\right] \times 100$$

   A 100-g portion of cheese contains a total of 300 μg RE and a total of 1200 IU, in which 1 IU_a has been *assumed* to equal 1 IU_c. Then,

   $$\%\ RE\ as\ retinol = \left[1.5 - \frac{0.15 \times 1200}{300}\right] \times 100 = 90\%$$

   $$\%\ RE\ as\ carotenoids = \left[\frac{0.15 \times 1200}{300} - 0.5\right] \times 100 \times 10\%$$

Continued

Table II.2   Continued

In this sample of cheese, therefore, 270 μg (270 μg RE) is present as retinol and 180 μg, or 30 μg RE, is present as β-carotene or its equivalent of other provitamin A carotenoids.

5. $$IU_a = \frac{10\ \mu g\ RE - total\ IU}{2}$$

   $$IU_c = \frac{3\ total\ IU - 10\ \mu g\ RE}{2}$$

In a cheese sample containing a total of 300 μg RE and a total of 1200 IU, in which 1 IU_a is *assumed* to equal 1 IU_c,

$$IU_a = \frac{10 \times 300 - 1200}{2} = 900$$

$$IU_c = \frac{3 \times 1200 - 10 \times 300}{2} = 300$$

Note: Assumptions used from revised sections of the United States Department of Agriculture's *Handbook 8* (i.e., 8.1–8.10) are (a) that 1 IU_a = 1 IU_c and (b) that 1 RE = 1 μg of retinol = 6 μg of β-carotene = 12 μg of other provitamin A carotenoids.

In some cases, small negative values for IU_c are obtained when the values for total IU and total RE are given for foods containing only preformed vitamin A_1 particularly in fortified foods like margarine. This aberrant calculation results from the rounding of analytic values. Similarly, small negative values for IU_a may result for foods containing only carotenoids. In both cases, the negative values should be taken as zero.
Prepared by J.A. Olson.

Table II.3   Weights and measures

VOLUMES:

Apothecaries' Measure	Metric	Household
1 fluid dram (fl dr)	4 milliliter (ml)	1 teaspoon (tsp)
2 fl dr	8 ml	1 dessert spoonful
$\frac{1}{2}$ fluid ounce (fl oz)	15 ml	1 tablespoon (Tbsp) (3 tsp)
1 fl oz	30 ml	2 Tbsp ($\frac{1}{8}$ cup)
$1\frac{1}{2}$ fl oz	45 ml	1 jigger
2 fl oz	58 ml	4 Tbsp ($\frac{1}{4}$ cup)
$2\frac{2}{3}$ fl oz	80 ml	$5\frac{1}{3}$ Tbs ($\frac{1}{3}$ cup)
4 fl oz	118 ml	8 Tbsp ($\frac{1}{2}$ cup)
8 fl oz	237 ml	1 cup
16 fl oz	473 ml	1 pint (pt)
32 fl oz	947 ml	1 quart (qt)
128 fl oz	3.785 ml	1 gallon (gal)
3.38 fl oz	1 deciliter (dl) (100 ml)	
2.11 pt	1 liter (L) (1,000 ml)	

Continued

Table II.3   Continued

WEIGHTS:

Avoirdupois	Metric
	1 femtogram (fg) $(10^{-15}$ g)
	1 picogram (pg) $(10^{-12}$ g)
	1 nanogram (ng) $(10^{-9}$ g)
	1 microgram (μg) $(10^{-6}$ g)
1 grain (gr)	0.065 g (65 mg)
1 gram (0.035 oz)	15.432 gr
1 scruple (20 gr)	1.296 g
1 dram (dr) (= drachm) (27.3 gr)	1.77 g
1 oz (16 dr)	28.35 g
1 lb (16 oz)	453.59 g
1 ton (2,000 lb)	0.91 metric tons
1.015 gr	1 milligram (mg) $(10^{-3}$ g)
	1 centigram (cg) $(10^{-2}$ g)
	1 decigram (dg) $(10^{-1}$ g)
15.4 gr (0.035 oz)	1 gram (g)
2.2 lb	1 kilogram (kg) $(10^3$ g)

LENGTH/AREA:

	Metric
1 angstrom (A)	10 millimeter (mm)
1/2500 inch (in)	1 micron (μ) $(10^{-3}$ mm) = micrometer (μm)
0.039 in	1 mm
0.39 in	1 centimeter (cm)
1 in	2.54 cm
1 foot (ft) (12 in)	30.5 cm
39.4 in	1 meter (m)
1 yard (yd) (3ft)	0.9 m
1 rod (5.5 yd)	4.85 m
1093.6 yd (0.62 mile)	1 kilometer (km)
1 mile (mi) (5280 ft)	1.61 km
1 acre (160 square rods)	0.4 hectare

TEMPERATURE CONVERSIONS:

F to C: 5/9 (F − 32)
C to F: (9/5 × C) + 32

ELECTROLYTE DATA:

Ion		Atomic Wt (1)	Valence (2)	Equivalent Wt* 1 ÷ 2
Bicarbonate	HCO_3^-	61.0	1	61.0
Calcium	Ca^{2+}	40.1	2	20.0
Chloride	Cl^-	35.5	1	35.5
Magnesium	Mg^{2+}	24.3	2	12.2
Phosphate†	HPO_4^{2-}	96.0	2	48.0†
Potassium	K^+	39.1	1	39.1
Sodium	Na^+	23.0	1	23.0
Sulfate	SO_4^{2-}	96.1	2	48.0

*Milliequivalent (mEq) = equivalent weight in milligrams (mg). To convert mg quantities of all electrolytes to mEq:

$$\frac{mg\ of\ electrolyte}{equivalent\ weight\ in\ mg} = mEq$$

To convert mEq quantities of all electrolytes to mg:
mEq × equivalent wt = mg

To convert mg/dl to mEq/L:

$$\frac{mg/dl \times 10}{equivalent\ wt\ in\ mg} = mEq/L$$

To convert mEq/L to mg/dl: mEq/L × equivalent wt in mg × 0.1

† At the normal pH of plasma, 20% of the total inorganic phosphate radical is combined with one equivalent of base as BH_2PO_4, and 80% with two equivalents of base as B_2HPO_4. Under these conditions, base equivalence is therefore 0.2 + (0.8 × 2) = 1.8, and the equivalent weight of 53.3 is obtained by dividing the ionic weight by 1.8 instead of by 2. For phosphorus content of phosphate solutions, 1 mEq provides approximately 15 mg, and 1 mmol provides approximately 31 mg.

Table II.4 Summary of examples of recommended nutrient intake based on age and body weight expressed as daily rates, Canada

Age	Sex	Weight (kg)	Protein (g)	Vit. A (RE)[a]	Vit. D (µg)	Vit. E (mg)	Vit. C (mg)	Folate (µg)	Vit. B_{12} (µg)	Calcium (mg)	Phosphorus (mg)	Magnesium (mg)	Iron (mg)	Iodine (µg)	Zinc (mg)
Months															
0–4	Both	6.0	12[b]	400	10	3	20	25	0.3	250[c]	150	20	0.3[d]	30	2[d]
5–12	Both	9.0	12	400	10	3	20	40	0.4	400	200	32	7	40	3
Years															
1	Both	11	13	400	10	3	20	40	0.5	500	300	40	6	55	4
2–3	Both	14	16	400	5	4	20	50	0.6	550	350	50	6	65	4
4–6	Both	18	19	500	5	5	25	70	0.8	600	400	65	8	85	5
7–9	M	25	26	700	2.5	7	25	90	1.0	700	500	100	8	110	7
	F	25	26	700	2.5	6	25	90	1.0	700	500	100	8	95	7
10–12	M	34	34	800	2.5	8	25	120	1.0	900	700	130	8	125	9
	F	36	36	800	2.5	7	25	130	1.0	1100	800	135	8	110	9
13–15	M	50	49	900	2.5	9	30[e]	175	1.0	1100	900	185	10	160	12
	F	48	46	800	2.5	7	30[e]	170	1.0	1000	850	180	13	160	9
16–18	M	62	58	1000	2.5	10	40[e]	220	1.0	900	1000	230	10	160	12
	F	53	47	800	2.5	7	30[e]	190	1.0	700	850	200	12	160	9
19–24	M	71	61	1000	2.5	10	40[e]	220	1.0	800	1000	240	9	160	12
	F	58	50	800	2.5	7	30[e]	180	1.0	700	850	200	13	160	9
25–49	M	74	64	1000	2.5	9	40[e]	230	1.0	800	1000	250	9	160	12
	F	59	51	800	2.5	6	30[e]	185	1.0	700	850	200	13	160	9
50–74	M	73	63	1000	5	7	40[e]	230	1.0	800	1000	250	9	160	12
	F	63	54	800	5	6	30[e]	195	1.0	800	850	210	8	160	9
75+	M	69	59	1000	5	6	40[e]	215	1.0	800	1000	230	9	160	12
	F	64	55	800	5	5	30[e]	200	1.0	800	850	210	8	160	9
Pregnancy (additional)															
1st trimester			5	0	2.5	2	0	200	0.2	500	200	15	0	25	6
2nd trimester			20	0	2.5	2	10	200	0.2	500	200	45	5	25	6
3rd trimester			24	0	2.5	2	10	200	0.2	500	200	45	10	25	6
Lactation (additional)			20	400	2.5	3	25	100	0.2	500	200	65	0	50	6

[a]Retinol Equivalents.
[b]Protein is assumed to be from breast milk and must be adjusted for infant formula.
[c]Infant formula with high phosphorus should contain 375 mg calcium.
[d]Breast milk is assumed to be the source of the mineral.
[e]Smokers should increase vitamin C by 50%.
(From Supply and Services Canada (1990) *Health and Welfare Canada: Nutrition Recommendations*. The Report of the Scientific Review Committee, Ottawa. Reproduced with permission of the Minister of Supply and Services Canada 1992.)

Table II.5 Estimated average requirements (EAR) for energy, United Kingdom

Age	EAR MJ/D (KCAL/D) Males	Females
0–3 months	2.28 (545)	2.16 (515)
4–6 months	2.89 (690)	2.69 (645)
7–9 months	3.44 (825)	3.20 (765)
10–12 months	3.85 (920)	3.61 (865)
1–3 years	5.15 (1,230)	4.86 (1,165)
4–6 years	7.16 (1,715)	6.46 (1,545)
7–10 years	8.24 (1,970)	7.28 (1,740)
11–14 years	9.27 (2,220)	7.92 (1,845)
15–18 years	11.51 (2,755)	8.83 (2,110)
19–50 years	10.60 (2,550)	8.10 (1,940)
51–59 years	10.60 (2,550)	8.00 (1,900)
60–64 years	9.93 (2,380)	7.99 (1,900)
65–74 years	9.71 (2,330)	7.96 (1,900)
75+ years	8.77 (2,100)	7.61 (1,810)
Pregnancy		+0.80*(200)
Lactation:		
1 month		+1.90 (450)
2 months		+2.20 (530)
3 months		+2.40 (570)
4–6 months (Group 1)		+2.00 (480)
4–6 months (Group 2)		+2.40 (570)
>6 months (Group 1)		+1.00 (240)
>6 months (Group 2)		+2.30 (550)

*last trimester only.
(From Report on Health and Social Subjects (1991) *Dietary Reference Values for Food and Energy and Nutrients for the United Kingdom*, Her Majesty's Stationery Office, London.)

Table II.6 Reference nutrient intakes for protein, United Kingdom

Age	Reference nutrient intake[a] (g/d)	
0–3 months	12.5[b]	
4–6 months	12.7	
7–9 months	13.7	
10–12 months	14.9	
1–3 years	14.5	
4–6 years	19.7	
7–10 years	28.3	
Males		
11–14 years	42.1	
15–18 years	55.2	
19–50 years	55.5	
50+ years	53.3	
Females		
11–14 years	41.2	
15–18 years	45.0	
19–50 years	45.0	
50+ years	46.5	
Pregnancy[c]		+6
Lactation[c]		
0–4 months		+11
4+ months		+8

[a]These figures, based on egg and milk protein, assume complete digestibility.
[b]No values for infants 0 to 3 months are given by WHO. The reference nutrient intake is calculated from the recommendations of Committee on Medical Aspects of Food Policy (COMA).
[c]To be added to adult requirement through all stages of pregnancy and lactation.
(From Report on Health and Social Subjects (1991) *No. 41, Dietary Reference Values for Food Energy and Nutrients for the United Kingdom*, Report of the Panel on Dietary Reference Values of the Committee on Medical Aspects of Food Policy. Her Majesty's Stationery Office, London.)

Table II.7   Reference nutrient intakes for vitamins, United Kingdom

Age	Thiamin (mg/d)	Riboflavin (mg/d)	Niacin (nicotinic acid equivalent) (mg/d)	Vitamin B_6 (mg/d^a)	Vitamin B_{12} (μg/d)	Folate (μg/d)	Vitamin C (mg/d)	Vitamin A (μg/d)	Vitamin D (μg/d)
0–3 months	0.2	0.4	3	0.2	0.3	50	25	350	8.5
4–6 months	0.2	0.4	3	0.2	0.3	50	25	350	8.5
7–9 months	0.2	0.4	4	0.3	0.4	50	25	350	7
10–12 months	0.3	0.4	5	0.4	0.4	50	25	350	7
1–3 years	0.5	0.6	8	0.7	0.5	70	30	400	7
4–6 years	0.7	0.8	11	0.9	0.8	100	30	500	–
7–10 years	0.7	1.0	12	1.0	1.0	150	30	500	–
Males									
11–14 years	0.9	1.2	15	1.2	1.2	200	35	600	–
15–18 years	1.1	1.3	18	1.5	1.5	200	40	700	–
19–50 years	1.0	1.3	17	1.4	1.5	200	40	700	–
50+ years	0.9	1.3	16	1.4	1.5	200	40	700	**
Females									
11–14 years	0.7	1.1	12	1.0	1.2	200	35	600	–
15–18 years	0.8	1.1	14	1.2	1.5	200	40	600	–
19–50 years	0.8	1.1	13	1.2	1.5	200	40	600	–
50+ years	0.8	1.1	12	1.2	1.5	200	40	600	**
Pregnancy	+0.1^b	+0.3	*	*	*	+100	+10	+100	10
Lactation									
0–4 months	+0.2	+0.5	+2	*	+0.5	+60	+30	+350	10
4+ months	+0.2	+0.5	+2	*	+0.5	+60	+30	+350	10

*No increment.
**After age 65 the RNI is 10 μg/d for men and women.
^{a}Based on protein providing 14.7% of EAR for energy.
^{b}For last trimester only.
(From Report on Health and Social Subjects (1991) *No. 41, Dietary Reference Values for Food Energy and Nutrients for the United Kingdom*. Report of the Panel on Dietary Reference Values of the Committee on Medical Aspects of Food Policy. Her Majesty's Stationery Office, London.)

Table II.8 Reference nutrient intakes for minerals, United Kingdom

Age	Calcium (mmol/d)	Phosphorus[1] (mmol/d)	Magnesium (mmol/d)	Sodium (mmol/d[2])	Potassium (mmol/d[3])	Chloride[4] (mmol/d)	Iron (μmol/d)	Zinc (μmol/d)	Copper (μmol/d)	Selenium (μmol/d)	Iodine (μmol/d)
0–3 months	13.1	13.1	2.2	9	20	9	30	60	5	0.1	0.4
4–6 months	13.1	13.1	2.5	12	22	12	80	60	5	0.2	0.5
7–9 months	13.1	13.1	3.2	14	18	14	140	75	5	0.1	0.5
10–12 months	13.1	13.1	3.3	15	18	15	140	75	5	0.1	0.5
1–3 years	8.8	8.8	3.5	22	20	22	120	75	6	0.2	0.6
4–6 years	11.3	11.3	4.8	30	28	30	110	100	9	0.3	0.8
7–10 years	13.8	13.8	8.0	50	50	50	160	110	11	0.4	0.9
Males											
11–14 years	25.0	25.0	11.5	70	80	70	200	140	13	0.6	1.0
15–18 years	25.0	25.0	12.3	70	90	70	200	145	16	0.9	1.0
19–50 years	17.5	17.5	12.3	70	90	70	160	145	19	0.9	1.0
50+ years	17.5	17.5	12.3	70	90	70	160	145	19	0.9	1.0
Females											
11–14 years	20.0	10.0	11.5	70	80	70	260[5]	140	13	0.6	1.0
15–18 years	20.0	20.0	12.3	70	90	70	260[5]	110	16	0.8	1.1
19–50 years	17.5	17.5	10.9	70	90	70	260[5]	110	19	0.8	1.1
50+ years	17.5	17.5	10.9	70	90	70	160	110	19	0.8	1.1
Pregnancy	*	*	*	*	*	*	*	*	*	*	*
Lactation											
0–4 months	+14.3	+14.3	+2.1	*	*	*	*	+90	+5	+0.2	*
4+ months	+14.3	+14.3	+2.1	*	*	*	*	+40	+5	+0.2	*
0–3 months	525	400	55	210	800	320	1.7	4.0	0.2	10	50
4–6 months	525	400	60	280	850	400	4.3	4.0	0.3	13	60
7–9 months	525	400	75	320	700	500	7.8	5.0	0.3	10	60
10–12 months	525	400	80	350	700	500	7.8	5.0	0.3	10	60
1–3 years	350	270	85	500	800	800	6.9	5.0	0.4	15	70
4–6 years	450	350	120	700	1,100	1,100	6.1	6.5	0.6	20	100
7–10 years	550	450	200	1,200	2,000	1,800	8.7	7.0	0.7	30	110
Males											
11–14 years	1,000	775	280	1,600	3,100	2,500	11.3	9.0	0.8	45	130
15–18 years	1,000	775	300	1,600	3,500	2,500	11.3	9.5	1.0	70	140
19–50 years	700	550	300	1,600	3,500	2,500	8.7	9.5	1.2	75	140
50+ years	700	550	300	1,600	3,500	2,500	8.7	9.5	1.2	75	140
Females											
11–14 years	800	625	280	1,600	3,100	2,500	14.8[5]	9.0	0.8	45	130
15–18 years	800	625	300	1,600	3,500	2,500	14.8[5]	7.0	1.0	60	140
19–50 years	700	550	270	1,600	3,500	2,500	14.8[5]	7.0	1.2	60	140
50+ years	700	550	270	1,600	3,500	2,500	8.7	7.0	1.2	60	140

Continued

Table II.9 Safe intakes, United Kingdom

Nutrient	Safe intake
Vitamins	
Pantothenic acid	
adults	3–7 mg/d
infants	1.7 mg/d
Biotin	10–200 µg/d
Vitamin E	
men	above 4 mg/d
women	above 3 mg/d
infants	0.4 mg/g polyunsaturated fatty acids
Vitamin K	
adults	1 µg/kg/d
infants	10 µg/d
Minerals	
Manganese	
adults	1.4 mg (26 µmol)/d
infants and children	16 µg (0.3 µmol)/d
Molybdenum	
adults	50–400 µg/d
infants, children, and adolescents	0.5–1.5 µg/kg/d
Chromium	
adults	25 µg (0.5 µmol)/d
children and adolescents	0.1–1.0 µg (2–20 µmol)/kg/d
Fluoride (for infants only)	0.05 mg (3 µmol)/kg/d

For some nutrients, which are known to have important functions in humans, the Panel found insufficient reliable data on human requirements and were unable to set any dietary reference values for these. However, they decided on grounds of prudence to set a safe intake, particularly for infants and children. The safe intake was judged to be a level or range of intake at which there is no risk of deficiency and below a level where there is risk of undesirable effects. They are not therefore intended as a "toxic level", and although exceeding these safe intakes would not necessarily result in undesirable effects, equally there is no evidence for any benefits. The Panel agreed that the safe range of intakes set for the nutrients need not be exceeded.

(From Report on Health and Social Subjects (1991) *No. 41, Dietary Reference Values for Food Energy and Nutrients for the United Kingdom.* Report of the Panel on Dietary Reference Values of the Committee on Medical Aspects of Food Policy, Her Majesty's Stationery Office, London.)

Table II.8 Continued

Age	Calcium (mmol/d)	Phosphorus[1] (mmol/d)	Magnesium (mmol/d)	Sodium (mmol/d)	Potassium (mmol/d[3])	Chloride[4] (mmol/d)	Iron (µmol/d)	Zinc (µmol/d)	Copper (µmol/d)	Selenium (µmol/d)	Iodine (µmol/d)
Pregnancy	*	*	*	*	*	*	*	*	*	*	*
Lactation											
0–4 months	+550	+440	+50	*	*	*	*	+6.0	+0.3	+15	*
4+ months	+550	+440	+50	*	*	*	*	+2.5	+0.3	+15	*

*No increment.

[1] Phosphorus RNI is set equal to calcium in molar terms.

[2] 1 mmol sodium = 23 mg.

[3] 1 mmol potassium 39 mg.

[4] Corresponds to sodium 1 mmol = 35.5 mg.

[5] Insufficient for women with high menstrual losses where the most practical way of meeting iron requirements is to take iron supplements.

(From Report on Health and Social Subjects (1991) *No. 41, Dietary Reference Values for Food Energy and Nutrients for the United Kingdom.* Report of the Panel on Dietary Reference Values of the Committee on Medical Aspects of Food Policy, Her Majesty's Stationery Office, London.)

Table II.10 Recommended dietary allowances for persons with low activity, Japan

Age	Energy (kcal) M	Energy (kcal) F	Protein (g) M	Protein (g) F	Fat (%)	Calcium (g) M	Calcium (g) F	Iron (mg) M	Iron (mg) F	Vitamin A (IU) M	Vitamin A (IU) F	Vitamin B₁ (mg) M	Vitamin B₁ (mg) F	Vitamin B₂ (mg) M	Vitamin B₂ (mg) F	Niacin (mg) M	Niacin (mg) F	Ascorbic acid (mg)	Vitamin D (IU)
15~	2,350	2,000	85	70	25~30	0.8		12	12			0.9	0.8	1.3	1.1	16	13	50	100
16~	2,400	1,950	80	70								1.0	0.8	1.3	1.1	16	13		
17~	2,400	1,900	80	70								1.0	0.8	1.3	1.0	16	13		
18~	2,350	1,850	75	65		0.7						0.9	0.7	1.3	1.0	16	12		
19~	2,300	1,850	75	60								0.9	0.7	1.3	1.0	15	12		
20~29	2,250	1,800	70	60		0.6		12	12	2,000	1,800	0.9	0.7	1.2	1.0	15	12		
30~39	2,200	1,750	70	60								0.9	0.7	1.2	1.0	15	12		
40~49	2,150	1,700	70	60								0.9	0.7	1.2	0.9	14	11		
50~59	2,000	1,650	70	60								0.8	0.7	1.1	0.9	13	11		
60~64	1,850	1,550	70	60	20~25	0.6		10				0.7	0.6	1.0	0.9	12	10		
65~69	1,800	1,500	70	60					†10			0.7	0.6	1.0	0.9	12	10		
70~74	1,650	1,450	65	55								0.7	0.6	1.0	0.9	12	10		
75~79	1,600	1,400	65	55								0.7	0.6	1.0	0.9	12	10		
80~	1,500	1,250	65	55								0.7	0.6	1.0	0.9	12	10		
1st Half Pregnancy*		+150		+10	25~30		+0.4		+3		+0		+0.1		+0.1		+1	+10	+300
Last Half Pregnancy		+350		+20			+0.4		+8		+200		+0.2		+0.2		+2	+10	+300
Lactation		+700		+20			+0.5		+8		+1,400		+0.3		+0.4		+5	+40	+300

*Pregnancy increases are shown for convenience; however, values apply to each activity level.
†Decrease to 10 mg after menopause.
(From the Health Promotion and Nutrition Division (1991) Health Policy Bureau, Ministry of Health and Welfare, Tokyo, Japan.)

Table II.11 Recommended dietary allowances for persons with medium activity or growth stages, Japan

Age	Average height (cm) M	F	Average weight (kg) M	F	Energy (kcal) M	F	Protein (g) M	F	Fat (%)	Calcium (g) M	F	Iron (mg) M	F	Vitamin A (IU) M	F	Vitamin B_1 (mg) M	F	Vitamin B_2 (mg) M	F	Niacin (mg) M	F	Ascorbic acid (mg)	Vitamin D (IU)
0~mo					120/kg		3.3/kg		45	0.4	0.4	6	6	1,300	1,300	0.2	0.2	0.3	0.3	4			400
2~mo					110/kg		2.5/kg		45	0.4	0.4	6	6	1,300	1,300	0.3	0.3	0.4	0.4	6			
6~mo					100/kg		3.0/kg		30~40	0.4	0.4	6	6	1,000	1,000	0.4	0.4	0.5	0.5	6			
1~yr	80.7	79.6	10.95	10.35	960	910	30	30								0.4		0.5		6	6		
2~	90.0	89.1	13.24	12.74	1,200	1,150	35	35				7	7					0.7		8	8		
3~	97.3	96.6	15.04	14.70	1,400	1,350	40	40								0.5				9	9		
4~	104.3	103.7	16.97	16.69	1,550	1,450	45	45		0.4	0.4	8	8	1,000	1,000		0.4	0.8		10		40	
5~	110.8	110.3	19.04	18.78	1,600	1,500	50	50								0.6			0.6		10		
6~	117.0	116.5	21.35	21.04	1,700	1,600	55	50										0.9		11			
7~	122.7	122.2	23.85	23.44	1,800	1,650	60	55		0.5	0.5	9	9	1,200	1,200	0.7	0.5						
8~	128.3	127.9	26.70	26.24	1,900	1,750	65	60										1.0	0.7	12			
9~	133.5	133.6	29.76	29.50	1,950	1,850	65	65								0.8				13	10		
10~	138.8	139.8	33.21	33.54	2,050	1,950	70	70	25~30	0.6	0.6	10	10				0.6	1.1					100
11~	144.6	146.5	37.26	38.46	2,150	2,100	75	75		0.7									0.8	14	11		
12~	151.4	151.9	42.29	43.31	2,350	2,250	80	80		0.8				1,500	1,500	0.9		1.2					
13~	159.0	155.4	48.34	47.43	2,500	2,300	85	80		0.9	0.7	12	12					1.3	0.9	15	12		
14~	164.9	157.1	53.87	50.32	2,600	2,300	85	75								1.0		1.4		16	13		
15~	168.5	157.6	57.98	51.99	2,700	2,250	85	70									0.7		1.0	17		50	
16~	169.9	158.0	60.21	52.87	2,700	2,200	80	70		0.8						1.1		1.5			14		
17~	170.8	158.1	61.55	52.92	2,700	2,150	80	70											1.1				
18~	171.3	158.1	62.18	52.52	2,650	2,100	75	65		0.7										18			
19~	171.5	158.1	62.41	52.02	2,600	2,050	75	60					12				0.8	1.4			15		
20~29	171.1	157.7	64.00	51.83	2,550	2,000	70	60	20~25														
30~39	169.8	156.7	65.48	54.09	2,500	2,000	70	60								1.0		1.3		17			
40~49	167.8	154.6	65.10	55.14	2,400	1,950	70	60					12										
50~59	164.2	151.9	61.93	54.13	2,250	1,850	70	60		0.6	0.6	10	*	2,000	1,800	0.9		1.2	1.1	16	15	50	
60~64	162.1	149.8	59.41	52.49	2,100	1,750	70	60															
65~69	160.8	148.3	57.61	51.02	2,000	1,700	70	60												15			
70~74	159.7	145.7	55.83	49.26	1,850	1,600	65	55					10			0.8	0.7	1.2	1.0	14	13		
75~79	158.7	145.0	54.07	47.22	1,750	1,550	65	55													12		
80~	157.6	142.4	52.38	44.53	1,650	1,400	65	55												14			

*Decrease to 10 mg after menopause.

(From the Health Promotion and Nutrition Division (1991) Health Policy Bureau. Ministry of Health and Welfare, Tokyo, Japan.)

Table II.12 Recommended dietary allowances for persons with medium-high activity, Japan

Age	Energy (kcal) M	F	Protein (g) M	F	Fat (%)	Calcium (g) M	F	Iron (mg) M	F	Vitamin A (IU) M	F	Vitamin B₁ (mg) M	F	Vitamin B₂ (mg) M	F	Niacin (mg) M	F	Ascorbic acid (mg)	Vitamin D (IU)
15~	3,200	2,650	100	85		0.8						1.3	1.1	1.8	1.5	21	17		
16~	3,200	2,600	95	80								1.3	1.0	1.8	1.4	21	17		
17~	3,200	2,550	95	80				12	12			1.3	1.0	1.8	1.4	21	17		
18~	3,150	2,500	90	75		0.7						1.3	1.0	1.7	1.4	21	17		
19~	3,100	2,450	90	70								1.2	1.0	1.7	1.3	20	16		
20~29	3,050	2,400	85	70	25~30	0.6				2,000	1,800	1.2	1.0	1.7	1.3	20	16	50	100
30~39	2,950	2,350	85	70				12				1.2	0.9	1.6	1.3	19	16		
40~49	2,850	2,300	85	70								1.1	0.9	1.6	1.3	19	15		
50~59	2,700	2,200	85	70		0.6		10	*			1.1	0.9	1.5	1.2	18	15		
60~64	2,450	2,050	80	70					10			1.0	0.8	1.3	1.1	16	14		
65~69	2,350	2,000	80	70								1.0	0.8	1.3	1.1	16	14		

*Decrease to 10 mg after menopause.
(From the Health Promotion and Nutrition Division (1991) Health Policy Bureau, Ministry of Health and Welfare, Tokyo Japan.)

Table II.13 Recommended dietary allowances for persons with high activity, Japan

Age	Energy (kcal) M	F	Protein (g) M	F	Fat (%)	Calcium (g) M	F	Iron (mg) M	F	Vitamin A (IU) M	F	Vitamin B₁ (mg) M	F	Vitamin B₂ (mg) M	F	Niacin (mg) M	F	Ascorbic acid (mg)	Vitamin D (IU)
15~	3,750	3,100	115	95		0.8						1.5	1.2	2.1	1.7	25	20		
16~	3,750	3,050	110	95								1.5	1.2	2.1	1.7	25	20		
17~	3,750	2,950	110	95				12	12			1.5	1.2	2.1	1.6	25	19		
18~	3,700	2,900	105	90		0.7						1.5	1.2	2.0	1.6	24	19		
19~	3,700	2,850	105	85								1.5	1.1	2.0	1.6	24	19		
20~29	3,550	2,800	100	85	25~30	0.6				2,000	1,800	1.4	1.1	2.0	1.5	23	18	50	100
30~39	3,450	2,750	100	85				12				1.4	1.1	1.9	1.5	23	18		
40~49	3,350	2,700	100	85								1.3	1.1	1.8	1.5	22	18		
50~59	3,150	2,600	100	85		0.6		10	*			1.3	1.0	1.7	1.4	21	17		
60~64	2,850	2,400	95	80					10			1.1	1.0	1.6	1.3	19	16		
65~69	2,750	2,300	95	80								1.1	1.0	1.6	1.3	19	16		

*Decrease to 10 mg after menopause.
(From the Health Promotion and Nutrition Division (1991) Health Policy Bureau, Ministry of Health and Welfare, Tokyo, Japan.)

Comments
1. These general guidelines are not for individual daily values. For individual nutrient requirements, other tables must be used.
2. An individual should take no more than 10 mg sodium daily.
3. Vitamin E: males should have at least 8 mg, females should have at least 7 mg.
4. For those in the low activity category, more exercise is recommended. The values in Table II.12 represent the ideal intake for adults. These values are reflective of individuals who exercise accordingly.

Table II.14 Recommended daily dietary allowances, Korea*

Category	Age (years)	Weight (kg)	Height (cm)	Energy (kcal)	Protein (g)	Vitamin A (re)[†]	Vitamin B_1 (mg)	Vitamin B_2 (mg)	Niacin (mg)	Vitamin C (mg)	Vitamin D (μg)[‡]	Calcium (mg)	Iron (mg)[§]
Infants													
	0–3 mo	5.5	58.5	800	25	350	0.40	0.48	6.4	35	10	400	10
	4–6 mo	8.4	67.5	900	25	350	0.45	0.54	7.2	35	10	400	10
	7–9 mo	9.5	76.0	1,000	30	350	0.50	0.60	8.0	35	10	400	15
	10–12 mo	10.4	79.0	1,100	30	350	0.55	0.66	8.0	35	10	400	15
Children													
	1–3	12.6	87.0	1,200	35	350	0.60	0.72	8.0	40	10	500	15
	4–6	19.0	110.0	1,300	40	400	0.75	0.90	10.0	40	10	600	10
	7–9	26.0	130.0	1,800	50	500	0.90	1.08	12.0	40	10	700	10
Males													
	10–12	36.0	144.0	2,100	60	600	1.05	1.26	14.0	50	10	800	15
	13–15	51.0	161.0	2,600	80	700	1.30	1.36	17.0	50	10	800	18
	16–19	59.0	169.0	2,500	75	700	1.25	1.50	16.5	55	10	800	18
	20–29	64.0	170.5	2,500	70	700	1.25	1.50	16.5	55	5	600	10
	30–49	65.0	168.5	2,500	70	700	1.25	1.50	16.5	55	5	600	10
	50–64	63.0	168.0	2,200	70	700	1.10	1.32	14.5	55	5	600	10
	65 or older	61.0	167.0	1,900	70	700	1.00	1.20	13.0	55	5	600	10
Females													
	10–12	37.0	145.0	2,000	60	600	1.00	1.20	13.0	50	10	800	18
	13–15	48.0	155.0	2,300	65	700	1.15	1.38	15.0	50	10	800	18
	16–19	52.0	158.0	2,200	60	700	1.10	1.32	14.5	55	10	700	18
	20–29	52.5	159.5	2,000	60	700	1.00	1.20	13.0	55	5	600	18
	30–49	55.0	158.0	2,000	60	700	1.00	1.20	13.0	55	5	600	18
	50–64	54.0	156.0	1,900	60	700	1.00	1.20	13.0	55	5	600	10
	65 or older	53.0	156.0	1,600	60	700	1.00	1.20	13.0	55	5	600	10
Pregnancy													
	First half			+150	+30	+ 0	+0.40	+0.30	+2.0	+15	+5	+400	+2
	Second half			+350	+30	+100	+0.40	+0.30	+2.0	+15	+5	+400	+2
Lactation													
				+700	+30	+300	+0.60	+0.50	+6.0	+35	+5	+500	+2

*The allowances for energy are based on individuals of moderate activity. Data in this table are intended to provide only a standard figure under usual environment and given conditions.

[†]Retinol equivalent: 1 RE = 1 μg retinol = 6 μg β-carotene.

[‡]Vitamin D: 10 μg = 400 IU.

[§]Supplemental iron should be taken to meet the increased requirement during pregnancy and lactation.

(From the Ministry of Health and Social Affairs (1989) Kyonggi, Korea.)

Table II.15   Equations for predicting basal metabolic rate from body weight (W)*

Age range (years)	KCAL_th/day	Correlation coefficient	SD[†]	MJ/day	Correlation coefficient	SD
Males						
0–3	60.9 W − 54	0.97	53	0.255 W − 0.226	0.97	0.222
3–10	22.7 W + 495	0.86	62	0.0949 W + 2.07	0.86	0.259
10–18	17.5 W + 651	0.90	100	0.0732 W + 2.72	0.90	0.418
18–30	15.3 W + 679	0.65	151	0.0640 W + 2.84	0.65	0.632
30–60	11.6 W + 879	0.60	164	0.0485 W + 3.67	0.60	0.686
> 60	13.5 W + 487	0.79	148	0.0565 W + 2.04	0.79	0.619
Females						
0–3	61.0 W − 51	0.97	61	0.255 W − 0.214	0.97	0.255
3–10	22.5 W + 499	0.85	63	0.0941 W + 2.09	0.85	0.264
10–18	12.2 W + 746	0.75	117	0.0510 W + 3.12	0.75	0.489
18–30	14.7 W + 496	0.72	121	0.0615 W + 2.08	0.72	0.506
30–60	8.7 W + 829	0.70	108	0.0364 W + 3.47	0.70	0.452
> 60	10.5 W + 596	0.74	108	0.0439 W + 2.49	0.74	0.452

*Since the present report was compiled, the data base for the equations contained in Schofield, W.N. et al. (1985) *Hum. Nutr. Clin. Nutr.* **39** (Suppl.), has been slightly expanded. They therefore differ from the equations shown in this table, but the differences are negligible.
[†]Standard deviation of differences between actual BMR and predicted estimates.
(From WHO (1985) *Energy and Protein Requirements: Report of a Joint FAO/WHO/UNU Expert Consultation*, Technical Report Series No. 724. World Health Organization, Geneva, p. 71.)

Table II.16   Examples of predicted basal metabolic rate (BMR) in subjects of the same height but different weights, predicted from actual weight and from median acceptable weight for height

	Man, age 40, height 1.8 m			Woman, age 25, height 1.5 m		
	Position in range*			Position in range*		
	Upper	Median	Lower	Upper	Median	Lower
BMI[†]	25	22	20	24	21	19
Wt (kg)	81.0	71.3	64.8	54.0	47.2	42.7
BMR[‡] from actual wt, kcal_th/day	1,820	1,710	1,630	1,290	1,190	1,120
MJ/day	7.61	7.15	6.82	5.39	4.98	4.68
BMR from median wt, kcal_th/day	1,710	1,710	1,710	1,190	1,190	1,190
MJ/day	7.15	7.15	7.15	4.97	4.97	4.97

*Acceptable range of BMI (see Annex 2A in original reference).
[†]Body mass index = wt(kg)/ht²(m).
[‡]Predicted from equations in Table II.15.
(From WHO (1985) *Energy and Protein Requirements: Report of a Joint FAO/WHO/UNU Expert Consultation*, Technical Report Series No. 724, World Health Organization, Geneva, p. 72.)

Table II.17   Basal metabolic rates of adolescent boys and girls

Age (years)	Height* (cm)	Weight[†] (kg)	BMR[‡] Total (kcal_th/day)	(MJ/day)	per kg (kcal_th/day)	(MJ/day)
Boys						
10–11	140	32.2	1215	5.08	37.7	0.16
11–12	147	37.0	1300	5.43	35.1	0.15
12–13	153	40.9	1370	5.73	33.4	0.14
13–14	160	47.0	1465	6.12	31.4	0.13
14–15	166	52.6	1570	6.57	29.9	0.12
15–16	171	58.0	1665	6.96	28.7	0.12
16–17	175	62.7	1750	7.32	27.9	0.12
17–18	177	65.0	1790	7.48	27.5	0.12

Continued

Table II.17   Continued

Age (years)	Height* (cm)	Weight† (kg)	BMR‡ Total ($kcal_{th}$/day)	(MJ/day)	per kg ($kcal_{th}$/day)	(MJ/day)
Girls						
10–11	142	33.7	1160	4.85	34.3	0.14
11–12	148	38.7	1220	5.10	31.5	0.13
12–13	155	44.0	1280	5.38	29.1	0.12
13–14	159	48.8	1340	5.60	27.5	0.12
14–15	161	51.4	1375	5.75	26.7	0.11
15–16	162	53.0	1395	5.83	26.3	0.11
16–17	163	54.0	1405	5.87	26.0	0.11
17–18	164	54.4	1410	5.89	25.9	0.11

*Median height for age from NCHS standards.
†Median weight for height and age from Baldwin's standards (Annex 2(B) of original reference.
‡Boys: BMR = 17.5 W + 651 $kcal_{th}$/day (2.72 MJ/day). Girls: 12.2 W + 746 $kcal_{th}$/day (3.12 MJ/day).
(From WHO (1985) *Energy and Protein Requirements: Report of a joint FAO/WHO/UNU Expert Consultation*, Technical Report Series No. 724. World Health Organization, Geneva, p. 72.)

Table II.18   Basal metabolic rate in adult men and women in relation to height and median acceptable weight for height* (values given in $kcal_{th}$ with MJ in parentheses)

Height (m)	Weight† (kg)	18–30 years Per kg per day	Per day	30–60 years Per kg per day	Per day	>60 years Per kg per day	Per day
Men							
1.5	49.5	29.0 (121)	1440 (6.03)	29.4 (123)	1450 (6.07)	23.3 (98)	1150 (4.81)
1.6	56.5	27.4 (115)	1540 (6.44)	27.2 (114)	1530 (6.40)	22.2 (93)	1250 (5.23)
1.7	63.5	26.0 (109)	1650 (6.90)	25.4 (106)	1620 (6.78)	21.2 (89)	1350 (5.65)
1.8	71.5	24.8 (104)	1770 (7.41)	23.9 (99)	1710 (7.15)	20.3 (85)	1450 (6.07)
1.9	79.5	23.9 (100)	1890 (7.91)	22.7 (95)	1800 (7.53)	19.6 (82)	1560 (6.53)
2.0	88	23.0 (96)	2030 (8.49)	21.6 (90)	1900 (7.95)	19.0 (80)	1670 (6.99)
Women							
1.4	41	26.7 (112)	1100 (4.60)	28.8 (120)	1190 (4.98)	25.0 (105)	1030 (4.31)
1.5	47	25.2 (105)	1190 (4.98)	26.3 (110)	1240 (5.19)	23.1 (97)	1090 (4.56)
1.6	54	23.9 (100)	1290 (5.40)	24.1 (101)	1300 (5.44)	21.6 (90)	1160 (4.85)
1.7	61	22.9 (96)	1390 (5.82)	22.4 (94)	1360 (5.69)	20.3 (85)	1230 (5.15)
1.8	68	22.0 (92)	1500 (6.28)	20.9 (87)	1420 (5.94)	19.3 (81)	1310 (5.48)

*BMR from equations in Table II.15 rounded to 10 $kcal_{th}$.
†Weight taken as median acceptable weight for height: body mass index (wt/ht^2) = 22 in men, 21 in women.
(From WHO (1985) *Energy and Protein Requirements: Report of a joint FAO/WHO/UNU Expert Consultation*, Technical Report Series No. 724. World Health Organization, Geneva, p. 72.)

Table II.19 Calculated energy requirements of infants from birth to 1 year

	Intake*		Calculated energy requirement[†]		Median body weight[‡]		Total requirement			
							Boys		Girls	
Age (months)	(kcal_{th}/kg per day)	(kJ/kg per day)	(kcal_{th}/kg per day)	(kJ/kg per day)	Boys (kg)	Girls (kg)	(kcal_{th}/day)	(kJ/day)	(kcal_{th}/day)	(kJ/day)
0.5	118	494	124	519	3.8	3.6	470	1,965	445	1,860
1–2	114	477	116	485	4.75	4.35	550	2,300	505	2,115
2–3	107	448	109	456	5.6	5.05	610	2,550	545	2,280
3–4	101	423	103	431	6.35	5.7	655	2,740	590	2,470
4–5	96	402	99	414	7.0	6.35	695	2,910	630	2,635
5–6	93	389	96.5	404	7.55	6.95	730	3,055	670	2,800
6–7	91	381	95	397	8.05	7.55	765	3,220	720	3,010
7–8	90	377	94.5	395	8.55	7.95	810	3,390	750	3,140
8–9	90	377	95	397	9.0	8.4	855	3,580	800	3,350
9–10	91	381	99	414	9.35	8.75	925	3,870	865	3,620
10–11	93	389	100	418	9.7	9.05	970	4,060	905	3,790
11–12	97	406	104.5	437	10.05	9.35	1,050	4,395	975	4,080
12	102	427								

*Observed intakes at ages indicated, from data of sources given in original publication. Average intake predicted from equation (age in months): 1 (kcal_{th}/kg) = 123 − 8.9 age + 0.59 age. See original reference.
[†]Requirement over interval indicated, calculated as predicted intake + 5%. See original reference.
[‡]NCHS median weights at midpoint of month.
(From WHO (1985) *Energy and Protein Requirements: Report of a Joint FAO/WHO/UNU Expert Consultation*, Technical Report Series No. 724. World Health Organization, Geneva, p. 91.)

Table II.20 Estimated average daily energy intakes and requirements, ages 1 to 10 years

	BOYS			
	Intake*		Requirement[†]	
Age (years)	(kcal_{th}/day)	(MJ/day)	(kcal_{th}/day)	(MJ/day)
1–2	1,140	4.76	1,200	5.02
2–3	1,340	5.60	1,410	5.89
3–4	1,490	6.23	1,560	6.52
4–5	1,610	6.73	1,690	7.07
5–6	1,720	7.19	1,810	7.57
6–7	1,810	7.57	1,900	7.94
7–8	1,895	7.92	1,990	8.32
8–9	1,970	8.24	2,070	8.66
9–10	2,045	8.55	2,150	8.99

Continued

Table II.20   Continued

Age (years)	GIRLS Intake* (kcal_th/day)	(MJ/day)	Requirement† (kcal_th/day)	(MJ/day)	REQUIREMENT BY WEIGHT‡ Boys (kcal_th/kg per day)	(kJ/kg per day)	Girls (kcal_th/kg per day)	(kJ/kg per day)
1–2	1,090	4.56	1,140	4.76	104	435	108	452
2–3	1,250	5.23	1,310	5.48	104	410	102	427
3–4	1,370	5.73	1,440	6.02	99	414	95	397
4–5	1,465	6.12	1,540	6.44	95	397	92	385
5–6	1,550	6.48	1,630	6.81	92	385	88	368
6–7	1,620	6.77	1,700	7.11	88	368	83	347
7–8	1,685	7.05	1,770	7.40	83	347	76	318
8–9	1,740	7.28	1,830	7.65	77	322	69	268
9–10	1,795	7.51	1,880	7.86	72	301	62	259

*From data of Ferro-Luzzi and Durnin, Rome, FAO, 1981 (Document ESN: FAO/WHO/UNU/EPR/81/9).
†Intakes +5%. See original reference.
‡From NCHS median weights at midyear.
(From WHO (1985) *Energy and Protein Requirements: Report of a Joint FAO/WHO/UNU Expert consultation*. Technical Report Series No. 724. World Health Organization, Geneva, pp. 94 and 95.)

Table II.21   Calculated average energy expenditure and observed intakes and comparison with recommendations of 1971 committee for adolescents aged 10 to 18 years

Age (years)	Expenditure (× BMR)*	Expenditure (kcal_th/day)	(MJ/day)	Intake† (kcal_th/day)	(MJ/day)	1971 committee‡ recommended requirement (kcal_th/day)	(MJ/day)
Boys							
10–11	1.76	2,140	8.95	2,110	8.82	2,500	10.46
11–12	1.73	2,240	9.37	2,170	9.07	2,600	10.87
12–13	1.69	2,310	9.66	2,200	9.20	2,700	11.29
13–14	1.67	2,440	10.20	2,280	9.53	2,800	11.71
14–15	1.65	2,590	10.83	2,340	9.79	2,900	12.13
15–16	1.62	2,700	11.29	2,390	9.99	3,000	12.55
16–17	1.60	2,800	11.71	2,440	10.20	3,050	12.76
17–18	1.60	2,870	12.0	2,490	10.41	3,100	12.97
Girls							
10–11	1.65	1,910	7.99	1,850	7.74	2,300	9.62
11–12	1.63	1,980	8.28	1,890	7.90	2,350	9.83
12–13	1.60	2,050	8.57	1,930	8.07	2,400	10.04
13–14	1.58	2,120	8.87	1,970	8.24	2,450	10.25
14–15	1.57	2,160	9.03	2,010	8.40	2,500	10.46
15–16	1.54	2,140	8.95	2,050	8.57	2,500	10.46
16–17	1.53	2,130	8.91	2,080	8.70	2,420	10.12
17–18	1.52	2,140	8.95	2,120	8.87	2,340	9.79

*Expenditure calculated as in original publication.
†Intakes from reference in original publication.
‡Reference in original 1971 publication. (cf ref. d)
(From WHO (1985) *Energy and Protein Requirements: Report of a Joint FAO/WHO/UNU Expert consultation*, Technical Report Series No. 724. World Health Organization, Geneva, p. 98.)

Table II.22   Derivation of average values of the energy cost of three grades of physical activity at work for women and men*

	Women[†]				Men[‡]			
	Cost/min (kcal_{th})	(kJ)	Average cost × BMR (gross)	(net)	Cost/min (kcal_{th})	(kJ)	Average cost × BMR (gross)	(net)
Light work								
75% of time sitting or standing	1.51	6.3			1.79	7.5		
25% of time standing and moving	1.70	7.1			2.51	10.5		
Average	1.56	6.5	1.7	0.7	1.99	8.3	1.7	0.7
Moderate work								
25% of time sitting or standing	1.51	6.3			1.79	7.5		
75% of time spent on specific occupational activity	2.20	9.2			3.61	15.1		
Average	2.03	8.5	2.2	1.2	3.16	13.2	2.7	1.7
Heavy work								
40% of time sitting or standing	1.51	6.3			1.79	7.5		
60% of time spent on specific occupational activity	3.21	13.4			6.22	26.0		
Average	2.54	10.6	2.8	1.8	4.45	18.6	3.8	2.8

*Times and energy costs of sitting, standing, moving around, and work tasks are composite values derived from published and unpublished data (Annex 5) in original reference.

[†]Based on young adult females (18–30 years). Wt 55 kg, BMR 0.90 kcal_{th}(3.8 kJ)/min (Table II.15).

[‡]Based on young adult males (18–30 years). Wt 65 kg, BMR 1.16 kcal_{th} (4.9 kJ)/min (Table II.15).

(From WHO (1985) *Energy and Protein Requirements: Report of a Joint FAO/WHO/UNU Expert Consultation*, Technical Report Series No. 724, World Health Organization, Geneva, p. 76.)

Table II.23   Average daily energy requirement of adults whose occupational work is classified as light, moderate, or heavy, expressed as a multiple of basal metabolic rate

	Light	Moderate	Heavy
Men	1.55	1.78	2.10
Women	1.56	1.64	1.82

(From WHO (1985) *Energy and Protein Requirements: Report of a Joint FAO/WHO/UNU Expert Consultation*, Technical Report Series No. 724, World Health Organization, Geneva, p. 78.)

Table II.24   Estimates of energy cost of weight gain*

	Energy cost	
Subjects	(kcal_{th}/g)	(kJ/g)
Premature infants	4.9	20.5
Premature infants	5.7	23.8
Normal infants	5.6	23.4
Infants recovering from malnutrition	5.55	23.2
	4.6	19.2
	3.5	14.6
	4.4	18.4
	7.1	29.7
Adults, recovering from anorexia nervosa	6.4	26.7
Adults, intentional overfeeding	8.2	34.3
Pregnancy Theoretic estimate[†]	6.4	26.7

*See original references for data sources.

[†]Calculated as 80,000 kcal_{th} (335 mJ) stored for 12.5 kg of weight gain.

(From WHO (1985) *Energy and Protein Requirements: Report of a Joint FAO/WHO/UNU Expert Consultation*, Technical Report Series No. 724, World Health Organization, Geneva, p. 185.)

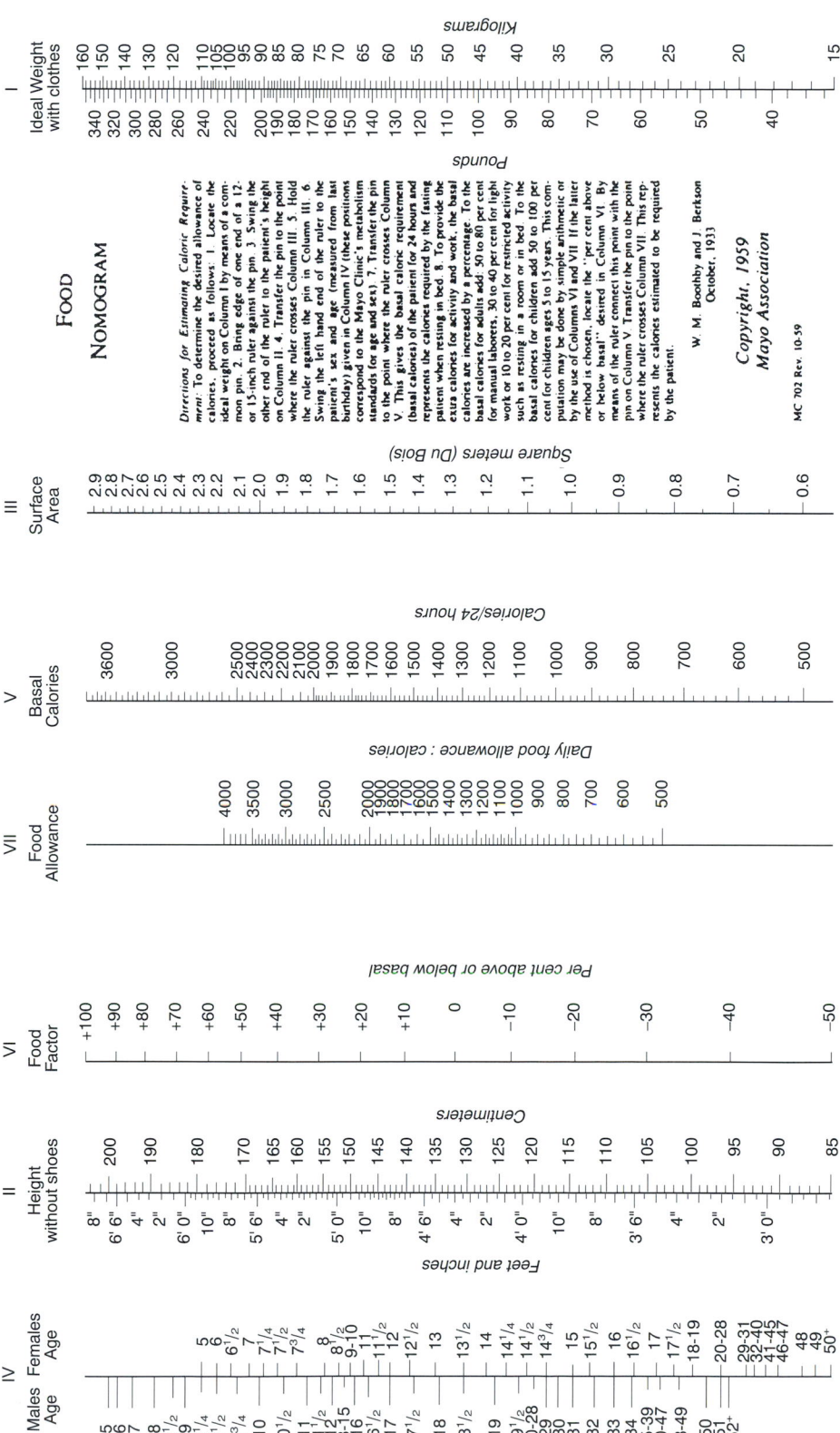

Figure II.1   Nomogram for estimation of caloric requirements. (From Pemberton, C. M., Gastineau, C. F.: *Mayo Clinic Diet Manual.* 5th Ed. W. B. Saunders, 1981, Philadelphia.)

Table II.25   Values for the digestibility of protein in man*

Protein source	True digestibility (mean ± SD)	Digestibility relative to reference proteins
Egg	97 ± 3	
Milk, cheese	95 ± 3 95	100
Meat, fish	94 ± 3	
Maize	85 ± 6	89
Rice, polished	88 ± 4	93
Wheat, whole	86 ± 5	90
Wheat, refined	96 ± 4	101
Oatmeal	86 ± 7	90
Millet	79	83
Peas, mature	88	93
Peanut butter	95	100
Soyflour	86 ± 7	90
Beans	78	82
Maize + beans	78	82
Maize + beans + milk	84	88
Indian rice diet	77	81
Indian rice diet + milk	87	92
Chinese mixed diet	96	98†
Brazilian mixed diet	78	82
Filipino mixed diet	88‡	93
American mixed diet	96‡	101
Indian rice + bean diet	78‡	82

*See original reference for data sources.
†Relative to egg measured in the same study.
‡Recalculated from apparent digestibility, using F_K = 12 mg N/kg (see original text).
(From WHO (1985) *Energy and Protein Requirements: Report of a Joint FAO/WHO/UNU Expert Consultation*, Technical Report Series No. 724, World Health Organization, Geneva, p. 119.)

Table II.27   Daily average energy requirements and safe level of protein intake for adolescents aged 10 to 18 years

Age (years)	Median weight (kg)	Energy requirement (kcal_th)	(kJ)	Safe level of protein intake (g/kg)*
Boys				
10–12	34.5	2,200	9,200	1.00
12–14	44.0	2,400	10,000	1.00
14–16	55.5	2,650	11,100	0.95
16–18	64.0	2,850	11,900	0.90
Girls				
10–12	36.0	1,950	8,200	1.00
12–14	46.5	2,100	8,800	0.95
14–16	52.0	2,150	9,000	0.90
16–18	54.0	2,150	9,000	0.80

*Minimum level considered safe.
(From WHO (1995) *Diet, Nutrition and the Prevention of Chronic Diseases: Report of a WHO Study Group*, Technical Report Series No. 797, World Health Organization, Geneva, pp. 167–8.)

Table II.26   Daily average (per kg) energy requirements and safe level of protein intake for infants and children aged 3 months to 10 years (sexes combined up to 5 years)

Age	Median weight (kg)	Energy requirement (kcal_th kg)		Energy requirement (kJ/kg)		Safe level of protein intake (g/kg)*
Months						
3–6	7.0	100		418		1.85
6–9	8.5	95		397		1.65
9–12	9.5	100		418		1.50
Years						
1–2	11.0	105		439		1.20
2–3	13.5	100		418		1.15
3–5	16.5	95		397		1.10
		Boys	Girls	Boys	Girls	
5–7	20.5	90	85	377	356	1.00
7–10	27.0	78	67	326	280	1.00

*Minimum level considered safe.
(From WHO (1990) *Diet, Nutrition and the Prevention of Chronic Diseases: Report of a WHO Study Group*, Technical Report Series No. 797, World Health Organization, Geneva, pp. 167–8.)

Table II.28   Daily average energy requirements and safe level of protein intake for adults*

Weight (kg)	Energy requirement						Safe level of protein intake (g/day)[†]
	18–30 years		30–60 years		Over 60 years		
	(kcal$_{th}$)	(kJ)	(kcal$_{th}$)	(kJ)	(kcal$_{th}$)	(kJ)	
Men							
50	2,300	9,700	2,350	9,700	1,850	7,700	37.5
55	2,400	10,100	2,450	10,100	1,950	8,300	41.0
60	2,550	10,600	2,500	10,400	2,100	8,600	45.0
65	2,700	11,300	2,600	10,900	2,200	9,100	49.0
70	2,800	11,700	2,700	11,200	2,300	9,600	52.5
75	2,900	12,300	2,800	11,800	2,400	10,000	56.0
80	3,050	12,900	2,900	12,000	2,500	10,400	60.0
Women							
40	1,700	7,200	1,900	7,900	1,650	6,800	30.0
45	1,850	7,700	1,950	8,300	1,700	7,100	34.0
50	1,950	8,200	2,050	8,500	1,800	7,500	37.5
55	2,100	8,600	2,100	8,800	1,900	7,900	41.0
60	2,200	9,200	2,200	9,000	1,950	8,200	45.0
65	2,300	9,800	2,250	9,400	2,050	8,500	49.0
70	2,450	10,300	2,300	9,600	2,150	8,900	52.5
75	2,550	10,800	2,400	10,000	2,200	9,300	56.0

*For a basal metabolic rate factor of 1.6.
[†]Minimum level considered safe.
(From WHO (1995) *Diet, Nutrition and the Prevention of Chronic Diseases: Report of a WHO Study Group*, Technical Report Series No. 797, World Health Organization, Geneva, pp. 167–8.)

Table II.29   Desirable weights for men and women aged 25 and over (in pounds by height and frame, in indoor clothing), 1959

Men (in shoes, one-inch heels)					Women (in shoes, two-inch heels)				
Height		Small frame	Medium frame	Large frame	Height		Small frame	Medium frame	Large frame
Feet	Inches				Feet	Inches			
5	2	112–120	118–129	126–141	4	10	92–98	96–107	104–119
5	3	115–123	121–133	129–144	4	11	94–101	98–110	106–122
5	4	118–126	124–136	132–148	5	0	96–104	101–113	109–125
5	5	121–129	127–139	135–152	5	1	99–107	104–116	112–128
5	6	124–133	130–143	138–156	5	2	102–110	107–119	115–131
5	7	128–137	134–147	142–161	5	3	105–113	110–122	118–134
5	8	132–141	138–152	147–166	5	4	108–116	113–126	121–138
5	9	136–145	142–156	151–170	5	5	111–119	116–130	125–142
5	10	140–150	146–160	155–174	5	6	114–123	120–135	129–146
5	11	144–154	150–165	159–179	5	7	118–127	124–139	133–150
6	0	148–158	154–170	164–184	5	8	122–131	128–143	137–154
6	1	152–162	158–175	168–189	5	9	126–135	132–147	141–158
6	2	156–167	162–180	173–194	5	10	130–140	136–151	145–163
6	3	160–171	167–185	178–199	5	11	134–144	140–155	149–168
6	4	164–175	172–190	182–204	6	0	138–148	144–159	153–173

(Data adapted from new weight standards for men and women. Stat. Bull. Metropol. Life Insur. Co. 40:1, 1959.)

Table II.30 Height–Weight Tables, 1983

Men					Women				
Height		Small frame	Medium frame	Large frame	Height		Small frame	Medium frame	Large frame
Feet	Inches				Feet	Inches			
5	2	128–134	131–141	138–150	4	10	102–111	109–121	118–131
5	3	130–136	133–143	140–153	4	11	103–113	111–123	120–134
5	4	132–138	135–145	142–156	5	0	104–115	113–126	122–137
5	5	134–140	137–148	144–160	5	1	106–118	115–129	125–140
5	6	136–142	139–151	146–164	5	2	108–121	118–132	128–143
5	7	138–145	142–154	149–168	5	3	111–124	121–135	131–147
5	8	140–148	145–157	152–172	5	4	114–127	124–138	134–151
5	9	142–151	148–160	155–176	5	5	117–130	127–141	137–155
5	10	144–154	151–163	158–180	5	6	120–133	130–144	140–159
5	11	146–157	154–166	161–184	5	7	123–136	133–147	143–163
6	0	149–160	157–170	164–188	5	8	126–139	136–150	146–167
6	1	152–164	160–174	168–192	5	9	129–142	139–153	149–170
6	2	155–168	164–178	172–197	5	10	132–145	142–156	152–173
6	3	158–172	167–182	176–202	5	11	135–148	145–159	155–176
6	4	162–176	171–187	181–207	6	0	138–151	148–162	158–179

Weight according to frame (ages 25 to 59) for men wearing indoor clothing weighing 5 lb, shoes with one-inch heels; for women, indoor clothing weighing 3 lb, shoes with one-inch heels.
(Reprinted with permission from the Metropolitan Life Insurance Company, New York.)

Table II.31 Height and elbow breadth for men and women*

Height in one-inch heels	Elbow breadth
Men	
5′2″–5′3″	$2\frac{1}{2}″$–$2\frac{7}{8}″$
5′4″–5′7″	$2\frac{5}{8}″$–$2\frac{7}{8}″$
5′8″–5′11″	$2\frac{3}{4}″$–3″
6′0″–6′3″	$2\frac{3}{4}″$–$3\frac{1}{8}″$
6′4″	$2\frac{7}{8}″$–$3\frac{1}{4}″$
Women	
4′10″–4′11″	$2\frac{1}{4}″$–$2\frac{1}{2}″$
5′0″–5′3″	$2\frac{1}{4}″$–$2\frac{1}{2}″$
5′4″–5′7″	$2\frac{3}{8}″$–$2\frac{5}{8}″$
5′8″–5′11″	$2\frac{3}{8}″$–$2\frac{5}{8}″$
6′0″	$2\frac{1}{2}″$–$2\frac{3}{4}″$

*See Table II.33; see Table II.34 for data on frame size by elbow breadth from NHANES I and II.
Extend your arm and bend the forearm upwards at a 90° angle. Keep fingers straight and turn the inside of your wrist towards your body. If you have a caliper, use it to measure the space between the two prominent bones on either side of your elbow. Without a caliper, place thumb and index finger of your other hand on these two bones. Measure the space between your fingers against a ruler or tape measure. Compare it with these tables that list elbow measurements for medium-frame men and women. Measurements lower than those listed indicate you have a small frame. Higher measurements indicate a larger frame.
(Reprinted with permission from Metropolitan Life Insurance Company, New York.)

Table II.32 Height–weight tables (metric units), 1983*

	Men				Women		
Height (cm)	Small frame (kg)	Medium frame (kg)	Large frame (kg)	Height (cm)	Small frame (kg)	Medium frame (kg)	Large frame (kg)
157.5	58.2–60.9	59.4–64.1	62.7–68.2	147.5	46.4–50.5	49.5–55.0	53.6–59.5
160	59.1–61.8	60.5–65.0	63.6–69.5	150	46.8–51.4	50.5–55.9	54.5–60.9
162.5	60.0–62.7	61.4–65.9	64.5–70.9	152.5	47.3–52.3	51.4–57.3	55.5–62.3
165	60.9–63.7	62.3–67.3	65.5–72.7	155	48.2–53.6	52.3–58.6	56.8–63.6
167.5	61.8–64.5	63.2–68.6	66.4–74.5	157.5	49.1–55.0	53.6–60.0	58.2–65.0
170	62.7–65.9	64.5–70.0	67.7–76.4	160	50.5–56.4	55.0–61.4	59.5–66.8
173	63.6–67.3	65.9–71.4	69.1–78.2	162.5	51.8–57.7	56.4–62.7	60.9–68.6
175	64.5–68.6	67.3–72.7	70.5–80.0	165	53.2–59.1	57.7–64.1	62.3–70.5
178	65.4–70.0	68.6–74.1	71.8–81.8	167.5	54.5–60.5	59.1–65.5	63.6–72.3
180	66.4–71.4	70.0–75.5	73.2–83.6	170	55.9–61.8	60.5–66.8	65.0–74.1
183	67.7–72.7	71.4–77.3	74.5–85.6	173	57.3–63.2	61.8–68.2	66.4–75.9
185.5	69.1–74.5	72.7–79.1	76.4–87.3	175	58.6–64.5	63.2–69.5	67.7–77.3
188	70.5–76.4	74.5–80.9	78.2–89.5	178	60.0–65.9	64.5–70.9	69.1–78.6
190.5	71.8–78.2	75.9–82.7	80.0–91.8	180	61.4–67.3	65.9–72.3	70.5–80.0
193	73.6–80.0	77.7–85.0	82.3–94.1	183	62.3–68.6	67.3–73.6	71.8–81.4

*The 1983 Metropolitan Height–Weight Tables are based on the 1979 Build Study.
The values are statistical computations from individuals ranging from 25 to 59 years of weights by height and body frame at which mortality has been found to be lowest or longevity the highest. Metropolitan Life does not advocate the use of the term "ideal", which has different meanings to various individuals, because the term was used originally in their 1942 to 1943 tables. If one wishes to use these tables in the sense that they are "ideal" in terms of lowest mortality, they are "appropriate" in that context. These tables do not provide weights related to minimizing illness, optimizing job performance, or creating the best appearance.
(Reprinted with permission from the Metropolitan Life Insurance Company, New York.)

Table II.33 Average weights by height and age group: 1959 and 1979 build and blood pressure studies

Men	Height														
	5'2"	5'3"	5'4"	5'5"	5'6"	5'7"	5'8"	5'9"	5'10"	5'11"	6'0"	6'1"	6'2"	6'3"	6'4"
15–16 years*															
1959 Study	107	112	117	122	127	132	137	142	146	150	154	159	164	169	†
1979 Study	112	116	121	127	133	137	143	148	153	159	162	168	173	178	184
Weight change	+5	+4	+4	+5	+6	+5	+6	+6	+7	+9	+8	+9	+9	+9	–
17–19 years															
1959 Study	119	123	127	131	135	139	143	147	151	155	160	164	168	172	176
1979 Study	124	129	132	137	141	145	150	155	159	164	168	174	179	185	190
Weight change	+5	+6	+5	+6	+6	+6	+7	+8	+8	+9	+8	+10	+11	+13	+14
20–24 years															
1959 Study	128	132	136	139	142	145	149	153	157	161	166	170	174	178	181
1979 Study	130	136	139	143	148	153	157	163	167	171	176	182	187	193	198
Weight change	+2	+4	+3	+4	+6	+8	+8	+10	+10	+10	+10	+12	+13	+15	+17
25–29 years															
1959 Study	134	138	141	144	148	151	155	159	163	167	172	177	182	186	190
1979 Study	134	140	143	147	152	156	161	166	171	175	181	186	191	197	202
Weight change	+0	+2	+2	+3	+4	+5	+6	+7	+8	+8	+9	+9	+9	+11	+12
30–39 years															
1959 Study	137	141	145	149	153	157	161	165	170	174	179	183	188	193	199
1979 Study	138	143	147	151	156	160	165	170	174	179	184	190	195	201	206
Weight change	+1	+2	+2	+2	+3	+3	+4	+5	+4	+5	+5	+7	+7	+8	+7

Continued

Table II.33 Continued

Men	Height														
	5'2"	5'3"	5'4"	5'5"	5'6"	5'7"	5'8"	5'9"	5'10"	5'11"	6'0"	6'1"	6'2"	6'3"	6'4"
40–49 years															
1959 Study	140	144	148	152	156	161	165	169	174	178	183	187	192	197	203
1979 Study	140	144	149	154	158	163	167	172	176	181	186	192	197	203	208
Weight change	+0	+0	+1	+2	+2	+2	+2	+3	+2	+3	+3	+5	+5	+6	+5
50–59 years															
1959 Study	142	145	149	153	157	162	166	170	175	180	185	189	194	199	205
1979 Study	141	145	150	155	159	164	168	173	177	182	187	193	198	204	209
Weight change	−1	+0	+1	+2	+2	+2	+2	+3	+2	+2	+2	+4	+4	+5	+4
60–69 years															
1959 Study	139	142	146	150	154	159	163	168	173	178	183	188	193	198	204
1979 Study	140	144	149	153	158	163	167	172	176	181	186	191	196	200	207
Weight change	+1	+2	+3	+3	+4	+4	+4	+4	+3	+3	+3	+3	+3	+2	+3

Women	Height														
	4'10"	4'11"	5'0"	5'1"	5'2"	5'3"	5'4"	5'5"	5'6"	5'7"	5'8"	5'9"	5'10"	5'11"	6'0"
15–16 years*															
1959 Study	97	100	103	107	111	114	117	121	125	128	132	136	†	†	†
1979 Study	101	105	109	112	117	121	123	128	131	135	138	142	146	149	152
Weight change	+4	+5	+6	+5	+6	+7	+6	+7	+6	+7	+6	+6	−	−	−
17–19 years															
1959 Study	99	102	105	109	113	116	120	124	127	130	134	138	142	147	152
1979 Study	103	108	111	115	119	123	126	129	132	136	140	145	148	150	154
Weight change	+4	+6	+6	+6	+6	+7	+6	+5	+5	+6	+6	+7	+6	+3	+2
20–24 years															
1959 Study	102	105	108	112	115	118	121	125	129	132	136	140	144	149	154
1979 Study	105	110	112	116	120	124	127	130	133	137	141	146	149	155	157
Weight change	+3	+5	+4	+4	+5	+6	+6	+5	+4	+5	+5	+6	+5	+6	+3
25–29 years															
1959 Study	107	110	113	116	119	122	125	129	133	136	140	144	148	153	158
1979 Study	110	112	114	119	121	125	128	132	134	138	142	148	150	156	159
Weight change	+3	+2	+1	+3	+2	+3	+3	+3	+1	+2	+2	+4	+2	+3	+1
30–39 years															
1959 Study	115	117	120	123	126	129	132	135	139	142	146	150	154	159	164
1979 Study	113	115	118	121	124	128	131	134	137	141	145	150	153	159	164
Weight change	−2	−2	−2	−2	−2	−1	−1	−1	−2	−1	−1	0	−1	0	0
40–49 years															
1959 Study	122	124	127	130	133	136	140	143	147	151	155	159	164	169	174
1979 Study	118	121	123	127	129	133	136	139	143	147	150	155	158	162	168
Weight change	−4	−3	−4	−3	−4	−3	−4	−4	−4	−4	−5	−4	−6	−7	−8
50–59 years															
1959 Study	125	127	130	133	136	140	144	148	152	156	160	164	169	174	180
1979 Study	121	125	127	131	133	137	141	144	147	152	156	159	162	166	171
Weight change	−4	−2	−3	−2	−3	−3	−3	−4	−5	−4	−4	−5	−7	−8	−9
60–69 years															
1959 Study	127	129	131	134	137	141	145	149	153	157	161	165	†	†	†
1979 Study	123	127	130	133	136	140	143	147	150	155	158	161	163	167	172
Weight change	−4	−2	−1	−1	−1	−1	−2	−2	−3	−2	−3	−4	−	−	−

*Height in shoes (feet and inches) and weight in indoor clothing (pounds).
†Averge weights omitted in classes with too few cases for analysis.
(Data from Association of Life Insurance Medical Directors of America and Society of Actuaries. Compiled by Seltzer, F. (1983) *Dietetic Currents*, **10** pp. 17–22. Reprinted with permission of Ross Laboratories, Columbus, Ohio.)

Table II.34 Frame size by elbow breadth (cm) of United States male and female adults derived from the combined NHANES I and II data sets

	Age (years)	Frame size		
		Small	Medium	Large
Men				
	18–24	≤6.6	>6.6 and <7.7	≥7.7
	25–34	≤6.7	>6.7 and <7.9	≥7.9
	35–44	≤6.7	>6.7 and <8.0	≥8.0
	45–54	≤6.7	>6.7 and <8.1	≥8.1
	55–64	≤6.7	>6.7 and <8.1	≥8.1
	65–74	≤6.7	>6.7 and <8.1	≥8.1
Women				
	18–24	≤5.6	>5.6 and <6.5	≥6.5
	25–34	≤5.7	>5.7 and <6.8	≥6.8
	35–44	≤5.7	>5.7 and <7.1	≥7.1
	45–54	≤5.7	>5.7 and <7.2	≥7.2
	55–64	≤5.8	>5.8 and <7.2	≥7.2
	65–74	≤5.8	>5.8 and <7.2	≥7.2

*The tenth and ninetieth percentiles, respectively, represent the predicted mean ± 1.282 times the SE. Similarly, the fifteenth and eighty-fifth percentiles are the predicted mean minus and plus, respectively, 1.036 times the SE of the regression equation. There were significant black–white population differences in weight and body composition when age and height were considered. However, when the comparisons were made with reference to age, height, and frame size, there were only minor interpopulation differences. For this reason, all races (white, black, and other) included in the NHANES I and II surveys were merged together for the purpose of calculating percentiles of anthropometric measurements.
(Combined NHANES I and II data sets from Frisancho, A.R. (1984) *Am. J. Clin. Nutr.*, **40**: pp. 808–19, with permission.)

Table II.35 Comparison of the weight-for-height tables from actuarial data (build study): non-age-corrected Metropolitan Life Insurance Company and age-specific Gerontology Research Center recommendations*

Height	Metropolitan 1983 weights for ages 25–59[†]		Gerontology Research Center Weight range for men and women by age (years)				
	Men	Women	25	35	45	55	65
ft–in			lb				
4–10	–	100–131	84–111	92–119	99–127	107–135	115–142
4–11	–	101–134	87–115	95–123	103–131	111–139	119–147
5–0	–	103–137	90–119	98–127	106–135	114–143	123–152
5–1	123–145	105–140	93–123	101–131	110–140	118–148	127–157
5–2	125–148	108–144	96–127	105–136	113–144	122–153	131–163
5–3	127–151	111–148	99–131	108–140	117–149	126–158	135–168
5–4	129–155	114–152	102–135	112–145	121–154	130–163	140–173
5–5	131–159	117–156	106–140	115–149	125–159	134–168	144–179
5–6	133–163	120–160	109–144	119–154	129–164	138–174	148–184
5–7	135–167	123–164	112–148	122–159	133–169	143–179	153–190
5–8	137–171	126–167	116–153	126–163	137–174	147–184	158–196
5–9	139–175	129–170	119–157	130–168	141–179	151–190	162–201
5–10	141–179	132–173	122–162	134–173	145–184	156–195	167–207
5–11	144–183	135–176	126–167	137–178	149–190	160–201	172–213
6–0	147–187	–	129–171	141–183	153–195	165–207	177–219
6–1	150–192	–	133–176	145–188	157–200	169–213	182–225
6–2	153–197	–	137–181	149–194	162–206	174–219	187–232
6–3	157–202	–	141–186	153–199	166–212	179–225	192–238
6–4	–	–	144–191	157–205	171–218	184–231	197–244

*Values in this table are for height without shoes and weight without clothes. To convert inches to centimeters, multiply by 2.54; to convert pounds to kilograms, multiply by 0.455.
[†]The weight range is the lower weight for small frame and the upper weight for large frame.
(Gerontology Research Center data from Andres, R. (1985) Mortality and obesity: the rationale for age-specific height–weight tables, in Andres, R., Bierman, E. and Hazzard, W.R. (eds), *Principles of Geriatric Medicine*, New York, McGraw-Hill, pp. 311–18.)

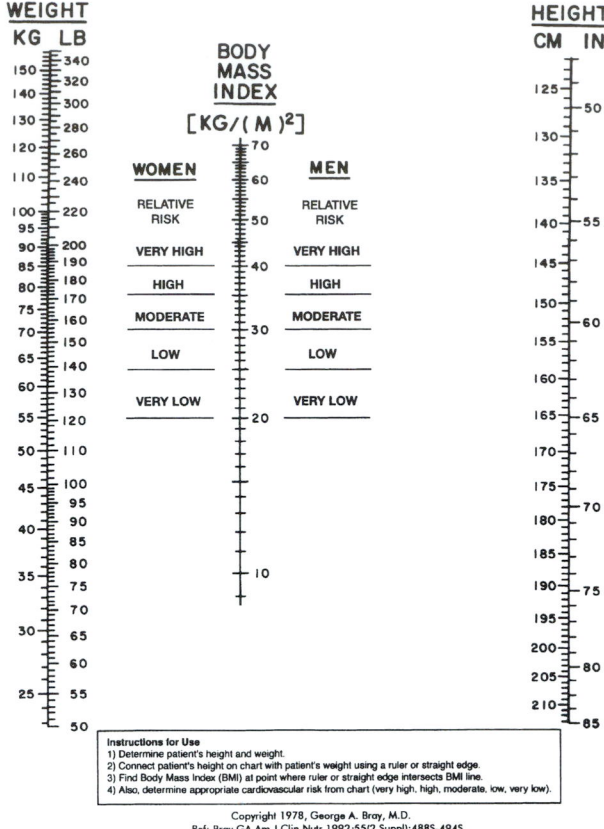

Figure II.2 Nomograph for estimating body mass index (kg/m²). The ratio of weight/height² emerges from varied epidemiologic studies are the most generally useful index of relative body mass in adults. This nomograph facilitates use of this insurance studies, the scale expresses relative weight as a continuous variable. This method encourages use of clinical judgment in interpreting "overweight" and "underweight" and in accounting for muscular and skeletal contributions to measured mass. (Copyright 1978 George A. Bray.)

Table II.36 Desirable body mass index (BMI) in relation to age

Age (years)	BMI (kg/m²)
19–24	19–24
25–34	20–25
35–44	21–26
45–54	22–27
55–65	23–28
>65	24–29

(From Committee on Diet and Health, Food and Nutrition Board, National Research Council (1989) *Diet and Health: Implications for Reducing Chronic Disease Risk*, National Academy Press, Washington, D.C., p. 564.)

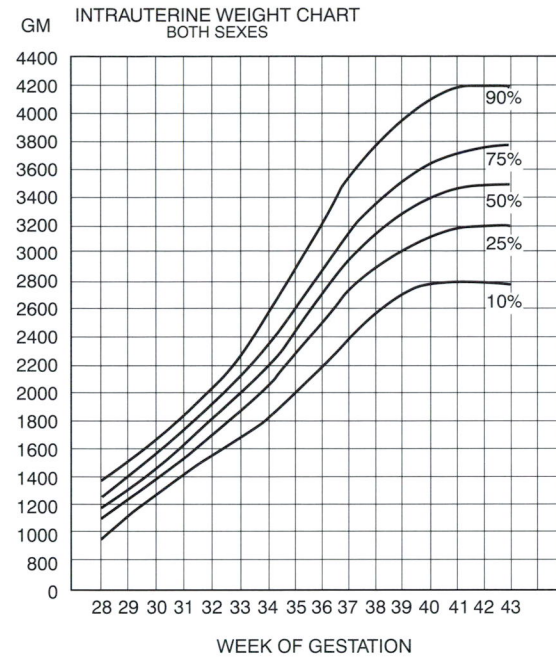
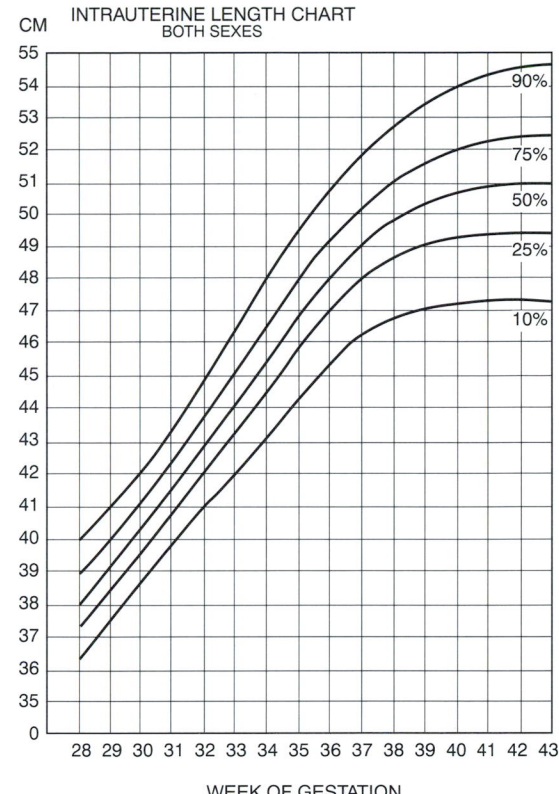

Figure II.3 Fetal growth standards: intrauterine weight* and length† charts.
*Fetal body weight percentiles from 28 to 43 weeks of gestation.
†Fetal body length percentiles from 28 to 43 weeks of gestation.
(From Naeye, R. L., Dixon, J. B.: *Pediatr. Res.,* **12**, p. 989, 1978.)

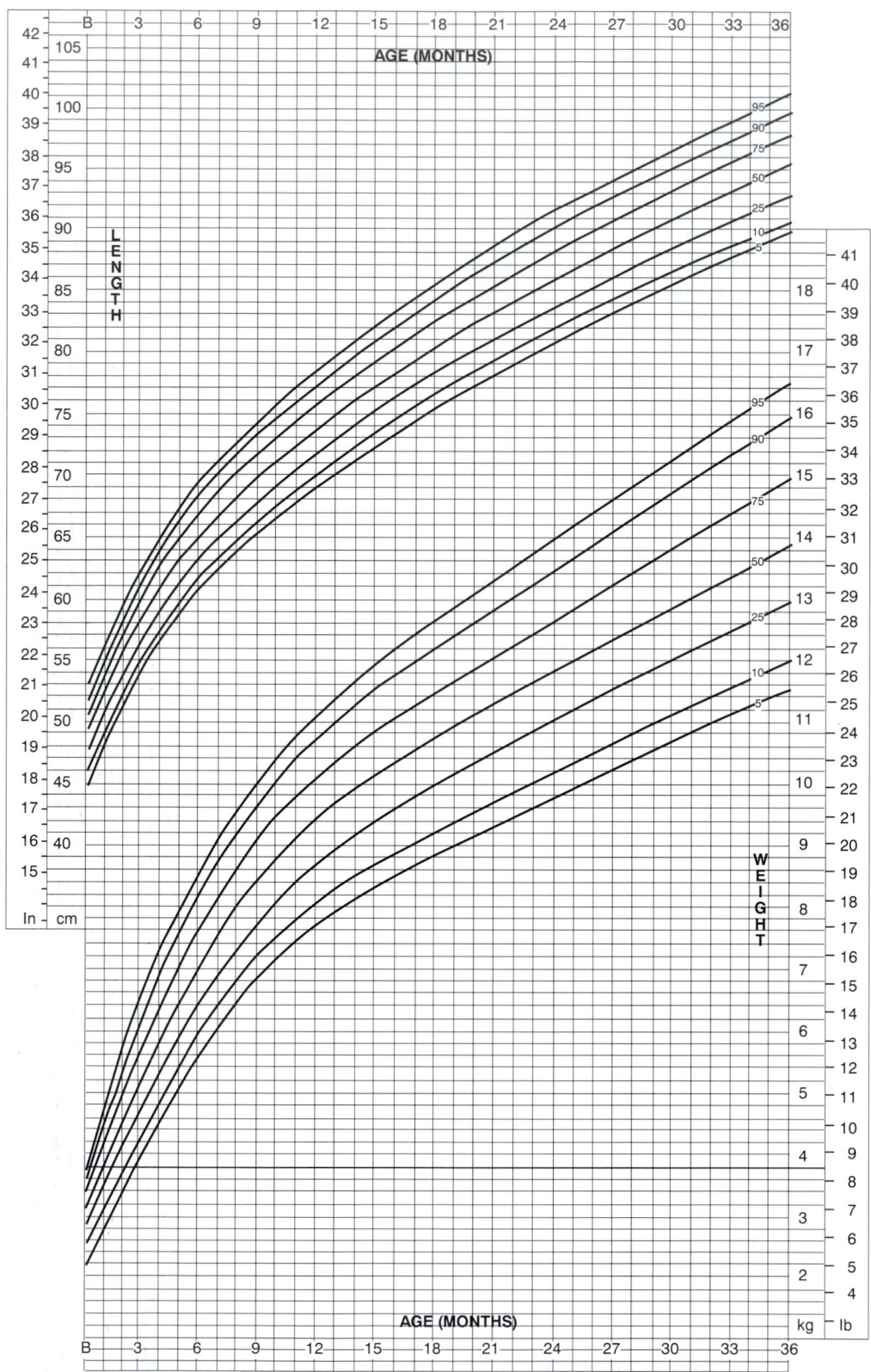

Figure II.4   Physical growth NCHS percentiles: girls from birth to 36 months. (Courtesy of Ross Laboratories, who adpated the growth curves from the original data: National Center for Health Statistics (1976) *NCHS Growth Charts. Monthly Vital Statistics Report* (1976) Vol. 25, No. 3, Suppl. (HRA) pp. 76–1120. Rockville, MD, Health Resources Administration, June. Data from The Fels Research Institute, Yellow Springs, Ohio.)

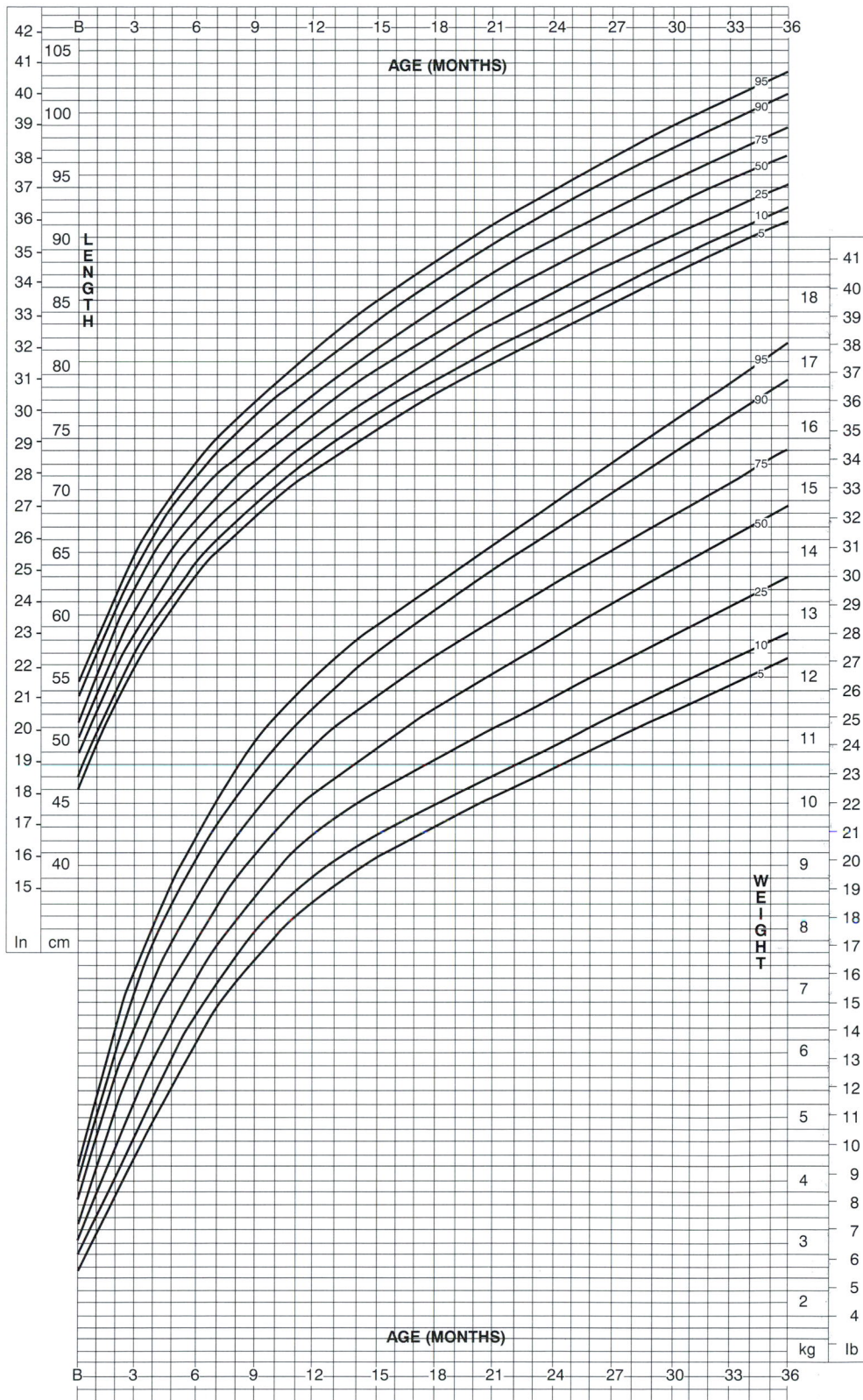

Figure II.5   Physical growth NCHS percentiles: boys from birth to 36 months. (Courtesy of Ross Laboratories, who adapted the growth curves from the original data: National Center for Health Statistics (1976) *NCHS Growth Charts. Monthly Vital Statistics Report* (1976) Vol. 25, No. 3, Suppl. (HRA) pp. 76–1120. Rockville, MD, Health Resources Administration, June. Data from The Fels Research Institute, Yellow Springs, Ohio.)

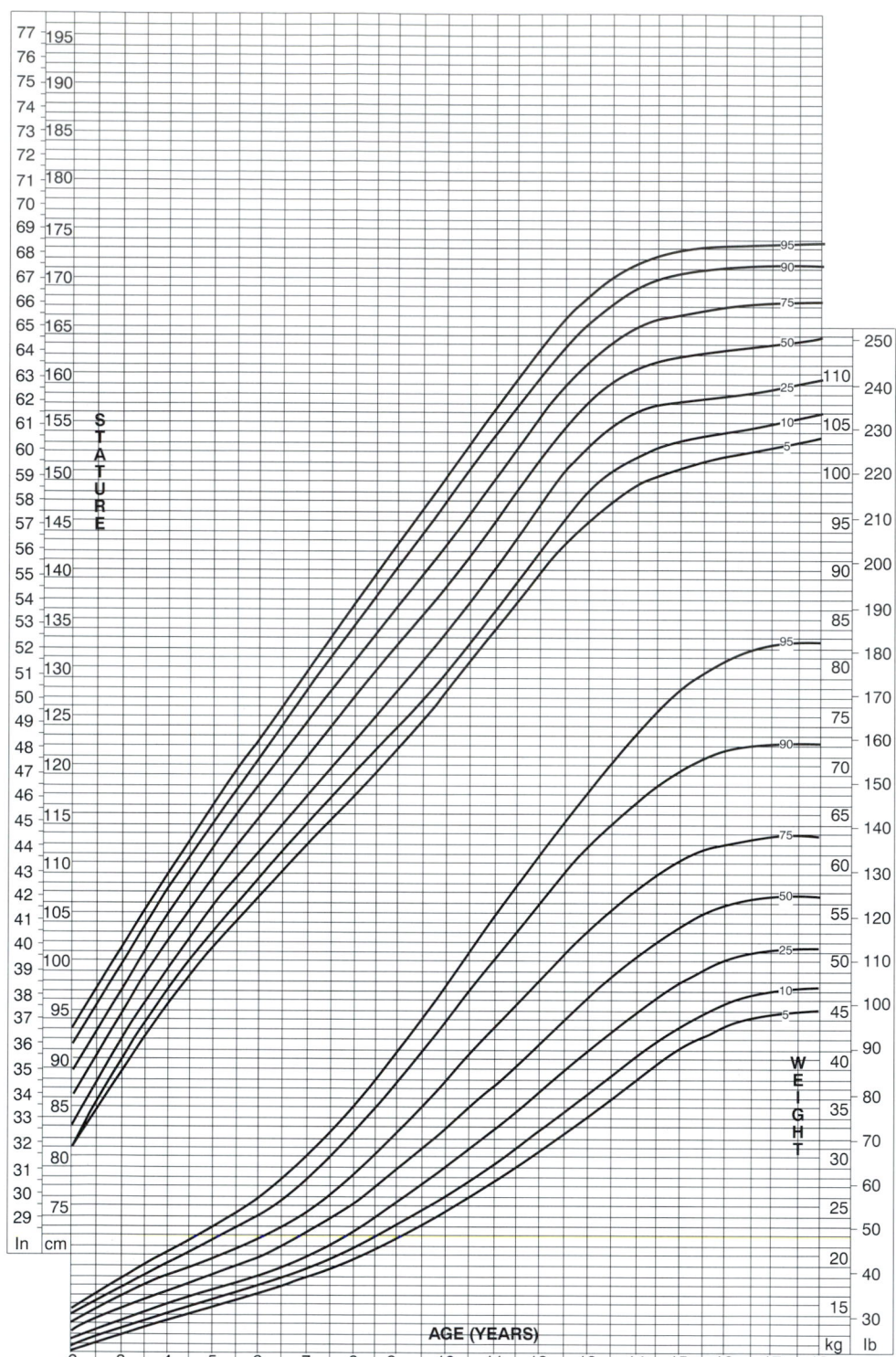

Figure II.6 Physical growth NCHS percentiles: girls from 2 to 18 years. (Courtesy of Ross Laboratories, who adpated the growth curves from the original data: National Center for Health Statistics (1976) *NCHS Growth Charts. Monthly Vital Statistics Report* (1976) Vol. 25, No. 3, Suppl. (HRA) pp. 76–1120. Rockville, MD, Health Resources Administration, June. Data from The Fels Research Institute, Yellow Springs, Ohio.)

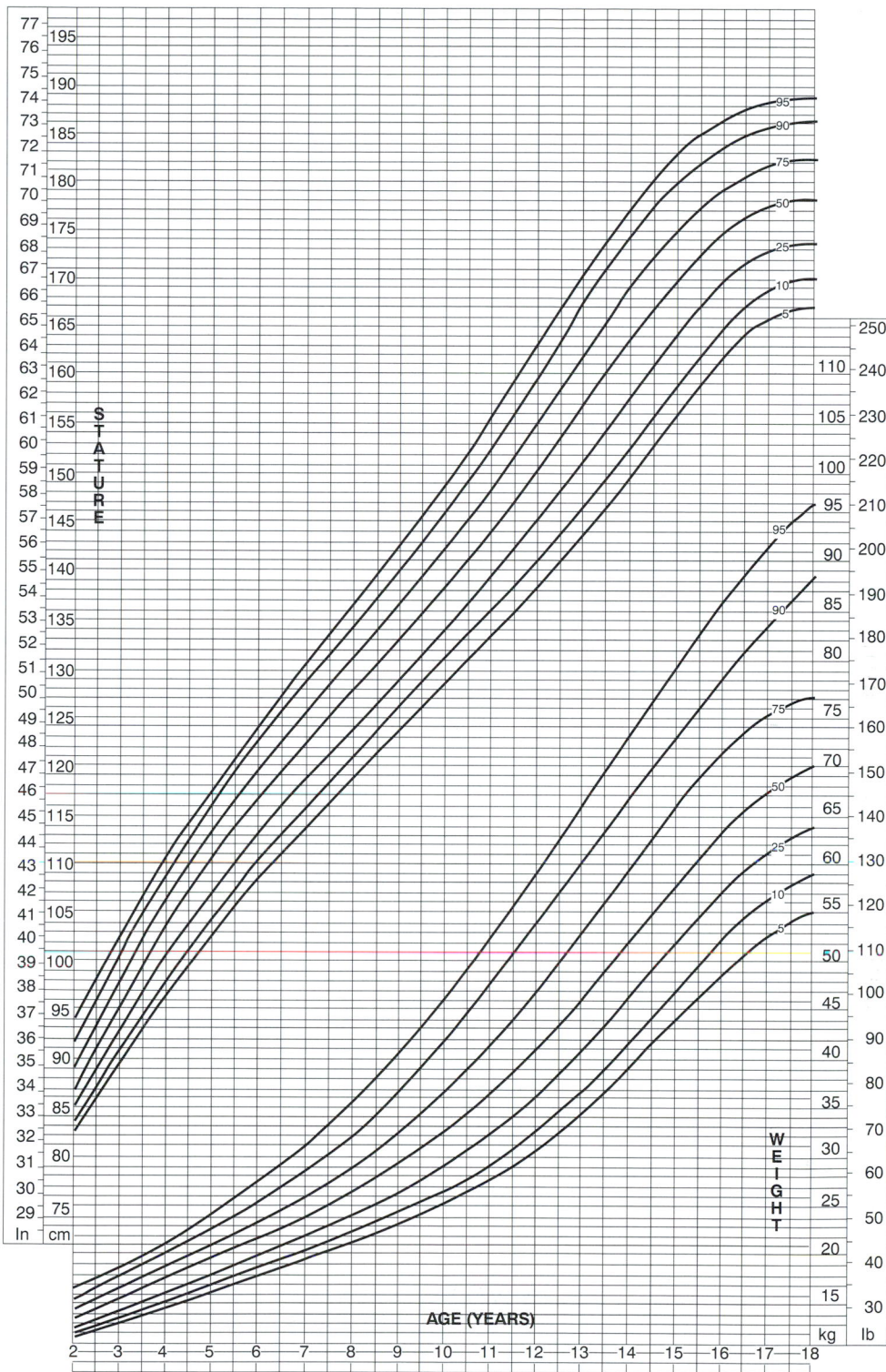

Figure II.7   Physical growth NCHS percentiles: boys from 2 to 18 years. (Courtesy of Ross Laboratories, who adpated the growth curves from the original data: National Center for Health Statistics (1976) *NCHS Growth Charts. Monthly Vital Statistics Report* (1976) Vol. 25, No. 3, Suppl. (HRA) pp. 76–1120. Rockville, MD, Health Resources Administration, June. Data from The Fels Research Institute, Yellow Springs, Ohio.)

Table II.37 Height in centimeters for persons 2 to 19 years of age: number examined, mean, standard deviation, and selected percentiles by sex and age, United States, 1976 to 1980*

Sex and age (years)	Number of examined persons	Mean	Standard deviation	Percentile								
				5th	10th	15th	25th	50th	75th	85th	90th	95th
Male												
2	375	91.2	4.3	84.5	85.8	85.5	88.2	91.3	94.2	95.8	96.6	97.6
3	418	99.2	4.5	92.0	94.3	94.9	96.5	98.8	102.0	103.9	105.0	107.0
4	404	106.0	5.2	97.8	99.5	100.5	102.5	106.4	109.2	111.0	112.4	115.0
5	397	112.6	5.4	104.0	105.8	107.2	109.4	112.6	115.6	118.1	119.6	121.2
6	133	119.5	5.1	111.2	112.6	114.5	115.9	120.1	122.6	124.7	125.5	126.8
7	148	125.1	5.9	115.4	117.6	119.1	121.8	125.9	128.1	130.2	131.5	133.6
8	147	129.9	7.0	118.6	122.0	123.5	125.3	130.6	134.1	136.5	138.0	142.0
9	145	135.5	5.8	125.9	126.4	129.4	131.2	136.1	139.6	141.2	143.1	144.7
10	157	141.6	7.3	130.3	132.8	134.0	137.0	141.5	146.4	149.6	150.6	153.0
11	155	146.0	7.8	133.1	135.9	138.0	141.1	145.6	151.2	153.9	155.2	160.2
12	145	152.5	7.9	139.0	142.6	144.9	147.5	152.0	158.0	160.5	162.0	164.4
13	173	158.9	8.3	144.4	147.6	149.7	152.6	159.7	165.0	168.7	169.5	171.6
14	186	167.5	8.3	153.9	156.5	159.1	162.5	167.5	173.1	176.5	178.7	180.6
15	184	170.8	6.7	160.1	162.0	162.6	165.7	171.1	175.5	177.5	178.2	181.9
16	178	173.8	6.4	163.0	164.7	167.4	169.8	173.7	178.1	180.3	182.6	186.1
17	173	175.1	7.1	164.1	167.3	168.4	170.6	174.9	179.7	182.8	184.3	187.5
18	164	176.9	6.7	166.5	168.8	169.9	172.3	176.9	180.9	183.9	185.1	189.6
19	148	176.5	6.7	164.5	168.2	169.4	171.8	176.9	181.1	183.5	184.8	187.2
Female												
2	336	89.7	4.2	83.1	84.4	85.5	86.7	89.8	92.2	93.6	94.9	97.2
3	366	97.5	4.8	89.6	91.1	92.5	94.5	97.6	100.8	102.5	103.4	104.5
4	396	104.6	5.0	96.1	98.2	99.5	101.5	104.5	108.2	109.8	110.7	112.4
5	364	111.6	5.3	103.0	105.1	106.4	108.1	111.6	115.2	116.5	118.8	120.3
6	135	118.4	6.1	109.9	111.1	111.5	113.3	118.5	122.2	124.5	126.5	128.7
7	157	123.7	6.7	113.3	116.6	117.4	119.6	124.1	128.1	130.1	132.2	134.7
8	123	130.2	5.7	120.8	123.4	124.4	125.8	130.6	133.2	135.4	137.5	140.5
9	149	134.4	7.6	124.0	126.4	127.8	129.0	134.8	139.0	140.7	142.6	147.1
10	136	141.9	6.5	131.6	133.6	135.1	137.6	141.6	146.3	148.1	150.4	153.8
11	140	147.9	7.8	134.7	139.3	140.6	142.2	147.9	152.2	154.7	156.9	162.7
12	147	154.4	7.2	143.9	145.7	146.7	149.2	154.8	158.6	161.9	164.7	165.9
13	162	158.9	6.6	149.0	150.3	152.7	155.3	159.0	163.0	164.5	166.9	170.3
14	178	160.8	6.4	151.0	152.7	154.5	156.7	160.9	165.1	166.9	168.2	172.3
15	145	163.2	6.2	153.0	155.2	157.1	159.1	163.1	167.1	170.2	172.4	173.5
16	170	162.9	6.1	152.0	154.5	157.2	159.1	163.2	166.4	169.4	171.4	173.3
17	134	163.5	5.7	153.8	156.8	158.5	160.4	163.1	166.7	169.7	170.7	172.2
18	170	162.4	6.8	150.7	154.2	155.6	158.0	162.7	166.2	169.1	171.5	174.0
19	158	163.5	5.6	153.8	156.8	157.7	159.7	163.7	167.2	169.5	170.4	172.1

*Height without shoes.
(From National Center for Health Statistics (1987) *Anthropometric Reference Data and Prevalence of Overweight, United States 1976–1980*, DHHS Publication No. 87-1688 (1987). U.S. Department of Health and Human Services, Public Health Service, Hyattsville, MD.

Table II.38 Weight in kilograms for persons 6 months to 19 years of age: number examined, mean, standard deviation, and selected percentiles by sex and age, United States, 1976 to 1980*

Sex and age (years)	Number of examined persons	Mean	Standard deviation	Percentile 5th	10th	15th	25th	50th	75th	85th	90th	95th
Male												
6–11 months	179	9.4	1.3	7.5	7.6	8.2	8.6	9.4	10.1	10.7	10.9	11.4
1 year	370	11.8	1.9	9.6	10.0	10.3	10.8	11.7	12.6	13.1	13.6	14.4
2 years	375	13.6	1.7	11.1	11.6	11.8	12.6	13.5	14.5	15.2	15.8	16.5
3 years	418	15.7	2.0	12.9	13.5	13.9	14.4	15.4	16.8	17.4	17.9	19.1
4 years	404	17.8	2.5	14.1	15.0	15.3	16.0	17.6	19.0	19.9	20.9	22.2
5 years	397	19.8	3.0	16.0	16.8	17.1	17.7	19.4	21.3	22.9	23.7	25.4
6 years	133	23.0	4.0	18.6	19.2	19.8	20.3	22.0	24.1	26.4	28.3	30.1
7 years	148	25.1	3.9	19.7	20.8	21.2	22.2	24.8	26.9	28.2	29.6	33.9
8 years	147	28.2	6.2	20.4	22.7	23.6	24.6	27.5	29.9	33.0	35.5	39.1
9 years	145	31.1	6.3	24.0	25.6	26.0	27.1	30.2	33.0	35.4	38.6	43.1
10 years	157	36.4	7.7	27.2	28.2	29.6	31.4	34.8	39.2	43.5	46.3	53.4
11 years	155	40.3	10.1	26.8	28.8	31.8	33.5	37.3	46.4	52.0	57.0	61.0
12 years	145	44.2	10.1	30.7	32.5	35.4	37.8	42.5	48.8	52.6	58.9	67.5
13 years	173	49.9	12.3	35.4	37.0	38.3	40.1	48.4	56.3	59.8	64.2	69.9
14 years	186	57.1	11.0	41.0	44.5	46.4	49.8	56.4	63.3	66.1	68.9	77.0
15 years	184	61.0	11.0	46.2	49.1	50.6	54.2	60.1	64.9	68.7	72.8	81.3
16 years	178	67.1	12.4	51.4	54.3	56.1	58.7	64.4	73.6	78.1	82.2	91.2
17 years	173	66.7	11.5	50.7	53.4	54.8	58.7	65.8	72.0	76.8	82.3	88.9
18 years	164	71.1	12.7	54.1	56.6	60.3	61.9	70.4	76.6	80.0	83.5	95.3
19 years	148	71.7	11.6	55.9	57.9	60.5	63.8	69.5	77.9	84.3	86.8	92.1
Female												
6–11 months	177	8.8	1.2	6.6	7.3	7.5	7.9	8.9	9.4	10.1	10.4	10.9
1 year	336	10.8	1.4	8.8	9.1	9.4	9.9	10.7	11.7	12.4	12.7	13.4
2 years	336	13.0	1.5	10.8	11.2	11.6	12.0	12.7	13.8	14.5	14.9	15.9
3 years	366	14.9	2.1	11.7	12.3	12.9	13.4	14.7	16.1	17.0	17.4	18.4
4 years	396	17.0	2.4	13.7	14.3	14.5	15.2	16.7	18.4	19.3	20.2	21.1
5 years	364	19.6	3.3	15.3	16.1	16.7	17.2	19.0	21.2	22.8	24.7	26.6
6 years	135	22.1	4.0	17.0	17.8	18.6	19.3	21.3	23.8	26.6	28.9	29.6
7 years	157	24.7	5.0	19.2	19.5	19.8	21.4	23.8	27.1	28.7	30.3	34.0
8 years	123	27.9	5.7	21.4	22.3	23.3	24.4	27.5	30.2	31.3	33.2	36.5
9 years	149	31.9	8.4	22.9	25.0	25.8	27.0	29.7	33.6	39.3	43.3	48.4
10 years	136	36.1	8.0	25.7	27.5	29.0	31.0	34.5	39.5	44.2	45.8	49.6
11 years	140	41.8	10.9	29.8	30.3	31.3	33.9	40.3	45.8	51.0	56.6	60.0
12 years	147	46.4	10.1	32.3	35.0	36.7	39.1	45.4	52.6	58.0	60.5	64.3
13 years	162	50.9	11.8	35.4	39.0	40.3	44.1	49.0	55.2	60.9	66.4	76.3
14 years	175	54.8	11.1	40.3	42.8	43.7	47.4	53.1	60.3	65.7	67.6	75.2
15 years	145	55.1	9.8	44.0	45.1	46.5	48.2	53.3	59.6	62.2	65.5	76.6
16 years	170	58.1	10.1	44.1	47.3	48.9	51.3	55.6	62.5	68.9	73.3	76.8
17 years	134	59.6	11.4	44.5	48.9	50.5	52.2	58.4	63.4	68.4	71.6	81.8
18 years	170	59.0	11.1	45.3	49.5	50.8	52.8	56.4	63.0	66.0	70.1	78.0
19 years	158	60.2	11.0	48.5	49.7	51.7	53.9	57.1	64.4	70.7	74.8	78.1

*Includes clothing weight, estimated as ranging from 0.09 to 0.28 kilogram.
(From National Center for Health Statistics (1987) *Anthropometric Reference Data and Prevalence of Overweight, United States 1978–1980*, DHHS Publication No. 87-1688. U.S. Department of Health and Human Services, Public Health Service, Hyattsville, MD.)

Table II.39 Weight in kilograms of youths aged 12 years at last birthday by sex and height group in centimeters: sample size, estimated population size, mean, standard deviation, standard error of the mean, and selected percentiles, United States, 1966 to 1970

Sex and height	n	N	$\bar{X}$	s	$s_{\bar{x}}$	5th	10th	25th	50th	75th	90th	95th
Male						in kilograms						
Under 130	5	15	*	*	*	*	*	*	*	*	*	*
130.0–134.9	4	8	*	*	*	*	*	*	*	*	*	*
135.0–139.9	34	111	32.50	3.741	0.727	26.6	27.6	30.2	31.6	34.7	37.7	39.4
140.0–144.9	80	241	34.28	3.635	0.601	28.1	30.0	31.8	34.1	36.5	38.6	40.7
145.0–149.9	123	386	39.27	6.243	0.615	32.1	33.2	35.7	38.2	40.9	46.1	52.5
150.0–154.9	156	513	42.90	6.314	0.480	34.9	36.1	38.2	42.1	46.0	51.6	56.3
155.0–159.9	135	432	47.35	7.551	0.769	38.3	39.4	41.9	46.2	50.5	57.4	61.9
160.0–164.9	65	201	50.82	8.735	1.388	42.1	42.7	44.9	48.4	56.0	61.1	67.1
165.0–169.9	29	88	55.75	8.811	2.031	43.3	46.4	49.0	54.4	59.9	68.3	76.6
170.0–174.9	8	21	62.37	4.503	1.993	54.0	58.1	60.1	61.0	66.0	69.1	69.5
175.0–179.9	3	10	*	*	*	*	*	*	*	*	*	*
180.0–184.9	1	2	*	*	*	*	*	*	*	*	*	*
185.0–189.9	–	–	–	–	–	–	–	–	–	–	–	–
190.0–194.9	–	–	–	–	–	–	–	–	–	–	–	–
195.0 and over	–	–	–	–	–	–	–	–	–	–	–	–
Female						in kilograms						
Under 130	–	–	–	–	–	–	–	–	–	–	–	–
130.0–134.9	3	10	*	*	*	*	*	*	*	*	*	*
135.0–139.9	12	44	29.41	3.372	0.914	25.0	25.0	26.4	28.9	32.1	34.1	34.2
140.0–144.9	32	116	38.30	7.314	1.194	28.8	30.6	33.3	36.8	41.4	49.2	55.1
145.0–149.9	72	258	39.78	6.205	0.975	31.8	32.8	35.5	38.5	42.8	48.3	50.6
150.0–154.9	147	517	44.00	7.421	0.677	34.4	35.8	38.9	42.8	47.4	52.9	57.4
155.0–159.9	144	525	48.74	8.369	0.714	37.9	39.2	43.0	46.8	53.8	60.7	63.5
160.0–164.9	95	336	53.06	8.010	0.658	42.5	43.9	47.2	51.1	57.2	65.6	69.6
165.0–169.9	31	117	54.89	7.022	1.384	43.9	47.1	50.4	53.1	59.7	64.5	71.3
170.0–174.9	11	42	63.66	14.501	6.214	48.7	50.1	50.8	56.7	82.2	86.0	86.1
175.0–179.9	–	–	–	–	–	–	–	–	–	–	–	–
180.0–184.9	–	–	–	–	–	–	–	–	–	–	–	–
185.0–189.9	–	–	–	–	–	–	–	–	–	–	–	–
190.0–194.9	–	–	–	–	–	–	–	–	–	–	–	–
195.0 and over	–	–	–	–	–	–	–	–	–	–	–	–

n, Sample size; N, estimated number of youths in population in thousands; $\bar{X}$, mean; s, standard deviation; $s_{\bar{x}}$, standard error of the mean.
(From National Center for Health Statistics (1973) Height and weight of youths 12–17 years, United States , in *Vital and Health Statistics*, Series 11, No. 124, Health Services and Mental Health Administration, U.S. Government Printing Office, Washington, D.C., pp. 282–8).

Table II.40   Weight in kilograms of youths aged 13 years at last birthday by sex and height group in centimeters: sample size, estimated population size, mean, standard deviation, standard error of the mean, and selected percentiles, United States, 1966 to 1970

Sex and height	n	N	$\bar{X}$	s	$s_{\bar{x}}$	Percentile 5th	10th	25th	50th	75th	90th	95th
Male						in kilograms						
Under 130	–	–	–	–	–	–	–	–	–	–	–	–
130.0–134.9	2	5	*	*	*	*	*	*	*	*	*	*
135.0–139.9	6	25	32.62	5.624	7.716	27.2	27.6	28.9	31.0	34.9	43.1	43.2
140.0–144.9	18	56	36.54	5.852	1.607	30.0	30.5	32.1	36.1	39.2	41.7	53.2
145.0–149.9	65	204	39.03	5.270	0.662	32.4	33.9	36.1	37.9	41.2	44.5	46.4
150.0–154.9	99	312	42.58	6.724	0.865	34.8	36.2	37.9	41.0	45.5	49.4	61.0
155.0–159.9	131	421	47.27	7.482	0.717	37.8	39.2	41.7	45.8	51.1	58.7	61.7
160.0–164.9	125	393	53.01	9.324	0.916	41.5	43.7	46.9	50.4	58.2	64.4	72.5
165.0–169.9	91	285	55.92	8.560	0.833	46.3	47.5	49.3	53.6	59.4	69.0	75.0
170.0–174.9	63	215	62.01	10.362	1.033	51.2	51.6	53.7	60.1	67.0	76.0	85.0
175.0–179.9	19	68	67.92	12.085	3.428	56.3	57.9	60.1	63.3	70.3	88.3	89.0
180.0–184.9	5	15	*	*	*	*	*	*	*	*	*	*
185.0–189.9	–	–	–	–	–	–	–	–	–	–	–	–
190.0–194.9	–	–	–	–	–	–	–	–	–	–	–	–
195.0 and over	–	–	–	–	–	–	–	–	–	–	–	–
Female												
Under 130	–	–	–	–	–	–	–	–	–	–	–	–
130.0–134.9	1	3	*	*	*	*	*	*	*	*	*	*
135.0–139.9	–	–	–	–	–	–	–	–	–	–	–	–
140.0–144.9	15	51	37.13	7.317	2.259	26.6	27.5	30.5	36.7	40.1	44.5	56.1
145.0–149.9	47	165	42.23	6.880	0.888	34.7	35.6	38.2	40.5	44.2	53.6	57.6
150.0–154.9	98	329	44.32	7.029	0.787	35.6	36.5	39.2	42.9	47.3	53.7	57.9
155.0–159.9	152	499	49.75	8.757	0.699	39.1	39.9	43.8	48.4	53.8	61.0	65.9
160.0–164.9	156	515	53.16	8.399	0.522	41.2	43.9	47.7	52.2	57.0	63.8	68.5
165.0–169.9	86	284	58.17	9.125	0.921	46.2	47.4	52.2	58.1	61.5	69.3	76.2
170.0–174.9	24	87	58.11	13.209	2.343	46.2	47.1	48.4	52.9	65.3	68.6	96.8
175.0–179.9	3	10	*	*	*	*	*	*	*	*	*	*
180.0–184.9	–	–	–	–	–	–	–	–	–	–	–	–
185.0–189.9	–	–	–	–	–	–	–	–	–	–	–	–
190.0–194.9	–	–	–	–	–	–	–	–	–	–	–	–
195.0 and over	–	–	–	–	–	–	–	–	–	–	–	–

n, Sample size; N, estimated number of youths in population in thousands; $\bar{X}$, mean; s, standard deviation; $s_{\bar{x}}$, standard error of the mean.
(From National Center for Health Statistics (1973). Health and weight of youths 12–17 years, United States, in *Vital and Health Statistics*, Series 11, No. 124, Health Services and Mental Health Administration. U.S. Government Printing Office, Washington, D.C., pp. 282–8.)

Table II.41   Weight in kilograms of youths aged 14 years at last birthday by sex and height group in centimeters: sample size, estimated population size, mean, standard deviation, standard error of the mean, and selected percentiles, United States, 1966 to 1970

Sex and height	n	N	$\bar{X}$	s	$s_{\bar{x}}$	Percentile 5th	10th	25th	50th	75th	90th	95th
Male						in kilograms						
Under 130	–	–	–	–	–	–	–	–	–	–	–	–
130.0–134.9	–	–	–	–	–	–	–	–	–	–	–	–
135.0–139.9	2	7	*	*	*	*	*	*	*	*	*	*
140.0–144.9	3	13	*	*	*	*	*	*	*	*	*	*
145.0–149.9	11	42	40.51	1.829	0.644	36.9	38.6	39.6	40.6	42.0	42.5	42.7
150.0–154.9	45	135	43.63	6.277	1.182	36.2	37.0	39.0	41.4	48.0	51.7	55.3
155.0–159.9	83	261	47.42	7.822	0.872	37.7	38.7	41.8	46.1	51.2	58.0	62.7

Continued

Table II.41 Continued

Sex and height	n	N	$\bar{X}$	s	$s_{\bar{x}}$	Percentile						
						5th	10th	25th	50th	75th	90th	95th
Male						in kilograms						
160.0–164.9	96	299	52.28	6.785	0.584	42.5	44.0	47.5	52.1	56.3	61.5	65.1
165.0–169.9	134	432	58.07	9.416	1.054	47.7	49.3	51.6	55.4	62.3	70.6	75.7
170.0–174.9	144	435	62.37	11.516	1.095	49.7	51.0	55.0	59.4	65.6	79.2	86.3
175.0–179.9	71	228	65.54	9.704	1.306	50.9	55.1	58.5	64.7	69.9	74.5	84.0
180.0–184.9	25	81	72.44	13.014	2.298	59.6	60.0	65.1	69.4	77.0	83.0	94.3
185.0–189.9	3	9	*	*	*	*	*	*	*	*	*	*
190.0–194.9	1	3	*	*	*	*	*	*	*	*	*	*
195.0 and over	–	–	–	–	–	–	–	–	–	–	–	–
Female												
Under 130	–	–	–	–	–	–	–	–	–	–	–	–
130.0–134.9	–	–	–	–	–	–	–	–	–	–	–	–
135.0–139.9	1	2	*	*	*	*	*	*	*	*	*	*
140.0–144.9	2	6	*	*	*	*	*	*	*	*		*
145.0–149.9	17	52	42.00	5.879	1.683	32.0	35.3	36.3	42.3	47.5	49.5	51.1
150.0–154.9	64	196	48.26	6.797	0.926	37.7	39.2	42.5	47.9	53.3	55.9	58.8
155.0–159.9	157	508	51.35	7.705	0.520	41.2	43.4	46.3	49.6	55.6	62.2	64.3
160.0–164.9	186	603	54.59	8.810	0.707	43.0	45.0	48.4	53.0	59.7	66.7	70.7
165.0–169.9	114	372	58.46	10.185	0.955	45.9	47.5	52.1	56.8	61.8	70.5	76.4
170.0–174.9	36	121	64.37	15.821	2.814	49.2	52.1	56.2	59.8	70.5	72.9	99.4
175.0–179.9	7	28	61.33	5.496	2.620	51.7	52.0	57.7	59.8	64.6	70.2	70.6
180.0–184.9	2	7	*	*	*	*	*	*	*	*	*	*
185.0–189.9	–	–	–	–	–	–	–	–	–	–	–	–
190.0–194.9	–	–	–	–	–	–	–	–	–	–	–	–
195.0 and over	–	–	–	–	–	–	–	–	–	–	–	–

n, Sample size; N, estimated number of youths in population in thousands; $\bar{X}$, mean; s, standard deviation; $s_{\bar{x}}$, standard error of the mean.
(From National Center for Health Statistics (1973) Height and weight of youths 12–17 years, United States, in *Vital and Health Statistics*, Series 11, No. 124, Health Services and Mental Health Administration. U.S. Government Printing Office, Washington, D.C., pp. 282–8.)

Table II.42 Weight in kilograms of youths aged 15 years at last birthday by sex and height group in centimeters: sample size, estimated population size, mean, standard deviation, standard error of the mean, and selected percentiles, United States, 1966 to 1970

Sex and height	n	N	$\bar{X}$	s	$s_{\bar{x}}$	Percentile						
						5th	10th	25th	50th	75th	90th	95th
Male						in kilograms						
Under 130	–	–	–	–	–	–	–	–	–	–	–	–
130.0–134.9	–	–	–	–	–	–	–	–	–	–	–	–
135.0–139.9	–	–	–	–	–	–	–	–	–	–	–	–
140.0–144.9	–	–	–	–	–	–	–	–	–	–	–	–
145.0–149.9	1	2	*	*	*	*	*	*	*	*	*	*
150.0–154.9	10	30	45.72	8.582	3.550	35.7	39.2	42.6	44.7	46.0	48.7	76.1
155.0–159.9	34	99	52.81	10.552	1.695	40.3	43.1	46.7	49.2	56.7	69.6	76.3
160.0–164.9	71	206	53.01	8.417	0.986	42.7	44.1	46.9	51.5	56.3	65.3	68.8
165.0–169.9	132	404	57.72	8.503	0.819	48.0	48.8	53.1	56.4	61.3	67.1	73.3
170.0–174.9	176	574	62.88	8.464	0.633	51.6	53.4	56.7	61.9	67.2	72.9	78.1
175.0–179.9	118	374	65.80	9.457	1.045	53.1	55.6	59.7	64.3	69.5	80.2	89.2
180.0–184.9	51	144	72.00	11.928	1.724	54.6	60.3	64.4	70.2	78.4	84.4	96.6
185.0–189.9	14	48	74.21	15.035	5.200	58.3	58.5	62.9	70.7	84.6	92.4	110.8
190.0–194.9	6	15	83.39	16.431	10.332	66.4	66.7	69.6	73.8	103.0	105.7	106.2
195.0 and over	–	–	–	–	–	–	–	–	–	–	–	–

Continued

Table II.42 Continued

Sex and height	n	N	$\bar{X}$	s	$s_{\bar{x}}$	Percentile						
						5th	10th	25th	50th	75th	90th	95th
Female						in kilograms						
Under 130	–	–	–	–	–	–	–	–	–	–	–	–
130.0–134.9	–	–	–	–	–	–	–	–	–	–	–	–
135.0–139.9	–	–	–	–	–	–	–	–	–	–	–	–
140.0–144.9	2	5	*	*	*	*	*	*	*	*	*	*
145.0–149.9	15	51	47.91	7.875	3.623	36.0	39.4	42.1	45.4	52.7	55.7	66.3
150.0–154.9	69	242	49.69	8.895	1.190	39.1	40.6	44.3	48.1	52.8	60.5	68.3
155.0–159.9	111	400	51.52	8.473	0.934	41.4	43.5	46.3	50.8	55.1	59.8	65.2
160.0–164.9	137	509	57.03	10.828	0.875	45.1	47.3	50.2	55.0	60.2	71.7	77.7
165.0–169.9	109	398	60.71	10.357	1.053	47.5	49.3	55.1	58.4	65.7	74.1	81.0
170.0–174.9	49	188	65.27	10.730	1.880	49.7	53.6	57.2	61.2	71.6	85.3	86.4
175.0–179.9	7	23	63.30	8.872	4.807	49.7	49.9	53.8	62.4	71.1	71.9	79.2
180.0–184.9	3	26	*	*	*	*	*	*	*	*	*	*
185.0–189.9	1	3	*	*	*	*	*	*	*	*	*	*
190.0–194.9	–	–	–	–	–	–	–	–	–	–	–	–
195.0 and over	–	–	–	–	–	–	–	–	–	–	–	–

n, Sample size; N, estimated number of youths in population in thousands; $\bar{X}$, mean; s, standard deviation; $s_{\bar{x}}$, standard error of the mean.
(From National Center for Health Statistics (1973) Height and weight of youths 12–17 years, United States, in *Vital and Health Statistics*, Series 11, No. 124, Health Services and Mental Health Administration, U.S. Government Printing Office, Washington, D.C., 1973, pp. 282–8.)

Table II.43 Weight in kilograms of youths aged 16 years at last birthday by sex and height group in centimeters: sample size, estimated population size, mean, standard deviation, standard error of the mean, and selected percentiles, United States, 1966 to 1970

Sex and height	n	N	$\bar{X}$	s	$s_{\bar{x}}$	Percentile						
						5th	10th	25th	50th	75th	90th	95th
Male						in kilograms						
Under 130	–	–	–	–	–	–	–	–	–	–	–	–
130.0–134.9	–	–	–	–	–	–	–	–	–	–	–	–
135.0–139.9	–	–	–	–	–	–	–	–	–	–	–	–
140.0–144.9	–	–	–	–	–	–	–	–	–	–	–	–
145.0–149.9	1	1	*	*	*	*	*	*	*	*	*	*
150.0–154.9	4	12	*	*	*	*	*	*	*	*	*	*
155.0–159.9	11	33	49.89	7.323	3.572	42.0	42.2	44.7	46.8	54.4	59.8	67.2
160.0–164.9	32	108	53.09	6.459	1.273	44.2	44.9	48.2	51.4	58.0	60.9	66.1
165.0–169.9	87	275	59.39	9.178	0.981	48.5	49.8	52.7	58.0	63.9	69.3	75.9
170.0–174.9	166	552	62.66	7.556	0.629	51.6	53.8	57.5	61.6	67.1	73.1	78.0
175.0–179.9	149	511	67.33	9.018	0.856	56.3	58.2	61.0	65.4	72.5	80.1	83.8
180.0–184.9	72	227	72.38	12.485	1.993	58.3	59.3	64.4	68.9	76.5	90.2	96.9
185.0–189.9	29	95	81.06	14.268	3.265	63.7	66.6	69.7	78.4	90.3	97.0	111.4
190.0–194.9	3	10	*	*	*	*	*	*	*	*	*	*
195.0 and over	2	7	*	*	*	*	*	*	*	*	*	*
Female												
Under 130	–	–	–	–	–	–	–	–	–	–	–	–
130.0–134.9	–	–	–	–	–	–	–	–	–	–	–	–
135.0–139.9	–	–	–	–	–	–	–	–	–	–	–	–
140.0–144.9	2	5	*	*	*	*	*	*	*	*	*	*
145.0–149.9	10	33	52.58	8.198	3.191	43.9	44.1	44.9	51.0	54.5	72.0	72.1
150.0–154.9	57	178	51.79	10.457	1.053	41.4	42.0	45.8	48.9	54.1	61.5	83.3
155.0–159.9	117	354	53.20	7.766	0.734	44.0	45.6	48.4	51.6	56.4	61.9	69.0
160.0–164.9	160	547	57.71	11.129	1.246	46.1	47.3	51.5	55.5	61.2	69.5	75.1

Continued

Table II.43   Continued

Sex and height	n	N	$\bar{X}$	s	$s_{\bar{x}}$	Percentile						
						5th	10th	25th	50th	75th	90th	95th
Female												
165.0–169.9	122	450	61.72	11.998	0.802	47.1	48.8	53.3	59.1	67.3	78.7	86.7
170.0–174.9	53	170	63.61	8.734	1.126	52.9	53.8	58.1	62.1	66.8	73.8	84.2
175.0–179.9	14	45	72.55	15.012	5.224	58.6	58.8	61.7	65.9	80.6	99.1	105.5
180.0–184.9	1	2	*	*	*	*	*	*	*	*	*	*
185.0–189.9	–	–	–	–	–	–	–	–	–	–	–	–
190.0–194.9	–	–	–	–	–	–	–	–	–	–	–	–
195.0 and over	–	–	–	–	–	–	–	–	–	–	–	–

n, Sample size; N, estimated number of youths in population in thousands; $\bar{X}$, mean; s, standard deviation; $s_{\bar{x}}$, standard error of the mean.
(From National Center for Health Statistics (1973) Height and weight of youths 12–17 years, United States, in *Vital and Health Statistics*, Series 11, No. 124, Health Services and Mental Health Administration, U.S. Government Printing Office, Washington, D.C., pp. 282–8.)

Table II.44   Weight in kilograms of youths aged 17 years at last birthday by sex and height group in centimeters: sample size, estimated population size, mean, standard deviation, standard error of the mean, and selected percentiles, United States, 1966 to 1970

Sex and height	n	N	$\bar{X}$	s	$s_{\bar{x}}$	Percentile						
						5th	10th	25th	50th	75th	90th	95th
Male						in kilograms						
Under 130	–	–	–	–	–	–	–	–	–	–	–	–
130.0–134.9	–	–	–	–	–	–	–	–	–	–	–	–
135.0–139.9	–	–	–	–	–	–	–	–	–	–	–	–
140.0–144.9	–	–	–	–	–	–	–	–	–	–	–	–
145.0–149.9	–	–	–	–	–	–	–	–	–	–	–	–
150.0–154.9	1	3	*	*	*	*	*	*	*	*	*	*
155.0–159.9	11	39	54.63	9.397	3.414	43.8	46.4	48.2	49.7	57.8	69.9	73.2
160.0–164.9	25	81	57.75	6.503	1.355	49.7	51.1	52.5	56.9	61.6	70.1	70.8
165.0–169.9	63	248	62.57	8.344	1.224	50.2	53.2	56.4	61.5	66.9	72.7	77.3
170.0–174.9	115	396	67.06	11.163	0.704	53.3	55.5	59.5	64.6	71.9	80.9	91.6
175.0–179.9	151	537	68.37	9.907	0.831	56.9	58.9	61.5	66.5	73.6	79.4	88.4
180.0–184.9	80	297	73.31	12.454	1.335	59.6	61.0	65.1	71.2	78.4	91.8	102.7
185.0–189.9	36	133	76.03	9.171	1.301	62.4	66.3	70.5	75.3	80.8	90.3	92.9
190.0–194.9	7	25	81.40	10.985	7.588	62.9	62.9	67.8	87.3	90.3	90.6	90.6
195.0 and over	–	–	–	–	–	–	–	–	–	–	–	–
Female												
Under 130	–	–	–	–	–	–	–	–	–	–	–	–
130.0–134.9	–	–	–	–	–	–	–	–	–	–	–	–
135.0–139.9	–	–	–	–	–	–	–	–	–	–	–	–
140.0–144.9	2	5	*	*	*	*	*	*	*	*	*	*
145.0–149.9	8	26	43.49	3.939	1.604	38.6	38.8	40.1	45.1	45.7	51.1	51.2
150.0–154.9	43	151	49.96	6.508	0.827	41.6	42.3	44.6	48.9	53.5	59.2	64.1
155.0–159.9	103	385	54.71	9.903	0.775	44.4	45.5	48.7	53.2	57.7	61.6	76.2
160.0–164.9	133	506	57.79	10.620	1.028	46.8	48.0	50.2	55.4	61.5	72.3	82.3
165.0–169.9	116	433	60.63	10.117	1.182	47.9	50.3	55.1	59.3	65.1	69.4	71.6
170.0–174.9	51	186	62.18	9.132	1.407	50.6	52.9	55.5	60.2	65.7	76.1	82.7
175.0–179.9	12	47	65.76	8.405	2.229	54.9	56.7	60.1	61.7	75.2	75.9	83.0
180.0–184.9	1	2	*	*	*	*	*	*	*	*	*	*
185.0–189.9	–	–	–	–	–	–	–	–	–	–	–	–
190.0–194.9	–	–	–	–	–	–	–	–	–	–	–	–
195.0 and over	–	–	–	–	–	–	–	–	–	–	–	–

n, Sample size; N, estimated number of youths in population in thousands; $\bar{X}$, mean; s, standard deviation; $s_{\bar{x}}$, standard error of the mean.
(From National Center for Health Statistics (1973) Height and weight of youths 12–17 years, United States, in *Vital and Health Statistics*, Series 11, No. 124, Health Services and Mental Health Administration, U.S. Government Printing Office, Washington, D.C., pp. 282–8.)

Table II.45   Weight in kilograms for women 18 to 74 years of age: number examined, mean, standard deviation, and selected percentiles by race and age, United States, 1976 to 1980*

Race and age (years)	Number of examined persons	Mean	Standard deviation	Percentile 5th	10th	15th	25th	50th	75th	85th	90th	95th
All races[†]												
18–74	6,588	65.4	14.6	47.7	50.3	52.2	55.4	62.4	72.1	79.2	84.4	93.1
18–24	1,066	60.6	11.9	46.6	49.1	50.6	53.2	58.0	65.0	70.4	75.3	82.9
25–34	1,170	64.2	15.0	47.4	49.6	51.4	54.3	60.9	69.6	78.4	84.1	93.5
35–44	844	67.1	15.2	49.2	52.0	53.3	56.9	63.4	73.9	81.7	87.5	98.9
45–54	763	68.0	15.3	48.5	51.3	53.3	57.3	65.5	75.7	82.1	87.6	96.0
55–64	1,329	67.9	14.7	48.6	51.3	54.1	57.3	65.2	75.3	82.3	87.5	95.1
65–74	1,416	66.6	13.8	47.1	50.8	53.2	57.4	64.8	73.8	79.8	84.4	91.3
White												
18–74	5,686	64.8	14.1	47.7	50.3	52.2	55.2	62.1	71.1	77.9	83.3	91.5
18–24	892	60.4	11.6	47.3	49.5	50.8	53.3	57.9	64.8	69.7	74.3	82.4
25–34	1,000	63.6	14.5	47.3	49.5	51.3	54.0	60.6	68.9	76.3	81.5	89.7
35–44	726	66.1	14.5	49.3	51.8	52.9	56.3	62.4	71.9	79.7	85.8	94.9
45–54	647	67.3	14.4	48.6	51.3	53.4	57.0	65.0	74.8	81.1	85.6	94.5
55–64	1,176	67.2	14.4	48.5	50.7	53.7	57.1	64.7	74.5	81.8	86.2	92.8
65–74	1,245	66.2	13.7	47.2	50.7	52.9	57.2	64.3	72.9	79.2	84.3	91.2
Black												
18–74	782	71.2	17.3	48.8	51.6	55.1	59.1	67.8	80.6	87.4	94.9	105.1
18–24	147	63.1	13.9	46.2	49.0	50.6	53.8	60.4	70.0	75.8	79.1	89.3
25–34	145	69.3	16.7	48.3	50.8	53.1	57.8	65.3	80.2	87.1	91.5	102.7
35–44	103	75.3	18.4	50.7	55.2	57.2	63.0	70.2	85.2	95.3	103.5	113.1
45–54	100	77.7	18.8	55.1	60.3	60.8	64.5	74.3	83.6	94.5	98.2	117.5
55–64	135	75.8	16.4	54.2	55.2	57.6	65.4	74.6	83.4	91.9	95.5	108.5
65–74	152	72.4	13.6	52.9	56.4	60.3	64.0	70.0	82.2	84.4	86.5	98.1

*Includes clothing weight, estimated as ranging from 0.09 to 0.28 kilogram.
[†]Includes all other races not shown as separate categories.
(From National Center for Health Statistics (1987) *Anthropometric Reference Data and Prevalence of Overweight, United States 1976–1980*, DHHS Publication No. 87-1688, U.S. Department of Health and Human Services, Public Health Service, Hyattsville, MD.)

Table II.46   Weight in kilograms for men 18 to 74 years of age: number examined, mean, standard deviation, and selected percentiles by race and age, United States, 1976 to 1980*

Race and age (years)	Number of examined persons	Mean	Standard deviation	Percentile 5th	10th	15th	25th	50th	75th	85th	90th	95th
All races[†]												
18–74	5,916	78.1	13.5	58.6	62.3	64.9	68.7	76.9	85.6	91.3	95.7	102.7
18–24	988	73.8	12.7	56.8	60.4	61.9	64.8	72.0	80.3	85.1	90.4	99.5
25–34	1,067	78.7	13.7	59.5	62.9	65.4	69.3	77.5	85.6	91.1	95.1	102.7
35–44	745	80.9	13.4	59.7	65.1	67.7	72.1	79.9	88.1	94.8	98.8	104.3
45–54	690	80.9	13.6	60.8	65.2	67.2	71.7	79.0	89.4	94.5	99.5	105.3
55–64	1,227	78.8	12.8	59.9	63.8	66.4	70.2	77.7	85.6	90.5	94.7	102.3
65–74	1,199	74.8	12.8	54.4	58.5	61.2	66.1	74.2	82.7	87.9	91.2	96.6
White												
18–74	5,148	78.5	13.1	59.3	62.8	65.5	69.4	77.3	85.6	91.4	95.5	102.3
18–24	846	74.2	12.8	56.8	60.5	62.0	65.0	72.4	80.6	85.5	91.0	100.0
25–34	901	79.0	13.1	59.9	63.7	65.9	69.8	78.0	85.6	91.3	95.3	102.7
35–44	653	81.4	12.8	62.3	66.6	68.8	72.9	80.1	88.2	94.6	98.7	104.1

Continued

Table II.46   Continued

Race and age (years)	Number of examined persons	Mean	Standard deviation	Percentile								
				5th	10th	15th	25th	50th	75th	85th	90th	95th
White												
45–54	617	81.0	13.4	62.0	66.1	67.3	71.9	79.0	89.4	94.2	99.0	104.5
55–64	1,086	78.9	12.4	60.5	64.5	66.6	70.6	78.2	85.6	90.4	94.5	101.7
65–74	1,045	75.4	12.4	55.5	59.5	62.5	67.0	74.7	83.0	87.9	91.2	96.0
Black												
18–74	649	77.9	15.2	58.0	61.1	63.6	67.2	75.3	85.4	92.9	98.3	105.4
18–24	121	72.2	12.0	58.3	60.9	62.3	64.9	70.8	77.1	81.8	83.7	93.6
25–34	139	78.2	16.3	58.7	63.4	64.9	68.4	75.3	84.4	90.6	92.2	106.3
35–44	70	82.5	15.4	*	61.7	65.2	69.7	83.1	94.8	100.4	104.2	*
45–54	62	82.4	14.5	*	64.7	67.0	73.2	81.8	93.0	100.0	102.5	*
55–64	129	78.6	14.7	56.8	61.4	64.3	68.0	77.0	86.5	93.8	98.6	104.7
65–74	128	73.3	15.3	52.5	56.7	58.0	61.0	71.2	81.1	90.8	97.3	105.1

*Includes clothing weight, estimated as ranging from 0.09 to 0.28 kilogram.
†Includes all other races not shown as separate categories.
(From National Center for Health Statistics (1987) *Anthropometric Reference Data and Prevalence of Overweight, United States 1976–1980*, DHHS Publication No. 87-1688, U.S. Department of Health and Human Services, Public Health Service, Hyattsville, MD.)

Table II.47   Height in centimeters for women 18 to 74 years of age: number examined, mean, standard deviation, and selected percentiles by race and age, United States, 1976 to 1980*

Race and age (years)	Number of examined persons	Mean	Standard deviation	Percentile								
				5th	10th	15th	25th	50th	75th	85th	90th	95th
All races†												
18–74	6,588	161.8	6.6	150.9	153.6	155.2	157.4	161.7	166.3	168.6	170.3	172.6
18–24	1,066	163.4	6.6	152.9	155.2	156.7	159.0	163.7	167.6	170.0	171.6	174.0
25–34	1,170	163.1	6.3	153.2	155.2	156.6	158.7	163.1	167.6	169.9	171.3	173.7
35–44	844	162.8	6.3	152.6	155.5	156.7	158.5	162.5	167.0	169.3	171.0	173.5
45–54	763	161.3	6.4	150.5	152.9	154.5	156.8	161.3	165.6	167.7	169.4	171.8
55–64	1,329	160.1	6.4	149.2	151.8	153.7	155.9	160.3	164.5	166.7	168.0	170.3
65–74	1,416	158.1	6.2	147.9	150.0	151.7	154.1	158.4	162.2	164.5	166.0	167.7
White												
18–74	5,686	161.9	6.5	151.3	153.8	155.4	157.6	161.9	165.4	168.7	170.3	172.7
18–24	892	163.7	6.4	153.1	155.7	157.1	159.4	163.9	167.7	170.1	171.8	174.0
25–34	1,000	163.3	6.2	153.5	155.4	156.6	158.9	163.3	167.8	170.1	171.5	173.7
35–44	726	162.9	6.3	152.6	155.6	156.7	158.4	162.6	167.0	169.4	171.2	173.5
45–54	647	161.5	6.2	151.5	153.6	155.2	157.2	161.3	165.7	167.6	169.4	171.7
55–64	1,176	160.1	6.3	149.6	151.9	153.9	156.1	160.3	164.4	166.5	167.7	170.1
65–74	1,245	158.1	6.2	147.8	150.1	151.7	154.1	158.5	162.2	164.5	166.0	167.7
Black												
18–74	782	162.1	6.7	150.6	154.2	155.2	157.6	162.2	166.6	168.9	170.4	173.0
18–24	147	163.2	6.9	152.8	155.1	156.4	158.6	163.0	168.1	170.2	171.1	174.8
25–34	145	162.3	6.3	151.3	154.8	156.3	158.1	162.5	166.2	168.6	170.4	174.1
35–44	103	163.3	5.5	155.2	156.9	157.3	159.7	162.5	167.0	168.7	170.1	171.7
45–54	100	161.7	6.9	150.4	152.6	154.4	155.2	162.1	167.5	169.3	170.5	171.9
55–64	135	161.0	7.4	148.7	149.2	153.4	155.8	161.8	166.5	169.1	171.0	174.5
65–74	152	158.8	6.2	148.2	150.4	152.6	155.6	159.1	163.0	164.7	166.4	169.4

*Height without shoes.
†Includes all other races not shown as separate categories.
(From National Center for Health Statistics (1987) *Anthropometric Reference Data and Prevalence of Overweight, United States 1976–1980*, DHHS Publication No. 87-1688, U.S. Department of Health and Human Services, Public Health Service, Hyattsville, MD.)

Table II.48　Height in centimeters for men 18 to 74 years of age: number examined, mean, standard deviation, and selected percentiles by race and age, United States, 1976 to 1980*

Race and age (years)	Number of examined persons	Mean	Standard deviation	Percentile 5th	10th	15th	25th	50th	75th	85th	90th	95th
All races[†]												
18–74	5,916	175.5	7.2	163.9	166.4	168.2	171.1	175.7	180.4	182.9	184.5	187.0
18–24	988	177.0	7.1	165.8	168.3	169.8	172.2	177.0	181.6	183.9	186.0	189.6
25–34	1,067	176.7	6.7	165.5	167.9	170.0	172.2	176.8	181.2	183.6	185.3	187.4
35–44	745	176.3	7.3	164.1	166.4	168.8	172.2	176.5	181.2	183.6	185.2	188.0
45–54	690	175.2	6.6	164.5	167.2	168.3	170.7	175.1	179.8	182.5	184.3	185.7
55–64	1,227	173.7	6.9	162.1	165.4	166.8	169.2	173.7	178.5	180.6	182.2	184.6
65–74	1,199	171.3	7.1	159.3	162.3	164.1	166.3	171.5	176.1	178.6	180.4	183.1
White												
18–74	5,148	175.7	7.1	164.2	166.7	168.6	171.2	175.9	180.5	183.0	184.6	187.2
18–24	846	177.2	7.0	166.3	168.6	170.1	172.4	177.1	181.9	184.1	186.4	189.7
25–34	901	177.0	6.6	165.8	168.2	170.6	172.5	177.0	181.4	183.8	185.4	187.7
35–44	653	176.7	7.3	164.5	166.7	169.6	172.6	176.8	181.7	183.7	185.8	188.0
45–54	617	175.4	6.8	164.6	167.3	168.9	171.2	175.3	179.8	182.5	184.3	185.7
55–64	1,086	173.8	6.8	163.1	165.6	167.2	169.5	173.6	178.5	180.7	182.2	184.5
65–74	1,045	171.6	6.9	159.6	162.9	164.6	166.9	171.6	176.4	178.7	180.5	183.3
Black												
18–74	649	175.5	7.0	164.3	166.5	168.1	171.1	175.7	180.3	183.0	184.5	186.5
18–24	121	176.7	7.0	165.1	167.6	169.9	172.5	177.9	181.0	183.8	185.0	186.4
25–34	139	176.7	6.9	165.5	168.5	169.6	172.4	177.1	181.8	183.2	184.7	187.1
35–44	70	176.5	6.4	*	167.6	170.7	172.8	175.2	179.9	181.9	185.1	*
45–54	62	174.2	6.7	*	167.6	167.7	169.1	172.8	178.4	183.2	184.5	*
55–64	129	174.2	6.9	162.7	165.3	166.8	168.6	174.6	178.8	180.7	182.8	186.8
65–74	128	171.2	6.5	161.2	162.6	163.8	165.9	171.6	175.3	177.7	180.8	182.2

*Height without shoes.
[†]Includes all other races not shown as separate categories.
(From National Center for Health Statistics (1987) *Anthropometric Reference Data and Prevalence of Overweight, United States 1976–1980*, DHHS Publication No. 87-1688, U.S. Department of Health and Human Services, Public Health Service, Hyattsville, MD.)

Table II.49　Provisional age- and sex-specific reference values for weight in kilograms (pounds) in elderly subjects*,[†]

Age group (years)	5%	50%	95%
	Men		
65	62.6 (138.0)	79.5 (175.0)	102.0 (224.9)
70	59.7 (131.6)	76.5 (168.7)	99.1 (218.5)
75	56.8 (125.2)	73.6 (162.3)	96.3 (212.3)
80	53.9 (118.8)	70.7 (155.9)	93.4 (205.9)
85	51.0 (112.4)	67.8 (149.5)	90.5 (199.5)
90	48.1 (106.0)	64.9 (143.1)	87.6 (193.1)
	Women		
65	51.2 (112.9)	66.8 (147.3)	87.1 (192.0)
70	49.0 (108.0)	64.6 (142.4)	84.9 (187.2)
75	46.8 (103.2)	62.4 (137.6)	82.8 (182.5)
80	44.7 (98.5)	60.2 (132.7)	80.6 (177.7)
85	42.5 (93.7)	58.0 (127.9)	78.4 (172.8)
90	40.3 (88.8)	55.9 (123.2)	76.2 (168.0)

*Data from 119 men and 150 women. The subjects were all ambulatory.
[†]See Tables II.54 through II.59 for data compiled by Frisancho A.R. (1984), *Am. J. Clin. Nutr.*, **40** pp. 808–19, from NHANES I and II.
(From Chumlea, W.C., Roche, A.F., Mukherjee, D. (1984) *Nutritional Assessment of the Elderly through Anthropometry*, Wright State University School of Medicine, Ohio.)

Table II.50 Triceps skinfold thickness: Girls, 1 to 17 years, United States, 1971 to 1974

Race and age in years	Number in sample	Estimated population in thousands	Mean†	Standard deviation	5th	10th	15th	25th	50th	75th	85th	90th	95th
					Percentile								

Race and age in years	Number in sample	Estimated population in thousands	Mean†	Standard deviation	5th	10th	15th	25th	50th	75th	85th	90th	95th
All Races*					Triceps Skinfold in Millimeters								
1	267	1,620	10.1	2.8	6.0	6.5	7.0	8.0	10.0	12.0	13.0	14.0	15.0
2	272	1,708	10.5	2.5	7.0	7.5	8.0	9.0	10.0	12.0	13.5	14.0	15.0
3	292	1,701	10.9	2.7	6.0	7.0	8.0	9.0	11.0	12.5	13.5	14.0	15.0
4	281	1,599	10.5	2.7	7.0	7.5	8.0	8.0	10.0	12.0	13.0	14.0	15.0
5	314	1,695	10.5	3.8	6.0	7.0	7.0	8.0	10.0	12.0	13.0	15.0	17.5
6	176	1,787	10.3	3.3	6.0	6.5	7.0	8.0	10.0	12.0	13.0	13.5	15.0
7	169	1,754	10.8	4.2	4.0	6.0	7.0	8.0	10.5	12.0	15.0	16.0	18.0
8	152	1,800	12.3	4.8	6.5	8.0	8.0	9.0	11.0	15.0	17.0	18.0	22.5
9	171	2,017	13.2	4.8	7.0	7.5	8.0	10.0	12.5	16.0	18.0	20.0	22.0
10	197	2,173	13.1	5.0	7.0	8.0	8.0	9.5	12.0	15.5	19.0	20.0	23.0
11	166	1,911	14.5	6.2	7.0	8.0	8.5	10.0	13.0	18.0	20.5	23.5	28.5
12	177	1,812	15.0	5.9	7.5	8.0	9.0	10.5	14.0	18.5	20.0	23.0	27.0
13	198	2,175	16.2	6.8	7.0	8.0	10.0	11.5	15.0	20.0	24.0	25.0	30.0
14	184	2,036	17.5	7.3	8.5	9.5	10.0	13.0	16.0	21.0	24.0	27.0	33.0
15	171	2,163	17.0	7.0	8.0	10.0	11.0	12.0	16.0	20.5	23.0	25.0	28.5
16	175	2,145	18.2	6.7	10.0	10.5	12.0	13.5	17.0	21.0	24.0	26.0	32.5
17	157	1,804	19.6	8.1	10.0	11.5	12.0	13.0	19.0	24.0	26.5	29.5	35.0
White													
1	189	1,328	10.2	2.8	6.0	7.0	7.0	8.0	10.0	12.0	13.0	13.5	15.5
2	203	1,434	10.6	2.6	7.0	7.5	8.0	9.0	10.0	12.0	13.5	14.0	15.0
3	211	1,438	11.1	2.6	7.0	8.0	8.5	9.0	11.0	13.0	13.5	14.0	15.0
4	204	1,339	10.8	2.6	7.5	8.0	8.0	9.0	10.5	12.0	13.0	14.5	16.0
5	224	1,416	10.7	3.7	6.0	7.0	8.0	8.5	10.0	12.0	13.0	15.0	17.5
6	125	1,445	10.6	3.3	6.5	7.0	7.5	8.0	10.5	12.0	13.0	14.0	16.0
7	122	1,507	10.9	4.2	4.0	6.0	7.0	8.0	11.0	12.0	15.0	15.5	17.5
8	117	1,507	12.4	4.7	7.0	8.0	8.0	9.0	11.5	15.0	16.5	18.0	22.0
9	129	1,751	13.6	4.6	7.5	8.0	9.0	10.0	13.0	16.0	18.0	20.0	22.0

10	148	13.4	4.8	7.5	8.0	8.5	10.0	12.5	15.5	19.0	20.0	23.0
11	122	14.9	6.1	8.0	8.5	9.0	10.0	13.0	17.5	20.5	24.5	28.5
12	128	15.2	5.6	8.0	9.0	10.0	11.0	14.0	18.5	20.0	23.0	26.0
13	153	16.2	6.8	7.0	8.0	10.0	11.5	15.0	20.0	24.0	25.0	28.5
14	132	17.8	7.3	9.0	9.5	10.5	13.0	16.7	21.0	24.0	28.5	33.0
15	125	17.7	6.7	9.0	10.5	11.0	13.0	17.0	21.0	24.0	25.0	28.5
16	141	18.2	6.6	10.0	10.5	12.5	14.0	17.0	21.0	24.0	26.0	32.1
17	117	19.8	8.0	10.0	12.0	12.5	13.5	19.0	24.0	26.5	29.5	35.0
Black												
1	73	10.0	3.0	5.5	5.5	7.0	8.0	10.0	12.0	13.0	14.0	15.0
2	66	10.0	2.3	7.0	8.0	8.0	8.0	10.0	11.0	12.0	14.0	15.5
3	78	9.7	2.9	6.0	7.0	7.0	8.0	10.0	11.0	12.0	13.0	14.0
4	73	8.8	2.7	5.0	6.0	7.0	7.0	8.0	10.5	12.0	13.0	14.0
5	88	9.4	3.9	5.0	5.0	6.5	7.0	8.0	10.0	12.0	13.5	17.0
6	50	9.0	3.1	5.5	6.0	6.0	8.0	8.0	10.0	11.5	12.0	13.0
7	46	10.1	4.0	5.0	6.0	7.0	7.5	9.0	11.0	17.5	18.0	18.0
8	35	11.5	5.1	5.0	6.5	7.0	8.0	10.0	13.5	18.0	18.0	23.0
9	41	10.2	5.1	5.5	6.0	6.0	6.5	8.0	12.0	18.0	18.0	20.0
10	48	11.7	5.6	6.5	6.5	7.0	7.5	10.0	16.0	18.0	19.0	24.0
11	42	12.7	6.4	4.0	5.0	6.5	7.5	10.0	18.0	22.0	23.0	23.0
12	47	13.6	7.6	5.5	6.0	6.0	7.5	12.0	17.0	22.0	25.0	30.0
13	44	16.1	7.0	7.0	8.5	10.0	11.0	14.0	18.0	24.0	24.0	33.5
14	50	15.9	6.7	8.0	8.0	9.0	10.5	14.0	20.5	24.0	24.5	24.5
15	46	14.0	7.6	6.5	6.5	8.0	10.0	12.5	16.0	16.5	20.0	32.8
16	33	18.9	8.0	8.0	8.0	10.0	12.0	19.0	24.0	24.5	33.0	33.1
17	39	16.9	6.6	7.5	9.0	11.0	12.0	14.5	20.0	24.0	28.0	31.0

*Includes data for races that are not shown separately.
†Measurements made in the right arm.
(From the National Center for Health Statistics, Department of Health and Human Services. See also Bishop, C.W., Bowen, P.E., Ritchey, S.J. (1981) *Am. J. Clin. Nutr.*, **34** pp. 2530–9.)

Table II.51   Subscapular skinfold thickness: Girls, 1 to 17 years, United States, 1971 to 1974

Race and age in years	Number in sample	Estimated population in thousands	Mean†	Standard deviation	Percentile 5th	10th	15th	25th	50th	75th	85th	90th	95th
All Races*					Subscapular Skinfold in Millimeters								
1	267	1,620	6.2	1.9	4.0	4.0	4.0	5.0	6.0	8.0	8.0	9.0	9.0
2	272	1,708	6.2	2.4	4.0	4.0	4.0	5.0	6.0	7.0	8.0	9.0	10.0
3	292	1,701	5.8	2.0	4.0	4.0	4.0	4.5	5.5	6.5	7.0	8.0	9.0
4	281	1,599	5.6	1.9	3.5	4.0	4.0	4.5	5.0	6.0	7.0	8.0	9.0
5	314	1,695	6.2	3.3	3.5	4.0	4.0	4.0	5.0	6.5	8.0	9.0	15.0
6	176	1,787	6.0	2.8	3.0	4.0	4.0	4.5	5.5	6.5	7.0	8.0	10.0
7	169	1,754	6.2	3.3	3.0	4.0	4.0	4.5	5.0	7.0	9.0	10.5	11.5
8	152	1,800	7.7	5.5	3.5	4.0	4.0	4.5	5.5	8.0	12.5	14.5	19.5
9	171	2,017	8.5	5.0	4.0	4.0	4.5	5.0	7.0	10.0	13.0	17.0	19.0
10	197	2,173	8.6	5.1	4.0	4.5	5.0	5.5	6.5	10.0	13.0	18.0	20.0
11	166	1,911	10.1	6.4	4.0	5.0	5.0	6.0	8.0	13.0	16.0	19.0	25.5
12	177	1,812	11.1	6.8	5.0	5.0	5.5	6.0	9.5	13.0	16.0	20.0	25.0
13	198	2,175	11.9	7.1	5.0	6.0	6.0	7.0	9.5	15.0	19.0	23.4	26.0
14	184	2,036	13.0	8.0	5.0	6.0	6.5	8.0	10.0	16.0	19.0	24.0	28.0
15	171	2,163	12.2	7.2	6.0	6.5	7.0	7.5	10.0	14.0	18.0	20.0	27.0
16	175	2,145	13.4	7.8	6.0	7.0	7.5	8.0	10.5	15.0	21.0	25.5	29.0
17	157	1,804	15.6	9.4	6.5	7.0	7.5	9.0	12.5	20.0	25.5	27.0	34.1
White													
1	189	1,328	6.3	1.9	3.5	4.0	4.0	5.0	6.0	8.0	8.0	9.0	9.5
2	203	1,434	6.0	2.1	4.0	4.0	4.0	5.0	6.0	7.0	8.0	8.5	10.0
3	211	1,438	5.8	1.9	4.0	4.0	4.0	5.0	5.5	6.5	7.0	8.0	9.0
4	204	1,339	5.7	1.9	3.5	4.0	4.0	4.5	5.0	6.0	7.0	8.0	9.0
5	224	1,416	6.2	3.2	3.5	4.0	4.0	4.5	5.5	6.5	8.0	10.0	15.0
6	125	1,445	6.0	2.7	3.0	3.5	4.0	4.5	6.0	6.5	7.0	8.0	10.0
7	122	1,507	6.2	3.4	3.0	3.5	4.0	4.5	5.0	7.0	8.5	10.0	12.5
8	117	1,507	7.6	5.6	3.5	4.0	4.0	4.5	6.0	8.0	10.0	13.0	21.0
9	129	1,751	8.5	4.7	4.0	4.5	5.0	5.0	7.0	10.0	13.0	16.0	18.0

10	148	8.8	5.1	4.0	4.5	5.0	5.5	7.0	10.0	13.0	18.0	20.0
11	122	10.3	6.7	4.0	5.0	5.0	6.0	8.0	13.0	16.5	20.5	25.5
12	128	11.1	6.4	5.0	5.0	6.0	6.5	9.5	13.5	17.0	20.0	22.0
13	153	11.6	6.9	5.0	5.5	6.0	7.0	9.0	15.0	19.0	21.0	25.0
14	132	13.2	8.2	5.0	6.0	6.5	8.0	10.5	16.0	20.0	24.0	30.0
15	125	12.4	6.9	6.0	7.0	7.0	8.0	10.0	14.5	18.0	20.0	27.0
16	141	12.9	7.3	6.0	7.0	7.5	8.0	10.0	15.0	20.5	25.0	28.5
17	117	15.2	9.3	6.0	7.0	7.5	8.0	12.5	18.0	25.0	26.5	34.0
Black												
1	73	6.1	2.0	4.0	4.0	4.0	5.0	5.5	8.0	8.5	9.0	9.0
2	66	6.8	3.3	4.0	4.0	4.5	5.0	6.0	7.5	9.5	12.0	15.5
3	78	5.5	2.0	4.0	4.0	4.0	4.5	5.0	6.0	7.0	7.0	8.0
4	73	5.2	1.7	3.0	3.5	4.0	4.0	5.0	6.0	6.0	8.0	8.5
5	88	5.8	3.5	4.0	4.0	4.0	5.0	5.0	6.0	6.5	7.0	13.0
6	50	6.0	3.3	3.0	4.0	4.5	5.0	5.0	7.0	7.5	7.5	10.0
7	46	6.4	2.6	3.0	4.0	5.0	5.5	5.5	8.0	11.0	11.0	11.0
8	35	8.2	5.2	4.0	4.0	4.5	5.0	5.0	14.0	15.0	16.0	17.5
9	41	8.3	6.4	4.0	4.0	4.5	4.5	5.5	7.5	14.5	24.0	24.0
10	48	8.1	5.5	4.0	4.0	5.0	5.0	6.0	8.0	12.5	14.3	22.0
11	42	9.2	4.5	4.0	5.0	5.5	5.5	8.0	11.0	14.5	14.5	15.5
12	47	10.7	8.6	4.5	5.0	5.5	7.0	11.5	15.0	16.0	28.0	31.0
13	44	13.9	8.1	6.0	6.0	8.0	12.0	15.0	26.0	26.0	28.4
14	50	12.5	7.3	6.0	6.0	6.5	7.0	10.0	16.5	23.0	23.0	25.0
15	46	11.2	8.4	5.5	5.5	6.0	6.5	7.5	10.5	19.0	20.0	33.4
16	33	17.8	10.7	6.0	7.0	8.0	10.5	15.0	24.5	31.0	38.0	38.0
17	39	16.4	8.4	7.0	7.5	8.0	9.0	12.5	23.5	27.0	28.0	30.0

*Includes data for races that are not shown separately.

†Measurements made in the right arm.

(From the National Center for Health Statistics, Department of Health and Human Services. See also Bishop, C.W., Bowen, P.E., Ritchey, S.J. (1981) *Am. J. Clin. Nutr.*, **34** pp. 2530–9.)

Table II.52   Triceps skinfold thickness: Boys, 1 to 17 years, United States, 1971 to 1974

Race and age in years	Number in sample	Estimated population in thousands	Mean†	Standard deviation	Percentile 5th	10th	15th	25th	50th	75th	85th	90th	95th
All Races*					Triceps Skinfold in Millimeters								
1	286	1,693	10.4	3.1	6.0	7.0	7.5	8.0	10.0	12.0	14.0	15.0	16.0
2	298	1,747	10.0	2.7	6.0	6.5	7.0	8.0	10.0	12.0	12.5	13.5	15.0
3	308	1,807	9.9	2.7	6.5	7.0	7.0	8.0	10.0	11.0	12.5	13.1	14.5
4	304	1,815	9.4	2.5	5.0	6.5	7.0	8.0	9.0	11.0	12.0	12.5	14.0
5	273	1,563	9.5	3.3	5.0	6.0	7.0	7.0	9.0	11.0	12.5	13.5	15.0
6	179	1,673	8.6	3.0	5.0	5.5	6.0	6.5	8.0	10.0	12.0	12.0	14.0
7	164	1,979	8.9	3.5	4.0	5.0	6.0	6.5	8.0	10.0	12.0	13.0	15.5
8	152	1,861	9.0	3.3	5.0	5.5	6.0	6.5	8.0	10.0	12.0	13.0	16.0
9	169	2,019	10.6	4.8	5.0	6.0	6.5	7.0	9.0	14.0	17.0	17.0	19.0
10	184	2,205	10.9	4.4	5.5	6.0	6.0	8.0	10.0	13.5	15.0	17.0	19.5
11	178	2,177	11.9	6.4	5.0	6.0	6.0	7.5	10.0	14.5	18.0	20.0	24.0
12	200	2,304	11.9	6.3	4.5	6.0	6.5	8.0	10.5	13.5	16.5	20.0	27.0
13	174	1,978	11.2	6.6	5.0	5.0	5.5	7.0	10.0	13.0	19.0	22.0	25.0
14	174	2,030	10.3	6.2	4.0	5.0	5.5	6.5	8.0	12.0	16.5	19.0	22.5
15	171	2,093	10.0	6.1	4.0	5.0	5.0	6.0	8.0	11.5	15.0	19.0	23.5
16	169	2,019	9.7	5.2	4.0	5.0	5.0	6.0	8.0	12.0	14.0	17.0	22.0
17	176	2,095	9.2	5.4	4.0	5.0	5.0	6.0	7.5	11.0	12.5	15.0	19.0
White													
1	211	1,402	10.7	3.0	7.0	7.0	7.5	8.0	10.0	12.0	14.0	15.0	16.5
2	217	1,461	9.9	2.6	6.0	6.5	7.0	8.0	10.0	12.0	12.5	13.0	14.7
3	226	1,536	9.9	2.6	6.5	7.0	7.0	8.0	10.0	11.0	12.5	13.5	14.5
4	229	1,547	9.6	2.4	6.0	7.0	7.0	8.0	10.0	11.0	12.0	12.5	14.0
5	207	1,319	9.8	3.2	6.0	6.5	7.0	7.5	9.0	11.0	12.5	13.5	15.0
6	126	1,343	8.9	3.1	5.5	5.6	6.0	7.0	9.0	10.0	12.0	12.5	14.0
7	125	1,718	9.1	3.5	5.0	6.0	6.0	7.0	8.0	10.5	12.0	13.5	17.0
8	116	1,644	9.1	3.3	5.0	5.5	6.0	7.0	8.5	10.5	12.0	13.0	16.0
9	117	1,636	11.1	4.8	5.5	6.5	6.5	7.5	10.0	14.0	17.0	17.0	19.0

Age	N	Mean	SD	5th	10th	15th	25th	50th	75th	85th	90th	95th
10	148	11.1	4.2	5.5	6.0	7.0	8.0	10.0	14.0	15.5	17.0	19.5
11	132	12.5	6.5	6.0	6.0	7.0	8.0	10.0	15.0	19.0	20.5	24.5
12	152	12.4	6.1	6.0	6.0	7.0	8.5	11.0	14.0	18.0	21.0	27.0
13	129	11.7	6.7	5.0	5.0	6.0	7.0	10.0	14.0	19.0	22.0	25.5
14	134	10.9	6.4	4.0	5.0	6.0	7.0	9.0	13.0	18.0	20.0	24.0
15	124	10.2	6.1	4.0	5.0	6.0	6.0	8.0	12.0	15.0	19.0	24.0
16	128	10.1	5.2	4.0	5.0	5.0	6.5	9.0	12.5	15.0	17.0	22.0
17	139	9.3	5.4	4.5	5.0	5.5	6.0	7.5	11.0	13.0	15.0	19.0

Black

Age	N	Mean	SD	5th	10th	15th	25th	50th	75th	85th	90th	95th
1	72	9.4	3.4	4.5	6.0	7.0	8.0	8.0	11.0	12.0	13.0	15.0
2	77	10.1	3.2	4.5	6.0	6.5	8.0	10.0	12.0	14.0	15.0	15.0
3	72	9.1	2.6	6.0	6.5	6.5	7.0	9.0	10.5	12.0	12.0	13.0
4	74	8.0	2.6	5.0	5.0	5.0	6.5	7.0	9.0	10.0	10.5	15.0
5	64	7.7	3.4	4.5	5.0	5.0	5.0	7.0	9.0	10.0	12.0	15.5
6	52	7.1	1.8	4.0	4.0	5.0	6.0	7.0	8.0	9.0	9.0	9.0
7	38	7.5	3.2	4.0	5.0	5.0	5.0	6.5	9.0	11.5	13.0	15.0
8	33	7.8	3.4	4.0	4.0	4.5	6.0	6.5	10.0	11.0	11.0	12.5
9	52	8.2	3.9	3.5	5.0	6.0	6.0	7.0	8.0	12.0	13.0	18.0
10	33	9.1	5.3	5.0	5.0	6.0	6.0	7.5	10.0	13.0	15.0	20.0
11	43	8.0	5.0	4.0	4.0	5.0	5.0	6.0	8.5	11.0	12.0	15.0
12	47	9.4	7.0	4.0	4.0	6.0	6.0	7.5	10.7	11.0	15.0	24.0
13	45	8.2	4.4	4.0	5.0	5.0	5.0	7.0	8.5	11.0	19.0	19.0
14	39	6.6	2.6	3.5	3.5	3.5	5.0	6.5	7.0	8.0	9.0	12.0
15	43	8.9	6.1	4.0	4.5	5.0	5.0	6.5	9.0	10.0	21.0	21.0
16	41	7.2	4.8	4.0	4.0	4.0	5.0	6.0	7.5	8.0	11.0	15.0
17	35	8.7	5.8	3.5	3.5	5.0	5.0	7.0	10.5	12.0	12.0	23.2

*Includes data for races that are not shown separately.
†Measurements made in the right arm.

(From the National Center for Health Statistics, Department of Health and Human Services. See also Bishop, C.W., Bowen, P.E., Ritchey, S.J. (1981) *Am. J. Clin. Nutr.*, **34** pp. 2530–9.)

Table II.53 Subscapular skinfold thickness: Boys, 1 to 17 years, United States, 1971 to 1974

Race and age in years	Number in sample	Estimated population in thousands	Mean†	Standard deviation	Percentile									
					5th	10th	15th	25th	50th	75th	85th	90th	95th
All Races*					Subscapular Skinfold in Millimeters								
1	286	1,693	6.2	1.9	4.0	4.0	4.0	5.0	6.0	7.0	8.0	8.5	10.0
2	298	1,747	5.7	2.0	3.0	4.0	4.0	4.5	5.0	6.5	7.0	8.0	10.0
3	308	1,807	5.4	2.0	3.5	4.0	4.0	4.0	5.0	6.0	6.8	7.0	9.5
4	304	1,815	5.1	1.7	3.0	3.5	4.0	4.0	5.0	6.0	6.0	7.0	7.0
5	273	1,563	5.3	2.7	3.0	3.5	4.0	4.0	5.0	6.0	7.0	7.0	8.0
6	179	1,673	5.1	2.4	3.0	3.0	3.5	4.0	4.5	5.0	6.0	7.0	9.0
7	164	1,979	5.5	3.0	3.0	3.0	3.5	4.0	4.5	6.0	7.0	9.0	11.0
8	152	1,861	5.1	2.3	3.0	3.0	3.5	4.0	4.5	6.0	6.0	7.5	9.0
9	169	2,019	7.1	5.1	3.5	3.5	4.0	4.0	5.0	8.0	11.0	14.0	14.0
10	184	2,205	6.8	4.5	3.5	4.0	4.0	4.0	5.5	7.0	10.0	12.0	18.0
11	178	2,177	8.0	6.2	4.0	4.0	4.0	4.5	6.0	8.5	13.0	15.0	19.0
12	200	2,304	8.0	6.0	3.5	4.0	4.5	5.0	6.0	9.0	11.0	14.0	20.5
13	174	1,978	8.8	6.9	3.5	4.0	4.5	5.0	6.5	9.0	13.5	17.0	26.0
14	174	2,030	8.5	6.1	4.0	4.5	5.0	5.0	6.5	9.0	13.0	16.0	20.0
15	171	2,093	9.1	6.5	4.0	5.0	5.0	5.5	7.0	10.0	13.0	15.5	23.0
16	169	2,019	9.8	6.2	5.0	5.5	6.0	6.5	8.0	10.5	13.5	16.5	23.5
17	176	2,095	9.7	5.9	5.0	5.5	6.0	7.0	8.0	10.0	13.0	16.0	23.0
White													
1	211	1,402	6.3	2.0	4.0	4.0	4.0	5.0	6.0	7.0	8.0	8.5	10.0
2	217	1,461	5.6	1.9	3.0	3.5	4.0	4.0	5.0	6.0	7.0	7.5	10.0
3	226	1,536	5.4	2.0	3.5	4.0	4.0	4.0	5.0	6.0	6.5	7.0	10.0
4	229	1,547	5.2	1.8	3.0	4.0	4.0	4.0	5.0	6.0	6.0	7.0	7.0
5	207	1,319	5.3	2.7	3.0	3.5	4.0	4.0	5.0	6.0	7.0	7.0	8.0
6	126	1,343	5.1	2.4	3.0	3.5	3.5	4.0	4.5	5.5	6.0	7.0	10.0
7	125	1,718	5.6	3.1	3.0	3.0	3.5	4.0	5.0	6.0	7.0	8.0	11.5
8	116	1,644	5.1	2.3	3.0	3.0	3.0	4.0	4.5	6.0	6.0	7.5	11.0
9	117	1,636	7.2	4.7	3.5	4.0	4.0	4.0	5.0	8.5	11.5	14.0	14.0
10	148	1,909	6.8	4.5	3.0	4.0	4.0	4.0	5.5	7.0	9.5	12.0	18.0
11	132	1,823	8.2	6.4	3.5	4.0	4.0	4.5	6.0	9.0	14.0	15.0	20.0
12	152	1,970	8.1	5.8	3.5	4.0	4.0	5.0	6.0	9.0	11.5	14.0	21.0
13	129	1,697	9.0	7.1	3.5	4.0	4.0	5.0	6.5	9.0	14.0	17.0	27.0
14	134	1,730	9.0	6.5	4.0	5.0	5.0	5.5	6.5	9.0	14.0	16.0	20.0
15	124	1,728	8.8	6.4	4.0	5.0	5.0	5.5	7.0	9.0	13.0	15.0	22.0
16	128	1,752	9.9	6.4	5.0	5.0	6.0	6.5	8.0	11.0	13.5	17.0	23.5
17	139	1,831	9.7	6.1	5.0	5.5	6.0	6.5	8.0	10.0	13.0	16.0	23.0

Table II.53   Continued

Race and age in years	Number in sample	Estimated population in thousands	Mean†	Standard deviation	Percentile								
					5th	10th	15th	25th	50th	75th	85th	90th	95th
Black													
1	72	280	6.0	1.6	4.0	4.0	4.0	5.0	6.0	7.0	7.5	8.0	9.0
2	77	267	6.5	2.4	4.0	4.0	4.0	5.0	5.5	7.0	10.0	11.5	11.5
3	72	212	5.3	1.6	3.5	4.0	4.0	4.0	5.0	6.0	6.5	6.5	9.0
4	74	260	4.8	1.2	3.0	3.0	3.5	4.0	5.0	5.1	6.0	6.0	8.0
5	64	226	5.1	2.5	2.5	3.0	3.0	4.0	4.5	5.0	7.0	7.0	8.5
6	52	321	4.9	2.1	3.0	3.0	3.5	4.0	5.0	5.0	5.5	7.0	7.0
7	38	253	5.2	2.4	3.0	3.5	3.0	3.5	4.0	6.0	8.0	10.0	11.0
8	33	203	5.5	2.1	3.5	3.0	4.0	4.0	5.0	6.0	7.5	9.0	9.0
9	52	383	6.6	6.3	3.0	3.0	3.0	4.0	5.0	6.0	8.0	8.0	30.0
10	33	251	6.7	3.8	4.0	4.0	4.0	4.5	5.0	7.0	9.0	12.0	18.5
11	43	313	6.7	4.9	4.0	4.0	4.0	5.0	5.5	6.5	8.0	8.0	12.5
12	47	316	7.4	6.9	4.0	4.0	4.5	4.5	5.0	7.0	7.0	17.0	19.0
13	45	281	7.6	5.9	4.0	4.5	4.5	5.0	6.0	7.0	8.0	18.5	26.0
14	39	282	6.1	2.1	4.0	4.0	5.0	5.0	6.0	7.0	7.0	7.5	12.0
15	43	310	10.6	6.7	4.0	5.0	5.5	7.0	9.0	12.0	12.0	24.0	24.0
16	41	267	8.5	4.2	5.5	5.5	6.5	6.5	7.0	9.0	9.5	10.0	16.0
17	35	235	9.6	5.2	6.0	6.0	6.0	7.0	8.0	10.0	12.0	16.0	16.0

*Includes data for races that are not shown separately.
†Measurements made in the right arm.
(From the National Center for Health Statistics, Department of Health and Human Services. See also Bishop, C.W., Bowen, P.E., Ritchey, S.J. (1981) *Am. J. Clin. Nutr.*, **34** pp. 2530—9.)

Table II.54 Selected percentiles of weight, triceps and subscapular skinfolds, and bone-free upper arm muscle area (AMA) for United States men and women with small frames (25 to 54 years old)

Ht in	cm	n	Wt (kg) 5	10	15	50	85	90	95	Triceps (mm) 5	10	15	50	85	90	95	Subscapular (mm) 5	10	15	50	85	90	95	Bone-free AMA (cm²) 5	10	15	50	85	90	95
Men																														
62	157	23	46*	50*	52*	64	71*	74*	77*				11							16							52			
63	160	43	48*	51*	53	61	70	75*	79*		6	10	17					8	12	20					32	48	54	
64	163	73	49*	53	55	66	76	76	80*	5	5	10	16	18			7	7	15	25	29			37	38	49	58	63
65	165	112	52	53	58	66	77	81	84	4	5	6	11	17	19	21	7	8	9	14	25	28	35	31	35	37	47	60	63	71
66	168	129	56	57	59	67	78	83	84	5	6	6	11	18	18	20	7	8	8	14	26	26	32	31	36	38	49	60	62	71
67	170	132	56	60	62	71	82	83	88	5	6	6	11	18	20	22	6	7	9	15	23	25	30	35	39	41	49	58	60	62
68	173	107	56	59	62	71	79	82	85	5	6	6	10	15	16	20	7	8	9	13	24	30	40	33	37	40	49	59	62	69
69	175	97	57*	62	65	74	84	87	88*		6	6	11	17	20			7	7	13	24	26			36	40	58	61	63
70	178	46	59*	62*	67	75	87	86*	90*			7	10	17					9	14	23				35	48	57	
71	180	49	60*	64*	70	76	79	88*	91*			7	10	16					8	13	22				39	47	52	
72	183	21	62*	65*	67*	74	87*	89*	93*				10							14						45		
73	185	9	63*	67*	69*	79*	89*	91*	94*																		
74	188	6	65*	68*	71*	80*	90*	92*	96*																		
Women																														
58	147	53	37*	43	43	52	58	62	66*		12	13	24	30	33			10	12	23	34	38			22	24	29	36	44	
59	150	108	42	43	44	53	63	69	72	8	11	14	21	29	36	37	6	9	10	17	29	32	34	17	20	22	28	38	39	43
60	152	142	42	44	45	53	63	65	70	8	11	12	21	28	29	33	6	7	8	18	27	32	39	19	21	22	28	36	40	44
61	155	218	44	46	47	54	64	66	72	11	12	14	21	28	31	34	7	8	9	16	28	32	36	20	21	23	28	38	39	42
62	157	255	44	47	48	55	63	64	70	10	12	14	20	28	31	34	6	7	8	14	22	27	32	20	21	21	27	33	35	37
63	160	239	46	48	49	55	65	68	79	10	11	13	20	27	30	36	6	7	7	14	27	29	31	20	21	22	27	33	35	38
64	163	146	49	50	51	57	67	68	74	10	13	13	20	28	30	34	6	7	8	13	24	27	34	22	23	23	28	34	38	42
65	165	113	50	52	53	60	70	72	80	12	13	14	22	29	31	34	7	8	8	15	26	30	33	21	22	23	28	37	39	47
66	168	47	46*	49*	54	58	65	71*	74*		12	19	30					9	12	25					23	27	35	
67	170	18	47*	50*	52*	59	70*	72*	76*		18							13							26		
68	173	18	48*	51*	53*	62	71*	73*	77*		20							15							25		
69	175	5	49*	52*	54*	63*	72*	74*	78*																		
70	178	1	50*	53*	55*	64*	73*	75*	79*																		

*Value estimated through linear regression equation.
(From Frisancho, A.R. (1984) *Am. J. Clin. Nutr.* **40** pp. 808–19, with permission.)

Table II.55 Selected percentiles of weight, triceps and subscapular skinfolds, and bone-free upper arm muscle area (AMA) for United States men and women with medium frames (25 to 54 years old)

Ht			Wt (kg)							Triceps (mm)							Subscapular (mm)							Bone-free AMA (cm^2)						
in	cm	n	5	10	15	50	85	90	95	5	10	15	50	85	90	95	5	10	15	50	85	90	95	5	10	15	50	85	90	95
Men																														
62	157	10	51*	55*	58*	68	81*	83*	87*				15							13							58			
63	160	30	52*	56*	59*	71	82*	85*	89*				11							18							55			
64	163	71	54*	60	61	71	83	84	90*		6	6	12	18	20			7	9	17	30	32			43	47	56	67	71	
65	165	154	59	62	65	74	87	90	94	5	7	8	12	20	22	25	8	9	10	16	26	29	32	40	43	45	56	67	69	70
66	168	212	58	61	65	75	85	87	93	5	6	7	11	16	18	22	7	7	9	16	25	27	33	38	42	44	55	69	72	78
67	170	409	62	66	68	77	89	93	100	5	7	7	13	21	23	28	8	9	10	18	26	30	33	39	42	44	53	66	69	73
68	173	478	60	64	66	78	89	92	97	4	5	7	11	18	20	24	7	8	9	16	25	28	31	41	44	45	55	67	71	76
69	175	464	63	66	68	78	90	93	97	5	6	7	12	18	20	24	7	8	9	16	25	27	31	38	41	44	54	66	69	73
70	178	419	64	66	70	81	90	93	97	5	6	7	12	18	20	23	7	8	9	15	24	27	30	39	42	43	55	65	68	72
71	180	282	62	68	70	81	92	96	100	4	5	7	12	19	21	25	7	8	9	14	24	27	30	37	41	44	54	67	68	73
72	183	231	68	71	74	84	97	100	104	5	7	7	12	20	22	26	7	8	9	15	26	30	32	40	42	44	56	65	67	74
73	185	106	70	72	75	85	100	101	104	6	7	8	12	20	24	27	8	9	9	15	25	29	32	39	42	43	55	67	69	73
74	188	50	68*	76	77	88	100	100	104*		6	9	13	21	23			7	9	14	25	30			43	43	55	62	63	
Women																														
58	147	40	41*	46*	50	63	77	75*	79*			20	25	40					15	23	38					24	35	42		
59	150	104	47	50	52	66	76	79	85	15	19	21	30	37	40	40	10	12	13	29	38	39	43	23	24	26	33	43	45	49
60	152	208	47	50	52	60	77	79	85	14	15	17	26	35	37	41	8	10	11	22	35	37	41	22	25	25	32	42	45	49
61	155	465	47	49	51	61	73	78	86	11	14	15	25	34	36	42	7	9	10	19	32	36	42	21	24	25	31	42	45	51
62	157	644	49	50	52	61	73	77	83	12	14	16	24	34	36	40	7	9	10	18	33	37	40	21	23	25	31	40	43	48
63	160	685	49	51	53	62	77	80	88	12	13	15	24	33	35	38	7	8	10	18	31	34	38	22	23	25	32	41	43	50
64	163	722	50	52	54	62	76	82	87	11	14	15	23	33	36	40	7	7	8	16	31	35	38	21	23	24	31	40	43	48
65	165	628	52	54	55	63	75	80	89	12	14	15	22	31	34	38	7	8	8	15	29	33	38	21	23	24	31	40	43	49
66	168	428	52	54	55	63	75	78	83	11	13	14	22	31	33	37	7	8	9	14	28	30	35	21	23	24	30	39	41	44
67	170	257	54	56	57	65	79	82	88	12	13	15	21	29	30	35	7	8	8	15	28	32	37	22	24	25	30	40	43	48
68	173	119	58	59	60	67	77	85	87	10	14	15	22	31	32	36	8	8	9	15	29	33	35	22	24	25	30	37	38	39
69	175	59	49*	58	60	68	79	82	87*		11	12	19	29	31			8	8	12	25	29			23	24	30	36	39	
70	178	15	50*	54*	57*	70	80*	83*	87*				19							20							32			

*Value estimated through linear regression equation.

(From Frisancho, A.R. (1984) *Am. J. Clin. Nutr.*, **40** pp. 808–19, with permission.)

Table II.56 Selected percentiles of weight, triceps and subscapular skinfolds, and bone-free upper arm muscle area (AMA) for United States men and women with large frames (25 to 54 years old)

Ht			Wt (kg)							Triceps (mm)							Subscapular (mm)							Bone-free AMA (cm²)						
in	cm	n	5	10	15	50	85	90	95	5	10	15	50	85	90	95	5	10	15	50	85	90	95	5	10	15	50	85	90	95
Men																														
62	157	1	57*	62*	66*	82*	99*	103*	108*																				
63	160	1	58*	63*	67*	83*	100*	104*	109*																				
64	163	5	59*	64*	68*	84*	101*	105*	110*																				
65	165	15	60*	65*	69*	79	102*	106*	111*			14							21							62			
66	168	37	60*	65*	75	84	103	106*	112*		9	14	30				13	22	36					48	58	76			
67	170	54	62*	70	71	84	102	111	113*	7	7	11	23	27			8	11	20	36	40			50	52	61	73	78	
68	173	84	63*	74	76	86	101	104	114*	9	10	14	22	23			12	14	20	31	35			51	53	65	78	86	
69	175	126	68	71	74	89	103	105	114	6	7	8	15	25	29	31	9	10	11	18	31	32	38	46	48	49	61	73	78	83
70	178	150	68	72	74	87	106	112	114	7	7	7	14	23	25	30	7	10	11	17	31	35	38	43	47	50	61	75	77	86
71	180	123	73	78	82	91	113	116	123	6	8	10	15	25	27	31	9	11	11	20	35	40	46	47	48	50	62	75	81	83
72	183	114	73	76	78	91	109	112	121	5	6	7	12	20	22	25	8	9	9	19	28	30	36	45	48	50	61	77	80	86
73	185	109	72	77	79	93	106	107	116	5	6	7	13	19	22	31	7	9	9	18	27	28	30	47	49	51	66	79	83	
74	188	37	69*	74*	82	92	105	115*	120*		8	12	19					9	18	32					53	66	78		
Women																														
58	147	6	56*	63*	67*	86*	105*	110*	117*																				
59	150	19	56*	62*	67*	78	105*	109*	116*			36							35						45			
60	152	32	55*	62*	66*	87	104*	109*	116*			38							42						44			
61	155	92	54*	64	66	81	105	117	115*		25	26	36	48	50			17	17	35	48	53			29	33	41	62	74	
62	157	135	59	61	65	81	103	107	113	16	19	22	34	48	48	50	13	16	18	32	48	51	55	26	28	31	44	56	63	72
63	160	162	58	63	67	83	105	109	119	18	20	22	34	46	48	51	11	14	16	32	44	48	50	27	30	32	43	60	65	77
64	163	196	59	62	63	79	102	104	112	16	20	21	32	43	45	49	10	12	15	28	42	46	50	26	28	29	39	50	55	63
65	165	242	59	61	63	81	103	109	114	17	20	21	31	43	46	48	10	12	14	29	42	48	52	27	28	29	39	56	59	67
66	168	166	55	58	62	75	95	100	107	13	17	18	27	40	43	45	8	9	11	25	36	40	45	23	24	27	35	49	53	69
67	170	144	58	60	65	80	100	108	114	13	16	17	30	41	43	49	7	10	11	25	41	46	55	25	28	30	37	50	53	55
68	173	81	51*	66	66	76	104	105	111*		16	20	29	37	40			10	12	21	45	48			28	30	38	51	54	
69	175	39	50*	57*	68	79	105	104*	111*		21	30	42					11	20	43					27	35	49			
70	178	17	50*	56*	61*	76	99*	104*	110*			20							16						37			

*Value estimated through linear regression equation.
(From Frisancho, A.R. (1984) *Am. J. Clin Nutr.,* **40** pp. 808–19, with permission.)

Table II.57 Selected percentiles of weight, triceps and subscapular skinfolds, and bone-free upper arm muscle area (AMA) for United States men and women with small frames (55 to 74 years old)

Ht in	cm	n	Wt (kg) 5	10	15	50	85	90	95	Triceps (mm) 5	10	15	50	85	90	95	Subscapular (mm) 5	10	15	50	85	90	95	Bone-free AMA (cm²) 5	10	15	50	85	90	95
Men
62	157	47	45*	49*	56	61	68	73*	77*			6	9	12					11	16	23					38	46	52		
63	160	78	47*	49	51	62	71	71	79*		5	5	10	16	17			6	6	12	21	22			34	35	43	54	55	
64	163	107	47	50	54	63	72	74	80	4	4	4	9	20	21	22	6	7	7	14	24	25	29	26	30	31	44	53	54	56
65	165	132	48	54	59	70	80	90	90	5	6	7	11	18	19	24	6	8	8	16	28	28	29	26	30	34	48	57	60	62
66	168	112	51	55	59	68	77	80	84	5	6	7	11	16	20	20	7	7	8	15	25	26	30	25	31	35	45	54	58	64
67	170	128	55	60	61	69	79	81	88	5	6	6	10	15	17	25	7	8	9	13	22	25	31	30	36	37	45	53	55	59
68	173	95	54*	54	58	70	79	81	86*		5	5	10	15	17			7	7	13	21	22			35	35	43	55	60	
69	175	47	56*	59*	63	75	81	84*	88*		8	10	15					10	16	27					38	47	62			
70	178	29	57*	61*	63*	76	83*	86*	89*			11							13							48			
71	180	14	59*	62*	65*	69	85*	87*	91*			9							10							43			
72	183	6	60*	64*	66*	76*	86*	89*	92*																				
73	185	1	62*	65*	68*	78*	88*	90*	94*																				
74	188	1	63*	67*	69*	77*	89*	92*	95*																				
Women
58	147	85	39*	46	48	54	63	65	71*		14	16	21	31	34			8	9	18	32	33			22	23	29	40	42	
59	150	122	41	45	48	55	66	68	74	11	13	15	21	30	31	33	6	7	9	19	29	30	33	22	23	24	30	39	40	44
60	152	157	43	45	47	54	67	70	73	10	11	13	20	29	31	35	5	7	8	15	27	32	36	20	22	23	30	37	41	44
61	155	145	43	43	45	56	65	70	71	10	12	14	22	29	29	32	6	7	8	17	29	31	34	18	21	23	28	36	40	42
62	157	158	47	49	52	58	67	69	73	11	11	12	21	29	30	32	7	8	9	17	25	26	30	20	23	24	30	37	40	43
63	160	89	42*	45	49	58	67	68	74*		12	13	20	29	30			6	7	14	25	27			19	20	27	35	36	
64	163	50	43*	47	49	60	68	70	75*		12	13	21	27	29			6	7	18	24	25			21	21	28	37	42	
65	165	26	43*	47*	49*	60	69*	72*	75*			18							13							28			
66	168	12	44*	48*	50*	68	70*	72*	76*			23							13							33			
67	170	1	45*	48*	51*	61*	71*	73*	77*																				
68	173	1	45*	49*	51*	61*	71*	74*	77*																				
69	175	0	46*	49*	52*	62*	72*	74*	78*																				
70	178	0	47*	50*	52*	63*	73*	75*	79*																				

*Value estimated through linear regression equation.
(From Frisancho, A.R. (1984) *Am. J. Clin. Nutr.*, **40** pp. 808–19, with permission.)

Table II.58 Selected percentiles of weight, triceps and subscapular skinfolds, and bone-free upper arm muscle area (AMA) for United States men and women with medium frames (55 to 74 years old)

Ht in	Ht cm	n	Wt (kg) 5	10	15	50	85	90	95	Triceps (mm) 5	10	15	50	85	90	95	Subscapular (mm) 5	10	15	50	85	90	95	Bone-free AMA (cm²) 5	10	15	50	85	90	95
Men																														
62	157	49	50*	54*	59	68	77	81*	85*			5	12	25					11	19	27						39	48	61		
63	160	89	51*	57	60	70	80	82	87*		7	7	11	20	23			8	10	15	26	28				36	38	50	60	63
64	163	210	55	59	62	71	82	83	91		6	6	10	17	20	26	6	7	9	15	25	27	35	35	39	40	51	64	66	71
65	165	335	56	60	64	72	83	86	89	5	6	7	11	17	19	24	7	8	9	17	25	29	31	35	38	41	52	63	65	72
66	168	405	57	62	66	74	83	84	89	5	6	7	12	18	19	22	7	9	10	16	25	28	31	34	39	42	51	60	62	67
67	170	509	59	64	66	78	87	89	94	6	6	7	12	18	20	23	7	9	10	17	26	29	34	35	39	42	52	65	67	70
68	173	413	62	66	68	78	89	95	101	5	7	8	12	18	21	23	7	9	10	17	26	29	32	37	40	42	52	65	67	72
69	175	366	62	66	68	77	90	93	99	6	6	7	12	19	22	25	6	8	9	16	25	28	30	31	36	40	51	62	65	68
70	178	248	62	68	71	80	90	95	101	6	7	7	11	18	19	21	7	9	10	16	25	27	30	36	41	44	53	63	65	72
71	180	146	68	70	72	84	94	97	101	5	6	6	11	16	17	20	7	9	10	15	25	26	31	36	42	44	56	65	67	71
72	183	81	66*	65	69	81	96	97	101*		6	8	11	19	20		8	10	16	28				27	39	50	58	59	
73	185	35	68*	72*	79	88	93	99*	103*			8	13	16			8	15	26					43	56	67		
74	188	11	69*	73*	76*	95	98*	101*	104*				11					18						56				
Women																														
58	147	105	40	44	49	57	72	82	85	5	13	17	28	40	40	41	3	7	10	25	37	43	48	21	23	25	32	46	47	51
59	150	198	47	49	52	62	74	78	86	12	15	18	26	34	38	41	8	9	11	23	32	36	43	24	26	27	35	44	48	48
60	152	358	47	50	52	65	76	79	86	13	17	18	25	33	34	38	8	10	12	22	34	36	40	21	24	26	35	45	49	57
61	155	543	49	51	54	64	78	81	86	13	16	18	25	35	37	42	8	10	10	20	33	36	42	22	24	26	34	44	49	52
62	157	576	49	53	54	64	78	82	88	13	15	17	24	33	36	39	7	8	10	20	33	36	38	24	25	26	35	45	47	54
63	160	551	52	54	55	65	79	83	89	12	14	16	24	32	35	38	8	8	10	18	32	37	41	24	26	27	35	44	45	51
64	163	406	51	54	57	66	78	81	87	12	14	16	25	33	34	37	7	9	10	17	30	33	38	21	24	26	33	44	46	49
65	165	307	54	56	59	67	78	84	88	14	16	17	24	33	35	39	7	8	9	17	30	35	37	24	25	27	34	44	45	50
66	168	119	54	57	57	66	79	85	88	12	13	16	24	33	33	36	6	7	8	16	30	31	34	24	26	27	33	41	43	49
67	170	63	51*	59	61	72	82	85	89*		17	17	27	35	35			9	10	19	35	35			27	28	32	41	43	
68	173	28	52*	56*	59*	70	83*	86*	90*				25						16							36			
69	175	5	53*	57*	60*	72*	84*	87*	91*																				
70	178	1	54*	58*	61*	73*	85*	88*	92*																				

*Value estimated through linear regression equation.
(From Frisancho, A.R. (1984) *Am. J. Clin Nutr.*, **40** pp. 808–19, with permission.)

Table II.59   Selected percentiles of weight, triceps and subscapular skinfolds, and bone-free upper arm muscle area (AMA) for United States men and women with large frames (55 to 74 years old)

Ht			Wt (kg)							Triceps (mm)							Subscapular (mm)							Bone-free AMA (cm²)						
in	cm	n	5	10	15	50	85	90	95	5	10	15	50	85	90	95	5	10	15	50	85	90	95	5	10	15	50	85	90	95
Men																														
62	157	7	54*	59*	63*	77*	91*	95*	100*				15							20										
63	160	12	55*	60*	64*	80	92*	96*	101*				21							31							57			
64	163	20	57*	62*	65*	77	94*	97*	102*				14						14	19							44			
65	165	36	58*	63*	73	79	89	98*	103*			11	14	22					11	20	27					44	59	66		
66	168	58	59*	67	73	80	101	102	105*		7	8	13	21	25	27		9	12	20	31	35	38		43	47	56	67	72	79
67	170	114	65	71	73	85	103	108	112	6	8	9	16	21	25	23	8	11	11	20	35	35	32	41	43	44	56	71	73	74
68	173	128	67	71	73	83	95	98	111	6	7	8	13	20	21	23	8	10	11	18	27	30	33	41	43	46	57	69	70	79
69	175	131	65	70	74	84	96	98	105	6	7	8	12	18	20		7	11	11	19	27	30	37	40	45	45	58	70	72	87
70	178	144	68	73	77	87	102	104	117	5	6	8	14	22	25	31	9	11	13	20	30	33		43	48	50	59	70	71	
71	180	95	65*	70	70	84	102	109	111*		6	6	13	18	22			8	9	15	30	30			46	47	54	70	75	
72	183	72	67*	76	81	90	108	112	112*		8	8	13	23	26			8	9	20	28	31			47	48	59	73	78	
73	185	23	68*	73*	76*	88	105*	108*	113*				11							19							59			
74	188	15	69*	74*	78*	89	106*	109*	114*				12							15							54			
Women																														
58	147	14	53*	59*	63*	92	95*	99*	104*				45	44	45	46				44							50			
59	150	26	54*	59*	63*	78	95*	99*	105*				36	40	44	50				31							49			
60	152	72	54*	65	69	78	87	88	105*		25	26	35	40	43	45			21	31	42	45	48		28	33	41	58	60	71
61	155	117	64	68	69	79	94	95	106	18	22	24	33	41	43	50	13	16	19	29	40	43	53	31	32	34	44	59	61	76
62	157	126	59	61	63	82	93	101	111	19	24	24	32	40	43	45	13	19	22	30	39	48	51	28	29	34	43	59	63	67
63	160	154	61	65	67	80	100	102	118	20	24	25	33	41	46	50	13	15	16	29	40	45	55	27	32	33	41	56	62	78
64	163	147	60	65	67	77	97	102	119	18	22	23	29	42	46	50	10	12	16	24	41	46	50	28	29	32	41	54	60	65
65	165	117	60	66	69	80	98	102	111	15	17	20	30	43	44	46	8	9	12	26	42	46	48	29	32	32	42	53	57	
66	168	64	57*	60	63	82	98	105	109*		18	18	27	35	44		8	9	12	26	34	36			31	31	40	57	58	
67	170	40	58*	64*	68	80	105	104*	109*			22	32	44	40				14	27	46					30	40	58		
68	173	17	58*	64*	68*	79	100*	104*	110*				26							25							48			
69	175	7	59*	65*	69*	85*	101*	105*	110*			14							14	21										
70	178	2	60*	65*	69*	85*	101*	105*	111*																					

*Value estimated through linear regression equation.

(From Frisancho, A.R. (1984) *Am. J. Clin. Nutr.,* **40** pp. 808–19, with permission.)

Table II.60   Midarm muscle circumference in adults (18 to 74 years), United States*†

Age group (years)	Sample size	Estimated population (millions)	Mean (cm)	Percentile						
				5th	10th	25th	50th	75th	90th	95th
Men										
18–74	5,261	61.18	28.0	23.8	24.8	26.3	27.9	29.6	31.4	32.5
18–24	773	11.78	27.4	23.5	24.4	25.8	27.2	28.9	30.8	32.3
25–34	804	13.00	28.3	24.2	25.3	26.5	28.0	30.0	31.7	32.9
35–44	664	10.68	28.8	25.0	25.6	27.1	28.7	30.3	32.1	33.0
45–54	765	11.15	28.2	24.0	24.9	26.5	28.1	29.8	31.5	32.6
55–64	598	9.07	27.8	22.8	24.4	26.2	27.9	29.6	31.0	31.8
65–74	1,657	5.50	26.8	22.5	23.7	25.3	26.9	28.5	29.9	30.7
Women										
18–74	8,410	67.84	22.2	18.4	19.0	20.2	21.8	23.6	25.8	27.4
18–24	1,523	12.89	20.9	17.7	18.5	19.4	20.6	22.1	23.6	24.9
25–34	1,896	13.93	21.7	18.3	18.9	20.0	21.4	22.9	24.9	26.6
35–44	1,664	11.59	22.5	18.5	19.2	20.6	22.0	24.0	26.1	27.4
45–54	836	12.16	22.7	18.8	19.5	20.7	22.2	24.3	26.6	27.8
55–64	669	9.98	22.8	18.6	19.5	20.8	22.6	24.4	26.3	28.1
65–74	1,822	7.28	22.8	18.6	19.5	20.8	22.5	24.4	26.5	28.1

*Measurements made in the right arm.
†See Tables II.54 through II.59 for data compiled by Frisancho, A.R. (1984) *Am. J. Clin. Nutr.*, **40** pp. 808–19, from NHANES I and II.
(From Bishop, C.W., Bowen, P.E., Ritchey, S.J. (1981) *Am. J. Clin. Nutr.*, **34** pp. 2530–9, [NHANES 1].)

Table II.61   Midarm muscle area in adults (18 to 74 years), United States*†

Age group (years)	Sample size	Estimated population (millions)	Mean (cm)	Percentile						
				5th	10th	25th	50th	75th	90th	95th
Men										
18–74	5,261	61.18	62.4	45.1	49.0	55.1	62.0	69.8	78.5	84.1
18–24	773	11.78	59.8	44.0	47.4	53.0	58.9	66.5	75.5	83.1
25–34	804	13.00	63.8	46.6	51.0	55.9	62.4	71.7	80.0	86.2
35–44	664	10.68	66.0	49.8	52.2	58.5	65.6	73.1	82.0	86.7
45–54	765	11.15	63.3	45.9	49.4	55.9	62.9	70.7	79.0	84.6
55–64	598	9.07	61.5	41.4	47.4	54.7	62.0	69.8	76.5	80.5
65–74	1,657	5.50	57.2	40.3	44.7	51.0	57.6	64.7	71.2	75.0
Women										
18–74	8,410	67.84	39.2	27.0	28.7	32.5	37.8	44.3	53.0	59.8
18–24	1,523	12.89	34.8	24.9	27.2	30.0	33.8	38.9	44.3	49.4
25–34	1,896	13.93	37.5	26.7	28.4	31.8	36.5	41.8	49.4	56.3
35–44	1,664	11.59	40.3	27.2	29.4	33.8	38.5	45.9	54.2	59.8
45–54	836	12.16	41.0	28.1	30.3	34.1	39.2	47.0	56.3	61.5
55–64	669	9.98	41.4	27.5	30.3	34.4	40.7	47.4	55.1	62.9
65–74	1,822	7.28	41.4	27.5	30.3	34.4	40.3	47.4	55.9	62.9

*Measurements made in the right arm.
†See Tables II.54 through II.59 for data compiled by Frisancho, A.R. (1984) *Am. J. Clin. Nutr.*, **40** pp. 808–19, from NHANES I and II.
(From Bishop, C.W., Bowen, P.E., Ritchey, S.J. (1981) *Am. J. Clin. Nutr.*, **34** pp. 2530–9, [NHANES 1].)

Table II.62 Age correction for estimates of weight, triceps and subscapular skinfold thicknesses, and bone-free upper arm muscle area (AMA)

Age group: Frame size	Median age	Weight	Triceps skinfold	Subscapular skinfold	Arm muscle area
Men					
25–54					
Small	39	0.074	0.016	0.080	0.030
Medium	39	0.080	0.005	0.083	0.055
Large	40	0.000	−0.024	0.049	0.026
55–74					
Small	66	−0.329	−0.036	−0.115	−0.407
Medium	67	−0.435	−0.040	−0.125	−0.521
Large	67	−0.562	−0.054	−0.185	−0.644
Women					
25–54					
Small	37	0.165	0.166	0.142	0.087
Medium	37	0.234	0.189	0.214	0.191
Large	37	0.284	0.191	0.233	0.270
55–74					
Small	67	−0.027	−0.072	−0.013	0.036
Medium	66	−0.196	−0.210	−0.221	−0.033
Large	67	−0.466	−0.370	−0.515	−0.378

(From Frisancho, A.R. (1984) *Am. J. Clin. Nutr.*, **40** pp. 808–19, with permission.)

Table II.63 Provisional percentiles for triceps skinfold thickness in the elderly*[†]

Age group (years)	Percentile		
	5th	50th	95th
Men			
65	8.6	13.8	27.0
70	7.7	12.9	26.1
75	6.8	12.0	25.2
80	6.0	11.2	24.3
85	5.1	10.3	23.4
90	4.2	9.4	22.6
Women			
65	13.5	21.6	33.0
70	12.5	20.6	32.0
75	11.5	19.6	31.0
80	10.5	18.6	30.0
85	9.5	17.6	29.0
90	8.5	16.6	28.0

*Data are from 119 men and 150 women. All subjects were ambulatory, and measurements were made in the recumbent position on the left side.
[†]See Tables II.54 and II.55 for data compiled by Frisancho, A.R. (1984) *Am. J. Clin. Nutr.*, **40** pp. 808–19, from NHANES I and II.
(From Chumlea, W.C., Roche, A.F., Mukherjee, D. (1984) *Nutritional Assessment of the Elderly Through Anthropometry*, Wright State University School of Medicine, Ohio.)

Table II.64 Provisional percentiles for midarm muscle area (cm²) in the elderly*[†]

Age group (years)	Percentile		
	5th	50th	95th
Men			
65	43.2	59.4	77.1
70	41.4	57.7	75.3
75	39.6	55.9	73.5
80	37.8	54.1	71.7
85	36.0	52.3	69.9
90	34.3	50.5	68.2
Women			
65	33.5	44.5	66.4
70	33.0	44.1	65.9
75	32.6	43.6	65.5
80	32.2	43.2	65.1
85	31.8	42.8	64.7
90	31.3	42.4	64.2

*Data are from 119 men and 150 women. All subjects were ambulatory, and measurements were made in the recumbent position on the left side.
[†]See Tables II.54 and II.55 for data compiled by Frisancho, A.R. (1984) *Am. J. Clin. Nutr.*, **40** pp. 808–19, from NHANES I and II.
(From Chumlea, W.C., Roche, A.F., Mukherjee, D. (1984) *Nutritional Assessment of the Elderly Through Anthropometry*, Wright State University School of Medicine, Ohio.)

Various investigators have developed equations for predicting the propotions of body fat by anthropometric measures of specific regions. Durnin and Womersley used four different skinfolds (Table II.66). Pollock, Schmidt, and Jackson have prepared tables based on three sites, including thigh skinfolds (Tables II.66 and II.67). Because some technicians have difficulty in obtaining consistent results with thigh skinfold measurements, data also are available based on other equations that do not use this skinfold. These data are included in the following sources:

Golding, L.A., Meyers, C.R., Sinning, W.E. (1989) *Y's Way to Physical Fitness: The Complete Guide to Fitness Testing and Instruction*, 3rd ed., Human Kinetics Publishers, Champaign, IL.

Pollock, M.L., Schmidt, D.H., Jackson, A.S. (1980) *Compr. Ther.*, **6**, pp. 12–27.

Jackson, A.S. and Pollock, M.L. (1985) *Phys. Sportsmed.*, **13**, pp. 76–90.

Table II.65 Equivalent fat content, as percentage of body weight, for a range of values for the sum of four skinfolds*

Skinfolds (mm)	Men (age in years)				Women (age in years)			
	17–29	30–39	40–49	50+	16–29	30–39	40–49	50+
15	4.8				10.5			
20	8.1	12.2	12.2	12.6	14.1	17.0	19.8	21.4
25	10.5	14.2	15.0	15.6	16.8	19.4	22.2	24.0
30	12.9	16.2	17.7	18.6	19.5	21.8	24.5	26.6
35	14.7	17.7	19.6	20.8	21.5	23.7	26.4	28.5
40	16.4	19.2	21.4	22.9	23.4	25.5	28.2	30.3
45	17.7	20.4	23.0	24.7	25.0	26.9	29.6	31.9
50	19.0	21.5	24.6	26.5	26.5	28.2	31.0	33.4
55	20.1	22.5	25.9	27.9	27.8	29.4	32.1	34.6
60	21.2	23.5	27.1	29.2	29.1	30.6	33.2	35.7
65	22.2	24.3	28.2	30.4	30.2	31.6	34.1	36.7
70	23.1	25.1	29.3	31.6	31.2	32.5	35.0	37.7
75	24.0	25.9	30.3	32.7	32.2	33.4	35.9	38.7
80	24.8	26.6	31.2	33.8	33.1	34.3	36.7	39.6
85	25.5	27.2	32.1	34.8	34.0	35.1	37.5	40.4
90	26.2	27.8	33.0	35.8	34.8	35.8	38.3	41.2
95	26.9	28.4	33.7	36.6	35.6	36.5	39.0	41.9
100	27.6	29.0	34.4	37.4	36.4	37.2	39.7	42.6
105	28.2	29.6	35.1	38.2	37.1	37.9	40.4	43.3
110	28.8	30.1	35.8	39.0	37.8	38.6	41.0	43.9
115	29.4	30.6	36.4	39.7	38.4	39.1	41.5	44.5
120	30.0	31.1	37.0	40.4	39.0	39.6	42.0	45.1
125	31.0	31.5	37.6	41.1	39.6	40.1	42.5	45.7
130	31.5	31.9	38.2	41.8	40.2	40.6	43.0	46.2
135	32.0	32.3	38.7	42.4	40.8	41.1	43.5	46.7
140	32.5	32.7	39.2	43.0	41.3	41.6	44.0	47.2
145	32.9	33.1	39.7	43.6	41.8	42.1	44.5	47.7
150	33.3	33.5	40.2	44.1	42.3	42.6	45.0	48.2
155	33.7	33.9	40.7	44.6	42.8	43.1	45.4	48.7
160	34.1	34.3	41.2	45.1	43.3	43.6	45.8	49.2
165	34.5	34.6	41.6	45.6	43.7	44.0	46.2	49.6
170	34.9	34.8	42.0	46.1	44.1	44.4	46.6	50.0
175	35.3					44.8	47.0	50.4
180	35.6					45.2	47.4	50.8
185	35.9					45.6	47.8	51.2
190						45.9	48.2	51.6
195						46.2	48.5	52.0
200						46.5	48.8	52.4
205							49.1	52.7
210							49.4	53.0

*Biceps, triceps, subscapular, and suprailiac of men and women of different ages.
(From Durnin, J.V.G.A., Womersley, J. (1974) *Br. J. Nutr.*, **32** pp. 77–97, with permission.)

Table II.66   Percentage of body fat estimation for women from age and triceps, suprailium, and thigh skinfolds*

Sum of skinfolds (mm)	Age to the last year								
	Under 22	23 to 27	28 to 32	33 to 37	38 to 42	43 to 47	48 to 52	53 to 57	Over 58
23–25	9.7	9.9	10.2	10.4	10.7	10.9	11.2	11.4	11.7
26–28	11.0	11.2	11.5	11.7	12.0	12.3	12.5	12.7	13.0
29–31	12.3	12.5	12.8	13.0	13.3	13.5	13.8	14.0	14.3
32–34	13.6	13.8	14.0	14.3	14.5	14.8	15.0	15.3	15.5
35–37	14.8	15.0	15.3	15.5	15.8	16.0	16.3	16.5	16.8
38–40	16.0	16.3	16.5	16.7	17.0	17.2	17.5	17.7	18.0
41–43	17.2	17.4	17.7	17.9	18.2	18.4	18.7	18.9	19.2
44–46	18.3	18.6	18.8	19.1	19.3	19.6	19.8	20.1	20.3
47–49	19.5	19.7	20.0	20.2	20.5	20.7	21.0	21.2	21.5
50–52	20.6	20.8	21.1	21.3	21.6	21.8	22.1	22.3	22.6
53–55	21.7	21.9	22.1	22.4	22.6	22.9	23.1	23.4	23.6
56–58	22.7	23.0	23.2	23.4	23.7	23.9	24.2	24.4	24.7
59–61	23.7	24.0	24.2	24.5	24.7	25.0	25.2	25.5	25.7
62–64	24.7	25.0	25.2	25.5	25.7	26.0	26.7	26.4	26.7
65–67	25.7	25.9	26.2	26.4	26.7	26.9	27.2	27.4	27.7
68–70	26.6	26.9	27.1	27.4	27.6	27.9	28.1	28.4	28.6
71–73	27.5	27.8	28.0	28.3	28.5	28.8	28.0	29.3	29.5
74–76	28.4	28.7	28.9	29.2	29.4	29.7	29.9	30.2	30.4
77–79	29.3	29.5	29.8	30.0	30.3	30.5	30.8	31.0	31.3
80–82	30.1	30.4	30.6	30.9	31.1	31.4	31.6	31.9	32.1
83–85	30.9	31.2	31.4	31.7	31.9	32.2	32.4	32.7	32.9
86–88	31.7	32.0	32.2	32.5	32.7	32.9	33.2	33.4	33.7
89–91	32.5	32.7	33.0	33.2	33.5	33.7	33.9	34.2	34.4
92–94	33.2	33.4	33.7	33.9	34.2	34.4	34.7	34.9	35.2
95–97	33.9	34.1	34.4	34.6	34.9	35.1	35.4	35.6	35.9
98–100	34.6	34.8	35.1	35.3	35.5	35.8	36.0	36.3	36.5
101–103	35.3	35.4	35.7	35.9	36.2	36.4	36.7	36.9	37.2
104–106	35.8	36.1	36.3	36.6	36.8	37.1	37.3	37.5	37.8
107–109	36.4	36.7	36.9	37.1	37.4	37.6	37.9	38.1	38.4
110–112	37.0	37.2	37.5	37.7	38.0	38.2	38.5	38.7	38.9
113–115	37.5	37.8	38.0	38.2	38.5	38.7	39.0	39.2	39.5
116–118	38.0	38.3	38.5	38.8	39.0	39.3	39.5	39.7	40.0
119–121	38.5	38.7	39.0	39.2	39.5	39.7	40.0	40.2	40.5
122–124	39.0	39.2	39.4	39.7	39.9	40.2	40.4	40.7	40.9
125–127	39.4	39.6	39.9	40.1	40.4	40.6	40.9	41.1	41.4
128–130	39.8	40.0	40.3	40.5	40.8	41.0	41.3	41.5	41.8

*Percentage of fat calculated by the formula of Siri: percentage of fat = $(4.95/D_b - 4.5) \times 100$, where D_b = body density. (Reprinted with permission from Pollock, M.L., Schmidt, D.H. and Jackson, A.S. (1980) Measurement of cardiorespiratory fitness and body composition in the clinical setting, *Compr. Ther.*, 6 pp. 12–27.)

Table II.67   Percentage of body fat estimation for men from age and the sum of chest, abdominal, and thigh skinfolds*

Sum of skinfolds (mm)	Age to the last year								
	Under 22	23 to 27	28 to 32	33 to 37	38 to 42	43 to 47	48 to 52	53 to 57	Over 58
23–25	9.7	9.9	10.2	10.4	10.7	10.9	11.2	11.4	11.7
26–28	11.0	11.2	11.5	11.7	12.0	12.3	12.5	12.7	13.0
29–31	12.3	12.5	12.8	13.0	13.3	13.5	13.8	14.0	14.3
32–34	13.6	13.8	14.0	14.3	14.5	14.8	15.0	15.3	15.5
35–37	14.8	15.0	15.3	15.5	15.8	16.0	16.3	16.5	16.8
38–40	16.0	16.3	16.5	16.7	17.0	17.2	17.5	17.7	18.0
41–43	17.2	17.4	17.7	17.9	18.2	18.4	18.7	18.9	19.2
44–46	18.3	18.6	18.8	19.1	19.3	19.6	19.8	20.1	20.3
47–49	19.5	19.7	20.0	20.2	20.5	20.7	21.0	21.2	21.5

Continued

Table II.67 Continued

Sum of skinfolds (mm)	Age to the last year								
	Under 22	23 to 27	28 to 32	33 to 37	38 to 42	43 to 47	48 to 52	53 to 57	Over 58
50–52	20.6	20.8	21.1	21.3	21.6	21.8	22.1	22.3	22.6
53–55	21.7	21.9	22.1	22.4	22.6	22.9	23.1	23.4	23.6
56–58	22.7	23.0	23.2	23.4	23.7	23.9	24.2	24.4	24.7
59–61	23.7	24.0	24.2	24.5	24.7	25.0	25.2	25.5	25.7
62–64	24.7	25.0	25.2	25.5	25.7	26.0	26.7	26.4	26.7
65–67	25.7	25.9	26.2	26.4	26.7	26.9	27.2	27.4	27.7
68–70	26.6	26.9	27.1	27.4	27.6	27.9	28.1	28.4	28.6
71–73	27.5	27.8	28.0	28.3	28.5	28.8	29.0	29.3	29.5
74–76	28.4	28.7	28.9	29.2	29.4	29.7	29.9	30.2	30.4
77–79	29.3	29.5	29.8	30.0	30.3	30.5	30.8	31.0	31.3
80–82	30.1	30.4	30.6	30.9	31.1	31.4	31.6	31.9	32.1
83–85	30.9	31.2	31.4	31.7	31.9	32.2	32.4	32.7	32.9
86–88	31.7	32.0	32.2	32.5	32.7	32.9	33.2	33.4	33.7
89–91	32.5	32.7	33.0	33.2	33.5	33.7	33.9	34.2	34.4
92–94	33.2	33.4	33.7	33.9	34.2	34.4	34.7	34.9	35.2
95–97	33.9	34.1	34.4	34.6	34.9	35.1	35.4	35.6	35.9
98–100	34.6	34.8	35.1	35.3	35.5	35.8	36.0	36.3	36.5
101–103	35.3	35.4	35.7	35.9	36.2	36.4	36.7	36.9	37.2
104–106	35.8	36.1	36.3	36.6	36.8	37.1	37.3	37.5	37.8
107–109	36.4	36.7	36.9	37.1	37.4	37.6	37.9	38.1	38.4
110–112	37.0	37.2	37.5	37.7	38.0	38.2	38.5	38.7	38.9
113–115	37.5	37.8	38.0	38.2	38.5	38.7	39.0	39.2	39.5
116–118	38.0	38.3	38.5	38.8	39.0	39.3	39.5	39.7	40.0
119–121	38.5	38.7	39.0	39.2	39.5	39.7	40.0	40.2	40.5
122–124	39.0	39.2	39.4	39.7	39.9	40.2	40.4	40.7	40.9
125–127	39.4	39.6	39.9	40.1	40.4	40.6	40.9	41.1	41.4
128–130	39.8	40.0	40.3	40.5	40.8	41.0	41.3	41.5	41.8

*Percentage of fat calculated by the formula of Siri: percentage of fat = $(4.95/D_b - 4.5) \times 100$, where D_b = body density. (Reprinted with permission from Pollock, M.L., Schmidt, D.H. and Jackson, A.S. (1980) Measurement of cardiorespiratory fitness and body composition in the clinical setting, *Compr. Ther.*, **6** pp. 12–27.)

Table II.68 Dietary recommendations in industrialized and developing countries, 1977 to 1989*

Country/region or source of recommendation	Target group(s)	Maintain appropriate body weight, exercise	Limit or reduce total fat (% energy)	Reduce saturated fatty acids (% energy)
Australia 1983	GP	Yes	Yes	NC
1987, targets for 1995	GP	Reduce obesity prevalence to 30%	35%	NS
1987, targets for 2000	GP	To 25%	33%	NS
Canada 1982	GP	Yes	35%	Yes
Czech Republic 1988	GP	Yes, reduce by 10–15%	Yes, reduce by 15 g/day	Yes
France 1981	GP	Yes	30–35%	Yes
Germany, Federal Republic of, 1985	GP	Yes	Yes	NS
Hungary 1988	GP	Yes	Avoid too much	Use vegetable oil
India 1988	HR (affluent people)	Yes	15–20%	NC
Ireland 1984	GP	Yes	≤35%	Yes
Japan 1985	GP	Yes	20–25%	Yes

Continued

Table II.68 Continued

Country/region or source of recommendation	Target group(s)	Maintain appropriate body weight, exercise	Limit or reduce total fat (% energy)	Reduce saturated fatty acids (% energy)	Increase polyunsaturated fatty acids (% energy)	Limit cholesterol (mg/day)	Limit free sugars (% energy)	Increase complex carbohydrates (% energy for total carbohydrates)
Latin America1988	GP	Yes	20–25%	≤8	NC	NC	Yes	Yes
Netherlands 1983–1984	GP	Yes	30–35%	Yes	NS	NS	<14%	Indirectly
1986	GP	Yes	30–35%	Yes	NS	NS	<12%	Indirectly
New Zealand 1982	GP, HR	Yes	Yes	Yes	Yes	No	Yes	Yes
Norway 1981–1982	GP	NC	<35%	Yes	No	NS	Yes	Yes, more plant foods, vegetables, cereals, legumes
Poland 1988	GP	Yes	≈30%	Yes	NS	NS	Yes	50–55%
Sweden 1981	GP	Yes	25–35%	Yes	NS	NS	Avoid excess	Yes; fresh fruits and vegetables, whole-grain cereals
1985	GP	Yes	Reduce by 5% energy by 1990; to ≈30% by 2000	NS	NS	NS	Yes	Yes, fresh vegetables, salads, whole-grains
United Kingdom 1983	GP	Yes	30%	10	Balance (n–3)/(n–6) ratio	NC	Yes	Yes; avoid refined and polished grains
United States of America 1977	GP	Yes	27–33%	Yes	NC	NC	Moderation; ≤7 g/day for weight reduction	Yes
1979	GP	Yes	Yes	Yes	Use vegetables and fish oils	NC	NC	NC
1985	GP	Yes	Yes	Yes	P/S ≈ 1.0	<100 mg/1000 $kcal_{th}$ in children, up to 300 mg/day	Yes	Yes
1988	GP, HR	Yes	Yes	Yes				
1989	GP	Balance energy intake and expenditure	≤30%	<10% for individuals, 7–8% population mean	Maximum 10%	Yes	Yes	NS
WHO 1988 Intermediate goals	GP	BMI	35%	15%	P/S = 1.0	<30 mg/MJ	Mono- and disaccharides 15–20%	45–55%
Ultimate goals		20–25	20–30%	10–15%	NS	NS	Yes	Yes

Continued

Table II.68 Continued

Increase polyunsaturated fatty acids (% energy)	Limit cholesterol (mg/day)	Limit free sugars (% energy)	Increase complex carbohydrates (% energy for total carbohydrates)
P/S = 0.5	NS	<10%	Yes; 50–60%
NS	Yes, <300 mg	≤10%	Yes
P/S = 0.5	Yes	<10%	Yes; 50–60%
P/S = >0.5	NS	Decrease by 3% energy by 1990	Yes; increase starch to 45–50% energy by 2000
NS	No	To 20 kg/year	Through whole grains, vegetables, cereals, fruits
Yes	250–350	Yes	Yes
NS	Yes	Yes	Yes
No	Yes	Yes	Adequate starch and fiber
No	Yes	Yes	Yes
Up to 10 for individuals and ≈7 population mean	<300	Yes	≥55%; ≥5 servings/day vegetables and fruits; ≥6 daily servings cereals, breads, and legumes
PS ≥0.5	<100 mg/1000 $kcal_{th}$	10%	>40%
P/S = 1.0			45–55%

Increase dietary fiber (g/day)	Restrict sodium chloride (g/day)	Moderate alcohol intake (% energy)	Other recommendations
Yes	Yes	Yes	Promote breast-feeding; variety
25	130 mmol/day	<5%	Promote water fluoridation, increase prevalence of breast-feeding
30	100 mmol/day	<5%	
Yes	Yes	Yes	Exercise
Yes	Yes	Yes	Increase vitamin C intake; more plant foods; nutrition education; variety
Yes	Yes	<10%	Water fluoridation
Yes	Yes	Yes	Variety; small, frequent meals, proper cooking; sufficient protein
Yes	Yes	Yes	Variety; focus on cooking methods; consume milk and cheese as skimmed-milk products; 4 or 5 even meals daily; food labeling
Include grains, leafy vegetables, and whole grains	Yes	NC	Breast-feeding; water fluoridation upper limit 1 mg/L; different recommendation for general, poorer population
To 20–35	<9	<5%	Reduce protein to 1 g/kg of body weight daily; more vegetable protein
NC	<10	NC	Varied diet (at least 30 different foods daily); home cooking; pleasant eating environment
>8 g/1000 $kcal_{th}$	≤5; in profuse sweating, up to 10	NC	Protein 10–12% energy; variety; dietary interactions; vitamin C with iron-containing foods; calcium intake
NC	NC	Yes	Variety
3 g/MJ	Yes	<9 g/day	Variety
Yes	Yes	Yes	Variety; less animal protein; water fluoridation
Yes	NC	NC	Maintain adequate nutrient intake
Yes	?	?	?
>30	≈7–8	Yes	Varied diet, exercise, regular meals
Increase by 7–8 g/day by 1990 and to 30–35 g by 2000	Reduce by 1–2 g/day by 1990 to 7–8 g by 2000	Yes	Year 1990 and year 2000 goals

Continued

Table II.68 Continued

Increase dietary fiber (g/day)	Restrict sodium chloride (g/day)	Moderate alcohol intake (% energy)	Other recommendations
To 30	Decrease by 3 g/day	<4%	Long-term proposals: food labeling; nutrition education; greater proportion of vegetable protein
Yes	<8	Yes	Limit additives and processed foods
NS	Yes	Yes	More fish, poultry, legumes; less red meat
Yes	Yes	Yes	Variety in diet; consider high-risk groups
Yes	Yes	Yes	Fluoridation of water; adolescent girls and women increase intake of calcium-rich foods; children, adolescents, and women of child-bearing age increase intake of iron-rich foods
Indirectly through vegetables, fruits, and cereals	≤6 with a goal of 4.5	<30 g of ethanol or <2 drinks/day	Population and individual goals; avoid dietary supplements in excess of RDAs; drink fluoridated water; limit protein intake to less than twice the RDA; comments on future goals
>30	7–8	Yes	Increase nutrient density of food; water fluoridation; iodine prophylaxis

*BMI = Body-mass index; GP = General population; HR = High-risk groups; NC = No comment; NS = Not specified; P/S = Ratio of polyunsaturated to saturated fatty acids; RDA = Recommended dietary allowance.
(From WHO (1990) *Diet, Nutrition and the Prevention of Chronic Diseases*, Report of a WHO Study Group, Technical Report Series No. 797, World Health Organization, Geneva, pp. 180–1.)

Table II.69 Dietary recommendations to reduce coronary heart disease risk in industrialized countries*

Country/region or source of recommendation	Target group(s)	Body weight/exercise	Total fat (% energy)
Australia			
1979	HR	Avoid obesity	Reduce to 30–35
Canada			
1977	GP	Maintain appropriate body weight	Reduce to 35
1988	GP	Adjust energy intake	<30
	HR	and expenditure	
Europe			
1987	GP	Control obesity;	≤30
	HR	increase exercise	
Finland			
1987	GP	Avoid excess weight;	<30
	HR	exercise	
Finland, Norway, Sweden			
1968	GP	Reduce energy intake to avoid obesity; exercise	Reduce to 25–35
Germany, Federal Republic of			
1975	GP	NC	Reduce
Japan			
1983	GP	NC	20–25
Netherlands			
1973	GP	Maintain appropriate body weight	33

Continued

Table II.69 Continued

Country/region or source of recommendation	Target group(s)	Body weight/exercise	Total fat (% energy)
New Zealand			
1976	GP	Maintain appropriate	35
	HR	body weight	
United Kingdom			
1982	GP	Avoid obesity; increase exercise	30
1984	GP	Avoid obesity; exercise	Reduce to 35
United States of America			
1984	GP	Control obesity	<30
1985	GP	Maintain appropriate	<30
	HR	body weight	
1988	GP	Maintain appropriate body weight	<30
WHO			
1982	GP	Avoid obesity	Reduce to 20–30
1988	HR	BMI 20–25, regular exercise	20–30

Saturated fat (% energy)	Polyunsaturated fat (% energy)	Cholesterol (mg/day)	Complex carbohydrates and fiber
P:S = 1.0	P:S = 1.0	Restrict	Eat enough
10	10	NC	Increase
<10	<10	Restrict through less meats and egg yolks; for HR <300	Increase
<10	Increase oleic and linoleic acids	<300	Increase, especially vegetables, fruits, cereals, legumes
<10	P:S >0.5	Reduce	NC
Reduce	Increase	NC	Increase vegetables, fruits, potatoes
Reduce	Increase	Reduce	NC
NC	Cook with vegetable oil	NC	Increase
Restrict	10–13	250–300	Increase to make up energy need
Reduce especially for HR	HR should substitute for saturated fatty acids	Reduce	NC
<10	NC	NC	Increase
Reduce to 15	P/S≈0.45	NS	Increase breads, cereals, vegetables, fruits
8	<10	<250	Increase to make up energy loss
10	Up to 10	250–300	Endorsed earlier recommendations
<10	Up to 10	<300	Increase, ≥50% energy from total carbohydrates
<10	Up to 10	<300	Increase
10	Up to 10	<100 mg/1000 kcal$_{th}$	45–55% energy
	P/S >1.0		>30 g fiber/day

Free sugars	Sodium chloride (g/day)	Alcohol intake	Other recommendations
Use less	Restrict	Moderation	Focus on HR groups; food labeling; recommendations safe for GP
NC	Restrict	NC	Variety of foods
NC	Limit	Limit	Focus on HR groups; limit protein to 10–15% energy
Reduce	Moderation	Moderation, <25–30 g/day	Nutrition education; collaboration among government and other groups; food labeling
NC	Reduce; for HR <5	Moderation	Avoid trace element deficiencies; food labeling; focus on HR groups

Continued

Table II.69 Continued

Free sugars	Sodium chloride (g/day)	Alcohol intake	Other recommendations
Decrease	NC	NC	10–12% of energy from protein; 30–50% of animal origin
NC	NC	NC	NC
Reduce	Limit to <10	Avoid too much	Variety; eat enough protein, half from vegetables and half from animal sources; eat enough potassium, especially from green vegetables; eat lean meat and fish and fewer sweets
Use little	NC	NC	NC
Restrict to reduce weight	NC	Restrict to reduce weight	NC
NC	NC	NC	Special attention to children
Do not increase	Decrease	Avoid excess; <90 ml/day men; <65 ml/day women	Special recommendations for governments, professionals, industry
NC	5	NC	NC
	NC	NC	Guidelines for health professionals, industry, and public
NS	<3 (as sodium)	30–50 g ethanol/day	Protein to make up remainder of energy; wide variety of foods
NC	<5	Drink less	Emphasis on plant foods, fish, poultry, lean meats, low-fat dairy products, and fewer whole eggs
10% energy	<5	Limit	Increase nutrient density; water fluoridation 0.7–1.2 mg/L; iodine prophylaxis; intermediate and ultimate goals

*BMI = Body-mass index; GP = General population; HR = High-risk groups; NC = No comment; NS = Not specified; P:S = Ratio of polyunsaturated to saturated fatty acids.
(From WHO (1990) *Diet, Nutrition and the Prevention of Chronic Diseases*, Report of a WHO Study Group. Technical Report Series No. 797, World Health Organization, Geneva, pp. 182–3. With permission.)

Table II.70 Dietary recommendations to reduce cancer risk in industrialized countries*

Country/region	Maintain appropriate body weight, exercise	Limit or reduce total fat (% energy)	Modify ratio of dietary fats	Promote fruit and vegetable intake	Increase complex carbohydrate/fiber intake
Canada 1985	Yes	Reduce	Decrease saturated fatty acids and cholesterol	Yes	More fiber-containing foods
Europe 1986	Yes	To ≈30	NC	Yes	Yes
Japan 1983	NC	Avoid excess	NC	Especially green/yellow vegetables, oranges, carotene, and fungi	Unrefined cereal, seafood, fiber-rich legumes
United States of America 1982	NC	To ≈30	NC	Especially citrus fruits, green and yellow and cruciferous vegetables	Whole-grain products, vegetables, and fruits

Continued

Table II.70 Continued

Country/region	Maintain appropriate body weight, exercise	Limit or reduce total fat (% energy)	Modify ratio of dietary fats	Promote fruit and vegetable intake	Increase complex carbohydrate/fiber intake
1984	Yes	To ≈30	NC	Especially vitamin A- and C-rich foods and cruciferous vegetables	High-fiber foods, whole-grain cereals
1987	Yes	To ≈30	NC	Vitamin A-rich, green and yellow vegetables, citrus fruits	Whole-grain products, 20–30 g fiber/day

Restrict sodium chloride	Food preparation methods	Alcohol intake	Other recommendations
NS	Minimize cured, pickled, and smoked foods	Two or fewer drinks per day, if any	NC
To <5 g/day	As above; avoid frying and high-temperature cooking	Drink less, if at all	Varied diet; no food supplements; recommendations to government, scientists, and industry
Yes	Avoid hot drinks and burned foods	Drink less, if at all	Varied diet, chew food well
Minimize cured and pickled foods	Minimize cured, pickled, and smoked foods	Drink less, if at all	Avoid food supplements; monitor and test mutagens and carcinogens; recommendations to government, scientists, and industry
NS	As above	As above	NC
NS	As above, avoid frying and high-temperature cooking	As above	Balanced diet; read labels

*NC = No comment; NS = Not specified.
(From WHO (1990) *Diet, Nutrition and the Prevention of Chronic Diseases*, Report of a WHO Study Group. Technical Report Series No. 797. World Health Organization, Geneva, pp. 184–5.)

Table II.71 National nutrition objectives for the year 2000

A. *Health Status Objectives*
1. Reduce deaths from coronary heart disease to no more than 100 per 100,000 persons (age-adjusted baseline: 135 per 100,000 in 1987).
2. Reverse the rise in deaths from cancer to achieve a rate of no more than 130 per 100,000 persons (age-adjusted baseline: 133 per 100,000 in 1987).
3. Reduce the overweight population to no more than 20% among adults aged 20 years and older and no more than 15% among adolescents aged 12 through 19 years (baseline: 26% for adults aged 20 through 74 years in 1976 to 1980, 24% for men and 27% for women; 15% for adolescents aged 12 through 19 years in 1976 to 1980).
4. Reduce growth retardation among low-income children aged 5 years and younger to less than 10% (baseline: up to 16% among low-income children in 1988, depending on age and race/ethnicity).

B. *Risk Reduction Objectives*
5. Reduce dietary fat intake to an average of 30% of calories or less and reduce average saturated fat intake to less than 10% of calories among persons aged 2 years and older (baseline: 36% of calories from total fat and 13% from saturated fat for persons aged 20 through 74 years in 1976 to 1980; 36% and 13% for women aged 19 through 50 years in 1985).
6. Increase complex carbohydrates and fiber-containing foods in the diets of adults to 5 or more daily servings for vegetables (including legumes) and fruits, and to 6 or more daily servings for grain products (baseline: 2.5 servings of vegetables and fruits and 3 servings of grain products for women aged 19 through 50 years in 1985).
7. Increase to at least 50% the proportion of overweight persons aged 12 years and older who have adopted sound dietary practices combined with regular physical activity to attain an appropriate body weight (baseline: 30% of overweight women and 25% of overweight men for people aged 18 years and older in 1985).
8. Increase calcium intake so that at least 50% of youth aged 12 through 24 years and at least 50% of pregnant and lactating women are consuming 3 or more servings daily of foods rich in calcium, and at least 50% of adults aged 25 years and older are consuming 2 or more servings daily (baseline: 7% of women and 14% of men aged 19 through 24 years and 24% of pregnant and lactating women consumed 3 or more servings daily, and 15% of women and 23% of men aged 25 through 50 years consumed 2 or more servings daily in 1985 to 1986).

Continued

Table II.71   Continued

9. Decrease salt and sodium intake so that at least 65% of those who prepare home-cooked meals do so without adding salt, at least 80% of persons avoid using salt at the table, and at least 40% of adults regularly purchase foods modified or lower in sodium (baseline: 54% of women aged 19 through 50 years who prepared most of the meals did not use salt in food preparation, and 68% of women aged 19 through 50 years did not use salt at the table in 1985; 20% of all persons aged 18 years and older regularly purchased foods with reduced salt and sodium content in 1988).

10. Reduce iron deficiency to less than 3% among children aged 1 through 4 years and among women of childbearing age (baseline: 9% for children aged 1 through 2 years, 4% for children aged 3 through 4 years, and 5% for women aged 20 through 44 years in 1976 to 1980).

11. Increase to at least 75% the proportion of mothers who breast-feed their babies in the early postpartum period and to at least 50% to the proportion who continue to breast-feed until their babies are 5 to 6 months old (baseline: 54% at discharge from birth site and 21% at 5 to 6 months in 1988).

12. Increase to at least 75% the proportion of parents and caregivers who use feeding practices that prevent baby-bottle tooth decay.

13. Increase to at least 85% the proportion of persons aged 18 years and older who use food labels to make nutritious food selections (baseline: 74% used labels to make food selections in 1988).

C. *Service and Protection Objectives*

14. Achieve useful and informative nutrition labeling for virtually all processed foods and for at least 40% of fresh meats, poultry, fish, fruits, vegetables, baked foods, and ready-to-eat carry-out foods (baseline: 60% of processed foods regulated by the Food and Drug Administration had nutrition labeling in 1988; baseline data on fresh and carry-out foods are unavailable).

15. Increase the available processed food products that are reduced in fat and saturated fat to at least 5000 brand items (baseline: 2500 brand items reduced in fat in 1986).

16. Increase to at least 90% the proportion of restaurants and institutional service operations that offer identifiable low-fat, low-calorie food choices, consistent with the nutrition principles in the *Dietary Guidelines for Americans*.

17. Increase to at least 90% the proportion of school lunch and breakfast services and child-care food services that offer menus consistent with the nutrition principles in the *Dietary Guidelines for Americans*.

18. Increase to at least 80% the receipt of home food services by people aged 65 years and older who cannot prepare their own meals or are otherwise in need of home-delivered meals.

19. Increase to at least 75% the proportion of schools in the United States that provide nutrition education from preschool through 12th grade, preferably as part of quality school health education.

20. Increase to at least 50% the proportion of worksites with 50 or more employees that offer nutrition education and/or weight management programs for employees (baseline: 17% offered nutrition education activities and 15% offered weight-control activities in 1985).

21. Increase to at least 75% the proportion of primary care providers who provide nutrition assessment and counseling and/or referral to qualified nutritionists or dietitians (baseline: physicians provided diet counseling for an estimated 40 to 50% of patients in 1988).

(From (1991) Nutrition in Healthy People 2000. *In* National Health Promotion and Disease Prevention Objectives. U.S. Government Printing Office, Washington, D.C.)

Table II.72   Beverages and alcoholic drinks: calories and selected electrolytes (per 100 ml)*

Beverage	Calories	Sodium (mg)	Sodium (mEq)	Potassium (mg)	Potassium (mEq)	Phosphorus (mg)
Cola (avg.)	48.1–55.0[†]	0.8–4.7 (mg)[†]		0–4.4 (mg)[†]		18.1–25[†]
Diet cola (avg.)	0.1–0.5[†]	0.8–13.0 (mg)[†]		0–33.2 (mg)[†]		8.5–17.6[†]
Patio grape/orange	52	11.2	0.5	4.1	0.1	–
Mountain Dew	49	8.7	0.4	2.7	0.1	–
Teem	41	8.6	0.4	–	–	–
Root beer	45	1	0.1	3.9	0.1	–
Club soda	0	21.9	1.0	–	–	0
Sprite	48	15.4	0.7	0.4	–	–
Fanta (avg.)	53	6.4	0.3	0.6	–	–
Fresca	1	12.1	0.5	–	–	–
Fanta ginger ale	42	9.4	0.4	–	–	–
Slice	45	3	0.1	27.6	0.7	–
Apricot nectar	56	3	0.1	114	2.9	9

Continued

Table II.72 Continued

Beverage	Calories	Sodium (mg)	Sodium (mEq)	Potassium (mg)	Potassium (mEq)	Phosphorus (mg)
Apple juice	47	3	0.1	119	3	7
Cranberry juice	58	4	0.2	24	0.6	1
Grape juice, canned	61	3	0.1	132	3.4	11
Grapefruit juice, unsweetened	38	trace	–	153	3.9	11
Orange juice, unsweetened or fresh	45	1	0.1	200	5.1	17
Pear nectar	60	4	0.2	13	0.3	3
Peach nectar	54	7	0.3	40	1	6
Pineapple juice, unsweetened	56	trace	–	134	3.4	8
Tomato juice	20	200.7	8.7	227	5.8	16.5
Fruit-flavored beverage	45	–	–	–	–	–
Beer, regular	41	5.3	0.2	25	0.6	12.4
Beer, light	28	2.8	0.1	18.1	0.5	12.1
Gin, rum, vodka, whiskey (86 proof)	250	trace	–	3.6	0.1	–
Table wine, 12.2% alcohol/vol.	86	3.5	0.1	93.1	2.4	10.3
Dessert wine, 18.5% alcohol/vol.	137	3.3	0.1	76.7	2	–

Alcoholic beverages are customarily served in special glassware, the size of which tends to standardize the alcoholic content:

1 cordial glass	= 20 ml	1 burgundy glass	= 120 ml
1 brandy glass	= 30 ml	1 champagne glass	= 150 ml
1 jigger	= 45 ml	1 tumbler	= 240–360 ml
1 sherry glass	= 60 ml	1 mixing glass	= 360 ml
1 cocktail glass	= 90 ml		

*Brand name data supplied by the commercial producer of the product. Other data obtained from Consumer Nutrition Center (1982) *Composition of Foods, Fruits, and Fruit Juices: Raw, Processed, Prepared*, Agriculture Handbook No. 8–9. U.S. Department of Agriculture, Washington.
†Range.

Table II.73 Dietary fiber content of selected foods*,† (g/100 g edible portion)

Food item	Moisture	Total dietary fiber (AOAC)‡
Breads, Crackers, and Cakes		
Bagels, plain	31.6	2.1
Biscuits, made from refrigerated dough, baked	28.7	1.5
Bread		
Bran	37.7	8.5
Cornbread mix, baked	34.4	2.4
Cracked-wheat	35.9	5.3
French	33.9	2.7
Hollywood-type, light	37.8	4.8
Italian	34.1	3.1
Mixed-grain	38.2	7.1
Oatmeal	36.7	3.9
Pita		
White	32.1	1.6
Whole-wheat	30.6	7.5
Pumpernickel	38.3	5.9
Reduced-calorie, high-fiber		
Wheat	43.7	11.3
White	41.8	9.3
Rye	37.0	6.2
Wheat	37.0	4.3
White	37.1	2.3
Whole-wheat	38.3	6.9

Table II.73 Continued

Food item	Moisture	Total dietary fiber (AOAC)‡
Bread crumbs, plain or seasoned	5.7	4.2
Bread stuffing, flavored, from dry mix	65.1	2.9
Cake mix		
Chocolate, prepared	33.3	2.2
Yellow, prepared	40.0	0.8
Cakes		
Boston cream pie	47.6	1.3
Coffeecake		
Crumb topping	22.3	3.3
Fruit	31.7	2.5
Fruitcake, commercial	22.0	3.5
Gingerbread, from dry mix	38.5	3.2
Cheesecake		
Commercial	44.6	2.1
From no-bake mix	44.4	1.9
Cookies		
Brownies	12.6	2.4
Brownies with nuts	12.6	2.6
Butter	4.7	2.4
Chocolate chip	4.0	2.7
Chocolate sandwich	2.2	3.0
Fig bar	16.7	4.6
Fortune	8.0	1.6
Oatmeal	5.7	3.1

Continued

Continued

Table II.73 Continued

Food item	Moisture	Total dietary fiber (AOAC)‡
Oatmeal, soft-type	–	2.7
Peanut butter	6.7	1.8
Shortbread with pecans	3.3	1.8
Vanilla sandwich	2.1	1.5
Crackers		
Cheese, sandwich with peanut butter filling	4.0	1.1
Crisp bread, rye	6.1	16.2
Graham		
Regular	4.1	2.7
Honey	4.1	2.7
Matzoh		
Plain	6.1	3.0
Egg/onion	8.0	5.0
Whole-wheat	3.0	11.6
Melba toast		
Plain	5.6	6.5
Rye	6.7	8.0
Wheat	6.1	7.4
Rye	7.2	15.8
Saltines	–	2.7
Snack-type	4.2	2.0
Wheat	3.2	5.5
Whole-wheat	2.7	10.4
Croutons, plain or seasoned	5.6	5.0
Doughnuts		
Cake	19.7	1.7
Yeast-leavened, glazed	26.7	2.1
English muffin, whole-wheat	45.7	6.3
French toast, commercial, ready-to-eat	48.1	2.8
Ice cream cones		
Sugar, rolled-type	3.0	4.6
Wafer-type	5.3	4.1
Muffins, commercial		
Blueberry	37.3	3.6
Oat bran	35.0	7.5
Pancake, waffle mix, prepared	50.4	1.3
Pastry, Danish		
Fruit	27.6	1.9
Plain	19.3	1.2
Pies, commercial		
Apple	51.7	1.7
Cherry	46.2	0.8
Chocolate, cream	43.5	2.0
Egg custard	46.5	1.2
Fruit and coconut	–	0.9
Lemon meringue	41.7	1.2
Pecan	19.8	3.5
Pumpkin	58.1	2.7
Rolls, dinner, egg	30.4	3.8
Taco shells	6.0	8.1
Toaster pastries	8.9	1.0
Tortillas		
Corn	43.6	5.2
Flour, wheat	26.2	3.1
Waffles, commercial, frozen, ready-to-eat	45.0	2.4

Continued

Table II.73 Continued

Food item	Moisture	Total dietary fiber (AOAC)‡
Breakfast Cereals, Ready-to-Eat		
Bran		
High-fiber	2.9	35.3
Extra fiber	–	45.9
Bran flakes	2.9	18.8
Bran flakes with raisins	8.3	13.4
Corn flakes		
Frosted or sugar-sparkled	1.9	2.2
Plain	2.8	2.0
Fiber cereal with fruit	–	14.8
Granola	3.3	10.5
Oat cereal	5.0	10.6
Oat flakes, fortified	3.1	3.0
Puffed wheat, sugar-coated	1.5	1.5
Rice, crispy	2.4	1.2
Wheat and malted barley		
Flakes	3.4	6.8
Nuggets	3.2	6.5
with raisins	–	6.0
Wheat flakes	4.3	9.0
Cereal Grains		
Barley	9.4	17.3
Bulgur, dry	8.0	18.3
Corn flour, whole-grain	10.9	13.4
Cornmeal		
Degermed	11.6	5.2
Whole-grain	10.3	11.0
Cornstarch	8.3	0.9
Farina, regular or instant, cooked	85.8	1.4
Hominy, canned	79.8	2.5
Millet, hulled, raw	–	8.5
Oat bran, raw	6.6	15.9
Oat flour	7.8	9.6
Oats, rolled or oatmeal, dry	8.8	10.3
Rice, brown, long-grain, cooked	73.1	1.7
Rice, white		
glutinous, raw	10.0	2.8
Long-grain		
Parboiled, cooked	–	0.5
Precooked or instant, cooked	76.4	0.8
Rye flour, medium or light	9.4	14.6
Semolina	12.7	3.9
Tapioca, pearl, dry	12.0	1.1
Wheat bran, crude	9.9	42.4
Wheat flour		
White, all-purpose	11.8	2.7
Whole-grain	10.9	12.6
Wheat germ, toasted	2.9	12.9
Wild rice, raw	7.8	5.2
Fruits and Fruit Products		
Apples, raw:		
With skin	83.9	2.2
Without skin	84.5	1.9
Apple juice, unsweetened	87.9	0.1
Applesauce, unsweetened	88.4	1.5
Apricots, dried	31.1	7.8
Apricot nectar	84.9	0.6
Bananas, raw	74.3	1.6

Continued

Table II.73   Continued

Food item	Moisture	Total dietary fiber (AOAC)‡
Blueberries, raw	84.6	2.3
Cantaloupe, raw	89.8	0.8
Figs, dried	28.4	9.3
Fruit cocktail, canned in heavy syrup, drained	–	1.5
Grapefruit, raw	90.9	0.6
Grapes, Thompson, seedless, raw	81.3	0.7
Kiwifruit, raw	83.0	3.4
Nectarines, raw	86.3	1.6
Olives		
Green	–	2.6
ripe	–	3.0
Orange, raw	86.8	2.4
Orange juice, frozen concentrate, prepared	88.1	0.2
Peach		
Canned in juice, drained	–	1.0
Dried	31.8	8.2
Raw	87.7	1.6
Pears, raw	83.8	2.6
Pineapple		
Canned in heavy syrup, chunks, drained	79.0	1.1
Raw	86.5	1.2
Prune		
Dried	32.4	7.2
Stewed	–	6.6
Prune juice	81.2	1.0
Raisins	15.4	5.3
Strawberries	91.6	2.6
Watermelon	91.5	0.4
Legumes, Nuts, and Seeds		
Almonds, oil-roasted	3.3	11.2
Baked beans, canned		
Barbecue-style	–	5.8
Sweet or tomato sauce, plain	72.6	7.7
Beans, Great Northern, canned, drained	69.9	5.4
Cashews, oil-roasted	5.4	6.0
Chickpeas, canned, drained	68.2	5.8
Coconut, raw	47.0	9.0
Cowpeas (black-eyed peas), cooked, drained	70.0	9.6
Hazelnuts, oil-roasted	1.2	6.4
Lima beans, cooked, drained	69.8	7.2
Miso	47.4	5.4
Mixed nuts, oil-roasted, with peanuts	–	9.0
Peanut		
Dry-roasted	1.6	8.0
Oil-roasted	2.0	8.8
Peanut butter		
Chunky	1.1	6.6
Smooth	1.4	6.0
Pecans, dried	4.8	6.5
Pistachio nuts	3.9	10.8
Sunflower seeds, oil-roasted	2.6	6.8
Tahini	3.0	9.3

Continued

Table II.73   Continued

Food item	Moisture	Total dietary fiber (AOAC)‡
Tofu	84.6	1.2
Walnuts, dried		
Black	4.4	5.0
English	3.6	4.8
Pasta		
Noodles, Chinese, chow mein	0.7	3.9
Noodles, egg, regular, cooked	68.7	2.2
Noodles, Japanese, dry		
Somen	9.2	4.3
Udon	8.7	5.4
Spaghetti and macaroni, cooked	64.7	1.6
Spaghetti, dry		
Spinach	8.7	10.6
Whole-wheat	7.1	11.8
Snacks		
Banana chips	4.3	7.7
Corn cakes	4.6	1.9
Corn-based, extruded		
Chips		
Barbecue-flavor	1.2	5.2
Plain	1.0	4.4
Puffs or twists, cheese-flavor	1.5	1.0
Cornnuts		
Barbecue-flavor	1.6	8.4
Nacho-flavor	2.1	8.0
Plain	1.3	6.9
Crisped rice bar		
Almond	6.7	3.6
Chocolate chip	7.0	2.2
Granola bars		
Hard		
Chocolate chip	2.4	4.4
Plain	3.9	5.3
Soft		
Milk-chocolate-coated, chocolate chip	3.6	3.4
Uncoated		
Chocolate chip	5.4	4.8
Chocolate chip, graham, and marshmallow	6.0	4.0
Nut and raisin	6.1	5.6
Peanut butter	7.3	4.3
Peanut butter and chocolate chip	5.9	4.2
Plain	6.4	4.6
Raisin	6.4	4.3
Popcorn		
Air-popped	4.1	15.1
Caramel-coated		
With peanuts	3.3	3.8
Without peanuts	2.8	5.2
Cheese-flavor	2.5	9.9
Oil-popped	2.8	10.0
Potato chips		
Barbecue-flavor	1.9	4.4
Plain	1.9	4.8
Sour-cream-and-onion-flavor	1.8	5.2

Continued

Table II.73 Continued

Food item	Moisture	Total dietary fiber (AOAC)‡
Potato chips, made from dried potatoes, plain	1.4	3.6
Potato sticks	2.2	3.4
Pretzels, hard, plain	3.3	2.8
Rice cakes, brown rice		
Buckwheat	5.9	3.8
Corn	5.9	2.9
Multigrain	6.3	3.0
Plain	5.8	4.2
Rye	6.8	4.0
Tortilla chips		
Nacho-flavor	1.7	5.3
Plain	1.8	6.5
Sweets		
Baking chocolate, unsweetened, squares	1.3	15.4
Candies		
Alpine White Bar with Almonds	1.1	5.4
Baby Ruth Bar	5.0	2.9
Butterfinger Bar	5.6	2.7
Caramels	8.5	1.2
Chunky Bar	2.9	4.8
Milk chocolate	1.3	2.8
Milk chocolate, with almonds	1.5	6.2
M&M's Plain Chocolate Candies	1.4	3.1
Nestle Crunch Milk Chocolate with Crisp Rice	1.7	2.6
O'Henry	5.9	3.5
Cocoa, dry powder, unsweetened	3.0	29.8
Jams and preserves	34.5	1.2
Jellies	28.4	0.6
Pie fillings, canned		
Apple	73.4	1.0
Cherry	69.7	0.6
Vegetables and Vegetable Products		
Artichokes, raw	84.4	5.2
Beans, snap		
Canned, drained, solids	93.3	1.3
Raw	90.3	1.8
Beets, canned, drained, solids	91.0	1.7
Broccoli		
Cooked	90.2	2.6
Raw	90.7	2.8
Brussels sprouts, boiled	87.3	4.3
Cabbage, Chinese		
Cooked	95.4	1.6
Raw	94.9	1.0
Cabbage, red		
Cooked	93.6	2.0
Raw	91.6	2.0
Cabbage, white, raw	91.5	2.4
Carrots		
Canned, drained, solids	93.0	1.5
Raw	87.8	3.2
Cauliflower		
Cooked	92.5	2.2
Raw	92.3	2.4

Table II.73 Continued

Food item	Moisture	Total dietary fiber (AOAC)‡
Celery, raw	94.7	1.6
Chives	92.0	3.2
Corn, sweet		
Canned		
Brine pack, drained, solids	76.9	1.4
Cream-style	78.7	1.2
Cooked	69.6	3.7
Cucumbers		
Raw	96.0	1.0
Pared	–	0.5
Lettuce		
Butterhead or Iceberg	95.7	1.0
Romaine	94.9	1.7
Mushrooms		
Boiled	91.1	2.2
Raw	91.8	1.3
Onions, raw	90.1	1.6
Parsley, raw	88.3	4.4
Peas, edible, podded		
Cooked	88.9	2.8
Raw	88.9	2.6
Peas, sweet, canned, drained, solids	81.7	3.4
Peppers, sweet, raw	92.8	1.6
Pickles		
Dill	93.8	1.2
Sweet	68.9	1.1
Potatoes		
Baked		
Flesh	75.4	1.5
Skin	47.3	4.0
Boiled	77.0	1.5
French-fried, home-prepared from frozen	52.9	4.2
Hashed brown	56.1	2.0
Spinach		
Boiled	91.2	2.2
Raw	91.6	2.6
Squash		
Summer, cooked	93.7	1.4
Winter, cooked	89.0	2.8
Sweet potatoes		
Canned, drained, solids	72.5	1.8
Cooked	72.8	3.0
Tomato, raw	94.0	1.3
Tomato products		
Catsup	–	1.6
Paste	74.1	4.3
Puree	87.3	2.3
Sauce	89.1	1.5
Turnip greens		
Boiled	93.2	3.1
Raw	91.1	2.4
Turnips, boiled	93.6	2.0
Vegetables, mixed, frozen, cooked	83.2	3.8
Water chestnuts, canned, drained, solids	87.9	2.2
Watercress	95.1	2.3

Continued

Footnote over page

*Modified from the Provisional Table on the Dietary Fiber Content of Selected Foods, HNIS/PT-106, 1988 and from updated Appendix Tables 8–19, Aug. 1991, and 8–20. Oct. 1989.

†Appreciation is expressed to the U.S. Department of Agriculture, Human Nutrition Information Service, Nutrition Monitoring Division for assistance in obtaining these data.

‡The total dietary fiber in foods is measured by the enzymatic-gravimetric method (the Association of Official Analytical Chemists (AOAC) official method of analysis). Duplicate samples of dried foods, with fat extracted if containing >10% fat, are gelatinized with Termamyl (heat-stable α-amylase) and then enzymatically digested with protease and amyloglucosidase to remove protein and starch. (When analyzing mixed diets, fat is always extracted prior to determining total dietary fiber.) Four volumes of ethyl alcohol (EtOH) are added to precipitated soluble dietary fiber. Total residue is filtered and then washed with 78% EtOH, 95% EtOH, and acetone. After drying, residue is weighed. One duplicate is analyzed for protein; the other is incinerated at 525° and ash is determined.

Total dietary fiber = weight residue − weight (protein + ash).

Table II.74 Nonstarch polysaccharide content of selected foods

Food item	Total g/100g fresh weight
Vegetables and Legumes	
Beans, baked, canned	3.5
Beans, French, cooked	3.1
Beans, red kidney, cooked	6.7
Cabbage, red, cooked	3.3
Carrots, raw	2.4
Lentils, red, cooked	1.9
Onion, cooked	1.8
Peas, garden, canned	4.0
Potato, boiled, fresh	1.1
Potato crisps	4.9
Sprouts, Brussels, boiled	4.8
Fruits and Nuts	
Apple, Golden Delicious with skin	1.7
Apricots, fresh	2.3
Avocado, fresh	4.4
Canteloupe	0.6
Coconut, fresh	7.3
Figs, dried	7.5
Kiwi fruit, no skin	1.7
Peanuts, roasted	6.2
Raisins, dried	2.1
Cereal Products	
Bran flakes	11.3
Corn flakes	0.9
Oatmeal, coarse	7.0
Popcorn	9.8
Pumpernickel bread	7.5
Shredded wheat	9.8
Spaghetti, white, cooked	1.7
Spaghetti, whole-wheat, cooked	3.5
White bread	1.6
Wholemeal bread (average)	5.0

From Schwartz, S.E., Levine, R.A., Singh, A. *et al.* (1982) *Gastroenterology* 83: 812; Edwards, C.A. (1990) Physiological Effects of Fiber, in Kritchevsky, D., Bonfield, C. and Anderson, J.W. (eds), *Dietary Fiber: Chemistry, Physiology and Health Effects*, Plenum Press, N.Y. (Courtesy of Dr. Barbara Schneeman.)

Table II.75 Average values for the triglycerides, fatty acids (FA), and cholesterol in selected foods and oils (including OMEGA-3 FA) (per 100 g edible portion)

	FAT (g)	SFA (g)	MFA (g)	PFA (g)	M18:1 (g)	P18:2 (g)	P18:3 (g)	P:S	CHOL (mg)	S14:0 (g)	S16:0 (g)	S18:0 (g)	P20:5 (g)	P22:5 (g)	P22:6 (g)
Meats															
Liver calf	6.90	2.56	1.49	1.09	1.28	0.61	0.08	0.43	561.00	0.00	1.40	1.16	0.00	0.00	0.00
Liver pork	4.40	1.41	0.63	1.05	0.56	0.42	0.04	0.74	355.00	0.02	0.53	0.84	0.00	0.04	0.03
Kidney, beef	3.44	1.09	0.74	0.74	0.61	0.40	0.01	0.68	387.00	0.06	0.47	0.51	0.00	0.00	0.00
Kidney, pork	4.70	1.51	1.55	0.38	1.40	0.25	0.01	0.25	480.00	0.05	0.85	0.60	0.00	0.00	0.00
Brains, beef	12.53	2.92	2.50	1.44	2.00	0.03	0.00	0.49	2054.00	0.06	1.51	1.27	0.00	0.00	0.67
Brains, pork	9.51	2.15	1.72	1.47	1.10	0.09	0.12	0.68	2552.00	0.04	1.06	1.03	0.00	0.30	0.46
Beef, 5% fat, cooked	4.90	1.68	1.90	0.22	1.75	0.17	0.02	0.13	84.00	0.11	1.02	0.54	0.00	0.00	0.00
Beef, 26% fat, cooked	25.98	10.52	11.16	0.90	10.04	0.61	0.27	0.09	84.00	0.85	6.45	3.07	0.00	0.00	0.00
Lamb, 9% fat, cooked	9.17	3.28	4.02	0.60	3.72	0.49	0.05	0.18	92.00	0.29	1.76	1.13	0.00	0.00	0.00
Lamb, 36% fat, cooked	36.00	16.80	14.68	2.10	13.80	1.36	0.68	0.13	98.00	1.45	8.28	6.18	0.00	0.00	0.00
Veal, 6% fat, cooked	5.81	2.31	2.16	0.43	1.87	0.32	0.04	0.19	109.00	0.21	1.23	0.77	0.00	0.00	0.00
Veal, 25% fat, cooked	21.20	9.21	9.24	1.30	7.82	0.87	0.33	0.14	101.00	0.94	4.84	3.19	0.00	0.00	0.00
Chicken, light meat, unknown part, skin removed before cooking	3.87	1.15	1.05	0.92	0.88	0.66	0.02	0.80	77.00	0.03	0.67	0.32	0.00	0.03	0.03
Duck, domestic, skin removed before cooking	11.94	4.37	4.02	1.49	3.56	1.34	0.15	0.34	92.50	0.05	2.53	1.34	0.00	0.00	0.00
Ground beef, unknown % fat	22.56	8.86	9.88	0.84	8.63	0.62	0.09	0.09	89.00	0.64	5.10	2.66	0.00	0.00	0.00
Bologna, beef, regular	28.49	12.07	13.80	1.09	12.16	0.85	0.24	0.09	58.00	0.87	6.64	4.05	0.00	0.00	0.00
Pork, fresh, 25% fat, cooked	25.13	9.08	11.52	2.84	10.59	2.29	0.45	0.31	82.00	0.32	5.60	2.94	0.00	0.00	0.00
Frankfurter, all beef (Kosher), regular	28.54	12.05	13.62	1.38	11.99	1.11	0.27	0.11	61.00	0.94	6.52	3.96	0.00	0.00	0.00
Frankfurter, chicken	17.70	5.89	5.58	5.00	5.30	6.46	0.36	0.85	107.00	0.30	3.62	1.83	0.00	0.00	0.00
Frankfurter, regular, beef and pork	29.15	10.76	13.67	2.73	12.36	2.34	0.39	0.25	50.00	0.53	6.45	3.65	0.00	0.00	0.00
Pork, cured, 23% fat, cooked	23.48	8.38	11.03	2.51	10.15	2.15	0.36	0.30	67.00	0.25	5.12	2.93	0.00	0.00	0.00
Salami, pork	33.72	11.89	16.00	3.74	14.67	3.27	0.28	0.31	79.00	0.52	7.64	3.56	0.00	0.00	0.00
Bacon, regular cut	49.24	17.42	23.69	5.81	21.96	4.89	0.79	0.33	85.00	0.62	10.98	5.67	0.00	0.00	0.00
Fish															
Mussel, cooked from fresh or frozen	1.95	0.19	0.17	0.55	0.07	0.03	0.01	2.89	67.00	0.03	0.12	0.04	0.14	0.10	0.15
Fish, 0 to 2.9% fat	1.53	0.36	0.31	0.63	0.15	0.01	0.02	1.75	68.00	0.06	0.23	0.05	0.24	0.05	0.26
Fish, 3.0 to 6.9% fat	4.31	0.83	1.33	1.54	0.79	0.32	0.15	1.86	73.00	0.09	0.49	0.17	0.18	0.13	0.55
Fish, 7.0 to 10.9% fat	7.54	1.39	2.61	2.20	1.52	0.32	0.24	1.58	49.00	0.35	0.79	0.24	0.41	0.27	0.62
Fish, 11.0 to 14.9% fat	12.14	4.50	3.31	1.46	0.75	0.05	0.00	0.32	64.00	0.21	0.95	0.35	0.13	0.11	0.03
Herring, smoked/kippered, canned and drained	12.37	2.79	5.11	2.92	2.07	0.18	0.14	1.05	82.00	0.76	1.85	0.15	0.97	0.07	1.18
Salmon, canned, drained, with salt	6.05	1.53	1.81	2.05	1.07	0.06	0.06	1.34	55.00	0.05	1.35	0.13	0.84	0.05	0.81
Sardines, canned in oil, drained	11.45	1.53	3.87	5.15	2.14	3.54	0.50	3.37	142.00	0.19	0.99	0.34	0.47	0.00	0.51

Continued

Table II.75   Continued

	FAT (g)	SFA (g)	MFA (g)	PFA (g)	M18:1 (g)	P18:2 (g)	P18:3 (g)	P:S	CHOL (mg)	S14:0 (g)	S16:0 (g)	S18:0 (g)	P20:5 (g)	P22:5 (g)	P22:6 (g)
Tuna, canned, oil pack, regular, drained	8.21	1.53	2.95	2.88	2.84	2.68	0.07	1.88	18.00	0.03	1.41	0.09	0.03	0.00	0.10
Tuna, canned, water pack, regular, drained, not rinsed	0.50	0.16	0.14	0.13	0.07	0.00	0.00	0.81	18.00	0.03	0.11	0.02	0.04	0.01	0.07
Clams, cooked from fresh or frozen	1.95	0.19	0.17	0.55	0.07	0.03	0.01	2.89	67.00	0.03	0.12	0.04	0.14	0.10	0.15
Crab, hardshell, Alaskan King	1.77	0.23	0.28	0.68	0.15	0.03	0.02	2.96	100.00	0.02	0.14	0.06	0.24	0.05	0.23
Lobster, cooked from fresh or frozen	0.59	0.11	0.16	0.09	0.09	0.00	0.00	0.82	72.00	0.01	0.08	0.02	0.05	0.00	0.03
Oyster, cooked from fresh or frozen, Pacific	4.95	1.26	0.50	1.48	0.19	0.10	0.07	1.17	109.00	0.22	0.87	0.12	0.42	0.10	0.46
Scallops	1.40	0.15	0.07	0.48	0.03	0.01	0.00	3.20	31.81	0.02	0.10	0.02	0.17	0.03	0.20
Shrimps, cooked from fresh or frozen	1.08	0.29	0.20	0.44	0.11	0.02	0.01	1.52	195.00	0.02	0.14	0.10	0.17	0.02	0.14
Caviar	17.90	4.21	5.86	5.66	2.94	0.99	0.55	1.34	588.00	0.90	1.87	0.72	1.03	0.81	1.35
Eggs, Dairy															
Eggs, whole, cooked	10.02	3.10	3.81	1.36	3.47	1.15	0.03	0.44	425.00	0.03	2.23	0.78	0.00	0.00	0.04
Eggs, yolk only, cooked	30.87	9.55	11.74	4.20	10.70	3.54	0.10	0.44	1281.00	0.10	6.86	2.42	0.01	0.00	0.11
Eggs, white only, cooked	0.00	0.00	0.00	0.00	0.00	0.00	0.00	0.00	0.00	0.00	0.00	0.00	0.00	0.00	0.00
Cream, coffee creamer, liquid/frozen	9.97	9.30	0.11	0.00	0.11	0.00	0.00	0.00	0.00	1.00	0.43	0.60	0.00	0.00	0.00
Cream, coffee creamer, powder, regular	35.48	32.52	0.97	0.01	0.97	0.00	0.01	0.00	0.00	5.99	3.75	6.34	0.00	0.00	0.00
Cream, coffee creamer, liquid/frozen	11.28	1.68	4.85	4.25	4.79	3.94	0.29	2.53	0.00	0.01	1.10	0.56	0.00	0.00	0.00
Cream, half and half, 10 to 12% fat	11.50	7.16	3.32	0.43	2.89	0.26	0.17	0.06	36.90	1.16	3.02	1.39	0.00	0.00	0.00
Cream, light/coffee cream, 20% fat	19.31	12.02	5.58	0.72	4.86	0.44	0.28	0.06	66.10	1.94	5.08	2.34	0.00	0.00	0.00
Milk, buttermilk, 1% fat	0.88	0.55	0.25	0.03	0.22	0.02	0.01	0.05	3.50	0.09	0.23	0.11	0.00	0.00	0.00
Milk, skim	0.18	0.12	0.05	0.01	0.04	0.00	0.00	0.08	1.80	0.02	0.05	0.02	0.00	0.00	0.00
Milk, 1% fat	1.06	0.66	0.31	0.04	0.27	0.02	0.01	0.06	4.00	0.11	0.28	0.13	0.00	0.00	0.00
Milk, 2% fat	1.92	1.19	0.55	0.07	0.48	0.04	0.03	0.06	7.50	0.19	0.50	0.23	0.00	0.00	0.00
Milk, whole, 3.5 to 4% fat	3.34	2.08	0.96	0.12	0.84	0.07	0.05	0.06	13.60	0.34	0.88	0.40	0.00	0.00	0.00
Parmesan cheese, dry	30.02	19.07	8.73	0.66	7.74	0.32	0.34	0.03	78.70	3.38	8.10	2.67	0.00	0.00	0.00
American cheese, processed	31.25	19.69	8.95	0.99	7.51	0.61	0.38	0.05	94.40	3.21	9.10	3.80	0.00	0.00	0.00
Cottage cheese, lowfat, 2% fat	1.93	1.22	0.55	0.06	0.45	0.04	0.02	0.05	8.40	0.20	0.58	0.22	0.00	0.00	0.00
Cottage cheese, regular or creamed, 4% fat	4.51	2.85	1.28	0.14	1.06	0.10	0.04	0.05	14.90	0.47	1.36	0.51	0.00	0.00	0.00
Cream cheese, Neufchatel	23.43	14.80	6.77	0.65	5.66	0.45	0.20	0.04	76.10	2.35	6.88	2.98	0.00	0.00	0.00
Cheddar cheese, natural	33.14	21.09	9.39	0.94	7.90	0.58	0.36	0.04	104.90	3.33	9.80	4.01	0.00	0.00	0.00
Swiss cheese, natural	27.45	17.78	7.27	0.97	6.02	0.62	0.35	0.05	91.70	3.06	7.79	3.25	0.00	0.00	0.00

Table II.75 Continued

	FAT (g)	SFA (g)	MFA (g)	PFA (g)	M18:1 (g)	P18:2 (g)	P18:3 (g)	P:S	CHOL (mg)	S14:0 (g)	S16:0 (g)	S18:0 (g)	P20:5 (g)	P22:5 (g)	P22:6 (g)
Monterey Jacke cheese, natural	30.04	19.11	8.71	0.66	7.34	0.43	0.23	0.03	95.60	3.07	9.22	3.57	0.00	0.00	0.00
Mozzarella cheese, part skim milk	17.12	10.88	4.85	0.51	4.17	0.36	0.15	0.05	54.00	1.72	5.22	2.08	0.00	0.00	0.00
Brie cheese	24.26	15.26	7.02	0.72	5.75	0.45	0.27	0.05	72.00	2.69	7.23	2.52	0.00	0.00	0.00
Cheese, Kraft Light 'N' Lively Singles, American flavor	15.50	9.77	4.44	0.49	3.73	0.30	0.19	0.05	52.91	1.59	4.51	1.88	0.00	0.00	0.00
Cheese, Borden Lite-Line Singles, American flavor	8.20	4.99	2.34	0.26	1.94	0.19	0.07	0.05	45.00	0.82	2.47	0.88	0.00	0.00	0.00
Yogurt, frozen, fruit or vanilla, whole milk, 3 to 4% fat	3.24	2.10	0.90	0.09	0.75	0.06	0.03	0.04	9.74	0.33	0.87	0.30	0.00	0.00	0.00
Yogurt, frozen, fruit or vanilla, low fat, 1 to 2% fat	1.08	0.70	0.30	0.03	0.25	0.02	0.01	0.04	4.20	0.11	0.29	0.10	0.00	0.00	0.00
Yoghurt, plain, lowfat, 1 to 2% fat	1.55	1.00	0.43	0.04	0.35	0.03	0.01	0.04	6.10	0.16	0.42	0.15	0.00	0.00	0.00
Yoghurt, fruit, nonfat, <1% fat	0.20	0.12	0.05	0.01	0.00	0.00	0.00	0.08	2.00	0.00	0.00	0.00	0.00	0.00	0.00
Yogurt, fruit, whole milk, 3 to 4% fat	3.24	2.10	0.90	0.09	0.75	0.06	0.03	0.04	9.74	0.33	0.87	0.30	0.00	0.00	0.00
Ice cream and frozen desserts, regular, 10% fat, other flavors include chocolate chip	10.77	6.70	3.11	0.40	2.71	0.24	0.16	0.06	44.70	1.08	2.83	1.30	0.00	0.00	0.00
Sherbet, plain	1.98	1.23	0.57	0.07	0.50	0.04	0.03	0.06	7.30	0.20	0.52	0.24	0.00	0.00	0.00
Ice cream and frozen desserts, regular 5% fat, other flavors include chocolate chip	4.30	2.68	1.24	0.16	1.08	0.10	0.06	0.06	13.90	0.43	1.13	0.52	0.00	0.00	0.00
Fats/Oils															
Oils, canola	100.00	7.10	58.90	29.60	56.10	20.30	9.30	4.17	0.00	0.00	4.00	1.80	0.00	0.00	0.00
Oils, corn	100.00	12.70	24.20	58.70	24.20	58.00	0.00	4.62	0.00	0.00	10.90	1.80	0.00	0.00	0.00
Oils, sunflower	100.00	10.30	19.50	65.70	19.50	65.70	0.00	6.38	0.00	0.00	5.90	4.50	0.00	0.00	0.00
Oils, cottonseed	100.00	25.90	17.80	51.90	17.00	51.50	0.20	2.00	0.00	0.80	22.70	2.30	0.00	0.00	0.00
Oils, safflower	100.00	9.10	12.10	74.50	11.70	74.10	0.40	8.19	0.00	0.10	6.20	2.20	0.00	0.00	0.00
Oils, sesame	100.00	14.20	39.70	41.70	39.30	41.30	0.30	2.94	0.00	0.00	8.90	4.80	0.00	0.00	0.00
Oils, soybean (partially hydrogenated)	100.00	14.90	43.00	37.60	42.50	34.90	2.60	2.52	0.00	0.10	9.80	5.00	0.00	0.00	0.00
Oils, olive	100.00	13.50	73.70	8.40	72.50	7.90	0.60	0.62	0.00	0.00	11.00	2.20	0.00	0.00	0.00
Oils, peanut	100.00	16.90	46.20	32.00	44.80	32.00	0.00	1.89	0.00	0.10	9.50	2.20	0.00	0.00	0.00

Continued

Table II.75 Continued

	FAT (g)	SFA (g)	MFA (g)	PFA (g)	M18:1 (g)	P18:2 (g)	P18:3 (g)	P:S	CHOL (mg)	S14:0 (g)	S16:0 (g)	S18:0 (g)	P20:5 (g)	P22:5 (g)	P22:6 (g)
Oils, coconut	100.00	86.50	5.80	1.80	5.80	1.80	0.00	0.02	0.00	16.80	8.20	2.80	0.00	0.00	0.00
Oils, palm	100.00	49.30	37.00	9.30	36.60	9.10	0.20	0.19	0.00	1.00	43.50	4.30	0.00	0.00	0.00
Oils, palm kernel	100.00	81.40	11.40	1.60	11.40	1.60	0.00	0.02	0.00	16.40	8.10	2.80	0.00	0.00	0.00
Shortening, vegetable	100.00	25.00	44.50	26.10	44.50	24.50	1.60	1.04	0.00	0.40	14.10	10.60	0.00	0.00	0.00
Margarine, regular, stick, salted, corn oil	80.50	19.85	36.48	18.62	36.48	18.62	0.00	0.94	0.00	1.08	11.54	7.23	0.00	0.00	0.00
Lard	100.00	39.20	45.10	11.20	41.20	10.20	1.00	0.29	95.00	1.30	23.80	13.50	0.00	0.00	0.00
Butter, regular, salted	81.11	50.49	23.43	3.01	20.40	1.83	1.18	0.06	218.90	8.16	21.33	9.83	0.00	0.00	0.00
Oils, medium chain triglyceride	100.00	94.50	0.00	0.00	0.00	0.00	0.00	0.00	0.00	0.00	0.00	0.00	0.00	0.00	0.00
Mayonnaise/mayo-type dressing, real, regular, commercial	79.40	11.80	22.70	41.30	22.50	37.10	4.20	3.50	59.00	0.10	8.50	3.10	0.00	0.00	0.00
Oils, rapeseed	100.00	6.80	55.50	33.30	53.80	22.10	11.10	4.90	0.00	0.00	4.80	1.60	0.00	0.00	0.00
Miscellaneous															
Peanuts, peanut butter, with salt	49.98	9.59	23.58	14.36	22.96	14.10	0.08	1.50	0.00	0.05	5.50	2.14	0.00	0.00	0.00
Almonds, roasted, dry roasted, salted	56.53	5.27	36.71	11.86	36.03	11.36	0.40	2.25	0.00	0.32	3.74	1.11	0.00	0.00	0.00
Cashews, roasted, dry roasted, salted	48.21	9.70	28.41	8.15	27.89	7.97	0.17	0.84	0.00	0.36	4.53	3.09	0.00	0.00	0.00
Peanuts, roasted, dry roasted, salted	49.30	6.84	24.46	15.58	23.79	15.58	0.00	2.28	0.00	0.02	5.16	1.10	0.00	0.00	0.00
Walnuts	61.87	5.59	14.17	39.13	13.30	31.76	6.81	7.00	0.00	0.19	4.24	1.08	0.00	0.00	0.00
Olives, black	10.68	1.41	7.89	0.91	7.77	0.85	0.06	0.65	0.00	0.00	1.18	0.24	0.00	0.00	0.00
Candy, chocolate pieces, fudge, plain	10.78	4.93	4.53	0.93	4.48	0.86	0.06	0.19	3.92	0.10	2.29	2.35	0.00	0.00	0.00
Avocado, unknown type	15.32	2.44	9.61	1.95	8.96	1.84	0.11	0.80	0.00	0.00	2.40	0.03	0.00	0.00	0.00
Coconut, fresh	33.49	29.70	1.42	0.37	1.42	0.37	0.00	0.01	0.00	5.87	2.84	1.73	0.00	0.00	0.00
Soybeans, cooked from dried	8.97	1.30	1.98	5.06	1.96	4.46	0.60	3.89	0.00	0.02	0.95	0.32	0.00	0.00	0.00
Peas, black-eyed, cooked from dried	0.53	0.14	0.04	0.22	0.04	0.14	0.08	1.57	0.00	0.00	0.11	0.02	0.00	0.00	0.00
Split peas, yellow or green, cooked from dried	0.39	0.05	0.08	0.16	0.08	0.14	0.03	3.20	0.00	0.00	0.04	0.01	0.00	0.00	0.00

SFA = saturated fatty acid, MFA = monounsaturated fatty acid, PFA = polyunsaturated fatty acid, M18:1 = oleic acid, P18:2 = linoleic acid, P18:3 = linolenic acid, S14:0 = myristic acid, S16:0 = palmitic acid, S18:0 = stearic acid, P20:5 = omega-3 (eicosapentaenoic acid), P22:5 = omega-3 (docosapentaenoic acid), P22:6 = omega-3 (docosahexaenoic acid).

(With appreciation to the Nutrition Coding Center, University of Minneapolis, Minneapolis, MN for the compilation and preparation of these tables. Data are based on Version 19 of the NCC Nutrient Data Base.)

Table II.76 Average values for triglycerides, fatty acids (FA), and cholesterol of marine foods and oils (including Omega-3 FA)

Fish (100 g)	Fat (g)	Chol (mg)	SFA (g)	MFA (g)	PFA (g)	M18:1 (g)	P18:2 (g)	P18:3 (g)	P20:5 (g)	P22:5 (g)	P22:6 (g)
Anchovy, European, raw	4.84	—	1.28	1.19	1.64	0.62	0.10	—	0.50	—	0.90
Bass, striped, raw	2.33	80.00	0.51	0.66	0.78	0.45	0.02	0.02	0.17	—	0.59
Bluefish, raw	4.24	58.82	0.92	1.79	1.06	0.68	0.06	trace	0.25	0.06	0.52
Burbot, raw	0.81	60.00	0.16	0.13	0.30	0.10	0.01	—	0.07	0.03	0.10
Carp, raw	5.60	65.88	1.08	2.33	1.44	1.15	0.52	0.27	0.24	0.08	0.11
Catfish, wild, raw	2.82	58.00	0.72	0.84	0.87	0.59	0.10	0.07	0.13	0.10	0.23
Catfish, farmed, raw	7.59	47.00	1.77	3.59	1.57	3.17	0.88	0.10	0.07	0.09	0.21
Cod, Atlantic, raw	0.67	43.53	0.13	0.09	0.23	0.06	0.01	trace	0.10	—	0.20
Eel, all varieties, raw	11.66	126.00	2.35	7.19	0.95	2.78	0.20	0.70	0.10	—	0.10
Flounder, unspecified, raw	1.00	46.00	0.20	0.30	0.30	—	—	trace	0.10	—	0.10
Haddock, raw	0.72	57.65	0.13	0.12	0.24	0.07	0.01	trace	0.10	—	0.10
Halibut, raw	2.29	31.77	0.33	0.65	0.84	0.36	0.03	0.07	0.07	0.09	0.29
Herring, Atlantic, raw	9.04	60.00	2.03	3.74	2.13	1.52	0.13	0.10	0.70	—	0.90
Mackerel, Atlantic, raw	13.87	70.07	3.26	4.06	4.76	2.28	0.22	0.16	0.90	0.21	1.40
Mussel, blue, raw	2.20	38.00	0.40	0.50	0.60	trace	—	—	0.20	1.03	0.37
Octopus, raw	1.01	—	0.30	0.10	0.30	—	—	—	0.10	—	0.10
Oyster, Eastern, wild, raw	2.46	53.00	0.77	0.31	0.97	0.12	0.06	0.05	0.27	0.06	0.29
Oyster, Eastern, farmed, raw	1.55	25.00	0.44	0.15	0.59	0.07	0.03	0.04	0.19	—	0.20
Perch, all varieties, raw	0.92	89.41	0.19	0.15	0.37	0.07	0.01	0.10	0.90	—	1.60
Pike, walleye, raw	1.21	85.88	0.25	0.29	0.45	0.20	0.03	0.01	0.09	0.04	0.23
Pollock, Atlantic, raw	0.98	71.06	0.14	0.11	0.48	0.07	0.01	—	0.07	0.02	0.35
Sablefish, raw	15.30	49.00	3.20	8.06	2.04	4.07	0.17	0.10	0.68	0.17	0.72
Salmon, Chinook, raw	10.45	65.88	2.51	4.48	2.08	2.80	0.11	0.09	0.79	0.23	0.57
Salmon, coho, wild, raw	5.93	45.00	1.26	2.13	1.99	1.20	0.21	0.16	0.43	0.23	0.66
Salmon, coho, farmed, raw	7.67	51.00	1.82	3.33	1.86	1.72	0.35	0.08	0.39	—	0.82
Sea bass, all, raw	2.00	41.18	0.51	0.42	0.74	0.29	0.02	trace	0.10	—	0.30
Smelt, rainbow, raw	2.58	75.00	0.48	0.68	0.94	0.43	0.05	0.10	0.30	—	0.40
Squid, short, finned, raw	1.50	0.40	0.42	0.09	0.52	—	—	trace	0.16	0.52	0.36
Red snapper, raw	1.34	37.06	0.29	0.25	0.46	0.17	0.02	trace	trace	—	0.20
Sole, European, raw	1.20	50.00	0.30	0.40	0.20	—	0.00	trace	trace	—	0.10
Sturgeon, all, raw	4.04	—	0.92	1.94	0.69	1.44	0.07	0.10	0.19	0.05	0.09
Swordfish, raw	4.01	38.82	1.10	1.54	0.92	1.09	0.03	—	0.10	0.00	0.10
Trout, rainbow, wild, raw	3.46	59.00	0.72	1.13	1.24	0.61	0.24	0.12	0.17	0.11	0.42
Trout, rainbow, farmed, raw	5.40	59.00	1.55	1.54	1.81	1.06	0.71	0.06	0.26	—	0.67
Tuna, bluefin, fresh, raw	4.91	37.65	1.26	1.37	1.67	0.92	0.05	—	0.40	—	1.20
Whitefish, all, raw	5.85	60.00	0.91	2.00	2.15	1.35	0.27	0.18	0.32	0.16	0.94
Cod liver oil	100.00	570.00	22.61	46.71	22.54	20.65	0.94	0.94	6.90	0.94	10.97
Herring oil	100.00	766.00	21.29	56.56	15.60	11.96	1.15	0.76	6.27	0.62	4.21
Menhaden oil	100.00	521.00	30.43	26.69	34.20	14.53	2.15	1.49	13.17	4.92	8.56
Max EPA conc fish body oil	100.00	600.00	25.40	28.30	41.10	—	—	0.00	17.80	—	11.60
Salmon oil	100.00	485.00	19.87	29.04	40.32	16.98	1.54	1.06	13.02	2.99	18.23

SFA = saturated fatty acid, MFA = monounsaturated fatty acid, PFA = polyunsaturated fatty acid, M18:1 = oleic acid, P18:2 = linoleic acid, P20:5 = omega-3 (eicosapentaenoic acid), P22:5 = omega-3 (docosapentaenoic acid), P22:6 = omega-3 (docosahexaenoic acid).

(From Human Nutrition Information Service (1988) Provisional Table on the Content of Omega-3 Fatty Acids and Other Fat Components in Selected Foods, U.S. Department of Agriculture, HNIS/PT-103. Other data obtained from Consumer Nutrition Center (1991) *Composition of Finfish and Shellfish Products*, Agriculture Handbook No. 8-15, 1991 Supplement. U.S. Department of Agriculture, Washington.)

Trace is less than 0.05 g/100 g food.

— denotes lack of reliable data for nutrient known to be present.

Table II.77   Protein, sodium, potassium, calcium, phosphorus, and magnesium content of selected common foods per serving portion

Food name	Serving portion	Pro (g)	Na (mg)	K (mg)	Ca (mg)	PO₄ (mg)	Mg (mg)
Dairy Products							
Egg, whole, raw, large	1.0 Item	6.250	63.000	60.000	25.000	89.000	5.000
Cheese, cottage, uncreamed	1.0 Oz	4.888	3.715	9.189	8.994	29.523	1.173
Cream, coffee, table, light	1.0 Tbsp	0.405	5.937	18.250	14.437	12.000	1.312
Cream, sour, cultured	1.0 Tbsp	0.454	7.687	20.687	16.750	12.187	1.625
Milk, buttermilk, fluid	1.0 Cup	8.110	257.000	371.000	285.000	219.000	27.000
Milk, whole, 3.3% fat, fluid	1.0 Cup	8.030	120.000	370.000	291.000	228.000	33.000
Milk, nonfat/skim, fluid	1.0 Cup	8.350	126.000	406.000	302.000	247.000	28.000
Milk, whole, low sodium	1.0 Cup	7.560	6.000	617.000	246.000	209.000	12.000
Fats							
Butter, regular	1.0 Tbsp	0.119	116.000	3.640	3.360	3.220	0.280
Vegetable oil, corn	1.0 Tsp	0.000	0.000	0.000	0.000	0.000	0.000
Vegetable oil, olive	1.0 Tsp	0.000	0.002	0.000	0.008	0.055	0.000
Shortening, veg. soybn/cottnsd	1.0 Tsp	0.000	0.000	0.000	0.000	0.000	0.000
Margarine, reg. hard, unsalted	1.0 Tsp	0.000	0.100	1.160	0.820	0.630	0.070
Mayonnaise, soy, commercial	1.0 Tsp	0.067	26.133	1.667	0.667	1.333	0.047
Cereals							
Bran flakes, Kellogg's	0.5 Cup	2.455	152.000	124.000	9.550	96.000	35.500
Corn flakes, Kellogg's	0.5 Cup	0.920	116.000	10.450	0.341	7.150	1.360
Cream of rice, cooked	1.0 Cup	2.200	2.440	48.800	7.320	41.500	7.320
Cream of wheat, instant	1.0 Cup	4.400	6.000	48.000	59.000	43.000	14.000
Farina, cooked, enriched	1.0 Cup	3.260	0.000	30.300	4.660	28.000	4.660
Oatmeal, cooked	1.0 Cup	6.080	2.340	131.000	18.700	178.000	56.200
Wheat, puffed, plain	0.5 Cup	0.880	0.240	20.900	1.680	21.300	8.700
Wheat, shredded, biscuit	1.0 Item	2.600	0.472	77.000	9.680	86.000	40.100
Rice Krispies	0.5 Cup	0.965	170.000	14.750	1.990	17.200	5.100
Breads, Cookies, Crackers							
Bread, white, soft	1.0 Slice	2.070	129.000	28.000	31.500	27.000	5.250
Bread, whole-wheat, soft	1.0 Slice	2.690	178.000	49.300	20.200	72.800	26.000
Crackers, graham, plain	1.0 Item	0.500	33.000	27.500	3.000	10.500	3.570
Crackers, sodium free/whole wheat	1.0 Serving	1.000	1.000	35.000	—	—	—
Crackers, saltines	1.0 Item	0.250	36.800	3.250	0.500	2.500	0.770
Muffin, English, plain	0.5 Item	2.215	179.000	157.000	45.350	31.350	5.300
Bread, Italian, enriched	1.0 Slice	3.000	152.000	22.000	5.000	23.000	—
Roll, hard, enriched	0.5 Item	2.500	156.000	24.500	12.000	23.000	5.750
Roll, hamburger/hotdog	1.0 Item	3.430	241.000	36.800	53.600	32.800	7.600
Cookies, vanilla wafer	5.0 Items	1.000	50.000	14.500	8.000	12.500	3.400
Meat, Fish							
Pot roast, arm, beef, cooked	1.0 Oz	9.355	18.711	81.931	2.551	75.978	6.804
Hamburger patty, beef/lean	1.0 Oz	7.004	21.679	85.384	3.002	44.693	6.004
Steak, sirloin, lean, broiled	1.0 Oz	8.606	18.731	114.000	3.119	69.356	9.062
Chicken, leg, no skin, roasted	1.0 Oz	7.669	25.963	68.637	3.402	51.925	6.864
Chicken, breast, roasted	1.0 Oz	8.447	19.961	69.429	4.050	60.750	7.811
Lamb, all cuts, lean/fat, cooked	1.0 Oz	6.971	20.345	87.718	4.669	53.365	6.671
Turkey, dark meat, no skin	1.0 Oz	8.100	22.275	82.215	9.113	57.915	6.885
Turkey, light, no skin, roasted	1.0 Oz	8.485	18.023	86.265	5.468	62.168	7.898
Veal, all cuts, lean, cooked	1.0 Oz	9.039	25.348	96.056	6.671	71.042	8.005
Bluefish	1.0 Oz	5.689	17.010	105.000	1.890	64.449	9.450
Flatfish, raw	1.0 Oz	5.336	23.014	102.000	5.003	52.031	9.005
Cod, cooked, dry heat	1.0 Oz	6.473	22.050	69.143	3.969	39.060	11.970
Halibut, broiled, dry	1.0 Oz	7.571	19.578	163.000	17.010	80.714	30.351
Shrimp, raw, mixed species	1.0 Oz	5.751	42.525	52.650	15.188	58.725	10.125
Tuna, can/oil, drained	1.0 Oz	8.272	100.000	58.701	3.702	88.052	8.805
Tuna, diet, low sodium	1.0 Oz	7.656	11.380	73.670	1.418	62.390	9.074
Sweets							
Honey, strained/extracted	1.0 Tbsp	0.000	1.000	11.000	1.000	1.000	0.630
Ice milk, van, hard, 4.3% fat	0.5 Cup	2.580	52.500	133.000	88.000	64.500	9.500

Continued

Table II.77   Continued

Food name	Serving portion	Pro (g)	Na (mg)	K (mg)	Ca (mg)	PO₄ (mg)	Mg (mg)
Ice cream, van, hard, 10% fat	0.5 Cup	2.400	58.000	129.000	88.000	67.000	9.000
Ice cream, van, hard, 16% fat	0.5 Cup	2.065	54.000	111.000	75.500	57.500	8.000
Jams/preserves, regular	1.0 Tbsp	0.000	2.000	18.000	4.000	2.000	—
Sherbet, orange, 2% fat	0.5 Cup	1.080	44.000	99.000	51.500	37.000	7.500
Sugar, brown, pressed down	0.5 Cup	0.000	33.000	379.000	93.500	21.000	—
Sugar, white, granulated	1.0 Tbsp	0.000	0.120	0.000	0.000	0.000	—
Juices							
Apple juice, can and bottle	3.5 Fl ozs	0.066	3.062	129.000	7.612	7.875	3.500
Apricot nectar, can	3.5 Fl ozs	0.402	3.937	125.000	7.700	9.887	5.687
Cranberry juice, bottle	3.5 Fl ozs	0.000	4.375	19.906	3.321	2.214	2.214
Grape juice, can	3.5 Fl ozs	0.000	0.000	38.500	3.500	3.500	—
Grapefruit juice, can, unsweetened	3.5 Fl ozs	0.560	1.081	165.000	7.569	11.900	10.806
Lemon juice, can and bottle	3.5 Fl ozs	0.427	22.400	109.000	11.725	9.625	8.531
Orange juice, can	3.5 Fl ozs	0.643	2.179	191.000	8.706	15.268	11.987
Pear nectar, can	3.5 Fl ozs	0.120	4.375	14.219	5.469	3.281	3.281
Pineapple juice, can	3.5 Fl ozs	0.350	1.094	147.000	18.593	8.750	14.219
Prune juice, can and bottle	3.5 Fl ozs	0.682	4.462	309.000	13.431	28.000	15.662
Tomato juice, can	3.5 Fl ozs	0.809	385.000	235.000	9.625	20.300	11.725
Tomato juice, low sodium	3.5 Fl ozs	0.809	10.675	235.000	9.625	20.300	11.725
Vegetables							
Asparagus, can, spears	0.5 Cup	2.590	472.000	208.000	19.350	52.000	12.100
Asparagus, can, low sodium	0.5 Cup	2.195	425.000	187.000	17.100	46.350	11.000
Beans, snap, green, can, cuts	0.5 Cup	0.775	170.000	73.500	17.550	12.850	8.800
Beans, green, can, low sodium	0.5 Cup	0.780	1.360	74.000	16.000	13.000	9.000
Beans, snap, wax, raw, boiled	0.5 Cup	1.180	1.875	187.000	28.750	24.000	15.650
Beets, can, whole	0.5 Cup	1.025	324.000	175.000	17.200	19.700	19.700
Beets, can, diet, low sodium	0.5 Cup	1.025	324.000	175.000	17.200	19.700	19.700
Broccoli, raw, boiled, drained	0.5 Cup	2.310	20.150	227.000	35.650	45.750	18.600
Cabbage, common, boiled, drained	0.5 Cup	0.695	13.800	149.000	23.950	18.150	10.900
Carrots, can, sliced, drained	0.5 Cup	0.467	176.000	131.000	18.250	17.500	5.850
Carrots, can, low sodium	0.5 Cup	0.750	47.950	213.000	30.750	24.600	11.050
Carrot, raw, whole, scraped	1.0 Item	0.740	25.200	233.000	19.400	31.700	10.800
Cauliflower, raw, boiled, drained	0.5 Cup	1.160	4.000	200.000	17.000	22.000	7.000
Celery, Pascal, raw, stalk	1.0 Item	0.300	34.800	115.000	16.000	10.000	4.400
Corn, sweet, can, drained	0.5 Cup	2.160	267.000	161.000	4.125	53.500	16.500
Corn, sweet, can, low sodium	0.5 Cup	2.480	3.840	196.000	5.100	65.500	20.500
Cucumber, raw, sliced	0.5 Cup	0.281	1.040	77.500	7.300	8.850	5.700
Peas, green, can, drained	0.5 Cup	3.755	186.000	147.000	17.000	57.000	14.450
Peas, green, can, low sodium	0.5 Cup	3.755	1.700	147.000	17.000	57.000	14.450
Tomato, raw, red, ripe	1.0 Item	1.050	11.100	273.000	6.150	29.500	13.500
Tomato, red, can, stewed	0.5 Cup	1.185	324.000	305.000	42.100	25.500	15.300
Tomato, can, low sodium, diet	0.5 Cup	1.115	15.600	265.000	31.200	22.800	14.400
Potato, boiled, peeled before cooked	1.0 Item	2.310	6.750	443.000	10.800	54.000	27.000
Noodles, egg, enriched, cooked	0.5 Cup	3.500	1.500	35.000	8.000	47.000	21.600
Rice, white, parboiled, cooked	0.5 Cup	2.005	2.625	32.400	16.650	36.750	10.500
Fruits							
Apples, raw, unpeeled	1.0 Item	0.262	1.000	159.000	10.000	10.000	6.000
Apples, raw, peeled	1.0 Item	0.190	0.000	144.000	5.000	9.000	4.000
Applesauce, can, unsweetened	0.5 Cup	0.208	2.440	91.500	3.660	8.550	3.660
Apricots, can, light syrup	0.5 Cup	0.675	5.000	175.000	13.900	17.000	10.500
Bananas, raw, peeled	1.0 Item	1.170	1.140	451.000	6.840	22.000	33.000
Blueberries, raw	0.5 Cup	0.486	4.350	64.500	4.350	7.250	3.625
Cherries, sweet, can/juice	0.5 Cup	1.140	3.750	164.000	17.500	27.500	15.000
Grapefruit, red/pnk/wht, raw	0.5 Cup	0.725	0.500	161.000	13.500	10.000	9.500
Oranges, raw, all varieties	1.0 Item	1.230	0.000	237.000	52.400	18.300	13.100
Peaches, raw, whole	1.0 Item	0.609	0.000	171.000	4.350	10.400	6.090
Peaches, can, light syrup	0.5 Cup	0.565	6.500	122.000	4.500	13.500	6.000
Pears, raw, bartlet, unpeeled	1.0 Item	0.647	0.000	208.000	18.300	18.300	9.960
Pineapple, can/juice	0.5 Cup	0.525	2.000	153.000	17.500	7.500	17.500
Strawberries, raw, whole	0.5 Cup	0.455	0.745	124.000	10.450	14.150	7.450

Pro = protein, Na = sodium, K = potassium, Ca = calcium, PO₄ = phosphorus, Mg = magnesium.
(Created on Nutritionist III, Version 7, N-Squared Computing, 1991. Data compiled from U.S. Department of Agriculture Handbook 8-Series, manufacturers' data, published journals, and industry sources. Appreciation expressed to Ms. Lori Cohen, M.S., R.D., for her assistance in preparing this table.)

Table II.78 Vitamin A, Vitamin E, α-Tocopherol (TOC), Vitamin C, Thiamin, Riboflavin, Niacin, Vitamin B₆, Vitamin B₁₂, and Folate content of selected common foods per serving portion

Food name	Serving portion	A* (RE)	E† (mg)	α-TOC (mg)	C (mg)	Thiamin (mg)	Ribo (mg)	Niacin (mg)	B_6 (mg)	B_{12} (µg)	Folate (µg)
Dairy Products											
Egg, whole, raw, large	1.0 Item	95.200	0.700	0.350	0.000	0.031	0.254	0.037	0.070	0.500	23.000
Cheese, cottage, uncreamed	1.0 Oz	2.581	—	0.181	0.000	0.007	0.040	0.044	0.023	0.235	4.106
Cream, coffee, table, light	1.0 Tbsp	32.437	0.094	—	0.114	0.005	0.022	0.009	0.005	0.033	0.375
Cream, sour, cultured	1.0 Tbsp	34.124	—	—	0.124	0.005	0.021	0.010	0.002	0.043	1.562
Milk, buttermilk, fluid	1.0 Cup	24.300	0.980	—	2.400	0.083	0.377	0.142	0.083	0.537	12.300
Milk, whole, 3.3% fat, fluid	1.0 Cup	92.200	0.220	0.146	2.290	0.093	0.395	0.205	0.102	0.871	12.000
Milk, nonfat/skim, fluid	1.0 Cup	150.000	0.221	0.147	2.400	0.088	0.343	0.216	0.098	0.926	13.000
Milk, whole, low sodium	1.0 Cup	95.200	0.220	0.146	2.290	0.049	0.256	0.105	0.083	0.876	12.200
Fats											
Butter, regular	1.0 Tbsp	105.000	0.221	0.221	0.000	0.001	0.005	0.006	0.000	0.018	0.420
Vegetable oil, corn	1.0 Tsp	0.000	3.771	0.650	0.000	0.000	0.000	0.000	0.000	0.000	0.000
Vegetable oil, olive	1.0 Tsp	0.000	0.569	0.535	0.000	0.000	0.000	0.000	0.000	0.000	0.000
Shortening, veg, soybn/cottnsd	1.0 Tsp	0.000	2.771	0.342	0.000	0.000	0.000	0.000	0.000	0.000	0.000
Margarine, reg. hard, unsalted	1.0 Tsp	47.000	2.710	0.423	0.004	0.000	0.001	0.001	0.000	0.003	0.030
Mayonnaise, soy, commercial	1.0 Tsp	3.900	2.667	0.967	0.000	0.000	0.000	0.000	0.027	0.012	0.360
Cereals											
Bran flakes, Kellogg's	0.5 Cup	258.000	0.412	0.082	0.000	0.254	0.293	3.430	0.351	1.050	69.000
Corn flakes, Kellogg's	0.5 Cup	150.000	—	0.012	6.000	0.148	0.171	2.000	0.205	0.000	40.050
Cream of rice, cooked	1.0 Cup	0.000	—	—	0.000	0.000	0.000	0.976	0.066	0.000	7.320
Cream of wheat, instant	1.0 Cup	0.000	—	—	0.000	0.200	0.100	1.800	0.029	0.000	11.000
Farina, cooked, enriched	1.0 Cup	—	2.190	—	—	0.186	0.117	1.280	0.023	0.000	4.660
Oatmeal, cooked	1.0 Cup	4.680	5.400	3.530	—	0.257	0.047	0.304	0.047	0.000	9.360
Wheat, puffed, plain	0.5 Cup	0.000	—	0.040	0.000	0.012	0.014	0.650	0.010	0.000	1.920
Wheat, shredded, biscuit	1.0 Item	0.000	0.508	0.085	0.000	0.070	0.060	1.080	0.060	0.000	12.000
Rice Krispies	0.5 Cup	188.000	0.040	0.006	7.550	0.185	0.213	2.500	0.256	0.000	50.000
Breads, Cookies, Crackers											
Bread, white, soft	1.0 Slice	0.000	0.298	0.030	0.000	0.118	0.078	0.938	0.009	0.000	8.750
Bread, whole-wheat, soft	1.0 Slice	0.000	0.252	0.028	0.000	0.098	0.059	1.070	0.052	0.000	15.400
Crackers, graham, plain	1.0 Item	0.000	0.128	0.026	0.000	0.010	0.040	0.250	0.006	0.000	0.910
Crackers, sodium free/whole-wheat	1.0 Serving	—	—	—	—	—	—	—	—	—	—
Crackers, saltines	1.0 Item	0.000	0.050	0.010	0.000	0.125	0.013	0.100	0.001	0.000	0.495
Muffin, English, plain	0.5 Item	0.000	—	—	0.000	0.129	0.090	1.050	0.011	0.000	8.950
Bread, Italian, enriched	1.0 Slice	0.000	0.357	0.036	0.000	0.120	0.070	1.000	0.016	0.000	10.500
Roll, hard, enriched	0.5 Item	0.000	0.133	0.010	0.000	0.100	0.060	0.850	0.009	0.000	14.750
Roll, hamburger/hotdog	1.0 Item	0.000	0.212	0.016	0.000	0.196	0.132	1.580	0.014	—	14.800
Cookies, vanilla wafer	5.0 Items	5.000	1.090	0.515	0.000	0.050	0.045	0.400	—	—	—
Meat, Fish											
Pot roast, arm, beef, cooked	1.0 Oz	0.000	—	0.040	0.000	0.023	0.082	1.055	0.094	0.964	3.118
Hamburger patty, beef, lean	1.0 Oz	3.005	0.172	0.101	0.000	0.014	0.060	1.464	0.073	0.667	2.668
Steak, sirloin, lean, broiled	1.0 Oz	1.519	0.156	0.037	0.000	0.036	0.084	1.215	0.128	0.810	2.835
Chicken, leg, no skin, roasted	1.0 Oz	5.372	0.156	0.099	0.000	0.021	0.066	1.791	0.104	0.093	2.387

Food	Serving										
Chicken, breast, roasted	1.0 Oz	0.868	0.093	0.156	3.602	0.034	0.019	0.000	0.099	0.156	7.912
Lamb, all cuts, lean/fat, cooked	1.0 Oz	5.003	0.724	0.037	1.888	0.073	0.027	—	0.181	—	—
Turkey, dark meat, no skin	1.0 Oz	2.552	0.105	0.101	1.035	0.070	0.018	0.000	0.026	—	0.000
Turkey, light, no skin, roasted	1.0 Oz	1.620	0.105	0.152	1.938	0.037	0.017	0.000	—	—	0.000
Veal, all cuts, lean, cooked	1.0 Oz	4.336	0.470	0.093	2.388	0.097	0.017	—	—	—	—
Bluefish	1.0 Oz	0.454	1.529	0.114	1.688	0.023	0.016	0.016	—	—	33.831
Flatfish, raw	1.0 Oz	—	0.430	0.059	0.820	0.022	0.025	—	—	—	2.668
Cod, cooked, dry heat	1.0 Oz	2.300	0.298	0.080	0.712	0.022	0.025	0.283	—	—	3.969
Halibut, broiled, dry	1.0 Oz	3.902	0.387	0.112	2.021	0.026	0.020	0.000	—	—	15.309
Shrimp, raw, mixed species	1.0 Oz	0.810	0.328	0.028	0.725	0.012	0.008	—	—	—	—
Tuna, can/oil, drained	1.0 Oz	1.504	0.624	0.031	3.502	0.034	0.011	0.000	0.474	—	6.537
Tuna, diet, low sodium	1.0 Oz	0.000	0.397	0.105	3.514	0.014	0.009	—	—	0.799	6.898
Sweets											
Honey, strained/extracted	1.0 Tbsp	—	0.000	0.004	0.100	0.010	0.000	0.000	—	—	0.000
Ice milk, van, hard, 4.3% fat	0.5 Cup	1.500	0.438	0.043	0.059	0.174	0.038	0.380	0.040	0.230	26.000
Ice cream, van, hard, 10% fat	0.5 Cup	1.500	0.313	0.031	0.067	0.165	0.026	0.350	0.040	0.233	66.500
Ice cream, van, hard, 16% fat	0.5 Cup	1.000	0.269	0.027	0.058	0.142	0.022	0.305	0.045	0.259	104.000
Jams, preserves, regular	1.0 Tbsp	1.600	0.000	0.004	0.000	0.010	0.010	0.000	0.018	—	0.000
Serbet, orange, 2% fat	0.5 Cup	7.000	0.079	0.013	0.066	0.045	0.016	1.930	—	—	19.500
Sugar, brown, pressed down	0.5 Cup	—	—	—	0.200	0.035	0.010	0.000	—	—	0.000
Sugar, white, granulated	1.0 Tbsp	—	—	—	0.000	0.000	0.000	0.000	—	—	0.000
Juices											
Apple juice, can and bottle	3.5 Fl ozs	0.108	0.000	0.032	0.108	0.018	0.023	1.006	0.011	—	0.087
Apricot nectar, can	3.5 Fl ozs	1.426	0.000	—	0.286	0.015	0.010	0.661	—	—	144.000
Cranberry juice, bottle	3.5 Fl ozs	0.221	0.000	0.021	0.039	0.010	0.010	39.199	—	—	0.000
Grape juice, can	3.5 Fl ozs	1.050	0.000	0.021	0.109	0.010	0.010	17.500	—	—	0.000
Grapefruit juice, can, unsweetened	3.5 Fl ozs	11.244	0.000	0.021	0.250	0.021	0.045	31.543	0.043	0.195	0.787
Lemon juice, can and bottle	3.5 Fl ozs	10.762	0.000	0.046	0.210	0.010	0.044	26.468	—	—	1.619
Orange juice, can	3.5 Fl ozs	19.731	0.000	0.096	0.342	0.031	0.065	37.493	0.044	0.218	19.118
Pear nectar, can	3.5 Fl ozs	1.312	0.000	0.015	0.140	0.014	0.002	1.203	—	—	0.044
Pineaplle juice, can	3.5 Fl ozs	25.287	0.000	0.105	0.281	0.024	0.060	11.725	—	—	0.525
Prune juice, can and bottle	3.5 Fl ozs	0.446	0.000	0.244	0.879	0.078	0.018	4.594	—	—	0.394
Tomato juice, can	3.5 Fl ozs	21.262	0.000	0.119	0.717	0.033	0.050	19.556	0.234	0.757	59.936
Tomato juice, low sodium	3.5 Fl ozs	21.262	0.000	0.119	0.717	0.033	0.050	19.556	0.235	0.757	59.936
Vegetables											
Asparagus, can, spears	0.5 Cup	116.000	0.000	0.133	1.155	0.121	0.074	22.250	0.460	—	64.000
Asparagus, can, low sodium	0.5 Cup	104.000	0.000	0.120	1.040	0.109	0.066	20.000	0.464	—	57.500
Beans, snap, green, can, cuts	0.5 Cup	21.450	0.000	0.025	0.135	0.038	0.010	3.240	0.021	0.034	23.650
Beans, green, can, low sodium	0.5 Cup	21.600	0.000	—	0.137	0.038	0.010	3.200	0.021	0.034	—
Beans, snap, wax, raw, boiled	0.5 Cup	20.800	0.000	0.035	0.384	0.061	0.047	6.050	0.182	—	41.900
Beets, can, whole	0.5 Cup	35.650	0.000	0.068	0.186	0.047	0.013	4.795	0.037	—	1.238
Beets, can, diet, low sodium	0.5 Cup	35.650	0.000	0.068	0.186	0.047	0.013	4.795	0.037	—	1.238
Broccoli, raw, boiled, drained	0.5 Cup	38.750	0.000	0.111	0.445	0.088	0.043	58.000	0.357	0.496	108.000
Cabbage, common, boiled drained	0.5 Cup	14.700	0.000	0.047	0.165	0.040	0.042	17.600	1.210	1.210	6.550

Continued

Table II.78 Continued

Food name	Serving portion	A* (RE)	E† (mg)	α-TOC (mg)	C (mg)	Thiamin (mg)	Ribo (mg)	Niacin (mg)	B₆ (mg)	B₁₂ (µg)	Folate (µg)
Carrots, can, sliced, drained	0.5 Cup	1005.000	0.336	0.307	1.970	0.013	0.022	0.403	0.082	0.000	6.700
Carrots, can, low sodium	0.5 Cup	1620.000	0.565	0.515	3.445	0.024	0.033	0.520	0.138	0.000	9.950
Carrot, raw, whole, scraped	1.0 Item	2025.000	0.367	0.317	6.700	0.070	0.042	0.668	0.106	0.000	10.100
Cauliflower, raw, boiled, drained	0.5 Cup	0.900	0.057	0.019	34.300	0.039	0.032	0.342	0.125	0.000	31.700
Celery, Pascal, raw, stalk	1.0 Item	5.200	0.292	0.144	2.800	0.018	0.018	0.129	0.035	0.000	11.200
Corn, sweet, can, drained	0.5 Cup	13.200	0.510	0.033	7.000	0.027	0.065	0.990	0.039	0.000	40.100
Corn, sweet, can, low sodium	0.5 Cup	15.350	0.795	0.051	8.600	0.033	0.078	1.200	0.048	0.000	48.750
Cucumber, raw, sliced	0.5 Cup	2.600	0.161	0.078	2.445	0.016	0.010	0.156	0.027	0.000	7.250
Peas, green, can, drained	0.5 Cup	65.500	2.235	0.017	8.150	0.103	0.066	0.620	0.055	0.000	37.650
Peas, green, can, low sodium	0.5 Cup	65.500	2.235	0.017	8.150	0.103	0.066	0.620	0.055	0.000	37.650
Tomato, raw, red, ripe	1.0 Item	76.300	0.603	0.418	23.500	0.073	0.059	0.772	0.098	0.000	18.500
Tomato, red, can, stewed	0.5 Cup	70.000	0.905	0.281	16.950	0.059	0.045	0.910	0.022	0.000	6.900
Tomato, can, low sodium, diet	0.5 Cup	72.000	—	0.264	18.150	0.054	0.037	0.080	0.108	0.000	9.350
Potato, boiled, peeled before cooked	1.0 Item	0.000	0.081	0.041	9.990	0.132	0.026	1.770	0.363	0.000	12.000
Noodles, egg, enriched cooked	0.5 Cup	5.500	—	—	0.000	0.110	0.065	0.950	0.071	0.000	9.600
Rice, white, parboiled, cooked	0.5 Cup	0.000	0.342	0.097	0.000	0.219	0.016	1.225	0.016	0.000	3.000
Fruit											
Apple, raw, unpeeled	1.0 Item	7.400	0.911	0.814	7.800	0.023	0.019	0.106	0.066	0.000	3.900
Apple, raw, peeled	1.0 Item	5.600	0.845	0.346	5.120	0.022	0.013	0.116	0.059	0.000	0.500
Applesauce, can, unsweetened	0.5 Cup	3.500	—	0.110	1.465	0.016	0.031	0.230	0.032	0.000	0.730
Apricots, can, light syrup	0.5 Cup	167.000	0.365	1.125	3.415	0.020	0.026	0.385	0.069	0.000	2.150
Bananas, raw, peeled	1.0 Item	9.200	0.365	0.308	10.400	0.051	0.114	0.616	0.659	0.000	21.800
Blueberries, raw	0.5 Cup	7.250	—	—	9.450	0.035	0.037	0.261	0.026	0.000	4.640
Cherries, sweet, can/juice	0.5 Cup	15.650	—	—	3.125	0.023	0.030	0.510	0.038	0.000	5.250
Grapefruit, red/pnk/wht, raw	0.5 Cup	14.500	—	—	39.550	0.042	0.023	0.288	0.049	0.000	11.700
Oranges, raw, all varieties	1.0 Item	26.900	0.314	0.314	69.700	0.114	0.052	0.369	0.079	0.000	39.700
Peaches, raw, whole	1.0 Item	46.500	—	0.087	5.740	0.015	0.036	0.861	0.016	0.000	2.960
Peaches, can, light syrup	0.5 Cup	44.500	—	—	2.950	0.012	0.032	0.745	0.024	0.000	4.100
Pears, raw, bartlet, unpeeled	1.0 Item	3.300	—	0.820	6.640	0.033	0.066	0.166	0.030	0.000	12.100
Pineapple, can/juice	0.5 Cup	4.750	0.125	0.125	11.900	0.119	0.024	0.355	0.093	0.000	6.000
Strawberries, raw, whole	0.5 Cup	2.050	0.194	0.090	42.250	0.015	0.049	0.172	0.044	0.000	13.200

*RE = µg retinol + µg β-carotene (0.167) + µg other carotenes (0.083).
  1 RE = 3.33 IU from vitamin A (retinol)
           10 IU from β-carotene

†mg of vitamin E represents mg of total tocopherol including α-tocopherol.
— denotes lack of reliable data for nutrient to be present.

(Created on Nutritionist III, Version 7, N-Squared Computing, 1991. Data compiled from U.S. Department of Agriculture Handbook 8-Series, manufacturers data, published journals, and industry sources. Appreciation expressed to Ms. Lori Cohen, M.S., R.D., for her assistance in preparing this table.)

Table II.79   Retention of nutrients in cooked vegetables[1]

	Ascorbic acid (%)	Thiamin (%)	Riboflavin (%)	Niacin (%)	Pantothenic acid[6] (%)	Vitamin B₆ (%)	Folacin[7] (%)	Vitamin A (%)
Potatoes								
Prepared from raw								
Baked in skin	80	85	95	95	90	95	90	—[8]
Boiled in skin	75	80	95	95	90	95	90	—
Boiled without skin	75	80	95	95	90	95	75	—
Fried	80	80	95	95	90	95	75	—
Hashed-brown[2]	25	40	85	80	—	—	65	—
Mashed	75	80	95	95	90	95	75	—
Scalloped and au gratin	80	80	95	95	90	95	75	—
Prepared from frozen								
French fried, heated	50	75	95	95	90	95	75	—
Baked, stuffed, heated	80	85	95	95	90	95	80	—
Hashed-brown	80	80	95	95	90	95	80	—
Sweet Potatoes								
Prepared from raw								
Baked in skin	80	85	95	95	90	95	90	90
Boiled in skin	75	80	95	95	90	95	90	85
Prepared from frozen								
Baked	80	80	95	95	90	95	80	90
Boiled	75	80	95	95	90	95	80	85
Tomatoes (prepared from raw, baked, boiled or stewed)	95	95	95	95	95	95	70	95
Other Vegetables (cooked in small or moderate amount of water until tender)								
Prepared from raw, drained								
Greens, dark and leafy[3]	60	85	95	90	95	90	65	95
Roots, bulbs, other vegetables of high starch and/or sugar content[4]	70	85	95	95	90	95	70	90
Other[5]	80	85	95	90	90	90	70	90
Prepared from frozen, drained								
Greens, dark and leafy[3]	60	90	95	90	95	90	55	95
Roots, bulbs, other vegetables of high starch and/or sugar content[4]	70	90	95	95	90	95	70	90
Other[5]	80	90	95	90	90	90	70	90

[1]% True Retention = $\dfrac{\text{Nutrient content per g of cooked food x g of food after cooking}}{\text{Nutrient content per g of raw food x g of food before cooking}} \times 100$

[2]Potatoes were pared, boiled, and held overnight before hashed-browning.

[3]Vegetables such as beet greens, Chinese cabbage, collards, mustard greens, spinach, Swiss chard, turnip greens, and other wild greens.

[4]Vegetables such as beets, carrots, green peas, lima beans, onions, parsnips, rutabagas, salsify, turnips, summer and winter squash, and other immature seeds of the legume group.

[5]Vegetables such as asparagus, bean sprouts, broccoli, brussels sprouts, cabbage, cauliflower, eggplant, kohlrabi, okra, and sweet peppers.

[6]Because of limited data, values are based on nutrient retention data from other cooked plant products.

[7]Values are based on limited data.

[8]Dashes denote lack of reliable data.

(From Human Nutrition Information Service (1990) *Composition of Foods, Raw, Processed, Prepared*, Supplement, Agriculture Handbook No. 8, U.S. Department of Agriculture, Washington, D.C.)

Table II.80 Iron, Zinc, Copper, Selenium, and Manganese content of selected foods, in MG (100 g = 3½ oz)*

Food name	Fe	Zn	Cu	Se	Mn
Dairy Products					
Egg, whole, raw, large	1.440	1.100	0.014	0.044	0.024
Cheese, cottage, uncreamed	0.228	0.469	0.028	0.023	0.003
Cream, coffee, table, light	0.042	0.271	0.008	0.000	0.001
Cream, sour, cultured	0.061	0.270	0.019	—	0.003
Milk, buttermilk, fluid	0.049	0.420	0.011	0.001	0.002
Milk, whole, 3.3% fat, fluid	0.049	0.381	0.010	0.001	0.004
Milk, nonfat/skim, fluid	0.041	0.400	0.011	0.003	0.002
Milk, whole, low sodium	0.050	0.380	0.010	0.001	0.004
Fats					
Butter, regular, tablespoon	0.157	0.050	0.014	0.000	0.007
Vegetable oil, corn	0.000	0.000	0.000	—	0.000
Vegetable oil, olive	0.384	0.060	0.074	—	—
Shortening, veg, soybn/cottnsd	0.000	0.000	0.000	—	0.000
Margarine, reg. hard, unsalted	0.000	0.000	—	0.000	—
Mayonnaise, soy, commercial	0.714	0.143	0.243	—	—
Cereals					
Bran flakes, Kellogg's	63.590	13.205	0.741	0.010	4.333
Corn flakes, Kellogg's	6.300	0.282	0.066	0.004	0.084
Cream of rice, cooked	0.200	0.160	0.034	—	0.144
Cream of wheat, instant	4.979	0.170	0.038	—	—
Farina, cooked, enriched	0.502	0.070	0.011	—	—
Oatmeal, cooked	0.679	0.491	0.055	0.009	0.585
Wheat, puffed, plain	4.733	2.358	0.408	—	1.758
Wheat, shredded, biscuit	3.136	2.500	0.500	—	3.072
Rice Krispies	6.303	1.690	0.250	0.014	0.989
Breads, Cookies, Crackers					
Bread, white, soft	2.840	0.620	0.140	0.028	0.280
Bread, whole-wheat, soft	3.373	1.655	0.338	0.046	—
Crackers, graham, plain	3.571	0.757	0.857	0.014	—
Crackers, sodium free/whole-wheat	—	—	—	—	—
Crackers, saltines	4.545	0.618	0.182	0.145	—
Muffin, English, plain	2.821	0.720	0.311	0.027	—
Bread, Italian, enriched	2.333	—	—	0.027	—
Roll, hamburger/hotdog	2.975	0.820	0.165	0.030	—
Cookies, vanilla wafer	1.500	—	—	0.000	—
Meat, Fish					
Pot roast, arm, beef, cooked	3.790	8.660	0.164	0.006	0.019
Hamburger patty, beef/lean	2.106	5.365	0.066	0.024	0.014
Steak, sirloin, lean, broiled	3.357	6.518	0.146	0.034	0.018
Chicken, leg, no skin, roasted	1.305	2.853	0.080	0.014	0.021
Chicken, breast, roasted	1.061	1.020	0.050	0.027	0.018
Lamb, all cuts, lean/fat, cooked	1.871	4.459	0.119	—	0.022
Turkey, dark meat, no skin	2.336	4.464	0.160	0.025	0.023
Turkey, light, no skin, roasted	1.343	2.036	0.042	—	0.020
Veal, all cuts, lean, cooked	1.165	5.094	0.120	—	0.038
Bluefish	0.480	0.807	0.053	—	0.021
Flatfish, raw	0.353	0.459	0.032	—	0.016
Cod, cooked, dry heat	0.490	0.578	0.036	0.045	0.020
Halibut, broiled, dry	1.071	0.529	0.035	0.060	0.020
Shrimp, raw, mixed species	2.400	1.114	0.271	—	0.057
Tuna, can/oil, drained	1.388	0.900	0.071	0.072	0.015
Tuna, diet, low sodium	1.201	0.500	0.060	0.116	0.039

Continued

Table II.80 Continued

Food name	Fe	Zn	Cu	Se	Mn
Sweets					
Honey, strained/extracted	0.476	0.095	0.038	0.005	0.029
Ice milk, van, hard, 4.3% fat	0.137	0.420	0.023	0.002	0.009
Ice cream, van, hard, 10% fat	0.090	1.060	0.019	0.002	0.006
Ice cream, van, hard, 16% fat	0.068	0.818	0.019	0.002	0.006
Jams/preserves, regular	1.000	—	0.310	0.000	—
Sherbet, orange, 2% fat	0.161	0.689	0.030	—	0.011
Sugar, brown, pressed down	3.409	—	0.350	0.001	—
Sugar, white, granulated	0.000	0.050	0.017	0.000	—
Juices					
Apple juice, can and bottle	0.371	0.028	0.022	0.001	0.113
Apricot nectar, can	0.382	0.092	0.073	—	0.032
Cranberry juice, bottle	0.150	0.070	0.018	0.000	0.183
Grape juice, can	0.098	—	—	—	—
Grapefruit juice, can, unsweetened	0.200	0.090	0.038	0.000	0.020
Lemon juice, can and bottle	0.130	0.060	0.037	0.000	0.020
Orange juice, can	0.442	0.070	0.057	0.000	0.014
Pear nectar, can	0.260	0.070	0.067	0.000	0.030
Pineapple juice, can	0.260	0.110	0.090	0.001	0.992
Prune juice, can and bottle	1.180	0.210	0.068	0.000	0.151
Tomato juice, can	0.582	0.140	0.101	0.000	0.077
Tomato juice, low sodium	0.582	0.140	0.101	0.000	0.077
Vegetables					
Asparagus, can, spears	1.831	0.400	0.096	0.004	0.170
Asparagus, can, low sodium	0.582	0.471	0.107	0.001	0.152
Beans, snap, green, can, cuts	0.904	0.290	0.038	0.001	0.200
Beans, green, can, low sodium	0.897	0.294	0.038	0.001	0.200
Beans, snap, wax, raw, boiled	1.280	0.360	0.103	0.001	0.294
Beets, can, whole	0.671	0.230	0.097	0.000	0.241
Beets, can, diet, low sodium	0.671	0.230	0.097	0.001	0.241
Broccoli, raw, boiled, drained	0.839	0.380	0.043	0.002	0.218
Cabbage, common, boiled, drained	0.390	0.160	0.028	0.002	0.129
Carrots, can, sliced, drained	0.640	0.260	0.104	0.001	0.450
Carrots, can, low sodium	0.610	0.290	0.103	0.001	0.451
Carrot, raw, whole, scraped	0.500	0.200	0.047	0.003	0.142
Cauliflower, raw, boiled, drained	0.419	0.242	0.090	0.001	0.177
Celery, pascal, raw, stalk	0.400	0.130	0.035	0.000	0.035
Corn, sweet, can, drained	0.861	0.390	0.058	0.001	0.173
Corn, sweet, can, low sodium	0.350	0.359	0.056	0.000	0.033
Cucumber, raw, sliced	0.280	0.230	0.040	0.001	0.061
Peas, green, can, drained	0.953	0.712	0.082	0.001	0.303
Peas, green, can, low sodium	0.953	0.712	0.082	0.001	0.303
Tomato, raw, red, ripe	0.450	0.089	0.074	0.001	0.105
Tomato, red, can, stewed	0.729	0.170	0.112	0.001	0.059
Tomato, can, low sodium, diet	0.608	0.160	0.110	0.001	—
Potato, boiled, peeled before cooked	0.310	0.270	0.167	0.001	0.140
Noodles, egg, enriched, cooked	0.875	—	0.169	0.059	—
Rice, white, parboiled, cooked	1.128	0.310	0.094	0.020	0.260
Fruits					
Apples, raw, unpeeled	0.181	0.036	0.041	0.001	0.045
Apple, raw, peeled	0.070	0.039	0.031	0.001	0.023
Applesauce, can, unsweetened	0.119	0.030	0.026	0.000	0.075
Apricots, can, light syrup	0.391	0.107	0.079	0.000	0.052
Bananas, raw, peeled	0.307	0.160	0.104	0.001	0.152

Continued

Table II.80   Continued

Food name	Fe	Zn	Cu	Se	Mn
Blueberries, raw	0.170	0.110	0.061	0.001	0.282
Cherries, sweet, can/juice	0.580	0.100	0.073	0.000	0.061
Grapefruit, red/pnk/wht, raw	0.087	0.070	0.047	—	0.012
Oranges, raw, all varieties	0.100	0.069	0.045	0.002	0.025
Peaches, raw, whole	0.110	0.140	0.068	0.001	0.047
Peaches, can, light syrup	0.359	0.088	0.052	—	0.046
Pears, raw, Bartlet, unpeeled	0.250	0.120	0.113	0.001	0.076
Pineapple, can/juice	0.280	0.100	0.086	0.001	1.120
Strawberries, raw, whole	0.380	0.130	0.049	0.001	0.290

*Values for five trace elements have been provided in this table. Other trace elements have been analyzed and can be found in the following article by Hunt and Mullen: Concentration of boron and other elements in the human foods and personal-care products (1991) *J. Am. Diet Assoc.,* **91** pp. 558–568. These authors report the analyzed concentrations of boron and molybdenum, as well as of calcium, copper, iron, magnesium, and manganese in selected foods and personal-care products (analgesics, antibiotics, decongestants, antihistamines, dental hygiene products, gastric antacids, and laxatives). For those interested in obtaining data on these nutrients, this article may serve as a helpful reference.

Fe = iron, Zn = zinc, Cu = copper, Se = selenium, Mn = manganese.

— denotes lack of reliable data for nutrient known to be present.

(Created on Nutritionist III, Version 7, N-Squared Computing, 1991. Data compiled from U.S. Department of Agriculture Handbook 8-Series, manufacturers' data, published journals, and industry sources. Appreciation expressed to Ms. Lori Cohen, M.S., R.D., for her assistance in preparing this table.)

INDEX